The SAGES Manual of Foregut Surgery

Jayleen Grams • Kyle A. Perry • Ali Tavakkoli
Editors

The SAGES Manual of Foregut Surgery

SAGES University MASTERS PROGRAM

Springer

Editors
Jayleen Grams
University of Alabama at Birmingham
Birmingham, AL
USA

Kyle A. Perry
The Ohio State University
Columbus, OH
USA

Ali Tavakkoli
Brigham and Women's Hospital
Boston, MA
USA

ISBN 978-3-319-96121-7 ISBN 978-3-319-96122-4 (eBook)
https://doi.org/10.1007/978-3-319-96122-4

This Springer imprint is published by the registered company Springer Nature Switzerland AG
The registered company address is: Gewerbestrasse 11, 6330 Cham, Switzerland

Contents

Contributors

Mohammed Al Mahroos, MD, FRCS(C) Department of General Surgery, McGill University, Montreal, QC, Canada

Mazen R. Al-Mansour, MD Department of General and Gastrointestinal Surgery, The Ohio State University, Wexner Medical Center, Columbus, OH, USA

Stanley W. Ashley, MD Brigham and Women's Hospital, Harvard Medical School, Boston, MA, USA

Dan E. Azagury, MD Bariatric & Minimally Invasive Surgery, Department of Surgery, Stanford University School of Medicine, Stanford, CA, USA

Ioana Baiu, MD, MPH Department of Surgery, Stanford Health Care, Stanford, CA, USA

Reginald C. W. Bell, MD SurgOne Foregut Institute, Englewood, CO, USA

Shanda Haley Blackmon, MD, MPH, FACS Department of Thoracic Surgery, Mayo Clinic, Rochester, MN, USA

Lawrence F. Borges, MD Department of Gastroenterology, Brigham and Women's Hospital, Boston, MA, USA

David C. Brooks, MD Division of General and Gastrointestinal Surgery, Brigham and Women's Hospital, Harvard Medical School, Boston, MA, USA

Miguel A. Burch, MD Department of Minimally Invasive Surgery, Cedars-Sinai Medical Center, Los Angeles, CA, USA

James Callaway, MD Division of Gastroenterology and Hepatology, University of Alabama, Birmingham, AL, USA

Michael Camilleri, MD Division of Gastroenterology and Hepatology, Mayo Clinic, Rochester, MN, USA

Amy Cha, MD Department of Surgery, Hospital of the University of Pennsylvania, Philadelphia, PA, USA

Matthew Cooper, MD Department of Surgery, Stanford Hospital and Clinics, Stanford, CA, USA

Britney L. Corey, MD Department of Surgery, University of Alabama at Birmingham, Birmingham Veteran's Affairs Medical Center, Birmingham, AL, USA

Brian Richard Davis, MD, FACS, FASGE Department of Surgery, Texas Tech Paul L. Foster School of Medicine, El Paso, TX, USA

Daniel T. Dempsey, MD Department of Surgery, Hospital of the University of Pennsylvania, Philadelphia, PA, USA

Daniel J. Deziel, MD Department of Surgery, Division of MIS and Bariatrics, Rush University Medical Center, Chicago, IL, USA

Adrian B. Dobrowolsky, MD Department of Upper GI, General, and Bariatric Surgery, USC Keck Medical Center, Los Angeles, CA, USA

James Patrick Dolan, MD, MCR Department of Surgery, Division of Gastrointestinal and General Surgery, Oregon Health and Science University, Portland, OR, USA

Matthew Dong, MD, MPH Department of Surgery, Icahn School of Medicine at Mount Sinai, New York, NY, USA

Joseph M. Drosdeck, MD, MS Department of General Surgery, The Everett Clinic, Everett, WA, USA

Kristoffel R. Dumon, MD Hospital of the University of Pennsylvania, Philadelphia, PA, USA

James C. Ellsmere, MD, MS, FRCS C, FACS Department of General Surgery, Dalhousie University, Halifax, NS, Canada

Gerald M. Fried, MD, FRCS(C), FACS, FCAHS Department of Surgery, McGill University Health Centre, Montreal, QC, Canada

Luke M. Funk, MD, MPH Division of Minimally Invasive, Foregut, and Bariatric Surgery; Department of Surgery, University of Wisconsin Hospital and Clinics, Madison, WI, USA

Victoria M. Gershuni, MD MSGM Department of Surgery, Hospital of the University of Pennsylvania, Philadelphia, PA, USA

Michael B. Goldberg, MD Department of Surgery, Brigham and Women's Hospital, Boston, MA, USA

Jon Gould, MD Department of Surgery, Medical College of Wisconsin, Milwaukee, WI, USA

Jacob A. Greenberg, MD, EdM Department of General Surgery, University Hospital, Madison, WI, USA

Daniela Guevara, MD Division of Metabolic, Endocrine and Minimally Invasive Surgery, Department of Surgery, Mount Sinai Hospital, Icahn School of Medicine at Mount Sinai, New York, NY, USA

Taher Gulamhusein, MD Department of Surgery, Stony Brook Medicine, Stony Brook University Hospital, Stony Brook, NY, USA

Rebecca L. Gunter, MD Department of Surgery, University of Wisconsin Hospital and Clinics, Madison, WI, USA

Shreya Gupta, MD Department of Surgery, University Hospitals Cleveland Medical Center, Cleveland, OH, USA

Jeffrey D. E. Hawel, MD, FRCSC Department of General Surgery, Dalhousie University, Halifax, NS, Canada

Mary Hawn, MD, MPH, FACS Department of Surgery, Stanford Hospital and Clinics, Stanford, CA, USA

Jeffrey W. Hazey, MD Division of General and Gastrointestinal Surgery, Department of Surgery, The Ohio State University, Wexner Medical Center, Columbus, OH, USA

Daniel M. Herron, MD, FACS, FASMBS Department of Surgery, Icahn School of Medicine at Mount Sinai, New York, NY, USA

William Hirsch Division of Gastroenterology, Department of Medicine, Beth Israel Deaconess Medical Center, Boston, MA, USA

Eric Hungness, MD Department of Surgery, Northwestern Memorial, Chicago, IL, USA

John G. Hunter, MD, FACS, FRCS Edin (Hon) Department of Surgery, World Journal of Surgery, OHSU, Portland, OR, USA

Andrew M. Ibrahim, MD, MSc Robertwood Johnson Clinical Scholar, Department of Surgery, University of Michigan, Ann Arbor, MI, USA

Jonathan Imran, MD University of Texas Southwestern Medical Center, Department of Surgery, Division of Burn, Trauma, and Critical Care, Dallas, TX, USA

Hope T. Jackson, MD University of Maryland School of Medicine, Baltimore, MD, USA

Terence Jackson, MD Department of Surgery, University Hospitals Cleveland Medical Center, Cleveland, OH, USA

Brian Jacob, MD Department of Surgery, Icahn School of Medicine at Mount Sinai, New York, NY, USA

Deepti Jacob, MD, FRCPC Division of Gastroenterology and Hepatology, Mayo Clinic, Rochester, MN, USA

Garth R. Jacobsen, MD Department of Surgery, University of California San Diego, Rancho Santa Fe, CA, USA

Kunal Jajoo, MD Department of Medicine, Division of Gastroenterology, Brigham and Women's Hospital, Boston, MA, USA

Lawrence F. Johnson, MD Department of Gastroenterology and Hepatology, University of Alabama-Birmingham, Birmingham, AL, USA

Daniel B. Jones Harvard Medical School, Division of Bariatric and Minimally Invasive Surgery, Beth Israel Deaconess Medical Center, Boston, MA, USA

Arinbjorn Jonsson, MD Emory Endosurgery Unit, Emory University Hospital, Atlanta, GA, USA

Jennifer A. Kalil, MD Department of Surgery, University Hospitals Cleveland Medical Center, Cleveland, OH, USA

Leena Khaitan, MD, MPH Metabolic and Bariatric Program, Department of Surgery, University Hospitals, Cleveland, OH, USA

Adil Haleem Khan, MD, FACS Department of Surgery, University Hospitals, Cleveland Medical Center, Cleveland, OH, USA

Anthony W. Kim, MD Department of Surgery, University of Southern California Keck School of Medicine, Los Angeles, CA, USA

Subhash Kini, MD, FACS, FRCS (Eng, Ed, Glas) Department of Surgery, Icahn School of Medicine at Mount Sinai St. Luke's, New York, NY, USA

Riley Katsuki Kitamura, MD Department of Surgery, Icahn School of Medicine at Mount Sinai, New York, NY, USA

Srinadh Komanduri, MD Department of Internal Medicine, Division of Gastroenterology, Northwestern University, Feinberg School of Medicine, Chicago, IL, USA

Kumar Krishnan, MD Division of Gastroenterology, Underwood Center for Digestive Disorders, Houston Methodist Hospital, Weill Cornell Medical College, Houston, TX, USA

Matthew D. Kroh, MD, FACS, FASMBS, FASGE Digestive Disease Institute, Cleveland Clinic Lerner College of Medicine, Department of General Surgery, Cleveland Clinic, Abu Dhabi, United Arab Emirates

Nathan G. LaFayette, MD Department of Surgery, The Ohio State University Wexner Medical Center, Columbus, OH, USA

Samuel Torres Landa, MD Hospital of the University of Pennsylvania, Philadelphia, PA, USA

Brian M. Lappas, MD, MPH Department of Internal Medicine, Vanderbilt University Medical Center, Nashville, TN, USA

Wayne S. Lee, MD Department of Minimally Invasive Surgery, Cedars-Sinai Medical Center, Los Angeles, CA, USA

Anthony Lembo, MD Division of Gastroenterology, Department of Medicine, Beth Israel Deaconess Medical Center, Boston, MA, USA

Feng Li, MD Division of Gastroenterology, Hepatology, and Nutrition, The Ohio State University Wexler Medical Center, Columbus, OH, USA

George Z. Li, MD Department of Surgery, Brigham and Women's Hospital, Boston, MA, USA

Paul Linsky, MD Department of Surgery, Division of Cardiothoracic Surgery, University of Alabama Birmingham, Birmingham, AL, USA

Brian E. Louie, MD Division of Thoracic Surgery, Swedish Cancer Institute, Seattle, WA, USA

Ran Bill Luo, MD Division of Minimally Invasive Surgery, Department of General Surgery, UC San Diego Health Systems, La Jolla, CA, USA

Minh B. Luu, MD, FACS Departments of General and Upper GI Surgery, Rush University Medical Center, Chicago, IL, USA

Tarik Madni, MD University of Texas Southwestern Medical Center, Department of Surgery, Division of Burn, Trauma, and Critical Care, Dallas, TX, USA

Jeffrey Marks, MD Department of Surgery, University Hospitals Cleveland Medical Center, Cleveland, OH, USA

Luis A. Martin del Campo, MD Department of Surgery, University Hospitals Cleveland Medical Center, Cleveland, OH, USA

Sarah Marucci, MD Division of Internal Medicine, University of Alabama, Birmingham, AL, USA

Patrick James McLaren, MD Department of Surgery, Division of Gastrointestinal and General Surgery, Oregon Health and Science University, Portland, OR, USA

Michael Paul Meara, MD, MBA, FACS Department of Surgery, The Ohio State University Wexner Medical Center, Columbus, OH, USA

W. Scott Melvin, MD Montefiore Medical Center, Albert Einstein College of Medicine, Bronx, NY, USA

Robert E. Merritt, MD The Division of Thoracic Surgery, Department of Surgery, The Ohio State University Wexner Medical Center, Columbus, OH, USA

Matias Mihura, MD Division of Thoracic Surgery, Swedish Cancer Institute, Seattle, WA, USA

Daniel Morrison, MD Department of Otolaryngology-Head and Neck Surgery, University of Alabama-Birmingham, Birmingham, AL, USA

Carmen L Mueller, BSc(Hon), MD, Med, FRCS(C) Department of General Surgery, McGill University, Montreal, QC, Canada

Kenric M. Murayama, MD Department of Surgery, University of Hawaii John A. Burns School of Medicine, Honolulu, HI, USA

Peter Nau, MD, MS Department of Surgery, The University of Iowa Hospitals and Clinics, Iowa City, IA, USA

Krzysztof Nowak, MD ENT and Allergy Associates, Yonkers, NY, USA

Nabeel R. Obeid, MD Department of Surgery, Stony Brook Medicine, Stony Brook, NY, USA

Brant K. Oelschlager, MD Department of Surgery, University of Washington, Seattle, WA, USA

Julia Park, MD Department of Surgery, Massachusetts General Hospital, Harvard Medical School, Boston, MA, USA

Abhishek D. Parmar, MD Division of Gastrointestinal Surgery, Department of Surgery, University of Alabama School of Medicine, Birmingham, AL, USA

Marco G. Patti, MD Department of Surgery and Center for Esophageal Diseases and Swallowing, University of North Carolina, Chapel Hill, NC, USA

Eric M. Pauli, MD, FACS Division of Minimally Invasive and Bariatric Surgery, Department of Surgery, Penn State Hershey Medical Center, Hershey, PA, USA

Luise I. M. Pernar, MD Department of Surgery, Division of Minimally Invasive and Weight Loss Surgery, Boston Medical Center, Boston, MA, USA

Kyle A. Perry Division of General and Gastrointestinal Surgery, The Ohio State University, Columbus, OH, USA

Thai Pham, MD, FACS Section Chief of General Surgery, North Dallas VA Medical Center, Surgical Services, Dallas, TX, USA

Stephanie Denise Pointer, MD Division of Gastroenterology, Hepatology, and Nutrition, The Ohio State University Wexler Medical Center, Columbus, OH, USA

Jeffrey L. Ponsky, MD, FACS Department of General Surgery, Cleveland Clinic, Cleveland, OH, USA

Aurora D. Pryor, MD, FACSFASMBS Department of Surgery, Stony Brook Medicine, Stony Brook University Hospital, Stony Brook, NY, USA

Gustavo Fernandez Ranvier, MD, PhD, FACS Division of Metabolic, Endocrine and Minimally Invasive Surgery, Department of Surgery, Mount Sinai Hospital, Icahn School of Medicine at Mount Sinai, New York, NY, USA

David W. Rattner, MD Department of Surgery, Massachusetts General Hospital, Harvard Medical School, Boston, MA, USA

Ali Rezaie, MD, MSc Department of Medicine, GI Motility Program, Cedars-Sinai Medical Center, Los Angeles, CA, USA

Marvin Ryou, MD Division of Gastroenterology, Hepatology, and Endoscopy, Brigham and Women's Hospital, Boston, MA, USA

Adham R. Saad, MD Minimally Invasive GI Surgery, Department of Surgery, University of Alabama at Birmingham, Birmingham, AL, USA

Sanjay Salgado, MD Division of Gastroenterology, Hepatology, and Endoscopy, Brigham and Women's Hospital, Boston, MA, USA

Barry Salky, MD, FACS Division of Metabolic, Endocrine and Minimally Invasive Surgery, Department of Surgery, Mount Sinai Hospital, Icahn School of Medicine at Mount Sinai, New York, NY, USA

Kamran Samakar, MD Department of Upper GI, General, and Bariatric Surgery, USC Keck Medical Center, Los Angeles, CA, USA

Francisco Schlottmann, MD Surgery and Center for Esophageal Diseases and Swallowing, University of North Carolina, Chapel Hill, NC, USA

Linda Schultz Society of American Gastrointestinal and Endoscopic Surgeons, Boston, MA, USA

Jennifer S. Schwartz, MD Department of Surgery, The Ohio State University Wexner Medical Center, Columbus, OH, USA

S. Scott Davis Jr, MD, FACS Emory Endosurgery Unit, Division of General and GI Surgery, Emory University Hospital, Atlanta, GA, USA

Anupamaa J. Seshadri, MD Department of Surgery, Brigham and Women's Hospital, Boston, MA, USA

Amber Shada, MD Department of Surgery, University of Wisconsin, Madison, WI, USA

Saurabh Sharma, MBBS, MS Department of Bariatric and Robotic Surgery Fortis Hospital, Mohali, Punjab, India

Saad Shebrain, MD, MMM, FACS Department of Surgery, Western Michigan University Homer Stryker MD School of Medicine, Kalamazoo, MI, USA

Eric G. Sheu, MD, PhD Assistant Professor of Surgery, Harvard Medical School; Associate Surgeon, Division of General and Gastrointestinal Surgery, Brigham and Women's Hospital, Boston, MA, USA

Kathleen Simon, MD Department of Surgery, Medical College of Wisconsin, Milwaukee, WI, USA

Matthew J. Skinner, MD Department of Surgery, Brigham and Women's Hospital, Harvard Medical School, Boston, MA, USA

Douglas S. Smink, MD, MPH Department of Surgery, Brigham and Women's Hospital, Boston, MA, USA

Cheyenne C. Sonntag, MD Division of Minimally Invasive and Bariatric Surgery, Department of Surgery, Penn State Hershey Medical Center, Hershey, PA, USA

Joel Sternbach, MD, MBA Department of Surgery, Northwestern Memorial Hospital, Chicago, IL, USA

Andrew T. Strong, MD Department of General Surgery, Cleveland Clinic, Cleveland, OH, USA

Andrea M. Stroud, MD University Hospital, Madison, WI, USA

Monisha Sudarshan, MD, MPH, FRCSC Department of Thoracic Surgery, Mayo Clinic, Rochester, MN, USA

Lowell S. Su, MD Department of Thoracic Surgery, Brigham and Women's Hospital, Boston, MA, USA

Lee L. Swanstrom, MD The Oregon Clinic, Portland, OR, USA

Ezra N. Teitelbaum, MD, MEd Northwestern University, Chicago, IL, USA

Dana A. Telem, MD, MPH Michigan Comprehensive Hernia Program, Department of Surgery, University of Michigan, Ann Arbor, MI, USA

Daniel C. Thomas, MD Yale School of Medicine, Yale University, New Haven, CT, USA

Christopher C. Thompson, MD Department of Surgery, Brigham and Women's Hospital, Harvard Medical School, Boston, MA, USA

Thadeus L. Trus, MD Geisel School of Medicine, Dartmouth Hitchcock Medical Center, Lebanon, NH, USA

Thomas C. Tsai, MD, MPH Department of Surgery, Brigham and Women's Hospital, Harvard Medical School, Boston, MA, USA

Michael B. Ujiki, MD Department of Surgery, NorthShore University Health System, University of Chicago Medical Center, Chicago, IL, USA

Michael F. Vaezi, MD, PhD, MSc (Epi) Division of Gastroenterology, Hepatology and Nutrition, Vanderbilt University Medical Center, Nashville, TN, USA

Oliver A. Varban, MD Department of General Surgery, Michigan Medicine, University Hospital, University of Michigan, Ann Arbor, MI, USA

Benjamin R. Veenstra, MD Department of Surgery, Division of MIS and Bariatrics, Rush University Medical Center, Chicago, IL, USA

Vic Velanovich, MD Department of Surgery, University of South Florida, Tampa, FL, USA

Ashley H. Vernon, MD Department of Surgery, Brigham and Women's Hospital, Harvard Medical School, Boston, MA, USA

Yalini Vigneswaran, MD Department of Surgery, NorthShore University Health System, University of Chicago Medical Center, Chicago, IL, USA

Jon P. Walker, MD Division of Gastroenterology, Hepatology, and Nutrition, The Ohio State University Wexler Medical Center, Columbus, OH, USA

Jon O. Wee, MD Department of Thoracic Surgery, Brigham and Women's Hospital, Boston, MA, USA

Benjamin Wei, MD Department of Surgery, University of Alabama-Birmingham Medical Center, Birmingham, AL, USA

Leonard K. Welsh Jr, MD Department of Surgery, University of Hawaii John A. Burns School of Medicine, Honolulu, HI, USA

Jaclyn Wierzbicki, MD Department of Surgery, The University of Iowa Hospitals and Clinics, Iowa City, IA, USA

Kirk Withrow, MD Department of Otolaryngology-Head and Neck Surgery, University of Alabama-Birmingham, Birmingham, AL, USA

Aric Wogsland, MD Department of Surgery, University Hospitals Cleveland Medical Center, Cleveland, OH, USA

Andrew S. Wright, MD University of Washington Medical School, Seattle, WA, USA

Mohammed Zakari, MD Division of Gastroenterology, Department of Medicine, Beth Israel Deaconess Medical Center, Boston, MA, USA

Jessica Zarzour, MD Department of Radiology, University of Alabama, Birmingham, AL, USA

SAGES University MASTERS PROGRAM: Foregut Pathway

1

Daniel B. Jones, Linda Schultz, and Brian Jacob

The Masters Program organizes educational materials along clinical pathways into discrete blocks of content which could be accessed by a surgeon attending the SAGES annual meeting or by logging into the online SAGES University (Fig. 1.1) [1]. The SAGES Masters Program currently has eight pathways including Acute Care, Biliary, Bariatrics, Colon, Foregut, Hernia, Flex Endoscopy, and Robotic Surgery (Fig. 1.2). Each pathway is divided into three levels of targeted performance: competency, proficiency, and mastery (Fig. 1.3). The levels originate from the Dreyfus model of skill acquisition [2], which has five stages: novice, advanced beginner, competency, proficiency, and expertise. The SAGES MASTERS Program is based on the three more advanced stages of skill acquisition: competency, proficiency, and expertise. Competency is defined as what a graduating general surgery chief resident or MIS fellow should be able to achieve; proficiency is what a surgeon approximately 3 years out from training should be able to accomplish; and mastery is what more experienced surgeons should be able to accomplish after several years in practice. Mastery is applicable to SAGES surgeons seeking in-depth knowledge in a pathway, including the

---

Adopted from Jones DB, Stefanidis D, Korndorffer JR, Dimick JB, Jacob BP, Schultz L, Scott DJ (2017) SAGES University Masters Program: a structured curriculum for deliberate, lifelong learning. Surg Endosc 31:3061–3071

D. B. Jones (✉)
Harvard Medical School, Division of Bariatric and Minimally Invasive Surgery, Beth Israel Deaconess Medical Center, Boston, MA, USA
e-mail: djones1@bidmc.harvard.edu

L. Schultz
Society of American Gastrointestinal and Endoscopic Surgeons, Boston, MA, USA

B. Jacob
Department of Surgery, Icahn School of Medicine at Mount Sinai, New York, NY, USA

J. Grams et al. (eds.), *The SAGES Manual of Foregut Surgery*,
https://doi.org/10.1007/978-3-319-96122-4_1

Fig. 1.1 MASTERS program logo

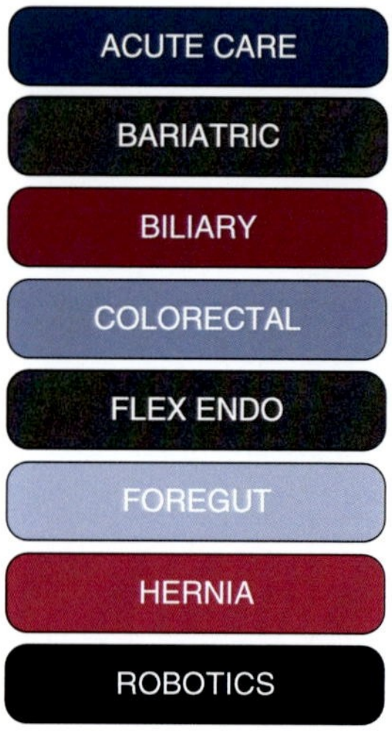

Fig. 1.2 MASTER program clinical pathways

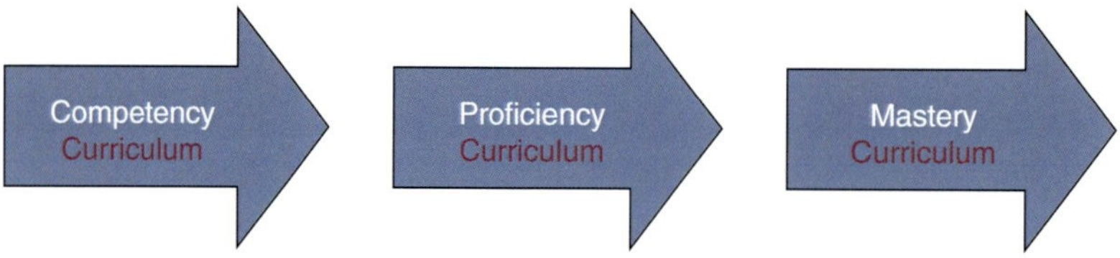

Fig. 1.3 MASTERS program progression

following: areas of controversy, outcomes, best practice, and ability to mentor colleagues. Over time, with the utilization of coaching and participation in SAGES courses, this level should be obtainable by the majority of SAGES members. This edition of the SAGES Manual – Foregut Surgery – aligns with the current version of the new SAGES University MASTERS Program Foregut Surgery Pathway (Table 1.1).

Foregut Curriculum

The key elements of the Foregut Surgery curriculum include a core lectures for the pathway, which provides a 45-minute general overview including basic anatomy, physiology, diagnostic work-up, and surgical management. As of 2018, all lecture

Table 1.1 Foregut surgery anchoring procedure by pathway

Curriculum elements	*Competency*
Anchoring procedure – competency	2
CORE LECTURE	1
CORE MCE 70%	1
Annual meeting content	5
Guidelines	1
SA CME hours	6
Sentinel articles	2
Social media	2
SAGES top 21 video	1
FLS	12
PEARLS	1
Motility module	1
Credits	**35**
Curriculum elements	*Proficiency*
Anchoring procedure – proficiency	2
CORE LECTURE	1
CORE MCE 70%	1
Annual meeting content	5
FUSE	12
Outcomes database enrollment	2
SA CME hours (ASMBS electives, SAGES or SAGES-endorsed)	6
Sentinel articles	2
Social media	2
SAGES top 21 video	1
PEARLS	1
Credits	**35**
Curriculum elements	*Mastery*
Anchoring procedure – mastery	2
CORE LECTURE	1
CORE MCE 70%	1
Annual meeting content	6
Fundamentals of surgical coaching	4
Outcomes database reporting	2
SA CME credits (ASMBS electives, SAGES or SAGES-endorsed)	6
Sentinel articles	2
Serving as video assessment reviewer and providing feedback (FSC)	4
Social media	6
SMART enhanced recovery	1
Credits	**35**

content of the annual SAGES meetings are labeled as follows: basic (100), intermediate (200), and advanced (300). This allows attendees to choose lectures that best fit their educational needs. Coding the content additionally facilitates online retrieval of specific educational material, with varying degrees of surgical complexity, ranging from introductory to revisional surgery.

SAGES identified the need to develop targeted, complex content for its mastery level curriculum. The idea was that these 25-min lectures would be focused on specific topics. It assumes that the attendee already has a good understanding of diseases and management from attending/watching competency and proficiency level lectures. Ideally, in order to supplement a chosen topic, the mastery lectures would also identify key prerequisite articles from *Surgical Endoscopy* and other journals, in addition to SAGES University videos. Many of these lectures will be forthcoming at future SAGES annual meetings.

The MASTERS Program has a self-assessment, multiple-choice exam for each module to guide learner progression throughout the curriculum. Questions are submitted by core lecture speakers and SAGES annual meeting faculty. The goal of the questions is to use assessment for learning, with the assessment being criterion-referenced with the percent correct set at 80%. Learners will be able to review incorrect answers, review educational content, and retake the examination until a passing score is obtained.

The MASTERS Program Foregut Surgery curriculum taps much of the SAGES existing educational products including FLS, FES, FUSE, SMART, Top 21 videos, and Pearls (Fig. 1.4). The Curriculum Task Force has placed the aforementioned modules along a continuum of the curriculum pathway. For example, FLS, in general, occurs during the Competency Curriculum, whereas the Fundamental Use of Surgical Energy (FUSE) is usually required during the Proficiency Curriculum. The Fundamentals of Laparoscopic Surgery (FLS) is a multiple-choice exam and a skills assessment conducted on a video box trainer. Tasks include peg transfer, cutting, intracorporeal and extracorporeal suturing, and knot tying. Since 2010, FLS has been required of all US general surgery residents seeking to sit for the American Board of Surgery qualifying examinations. The Fundamentals of Endoscopic Surgery (FES) assesses endoscopic knowledge and technical skills in a simulator. FUSE teaches about the safe use of energy devices in the operating room and is available at FUSE.didactic.org. After learners complete the self-paced modules, they may take the certifying examination.

The SAGES Surgical Multimodal Accelerated Recovery Trajectory (SMART) Initiative combines minimally invasive surgical techniques with enhanced recovery pathways (ERPs) for perioperative care, with the goal of improving outcomes and patient satisfaction. Educational materials include a website with best practices, sample pathways, patient literature, and other resources such as videos, FAQs, and an implementation timeline. The materials assist surgeons and their surgical team with implementation of an ERP.

Top 21 videos are edited videos of the most commonly performed MIS operations and basic endoscopy. Cases are straightforward with quality video and clear anatomy.

Pearls are step-by-step video clips of ten operations. The authors show different variations for each step. The learner should have a fundamental understanding of the operation.

SAGES Guidelines provide evidence-based recommendations for surgeons and are developed by the SAGES Guidelines Committee following the Health

Fig. 1.4 SAGES educational content: FLS, FES, FUSE, SMART and Medicine Division of the National Academies of Sciences, Engineering, and Medicine standards (formerly the Institute of Medicine) for guideline development [3]. Each clinical practice guideline has been systematically researched, reviewed, and revised by the SAGES Guidelines Committee and an appropriate multidisciplinary team. The strength of the provided recommendations is determined based on the quality of the available literature using the GRADE methodology [4]. SAGES Guidelines cover a wide range of topics relevant to the practice of SAGES surgeon members and are updated on a regular basis. Since the developed guidelines provide an appraisal of the available literature, their inclusion in the MASTERS Program was deemed necessary by the group.

The Curriculum Task Force identified the need to select required readings for the MASTERS Program based on key articles for the various curriculum procedures. Summaries of each of these articles follow the American College of Surgeons (ACS) Selected Readings format.

Facebook™ Groups

While there are many great platforms available to permit online collaboration by user-generated content, Facebook(™) offers a unique, highly developed mobile platform that is ideal for global professional collaboration and daily continuing surgical education (Fig. 1.5). Facebook groups allow for video assessment, feedback, and coaching as a tool to improve practice.

Based on the anchoring procedures determined via group consensus (Table 1.2), participants in the MASTERS Program will submit video clips on closed Facebook groups, with other participants and/or SAGES members providing qualitative feedback. For example, for the Foregut Curriculum, surgeons would submit the critical views during a laparoscopic paraesophageal hernia repair such as identification of the anterior and posterior vagus nerves. Using crowdsourcing, other surgeons would comment and provide feedback.

Eight unique vetted membership-only closed Facebook groups were created for the MASTERS Program, including a group for bariatrics, hernia, colorectal, biliary, acute care, flexible endoscopy, robotics, and foregut. The Foregut Surgery Facebook group is independent of the other groups and will be populated only by physicians, mostly surgeons or surgeons in training interested in foregut surgery.

The group provides an international platform for surgeons and healthcare providers interested in optimizing outcomes in a surgical specialty to collaborate, share, discuss, and post photos, videos, and anything related to a chosen specialty. By embracing social media as a collaborative forum, we can more effectively and transparently obtain immediate global feedback that potentially can improve patient outcomes, as well as the quality of care we provide, all while transforming the way a society's members interact.

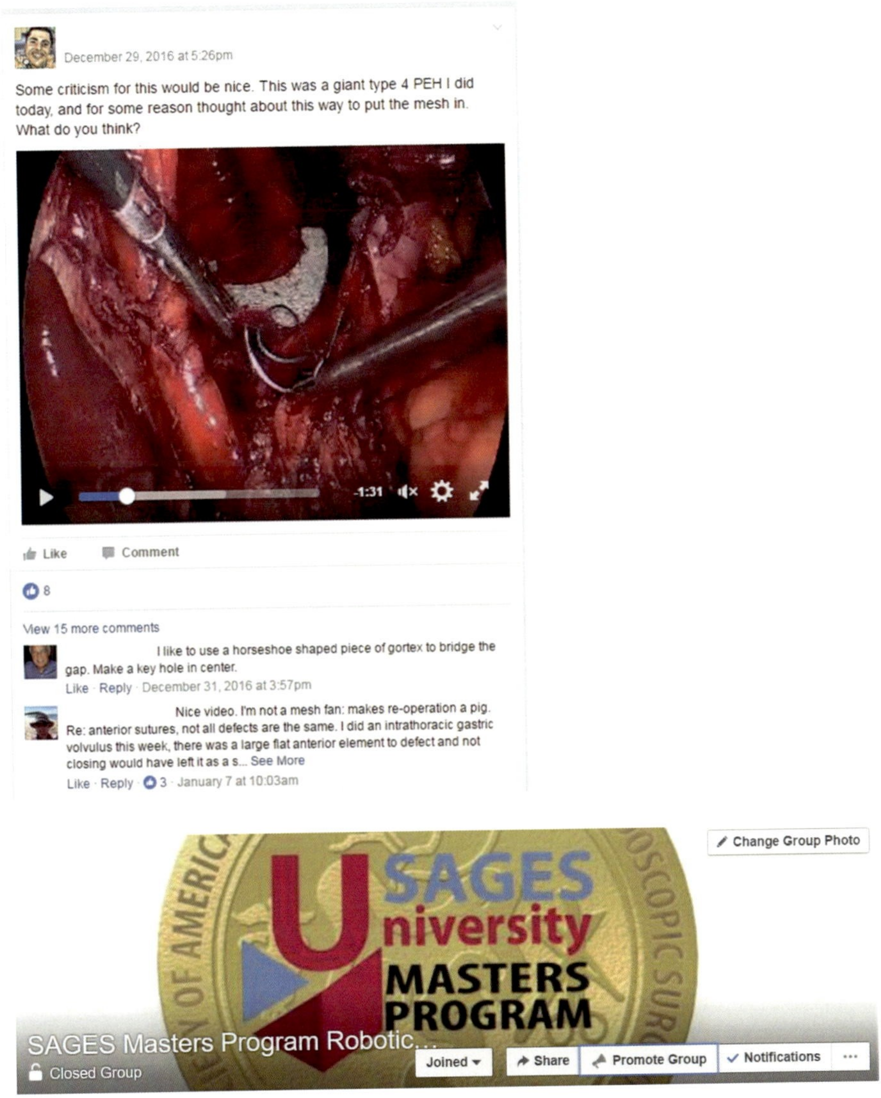

Fig. 1.5 Foregut surgery facebook Facebook(TM)group

Table 1.2 MASTERS program colon curriculum outline

Anchoring procedure by pathway	Level
Foregut Surgery	
Lap Nissen	Competency
Lap Paraesophageal or Heller Myotomy	Proficiency
Lap Redo Nissen	Mastery

For the first two levels of the MASTERS Program, competency and proficiency, participants will be required to post videos of the anchoring procedures and will receive qualitative feedback from other participants. However, for the mastery level, participants will submit a video to be evaluated by an expert panel. A standardized video assessment tool, depending on the specific procedure, will be used. A benchmark will also be utilized to determine when the participant has achieved the mastery level for that procedure.

Once the participant has achieved mastery level, s/he will participate as a coach by providing feedback to participants in the first two levels. MASTERS Program participants will therefore need to learn the fundamental principles of surgical coaching. The key activities of coaching include goal setting, active listening, powerful inquiry, and constructive feedback [5, 6]. Importantly, peer coaching is much different than traditional education, where there is an expert and a learner. Peer coaching is a "co-learning" model where the coach is facilitating the development of the coachee by using inquiry (i.e., open-ended questions) in a noncompetitive manner.

Surgical coaching skills are a crucial part of the MASTERS curriculum. At the 2017 SAGES Annual Meeting, a postgraduate course on coaching skills was developed and video recorded. The goal is to develop a "coaching culture" within the SAGES MASTERS Program, wherein both participants and coaches are committed to lifelong learning and development.

The need for a more structured approach to the education of practicing surgeons as accomplished by the SAGES MASTERS Program is well recognized [7]. Since performance feedback usually stops after training completion and current approaches to MOC are suboptimal, the need for peer coaching has recently received increased attention in surgery [5, 6]. SAGES has recognized this need, and its MASTERS Program embraces social media for surgical education to help provide a free, mobile, and easy to use platform to surgeons globally. Access to the MASTERS Program groups enables surgeons at all levels to partake in the MASTERS Program curriculum and obtain feedback from peers, mentors, and experts. By creating surgeon-only private groups dedicated to this project, SAGES can now offer surgeons posting in these groups the ability to discuss preoperative, intraoperative, and postoperative issues with other SAGES colleagues and mentors. In addition, the platform permits transparent and responsive dialogue about technique, continuing the theme of deliberate, lifelong learning.

To accommodate the needs of this program, SAGES University is upgrading its web-based features. A new learning management system (LMS) will track progression and make access to SAGES University simple. Features of the new IT infrastructure will provide the ability to access a video or lecture on-demand in relation to content, level of difficulty, and author. Once enrolled in the MASTERS Program, the LMS will track lectures, educational products, MCE, and other completed requirements. Participants will be able to see where they stand in relation to module completion, and SAGES will alert learners to relevant content they may be interested in pursuing. Until such time that the new LMS is up and running, it is hoped that the SAGES Manual will help guide learners through the Masters Program Curriculum.

Conclusions

The SAGES MASTERS Program Foregut Surgery Pathway facilitates deliberate, focused postgraduate teaching and learning. The MASTERS Program certifies completion of the curriculum but is *not* meant to certify competency, proficiency, or mastery of surgeons. The MASTERS Program embraces the concept of lifelong learning after fellowship, and its curriculum is organized from basic principles to more complex content. The MASTERS Program is an innovative, voluntary curriculum that supports MOC and deliberate, lifelong learning.

References

1. Jones DB, Stefanidis D, Korndorffer JR, Dimick JB, Jacob BP, Schultz L, Scott DJ. SAGES University masters program: a structured curriculum for deliberate, lifelong learning. Surg Endosc. 2017;31:3061–71.
2. Dreyfus SE. The five-stage model of adult skill acquisition. Bull Sci Technol Soc. 2004;24: 177–81.
3. Graham R, Mancher M, Miller Woman D, Greenfield S, Steinberg E. Institute of Medicine (US) committee on standards for developing trustworthy clinical practice guidelines. Clinical practice guidelines we can trust. Washington, DC: National Academies Press (US); 2011.
4. Guyatt GH, Oxman AD, Vist GE, Kunz R, Falck-Ytter Y, Alonso-Coello P, Schünemann HJ, GRADE Working Group. GRADE: an emerging consensus on rating quality of evidence and strength of recommendations. BMJ. 2008;336:924–6.
5. Greenberg CC, Ghousseini HN, Pavuluri Quamme SR, Beasley HL, Wiegmann DA. Surgical coaching for individual performance improvement. Ann Surg. 2015;261:32–4.
6. Greenberg CC, Dombrowski J, Dimick JB. Video-based surgical coaching: an emerging approach to performance improvement. JAMA Surg. 2016;151:282–3.
7. Sachdeva AK. Acquiring skills in new procedures and technology: the challenge and the opportunity. Arch Surg. 2005;140:387–9.

Anatomy and Physiology of the Esophagus and Lower Esophageal Sphincter

2

Lawrence F. Johnson

As surgeons address foregut disease in their patients with different procedures, a review of relevant anatomy and physiology of the esophagus and LES will complement discussion with their patients and decision-making. As will be apparent in this chapter, the esophagus is more than a conduit that directs liquids and food to other organs, deters reflux, or serves as a passageway for radiographic contrast, or endoscopes to define more distant foregut disease/disorders. Instead, the esophagus is a very complex organ whose function is directed by CNS and intrinsic esophageal control that is implemented by skeletal and smooth muscle. In preparing this manuscript rather than use time-tested anatomical illustrations by Frank Netter, MD, I chose where possible to use operative photographs, anatomical dissections undertaken by interested clinicians addressing perplexing problems, as well as illustrations from 3D printers, dissections, and combined techniques. Animal models were held to a minimum and only used to confirm a clinical point in humans or when these studies lead to important discoveries in humans. In some instances, the reader will need to refer to the original references since permissions could not be obtained for all of the intended figures. While this text was limited to anatomy and physiology, I could not resist the temptation for brief clinical departures to emphasize the importance of learning the anatomy and physiology so that it might be implemented in every day practice.

Introduction

Measurements in adult human cadavers have shown the esophageal length when measured from cricoid cartilage/bone to stomach opening ranges from 24 to 34 cm with an average of 27.6 cm [1]. While the cricoid cartilage or bone if calcified can be identified radiographically on the lateral barium swallow [2, 3] and at

L. F. Johnson
Department of Gastroenterology and Hepatology, University of Alabama-Birmingham, Birmingham, AL, USA

J. Grams et al. (eds.), *The SAGES Manual of Foregut Surgery*,
https://doi.org/10.1007/978-3-319-96122-4_2

laryngoscopy [4], this orad landmark has not been clinically popular even though it could be anatomically justified because the cricopharyngeus muscle inserts into the cricoid cartilage or bone [5]. Instead, endoscopists use the incisors teeth as the orad landmark and termination of the gastric rugal folds and/or distal margin of the esophageal palisade veins as a close approximation of the esophagogastric junction (approximately 40 cm) [6]. Using this definition and subtracting 15 cm (distance incisor teeth to UES) [7], the esophageal length again measures 25 cm. When esophageal length is measured using high-resolution esophageal motility from the inferior margin of the UES to the superior margin of the LES in patients without a hiatal hernia, the mean distance is again 25 cm [8]. Thus, the adult human esophagus appears to be approximately 25 cm long when measured by different techniques in vivo or cadavers.

As one would expect, the esophagus grows in length as the individual ages and gains height [9]. For instance, esophageal length when measured at the superior border of the LES directly correlates with height. When all age groups from infancy to adulthood are combined, a regression analysis shows that the esophagus grows in length as the individual grows in height [9]. However, only in children less than 2 years old can their height accurately predict LES location (90% of predictions within 1 cm of actual location). Unfortunately, in all other age groups, height poorly predicts LES location probably because some individuals are developing hiatal hernias and/or esophageal shortening.

UES and Proximal Esophagus

The esophageal body is a muscular tube composed of an inner layer of circular and an outer layer of longitudinal muscle and includes a sphincter at either end. The proximal or upper esophageal sphincter is more macroscopically defined than that of the distal or lower esophageal sphincter, which some think is primarily a manometric phenomenon. While we think of the upper esophageal sphincter as the cricopharyngeus muscle, the anatomy is more complex (Fig. 2.1). For instance, the cricopharyngeus muscle inserts into the posterior surface of the cricoid cartilage, and as a result the anterior wall of the sphincter is the cricoid lamina or posterior surface of the cricoid cartilage, which encircles the airway as opposed to tracheal rings. In turn, the cricopharyngeal muscle forms a horseshoe or C-like sphincter with the posterior surface of the cricoid cartilage closing the anterior gap [10]. The attachment of the cricopharyngeus muscle or UES to the cricoid cartilage is so tight that any movement of the larynx reflects that of the cricopharyngeus muscle or upper esophageal sphincter [11]. Contrary to common thought, there is no connection between the UES and pre-cervical vertebral fascia because this space in human dissections shows only loose adipose tissue and pools of amorphous substance (Fig. 2.2), but no dense connective tissue strands between

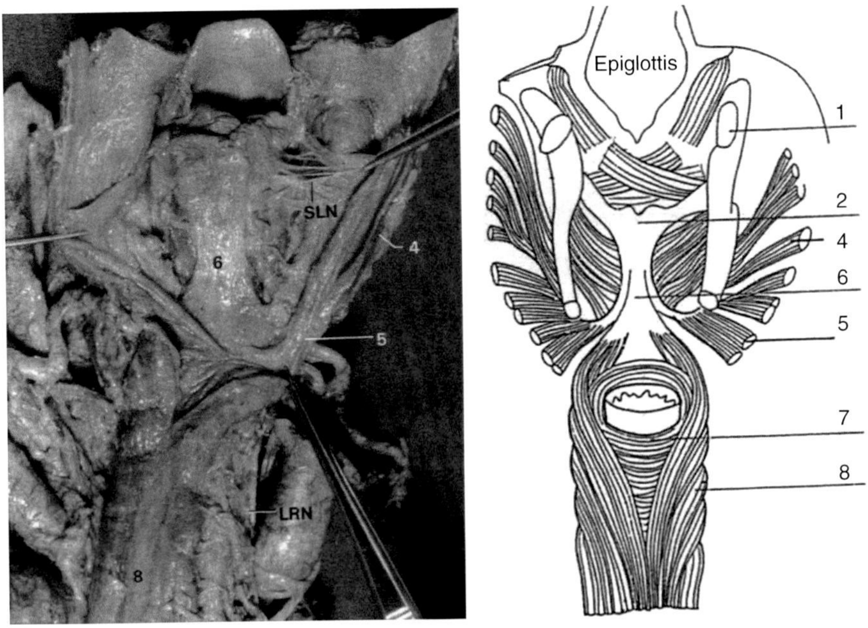

Fig. 2.1 Dissection and schematic drawing of the pharyngoesophageal junction viewed from the dorsal aspect, with the pharynx and esophageal wall both opened in the midline. Note broad-based exposed cricopharyngeal tendon (6) that attaches to the posterior surface of cricoid cartilage (2) and thereby serves to attach the left and right branching of the outer longitudinal esophageal muscle wall (8) to the lateral aspect of the cricoid cartilage. The tip of the metal forceps is attached to the upper esophageal sphincter [cricopharyngeus muscle (5), a component of the inferior pharyngeal constrictor (4)]. If not cut, the UES would have a U appearance when attached to the flat lateral surface of the post-cricoid cartilage, its anterior wall. Components: 1 = thyroid cartilage, 2 = cricoid cartilage, 3 = trachea, 4 = inferior pharyngeal constrictor, 5 = cricopharyngeus muscle, 6 = cricopharyngeal tendon, 7 = inner circular wall of the esophagus, 8 = outer longitudinal wall of the esophagus, 9 = arytenoid muscle, and 10 = aryepiglottic muscle. *SLN* superior laryngeal nerve, *RLN* recurrent laryngeal nerve. (With permission from Liebermann-Meffert [10])

UES and pre-cervical vertebral fascia [11]. In contrast, at C1–C4 the pharyngeal and cervical vertebral fascia intertwines and stabilizes the pharynx to the cervical spine [12]. More caudad, the cricopharyngeal muscle continues into the internal circular muscle of the esophagus without any attachment to the cricoid cartilage. However, to make up for this lack of attachment, the outer longitudinal muscle of the esophagus inserts into the cricoid cartilage via the cricoesophageal tendon, thereby giving the proximal esophagus a stability point. The cricoid cartilage is unique for it is only one of a few instances in which skeletal muscle directly inserts on cartilage.

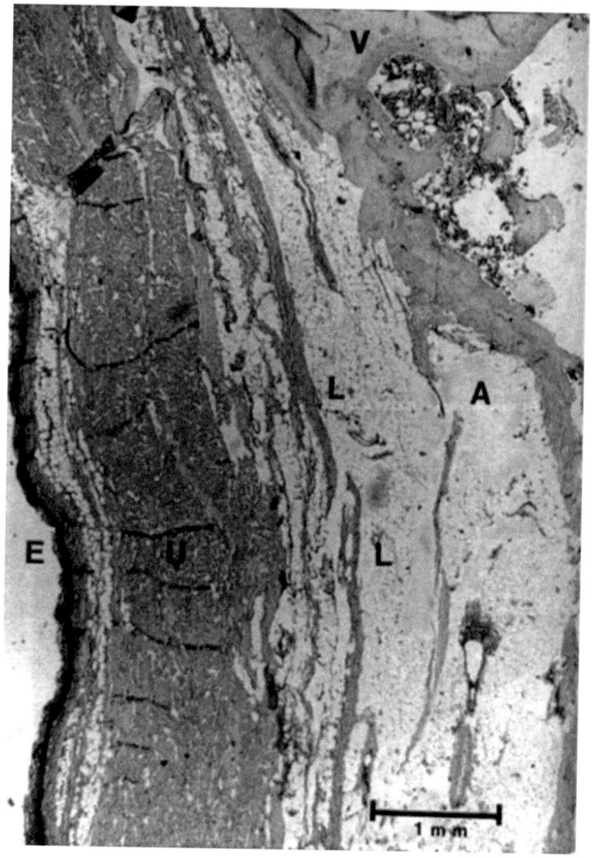

Fig. 2.2 This cross section of the prevertebral space in region of the upper esophageal sphincter (U) shows loose fatty tissue (L) with pools of an amorphous substance (A). Note esophageal epithelium (E) and the vertebral body (V). This paraffin section was stained with hematoxylin-eosin. (With permission from Nilsson et al. [11])

The change in direction of skeletal muscle fibers both above and below the cricoid cartilage causes weakness in the wall of the pharyngoesophageal junction [13]. Above the cricoid cartilage, when oblique muscle fibers of the inferior pharyngeal sphincter meet more horizontal muscle fibers of the cricopharyngeal muscle, the wall is weakened resulting in Killian's triangle, which is the site of Zenker's diverticulum that develops posterior above the cricopharyngeus muscle. In contrast, below the cricoid cartilage when the outer layer of longitudinal esophageal muscle begins to separate in order to join the cricoesophageal tendon for insertion into the cricoid cartilage, gaps in the muscle area are created where only the inner circular esophageal muscle is left to constitute the esophageal wall, and as a result the wall is weakened. This area is known as Laimer's triangle [14] that predisposes to the formation of Killian-Jamieson diverticula that develop lateral or anterolateral [15] located below the cricopharyngeus muscle. While weakness in the pharyngoesophageal junction wall causes both diverticula to form, Zenker's is the more common, i.e., 4:1 [15]. While pharyngosphincteric incoordination or lack of sphincter relaxation was thought to cause Zenker's diverticula, investigators have shown increased intrabolus pressure correlated with reduced sphincter opening [16, 17] and the latter appeared caused by replacement of cricopharyngeal muscle fibers by fibrous adipose tissue and degenerative changes, which appears to cause lack of sufficient sphincter elasticity [18]. This diminished elasticity or alteration in the composition of the sphincter causes increased hypopharyngeal pressure that result in the diverticulum subsequently causing symptoms such as dysphagia and overflow aspiration. These patients may benefit from a myotomy [19]. However, the therapeutic benefit of a myotomy might not apply to patients with Killian-Jamieson diverticula. These diverticula are small and often cause no symptoms, because they occur below the cricopharyngeus muscle [15], and a myotomy may not be of similar benefit. Most important, anatomically – the recurrent laryngeal nerve (right or left) may travel across the base of the diverticulum (Fig. 2.3) as the nerve passes between the cricopharyngeus muscle and the cricoid cartilage in the region of the articulation between thyroid and cricoid cartilage [20, 21]. These nerves innervate all intrinsic muscles of the larynx (except for the cricothyroid) and provide sensory input to the mucosa of the larynx below the vocal fold including the inferior surface of the vocal fold, as well as mucosa of the upper trachea and esophagus. Thus, the anatomic relationship between the base of the diverticulum and recurrent laryngeal nerve in the region of the cricoid cartilage suggest a direct approach to addressing Killian-Jamieson diverticula if indicated [22] and even sometimes sensory testing of the nerve during the conduct of the procedure [23].

While with conventional manometry, we think of the UES as a bell-shaped curve with two slopes that culminate at the apex showing the peak pressure or with high-resolution manometry, a horizontal pressure bar of various colors with the highest displayed in the center of the bar, the UES is anatomically complex. For instance, when 360 degree circumferential unidirectional pressure probes are used to determine resting basal LES pressure over the length of the sphincter, the pressure profile is asymmetrical

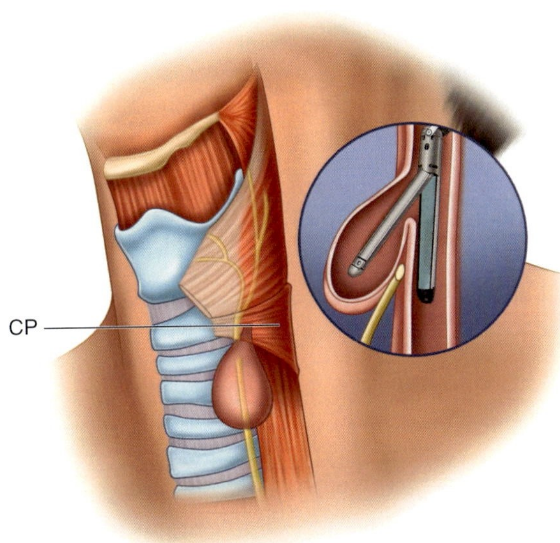

Fig. 2.3 Illustration depicting the location of the Killian-Jamieson diverticulum, which is closely related to the recurrent laryngeal nerve (RLN), seen in yellow. Inset, illustration showing how endoscopic diverticulotomy might damage the RLN [20]. CP cricopharyngeus muscle

over the 3 cm UES length [24]. This asymmetry occurs because the cricopharyngeal muscle attaches to both the right and left lateral margin of the cricoid lamina [25] so that the sustained basal contraction is greatest in the anterior and posterior dimension rather than lateral. That the cricoid cartilage is instrumental in causing this pressure asymmetry is evident by its removal following laryngectomy. For instance, when the cricopharyngeus muscle is closed in a three-layer manner after laryngectomies, the basal pressure decreases because of the myotomy and now becomes symmetrical because the muscle lost its bilateral attachment to the lamina of the cricoid cartilage [24].

That the length of the post-cricoid lamina and manometric UES are comparable in length (approximately 3 cm) [25, 26] yet the cricopharyngeus muscle is only 1 cm in longitudinal length [2] suggests other muscle(s) may be measured in the UES pressure profile. The muscle best documented to contribute to the UES pressure profile concerns the caudad portion of the inferior pharyngeal sphincter sometimes known as the thyropharyngeal muscle [26] with oblique fibers that attach to the cricoid and thyroid cartilages and a ligament that spans between these cartilages [27]. In support of the above assertion, the cricopharyngeus muscle occupies only the distal 3rd of the cricoid cartilage and appears best to represent the descending slope of the bell-shaped curve. In several studies the apex of the bell curve is above the cricopharyngeus and in the region of the thyropharyngeal, which correlates with the ascending portion of the bell shape curve and indeed is located in the region of the apex of that curve [26]. There is no apparent data to support a contribution to the pressure curve by circular muscle from the proximal esophagus that at best is controversial [26].

Anatomic markers on the lateral x-ray of the pharynx that correlate with the length and apex of the UES bell-shaped pressure curve (a distance of 2–4 cm) [26] are as follows: the orad margin consists of the arytenoid cartilage (arytenoid mass) [12], which also serves for the opening of the laryngeal airway and the caudad margin of the UES, the terminus of the cricoid cartilage, which can also be seen radiographically [2, 3, 12]. Alternatively, one might use the superior surface of the tracheal air column seen on the lateral x-ray of the pharynx, which represents the level of the vocal folds that in turn marks the start or ascending limb of the bell-shaped UES pressure curve, and the caudad margin of the descending UES curve would be the caudad margin of the cricopharyngeus muscle, if observed (Fig. 2.4), or pick a location 2–4 cm below the laryngeal opening [26]. To anatomically identify the area related to the apex of the UES bell-shaped pressure curve, one might use an area 1.6 cm below the vocal folds, i.e., tracheal air column [5] or the mid-cricoid cartilage region [28].

In support of other muscle(s) contributing to the UES pressure curve other than the cricopharyngeus concerns a study [29] that measured changes in sequential UES pressure before anesthesia and then during different stages of a 6 cm myotomy at the pharyngoesophageal junction. The initial incision was 2 cm on the proximal cervical esophagus, then a 2 cm incision on the cricopharyngeus identified by cricoid cartilage, followed by a 2 cm incision on the hypopharynx (i.e., presumed inferior sphincter or thyropharyngeal muscle), and after anesthesia recovery for a final pressure determination (Fig. 2.5). After controlling for changes related to anesthesia, they found that the cervical esophageal incision did not alter UES pressure. However, that of the cricopharyngeus did significantly

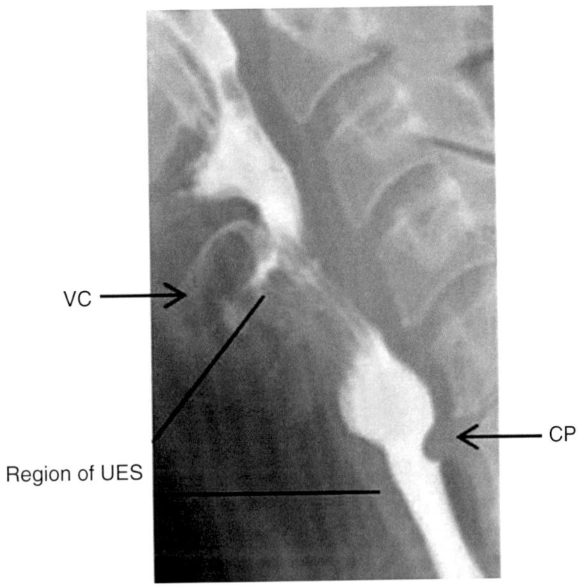

Fig. 2.4 Lateral radiograph of a barium esophagram in a patient with a prominent cricopharyngeal bar (arrow). Note that cricopharyngeus muscle is present in the lower part of the cricoid cartilage. Measured in this manner, the upper esophageal sphincter (UES) would extend from the level of the vocal folds to the lower border of the cricoid cartilage. VC vocal cords, CP cricopharyngeus muscle. (Photo courtesy of Michelle McNamara, MD)

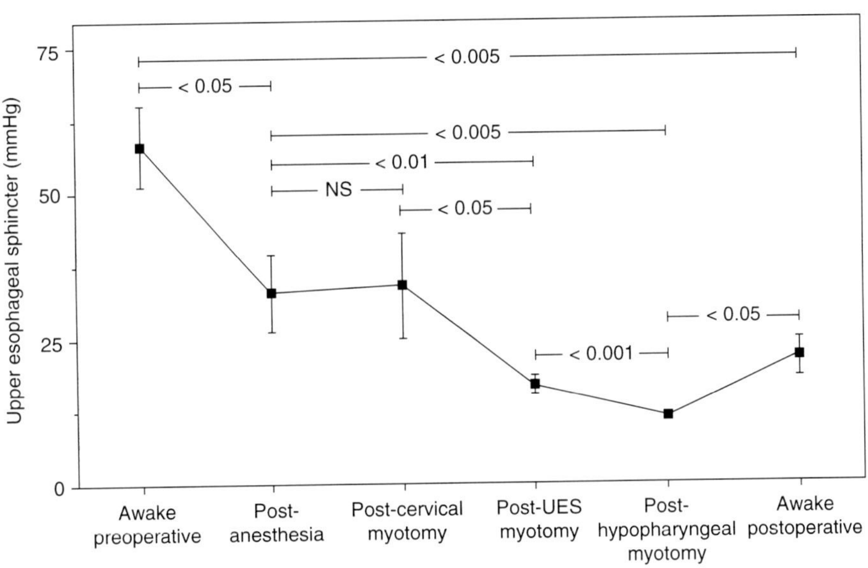

Fig. 2.5 The effects of myotomy on the resting pressure when staged at the cricopharyngeal junction [29]. Post-cervical myotomy denotes 2 cm incision on proximal esophagus

lower UES pressure, and a further significant reduction in pressure occurred after the hypopharyngeal incision. After recovery from anesthesia, the 6 cm myotomy significantly lowered LES pressure over that noted prior to anesthesia. Most importantly, the reduction in pressure appeared to result from the incision on the cricopharyngeus and the thyropharyngeal muscles rather than that on the proximal cervical esophagus.

While the inferior pharyngeal constrictor (thyropharyngeal) and the cricopharyngeus muscles insert on the thyroid and cricoid cartilages helping to form the bell-shaped curve of the UES, both muscles and cartilages have very dissimilar anatomy. For instance, the thyroid cartilage has no posterior surface as does the cricoid cartilage with its posterior lamina. As a result, the pharyngeal constrictor muscle itself serves as the anterior wall, and these muscle fibers insert posteriorly into a median raphe, not present in the cricopharyngeus muscle that inserts into the cricoid cartilage, its anterior wall. Thus, the UES is a more anatomically complex structure than that depicted by a bell-shaped pressure curve with an apex as observed during conventional manometry or that of a multicolor bar seen during high-resolution motility.

Esophageal Body

In the forthcoming discussion of the esophageal body, when necessary, the UES and LES will be included, especially, since the terminal esophagus joins the stomach as much as 3–6 [30] or 0.5–2.5 [31] cm below the diaphragmatic hiatus and this esophageal "submerged segment" can be seen on retroflexion at endoscopy (Fig. 2.6a) [6] or x-ray (Fig. 2.6b) [32]. However, because the esophagogastric junction inclusive of the LES has equally complex anatomy as that of the pharyngoesophageal junction, the former junction deserves special attention in a dedicated section and that will follow a general discussion of the esophageal body.

In traveling from the neck through the chest and into the abdomen below the diaphragm to join the stomach, the esophagus is not a straight open organ as sometimes depicted anatomically in the anterior-posterior dimension. For instance, at the pharyngoesophageal junction, the esophagus is immediately posterior to the cricoid cartilage as previously discussed. Immediately below that location in the neck, the esophagus deviates to the left of the trachea down to the base of the neck. At the level of the seventh cervical vertebra, the esophagus deviates to the right of the spine and continues on that course to the diaphragmatic hiatus. Just below the hiatus, the terminal esophagus turns to the left and joins the stomach in a left lateral position. Surface markers for the EG junction include a position just left of the xiphoid process and lateral to the 12th thoracic vertebral body [13]. In the upper mediastinum, the esophagus is positioned between the trachea and heart [33]. The esophagus in the oblique and lateral positions follows the thoracic vertebrae [34, 35]. Contrary to common anatomical depiction, the

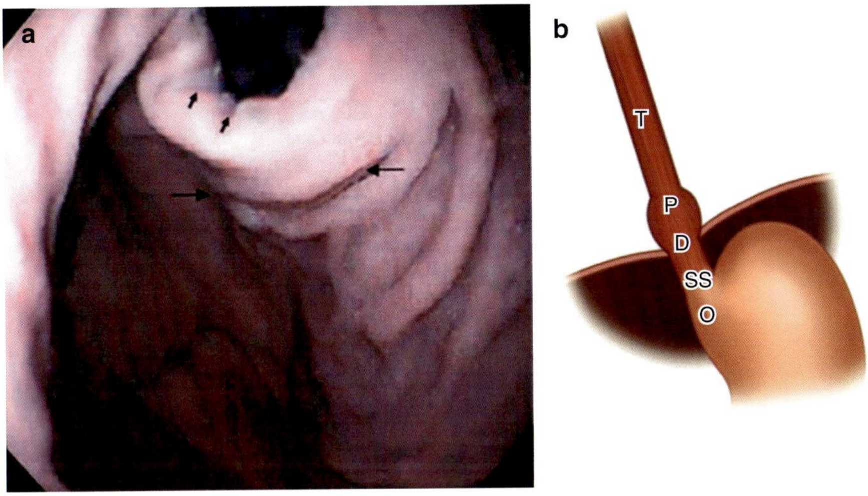

Fig. 2.6 (**a**) The submerged or intra-abdominal segment of the distal esophagus that shows the squamocolumnar junction (SCJ, upper arrows) and the crural segment of the lower esophageal sphincter (the two lower arrows). (With permission from Boyce [6]). (**b**) Normal EG junction anatomy when all segments are maximally distended. T tubular esophagus, P phrenic ampulla, D upper border of hiatus, SS submerged segment, O cardiac orifice [13]

esophagus is collapsed in the resting state and flat or oval in symmetry in the upper and middle regions (2.5–1.6 cm) and rounded in the distal region (2.5–2.4 cm) [13]. While the above anatomical deviations might sound trivial, they influence incision sites such as left cervical incision when performing an intestinocervical anastomosis after esophagectomy [33] or positioning for radiographic studies such as the left lateral decubitus position when using computerized tomography to differentiate pseudo masses from true masses at the esophagogastric junction [36]. Moreover, the advent of 3D imaging and models through esophageal segmentation has facilitated radiologist localization of the esophagus with respect to mediastinal lymphomas so that if possible the esophagus and trachea might be better removed out of the radiation field in individual patients [34]. Also, exact esophageal location posterior to the atrium when delivering thermal energy to treat atrial fibrillation with radio frequency ablation may prevent esophageal injury (Fig. 2.7) [37, 38].

That the esophagus has no serosa makes this lack of an outside barrier or covering clinically relevant in its close anatomical contact with other organs as it courses from neck through chest to the abdomen. For instance, the membranous posterior surface of the trachea also has no definitive covering, and only loose alveolar tissue separates the close intimate contact between the esophagus and trachea above its bifurcation. The absence of a barrier tissue between these two organs probably accounts for the formation of T–E fistula resulting from blunt dissection, chemotherapy, or radiation [13]. Another example of close contact

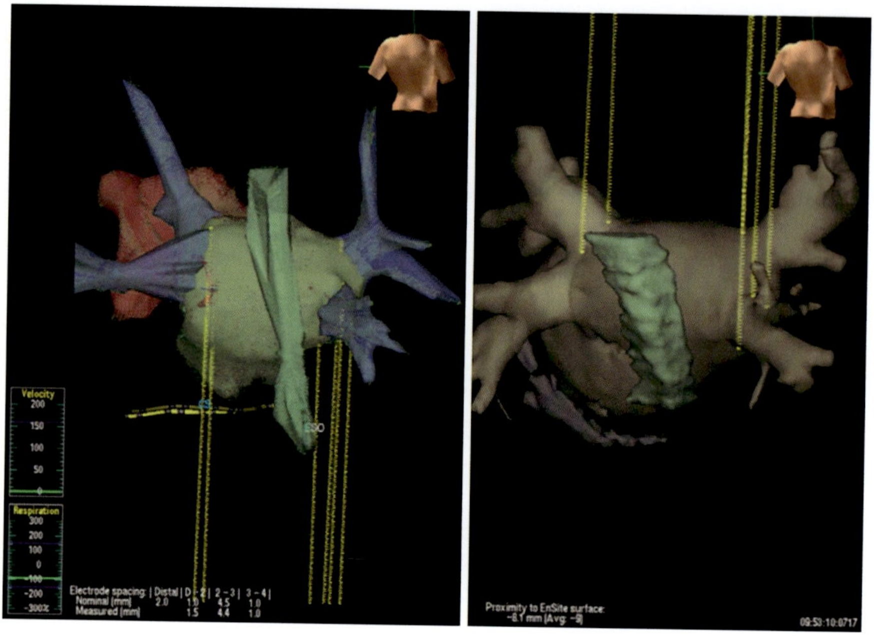

Fig. 2.7 Posterior view of 3D reconstruction images created by electro-anatomical mapping (left) and CT (right). The esophagus is colored green with the globular left atrium immediately anterior. Variable esophageal positioning influences the conduct of radiofrequency ablation of left atrial arrhythmias. The yellow lines represent points of alignment used as a reference to perform image fusion. (With permission from Scazzuso et al. [37])

concerns that between the esophagus without a tissue barrier and the left atrium such that caution needs to be taken in preventing thermal injuries to the esophagus during radiofrequency ablation for atrial fibrillation [37, 38] or caustic pills that might stop in the esophagus related to vascular compression and perforate into the aorta [39].

While the esophagus lacks an outer serosa, fascial tissue planes within the neck and mediastinum provide some barrier function by compartmentalization of various structures including the esophagus [26, 40, 41]. At different esophageal locations, the spaces created between these compartments are relevant. To properly understand these compartments and spaces with respect to the esophagus, one must begin with an appreciation of cervical fascial planes (see sagittal and cross section of neck in 41). These fascial planes begin at the skull base and can be divided into an investing or superficial fascia that surrounds the entire neck and the deep cervical fascia within the neck that divides into the pretracheal (anterior, ventral, or visceral) fascia and prevertebral (posterior or dorsal fascia) [42–44]. The pretracheal fascia contains the larynx, trachea, esophagus, thyroid, parathyroid glands, recurrent laryngeal nerves, and the cranial sympathetic trunk as well as the vascular structures of the anterior mediastinum and becomes known as the pretracheal compartment, which is limited more caudad by the fibrous tissue of the pericardium. The other branch of the deep cervical fascia becomes the prevertebral fascia that surrounds the cervical spine and attached muscles and becomes known as the prevertebral compartment. The deep cervical fascia also forms a carotid sheath that surrounds the carotid artery, internal jugular vein, vagus nerve, and ansa cervicalis (loop of nerves from the cervical plexus in the carotid triangle supplying infrahyoid muscles).

As the esophagus travels from the neck through chest to diaphragm, additional cervical fascia planes become relevant and some merge. New to our discussion concerns the buccopharyngeal fascia that covers the posterior surface of the pharynx and more caudad the esophagus and merges into the pretracheal or visceral fascia that is tightly adherent to the esophagus in its extension inferiorly into the thoracic cavity where it separates the esophagus from the prevertebral fascia [27]. Another fascial plane relevant to the esophagus concerns the alar fascia that begins from medial extensions of the carotid sheath with minor contributions from lateral slips of the prevertebral fascia and extends from the skull base to the superior mediastinum where it fuses with the buccopharyngeal fascia [41]. At this point, the prevertebral fascia becomes relevant to the esophagus and anatomically unique. For uniqueness, the prevertebral fascia splits into two layers in passing between its attachment points on the transverse process of the vertebra, thereby creating a cylindrical longitudinal fascial space containing loose connective tissue that extends from its circular attachment at the base of the skull through the thorax and posterior to the esophagus to the diaphragm [27].

Now that cervical fascia from skull through chest has been reviewed, one can understand how spaces between these planes might be relevant to esophageal disorders or diseases. From anterior to posterior, these spaces include that contained within the pretracheal compartment now thought of as space that runs from the hyoid cartilage to the pericardium. Next is the retropharyngeal space formed by the buccopharyngeal fascia and alar fascia both of which begin at the skull base and extend down to approximately the C6–T6 where both fasciae fuse and the space ends [42, 43]. The alar fascia also serves as a landmark for resection of cervical lymph nodes [45]. Lateral margins for this space include the carotid sheath and superiorly the skull base. Posterior to the retropharyngeal space is the cylindrical prevertebral space that runs uninterrupted from the skull base to diaphragm and thought of as “danger space” because of the potential to spread infection [42]. A plastination study shows all three fascial planes that form the retropharyngeal and danger space and their relationship to the esophagus (Fig. 2.8) [46]. In health, all the above spaces contain adipose tissue.

While one might think that strap muscles within the neck might protect against the spread of noxious cervical infections such as a tooth or tonsillar abscess or instrument perforation in the hypopharynx, that is not the case. The above anatomical spaces provide a potential path for the spread of infection to the pericardium, retropharyngeal space, and even down to the inferior mediastinum. Central to the spread of infection concerns the oropharyngeal flora, a mixture of aerobic and anaerobic organisms that can include streptococci, which are capable of producing proteolytic enzymes that can digest loose connective tissue and open tissue spaces [40]. With respect to the esophagus and mediastinum, the physiologic

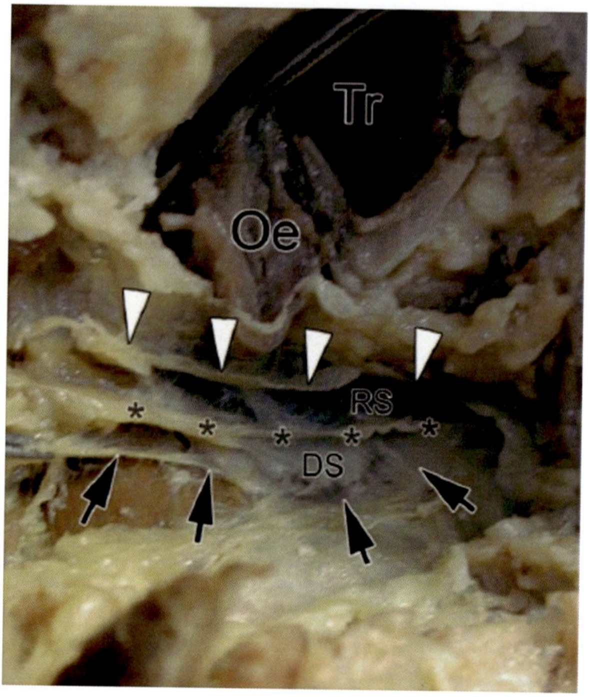

Fig. 2.8 Transverse cut of the cervical spine using a plastination process to illustrate cervical fascia and spaces. Note trachea (Tr) and esophagus (Oe) at top of photograph. Buccopharyngeal fascia denoted by white arrowheads, retropharyngeal space by RS, alar fascia by *, danger space by DS and prevertebral fasciae (black arrows). All layers appear similar in thickness and consistency when traction was applied. (With permission from Scali et al. [46])

narrowing at the pharyngoesophageal junction created by the cricoid cartilage and more caudad the "sling-shaped" attachment of the cricopharyngeus muscle inserting onto the lateral margins of the cricoid cartilage, i.e., "lips of the esophagus," create a physiologic narrowing (23–17 mm) [47], which along with weak walls in the lower pole of pyriform sinus [48] creates a potential area of risk. Misdirection in passing an endoscope or other instrument can cause a hypopharyngeal perforation above the UES [48] that might lead to an abscess contained in the retropharyngeal space. If the junction of the buccopharyngeal and alar fascia fusion is breached or digested at the C6–T6 region, then the inflammatory process can extend into the cylindrical prevertebral space that runs from the skull base to inferior mediastinum at the diaphragmatic hiatus. In regard to perforations, even professional sword swallowers are not exempt from this potential complication [49, 50]. Assigning a lesion to a cervical space aids in differential diagnosis [44, 51]. The esophagus to a lesser extent is influenced by lesions within the pretracheal space, i.e., thyroid enlargement or the prevertebral space, i.e., cervical vertebral spurs [44].

As the esophagus travels through the chest in the mediastinum contained in a bed of loose areolar connective tissue, tiny fibroelastic membranes of elastic or collagen fibers sometimes mixed with skeletal or smooth muscle fibers known as bronchoesophageal, or pleuroesophageal membranes connect the proximal esophagus to the membranous posterior surface of the trachea, as well as pleura, and retroperitoneum [13, 41]. These tiny membranes may range in thickness from 30 to 300 μm and in length from 0.5 to 3 cm and can be seen at mediastinoscopy [13].

However, these tiny membranes are absent below the tracheal bifurcation, and only a continuation of the buccopharyngeal fascia that ultimately becomes the pretracheal fascia separates the esophagus from the prevertebral fascia below the tracheal bifurcation. Thus, above the tracheal bifurcation, the esophagus is loosely tethered to surrounding structures, and below the bifurcation, there is an absence of tethering until the phrenoesophageal ligament at the diaphragm and EG junction. Therefore, this limited attachment allows the esophagus to move vertically approximately 2 cm [52] or 7% of total length and 18% for the distal segment during a swallow [53] or be displaced transversely by large vessels, enlarged heart chambers, or neoplasms [13]. Also, that the esophagus is contained in a loose connective tissue bed in the mediastinum allows for its stripping or blunt pull-through from the mediastinum providing there is no periesophageal tumor invasion. However, blood supply [1] and the unpredictable course of the recurrent laryngeal nerve in the groove between trachea and esophagus (Fig. 2.9) [54] are possible confounding factors to esophageal resection performed in the above matter [55].

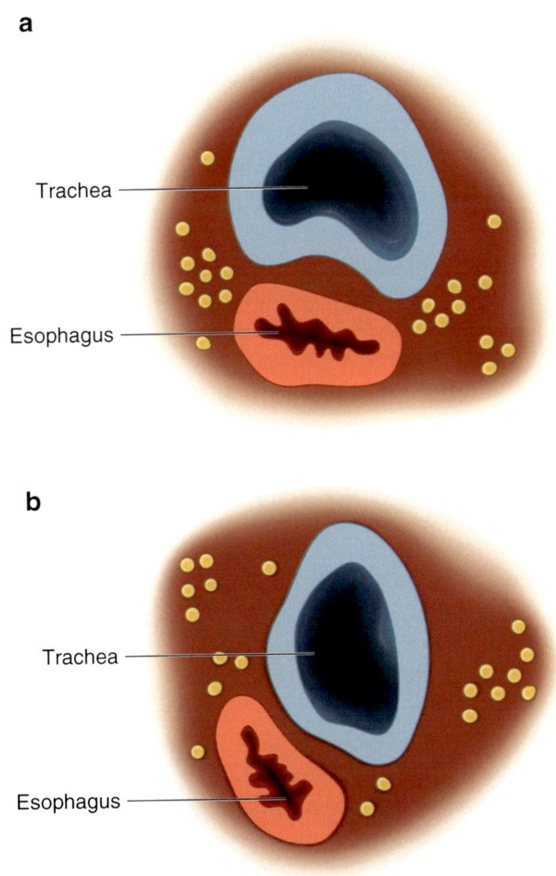

Fig. 2.9 Variation in recurrent laryngeal nerve position in relation to the trachea and esophagus in transverse sections at 1 (**a**) and 4 cm (**b**) caudal to the cricoid cartilage in ten specimens (fixation shrinkage 22%) [54]

As previously commented, the esophageal body is a muscular tube that is the narrowest of the intestinal tract. It is oval in shape in the 1st half and circular in the distal 2nd half, and both halves are lined by a mucosa of squamous epithelium [30]. The muscular wall of the esophagus is approximately 3 mm thick and includes an inner layer of circular and an outer layer of longitudinal muscle each 1.5 mm in thickness [13]. The proximal attachments of the esophagus have been discussed. Distally, the esophageal muscular tube contains an LES attached by the phrenoesophageal ligament, diaphragm, and subdiaphragmatic ligaments. As previously commented, the esophageal body contains no serosa as opposed to other hollow viscus. This unique feature of the esophagus is important when considering manipulations that involve the esophagus such as dilation, delivery of thermal energy, and operative handling. For instance, with circumferential expansion, the esophageal mucosa is approximately six times more stress resistant than that of the muscular wall of the esophagus [56]. In support of this observation, compressed air experiments in vitro on human hollow viscus tissue such as intestine and colon show the mucosa to be more resistant to perforation than the muscular bowel wall with the latter and serosa comparable in their propensity to injury [57]. Some air compression experiments showed a perforation of the serosa and muscular wall with still intact intestinal mucosa, that subsequently blows out of the perforation and busts. That the esophagus has no serosa on the outside wall and the muscular wall is only 3 mm thick leaves the esophageal mucosa as the main guard against manipulations that might cause perforation.

While the muscular tubular wall of the esophagus contains an inner circular layer and an outer longitudinal layer with thin adventitial connective tissue separating both layers, either muscular layer, depending on location can be composed of skeletal or smooth muscle. At the most proximal 2 cm portion of each esophageal specimen, both the inner circular and outer muscle layers contain skeletal muscle [30, 58]. In contrast, below the tracheal bifurcation, both layers only contain smooth muscle that ultimately joins that at the esophagogastric junction [58]. Said another way, if all esophageal specimens in length were made to be 100%, the conversion point between skeletal to smooth muscle appears to be complete at 46% of total esophageal length (Fig. 2.10) [58]. This location is consistent with that published by others [59]. Interestingly, the muscle that composes the superficial muscularis mucosa appears to be smooth muscle for the entire length of the esophagus [30].

The esophageal transition from skeletal to smooth muscle has many important implications that deserve attention. For instance, skeletal muscles at the pharyngo-esophageal junction and upper part of the cervical esophagus receive their innervation from the nucleus ambiguus of the brainstem [60, 61]. Myelinated neurons from this nucleus contain choline acetyltransferase and make direct synaptic contact to motor end plates on individual skeletal muscle cells. On these end plates, acetylcholine is the main excitatory neurotransmitter that acts on nicotinic cholinergic receptors to cause a contraction. It appears that sequential activation of upper motor neurons in the nucleus ambiguus in the brainstem leads to peristalsis in the striated muscle portion of the esophagus. That swallow-induced peristalsis is due to sequential activation of lower motor neurons in the nucleus ambiguus is evident

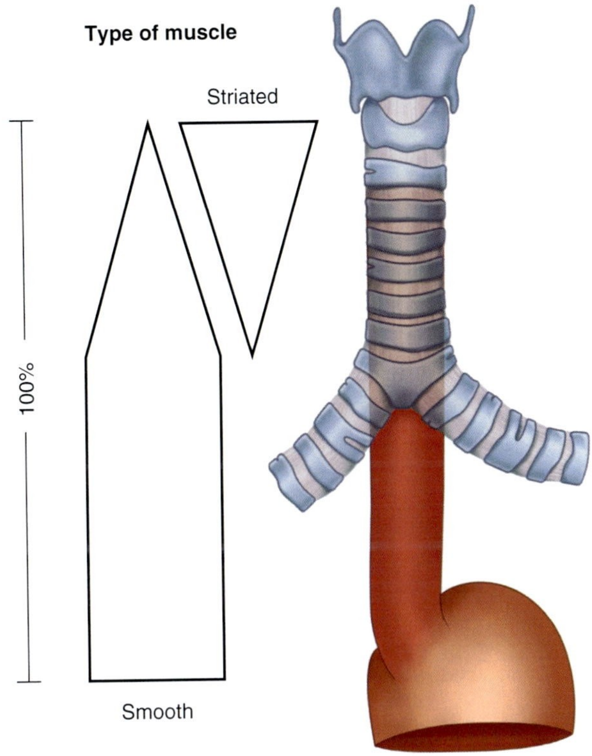

Fig. 2.10 Transition between esophageal striated and smooth muscle. Graphic of the proportion of esophagus each type of muscle occupies when each specimen length is made 100% [58]

when the peripheral end of the decentralized vagus nerve is electrically stimulated – all segments of the cervical esophagus contract simultaneously [61]. Also, because of the unique anatomy described above, a bilateral vagotomy above the origin of the pharyngoesophageal nerve branches renders the proximal esophagus aperistaltic.

The esophageal smooth muscle, in contrast, receives innervation by way of preganglionic neurons from the dorsal motor nucleus of the 10th cranial nerve (the vagal nerve) that synapses on postganglionic neurons of the myenteric ganglia [60, 61]. These ganglia lie in the connective tissue between the circular and longitudinal esophageal (Auerbach) and submucosa (Meissner) plexuses. These plexuses innervate smooth muscle peristalsis and secretion [13, 30]. Postganglionic neurons in both plexuses may be motor, sensory, or interconnecting as well as excitatory (contractile) or inhibitory (relaxatory). Excitatory neurons in both plexuses are considered cholinergic because they contain choline acetyltransferase and substance P that fosters smooth muscle contraction by releasing acetylcholine. In contrast, inhibitory (relaxatory) neurons are considered nitrergic because they contain nitrous oxide (NO), vasoactive intestinal peptide (VIP), and adenosine triphosphate (ATP). Neuronal nitric oxide synthase (nNOS) is also present in these neurons and releases NO a neurotransmitter that is relaxatory. Thus, with swallowing, preganglionic neurons in the caudal DMN (cDMN) are activated first and cause simultaneous inhibition of all parts of the smooth muscle esophagus, which is longer in the lower than in the upper part. When inhibition ends, sequential activation of excitatory neurons in the rostral DMN (rDMN) elicits a peristaltic contraction wave [60, 61].

As outlined above, knowledge of esophageal musculature and its innervation is important, for that serves as a basis for understanding esophageal peristaltic pressure phenomena, classifying motility disorders, and understanding some diseases. For instance, even though most of the time esophageal peristaltic waves triggered by swallowing when viewed radiographically appear continuous for the entire esophagus (traveling at 2–4 cm/second) and manometric peristaltic contractions between striated and smooth muscle phenotypically appear similar [62], important regional physiologic phenomenon might still occur. For example, in the region of the aortic knob [62, 63] or the junction of the 1st and 2nd third of the esophagus [62], there is a demonstrable decrease in peristaltic pressure amplitude over a 5–8 cm segment of esophagus using a 20 mm isobaric contour [64, 65]. This segment appears to correlate with the transition zone (50% striated and 50% smooth) located approximately 5 cm below the UES and may occur over a 6–8 cm segment of esophagus [59]. This pressure trough occurs in the region where the first 2–3 cm of all striated esophageal muscle immediately below the cricopharyngeus begins changing to all smooth muscle by the location of the tracheal bifurcation, a length of approximately 6–8 cm [59]. With the advent of high-resolution esophageal manometry, this transition zone has received much attention; especially, since sometimes there is proximal escape of a small portion of bolus content as the majority of the bolus passes from this region [66]. From simultaneous videos of barium esophagrams and high-resolution esophageal motility performed in patients with dysphagia, a computer model was made that proposed two different rates of peristalsis through this region as well as a "jump zone" between these two different peristaltic rates [67, 68]. That is, a region where proximal esophageal contractions stops and momentarily that for the distal esophagus begins. This hypothesis was confirmed in a follow-up study in patients that showed the CNS control center for the skeletal muscle defined above hand off of the bolus to that of the smooth muscle [69]. This phenomenon is not just of academic curiosity. For instance, approximately 6% of individuals with otherwise normal high-resolution motility studies, but a gap of more than 2 cm and/or delay of longer than 1 second between the proximal and distal contraction using a 20 mm isobaric contour will have a definable cause of dysphagia [64, 70]. Thus, the "drop zone" or hand off between the two CNS areas of control sometimes appears analogous to the fumble in football between the center and quarterback.

In addition, the CNS – innervation of skeletal muscle and that of parasympathetic smooth muscle influences the expression of disease. For example, myasthenia gravis is an autoimmune disease with antibodies thought to originate in the thymus that attach to the neuromuscular junction and block postsynaptic transmission to skeletal muscle of the pharynx, UES, and most proximal esophagus [71]. Approximately, 6% of patients with myasthenia gravis will present with dysphagia [72]. Others might present during the postoperative period with a sudden need for ventilation therapy [73] or have dysphagia associated with other conditions known to cause dysphagia such as a Zenker's diverticulum [74]. In contrast, scleroderma is a connective tissue disease that causes smooth muscle atrophy in the distal 2/3 of the esophagus involving both circular and longitudinal muscles [75] that in turn causes dysphagia by weakening esophageal peristalsis in that region and LES pressure tone [76].

The inhibitory and stimulatory activity of the CNS parasympathetic system on smooth muscle previously discussed also has clinical relevance for it serves as a classification for describing and understanding motility disorders of the distal 2/3 of the esophagus and LES (Fig. 2.11). For instance, loss of inhibitory activity leads to achalasia involving the LES and smooth muscle esophageal body by loss of deglutitive inhibition of the LES or a short inhibition latency that causes esophageal spasm [61, 77]. In support of this observation and classification, an inhibitory nitrergic neural network occurs in the region of Meissner plexus known as the interstitial cells of Cajal. These cells are present in the esophagus and concentrated in the LES [78, 79]. These cells were first described by a physician and neuropathologist Santiago Ramon y Cajal in 1893 and later found to be a major source of nitric oxide that relaxes smooth muscle [80], which has implications in patients with achalasia. For instance, staining and counting the interstitial cells of Cajal and measuring the amount of the enzyme nitric oxide synthase, which these cells produce are both reduced in patients with achalasia [81]. In support of this neurologic biochemical observation, the number of interstitial cells of Cajal present in the achalasia patients significantly correlated with their Eckardt scores that measured the severity of their achalasia. Thus, reduced nitric oxide inhibition on the LES appears to cause unopposed cholinergic stimulation that result in a hypertensive sphincter that fails to relax, i.e., characteristics of achalasia. Alternatively, a hypoactive excitatory innervation leads to hypotensive LES and hypotensive peristalsis [61]. That the interstitial nerves of Cajal are found from the esophagus to internal anal sphincter raises the question of their involvement in other foregut motility disorders [82].

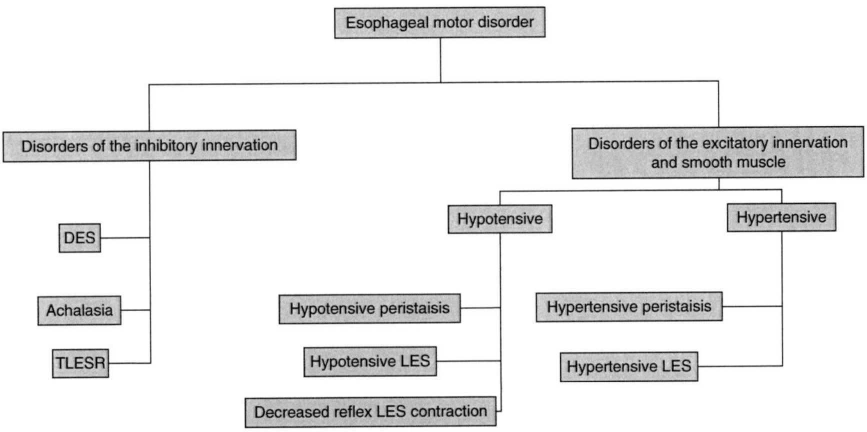

Fig. 2.11 Esophageal motility disorders can be classified on basis of pathophysiology: disorders of inhibitory or excitatory innervation and smooth muscle status

Peristalsis is another physiologic phenomenon caused by skeletal and smooth muscle contained within the inner circular and outer longitudinal muscle walls of the esophageal body deserving comment. For years, peristalsis has been recognized as an integrated, progressive contraction of circular esophageal muscle whose amplitude can be measured in mm Hg as it proceeds down the esophagus. While the outer longitudinal muscle wall has been anatomically defined for a long time, the functional purpose of that outer anatomical wall has not been well defined. Dodds et al. [83, 84] first emphasized the role of longitudinal muscle in esophageal peristalsis. They showed in cats with percutaneously placed metallic clips in the outer muscular wall of their esophagi ($n = 6$) that the initial movement of peristalsis was orad obviously caused by outer longitudinal muscle to receive the bolus. After esophageal shortening, the focused horizontal contraction occurred and progressed down the esophagus causing symmetry that like a "P or D" shape or loop depending on esophageal location. Most importantly for this and later studies that followed motility, catheters did not appear to impair this movement phenomenon. This initial orad motion was later confirmed in possums that have a better skeletal to smooth muscle ratio (2/3 smooth) more like that of humans rather than cats [85, 86]. This orad movement by longitudinal muscle was later proven with metallic clips placed in the esophageal mucosa of humans at endoscopy, which showed 7% total shortening with that in the distal esophagus showing the most change [53]. However, endoscopically placed clips and intraluminal motility catheters do not definitively point to the precise layer, i.e., contraction of the circular or longitudinal muscular wall. Also confounding the problem in humans, some circular muscle in the distal esophagus was found to be spiral or helical and conceivably might contribute to longitudinal muscle [87].

Synchrony between these two muscular walls influences effective propulsion, and disorganization between the walls sometimes results in dysphagia and chest pain in patients without an apparent anatomical cause. Also, one wall and not the other may dominate in certain esophageal disease conditions. Hence, the physiologic interaction between these two muscular walls appears to be emerging as insight and basis for understanding motility disorders [87, 88]. Fortunately to resolve the above problem, a major breakthrough occurred in elucidating the contribution of circular and longitudinal muscular layers in peristalsis. That is, the use of esophageal synchronized high-frequency M-mode ultrasound imaging and manometry, which allows for direct measure of longitudinal and circular muscle wall thickness in conjunction with point pressure at that location [89]. Now the contraction of longitudinal muscle in the outer wall and circular muscle in the inner wall can be directly measured and related to pressure recorded at that location, i.e., circular or longitudinal muscle thickness equates to high pressure and thinness to low pressure [90]. Moreover, just like circular muscle produces progressive amplitude of peristaltic contraction that propels content down the esophagus, so does the longitudinal muscle. Essentially, both the bell-shaped curves of longitudinal and circular muscle move in a synchronous manner at any location as the wave progresses down the esophagus [89]. Even though with swallowing transient neurologic esophageal inhibition occurs as previously discussed, the swallowed bolus does not disperse in the form of a cylinder or have a sausage shape as one would expect. Instead, the bolus transits the esophagus in the shape of an American football with wide girth and tapered ends [87] or upright V for the leading edge and inverted Λ for the trailing edge [62]. This observation implies progressive synchronous relaxation between the circular and smooth muscle wall for the leading bolus edge just like there is progressive synchronous contraction between the longitudinal and circular smooth muscle wall propelling the trailing bolus edge. This assertion is supported by ultrasound imaging showing progressive thinning of the circular and longitudinal muscle walls preceding the bolus in esophageal descent [91]. The biomechanical advantage of esophageal shortening with synchronous circular muscular contraction fosters concentration of circular muscle fibers for propulsion. As a result of this action, thinning of the esophageal wall in the caudad receiving segment occurs with increased compliance, which is needed for bolus accommodation or filling [87]. That the two walls could have a synchronous relationship is fostered by the interstitial layer of connective tissue laying between the longitudinal and circular muscle that allows these muscular walls to slide on each other and in turn deliver the mechanical advantage just described [92].

Just as the interstitial tissue between the two muscle walls affords synchrony, it also facilitates asynchrony. For instance, in patients with nutcracker esophagus, when longitudinal muscle contractions precede circular muscle contractions, the potential downstream receiving esophageal segment has diminished cross-sectional area due to the contraction of the longitudinal muscle. Consequently, when the circular muscle contraction occurs, the receiving segment is less accommodating, thereby causing greater peristaltic pressure to propel the bolus through the narrow and less compliant receiving segment [93]. In support of this observation, the peak peristaltic amplitude and duration significantly correlated directly with the duration of latency between longitudinal and circular muscle contractions [93]. Also, in chronic distal esophageal obstruction, an animal model showed that over time possums develop an increase in their circular muscular wall due to hypertrophic smooth muscle cells [94]. Asynchrony between the two esophageal muscular walls also raises other clinically relevant concerns. For instance, asynchrony might cause functional dysphagia or create the potential for esophageal diverticula in areas of the esophageal wall that cannot tolerate the chronic stress of increased peristaltic amplitudes, especially when not bolstered by synchronous longitudinal muscle contractions [87]. That the esophageal wall is thickened in all major motility disorders [95] some of which are associated with diverticula [96, 97] fosters attention to elucidate the role of circular, longitudinal, or both in the pathophysiology of these disorders.

Distal Esophagus and Lower Esophageal Sphincter

Interest in esophageal peristaltic velocity and the role of the esophageal ampulla has been further extended by conventional manometry [98] and the advent of high-resolution manometry (HRM) used in conjunction with simultaneous fluoroscopy and radiopaque markers placed in the motility probe [98] or endoclip attached at the squamocolumnar junction [99]. Also, HRM defined a new marker to diagnose dysmotility and distinguish the tubular esophagus from the esophageal ampulla and differentiate their functional differences. For instance, HRM showed that peristaltic velocity traveling at approximately 4.5 cm/s abruptly slowed to 1.1 cm/s at a point approximately 4 cm above the squamocolumnar junction located in the center of the diaphragmatic hiatus determined fluoroscopically and the caudad margin the LES high-pressure zone [99]. This precise point of slowing was manometrically designated the contractile deceleration point (CDP) [100]. Radiographically, this point of slowing coincides with a pronounced change in the inverted V of the propelling stripping wave (Λ) of less than 90 degrees from the tubular esophagus to an obtuse angle of 120 or more degrees caused by the wave slowing and the formation of the globular and more distensible appearing ampulla now receiving the bolus content propelled by peristalsis in the tubular esophagus (Fig. 2.12) [99]. Ampulla filling in part accounts for wave slowing at the terminal aspect of the esophageal ampulla, i.e., last 4 cm before the esophagogastric junction. At this point the propelling contraction from the tubular esophagus has driven the bolus into the more distensible globular-shaped esophageal ampulla which suddenly appears in the distal esophageal radiographic morphology.

The sudden appearance of the esophageal ampulla raises the question: where did it come from, and why is it not always present? It is certainly not a static structure [101]. The two studies cited above addressed that question [98, 99]. That is, the distal esophageal ampulla appears to originate from the lower esophageal sphincter initially contained within the diaphragmatic hiatus. Elongation of the LES appears to occur by shortening of the esophagus above the ampulla as the peristaltic wave travels to a location just above the ampulla and perhaps by relaxation of the longitudinal muscle within the LES that permits the elongation with loss of LES pressure [99]. Evidence of LES elongation through stretching and effacement is supported by orad migration of radiopaque clips attached to the radiographic LES and clips attached to the stationary anatomical EG junction [101] or clips attached to the squamocolumnar junction at the caudad margin of the diaphragmatic hiatus that migrate to a location above the diaphragmatic hiatus (1.9–4 cm) [99]. This distension permits the globular appearance of the ampulla so that it might act as a receptacle for the bolus driven by peristalsis from the tubular esophagus.

Interestingly, once distended, the ampulla we recognize radiographically appears as a closed chamber, sealed by the propelling tubular peristaltic contraction above, the crural diaphragm below and laterally by the effaced and elongated ampulla or LES [99]. These circumstances cause hydrostatic pressure to develop within the ampulla, which is distributed in a radial, equilateral, and isometric manner. That the potential propelling force for ampullary emptying is much lower than that found in the tubular esophagus (<40 vs 80 mm Hg, respectively) shows that tubular esophageal peristalsis does not empty the esophageal ampulla [99]. Instead, the ampulla empties because of sustained contraction from the effaced circular muscle of the LES, longitudinal esophageal muscle contraction immediately above the ampulla, and perhaps contraction of longitudinal muscle within the LES whose relaxation facilitated effacement and elongation. That the SC junction remains 1.5 cm above

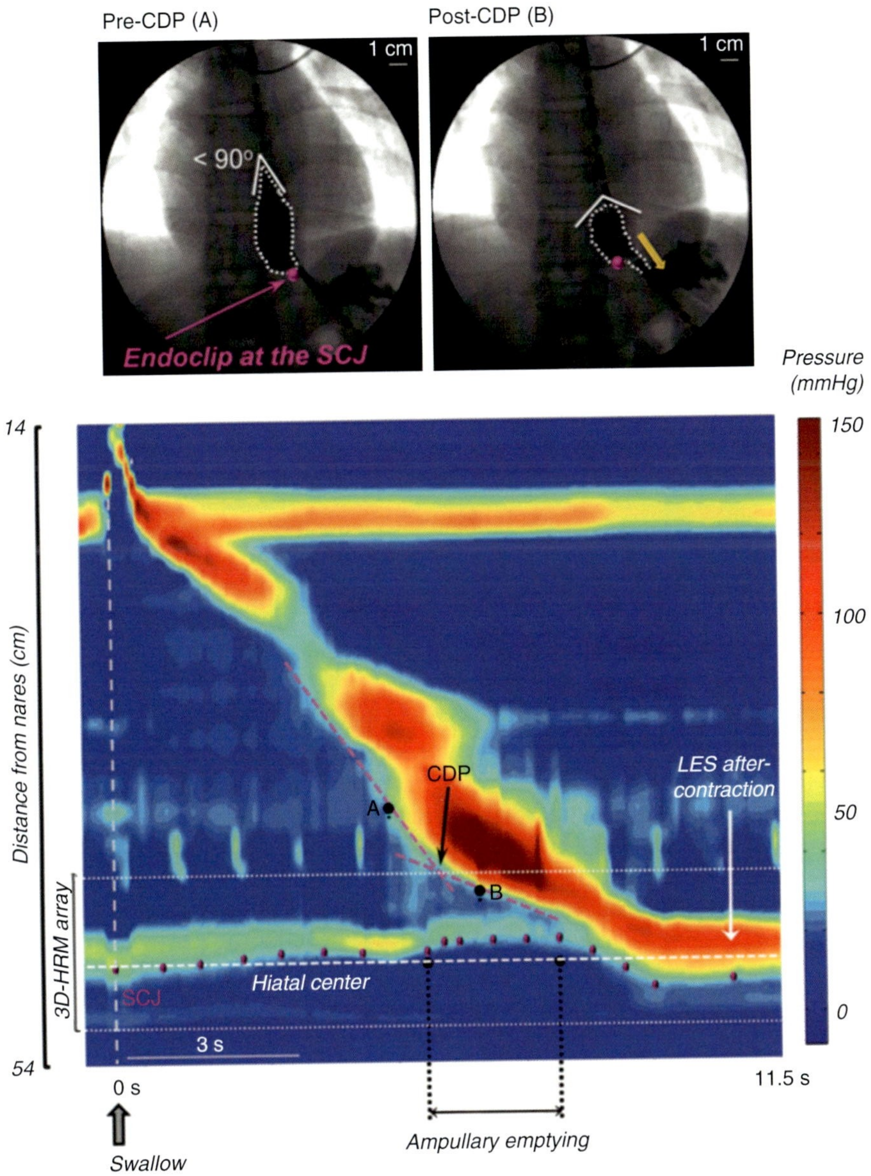

Fig. 2.12 Videofluoroscopic images (top) correlated with esophageal pressure topography (EPT) illustrating the transition from tubular esophageal peristalsis to esophageal ampullary filling and emptying. Key landmarks are identified in both illustrations: pre-contractile deceleration point (Pre-CDP A), Post-contractile deceleration point (Post-CDP B), inverted V of the peristaltic clearing wave (Λ), shape of ampulla (dotted white lines), location of Endoclip at the squamocolumnar junction (SCJ) and ampullary emptying by the down arrow. Below the radiograph, a high-resolution manometry (HRM) study shows location from nares, color codes for pressures, and hiatal center (dashed white lines) with super imposed SCJ. Note slowdown in peristaltic velocity at the CDP (region A vs B) related to ampulla filling and then emptying during LES relaxation after a swallow. (With permission from Kwiatek et al. [99])

the diaphragmatic hiatus while the ampulla empties supports the assertion that esophageal longitudinal muscle contraction supports the radial and axial collapse of the ampulla during emptying. As a result of the above ampullary contraction, content empties through the diaphragmatic hiatus by a favorable hydrostatic intrabolus pressure gradient between ampulla and stomach (13 vs 5 mm Hg). Also, ampullary emptying predominantly occurs during expiration [98] and appeared facilitated by minimal inhibition of the crural diaphragm as shown by EMG [102]. Thus, differences between the tubular and ampullary esophagus account for the slower emptying velocity found in high-resolution manometry caudad to the contractile deceleration point (CDP). Once content has been emptied from the stretched, effaced, and axially displaced LES that formed the ampulla, the LES now returns to its original length or high-pressure zone within the diaphragmatic hiatus. The return of the LES to original location and length with the diaphragmatic hiatus occurs because of esophageal longitudinal muscle relaxation above the ampulla and perhaps contraction of LES longitudinal muscle, as well as passive elasticity from the stretched phrenoesophageal ligament anchored to the diaphragmatic hiatus [98, 99].

After reviewing the above physiologic interaction between tubular and ampullary esophagus, it is important clinically to distinguish the esophageal ampulla from a small adjacent hiatal hernia, especially since that distention is sometimes confusing [98, 103, 104]. Also, might the previously discussed contractile deceleration point (CDP) serve a diagnostic purpose? Fortunately, for the first question, several clinical studies have shown that a phrenic ampulla with an adjoining small sliding hiatal hernia that reduces by returning to the diaphragmatic hiatus after completion of the primary peristaltic contraction wave empties almost as well as the phrenic ampulla without a small adjoining sliding hiatal hernia [98]. Nevertheless, there appears to be a gradual degradation in ampullary emptying as the hiatal hernia increases in size and fails to reduce after completion of the primary peristaltic contraction [105]. For those who might wonder whether ampullary emptying is clinically relevant, the dominant cause of impaired esophageal emptying in patients with gastroesophageal reflux and esophagitis is not deficient tubular esophageal peristalsis but impaired ampulla emptying [106]. Unfortunately, in my experience, while radiologists diligently follow and document the tubular esophageal peristaltic stripping wave in the recumbent position and look for proximal escape, the fluoroscopic videotape often terminates with ampullary filling, and the quality of ampullary emptying is not evaluated. This phenomenon probably occurs to save the patient radiation exposure. However, a compromise to evaluate ampullary emptying might include infrequent short fluoroscopic observations of ampullary emptying, especially, since ampullary contraction occurs over a longer period of time. Lastly, the recently discussed contractile deceleration point (CDP) when temporally measured from the onset of UES relaxation serves as an important marker to help distinguish normal esophageal peristaltic contractions (latency >4.5 s from spastic contractions seen in those with distal esophageal spasm or spastic achalasia (latency <4.5 s). A shortened latency is thought to represent deficient inhibitory ganglionic neurons that program primary peristalsis resulting in the above dysmotility [77].

The lower esophageal sphincter (LES) or high-pressure zone in humans that straddles the diaphragmatic hiatus resulting in opposite deflections on inspiration and relaxation on swallowing has for many years been considered a manometric phenomenon more than an anatomical sphincter like the UES. That assumption appears wrong related to the work of Dorothy Lieberman-Meffert et al. [107] who took stomachs, a 2 cm cuff of diaphragm, and the lower half of the esophagi from circulatory perfused kidney donors prior to their demise and cadaver specimens taken within 10 h of death. These specimens were emerged in large containers, which allowed retention of their original 3D shape so that the esophagogastric junction might be later sectioned in a manner to represent lesser curve, greater curve, anterior, and posterior walls of the EG junction (Fig. 2.13). To examine the muscular architecture, other specimens underwent the above process but in addition were subjected to a stain that distinguished muscle fibers from connective tissue, and the specimens were then dehydrated. This process then allowed microdissection of dried muscle fiber architecture in a region of the esophagogastric junction likely responsible for the LES or high-pressure zone. The authors found an increase in muscle mass at the esophagogastric junction caused by fiber aggregation of the inner muscular coat (Fig. 2.14). The increase in muscle mass tapered both above and below the EG junction over a distance comparable to that of the LES or high-pressure zone, i.e., approximately 3 cm.

The detail study of muscle fibers that comprise the outer longitudinal and inner circular walls at the esophagogastric junction by Liebermann-Meffert et al. [107] has surgical relevance that will become evident later. The longitudinal muscle fibers

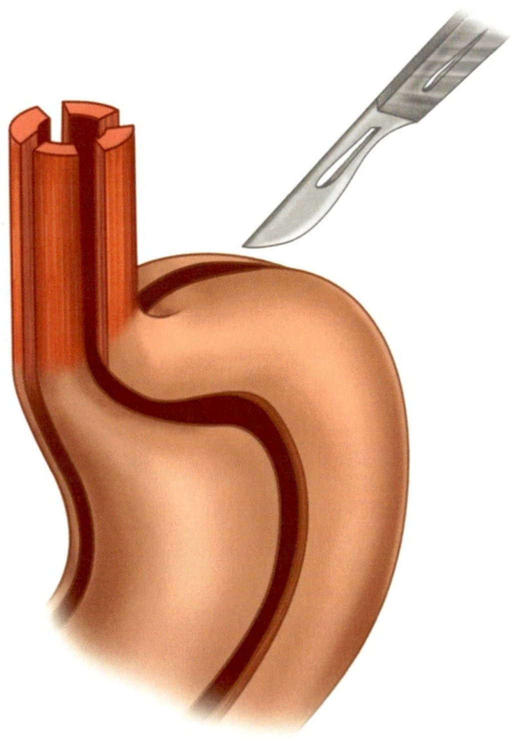

Fig. 2.13 Incision lines made at the EG junction to define lesser curve, anterior wall, greater curvature and posterior wall of the stomach [107]. To better conceptualize measurements made at the lesser curve, greater curve, anterior and posterior walls, the greater curvature in situ faces the left dorsolateral direction. Therefore, in the abdominal cavity, the upper part of the stomach including, the anterior wall, greater curvature, posterior wall, and lesser curvature wall are rotated by 45°. This rotation results in movement of the anterior wall, left; greater curvature, posterior; posterior wall, right; and lesser curve to the anterior side of the vertebral axis

of the outer muscular wall of the esophagus run parallel with its long axis and continue longitudinally onto the lesser and greater curvature of the EG junction and stomach. However, the longitudinal muscle fibers that comprise the anterior and posterior wall of the esophagus just below the esophagogastric junction turn at a right angle and head upward toward the fundus and terminate on either the underlying inner muscle bundles or serosa at the EG junction (Fig. 2.15).

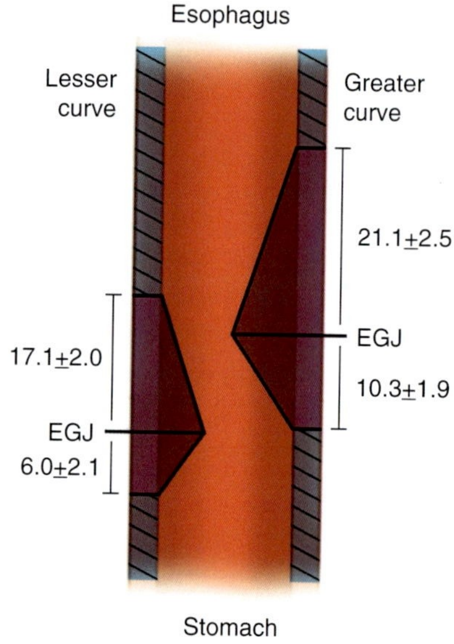

Fig. 2.14 Muscle thickness on the lesser and greater curve of the EG junction [107]

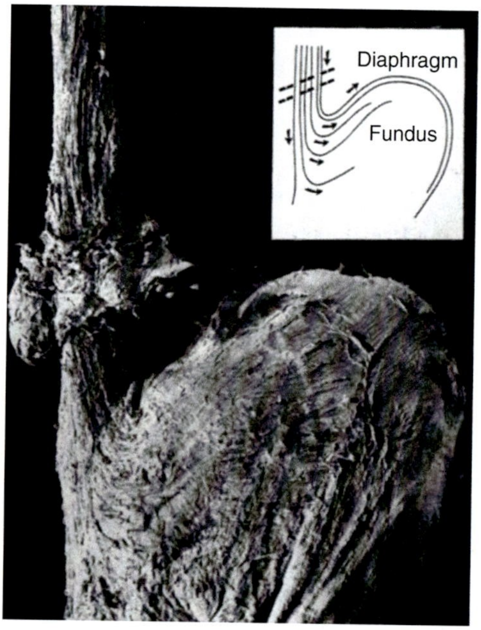

Fig. 2.15 Outer longitudinal muscle fiber arrangement on the anterior wall of the EG junction. Note the change of muscle fiber direction on the anterior wall of the anatomical specimen just below the EG junction, which is also depicted in the above illustration. Diaphragm location shown on the anatomical specimen and in top illustration (//). (With permission from Liebermann-Meffert [107])

As opposed to muscle fibers that form the outer longitudinal smooth muscle coat at the esophagogastric junction, the inner circular muscle anatomy is more complex. For instance, at the orad margin of the EG junction, the inner circular muscle that surrounds the esophageal body by 360° degrees ends (Fig. 2.16) and is replaced by semicircular muscle loops or clasps of 180°, which are located anterior and posterior so that their open ends join or interdigitate with each other to complete 360°. Further caudad on the lesser curve of the EG junction, the posterior transverse semicircular loop or clasp muscles drop out and are replaced by the presence of thickened oblique muscle fibers that come down from the circular muscle of the fundus. These thickened oblique muscles now interdigitate with the anterior transverse semicircular loops or clasps. This arrangement persists for several cm caudad on the lesser curve of the junction. Then the transverse clasp muscle fibers stop, and the thickened oblique muscles thin. In concert, the above-described inner muscle arrangement provides a potential circular contraction ability for the EG junction, but not from a single muscle or organ. While one cannot predict function from structure, some correlations between this anatomical study and functional

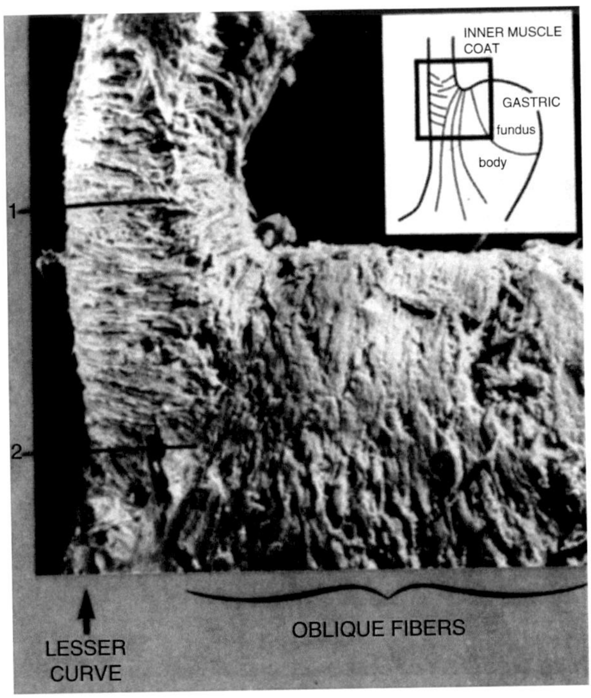

Fig. 2.16 The arrangement of the inner muscle coat at the esophagogastric junction. Numeral 1 denotes the region where complete 360 degree circular muscle loops characteristic of the esophageal body end. Now beginning at 1 and extending to 2, semicircular muscle loops or clasps (180 degrees) are located anterior and posterior and in turn their open ends intersect with each other as shown. Further caudad on the lesser curve, the posterior loops drop out because of the influence of the fundic angle or (angle of His). At this point, the anterior loops or clasps begin to intersect with oblique circular muscle related to the influence of the fundus. Anterior semicircular muscle loops or clasps intersect caudad with oblique circular muscle fibers on the lesser curve down to the region denoted by numeral 2. In concert, this inner muscle arrangement provides the EG junction an ability for circular constriction. (With permission from Liebermann-Meffert [107])

observations seem relevant. For instance, the location of muscle thickening at the esophagogastric junction and the manometrically defined LES high-pressure zone correlate, and the highest manometric pressure correlates with the area of the most muscle thickening. Also, in terms of injuring the EG junction and causing complications from reflux, an animal study showed that an anterior incision involving the anterior semicircular clasp muscles was not as damaging as that of a more lateral or lateral posterior incision that involved the thicker oblique muscles that formed the EG Junction [108]. Clearly, there seems to be some correlation between anatomical form and function at the EG junction.

The above work of EG junction muscular architecture was later extended by using a special 3D manometric assembly with eight radial ports that measured LES pressure along a linear axis above and below the respiratory inversion point. In turn, this 3D expression of LES pressure was compared to the width of the EG junction wall at a comparable location on especially prepared anatomical specimens or to different aspects of a microdissection of the inner circular wall at that location (Fig. 2.17) [109]. The authors found that pressures peaked in all directions at the respiratory inversion point and that the LES was asymmetrical. Most importantly, along the axis of the EG junction, the longitudinal and radial

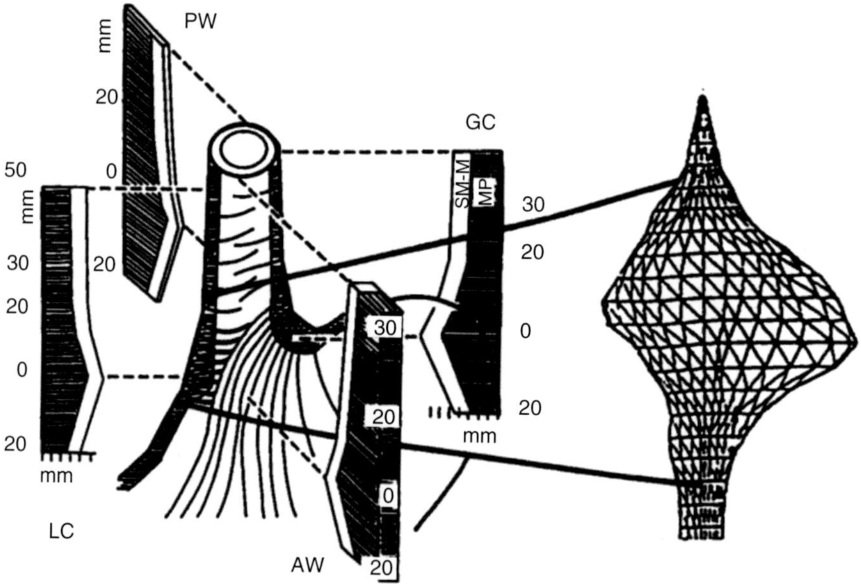

Fig. 2.17 Correlation between radial muscle thickness (left) and 3D manometric pressure image (right) for the human EG junction. Muscle wall thickness shown for greater curve (GC), lesser curve (LC), posterior wall (PW), and anterior wall (AW) with scale given for all walls at bottom of LC and GC (mm). Height of wall in mm denotes distance above and below the respiratory inversion point (0) for all four walls. Radial pressures in mm Hg for EG junction on right side of drawing are plotted around an axis representing atmospheric pressure and portrayed on four quadrant walls in proportion to each other. The 3D aspect of the wall (white area) is draw in proportion to wall thickness. (With permission from Stein et al. [109])

pressures of the 3D LES and muscular wall thickness showed congruence. The highest-pressure values and thickest circular muscle wall width were located left posterior, which is the location of the EG junction and gastric fundus from which the bilateral oblique or sling muscle emanate especially since these structures are located left posterior to the adjacent spine in situ. The next highest pressures and muscle thickness occurred on the lesser curve of the junction where the semicircular or clasp muscle fibers interdigitated with the oblique or sling muscle fibers. Again, this study showed the LES is not a single anatomical muscular structure but composed of different muscular components, i.e., the gastric sling or oblique muscle fibers from the greater curvature of the stomach and the anterior semicircular or clasp muscle fibers from the esophagus. The location of these muscular components is surgically relevant [110].

As cited above, especially processed anatomic specimens of circular musculature from the esophagogastric junction were compared to 3D basal LES pressure in asymptomatic controls. That the authors found circular muscle thickness directly related with basal LES pressure in this association was a helpful concept to carry forward. Now, with the availability of high-frequency, catheter-based intraluminal ultrasonography probes, Liu et al. [111] added a 3D motility probe. This combination of probes afforded the simultaneous study and comparison of muscular anatomy during esophageal peristalsis, basal LES pressure, and the LES contraction that follows a normal swallow-induced relaxation – now all in the same control subject. Measured from the middle of the LES, both longitudinal and circular muscles had axial asymmetry (bell-shaped curve) as the catheter was pulled through the LES. Also, there was a strong linear correlation between circular and longitudinal muscle thickness and pressure ($r = 0.86$ and 0.72, respectively). At basal conditions, longitudinal and circular muscles are thicker in the mid-LES than in the esophagus 5 cm orad to the LES, and circular muscle in the LES is approximately 2–3× as thick as that in the esophagus. When circumferential asymmetry was examined, the peak pressure in the axial LES was selected to compare pressure to muscle thickness. Both the circular and longitudinal muscles showed asymmetry in their thicknesses. The circular muscle was thicker in the left and posterior quadrants. Interestingly, during the LES hypercontraction that follows a normal swallow, the axial radial pressure appeared symmetrical and consistent with that found within the esophagus [109]. Since the authors sometimes observed the aorta and vertebra influence LES asymmetry in the basal state, they felt that during swallow-induced contraction, the LES walls not being fixed could become less compliant and resist any extrinsic compression and assume the same symmetry as observed in the esophageal body. This finding as do others in the paper supports the above dissection studies.

To elucidate the cause of LES pressure asymmetry, determine the location and symmetry of the skeletal muscle crural diaphragm (CD) with respect to the smooth muscle LES, and to see if these findings related to muscular dissection of the LES [107], Mittal et al. [112] used a 3D high-resolution motility catheter in conjunction with computer tomography. These observations are of interest to surgeons. While a 3D motility catheter renders longitudinal symmetry, it does not address circumferential symmetry, and for that reason, computer tomography was added to the study to determine the circumferential orientation of the LES and CD pressure profiles. To complement that anatomical orientation, the equivalent of a flattened BB was attached to the surface of 3D catheter to orientate the catheter to known anatomical reference points: anterior (sternum) and posterior (vertebrae) as well as individuals' right and left directions. This direct orientation permitted using a clock face for orientation. Respiratory maneuvers were used to determine baseline circumferential pressures for the LES and judge circumferential pressure contribution for the CD. They found the length of the basal LES cranial-caudad pressure profile was longer, and the pressures were lower toward the lesser curvature of the stomach on the right as opposed to the shorter cranial-caudad length with higher pressure on the greater curve of the stomach on the left close to the angle of His (Fig. 2.18 a, b, e). The contribution of the crural diaphragmatic contraction was determined by forced inspiration and tidal inspiration (Fig. 2.18 c d, respectively). All LES pressure profiles (Fig. 2.18 a–e) showed increased pressure in the cranial half of their profile. Also, the asymmetrical basal LES end expiratory profiles have the same horizontal orientation as did the accentuated pressures from the crural

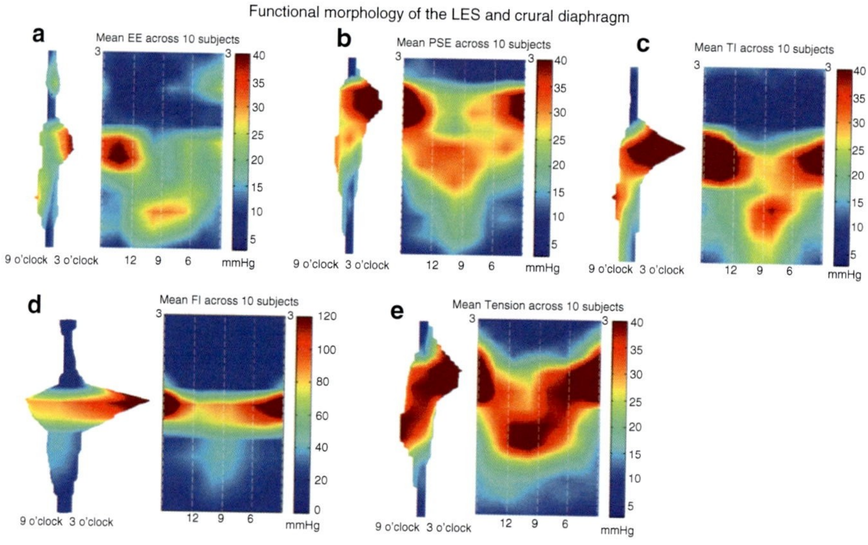

Fig. 2.18 The 3D pressure profile of basal LES without the influence of the crural diaphragm (CD) in ten subjects: (**a**) end-expiration (EE); (**b**) post-swallow end-expiration (PSE); and E, post-Tensilon during end-expiration. LES pressure profiles C and D show two different strengths of crural diaphragm contractions in the same individuals: (**c**) tidal inspiration (TI); and (**d**) forced inspiration (FI). The 9 o'clock and 3 o'clock positions are toward the lesser and greater curvature of the stomach, respectively. Each profile (**a–e**) has an adjacent rectangle that shows the LES pressure profile on a flat surface with an adjacent color code. To conceptualize the flat rectangular surface as a tubular structure join the 3 o'clock position shown on the upper left and right corner of the rectangle. The 12 o'clock and 6 o'clock positions at the bottom of each rectangle represent the anterior (sternum) and posterior (vertebral) direction of the study subjects, respectively. (With permission from Mittal et al. [112])

diaphragm caused by tidal and forced inspiration, i.e., horizontal and asymmetrical with their respective greater pressure on the left side toward the greater curvature of the stomach. Placing this asymmetry on a clock face shows the greatest pressure occurs at 3 o'clock (left side, greater curve, angle of His) followed by 9 o'clock (right side, lesser curve), and the least pressure was noted at 6 and 12 o'clock (anterior – substernal and posterior – spine, respectively). Interestingly, pressures from the crural diaphragm appear oblique with greater pressure on the left upper and less on the right lower crus, which will be addressed later.

At this point, the CT study that allowed 3D construction of the esophagus, CD, and stomach becomes helpful (Fig. 2.19) in understanding the results of the 3D EG junction motility study that defined axial and circumferential asymmetry of the LES and crural diaphragm. From results of the CT study, the authors [112] felt that the CD contraction-related pressure profile was horizontal rather than oblique like the anatomical diaphragmatic hiatus because the upper margin of the LES makes a sharp turn to the left at the upper edge of the esophageal hiatus on the left, thus placing the LES and esophageal hiatus at a right angle to the pressure transducers of the 3D manometric catheter. This phenomenon causes diaphragmatic crural pressure to be horizontal rather than oblique like the anatomical hiatus. In a similar manner, they felt that since the LES is longer toward the lesser curvature side of the stomach as opposed to the greater curvature side, it provides reason for the axial and circumferential asymmetry of the LES. Thus, the authors' findings appear in agreement with earlier reports showing the LES is circumferentially asymmetrical with greater

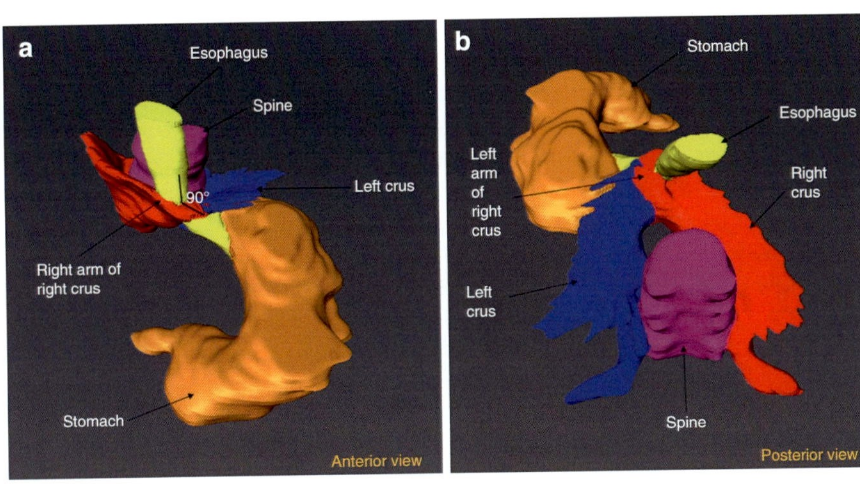

Fig. 2.19 CT scan images of the anterior (**a**) and posterior views (**b**) of the EG junction. The esophagus is colored (yellow), the stomach (beige), right crural diaphragm (red), and the left (blue). Note that the esophageal hiatus is mainly formed by the right crus of the diaphragm dividing into two bundles, which surround the esophagus with its left bundle joining the left crus to enforce the esophagus on the left side. Also, note the upper edges of the LES and CD are located where the esophagus makes a sharp turn to the left as it enters the abdomen from the thorax, and the crus is placed at a right angle to the esophagus. (With permission from Mittal et al. [112])

pressure on the left, greater curvature angle of His side compared to the right lesser curve side [109]. Also, their findings appear to conform to the smooth muscle findings found on LES dissection, i.e., semicircular muscle clasps/oblique fibers [107]. Most important, these physiologic and morphologic findings shed light on the placement of myotomy incisions in the treatment of patients with achalasia. For instance, Heller myotomy incisions are sometimes placed at the 12 o'clock or 3 o'clock position at the esophagogastric junction position because the exposure is ideal; however, according to the above discussion, the 12 o'clock position might be less than an ideal location. Also, experience has taught that the myotomy should be extended onto the stomach, an observation supported by the above data, especially, if it involved the sling fibers on the greater curve close to the angle of His. In support of this observation, a recent study showed that achalasia patients with a marginal response from a POEM procedure performed at the 9 o'clock position had marked improvement when performed at the 3 o'clock position; especially, since the angle of His could be identified and sling fibers addressed [113].

Summary

In conclusion, this review shows that over time even though human anatomy remains unchanged, new innovations and interventions have advanced our understanding of the biomechanics of esophageal physiology as well as fostered new theories. For instance, microdissections, 3D printers, intraluminal ultrasound, and high-resolution manometry alone, and in conjunction with impedance and CT imaging as well as animal models, have impacted clinical medicine and surgical practice. As an example, a recent publication in the *Archives of Surgery* entitled "Effects of Large Hiatal Hernias on Esophageal Peristalsis" along with an accompanying editorial by Jeffrey H. Peters, MD, entitled "What Do the Esophagus and a Jump Rope Have in Common?" [8, 114] emphasizes the above points. In the article, the authors showed how large hiatal hernias (>5 cm) resulted in a shortened esophagus and that in turn adversely affected manometric phenomenon directly affected by esophageal length but still purported to be accepted markers for the quality of esophageal peristaltic strength and effectiveness and might cause dysphagia not examined in the article. From this article, the editorial writer made a biomechanical observation that the esophagus benefits if tethered or anchored at both ends so that at a proper length it might have the functional qualities of an ideal "jump rope" length. There is anatomical precedent for this analogy; the circular muscle of the esophagus joins that of the pharynx, which is firmly attached to cervical vertebrae (C1–C4) [12], but not in the region of the UES (C5–6) [115] because a recent dissection showed this prevertebral space contains loose fatty tissue with pools of amorphous substance to facilitate hyolaryngeal elevation [11]. As previously covered, for additional proximal attachment, the longitudinal muscle of the esophagus attaches to the cricoid cartilage. Further caudad, the esophagus shares the same adventitia with the trachea and loose elastic and/or collagen fiber strands also connect the esophagus to the trachea. So, firm anchor points are present for the proximal esophagus. However, beyond the tracheal bifurcation, the esophagus is rather loose and devoid of strong attachments. At the caudad end of the esophagus, the phrenoesophageal ligament firmly attaches the esophagus to the hiatus of the diaphragm. Hence, the "jump rope" analogy has anatomical merit in the form of anchor points at both ends of the esophagus and as pointed out in the above editorial; hiatal hernia patients are deficient in a distal anchor point.

If the "jump rope" analogy to esophageal function has clinical merit, one might expect an esophagus stretched too tightly or loosely between anchor points might also be associated with dysfunction or dysphagia. A case can be made for both alternatives. For instance, the esophagus has been shown to be lengthened by three types of antireflux procedures when measured by its initial length prior to surgery and then compared to that approximately 5 months after surgery [116]. The Hill procedure (a posterior esophagogastropexy performed by suturing the phrenoesophageal membrane and gastroesophageal junction to the median arcuate ligament of the aortic hiatus had no formal fundoplication and was lengthened the most 7.7% or 1.9 cm [116]. In contrast, that of the Belsey Mark IV (270° wrap) was the least (0.4%) and that of the 360° Nissen fundoplication between the two (6% or 1.5 cm). When we published this study in 1974, Wylie J. Dodds et al. had just published their cat study earlier showing that the initial esophageal movement associated with swallowing was orad to accept the bolus [83]. For that reason, this animal study was referenced in the 1974 paper, and concern was expressed that antireflux procedures might put the esophagus on a stretch when the first movement required for swallowing was orad. This concern was validated because patients having the Hill procedure with almost no fundoplication had comparable dysphagia to that of the Nissen fundoplication with a 360° wrap (both procedures 83%). Later, in 1991 Clouse et al. [53] showed in humans the initial orad esophageal movement associated with swallowing was approximately 7% of pre-swallow esophageal length, and most of this shortening occurred in the distal segment of esophagus where approximately 18% shortening occurred before the manometric contraction or circular muscle contraction wave. If one takes the mean length of the human esophagus in men measured from cricopharyngeus to esophagogastric junction as 22 cm [117] and determines 7% shortening, the value (1.5 cm) is comparable to that found in the above antireflux study. While one might say a mean stretch of 1.5 is not that much, the volitional swallow in a patient with a Nissen fundoplication begins at a disadvantaged position, i.e., 6% stretched due to the fundoplication procedure and now must shorten an additional 7% related to the volitional swallow before the circular muscular contraction begins. Actually, the patient with a fundoplication may be more disadvantaged than that just portrayed. For example, the distal esophageal segment shortens 18% of its pre-swallow length [53]. Also as previously discussed, this esophageal segment includes the LES, which on swallowing moves orad to become the ampulla, and in turn accepts the bolus with distension, then has its own rate of slower contraction on emptying before returning to its original length and position within the diaphragmatic hiatus [99]. That the Nissen fundoplication has been shown to significantly increase the segment of LES in the positive pressure of the abdomen below the respiratory inversion point by 0.9 cm or 33% over that measured before surgery further confounds the stretching problem.

The stretching caused by fundoplication also concerns others, especially, since swallowing causes an initial axial orad esophageal movement, which fundoplication restricts [118]. Also, this axial movement in animals appears by neurologic means to directly trigger LES relaxation [119]. Lastly, orad axial movement caused by longitudinal muscle contraction occurs with transient LES relaxations (TLESRs) that vent the stomach [87] and fundoplications markedly diminish these contractions [120]. Without question, to place more of the LES below the respiratory inversion point in the positive pressure environment of the abdomen significantly increases LES pressure and deters reflux by both pH and impedance [116, 121]. However, this benefit to reflux appears at the expense of dysphagia. While most studies show a major portion of dysphagia associated with a fundoplication is gone by 6 months, others do not share this observation [122]. Perhaps, if surgical strategies could be developed to address the conflict in movement between the physiologic need for axial orad distal esophageal segment movement needed for swallowing and the caudad stretching associated with fundoplication, this highly effective antireflux procedure would be more tolerable and acceptable to a larger population of symptomatic reflux patients. I do not sense that the dysphagia problem with fundoplication will be eliminated by varying the degree of fundoplication and length of fundoplication or even performing floppy fundoplications based on the data just presented. Lastly, a clinical esophageal example of a loose jump rope occurs in achalasia patients with dysphagia from an elongated or S-shaped esophagus.

In conclusion, I hope the reader has learned as much from this manuscript as I have in its preparation.

References

1. Liebermann-Meffert DM, Luescher U, Neff U, Ruedi TP, Allgower M. Esophagectomy without thoracotomy: is there a risk of intramediastinal bleeding? A study on blood supply of the esophagus. Ann Surg. 1987;206(2):184–92.
2. Gates GA. Upper esophageal sphincter: pre and post-laryngectomy--a normative study. Laryngoscope. 1980;90(3):454–64.
3. Pitman R, Fraser G. The post-cricoid impression on the oesophagus. Clin Radiol. 1965;16(1):34–9.
4. Chiu M-J, Chang Y-C, Hsiao T-Y. Prolonged effect of botulinum toxin injection in the treatment of cricopharyngeal dysphagia: case report and literature review. Dysphagia. 2004;19(1):52–7.
5. Cook IJ, Dodds WJ, Dantas RO, Massey B, Kern MK, Lang IM, Brasseur JG, Hogan WJ. Opening mechanisms of the human upper esophageal sphincter. Am J Phys. 1989;257(5 Pt 1):G748–59.
6. Boyce HW. The normal anatomy around the oesophagogastric junction: an endoscopic view. Best Pract Res Clin Gastroenterol. 2008;22(4):553–67. https://doi.org/10.1016/j.bpg.2008.02.003.
7. Tang SJ, Wu R. Esophageal introitus (with videos). Gastrointest Endosc. 2015;81(2):270–81. https://doi.org/10.1016/j.gie.2014.09.065.
8. Roman S, Kahrilas PJ, Kia L, Luger D, Soper N, Pandolfino JE. Effects of large hiatal hernias on esophageal peristalsis. Arch Surg. 2012;147(4):352–7. https://doi.org/10.1001/archsurg.2012.17.

9. Staiano A, Clouse RE. Value of subject height in predicting lower esophageal sphincter location. Am J Dis Child. 1991;145(12):1424–7.
10. Liebermann-Meffert D. The Pharyngoesophageal segment: anatomy and innervation. Dis Esophagus. 1995;8:242–51.
11. Nilsson ME, Isacsson G, Isberg A, Schiratzki H. Mobility of the upper esophageal sphincter in relation to the cervical spine: a morphologic study. Dysphagia. 1989;3(3):161–5. https://doi.org/10.1007/bf02407135.
12. Curtis DJ. Radiographic anatomy of the pharynx. Dysphagia. 1986;1(2):51–62.
13. Liebermann-Meffert D. Clinically oriented anatomy, embryology, and histology. In: Pearson FG, Patterson GA, editors. Pearson's thoracic and esophageal surgery. London: Churchill Livingstone; 2008.
14. Kumoi K, Ohtsuki N, Teramoto Y. Pharyngo-esophageal diverticulum arising from Laimer's triangle. Eur Arch Otorhinolaryngol. 2001;258(4):184–7.
15. Rubesin SE, Levine MS. Killian-Jamieson diverticula: radiographic findings in 16 patients. AJR Am J Roentgenol. 2001;177(1):85–9. https://doi.org/10.2214/ajr.177.1.1770085.
16. Cook IJ, Gabb M, Panagopoulos V, Jamieson GG, Dodds WJ, Dent J, Shearman DJ. Pharyngeal (Zenker's) diverticulum is a disorder of upper esophageal sphincter opening. Gastroenterology. 1992;103(4):1229–35.
17. McConnel FM, Hood D, Jackson K, O'Connor A. Analysis of intrabolus forces in patients with Zenker's diverticulum. Laryngoscope. 1994;104(5 Pt 1):571–81.
18. Cook IJ, Blumbergs P, Cash K, Jamieson GG, Shearman DJ. Structural abnormalities of the cricopharyngeus muscle in patients with pharyngeal (Zenker's) diverticulum. J Gastroenterol Hepatol. 1992;7(6):556–62.
19. Achkar E. Zenker's diverticulum. Digest Dise (Basel, Switzerland). 1998;16(3):144–51.
20. Undavia S, Anand SM, Jacobson AS. Killian-Jamieson diverticulum: a case for open transcervical excision. Laryngoscope. 2013;123(2):414–7. https://doi.org/10.1002/lary.23639.
21. Siow SL, Mahendran HA, Hardin M. Transcervical diverticulectomy for Killian-Jamieson diverticulum. Asian J Surg. 2015;40:324. https://doi.org/10.1016/j.asjsur.2015.01.007.
22. Orzell SFT, Grillone G. Killian-Jamieson diverticulum: a case report and argument for Transcervical Diverticulectomy. J Otolaryngol Rhinol. 2016;2(4):1–4.
23. Coughlan CA, Verma SP. The utility of recurrent laryngeal nerve monitoring during open pharyngeal diverticula procedures. Ann Otol Rhinol Laryngol. 2016;125(8):648–51. https://doi.org/10.1177/0003489416642815.
24. Welch RW, Luckmann K, Ricks PM, Drake ST, Gates GA. Manometry of the normal upper esophageal sphincter and its alterations in laryngectomy. J Clin Invest. 1979;63(5):1036–41. https://doi.org/10.1172/JCI109372.
25. Standring S. Larynx. In: Standring S, editor. Gray's anatomy: the anatomical basis of clinical practice. Philadelphia, PA: Elsevier Health Sciences; 2015. p. 586–604.
26. Sivarao DV, Goyal RK. Functional anatomy and physiology of the upper esophageal sphincter. Am J Med. 2000;108(Suppl 4a):27s–37s.
27. Drake R, Vogl AW, Mitchell AW. Head and neck. In: Drake R, Vogl AW, Mitchell AW, editors. Gray's anatomy for students. Philadelphia, PA: Elsevier Health Sciences; 2009. p. 1–455.
28. Goyal RK, Martin SB, Shapiro J, Spechler SJ. The role of cricopharyngeus muscle in pharyngoesophageal disorders. Dysphagia. 1993;8(3):252–8.
29. Pera M, Yamada A, Hiebert CA, Duranceau A. Sleeve recording of upper esophageal sphincter resting pressures during cricopharyngeal myotomy. Ann Surg. 1997;225(2):229–34.
30. Liebermann-Meffert D, Duranceau A. Embryology, anatomy and physiology of the esophagus. In: Shackelford's surgery of the alimentary tract, vol. 1. Philadelphia, PA: Elsevier; 1991. p. 3–49.
31. Boyce H, Boyce G. Esophagus. In: Tadataka Y, David H, Alpers H, editors. Textbook of gastroenterology. Phidelphia: Lippencott; 2003. p. 1148–65.
32. Wolf BS. Heartburn: the role of radiology. JAMA. 1976;235(12):1244–7. https://doi.org/10.1001/jama.1976.03260380038023.

33. Liebermann-Meffert D. Anatomical basis for the approach and extent of surgical treatment of esophageal cancer. Dis Esophagus. 2001;14(2):81–4.
34. Feulner J, Zhou SK, Cavallaro A, Seifert S, Hornegger J, Comaniciu D. Fast automatic segmentation of the esophagus from 3d ct data using a probabilistic model. In: International conference on medical image computing and computer-assisted intervention. New York, NY: Springer; 2009. p. 255–62.
35. Feulner J, Zhou SK, Hammon M, Seifert S, Huber M, Comaniciu D, Hornegger J, Cavallaro A. A probabilistic model for automatic segmentation of the esophagus in 3-D CT scans. IEEE Trans Med Imaging. 2011;30(6):1252–64. https://doi.org/10.1109/TMI.2011.2112372.
36. Thompson WM, Halvorsen RA, Foster W Jr, Roberts L, Korobkin M. Computed tomography of the gastroesophageal junction: value of the left lateral decubitus view. J Comput Assist Tomogr. 1984;8(2):346–9.
37. Scazzuso FA, Rivera SH, Albina G, de la Paz Ricapito M, Gomez LA, Sanmartino V, Kamlofsky M, Laino R, Giniger A. Three-dimensional esophagus reconstruction and monitoring during ablation of atrial fibrillation: combination of two imaging techniques. Int J Cardiol. 2013;168(3):2364–8. https://doi.org/10.1016/j.ijcard.2013.01.026.
38. Lemola K, Sneider M, Desjardins B, Case I, Han J, Good E, Tamirisa K, Tsemo A, Chugh A, Bogun F. Computed tomographic analysis of the anatomy of the left atrium and the esophagus. Circulation. 2004;110(24):3655–60.
39. Kikendall JW, Friedman AC, Oyewole MA, Fleischer D, Johnson LF. Pill-induced esophageal injury. Case reports and review of the medical literature. Dig Dis Sci. 1983;28(2): 174–82.
40. Standring S. Neck. In: Gray's anatomy: the anatomical basis of clinical practice. 39th ed. Philadelphia, PA: Elsevier Health Sciences; 2015. p. 49.
41. Frank H Netter M. Netter basic science : atlas of human anatomy : with student consult online access. 6th ed. Philadelphia, PA: Saunders Elsevier; 2014.
42. Guidera AK, Dawes PJ, Stringer MD. Cervical fascia: a terminological pain in the neck. ANZ J Surg. 2012;82(11):786–91. https://doi.org/10.1111/j.1445-2197.2012.06231.x.
43. Guidera AK, Dawes PJ, Fong A, Stringer MD. Head and neck fascia and compartments: no space for spaces. Head Neck. 2014;36(7):1058–68. https://doi.org/10.1002/hed.23442.
44. Som PM, Curtin HD. Fascia and spaces of the neck. In: Som PM, Curtin HD, editors. Head and neck imaging. 5th ed. St Louis, MO: Mosby; 2011. p. 2203–34. https://doi.org/10.1016/b978-0-323-05355-6.00036-7.
45. Ozlugedik S, Ibrahim Acar H, Apaydin N, Firat Esmer A, Tekdemir I, Elhan A, Ozcan M. Retropharyngeal space and lymph nodes: an anatomical guide for surgical dissection. Acta Otolaryngol. 2005;125(10):1111–5. https://doi.org/10.1080/00016480510035421.
46. Scali F, Nash LG, Pontell ME. Defining the morphology and distribution of the alar fascia: a sheet plastination investigation. Ann Otol Rhinol Laryngol. 2015;124(10):814–9. https://doi.org/10.1177/0003489415588129.
47. Skandalakis JE, Ellis H. Embryologic and anatomic basis of esophageal surgery. Surg Clin North Am. 2000;80(1):85–155. x
48. Miller MSaG The Esophagus, Hand book and Atlas of Endoscopy (trans: Duncan Colin-Jones M). Grassmann AG, Solothurn, Switzerland.
49. Witcombe B, Meyer D. Sword swallowing and its side effects. BMJ. 2006;333(7582):1285–7. https://doi.org/10.1136/bmj.39027.676690.55.
50. Martin M, Steele S, Mullenix P, Long W, Izenberg S. Management of esophageal perforation in a sword swallower: a case report and review of the literature. J Trauma. 2005;59(1):233–5.
51. Smoker W, Harnsberger H. Differential diagnosis of head and neck lesions based on their space of origin. 2. The infrahyoid portion of the neck. AJR Am J Roentgenol. 1991;157(1):155–9.
52. Pouderoux P, Lin S, Kahrilas PJ. Timing, propagation, coordination, and effect of esophageal shortening during peristalsis. Gastroenterology. 1997;112(4):1147–54.
53. Edmundowicz SA, Clouse RE. Shortening of the esophagus in response to swallowing. Am J Phys. 1991;260(3 Pt 1):G512–6.

54. Liebermann-Meffert DM, Walbrun B, Hiebert CA, Siewert JR. Recurrent and superior laryngeal nerves: a new look with implications for the esophageal surgeon. Ann Thorac Surg. 1999;67(1):217–23.
55. Orringer MB, Orringer JS. Esophagectomy without thoracotomy: a dangerous operation? J Thorac Cardiovasc Surg. 1983;85(1):72–80.
56. Gregersen H, Liao D, Fung YC. Determination of homeostatic elastic moduli in two layers of the esophagus. J Biomech Eng. 2008;130(1):011005. https://doi.org/10.1115/1.2838031.
57. Burt AV. Pneumatic rupture of the intestinal canal: with experimental data showing the mechanism of perforation and the pressure required. Arch Surg. 1931;22(6):875–902.
58. Liebermann-Meffert D, Geissdörfer K. Is the transition of striated into smooth muscle precisely known. In: Giuli RM, Skinner DB, editors. Primary motility disorders of the esophagus: 450 Questions-450 Answers. Paris, Londres, RomeParis: Libbey Eurotext; 1991. p. 108–12.
59. Meyer G, Austin R, Brady C III, Castell D. Muscle anatomy of the human esophagus. J Clin Gastroenterol. 1986;8(2):131–4.
60. Mashimo HMD, Goyal RK. Physiology of esophageal motility. 2006;2017. www.GIMotilityonline.com.
61. Goyal RK, Chaudhury A. Physiology of normal esophageal motility. J Clin Gastroenterol. 2008;42(5):610–9. https://doi.org/10.1097/MCG.0b013e31816b444d.
62. Dodds WJ. 1976 Walter B. Cannon lecture: current concepts of esophageal motor function: clinical implications for radiology. AJR Am J Roentgenol. 1977;128(4):549–61. https://doi.org/10.2214/ajr.128.4.549.
63. Karamanolis G, Stevens W, Vos R, Tack J, Clave P, Sifrim D. Oesophageal tone and sensation in the transition zone between proximal striated and distal smooth muscle oesophagus. Neurogastroenterol Motil. 2008;20(4):291–7. https://doi.org/10.1111/j.1365-2982.2007.01028.x.
64. Ghosh SK, Pandolfino JE, Zhang Q, Jarosz A, Shah N, Kahrilas PJ. Quantifying esophageal peristalsis with high-resolution manometry: a study of 75 asymptomatic volunteers. Am J Physiol Gastrointest Liver Physiol. 2006;290(5):G988. https://doi.org/10.1152/ajpgi.00510.2005.
65. Weijenborg PW, Kessing BF, Smout AJ, Bredenoord AJ. Normal values for solid-state esophageal high-resolution manometry in a European population; an overview of all current metrics. Neurogastroenterol Motil. 2014;26(5):654–9. https://doi.org/10.1111/nmo.12314.
66. Massey BT, Dodds WJ, Hogan WJ, Brasseur JG, Helm JF. Abnormal esophageal motility. An analysis of concurrent radiographic and manometric findings. Gastroenterology. 1991;101(2):344–54.
67. Li M, Brasseur JG, Dodds WJ. Analyses of normal and abnormal esophageal transport using computer simulations. Am J Phys. 1994;266(4 Pt 1):G525–43.
68. Kahrilas P, Dodds W, Hogan W. Effect of peristaltic dysfunction on esophageal volume clearance. Gastroenterology. 1988;94(1):73–80.
69. Ghosh SK, Janiak P, Schwizer W, Hebbard GS, Brasseur JG. Physiology of the esophageal pressure transition zone: separate contraction waves above and below. Am J Physiol Gastrointest Liver Physiol. 2006;290(3):G568–76. https://doi.org/10.1152/ajpgi.00280.2005.
70. Ghosh SK, Pandolfino JE, Kwiatek MA, Kahrilas PJ. Oesophageal peristaltic transition zone defects: real but few and far between. Neurogastroenterol Motil. 2008;20(12):1283–90. https://doi.org/10.1111/j.1365-2982.2008.01169.x.
71. Breen E, Bleich L, Loeser C. Myasthenia gravis presenting with dysphagia in an elderly male: a case report. Am J Med. 2014;127(9):e7–8. https://doi.org/10.1016/j.amjmed.2014.05.028.
72. Grob D, Brunner NG, Namba T. The natural course of myasthenia gravis and effect of therapeutic measures. Ann N Y Acad Sci. 1981;377:652–69.
73. Haider-Ali AM, MacGregor FB, Stewart M. Myasthenia gravis presenting with dysphagia and postoperative ventilatory failure. J Laryngol Otol. 1998;112(12):1194–5.

74. Khan OA, Campbell WW. Myasthenia gravis presenting as dysphagia: clinical considerations. Am J Gastroenterol. 1994;89(7):1083–5.
75. Roberts CG, Hummers LK, Ravich WJ, Wigley FM, Hutchins GM. A case-control study of the pathology of oesophageal disease in systemic sclerosis (scleroderma). Gut. 2006;55(12):1697–703. https://doi.org/10.1136/gut.2005.086074.
76. Sjogren RW. Gastrointestinal motility disorders in scleroderma. Arthritis Rheum. 1994;37(9):1265–82.
77. Pandolfino JE, Roman S, Carlson D, Luger D, Bidari K, Boris L, Kwiatek MA, Kahrilas PJ. Distal esophageal spasm in high-resolution esophageal pressure topography: defining clinical phenotypes. Gastroenterology. 2011;141(2):469–75. https://doi.org/10.1053/j.gastro.2011.04.058.
78. Mostafa RM. Interstitial cells of Cajal, the maestro in health and disease. World J Gastroenterol. 2010;16(26):3239. https://doi.org/10.3748/wjg.v16.i26.3239.
79. Faussone-Pellegrini M, Cortesini C. Ultrastructural features and localization of the interstitial cells of Cajal in the smooth muscle coat of human esophagus. J Submicrosc Cytol. 1985;17(2):187–97.
80. Ward SM, Morris G, Reese L, Wang X-Y, Sanders KM. Interstitial cells of Cajal mediate enteric inhibitory neurotransmission in the lower esophageal and pyloric sphincters. Gastroenterology. 1998;115(2):314–29.
81. Gockel I, Bohl JR, Eckardt VF, Junginger T. Reduction of interstitial cells of Cajal (ICC) associated with neuronal nitric oxide synthase (n-NOS) in patients with achalasia. Am J Gastroenterol. 2008;103(4):856–64. https://doi.org/10.1111/j.1572-0241.2007.01667.x.
82. Streutker CJ, Huizinga JD, Driman DK, Riddell RH. Interstitial cells of Cajal in health and disease. Part I: normal ICC structure and function with associated motility disorders. Histopathology. 2007;50(2):176–89. https://doi.org/10.1111/j.1365-2559.2006.02493.x.
83. Dodds WJ, Stewart ET, Hodges D, Zboralske FF. Movement of the feline esophagus associated with respiration and peristalsis. An evaluation using tantalum markers. J Clin Invest. 1973;52(1):1–13. https://doi.org/10.1172/jci107152.
84. Stewart ET, Dodds WJ. Marking the feline esophagus with small tantalum wires an experimental technic. Radiology. 1969;93(1):176–7.
85. Sugarbaker DJ, Rattan S, Goyal RK. Mechanical and electrical activity of esophageal smooth muscle during peristalsis. Am J Phys. 1984;246(2 Pt 1):G145–50.
86. Christensen J, Lund GF. Esophageal responses to distension and electrical stimulation. J Clin Invest. 1969;48(2):408–19. https://doi.org/10.1172/jci105998.
87. Mittal RK. Regulation and dysregulation of esophageal peristalsis by the integrated function of circular and longitudinal muscle layers in health and disease. Am J Physiol Gastrointest Liver Physiol. 2016;311(3):G431–43. https://doi.org/10.1152/ajpgi.00182.2016.
88. Mittal RK. Longitudinal muscle of the esophagus: its role in esophageal health and disease. Curr Opin Gastroenterol. 2013;29(4):421–30. https://doi.org/10.1097/MOG.0b013e3283622b57.
89. Mittal RK, Padda B, Bhalla V, Bhargava V, Liu J. Synchrony between circular and longitudinal muscle contractions during peristalsis in normal subjects. Am J Physiol Gastrointest Liver Physiol. 2006;290(3):G431–8. https://doi.org/10.1152/ajpgi.00237.2005.
90. Miller LS, Liu JB, Colizzo FP, Ter H, Marzano J, Barbarevech C, Helwig K, Leung L, Goldberg BB, Hedwig K. Correlation of high-frequency esophageal ultrasonography and manometry in the study of esophageal motility. Gastroenterology. 1995;109(3):832–7.
91. Yamamoto Y, Liu J, Smith TK, Mittal RK. Distension-related responses in circular and longitudinal muscle of the human esophagus: an ultrasonographic study. Am J Phys. 1998;275(4 Pt 1):G805–11.
92. Patel N, Jiang Y, Mittal RK, Kim TH, Ledgerwood M, Bhargava V. Circular and longitudinal muscles shortening indicates sliding patterns during peristalsis and transient lower esophageal sphincter relaxation. Am J Physiol Gastrointest Liver Physiol. 2015;309(5):G360–7. https://doi.org/10.1152/ajpgi.00067.2015.

93. Jung HY, Puckett JL, Bhalla V, Rojas-Feria M, Bhargava V, Liu J, Mittal RK. Asynchrony between the circular and the longitudinal muscle contraction in patients with nutcracker esophagus. Gastroenterology. 2005;128(5):1179–86.
94. Tung HN, Schulze-Delrieu K, Shirazi S, Noel S, Xia Q, Cue K. Hypertrophic smooth muscle in the partially obstructed opossum esophagus. The model: histological and ultrastructural observations. Gastroenterology. 1991;100(4):853–64.
95. Mittal R. Hypertrophy of the muscularis propria of the lower esophageal sphincter and the body of the esophagus in patients with primary motility disorders of the esophagus. Am J Gastroenterol. 2003;98(8):1705–12. https://doi.org/10.1016/s0002-9270(03)00436-2.
96. Nehra D, Lord RV, DeMeester TR, Theisen J, Peters JH, Crookes PF, Bremner CG. Physiologic basis for the treatment of epiphrenic diverticulum. Ann Surg. 2002;235(3):346–54.
97. Carlson DA, Gluskin AB, Mogni B, Koo J, Sood R, Lin Z, Pandolfino JE. Esophageal diverticula are associated with propagating peristalsis: a study utilizing high-resolution manometry. Neurogastroenterol Motil. 2015;28:392. https://doi.org/10.1111/nmo.12739.
98. Lin S, Brasseur JG, Pouderoux P, Kahrilas PJ. The phrenic ampulla: distal esophagus or potential hiatal hernia? Am J Phys. 1995;268(2 Pt 1):G320–7.
99. Kwiatek MA, Nicodeme F, Pandolfino JE, Kahrilas PJ. Pressure morphology of the relaxed lower esophageal sphincter: the formation and collapse of the phrenic ampulla. Am J Physiol Gastrointest Liver Physiol. 2012;302(3):G389–96. https://doi.org/10.1152/ajpgi.00385.2011.
100. Pandolfino JE, Leslie E, Luger D, Mitchell B, Kwiatek MA, Kahrilas PJ. The contractile deceleration point: an important physiologic landmark on oesophageal pressure topography. Neurogastroenterol Motil. 2010;22(4):395. https://doi.org/10.1111/j.1365-2982.2009.01443.x.
101. Berridge FR, Friedland GW, Tagart RE. Radiological landmarks at the oesophago-gastric junction. Thorax. 1966;21(6):499–510.
102. Mittal RK, Fisher MJ. Electrical and mechanical inhibition of the crural diaphragm during transient relaxation of the lower esophageal sphincter. Gastroenterology. 1990;99(5):1265–8.
103. Heitmann P, Wolf BS, Sokol EM, Cohen BR. Simultaneous cineradiographic-manometric study of the distal esophagus: small hiatal hernias and rings. Gastroenterology. 1966;50(6):737–53.
104. Wolf BS. The definition of a sliding hiatal hernia. A radiologist's point of view. Am J Dig Dis. 1960;5:168–73.
105. Sloan S, Kahrilas PJ. Impairment of esophageal emptying with hiatal hernia. Gastroenterology. 1991;100(3):596–605.
106. Lin S, Ke M, Xu J, Kahrilas PJ. Impaired esophageal emptying in reflux disease. Am J Gastroenterol. 1994;89(7):1003–6.
107. Liebermann-Meffert D. Muscular equivalent of the lower esophageal sphincter. Gastroenterology. 1978;76:31.
108. Gahagan T. The function of the musculature of the esophagus and stomach in the esophagogastric sphincter mechanism. Surg Gynecol Obstet. 1962;114:293–303.
109. Stein HJ, Liebermann-Meffert D, DeMeester TR, Siewert JR. Three-dimensional pressure image and muscular structure of the human lower esophageal sphincter. Surgery. 1995;117(6):692–8.
110. Mattioli S, Pilotti V, Felice V, Di Simone MP, D'Ovidio F, Gozzetti G. Intraoperative study on the relationship between the lower esophageal sphincter pressure and the muscular components of the gastro-esophageal junction in achalasic patients. Ann Surg. 1993;218(5):635–9.
111. Liu J, Parashar VK, Mittal RK. Asymmetry of lower esophageal sphincter pressure: is it related to the muscle thickness or its shape? Am J Phys. 1997;272(6 Pt 1):G1509–17.
112. Mittal RK, Zifan A, Kumar D, Ledgerwood-Lee M, Ruppert E, Ghahremani G. Functional morphology of the lower esophageal sphincter and crural diaphragm determined by three-dimensional high-resolution esophago-gastric junction pressure profile and CT imaging. Am J Physiol Gastrointest Liver Physiol. 2017;313(3):G212–9. https://doi.org/10.1152/ajpgi.00130.2017.

113. Onimaru M, Inoue H, Ikeda H, Sato C, Sato H, Phalanusitthepha C, Santi EG, Grimes KL, Ito H, Kudo SE. Greater curvature myotomy is a safe and effective modified technique in peroral endoscopic myotomy (with videos). Gastrointest Endosc. 2015;81(6):1370–7. https://doi.org/10.1016/j.gie.2014.11.014.
114. Peters J. What do the esophagus and a jump rope have in common. Arch Surg. 2012;147(4):357.
115. Curtis DJ, Cruess DF, Berg T. The cricopharyngeal muscle: a videorecording review. Am J Roentgenol. 1984;142(3):497–500.
116. Demeester TR, Johnson LF, Kent AH. Evaluation of current operations for the prevention of gastroesophageal reflux. Ann Surg. 1974;180(4):511–25.
117. Hagen JA, DeMeester TR. Anatomy of the esophagus. In: Shields TW, LoCicero J, Ponn RB, et al., editors. General thoracic surgery. International textbook of medicine, vol. 2. 6th ed. Philadelphia: Lippincott Williams & Wilkins; 2005. p. 1885–93.
118. Kahrilas PJ, Lin S, Spiess AE, Brasseur JG, Joehl RJ, Manka M. Impact of fundoplication on bolus transit across esophagogastric junction. Am J Phys. 1998;275(6 Pt 1):G1386–93.
119. Jiang Y, Sandler B, Bhargava V, Mittal RK. Antireflux action of Nissen fundoplication and stretch-sensitive mechanism of lower esophageal sphincter relaxation. Gastroenterology. 2011;140(2):442–9. https://doi.org/10.1053/j.gastro.2010.10.010.
120. Scheffer RC, Tatum RP, Shi G, Akkermans LM, Joehl RJ, Kahrilas PJ. Reduced tLESR elicitation in response to gastric distension in fundoplication patients. Am J Physiol Gastrointest Liver Physiol. 2003;284(5):G815–20. https://doi.org/10.1152/ajpgi.00247.2002.
121. del Genio G, Tolone S, del Genio F, Rossetti G, Brusciano L, Pizza F, Fei L, del Genio A. Total fundoplication controls acid and nonacid reflux: evaluation by pre- and postoperative 24-h pH-multichannel intraluminal impedance. Surg Endosc. 2008;22(11):2518–23. https://doi.org/10.1007/s00464-008-9958-0.
122. Blom D, Peters JH, DeMeester TR, Crookes PF, Hagan JA, DeMeester SR, Bremner C. Physiologic mechanism and preoperative prediction of new-onset dysphagia after laparoscopic Nissen fundoplication. J Gastrointest Surg. 2002;6(1):22–7. discussion 27-28

Anatomy and Physiology of the Stomach and Pylorus

3

Samuel Torres Landa, Kristoffel R. Dumon, and Daniel T. Dempsey

Anatomy of the Stomach

The stomach is an organ of digestion situated in the abdomen between the termination of the esophagus and the beginning of the duodenum. The stomach develops from the caudal portion of the embryonic foregut during the 5th week of gestation, as a primitive structure located within the ventral and dorsal mesenteries [1]. Due to the rotation of the gut, the left vagal trunk ends up in an anterior location, and the right vagal trunk ends up in a posterior location. Due to the movement of the foregut toward the embryo's left side, the stomach ends up occupying most of the left upper quadrant of the abdomen.

In the adult, the stomach rests between the 10th thoracic and the 3rd lumbar vertebral segments, and it is suspended and fixed by four ligaments despite its intraperitoneal location: (1) gastrosplenic or gastrolienal (from the stomach to the spleen), (2) gastrophrenic (from the stomach to the diaphragm), (3) hepatogastric or lesser omentum (from the stomach to the liver), and (4) gastrocolic or greater omentum (from the stomach to the transverse colon). The borders of the stomach are (1) the liver (superiorly and laterally to the right), (2) the spleen (laterally to the left), (3) the pancreas (posteriorly), and (4) the transverse colon inferiorly.

The stomach is divided into four segments that are important guides when planning a surgical resection: (1) the *cardia*, (2) the *fundus*, (3) the *corpus* or *body*, and (4) the *antrum* (Fig. 3.1). The *cardia* is the most proximal part of the stomach located immediately after the gastroesophageal junction. The *fundus* is the region of

S. T. Landa · K. R. Dumon (✉)
Hospital of the University of Pennsylvania, Philadelphia, PA, USA
e-mail: SamuelTorreslanda@uphs.upenn.edu; Kristoffel.dumon@uphs.upenn.edu

D. T. Dempsey
Department of Surgery, Hospital of the University of Pennsylvania, Philadelphia, PA, USA
e-mail: Daniel.dempsey@uphs.upenn.edu

J. Grams et al. (eds.), *The SAGES Manual of Foregut Surgery*,
https://doi.org/10.1007/978-3-319-96122-4_3

Fig. 3.1 Stomach segmental division

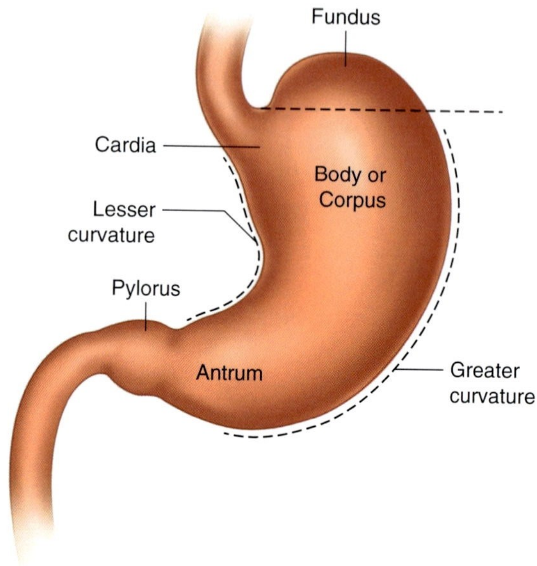

the stomach that extends above the gastroesophageal junction. The *corpus* or *body* lies between the fundus and the antrum and is marked distally by the *angularis incisura*, a notch on the lesser curvature of the stomach located near to the pyloric end. The last segment is the *antrum*, which extends from the corpus or body to the pyloric sphincter, a thick muscular valve that separates the antrum from the duodenum [1]. Each of these segments has histologic differences and is involved in unique roles in the process of digestion [2].

The stomach has four layers from the outermost to the innermost: (1) the *peritoneum* or *serosa*; (2) the *muscularis propria*, also known as *muscularis externa* that is composed of three layers of muscles (longitudinal, circular, and oblique) (Fig. 3.2), which contains the myenteric plexus of Auerbach; (3) *the submucosa*, which represents the strongest layer of the stomach; and (4) the *mucosa*, which is subdivided into muscularis mucosae, lamina propria, and surface epithelium.

Arterial Blood Supply and Venous Drainage of the Stomach

Five major sources contribute to the rich vascular supply of the stomach, all of which arise from the celiac trunk forming multiple anastomoses that protect the stomach from ischemic events. In a clockwise matter, the *left gastric artery* (a direct branch from the celiac trunk) supplies the upper portion of the lesser curvature of the stomach; the *vasa brevia* or *short gastric arteries* (direct branches from the splenic artery) supply the fundus and upper portion of the corpus; the

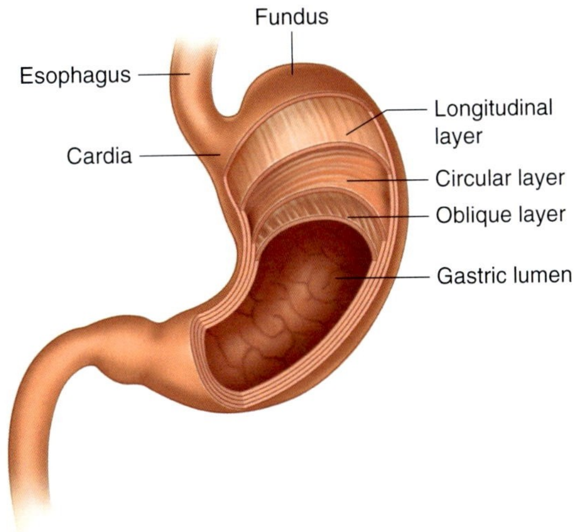

Fig. 3.2 Outermost to the innermost muscular layer division of the stomach

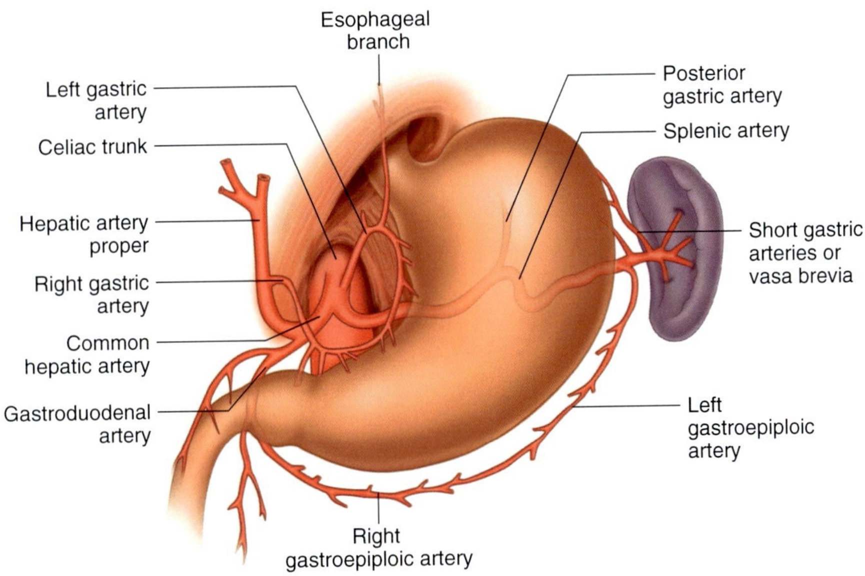

Fig. 3.3 Arterial blood supply to the stomach

left gastroepiploic artery (branch from the splenic artery) supplies the upper corpus; *the right gastroepiploic artery* (branch from the gastroduodenal) supplies the lower corpus and the antrum; and the *right gastric artery* (branch from the common hepatic artery) supplies the lower portion of the lesser curvature (Fig. 3.3) [2].

The venous drainage of the stomach parallels the arterial blood supply. The short gastric veins and left gastroepiploic, via the splenic vein, drain to the portal vein. The right gastroepiploic, via the superior mesenteric vein, drains to the portal vein. Lastly, both right and left gastric (coronary vein) veins drain directly to the portal system [1]. The vein drainage of the stomach is important to understand the pathophysiology of portal hypertension and its complications [3].

Innervation

The stomach has both parasympathetic and sympathetic innervation. Sympathetic nerves are in charge of transmitting pain via the greater splanchnic nerve and celiac plexus. Parasympathetic innervation is characterized by afferent signals of the two anterior and posterior vagal trunks that descend laterally through the esophageal hiatus of the diaphragm, adherent to the muscularis of the esophagus. The right vagal trunk runs posteriorly between the aorta and the esophagus, gives off a celiac branch, and continues its way through the lesser curvature of the stomach (*posterior nerve of Latarjet*), innervating the posterior wall of the stomach. Near the gastroesophageal junction, there is a branch known as the *criminal nerve of Grassi*. Its identification during a truncal vagotomy is very important, as it is thought to be related to recurrent symptoms (Fig. 3.4) [2]. The left vagal trunk runs anteriorly through the esophagus, gives off a hepatic branch, and continues its way throughout the anterior lesser curvature of the stomach (*anterior nerve of Latarjet*), innervating the anterior wall of the stomach and pylorus.

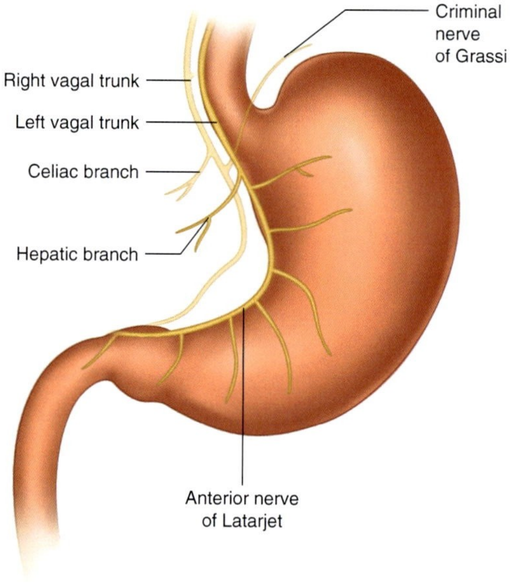

Fig. 3.4 Vagal innervation of the stomach

Lymphatic Drainage

The lymphatic drainage of the stomach also runs near the arterial blood supply. The anatomical importance of lymphatic drainage and the location of the gastric lymph nodes (LNs) relies on its relationship with gastric cancer and gastric metastasis [4]. The anatomical description of lymph node stations has been defined by the Japanese Gastric Cancer Association [5]. The lymph node stations in closer proximity to the stomach that correspond to N1 and N2 lymph node metastasis of the TNM classification include (1) right paracardial LNs, (2) left paracardial LNs, (3) lesser curvature LNs, (4) left and right greater curvature LNs, (5) suprapyoric LNs, and (6) infrapyloric LNs (Fig. 3.5). However, due to the extensive lymphatic communications, metastatic disease can bypass primary lymph node groups [5].

Gastric Physiology

The main function of the stomach is to prepare the ingested food for digestion and absorption. The solid food components need to be broken down to its basic metabolic components in order be absorbed. Thus, the stomach serves as a storage organ to enable this process that takes approximately 3–4 h (transit time). This process

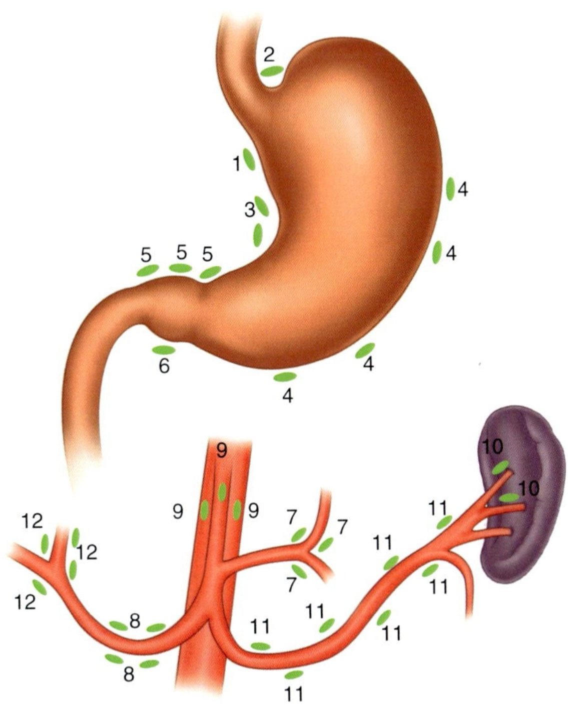

Fig. 3.5 *Lymphatic node stations of the stomach according to the Japanese Gastric Cancer Association 2011. 1 = right paracardial lymph nodes; 2 = left paracardial lymph nodes; 3 = lesser curvature lymph nodes; 4 = greater curvature lymph nodes; 5 = suprapyloric lymph nodes; 6 = infrapyloric lymph nodes; 7 = lymph nodes along the trunk of the left gastric artery; 8 = lymph nodes along the common hepatic artery; 9 = celiac artery lymph nodes; 10 = splenic hilar lymph nodes; 11 = distal splenic artery lymph nodes; 12 = hepatoduodenal ligament lymph nodes*

also involves the release of hydrochloric acid and other peptides from the gastric glands that mixed with the food content (*chyme*) passes from the stomach to the first portion of the small intestine, through the pyloric sphincter to be absorbed.

The stomach contains a glandular epithelium divided into two functional areas: the oxyntic area that corresponds to 80% of the stomach and the pyloric area. The oxyntic area is located in the fundus and corpus (Fig. 3.1). This area is characterized by gastric glands (the acid-secreting unit of the mucosa) (Fig. 3.6) that contain (1) mucus neck cells; (2) parietal cells, in charge of the production and secretion of hydrochloric acid and intrinsic factor; (3) chief cells, in charge of the production of pepsinogen; and (4) enterochromaffin-like cells (ECL cells) that express the enzyme in charge of the production of histamine (histidine decarboxylase). The pyloric area is located in the antrum of the stomach and is mainly composed of G cells that secrete gastrin. Somatostatin releasing cells (D cells) are present in both oxyntic and pyloric glands, and its function is to inhibit gastrin and acid release. Endoscopically, the acid-secreting cells area and the non-acid-secreting cells area are relatively distinguished by the rugal pattern. In the antrum, the rugae are linear and aligned with the long axis of the stomach. In the corpus, the rugae are oriented obliquely and have a convoluted pattern [2].

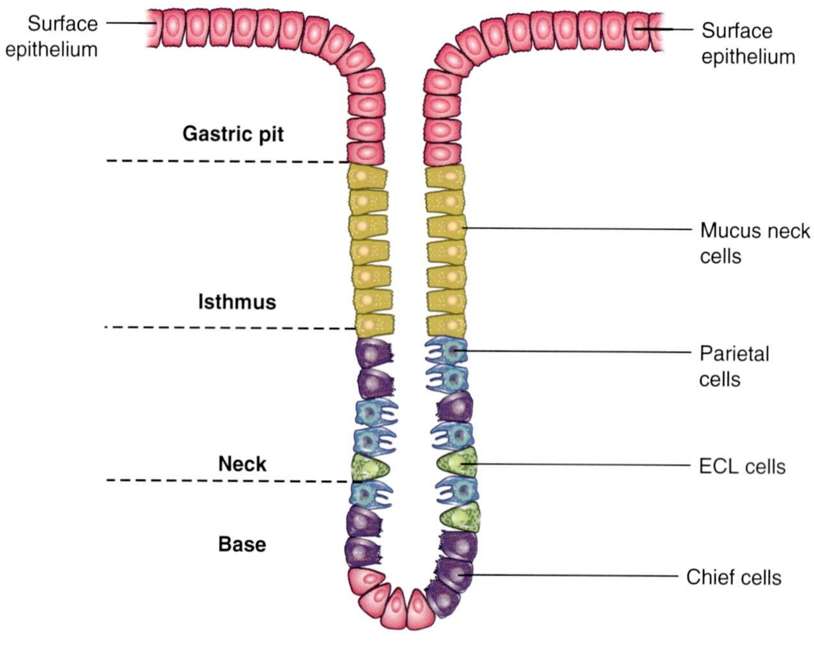

Fig. 3.6 Gastric gland. *ECL enterochromaffin-like cells*

Gastric Acid Secretion

Gastric acid secretion is divided into three phases. First, a *cephalic phase* that originates through sight of food, smell, thought, taste, or swallowing, which accounts for 20–30% of the total acid secretion. This phase is mainly mediated by cholinergic mechanisms. Second, a *gastric phase* stimulated by gastric distention and chemical effects of food in the gastric lumen, which accounts for 60–70% of the total acid secretion. This phase appears to be mainly mediated by gastrin. Finally, a primarily inhibitory *intestinal phase* that is thought to start with the entry of chyme into the first portion of the intestine. However, its mediation is still controversial, and it only accounts for 10% of the total acid secretion [6, 7].

Gastric acid physiologic secretion regulation consists of three stimulating pathways, two inhibitory pathways, and other regulators (Fig. 3.7). The three stimulating pathways in charge of acid secretion in the stomach include (1) acetylcholine, released by cholinergic cells from the vagal trunks; (2) histamine, released by ECL cells; and (3) gastrin, released by G cells [8, 9]. The two inhibitory pathways include extrinsic signals: (1) somatostatin, released by D cells and (2) prostaglandins (E and I) [10]. There have been proposed other types of intrinsic cell signals like the

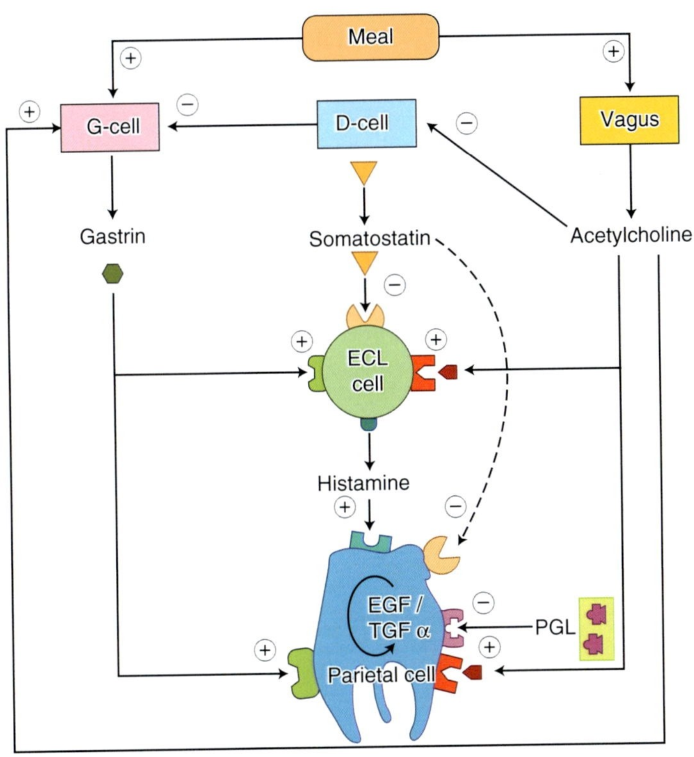

Fig. 3.7 Physiology control of acid secretion. *PGL prostaglandins, EGF epidermal growth factor, TGFα transforming growth factor alpha*

epidermal growth factor and the transforming growth factor alpha (EGF/TGFα) that may play an important role in acid secretion by modulating intracellular tyrosine kinase activity [11].

The stomach has a basal acid secretion level of 1–5 mmol/h of HCL and a total of 1–2 L of HCL acid secretion every 24 hours that maintain a luminal concentration of 150–160 mmol/L. The basal acid secretion can be decreased with medical (H2 blockers) or surgical (vagotomy) interventions. Thus, this basal acid secretion is thought to be stimulated by cholinergic as well as histaminergic output [1].

Intracellular Signals for Acid Secretion

Gastrin, histamine, and acetylcholine stimulate the parietal cell through intracellular pathways that involve second messengers (Fig. 3.8) (1). Gastrin binds to the CCK-2 receptors located in the parietal cell membrane. This process activates phospholipase C that activates phosphatidylinositol triphosphate through phosphorylation, which increases cytosolic calcium release, that act on calmodulin kinases that ultimately stimulate the hydrogen potassium ATPase pump (H+/K+ ATPase pump) (2). Histamine binds to the H2 receptors that activates adenylate cyclase, increasing cAMP, which activates protein kinase A that ultimately stimulates the H+/K+ ATPase pump (3). Acetylcholine binds to type 3 muscarinic receptors (M3) that also act through the activation of the phospholipase C pathway mentioned above (4). Somatostatin represents the main inhibitor of acid secretion. Its major role has been the indirect inhibition of histamine release through SSTR2 receptors in the ECL cells. However, this hormone may also bind to SSTR2 receptors located in the parietal cell membrane [12].

Potassium plays a critical and essential role in the activation of the H+/K+ ATPase pump (Fig. 3.9). During the resting state, the parietal cell stores the H+/K+ ATPase pump within tubulovesicular intracellular elements that have a low K+ concentration and an impermeable membrane to K+ ions. After parietal cell stimulation, cellular relocation of the H+/K+ ATPase pump to the apical membrane occurs through cytoskeletal mobilization. This process leads to the exposure of the H+/K+ ATPase pump to K+ ions, which starts exchanging H+ ions. The process is in charge of ion transport to maintain electroneutrality within the membranes. For each H+ ion transported into the canaliculus by the H+/K+ ATPase pump, the basolateral CL-/HC03- exchanger delivers a HCO3- out the parietal cell and a Cl- into the cell. Moreover, in the apical membrane, Cl- is secreted into the canaliculus through Cl-channels (C1C-2 channel). In order to maintain electroneutrality, the Cl- excreted accounts as a counter for the K+ flux across the membrane. The Na+/K+ ATPase

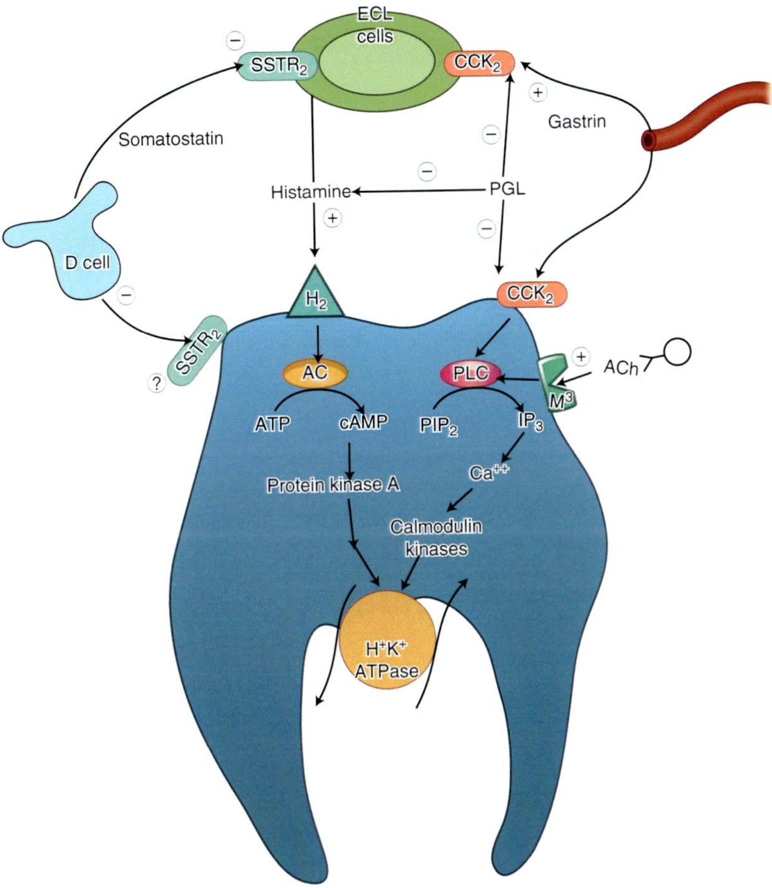

Fig. 3.8 Intracellular control of acid secretion in the parietal cell. *ECL enterochromaffin-like cells, PGL prostaglandins,* $SSTR_2$ *somatostatin receptor type 2,* CCK_2 *cholecystokinin type 2 receptor,* H_2 *histamine type 2 receptor,* M^3 *muscarinic acetylcholine receptor type 3, Ach acetylcholine, AC adenylate cyclase, ATP adenosine triphosphate, cAMP cyclic adenosine monophosphate, PLC phospholipase C,* PIP_2 *phosphatidyl 4,5-bisphosphate,* IP_3 *inositol triphosphate,* Ca^{++} *calcium ion,* K^+ *potassium ion,* H^+ *hydrogen ion,* H^+K^+ *ATPase hydrogen potassium ATPase*

located in the basolateral membrane also plays a major role in the parietal cell by exchanging intracellular Na + for extracellular K+. Furthermore, also in the basolateral membrane, K+ channels allow the efflux of K+ ion to create a negative cell membrane potential [13].

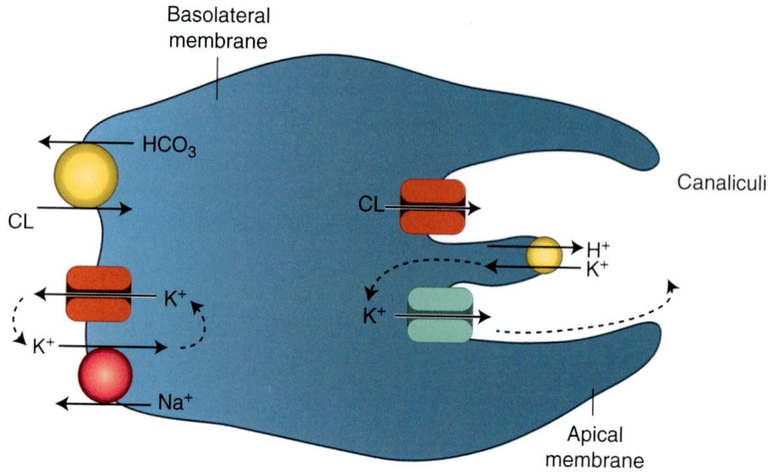

Fig. 3.9 Intracellular ion movement in the parietal cell. *Cl⁻ chloride ion, HCO_3^- bicarbonate ion, K^+ potassium ion, Na^+ sodium ion, H^+ hydrogen ion*

Medical and Surgical Approaches to Decrease Gastric Acid Secretion

The complex physiological acid secretion control led to the creation of multiple drugs that act through different mechanisms. The most commonly used groups of drugs for patients with increased acid secretion and further symptomatology are proton pump inhibitors (PPIs) (omeprazole, pantoprazole, esomeprazole, dexlansoprazole) and H2 receptor antagonists (famotidine, ranitidine, nizatidine, cimetidine). PPIs act through an irreversible inhibition of the H+/K+ ATPase pump, and H2 receptor antagonists act as competitive antagonists of the H2 receptor. Rebound acid hypersecretion occurs after the cessation of both types of medications. Thus, the abrupt discontinuation of these medications in patients with high risk of recurrence or complications might not be the best approach. It is also important to know that H2 receptor antagonists, but not proton pump inhibitors, have been related to the development of tolerance as soon as 7 days after therapy. Lastly, PPI are among the most commonly prescribed classes of drugs. However, it is important to acknowledge that the chronic use of this class of drugs have been (1) consistently related to the development of fundic gland polyps; (2) have a weak association (Odds ratio <2) with an increased risk of fracture, hypomagnesemia, vitamin B 12 deficiency, cardiovascular risk, *C. difficile* infection, and pneumonia; and (3) have an uncertain and modest association with dementia and renal disease, respectively [14].

H. pylori, a pathogen that is transmitted from human to human, has been implicated in the development of chronic active gastritis, and its eradication cures this disease, altering the progression of its complications. Moreover, *H. pylori* can both increase and decrease acid secretion by different mechanisms. The treatment for *H. pylori* in patients with non-atrophic antral-predominant gastritis and atrophic gastritis, but not in patients with extensive atrophic changes, leads to a partial correction of the low or high acid state of these patients. However, the treatment for "acid correction" should not be used as an argument to treat this infection as it has not been proven to be of clinical relevance [15].

The surgical approaches to control gastric acid secretion include (1) gastrectomy, (2) antrectomy, and (3) vagotomy. These three approaches act through different mechanisms that each serve to decrease acid secretion. Parietal ECL cells are removed in a gastrectomy. A decrease in both G and ECL cells occurs as part of an antrectomy. Cholinergic stimulation of the parietal cells is interrupted by a vagotomy [2].

Non-Acid Gastric Secretion

Mucus and HC03- are constantly secreted by mucus glands located throughout the entire gastric mucosa, which help to neutralize acid levels and provide a mechanical barrier that protects against mucosal injury. Mucus production is stimulated by cholinergic stimuli and prostaglandins. Thus, nonsteroidal anti-inflammatory drugs and anticholinergics can inhibit mucus secretion, making the gastric mucosa susceptible to injury. *H. pylori* infection has also been related to the secretion of lipases and proteases that cleave mucin, therefore affecting the protective mucosal barrier. Another important role of the gastric mucus that protects the apical cell membrane is its relative impermeability to pepsin and its intrinsic resistance to the diffusion of H+ ions. Lastly, the mucosal blood flow that can be affected by multiple factors is also crucial to maintain a healthy mucosa by delivering the appropriate oxygen and nutrients needed for cytoprotection and cellular function.

Gastric Digestion

The stomach is implicated in the preparation of the ingested food for its digestion and absorption in the small intestine by mixing the ingested food with acid (chyme) and releasing pepsinogen that is consequently activated into pepsin, cleaving peptides into their basic metabolic constituents. The parietal cell also secretes intrinsic factor that helps with the absorption of vitamin B12 in the terminal ileum. Thus, patients with intrinsic factor deficiency secondary to a gastrectomy or pernicious anemia require vitamin B12 supplementation. Gastric acid also promotes the absorption of iron and calcium cations [2, 16]. Therefore, the alteration of gastric pH through medications like proton pump inhibitors can alter the absorption of these types of molecules.

Gastric Motility

Intrinsic and extrinsic neural mechanisms control and modulate gastric motility. The extrinsic control is carried through sympathetic and parasympathetic pathways, and the intrinsic control is mediated by the enteric nervous system. Gastric motility differs in the fasting and postprandial state. The *gastric electrical pacemaker* responsible for the motor functions is located in the midportion of the greater curvature. In the fasting state, slow waves travel circumferentially and distally toward the pylorus at three cycles per minute, and a cyclical pattern of slow waves and electrical spikes, also known as the *myoenteric migrating complex*, run through the stomach and help the clearance of gastric content. In anticipation of food intake, the proximal portion of the stomach relaxes, through a process called *receptive relaxation*. This relaxation settles the solid food in the fundus and greater curvature of the stomach, while liquids pass without difficulty through the lesser curvature [16]. In the postprandial state, the proximal and fundus tone relaxes to enable its storage function, and the midportion and antrum create repetitive forceful contractions that help to mix and grind the food into small particles. Even though most gastric motility disorders causing delayed gastric emptying are idiopathic, diseases like diabetes or postsurgical vagotomy and/or iatrogenic vagal injuries are commonly associated with gastric motility disorders.

Gastric Implication in Appetite Control

During the last decades, appetite control has been broadly studied as it has been shown to have an important role after bariatric procedures. However, it has not been completely understood as it involves a complex neurohormonal mechanism. Even though the small and large intestine significantly contribute to appetite control through the release of multiple hormones implicated in this process (GLP-1, PYY, GIP, and oxyntomodulin), the stomach also plays an important role [17]. Ghrelin and gastrin, hormones that are mainly released by the stomach, have also been associated with increased and decreased appetite, respectively. Ghrelin is secreted in a diurnal rhythm that stimulates appetite and food intake. This peptide is released during fasting states to the portal circulation and travels through the systemic circulation to finally stimulate hypothalamic appetite centers. Ghrelin levels decrease dramatically when the stomach begins to fill [18]. Thus, after bariatric procedures (sleeve gastrectomy and Roux-en-Y gastric bypass) that create small pouches that are easily stretched, a dramatic fall of the levels of this hormone is detected. Therefore, decreasing appetite is thought to benefit patients by promoting weight loss and theoretically affecting metabolic status [19].

Gastric Secreted Peptides and Compounds

Gastrin

Gastrin is a peptide produced by G cells located in the antrum of the stomach. Several molecular forms have identified (G-34, G17, and G-14). Most of the antral gastrin is released as G-17. However, G-34 predominates in the circulation due to the longer metabolic half-life, compared to that of G-17. Gastrin is released by stomach muscle distention and by the presence of food (especially by peptides) in the lumen. Moreover, luminal acid and somatostatin decrease its release. Gastrin functions include (1) an increase production of HCL acid, pepsinogen, intrinsic factor, pancreatic secretions, and bile; (2) the promotion of satiety; and (3) a trophic regulation of the parietal and ECL cells [16, 17, 20].

Ghrelin

Ghrelin is a peptide produced by ghrelin release cells mainly located in the oxyntic area of the stomach. It is secreted during fasting states and its levels decrease after the stomach starts to fill. Ghrelin functions include (1) an increase in appetite, (2) an increase of gastric emptying and motility, (3) the induction of growth hormone release, and (4) inhibition of glucose-stimulated insulin production [17, 18].

Somatostatin

Somatostatin is a peptide produced by D cells located throughout the entire gastric mucosa. It is secreted by the increase in gastric acid, gastrin itself, and vasoactive intestinal peptide and decreases after cholinergic activation. Somatostatin functions include (1) inhibition of histamine release (ECL cells) and may directly inhibit parietal cells, therefore decreasing acid secretion and (2) a decrease of gastrin release [10, 17].

Pepsin

Pepsinogen is released by chief cells located in the oxyntic area of the stomach. Pepsinogen is activated to pepsin (its active protease state) by low gastric pH and inactivated by pH above 4. It is secreted by gastrin, cholecystokinin, and acetylcholine stimuli. Pepsin functions include (1) protease activity and (2) mucolytic activity [21, 22].

Histamine

Histamine is nitrogenous compound released by ECL cells and mastocytes located in the oxyntic area of the stomach. It is secreted by gastrin, acetylcholine, adenylate cyclase-activating polypeptide, and vasoactive intestinal peptide, and its secretion decreases by somatostatin, calcitonin, gene-related peptide, PYY, prostaglandins, and galanin. Histamine is the major paracrine stimulator of acid secretion through the stimulation of the parietal cell [16, 23].

Prostaglandins

Prostaglandins are autocrine factors mainly released by macrophages and capillary endothelial cells [24]. Its functions include (1) inhibition of acid secretion, (2) inhibition of histamine-stimulated parietal cell function, (3) inhibition of gastrin-stimulated histamine release, and (4) stimulation of mucus production [25].

Pylorus Anatomy and Physiology

The pyloric sphincter represents a zone of high resting pressure that is easily identified endoscopically (by the underlying muscular ring) and is easily palpated during surgery as a muscular ring on the gastroduodenal junction. The pyloric area is defined by a *proximal pyloric loop* (3 cm lumen) and a *distal pyloric loop* (1 cm lumen) that are not easily identified. However, this entire segment (proximal and distal pyloric loops) contracts as a unit and differs structurally and functionally from the adjacent antrum and duodenum. The proximal loop participates in gastric phasic contractions (every 3 minutes) that lead to a forceful closure of the pyloric lumen, this way, controlling the passage of the chyme from the stomach to the duodenum [26].

The pylorus receives blood supply mainly from the gastroduodenal artery, a branch of the common hepatic artery. The pylorus is innervated by intrinsic (myenteric plexus) and extrinsic (vagal branches and adrenergic fiber) nerves. The myenteric plexus nerve cells contain excitatory (enkephalins and substance P) and inhibitory (vasoactive intestinal peptide and nitric oxide) transmitters. The vagal innervation is mechanosensitive, responding to muscle stretch. However, vagal motor fibers have been also found to mediate excitatory (enkephalins and acetylcholine) and inhibitory responses (vasoactive intestinal peptide and nitric oxide) [26]. Therefore, the stimulation of the pyloric nerves can trigger both phasic contractions and/or relaxation of this segment.

The importance of the pyloric sphincter is not fully appreciated until pathology is encountered, such as in a patient with an intrinsic pyloric disease like infantile hypertrophic pyloric stenosis or patients with destruction or bypass of the pyloric sphincter who present to clinic with dumping syndrome.

Gastric Microbiome

The discovery of *H. pylori* in 1982 by Marshall and Warren led to the consideration of other commensal organisms in the stomach (gastric microbiota), shifting the belief of a “sterile stomach.” *H. pylori* is mainly transmitted person to person (fecal/oral or oral/oral), and once it has colonized the stomach, it becomes the predominant gastric microbiota species. The prevalence of *H. pylori* differs between regions, reaching 80% in developing countries [27]. In developed countries, such as the USA, its prevalence has been declining through the years, with a reported prevalence of 50% in 1991 and 17% in 2010 [28]. *H. pylori*'s urease activity, its ability to penetrate through the gastric mucus layer, and then binding to specific gastric receptors explain its adaptation to the gastric hazardous environment and predilection to the gastric mucosa. Moreover, most of the *H. pylori* positive patients are asymptomatic. However, all carriers will ultimately develop chronic gastritis. The location of the affected part of the stomach has different patterns of gastritis and therefore different changes in gastric acid secretion. Antrum-predominant gastritis, which decreases somatostatin production, is related to gastrin-induced increased acid secretion, and pangastritis or corpus-predominant gastritis, which is associated with extensive gastric atrophy, causes hypo- or achlorhydria and thus a decrease in acid secretion [27].

Other possible commensal organisms of the stomach have also been studied in recent years. Bik et al. characterized bacterial diversity of the gastric mucosa of 23 gastric endoscopy biopsies and found 128 phylotypes, the majority assigned to the *Proteobacteria*, *Firmicutes*, *Actinobacteria*, *Bacteroidetes*, and *Fusobacteria* phyla. This finding suggests that the stomach may have a distinct microbiota, and its role in human health still needs to be studied and elucidated [29].

References

1. Porrett PM, Drebin J. The surgical review: an integrated basic and clinical science study guide. Books Express (Portsmouth, NH, U.S.A): Lippincott Williams & Wilkins; 2015.
2. Soybel DI. Anatomy and physiology of the stomach. Surg Clin North Am. 2005;85(5): 875–94.
3. Garcia-Tsao G. Portal hypertension. Curr Opin Gastroenterol. 2006;22(3):254–62.
4. Ikoma N, Blum M, Estrella JS, Wang X, Fournier KF, Mansfield PF, et al. Left gastric artery lymph nodes should be included in D1 lymph node dissection in gastric cancer. J Gastrointest Surg. 2017;21:1563.
5. Japanese Gastric Cancer A. Japanese classification of gastric carcinoma: 3rd English edition. Gastric Cancer. 2011;14(2):101–12.
6. Lloyd KK. Peripheral regulation of gastric acid secretion. Physiol Gastrointest Tract. 1994;1:1185–226.
7. Ramsay PT, Carr A. Gastric acid and digestive physiology. Surg Clin North Am. 2011;91(5):977–82.
8. Schubert ML, Peura DA. Control of gastric acid secretion in health and disease. Gastroenterology. 2008;134(7):1842–60.
9. Schubert ML, Makhlouf GM. Gastrin secretion induced by distention is mediated by gastric cholinergic and vasoactive intestinal peptide neurons in rats. Gastroenterology. 1993;104(3):834–9.
10. Saffouri B, DuVal JW, Arimura A, Makhlouf GM. Effects of vasoactive intestinal peptide and secretin on gastrin and somatostatin secretion in the perfused rat stomach. Gastroenterology. 1984;86(5 Pt 1):839–42.
11. Yao X, Forte JG. Cell biology of acid secretion by the parietal cell. Annu Rev Physiol. 2003;65:103–31.
12. Schubert ML. Functional anatomy and physiology of gastric secretion. Curr Opin Gastroenterol. 2015;31(6):479–85.
13. Geibel JP. Role of potassium in acid secretion. World J Gastroenterol. 2005;11(34):5259–65.
14. Eusebi LH, Rabitti S, Artesiani ML, Gelli D, Montagnani M, Zagari RM, et al. Proton pump inhibitors: risks of long-term use. J Gastroenterol Hepatol. 2017;32(7):1295–302.

15. Malfertheiner P, Megraud F, O'Morain CA, Gisbert JP, Kuipers EJ, Axon AT, et al. Management of Helicobacter pylori infection-the Maastricht V/Florence Consensus Report. Gut. 2017;66(1):6–30.
16. Townsend CM, Beauchamp RD, Evers BM, Mattox KL. Sabiston textbook of surgery E-book. Elsevier (New York, NY, U.S.A.): Elsevier Health Sciences; 2016.
17. Meek CL, Lewis HB, Reimann F, Gribble FM, Park AJ. The effect of bariatric surgery on gastrointestinal and pancreatic peptide hormones. Peptides. 2016;77:28–37.
18. Yakabi K, Kawashima J, Kato S. Ghrelin and gastric acid secretion. World J Gastroenterol. 2008;14(41):6334–8.
19. Mechanick JI, Youdim A, Jones DB, Garvey WT, Hurley DL, McMahon MM, et al. Clinical practice guidelines for the perioperative nutritional, metabolic, and nonsurgical support of the bariatric surgery patient--2013 update: cosponsored by American Association of Clinical Endocrinologists, The Obesity Society, and American Society for Metabolic & Bariatric Surgery. Obesity (Silver Spring). 2013;21(Suppl 1):S1–27.
20. Chen D, Monstein HJ, Nylander AG, Zhao CM, Sundler F, Hakanson R. Acute responses of rat stomach enterochromaffinlike cells to gastrin: secretory activation and adaptation. Gastroenterology. 1994;107(1):18–27.
21. Samloff IM. Pepsins, peptic activity, and peptic inhibitors. J Clin Gastroenterol. 1981;3(Suppl 2):91–4.
22. Allen A, Pearson JP, Blackburn A, Coan RM, Hutton DA, Mall AS. Pepsins and the mucus barrier in peptic ulcer disease. Scand J Gastroenterol Suppl. 1988;146:50–7.
23. Waldum HL, Hauso O, Fossmark R. The regulation of gastric acid secretion - clinical perspectives. Acta Physiol (Oxf). 2014;210(2):239–56.
24. Chen MC, Sanders MJ, Amirian DA, Thomas LP, Kauffman G, Soll AH. Prostaglandin E2 production by dispersed canine fundic mucosal cells. Contribution of macrophages and endothelial cells as major sources. J Clin Invest. 1989;84(5):1536–49.
25. Lindstrom E, Hakanson R. Prostaglandins inhibit secretion of histamine and pancreastatin from isolated rat stomach ECL cells. Br J Pharmacol. 1998;124(6):1307–13.
26. Ramkumar D, Schulze KS. The pylorus. Neurogastroenterol Motil. 2005;17(Suppl 1):22–30.
27. Minalyan A, Gabrielyan L, Scott D, Jacobs J, Pisegna JR. The gastric and intestinal microbiome: role of proton pump inhibitors. Curr Gastroenterol Rep. 2017;19(8):42.
28. Lender N, Talley NJ, Enck P, Haag S, Zipfel S, Morrison M, et al. Review article: associations between helicobacter pylori and obesity--an ecological study. Aliment Pharmacol Ther. 2014;40(1):24–31.
29. Bik EM, Eckburg PB, Gill SR, Nelson KE, Purdom EA, Francois F, et al. Molecular analysis of the bacterial microbiota in the human stomach. Proc Natl Acad Sci U S A. 2006;103(3):732–7.

4 Anatomic and Physiologic Tests of Esophageal and Gastric Function

Sarah Marucci, Jessica Zarzour, and James Callaway

Introduction

Both the medical and surgical management of chronic and acute disease require an accurate diagnosis and understanding of the underlying physiology and pathology. Physiology is often thought of in global terms, but scientific discovery and innovation over the last millennia have enabled the scientific community to accurately describe, quantify, and manipulate human physiology in a way that allows clinicians to tailor treatment plans and interventions in an individual fashion.

The foregut is at the forefront of intestinal transit and motility as well as digestion and absorption. Thus the manipulation of these processes during the treatment of disease, both medically and surgically, allows for both treatment success and treatment consequences. This chapter will review the various methods for the evaluation of esophageal and gastric transit, motility, acid physiology, as well as anatomic considerations and evaluations. It will review the basic procedural elements to each testing method and review salient features to each test.

S. Marucci
Division of Internal Medicine, University of Alabama, Birmingham, AL, USA

J. Zarzour
Department of Radiology, University of Alabama, Birmingham, AL, USA

J. Callaway (✉)
Division of Gastroenterology and Hepatology, University of Alabama, Birmingham, AL, USA
e-mail: jcallaway@uabmc.edu

J. Grams et al. (eds.), *The SAGES Manual of Foregut Surgery*,
https://doi.org/10.1007/978-3-319-96122-4_4

Esophageal Motility

Barium Swallow

The barium esophagram is a useful diagnostic tool in the real-time evaluation of esophageal anatomy, motility, and physiology. It is often the initial test used in the evaluation of dysphagia given its ability to identify both mechanical and functional causes, but it is also widely used in the evaluation of gastroesophageal reflux disease, hiatal hernias, peristalsis, and postoperative functional and structural evaluations. A barium swallow is used in patients with a suspected proximal esophageal lesion such as Zenker's diverticulum or stricture, both of which may carry a risk of perforation with initial evaluation by upper endoscopy. It is also used following an unrevealing upper endoscopy when a subtle mechanical obstruction is still suspected. Though high-resolution manometry and impedance technology are now commonly available for assessment of esophageal motility and bolus transit, the barium esophagram can be used in conjunction with these tests for further evaluation and confirmation.

Basic Procedure Prior to performing the barium esophagram, the patient should have nothing by mouth for 2 h. The exam begins by examining the pharynx and upper esophageal sphincter in the upright lateral and anteroposterior (AP) positions. Esophageal emptying is assessed in the upright positions. If esophageal emptying is impaired in the upright position, the exam is then converted to a timed barium swallow to assess for the possibility of achalasia. Spot images of the esophagus are obtained at 1, 2, and 5 min with times denoted on the image [1]. The gastroesophageal junction (GEJ) and the air-fluid column should be included in each image. In a normal individual, the barium should empty within 1 min. This timed study can be used to confirm an achalasia diagnosis or used after treatment to monitor success of treatment and detect disease [2].

If esophageal emptying is normal in the upright position, then the exam continues with the double-contrast portion. The patient is placed in the erect left posterior oblique position and swallows a sodium bicarbonate effervescent agent dissolved in 10 cc of water in order to distend the esophagus. This is followed by rapidly swallowing of 2 ounces of "thick" (high-density) barium, and spot images are obtained to assess the esophageal mucosa.

To observe the motility phase without the effect of gravity, the patient is then placed in the horizontal right anterior oblique position and is asked to swallow single sips of "thin" (low-density) barium. Three to five individual sips should be observed, as motility disorders can be intermittent. The patient then drinks the barium continuously to fully distend the esophagus, and then single-contrast spot images of the entire esophagus are obtained. This distention is useful to detect strictures, rings, and contour abnormalities from extrinsic compression and to evaluate the GEJ [3].

Gastroesophageal reflux is then assessed. The patient is rolled into the left lateral position to allow barium to move into the gastric fundus. Then the patient is observed as he or she is rolled into the right posterior oblique position. If no reflux is seen, several maneuvers can be used to provoke gastroesophageal reflux including the Valsalva maneuver, strong cough, and the water siphon test. The degree of esophageal injury depends on the amount of reflux, the superior extent of the reflux, and the time it takes to clear. The sole purpose of the barium swallow is not to determine the presence or absence of reflux but to assess for the complications from reflux (strictures, erosions, hiatal hernias). As compared to pH and impedance monitoring in the evaluation of reflux, barium esophagography is the only method available to measure reflux volume.

A 13 mm barium tablet is given to patients with dysphagia unexplained by the findings on the routine study or to evaluate possible strictures and assess its clinical significance. The barium tablet can be used to localize the site of subtle obstruction such as a ring or stricture that the patient could have compensated for in earlier tests by smaller and slower ingestion of liquids. Barium meals can also be useful in order to provoke the patient's symptoms. This form of provocative testing can help distinguish the actual site for symptom development in patients who may have more than one potential contributor.

Motor Function/Peristalsis Esophageal peristalsis normally occurs in three distinct phases which can be elicited and observed using the barium esophagram. With intake of a bolus, the upper esophageal sphincter (UES) relaxes allowing the bolus to pass from the pharynx to the cervical esophagus. A primary peristaltic wave then occurs with the contraction of the inner circular muscles and propagation of the contraction to the distal esophagus. During normal peristalsis the barium column will rapidly progress distally as an inverted *V* [4]. This coordinated and stepwise progression down the esophageal body results in a primary stripping wave that can be observed on barium esophagography. The lower esophageal sphincter (LES) then relaxes and allows the bolus to pass through the GEJ into the stomach. A secondary peristaltic wave, which is induced by esophageal distention from any retained barium bolus or refluxed material, may occur in up to 30% of normal swallows and clears any remaining bolus without the need for an additional swallow triggered by a conscious effort [5]. Tertiary contractions are simultaneous, isolated, and dysfunctional contractions with no peristaltic or physiologic function. Barium esophagography can also be used to visualize "proximal escape," in which a small volume of barium escapes proximally from the inverted *V* to an area previously cleared. This can be a normal variant and is typically cleared by secondary peristalsis; however, substantial (>10 cm) retrograde escape has also been shown to be due to hypotensive peristaltic waves in patients with incompetent peristaltic contractions or occurring prior to the next swallow due to obstruction [6]. Proximal escape can also result from breaks in the peristaltic wave, typically occurring in the transition zone between the striated muscle of the proximal esophagus and the smooth muscle distally. These peristaltic breaks may appear as an incomplete stripping wave during peristalsis evaluation.

Motility Disorders

With the capability of assessing bolus transit and structural characteristics with fluoroscopy, the barium swallow can aid in the diagnosis of motility disorders. Classical achalasia (type I), characterized by failure of LES relaxation and aperistalsis, may show a smooth taper of the esophageal lumen toward the LES, giving the classic "bird beak" appearance. A dilated and tortuous esophagus may be seen proximally along with aperistalsis of the lower two-thirds of the esophagus, and delayed barium emptying (Fig. 4.1) [3]. It is important to note that a barium esophagram cannot always distinguish between primary achalasia and secondary achalasia, and thus direct endoscopic evaluation as well as esophageal manometry should be used as conjunctive studies [7]. Also, if esophageal manometry shows equivocal results, an esophagram should be performed to assess esophageal morphology and emptying [8].

Spastic esophageal motility disorders may be seen on a barium esophagram as lumen-obliterating contractions or tertiary contractions seen during peristalsis evaluation in the setting of distal esophageal spasm or hypertensive peristalsis. Distal esophageal spasm can have a "corkscrew appearance" as the esophagus is compartmentalized with repetitive and simultaneous lumen-obliterating contractions (Fig. 4.2) [9]. Secondary esophageal motility disorders such as those due to scleroderma, diabetes mellitus, or gastroesophageal reflux disease may be characteristically identified and suggested with fluoroscopy. In patients with scleroderma, the GEJ is often patulous with free gastroesophageal reflux. Barium may be ineffectively cleared due to poor LES tone and ineffective contractions

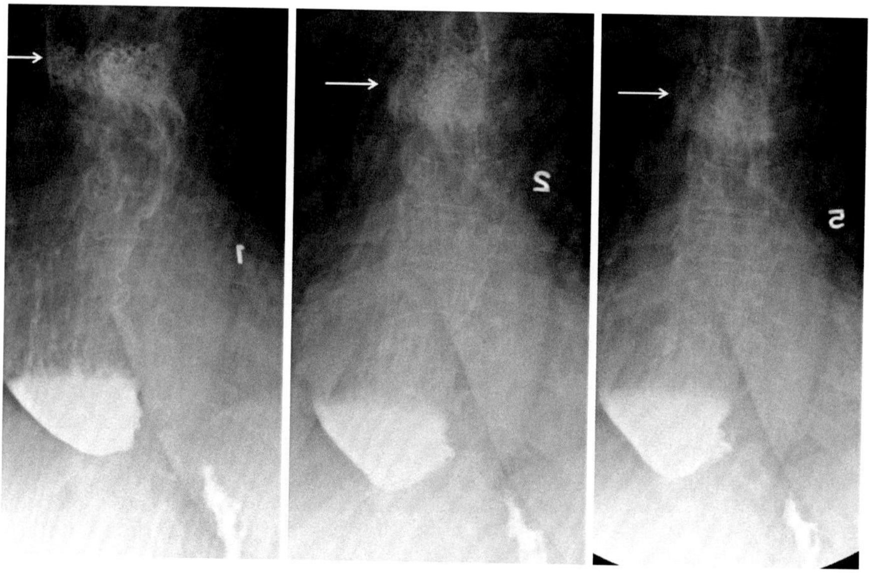

Fig. 4.1 Timed barium esophagram at 1, 2, and 5 min demonstrates a static column of fluid (arrow) within the dilated esophagus and a birds beak appearance of the lower esophageal sphincter. This is a classic appearance of type 1 achalasia

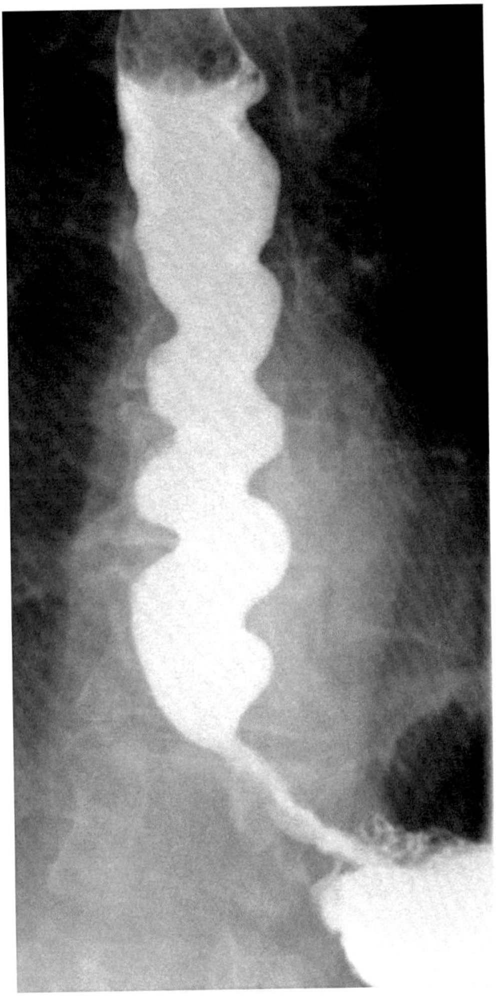

Fig. 4.2 Single-contrast barium esophagram in a patient with distal esophageal spasm shows tertiary contractions throughout the mid and distal esophagus. The contractions delay emptying of the esophagus

from atrophied smooth muscle in the distal esophagus. Patients with scleroderma are at particularly high risk of esophageal stricture formation due to persistent reflux [4, 10].

Anatomic Considerations

Barium esophagography evaluates structural components of the esophagus that may be contributing to symptoms of dysphagia such as strictures, rings and webs, ulcers, hernias, diverticula, and neoplasms. The double-contrast barium esophagram allows for enhanced mucosal evaluation and provides detail for diagnosing mucosal pathology. Radiographic findings of esophagitis are typically seen in the distal one-third of the esophagus. Findings can include granularity of the mucosa (due to edema and inflammation), fold thickening, erosions, ulcerations, and stricture [11]. Barrett's esophagus, a premalignant complication of GERD, may be suggested on barium testing as a delicate reticular pattern in the distal esophagus or as a stricture in the mid-esophagus, although endoscopy and histology are still required for diagnosis [12, 13]. GERD may also be suggested by the presence of a "feline esophagus" where transient transverse folds are present in the distal esophagus on barium esophagography (Fig. 4.3a).

The barium esophagram allows for a more accurate diagnosis of esophageal rings and webs, as these can be subtle and overlooked by endoscopy. Esophageal webs may be seen in the cervical esophagus, often occurring anteriorly and are usually eccentric. The esophageal vestibule is bordered superiorly by the muscular "A" ring and inferiorly by the mucosal "B" ring at the squamocolumnar junction (Fig. 4.3b). A Schatzki's ring is a weblike narrowing of the "B" ring that causes dysphagia. The "B" ring is located at the EGJ and is a thin concentric protrusion covered by squamous epithelium proximally and gastric columnar cells distally (Fig. 4.3c). A "C" ring may also be identified, and this denotes a ring formed by diaphragmatic crural pressure. A "ringed" esophagus has been described as multiple circumferential rings occurring most commonly in the mid-esophagus and is associated with eosinophilic esophagitis (Fig. 4.3d) [14].

Identification of the GEJ on the barium swallow is important to diagnose a hiatal hernia. Inspiration while lying prone can accentuate subtle sliding-type hiatal hernias (Fig. 4.3e). The barium swallow can characterize and subtype hiatal hernias. Identification of a shortened esophagus is critical in the preoperative evaluation of patients with GERD as it may alter surgical planning [15, 16]. Esophageal diverticula can also be identified with barium swallows.

In the immediate postoperative exam, water-soluble contrast can be used to assess for leak. Postoperative barium swallows may also be helpful to assess to integrity and position of the fundoplication wrap as well as for recurrent hiatal hernia [17].

Esophageal Manometry

The evaluation of esophageal motility, in a dynamic fashion, was initially only able to be completed with the barium esophagram. With the advent of esophageal pressure monitoring in the 1940s, scientists have had an additional method to clarify and quantify esophageal motility in both health and disease. Catheters, placed transnasally into the stomach, were initially water-perfused and had between four and eight pressure sensors that were spaced apart every few centimeters. Each of these sensors is connected to a transducer and an external data recording device which allows pressure amplitudes to be logged and displayed over time in a continuum along the esophageal body. This technology has been largely replaced by high-resolution esophageal manometry (HRM) which utilizes pressure monitors in a solid-state catheter which are spaced out approximately every 1 cm. (Fig. 4.4). There are numerous brands and configurations, but most esophageal catheters have between 32 and 36 sensors which allow for a more detailed analysis of both the esophageal body and the LES than was previously seen with conventional manometry. The resultant pressure tracings are converted to Clouse plots, termed

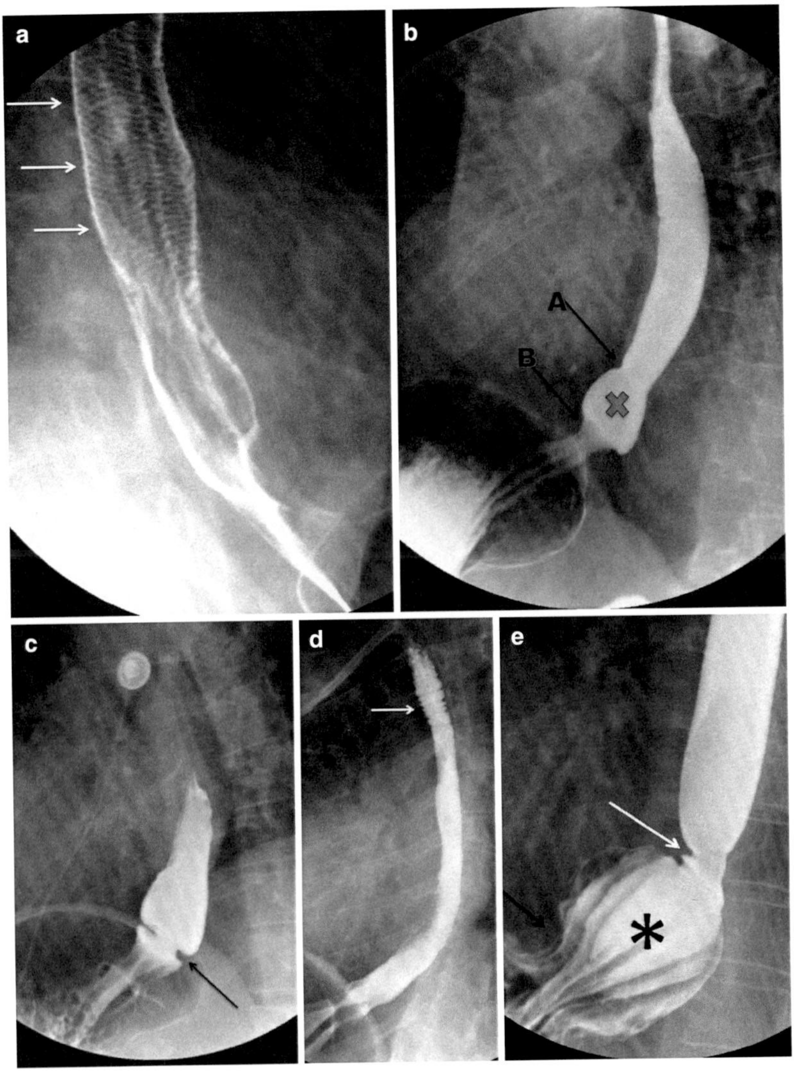

Fig. 4.3 (**a**) Top left, double-contrast barium esophagram demonstrates thin, transient transverse folds in the distal esophagus, consistent with "feline esophagus." This appearance is almost always consistent with gastroesophageal reflux and occurs transiently in response to reflux. (**b**) Top right, GEJ anatomy: right anterior oblique image of a barium filled esophagus in a patient with a normal gastroesophageal junction. "A" designates the muscular A ring. "B" designates the mucosal B ring. "X" designates the esophageal vestibule. (**c**) Bottom left, Schatzki's ring: right anterior oblique image of the gastroesophageal junction in a 42-year-old man with dysphagia. The B ring narrows the gastroesophageal junction to 1 cm and is the cause of the patient's dysphagia. This Schatzki's ring prevented the passage of the barium tablet. (**d**) Bottom center, single-contrast barium esophagram image obtained in the right anterior oblique position in a patient presenting with dysphagia shows a "ringed" appearance of the upper thoracic esophagus *(arrow)* where there is mild narrowing. This was confirmed to represent eosinophilic esophagitis. (**e**) Bottom right, hiatal hernia: this is a 49-year-old woman with history of reflux and increasing dysphagia. A peptic stricture is present at the gastroesophageal junction *(white arrow)*. The patient has a sliding-type hiatal hernia *(black star)*. The hiatus is widened in the patient *(black arrow)*, making her more prone to reflux

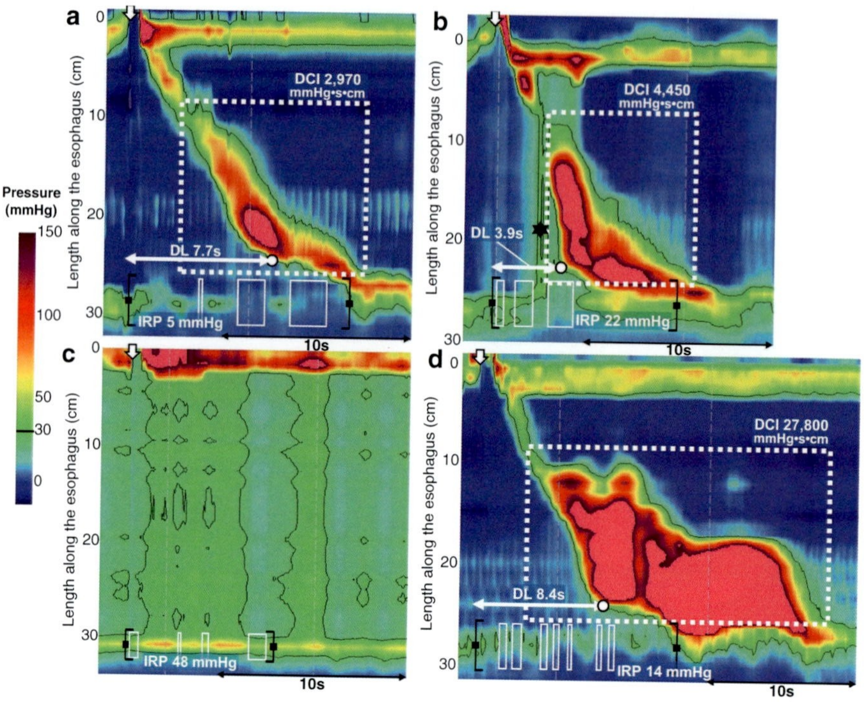

Fig. 4.4 High-resolution esophageal manometry metrics: examples of (**a**) a normal swallow, (**b**) a premature swallow, (**c**) a failed swallow with pan-esophageal pressurization, and (**d**) a hypercontractile swallow are displayed. Swallow onset (relaxation of the UES) is represented by a white arrow. The contraction deceleration point is represented by a white dot. Compartmentalized pressurization (star) can be appreciated in B. DCI, distal contractile integral; DL, distal latency; IRP, integrated relaxation pressure. (From Kahrilas [88])

esophageal pressure topography, which display a vivid representation of pressure amplitude over time and space [18]. The HRM computer software also allows for a virtual sleeve to be created to accurately characterize the LES by grouping 5–6 sensors together in the distal esophagus.

The manometry catheter can be placed transorally but is typically placed transnasally due to patient tolerability. The catheter is passed down the esophagus and positioned across the LES, 2–3 cm into the stomach. The study is typically performed in the supine position, similar to barium esophagography, to reduce the effects of gravity and allow for isolated measurement of esophageal peristalsis and motility. Either before or after the assessment of esophageal peristalsis, baseline characteristics of the esophagus are recorded including basal/resting LES and UES pressures, the presence or absence of a hiatal hernia, and the relationship between the LES and diaphragm. To evaluate peristalsis, the patient is given 5 cc boluses of saline, separated by at least 30 s between swallows to allow for a return of baseline muscle potential. Typical protocols involve the recording and analysis of ten individual swallows. Variations can be performed, including the use of viscous or solid foods instead of saline or using the semi-erect or erect posture depending on patient tolerability of the supine position.

High-resolution manometry testing provides quantifiable, objective measurements which allow for standardized interpretation. The Chicago Classification for Esophageal Motility Disorders, currently in its third edition, is the most widely used classification scheme for defining esophageal motility disorders [19] (see Chapter 32). This system utilizes an approach in which each swallow is analyzed with regard to esophageal body contraction vigor, esophageal contraction pattern, LES relaxation, and the intrabolus pressure pattern (Table 4.1).

The contraction vigor of esophageal peristalsis is measured by a software algorithm of the contraction pressure from the start of the transition zone, where the esophageal muscle composition changes from striated to smooth muscle, to the LES (Clouse segments 2 and 3) [18]. This is termed the distal contractile integral (DCI) and is measured in terms of mmHg × cm × s. Normative values for the DCI and the other definitions listed below have been suggested by the International HRM Working Group and are based on studies primarily performed on the Medtronic (formerly Sierra Scientific) apparatus [19]. Contraction vigor is defined as weak

Table 4.1 Esophageal manometry keywords and measurements

Keyword	Definition	Application
Distal contractile integral (DCI)	The contraction pressure (measured by mmHg × cm × sec) from the start of the transition zone to the LES	Failed contraction (DCI <100) Weak (DCI <450) Normal (DCI 450–8000) Hypercontractile (DCI >8000)
Contractile deceleration point (CDP)	The inflection point where propagation velocity slows as it approaches the LES at the phrenic ampulla	Allows for measurement of distal latency
Distal latency (DL)	The time interval (measured in amplitude × duration × length) between UES relaxation and the peristaltic wave reaching the CDP	Normal >4.5 s Premature contraction is <4.5 s Helps define distal esophageal spasm and type III achalasia
Peristaltic breaks	Gaps in the 20 mmHg isobaric contour of the peristaltic contraction between the UES and EGJ, measured in axial length	Swallow is termed "fragmented" if breaks are present >5 cm in length
Integrated relaxation pressure (IRP)	The average lowest EGJ pressure measured for 4 contiguous or noncontiguous seconds of relaxation in the 10 s window following deglutitive UES relaxation	Normal IRP < 15 mmHg Impaired EGJ relaxation is an IRP >15 mmHg which is a defining characteristic of achalasia
Esophageal pressurization	Intrabolus pressure measurement within the esophagus	Normal: No bolus pressurization >30 mmHg Panpressurization: Uniform pressure > 30 mmHg from UES to EGJ Compartmentalized: pressurization extending from contractile front to EGJ

(DCI <450), failed (DCI <100), hypercontractile (DCI >8000), or normal (DCI 450–8000). Similar metrics have been defined on other platforms [20, 21].

To evaluate for premature contractions, the time interval between UES relaxation and the peristaltic wave reaching the contraction deceleration point (CDP) is measured. The CDP demarcates the inflection point where esophageal peristaltic velocity slows as it approaches the LES at the esophageal vestibule [22, 23]. This time elapse is termed the distal latency (DL), and normal values have been determined for each of the software apparatuses [20, 21, 24]. Swallows with a value less than 4.5 s are considered premature. This metric is primarily used in defining distal esophageal spasm and type III achalasia (see Chapter 31).

When evaluating the LES, the metric used to define appropriate deglutitive EGJ relaxation is called the Integrated Relaxation Pressure or IRP. The IRP, measured in mmHg, is the average lowest pressure in four contiguous or noncontiguous seconds of deglutitive relaxation in the 10-s relaxation window which begins at UES relaxation. This metric is expressed as the median value of the 10 analyzed swallows and is normal if <15 mmHg on the Medtronic apparatus. Impaired LES relaxation is defined as an IRP >15 mmHg (>20 mmHg on Sandhill software), and this is one of the defining characteristics of achalasia.

Breaks in peristalsis, where circular muscle contractions do not occur contiguously, can be seen on esophageal pressure topography. Breaks are considered clinically significant if they are greater than 5 cm in axial length. If present, these swallows are termed fragmented and may be associated with impaired bolus transit [19, 25]. Intrabolus pressurization patterns are also defined by the Chicago Classification [19]. Pressurization within the esophagus greater than 30 mmHg is considered abnormal and is classified into "panpressurization" if this occurs from the UES to the EGJ or "compartmentalized" if this extends from the contractile front to the EGJ.

Each swallow is analyzed individually based on the above parameters, and then the Chicago Classification is applied to determine if a major or minor disorder of peristalsis is present. Also, the presence of a hiatal hernia can be determined as well as characteristics of EGJ morphology. When esophageal manometry is coupled with impedance monitoring, bolus transit abnormalities can also be described.

Assessment of Esophageal Bolus Transit

Clinically, patients with dysphagia will often describe the sensation of food "sticking" or slowing in their neck, chest, or epigastrium. Dysphagia symptoms may also develop after esophageal or gastric surgery. In addition to describing esophageal peristalsis and motor function, assessment of bolus transit through the esophagus may also provide clinically useful information. To describe and quantify this, multiple diagnostic methods have been developed including fluoroscopy, luminal impedance testing, and scintigraphy. Each of these tools has different characteristics which provide insight into transit time, the direction of flow, and potential quantification of bolus retention or reflux.

Fluoroscopy

The barium swallow is the gold standard for assessing esophageal bolus transit. It is useful in evaluation of bolus transit and has been shown to have excellent correlation with impedance monitoring [5]. Bolus transit can be assessed in both the erect and horizontal positions. In addition to assessment of bolus transit of liquid barium, the patient can also be tested with provocative foods coated in barium. In patients with a major motility disorder such as achalasia or scleroderma, a barium esophagram may be useful to assess bolus transit because of the low baseline impedance values [26].

Intraluminal Impedance Testing

Impedance is the effective resistance of an electrical circuit. Intraluminal esophageal impedance testing measures the changes in resistance over time due to the conductance of a substance as it passes through the esophagus [27]. Data is gathered via a catheter which has metal electrodes which are positioned at 3, 5, 7, 9, 15, and 17 cm above the GEJ [27]. Changes in impedance, when measured in a sequential fashion, can determine the direction and time of bolus transit without the use of radiation. Impedance monitoring can detect both air and liquid as these substances change the electrical conductivity along the catheter. The baseline impedance of the esophagus is lowered as liquid-containing boluses pass each sensor due to increased ion conductivity, whereas air has high impedance due to poor conductivity [27]. A decrease in impedance from proximal to distal indicates anterograde bolus transit. On the other hand, a change in impedance moving from the distal to proximal esophagus indicates retrograde transit of a refluxed material. A potential limitation of this technology is that liquid boluses of varying volumes may produce similar amounts of changes in impedance within the esophagus; thus, impedance testing cannot be used to accurately measure the volume of swallowed boluses with currently available software. However, preliminary work has been completed using novel, proprietary software, which may allow quantification of bolus transit with this technology [28].

Intraluminal impedance testing is almost exclusively completed on a multichannel device which allows for esophageal motility testing to be completed simultaneously. As previously described, the catheter is placed transnasally down the esophagus into the stomach. Patients are then asked to complete 10 liquid or 10 viscous swallows with each swallow separated by 30 s. The impedance at each electrode is then measured and recorded to show the path and extent of bolus transit. Viscous solutions are important to include in the impedance evaluation as studies have shown that patients being evaluated for nonobstructive dysphagia with normal liquid manometry could actually have a motility disorder as seen by abnormal bolus transit on viscous impedance testing [29–31]. Esophageal transit is deemed abnormal if more than 30% of liquid or 40% of viscous swallows show incomplete bolus transit [28, 32].

Esophageal emptying, as measured by intraluminal impedance monitoring, has been validated against videofluoroscopy with a 97% concordance rate among healthy individuals [5, 33]. The esophageal impedance integral (EII) and bolus flow time (BFT) are additional metrics being evaluated as surrogates for esophageal emptying [28, 34].

Impedance technology has also been applied to the study of gastroesophageal reflux disease as a way to recognize and identify weakly acidic (pH 4–7) and non-acid (pH >7) reflux, which also may contribute to GERD symptoms [35–38] (see combined pH/impedance monitoring).

Esophageal Scintigraphy

Esophageal scintigraphy was initially developed in 1972 and is designed to evaluate esophageal bolus transit in the workup of GERD and nonspecific motility disorders by providing quantitative data on transit through the entire esophagus or in separate regions. In addition, when the scanning area is widened to include the lungs, scintigraphy can help detect episodes of aspiration [39, 40]. Radionucleotide esophageal testing is noninvasive, has a low radiation burden, and is generally well tolerated by patients. After a period of fasting, patients in the upright or supine position are asked to swallow a 10–15 cc bolus, liquid, or in some cases solid, labeled with Tc-99 m sulfur colloid [41]. The volume of radioactive isotopes is detected by a gamma camera. Data are recorded every 0.1–0.15 s and generate time activity curves showing bolus passage time and time to maximal clearance. Normal transit time of a liquid bolus is approximately 7 s in the upright position and 10 s in the supine position, while normal isotope clearance averages 96 percent in either position [42, 43]. Currently, the use of esophageal scintigraphy is limited and may serve in a complementary role to barium swallows and manometry [44].

Physiologic Esophageal Testing

pH Monitoring

Ambulatory esophageal pH monitoring has allowed for easier, more sensitive, and more specific diagnosis of GERD, especially in patients who have failed an empiric proton pump inhibitor trial or those with atypical symptoms. The Tuttle test in 1958 was the first widely used pH test where a probe was inserted into the patient's esophagus and instantly determined the pH to diagnose GERD [45]. As expected, this test had low sensitivity and specificity so in 1974, Johnson and DeMeester performed 24-h pH testing in hospitalized patients [46]. Their research established normal and abnormal standards for esophageal reflux frequency and duration based on a composite score with six parameters: percentage of total time pH < 4, percentage supine time pH < 4, percentage upright time pH < 4, total number of reflux episodes, number of reflux episodes >5 min, and duration of the longest reflux episode.

Thus with baseline values that could be used for more accurate diagnosis, ambulatory pH testing was established in the 1980s [47]. Since then, advancements have been made to pH monitoring, and there are now two widely used methods: catheter-based monitoring and the wireless pH monitor (Bravo™, Medtronic, Minneapolis, MN) [48, 49]. For both methods, prior to placement of the pH monitor, patients should not eat anything after midnight the night before the test. For those patients on proton pump inhibitor or H2 blocker therapy, medications should be stopped for 7 and 3 days, respectively, prior to the test. In catheter-based pH monitoring, the antimony catheter is advanced through the nasopharynx into the esophagus, which can be facilitated by the patient drinking sips of water. The probe is advanced until the pH reads less than 4, indicating entry into the stomach, and then is pulled back so that it rests 5 cm above the LES. The gold standard for pH probe placement is coordinating with esophageal manometry to locate the LES and then pulling the pH catheter back by 5 cm. Some esophageal catheter probes also have proximal sensors to detect acid reflux that may contribute to laryngeal or upper airway irritation. Additionally, an oropharyngeal catheter-based pH probe, Restech (Respiratory Technology Corporation, Houston, TX), is placed in the posterior oropharynx and measures pH of liquid or aerosolized droplets [50]. During the 24-h monitoring period, patients should perform their normal daily activities while keeping a journal indicating the start and end times of meals, any supine positioning, as well as the onset of any symptoms thought to be reflux related. Another technique, wireless pH monitoring, uses the Bravo™ capsule which contains an antimony pH electrode and measures pH at 6-s intervals [48]. As compared to the catheter approach, wireless pH testing is better tolerated by patients and allows for longer testing (up to 96 h) to capture the day-to-day variance in reflux symptoms [48, 51, 52]. The capsule is placed endoscopically 6 cm above the squamocolumnar junction with attachment to the esophageal wall using a special vacuum pump and then communicates by radio transmitter with an external data logger worn by the patient [48]. Typically, the capsule will fall off by itself within 5 days, though the capsule can detach early from esophageal mucosa and enter the stomach, thus recording the acidic gastric contents resulting in a false-positive study.

During the typical 24- to 48-h pH monitoring period, statistical metrics are often used to quantify the association between a patient's symptoms and reflux using three indices: symptom association probability (SAP), symptom index (SI), and symptom sensitivity index (SSI) (Table 4.2) [53–55]. During pH testing, a reflux episode is defined as a drop in pH below 4 that lasts for at least 10 s. The SI is the percentage of reflux-associated symptom episodes [54]. It is calculated by dividing the number of reflux-related symptom episodes by the total number of symptom episodes × 100 and is considered positive if >50% [54]. This index does have drawbacks however as it does not factor in the total number of reflux events. The SSI is defined as the number of symptom-associated reflux episodes divided by the total number of reflux episodes × 100. It is the percentage of symptom-associated reflux episodes and is considered positive if >10% [55]. This metric also has disadvantages as it does not take the total number of symptom episodes into account. The SAP measurement was created to avoid the shortcomings of the SI and SSI by

Table 4.2 Symptom indices for GERD using pH monitoring

Keyword	Definition	Application
Symptom index (SI)	The percentage of reflux-associated symptom episodes Calculation: (# reflux-related symptom episodes)/(# symptom episodes) × 100	Positive if >50% Does not factor in total # of reflux events
Symptom sensitivity index (SSI)	The percentage of symptom-associated reflux episodes Calculation: (# symptom-associated reflux episodes)/(# reflux episodes)×100	Positive if >10% Does not factor in total # of symptom episodes
Symptom association probability (SAP)	The cross-tabulation statistical analysis using the Fisher's exact test of a contingency table consisting of 4 possible combinations of reflux and symptoms (reflux being present or absent and symptoms being present or absent) compiled from the 24-h data divided into consecutive 2-min segments	Created to avoid the shortcomings of the SI and SSI Result ≥95% is considered statistically significant association, though it cannot definitively imply causality

using cross-tabulation statistical analysis of a contingency table consisting of four possible combinations of reflux and symptoms (reflux being present or absent and symptoms being present or absent) compiled from the 24-hr data divided into consecutive 2-min segments [53]. The Fisher's exact test is then used to calculate the probability that the observed distribution of results could have been the result of chance alone or is statistically significant. A result ≥95% is considered statistically significant association, though it cannot definitively imply causality [56]. The SI, SSI, and SAP are typically used in a complementary fashion as direct comparisons may lead to inaccurate conclusions (Table 4.2).

Ambulatory pH monitoring establishes a temporal correlation between symptoms and episodes of reflux, which may be helpful in cases of atypical symptoms of GERD such as cough. Moreover, pH monitoring can stratify patients on the basis of its severity. More severe GERD, which places patients at higher risk for Barrett's metaplasia or other complications, can be seen during pH testing as more acid reflux in the distal and proximal esophagus and slower acid clearance.

Combined pH and Impedance Monitoring

By combining multichannel intraluminal impedance (MII) monitoring with ambulatory pH monitoring, clinicians can characterize the physical properties of the reflux material. MII-pH monitoring can not only determine whether the reflux is acidic (pH <4), weakly acidic (pH 4–7), or non-acid (pH >7), it can also differentiate between gas, liquid, and mixed (liquid-gas) reflux based on impedance values. Additionally, since impedance testing measures reflux independent of pH, a bolus exposure time (BET) is measured which is akin to acid exposure time in pH testing, but it also includes weakly or non-acid reflux [57]. Impedance monitoring also determines the proximal extent of reflux as there are two impedance channels positioned at 15 and 17 cm above the lower esophageal sphincter. This provides insight into the extent of reflux and may have implications in the management of extraesophageal reflux symptoms. In addition to gastroesophageal reflux disease, MII-pH also has implications in the diagnosis and treatment of other foregut disorders including rumination, aerophagia, supragastric belching, esophageal hypersensitivity, and functional heartburn.

The ability to detect reflux independent of pH helps identify patients with continued symptoms despite PPI therapy. In patients on PPI therapy, the key measurement is the number of acid and non-acid reflux episodes and their relationship with the symptoms using the SI, SSI, or SAP. When patients with persistent symptoms while on acid-suppressive therapy show a positive symptom association between symptoms and reflux, this modality can help the clinician determine if the refractory symptoms are due to uncontrolled acid exposure, ongoing weakly acidic reflux which may denote a hypersensitive esophagus, or if the symptoms are functional in nature. Fundoplication may have a role in the treatment of patients with ongoing reflux and large-volume regurgitation which has been determined to be of weakly or non-acidic in origin as determined by MII-pH testing [56].

Gastric Function and Physiologic Testing

Gastric Emptying

Gastric emptying is frequently assessed in patients with unexplained nausea and/or vomiting, refractory gastroesophageal reflux disease, suspected chronic intestinal pseudo-obstruction, or suspected dumping or stasis syndrome following gastric surgery. Prior to assessing for abnormal gastric emptying, a mechanical obstruction should be excluded with upper endoscopy and/or barium swallow or CT/MRI enterography [58]. In addition, gastric emptying tests can be useful to evaluate response to treatment.

Gastric Scintigraphy Gastric scintigraphy is the most commonly utilized and cost-effective test to evaluate for delayed or rapid gastric emptying. Given the standardization and ease of quantifying gastric retention, scintigraphy has become the gold standard for measuring gastric emptying [58, 59]. A standard test meal is labeled with radioactive isotope, specifically 99mTc for solids and 111 indium for liquids. Ideally, the test meal is standard solid food, usually a low-fat egg-white meal, since liquids will often empty normally from the stomach when solids are abnormally retained and also the fat content of the meal will impact the rate of emptying [60, 61]. Medications that affect gastric emptying should be stopped at least 48 h prior to the test, premenopausal women should have the test done within the first 10 days of their menstrual cycle, and patients with diabetes should have blood glucose checked and hyperglycemia (fasting glucose >275 mg/dL) treated before the test meal is consumed [58]. After an overnight fasting, the patient ingests the meal within 10 min, and preferably while patient is standing, scans are obtained immediately ($t = 0$) and then 1, 2, and 4 h afterward so that the percentage of gastric emptying can be measured. Anterior and posterior images are obtained to help adjust for depth attenuation as solid food migrates from the posterior fundus to the more anterior gastric antrum and to help distinguish isolated fundal or antral dysmotility. The radioactive counts, expressed as a percent of maximal gastric counts at the beginning of the study, are directly proportional to the volume and amount of solid or liquid remaining in the stomach [62]. Sensitivity for delayed gastric emptying increases over a 4-h evaluation, and thus this time duration is typically preferred over a 2-h evaluation. Delayed gastric emptying using the standard low-fat egg meal is defined as greater than 10% retention of gastric contents at 4 h and/or > 60% at 2 h. Rapid gastric emptying is present when less than 35% or the meal is retained at 1 h [63]. Scintigraphy images may sometimes reveal gastroesophageal reflux. Throughout the evaluation process, it is important to realize that the severity of symptoms does not always correlate with the rate of gastric emptying.

Smart Pill Though scintigraphy is widely used for evaluating gastric emptying, another approach in the ambulatory setting is with the wireless motility capsule, known as the SmartPill™(Medtronic, Minneapolis, MN), which was FDA approved in 2006 for evaluation of gastroparesis. In addition to documenting the time required for the capsule to traverse the gastrointestinal tract via gut peristalsis, the SmartPill™ can simultaneously gather information on phasic pressure amplitudes, temperature, and pH [64]. After an overnight fast, the 26.8 × 11.7 mm SmartPill™ capsule is ingested in conjunction with a standard nutrient bar or meal, and the patient then must fast for the following 6 h to allow for accurate measurement. The SmartPill™ can continue to record data for the transit of the entire GI tract over the next 3–5 days in intervals of 20 s during the first 24 h and every 40 s thereafter. During this time, patients record mealtimes, sleep, and bowel movements, all while avoiding strenuous exercise. Gastric emptying time (GET) is defined as the time of the capsule's ingestion to its departure from the stomach [65]. An abrupt change in pH (pH >4 or ≥ 2 pH units from baseline) signifies the transition from the acidic stomach to the alkaline duodenum to calculate the GET. The SmartPill™ capsule will empty from the stomach with the return of phase 3 of the migrating motor complex, which occurs upon complete emptying of solid food from the stomach [64]. A GET of 5 h or less is defined as normal; a GET greater than 5 h is determined delayed gastric emptying [65]. When comparing the GET simultaneously in healthy and symptomatic patients using scintigraphy and the wireless motility capsule, a strong correlation (>0.7) at 4 h exists between the two tests, suggesting that the capsule method can be a useful determination of clinically significant delayed gastric emptying [66, 67].

Gastroduodenal Manometry

Gastroduodenal manometry, a similar technology to esophageal manometry, can be used to assess the coordination and amplitude of contractions spanning the transition from the gastric antrum to the duodenum. Although this technology is primarily limited to quaternary referral centers and research institutions, gastroduodenal manometry may be used to clarify conditions such as intestinal pseudo-obstruction, partial mechanical obstruction, rumination, gastroparesis, and pylorospasm [68–72]. When dysmotility is suspected, gastroduodenal manometry can help differentiate between myopathic and neuropathic etiologies as myopathic conditions will lead to low-amplitude contractions, while neuropathic disorders will be typically associated with normal to increased amplitude but an unorganized contractile response [71]. From a surgical perspective, gastroduodenal manometry may have the most utility in excluding dysmotility as a contributor to a patient's symptoms and thus can have a major impact on the physician's choice of medical or surgical intervention for patients.

To perform the procedure, patients should fast at least 8 h prior to having one of two different types of motility catheters – water-perfused or solid-state – placed either by endoscopic or nasoenteric placement via fluoroscopic guidance. Antroduodenal motility is recorded in the fasting state for 3 h to assess the 3 phases of the migrating motor complexes. Then, the patient is stimulated, either pharmacologically with erythromycin or octreotide or by meal ingestion, and the postprandial amplitude and frequency of contractions are recorded for an additional hour [3, 73]. Solid-state catheters are typically used because of increased sensitivity due to rapid response to pressure events; in addition, they can now measure contractility patterns over a 24-h ambulatory period. However, it is important to note that these ambulatory results can be affected by motion artifact and vomiting since they can mimic abnormal duodenal contraction patterns or cause the catheter to migrate from its original position [3, 74].

Anatomical Tests

Upper Gastrointestinal Examination

The most common indications for an upper GI include epigastric pain, symptoms of gastroesophageal reflux, anemia, and suspected hiatal hernia. A technique combining double- and single-contrast portions is most commonly used. A single-contrast upper GI study may be used in postoperative settings, immobile patients, in patients with food or fluid in the stomach, or gastric distention (gastric outlet obstruction). The patient should be NPO for 4–6 h before the exam.

The exam begins with the patient in the upright left posterior oblique position. The patient drinks a sodium bicarbonate effervescent agent dissolved in 10 cc of water followed by 2 ounces of “thick” barium. Three air-distended views of the esophagus are obtained, and then the patient is quickly put in the horizontal position prior to barium entering the duodenum. The patient is rolled to ensure coating of the stomach, and double-contrast images are obtained of the stomach and duodenum. After the double-contrast portion of the exam is over, the patient is then evaluated using single-contrast technique. Esophageal motility is assessed with the patient drinking “thin” barium in the horizontal right anterior oblique position, but videos are generally not recorded in upper GI exams (as they are in barium swallows). Next, single-contrast images of the stomach and duodenum are obtained using paddle compression of the gastric antrum and duodenum. Final spot images are obtained including the stomach, duodenum, and proximal jejunum. Gastroesophageal reflux may then be assessed using provocative maneuvers as previously described.

The gastric cardia is characterized by a stellate fold pattern radiating to the gastroesophageal junction, also known as the cardiac “rosette” [75]. The gastric fundus is defined as the portion of the stomach cranial to the gastric cardia. The gastric body is the portion of the stomach between the gastric cardia and the bend in the mid-lesser curvatures known as the incisura angularis. The gastric antrum is the portion of the stomach extending distal to the incisura angularis to the pylorus (Fig. 4.5) [76]. The rugal folds are most prominent in the gastric fundus and body and are straighter along the lesser curvature and more undulating on the greater curvature. The mucosal surface of the stomach consists of areae gastricae, which are flat polygonal-shaped tufts of mucosa separated by narrow grooves. Enlarged areae gastricae have been reported in the setting of *Helicobacter pylori* gastritis and small or absent areae gastricae have been seen in patients with atrophic gastritis or pernicious anemia [76]. Other pathology seen within the stomach includes rugal fold thickening, erosions, ulcers, polyps, masses, diverticula, or gastric narrowing.

While the esophagus is evaluated in an upper GI exam, images of the pharynx and entire esophagus are not taken with every upper GI exam. Barium swallows are better for the evaluation of dysphagia, gastroesophageal reflux, and esophageal motility, and upper GI exams are better for the evaluation of epigastric pain. Hiatal hernias can be assessed with either exam.

Endoscopy

The advent of fiber-optic endoscopy in the 1950s by Basil Hirschowitz paved the way for focused intraluminal evaluation of the foregut. The esophagogastroduodenoscopy (EGD) is now one of the most commonly performed procedures during the workup and treatment of foregut disorders. Endoscopy is typically performed under moderate sedation or can be performed with deep sedation or general anesthesia with appropriate anesthesia support and personnel.

From an anatomic standpoint, an EGD allows for complete intraluminal visualization of the esophagus, stomach, and proximal duodenum. In the esophagus, the

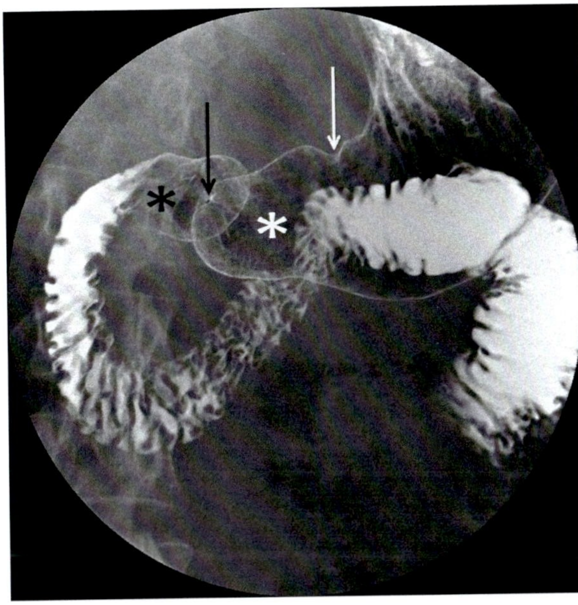

Fig. 4.5 Double-contrast image of the stomach and duodenum. The incisor angularis *(white arrow)* is a bend in the stomach between the lesser curve and antrum *(white star)*. The pylorus is designated by the black arrow and the duodenal bulb by the black star. The normal duodenum has a "C shape" and then extends superiorly to the ligament of Treitz

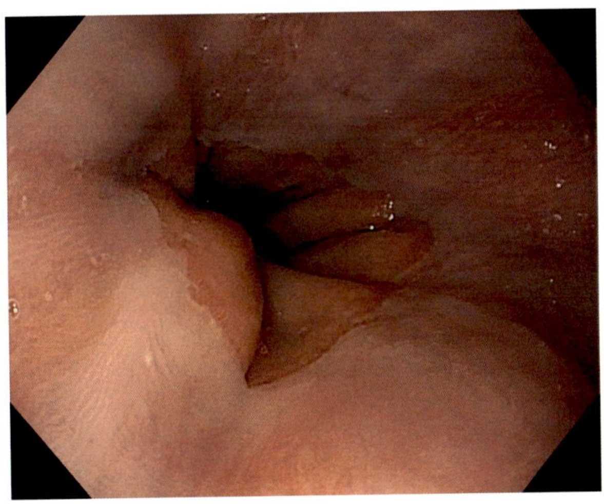

Fig. 4.6 Endoscopic view of the gastroesophageal junction. The white squamous mucosa of the esophagus extends completely to the top of the gastric folds. The GEJ narrows at this level signifying external compression from the diaphragm

presence of complicated gastroesophageal reflux disease can be identified in the form of erosive esophagitis, Barrett's esophagus or stricture. Esophageal tumors, both intraluminal or submucosal, are readily evident on white light endoscopy. The appearance of the GEJ, noted as the transition point between the tubular esophagus and proximal extent of the gastric folds and its relationship to the diaphragmatic hiatus/pinch are easily identifiable (Fig. 4.6). This relationship defines the presence or absence of a hiatal hernia, and retroflexed views of the GEJ/hiatus from within the stomach can help characterize this relationship even further. Classification schemes, including the Hill classification (flap valve), are used to standardize the reporting of the diaphragmatic hiatus on retroflexed views, and the different grades (Hill/flap valve I–IV) have been shown to directly correlate with the presence and amount of reflux (Fig. 4.7) [77]. Standardized descriptions of the hiatus should be routinely used in endoscopy reports as they can help with operative planning. Endoscopy is also useful in the diagnosis of achalasia or pseudoachalasia as the muscular LES, if not relaxing appropriately, can be felt as the endoscope is passed through the GEJ. Additionally, advanced imaging techniques, such as narrowband imaging (NBI), can be used to better clarify mucosal conditions such as Barrett's esophagus by providing visual contrast during routine endoscopy.

In the stomach, inspection is performed of the body, antrum, incisura, and pylorus, and retroflexed views are utilized for the fundus, cardia, and hiatus. With a typical adult gastroscope, the duodenal bulb and the second/third portions of the duodenum are accessible for inspection, and mucosal sampling is easily performed through the working channel of the endoscope in any location if indicated.

Although endoscopy is not the test of choice for the characterization of upper gastrointestinal motility, it can provide useful information. In the absence of a mechanical obstruction, a dilated esophagus may suggest achalasia, and stasis changes in the form of esophagitis, or retained food/liquid may also suggest hypomotility. Tertiary esophageal contractions may also be visualized in spastic motility disorders. In the stomach, antral contractility is visible, and gross motor dysfunction may be suggested by the presence of retained food/liquid or in the form of a gastric bezoar. Pylorospasm may also be suggested on endoscopy, although gastroduodenal manometry is more specific.

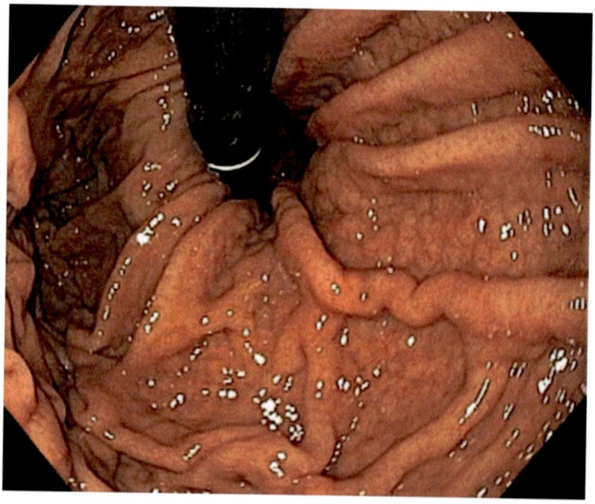

Fig. 4.7 Endoscopic view of an open diaphragmatic hiatus as seen from the retroflexed position. The gastric folds extend cephalad through the hiatus which defines the presence of a hiatal hernia. A muscular ridge is not present. (Hill grade IV flap valve)

Endoscopic Ultrasound

Endoscopic ultrasound (EUS) provides an additional diagnostic dimension to the standard fiber-optic endoscopic evaluation. Performed with an echoendoscope, EUS is indicated in the staging of malignancy for lung, esophageal, GEJ, and gastric malignancies and provides access to structures both within and beyond the luminal wall of the gastrointestinal tract. Submucosal lesions in the esophagus, stomach, and the proximal small bowel can be defined by which layer they originate, and sampling can be performed with fine needle aspiration (FNA). Mediastinal and hilar structures are readily accessible with EUS via the esophagus. When EUS is performed in the stomach and small intestine, the liver, kidneys, adrenal glands, pancreas, biliary tree, and gall bladder as well as adjacent structures (vasculature, lymph nodes, and nerve plexuses) can be characterized based on sonographic features and fine needle aspiration. Although not routinely used in achalasia, EUS can provide additional information regarding the thickness of the inner circular muscles at the level of the LES [78]. In patients with manometrically defined EGJ outflow obstruction, EUS can evaluate for pseudoachalasia or external compression from adjacent structures which may mimic achalasia, although this is infrequently encountered [79].

Emerging Technologies: Functional Luminal Imaging Probe (FLIP)

The functional luminal imaging probe (FLIP) is an FDA-approved device (EndoFLIP, Crospon, Galway, Ireland) which can simultaneously obtain pressure and luminal diameter measurements within the gastrointestinal tract (Fig. 4.8). It is gaining clinical trial data primarily in disorders of the esophagogastric junction, such as achalasia. Applications in the evaluation of esophageal dysmotility and eosinophilic esophagitis are also emerging [80–83]. Commercially available since 2009, the FLIP catheter is positioned across the EGJ, and utilizes high-resolution impedance planimetry sensors housed within a volume-controlled distensible balloon which allows cross-sectional area to be measured. A solid-state pressure transducer is also housed within the apparatus which allows for simultaneous pressure measurements as well as distensibility of the lumen and most notably, the EG junction. Software analysis allows for determination of a distensibility index (DI) which provides complementary diagnostic value preoperatively to high-resolution esophageal manometry, and may have predictive value both intraoperatively and postoperatively as a measure of the effectiveness of myotomy [84–87].

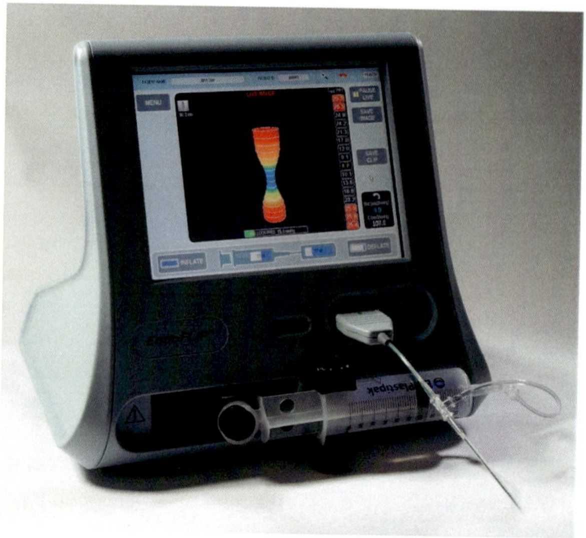

Fig. 4.8 EndoFLIP system (EF-100) with three-dimensional image of the EGJ. (Image courtesy of Crospon, Galway, Ireland)

References

1. de Oliveira JM, et al. Timed barium swallow: a simple technique for evaluating esophageal emptying in patients with achalasia. Am J Roentgenol. 1997;169(2):473–9.
2. Allen BC, Baker ME, Falk GW. Role of barium esophagography in evaluating dysphagia. Cleve Clin J Med. 2009;76(2):105–11.
3. Parkman HP, McCallum RW, Rao SSC. GI motility testing: a laboratory and office handbook. Thorofare, NJ: SLACK; 2011.
4. Massey BT, et al. Abnormal esophageal motility. An analysis of concurrent radiographic and manometric findings. Gastroenterology. 1991;101(2):344–54.
5. Imam H, et al. Bolus transit patterns in healthy subjects: a study using simultaneous impedance monitoring, videoesophagram, and esophageal manometry. Am J Physiol Gastrointest Liver Physiol. 2005;288(5):G1000–6.
6. Kahrilas PJ, Dodds WJ, Hogan WJ. Effect of peristaltic dysfunction on esophageal volume clearance. Gastroenterology. 1988;94(1):73–80.
7. Kahrilas PJ, et al. Comparison of pseudoachalasia and achalasia. Am J Med. 1987;82(3):439–46.
8. Howard PJ, et al. Five year prospective study of the incidence, clinical features, and diagnosis of achalasia in Edinburgh. Gut. 1992;33(8):1011–5.
9. Patti MG, Herbella FA. Achalasia and other esophageal motility disorders. J Gastrointest Surg. 2011;15(5):703–7.
10. Ebert EC. Esophageal disease in scleroderma. J Clin Gastroenterol. 2006;40(9):769–75.
11. Canon CL, et al. Surgical approach to gastroesophageal reflux disease: what the radiologist needs to know. Radiographics. 2005;25(6):1485–99.
12. Baker ME, et al. Gastroesophageal reflux disease: integrating the barium esophagram before and after Antireflux surgery. Radiology. 2007;243(2):329–39.
13. Gore RM, Levine MS. Textbook of gastrointestinal radiology. Philadelphia, PA: Elsevier Health Sciences; 2014.
14. Smith MS. Diagnosis and Management of Esophageal Rings and Webs. Gastroenterol Hepatol. 2010;6(11):701–4.

15. Kahrilas PJ. The role of hiatus hernia in GERD. Yale J Biol Med. 1999;72(2–3):101–11.
16. Kahrilas PJ, Kim HC, Pandolfino JE. Approaches to the diagnosis and grading of hiatal hernia. Best Pract Res Clin Gastroenterol. 2008;22(4):601–16.
17. Jobe BA, et al. Preoperative diagnostic workup before antireflux surgery: an evidence and experience-based consensus of the esophageal diagnostic advisory panel. J Am Coll Surg. 2013;217(4):586–97.
18. Clouse RE, Staiano A, Alrakawi A. Development of a topographic analysis system for manometric studies in the gastrointestinal tract. Gastrointest Endosc. 1998;48(4):395–401.
19. Kahrilas PJ, et al. The Chicago classification of esophageal motility disorders, v3.0. Neurogastroenterol Motil. 2015;27(2):160–74.
20. do Carmo GC, et al. Normal esophageal pressure topography metrics for data derived from the Sandhill-Unisensor high-resolution manometry assembly in supine and sitting positions. Neurogastroenterol Motil. 2015;27(2):285–92.
21. Kessing BF, et al. Water-perfused esophageal high-resolution manometry: normal values and validation. Am J Physiol Gastrointest Liver Physiol. 2014;306(6):G491–5.
22. Pandolfino JE, et al. The contractile deceleration point: an important physiologic landmark on oesophageal pressure topography. Neurogastroenterol Motil. 2010;22(4):395–400. e90
23. Ghosh SK, et al. Quantifying esophageal peristalsis with high-resolution manometry: a study of 75 asymptomatic volunteers. Am J Physiol Gastrointest Liver Physiol. 2006;290(5):G988–97.
24. Roman S, et al. Distal contraction latency: a measure of propagation velocity optimized for esophageal pressure topography studies. Am J Gastroenterol. 2011;106(3):443–51.
25. Li YW, et al. Motility characteristics in the transition zone in Gastroesophageal Reflux Disease (GORD) patients. BMC Gastroenterol. 2016;16:106.
26. Cho YK, et al. Comparison of bolus transit patterns identified by esophageal impedance to barium esophagram in patients with dysphagia. Dis Esophagus. 2012;25(1):17–25.
27. Silny J. Intraluminal multiple electric impedance procedure for measurement of gastrointestinal motility. Neurogastroenterol Motil. 1991;3(3):151–62.
28. Lin Z, et al. Parameters for quantifying bolus retention with high-resolution impedance manometry. Neurogastroenterol Motil. 2014;26(7):929–36.
29. Clayton SB, et al. Viscous impedance is an important indicator of abnormal esophageal motility. Neurogastroenterol Motil. 2013;25(7):563–e455.
30. Blonski W, et al. Impedance manometry with viscous test solution increases detection of esophageal function defects compared to liquid swallows. Scand J Gastroenterol. 2007;42(8):917–22.
31. Chen CL, Yi CH. Clinical correlates of dysphagia to oesophageal dysmotility: studies using combined manometry and impedance. Neurogastroenterol Motil. 2008;20(6):611–7.
32. Tutuian R, et al. Esophageal function testing with combined multichannel intraluminal impedance and manometry: multicenter study in healthy volunteers. Clin Gastroenterol Hepatol. 2003;1(3):174–82.
33. Simren M, et al. Relevance of ineffective oesophageal motility during oesophageal acid clearance. Gut. 2003;52(6):784–90.
34. Carlson DA, et al. High-resolution impedance manometry parameters enhance the esophageal motility evaluation in non-obstructive dysphagia patients without a major Chicago Classification motility disorder. Neurogastroenterol Motil. 2017;29(3).
35. Hila A, Agrawal A, Castell DO. Combined multichannel intraluminal impedance and pH esophageal testing compared to pH alone for diagnosing both acid and weakly acidic gastroesophageal reflux. Clin Gastroenterol Hepatol. 2007;5(2):172–7.
36. Mainie I, et al. Acid and non-acid reflux in patients with persistent symptoms despite acid suppressive therapy: a multicentre study using combined ambulatory impedance-pH monitoring. Gut. 2006;55(10):1398–402.
37. Vela MF, et al. Simultaneous intraesophageal impedance and pH measurement of acid and non-acid gastroesophageal reflux: effect of omeprazole. Gastroenterology. 2001;120(7):1599–606.
38. Boeckxstaens GE, Smout A. Systematic review: role of acid, weakly acidic and weakly alkaline reflux in gastro-oesophageal reflux disease. Aliment Pharmacol Ther. 2010;32(3):334–43.
39. Velasco N, et al. Measurement of esophageal reflux by scintigraphy. Dig Dis Sci. 1984;29(11):977–82.

40. Ferguson MK, et al. Esophageal emptying and acid neutralization in patients with symptoms of esophageal reflux. Ann Surg. 1985;201(6):728–35.
41. Taillefer R, et al. Nuclear medicine and esophageal surgery. Clin Nucl Med. 1986;11(6):445–60.
42. Tolin RD, et al. Esophageal scintigraphy to quantitate esophageal transit (quantitation of esophageal transit). Gastroenterology. 1979;76(6):1402–8.
43. Mariani G, et al. Radionuclide gastroesophageal motor studies. J Nucl Med. 2004;45(6):1004–28.
44. Maurer AH. Gastrointestinal motility, part 1: esophageal transit and gastric emptying. J Nucl Med. 2015;56(8):1229–38.
45. Tuttle SG, Grossman MI. Detection of gastro-esophageal reflux by simultaneous measurement of intraluminal pressure and pH. Proc Soc Exp Biol Med. 1958;98(2):225–7.
46. Johnson LF, Demeester TR. Twenty-four-hour pH monitoring of the distal esophagus. Am J Gastroenterol. 1974;62(4):325–32.
47. Falor W, et al. Outpatient 24 hour esophageal pH monitoring by telemetry. In: Gastroenterology. Philadelphia, PA: WB Saunders Co Independence Square West Curtis Center, Ste 300; 1980. p. 19106–3399.
48. Pandolfino JE, et al. Ambulatory esophageal pH monitoring using a wireless system. Am J Gastroenterol. 2003;98(4):740–9.
49. Hirano I, Richter JE. ACG practice guidelines: esophageal reflux testing. Am J Gastroenterol. 2007;102(3):668–85.
50. Ayazi S, et al. A new technique for measurement of pharyngeal pH: normal values and discriminating pH threshold. J Gastrointest Surg. 2009;13(8):1422–9.
51. Sweis R, et al. Patient acceptance and clinical impact of Bravo monitoring in patients with previous failed catheter-based studies. Aliment Pharmacol Ther. 2009;29(6):669–76.
52. Wong WM, et al. Feasibility and tolerability of transnasal/per-oral placement of the wireless pH capsule vs. traditional 24-h oesophageal pH monitoring--a randomized trial. Aliment Pharmacol Ther. 2005;21(2):155–63.
53. Weusten BL, et al. The symptom-association probability: an improved method for symptom analysis of 24-hour esophageal pH data. Gastroenterology. 1994;107(6):1741–5.
54. Wiener GJ, et al. The symptom index: a clinically important parameter of ambulatory 24-hour esophageal pH monitoring. Am J Gastroenterol. 1988;83(4):358–61.
55. Breumelhof R, Smout AJ. The symptom sensitivity index: a valuable additional parameter in 24-hour esophageal pH recording. Am J Gastroenterol. 1991;86(2):160–4.
56. Bredenoord AJ, Weusten BLAM, Smout AJPM. Symptom association analysis in ambulatory gastro-oesophageal reflux monitoring. Gut. 2005;54(12):1810–7.
57. Shay S, et al. Twenty-four hour ambulatory simultaneous impedance and pH monitoring: a multicenter report of normal values from 60 healthy volunteers. Am J Gastroenterol. 2004;99(6):1037–43.
58. Camilleri M, et al. Clinical guideline: management of gastroparesis. Am J Gastroenterol. 2013;108(1):18–37. quiz 38
59. Camilleri M, Shin A. Novel and validated approaches for gastric emptying scintigraphy in patients with suspected gastroparesis. Dig Dis Sci. 2013;58(7):1813–5.
60. Tougas G, et al. Assessment of gastric emptying using a low fat meal: establishment of international control values. Am J Gastroenterol. 2000;95(6):1456–62.
61. Abell TL, et al. Consensus recommendations for gastric emptying scintigraphy: a joint report of the American Neurogastroenterology and Motility Society and the Society of Nuclear Medicine. J Nucl Med Technol. 2008;36(1):44–54.
62. Parkman HP, Hasler WL, Fisher RS. American Gastroenterological Association technical review on the diagnosis and treatment of gastroparesis. Gastroenterology. 2004;127(5):1592–622.
63. Camilleri M, et al. Performance characteristics of scintigraphic measurement of gastric emptying of solids in healthy participants. Neurogastroenterol Motil. 2012;24(12):1076–e562.
64. Cassilly D, et al. Gastric emptying of a non-digestible solid: assessment with simultaneous SmartPill pH and pressure capsule, antroduodenal manometry, gastric emptying scintigraphy. Neurogastroenterol Motil. 2008;20(4):311–9.
65. Saad RJ, Hasler WL. A technical review and clinical assessment of the wireless motility capsule. Gastroenterol Hepatol (NY). 2011;7(12):795–804.

66. Kuo B, et al. Comparison of gastric emptying of a nondigestible capsule to a radio-labelled meal in healthy and gastroparetic subjects. Aliment Pharmacol Ther. 2008;27(2):186–96.
67. Tran K, Brun R, Kuo B. Evaluation of regional and whole gut motility using the wireless motility capsule: relevance in clinical practice. Ther Adv Gastroenterol. 2012;5(4):249–60.
68. Absah I, et al. Rumination syndrome: pathophysiology, diagnosis, and treatment. Neurogastroenterol Motil. 2017;29(4)
69. Mearin F, Camilleri M, Malagelada JR. Pyloric dysfunction in diabetics with recurrent nausea and vomiting. Gastroenterology. 1986;90(6):1919–25.
70. Camilleri M, Brown ML, Malagelada JR. Relationship between impaired gastric emptying and abnormal gastrointestinal motility. Gastroenterology. 1986;91(1):94–9.
71. Stanghellini V, Camilleri M, Malagelada JR. Chronic idiopathic intestinal pseudo-obstruction: clinical and intestinal manometric findings. Gut. 1987;28(1):5–12.
72. Frank JW, Sarr MG, Camilleri M. Use of gastroduodenal manometry to differentiate mechanical and functional intestinal obstruction: an analysis of clinical outcome. Am J Gastroenterol. 1994;89(3):339–44.
73. Camilleri M, et al. Measurement of gastrointestinal motility in the GI laboratory. Gastroenterology. 1998;115(3):747–62.
74. Nguyen LPS, Snape WJ Jr. Utility of antroduodenal manometry in clinical practice. Gastroenterology. 2003;128:A-675.
75. Freeny PC. Double-contrast gastrography of the fundus and cardia: normal landmarks and their pathologic changes. AJR Am J Roentgenol. 1979;133(3):481–7.
76. Rubesin SE, Levine MS, Laufer I. Double-contrast upper gastrointestinal radiography: a pattern approach for diseases of the stomach. Radiology. 2008;246(1):33–48.
77. Hill LD, et al. The gastroesophageal flap valve: in vitro and in vivo observations. Gastrointest Endosc. 1996;44(5):541–7.
78. Minami H, et al. Clinical application of endoscopic ultrasonography for esophageal achalasia. Dig Endosc. 2015;27(Suppl 1):11–6.
79. Okeke FC, et al. What is the clinical significance of esophagogastric junction outflow obstruction? evaluation of 60 patients at a tertiary referral center. Neurogastroenterol Motil. 2017;(6):29.
80. Carlson DA, et al. Evaluation of esophageal motility utilizing the functional lumen imaging probe. Am J Gastroenterol. 2016;111(12):1726–35.
81. Carlson DA, et al. Evaluation of esophageal distensibility in eosinophilic esophagitis: an update and comparison of functional lumen imaging probe analytic methods. Neurogastroenterol Motil. 2016;28(12):1844–53.
82. McMahon BP, et al. The functional lumen imaging probe (FLIP) for evaluation of the esophagogastric junction. Am J Physiol Gastrointest Liver Physiol. 2007;292(1):G377–84.
83. Pandolfino JE, et al. Distensibility of the esophagogastric junction assessed with the functional lumen imaging probe (FLIP) in achalasia patients. Neurogastroenterol Motil. 2013;25(6):496–501.
84. Rieder E, et al. Intraoperative assessment of esophagogastric junction distensibility during per oral endoscopic myotomy (POEM) for esophageal motility disorders. Surg Endosc. 2013;27(2):400–5.
85. Teitelbaum EN, et al. Comparison of esophagogastric junction distensibility changes during POEM and Heller myotomy using intraoperative FLIP. Surg Endosc. 2013;27(12):4547–55.
86. Teitelbaum EN, et al. An extended proximal esophageal myotomy is necessary to normalize EGJ distensibility during Heller myotomy for achalasia, but not POEM. Surg Endosc. 2014;28(10):2840–7.
87. Teitelbaum EN, et al. The effect of incremental distal gastric myotomy lengths on EGJ distensibility during POEM for achalasia. Surg Endosc. 2016;30(2):745–50.
88. Kahrilas P. How to Effectively Use High-Resolution Esophageal Manometry. Gastroenterology. 2016;151:789–92.

The History of Hiatal Hernia and Antireflux Surgery

5

Thadeus L. Trus

The history of diaphragmatic hernias dates back as far as the sixteenth century. Interestingly, hiatal hernia was thought to be clinically irrelevant. The link between hiatal hernia and gastroesophageal reflux did not warrant any attention until the mid-twentieth century. This understanding seemed to be biphasic; the first being in the 1950s and the second in the era of laparoscopic surgery where visualization of the hiatus was unprecedented. The revitalization of laparoscopic fundoplication spurred a resurgence of interest and research in the pathophysiology of reflux disease. This chapter will outline the evolution of hiatal hernia and antireflux surgery from thoracic to abdominal to laparoscopic and endoscopic approaches.

There are numerous descriptions of diaphragmatic defects, both congenital and posttraumatic. The earliest reports date back to 1579 (Ambroise Pare). Perhaps the most well known of these congenital defects still carry the names of those who first described them in the eighteenth and nineteenth centuries. Anterior diaphragmatic, Morgagni, hernia was first described by Giovanni Battista Morgagni in 1761. Posterior diaphragmatic, Bochdalek, hernia was first described by Vincent Alexander Bochdalek in 1848. It is possible that little attention was paid to hiatal hernias due to the autopsy practice at the time where the esophagus was sectioned en bloc with the thoracic organs above the diaphragm [1].

There were several references to herniation through natural apertures in the diaphragm, but they were sporadic and still thought to be posttraumatic or variants of malformations. It was not until 1853 that Henry Ingersoll Bowditch published a comprehensive review of all published cases of diaphragmatic hernia from 1610 to 1846 [2]. Within this series were three cases which intrigued Bowditch and, by descriptions, were most likely true paraesophageal hernias (type II hiatal hernia). The advent of radiography in the late 1800s allowed the study of swallowing, and in 1904, H. Eppinger successfully radiographically confirmed a hiatal hernia in a

T. L. Trus
Geisel School of Medicine, Dartmouth Hitchcock Medical Center, Lebanon, NH, USA
e-mail: thadeus.trus@hitchcock.org

J. Grams et al. (eds.), *The SAGES Manual of Foregut Surgery*,
https://doi.org/10.1007/978-3-319-96122-4_5

patient he suspected had hiatal herniation based on auscultation [3]. Eppinger's review of the literature in 1911 in which he described 11 herniations through the esophageal hiatus out of 635 cases is frequently cited as the first published description of hiatal hernias in a series [4]. Akerlund introduced the term "hiatus hernia" in 1926 and quite eloquently described an early classification of the types of hiatal hernia as well as associated symptoms of heartburn and dysphagia [5].

The association of gastroesophageal reflux and esophagitis was described in the early 1800s. Several published reports throughout the 1800s speculated the cause of esophagitis to be reflux of gastric contents [6–8]. The association was controversial since many, including Friedrich Albert Zenker, thought gastric reflux into the esophagus was clinically irrelevant [9]. The early twentieth century saw a growth of publications describing both symptoms and clinical findings of reflux esophagitis [10–12]. In 1935, peptic esophagitis was introduced as a new clinical entity in the literature [13].

Early reports of surgery for hiatal hernia focused on closure of the hiatus and restoration of the stomach below the diaphragm with little focus on the lower esophageal sphincter. In fact, the symptoms were felt to be secondary to the presence of the hernia [14]. The phrenic nerve was even divided to facilitate difficult closures! [15]. It was not until the 1950s that the hiatal hernia was implicated as a contributor to the development of reflux by altered hiatal anatomy.

Two earlier pioneers of antireflux surgery focused on the correction of two different anatomic aspects of the hiatal region. Philip Allison postulated that hiatal hernias resulted in the loss of the crural pinch of the lower esophagus which in turn led to symptoms of heartburn and indigestion [16]. He emphasized the reduction of the herniated stomach, fixation of the phrenoesophageal ligaments to the diaphragm, and closure of the crura. Norman Barrett felt the key to repair rested with the restoration of the cardioesophageal or "esophagogastric" angle which would augment the function of an antireflux flapper valve at the gastroesophageal junction [17]. The early work of these two individuals led to the development of a variety of gastropexy operations most of which were abandoned due to high recurrence rates.

Ronald Belsey embarked on a long journey of endoscopic observation and surgical trials to perfect his antireflux operation. Through endoscopic observations starting in the 1940s, Belsey concluded that the key to success was reduction of the cardia below the diaphragm and adequate esophageal length (hence the thoracic approach) to maintain a proper cardioesophageal angle below the diaphragm without tension. He evolved his procedure from a Belsey Mark I, very similar to Allison's initial procedure, to a Belsey Mark IV. His meticulous study and follow-up led to a publication with Skinner in 1967 of long-term follow-up of over 1000 patients with 85% successful reflux control. Their paper remains a hallmark publication in reflux surgery [18].

This same year, Lucius Hill published his experience with a procedure he developed after extensive study of manometry, pH, and anatomy of the gastroesophageal junction [19]. Hill's repair focused on restoration of the angle of His by anchoring the phrenoesophageal bundles to the median arcuate ligament. The Hill repair is essentially the only gastropexy procedure that has withstood the test of time. Hill's other contributions to antireflux surgery include the use of intraoperative manometry and a grading system of the antireflux "flap valve" that is still used to this day [20].

Arguably the most well-known name associated with antireflux surgery is Rudolph Nissen. Nissen, like many of his contemporaries in the mid-1940s, approached problematic diaphragmatic hernia repair through a transthoracic approach. In 1946 the famous American radiologist, Gustav Bucky, developed an incarcerated paraesophageal hernia. Due to Bucky's frail health, Nissen approached the repair transabdominally thus avoiding the riskier thoracotomy. He managed to safely reduce the hernia and fix the stomach to the anterior abdominal wall. The patient recovered and remained symptom free for over 15 years. This transabdominal "gastropexy" became a common procedure for hiatal hernias [21]. Longer follow-up of these patients however showed a high recurrence rate.

In the mid-1930s, Nissen encountered a patient with a distal esophageal ulcer penetrating into the pericardium. He resected the distal esophagus and cardia and anastomosed the esophagus to the proximal gastric body. To protect the anastomosis, Nissen wrapped the anastomosed area with the body of the stomach using a Witzel technique [22] (Fig. 5.1). He later learned that the patient remained well and free from reflux 15 years after the original procedure. Faced with the frustrating recurrence rate of gastropexy, Nissen combined the two procedures in 1955 on a patient

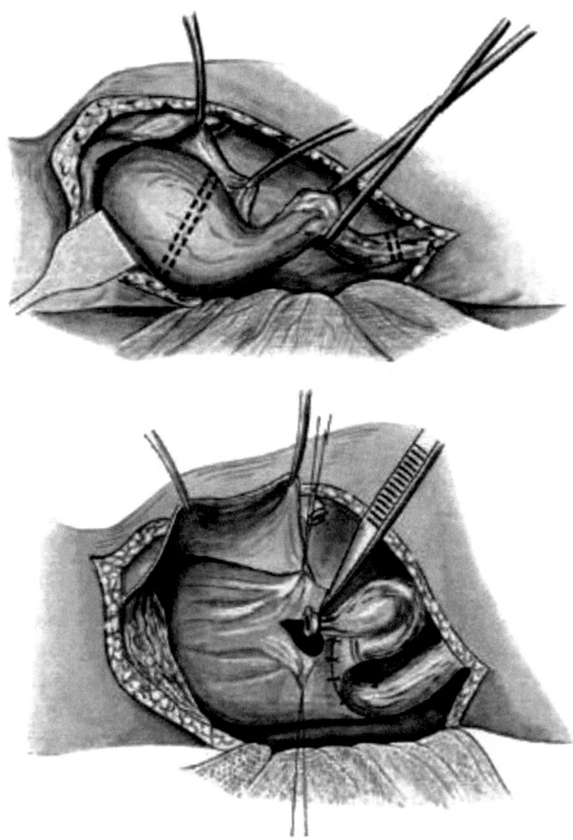

Fig. 5.1 Nissen [22]

with severe reflux disease and no hiatal hernia. He essentially performed a division of the phrenoesophageal ligament, mobilized the fundus behind the esophagus, and plicated the fundus to itself around the esophagus using 4 or 5 sutures for a length of 6 cm. After duplicating the excellent result in a second patient, he published his experience with "gastroplication" [23] (Fig. 5.2).

Nissen fundoplication quickly became the standard operation for gastroesophageal reflux. Dramatic improvements in lower esophageal sphincter competence were achieved by utilizing the anterior wall of the fundus to create the fundoplication. This development was achieved after extensive study by Mario Rossetti, Nissen's well-known understudy and collaborator [24]. Other investigators suggested partial fundoplication to avoid problematic dysphagia, specifically Dor (anterior partial fundoplication) and Toupet (posterior fundoplication) [25, 26]. Demeester and Johnson populated the literature with extensive pH and manometry evaluations of various iterations of fundoplication and concluded that a short, loose fundoplication provides the ultimate reflux control [27, 28]. Despite this body of data, many surgeons continued to create fundoplications which were too long and too tight causing the procedure to decline in popularity due to higher-than-expected complication rates.

The development of laparoscopic surgery rekindled the popularity of Nissen's fundoplication. The first description of laparoscopic fundoplication was by Bernard Dallemagne in 1991 [29]. North American laparoscopic pioneers quickly adopted this procedure, studied it extensively, and advocated again for short, loose floppy fundoplication as the key to successful, durable antireflux control with low complication rates. Hunter, Swanstrom, Demeester, and others were instrumental in perfecting safe reliable fundoplications.

Although the availability of proton pump inhibitors has led to fewer fundoplications, the interest in antireflux surgery remains strong. Endoscopic therapies have been numerous, but most have come and gone either due to ineffectiveness, poor reimbursement, or unacceptable complications. Few still exist but are not as popular as surgery. New procedures have also emerged such as magnetic sphincter

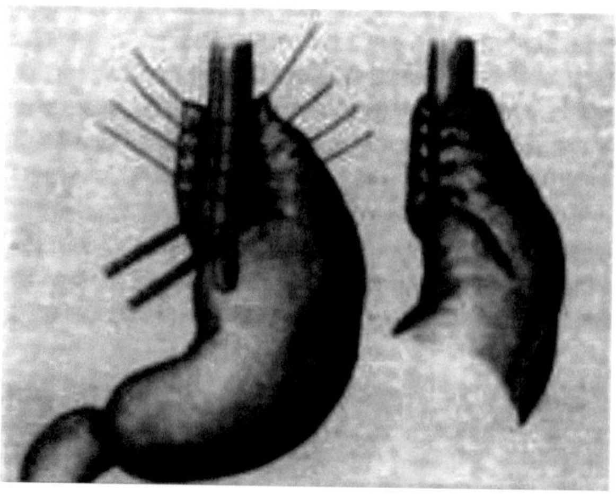

Fig. 5.2 Nissen [23]

augmentation which show great promise in the early stages. The early forges of antireflux surgery have set the example of meticulous study and attention to detail to improve the procedures. Hopefully future antireflux technology investigators will follow the practice of these pioneers.

References

1. Stylopoulos N, Rattner DW. The history of hiatal hernia surgery from Bowditch to laparoscopy. Ann Surg. 2005;241(1):185–93.
2. Bowditch HI. A treatise on diaphragmatic hernia. Buffalo: Jewett Thomas; 1853.
3. Schwarz GS. Historical aspects of the anatomy of the cardia with special reference to hiatus hernia. Bull NY Acad Med. 1967;43:112–25.
4. Eppinger H. Allgemeine und spezielle pathologie des Zwerchfells. In: Frankl-Hochwart L, editor. Supplemente zu H. Nothnagel, Spezielle Pathologie und Therapie. Wein: Holder; 1911.
5. Akerlund A, Onnell H, Key E. Hernia diaphragmatica hiatus oesophagei vom anastomischen und roentgenologischen gesichtspunkt. Acta Radiol. 1926;6:3–22.
6. Billard CM. Traite des Maladies des Enfans Nouveaux-Nes et a la Mamelle: Fonde sur de Nouvelles Observations Cliniques et d'Anatomie Pathologique, faites a l'Hopital des Enfans-Trouves de Paris, dans le Service de M. Baron. Paris: JB Bailliere; 1828.
7. Rìíokitansky C. Referenced by Nissen R. In: Fundoplication und Gastropexie Bei Refiuxkrankheit und Hiatushernie. New York: G Thieme Verlag Stuggart; 1981.
8. Quincke H. Esophageal ulcers from digestive juice (ulcus oesophagi ex digestione). Dtsch Arch Klin Med. 1879;24:72.
9. Zenker FA von Ziemsen H. Diseases of the esophagus. In: Cyclopedia of the practice of medicine, vol. 8. New York: William Wood; 1878. p. 1–214.
10. Vinson PP. Oesophageal stricture following the vomiting of pregnancy. Surg Gynecol Obstet. 1921;33:412.
11. Tileston W. Peptic ulcer of the oesophagus. Am J Med Sci. 1906;132:240–65.
12. Sheehan JE. Ulcer of the esophagus from the standpoint of an endoscopist. Med Rec. 1920;97:319.
13. Winkelstein A. Peptic esophagitis: a new clinical entity. JAMA. 1935;104:906.
14. Soresi AL. Diaphragmatic hernia: its unsuspected frequency: diagnosis and technique for radical cure. Ann Surg. 1919;69:254–70.
15. Harrington SW. The surgical treatment of the more common types of diaphragmatic hernia: esophageal hiatus, traumatic, pleuroperitoneal hiatus, congenital absence and foramen of Morgagni: report of 404 cases. Ann Surg. 1945;122:546–68.
16. Allison PR. Reflux esophagitis, sliding hiatal hernia and anatomy of repair. Surg Gynecol Obstet. 1951;92:419–31.
17. Barrett NR. Hiatus hernia. Br J Surg. 1954;42:231–43.
18. Skinner DB, Belsey RH. Surgical management of esophageal reflux and hiatus hernia; long-term results with 1030 patients. J Thorac Cardiovasc Surg. 1967;53:33–54.
19. Hill LD. An effective operation for hiatal hernia: an eight year appraisal. Ann Surg. 1967;166:681–92.
20. Hill LD, Kozarek RA, Kraemer SJ, et al. The gastroesophageal flap valve: in vitro and in vivo observations. Gastrointest Endosc. 1996;44:541–7.
21. Nissen R. Gastropexy as the lone procedure in the surgical repair of hiatus hernia. Am J Surg. 1956;92:389–92.
22. Nissen R. Die transpleurale Reseftion der Kardia. Dtsch Z Chir. 1937;249:311–6.
23. Nissen R. Eine einfache Operation zur Beeinflusung der Refluxeosophagitis. Schweiz Med Wochenschr. 1956;86:590–2.

24. Rossetti ME, Liebermann-Meffert DMI. Nissen-Rossetti Antireflux Fundoplication (open Procedure). In: Baker RJ, Fischer JE, editors. Mastery of surgery. 4th ed. Philadelphia: Lippincott Williams & Wilkins; 2001. p. 764–76.
25. Dor J, Humbert P, Dor V, et al. The role of the modified Nissen cardiomyotomy. Mem Acad Chir. 1962;88:877–82.
26. Toupet A. Technique d'eosophago-gastroplastie avec phreno-gastropexie dan la cure radicales des hernies hiatales et comme complement de l'operation de Heller dans les cardiospsmes. Mem Acad Chir. 1963;89:394–9.
27. DeMeester TR, Johnson LF. Evaluation of Nissen antireflux procedure by esophageal manometry and 24 hour pH monitoring. Am J Surg. 1975;129:94–100.
28. DeMeester TR, Bonavina L, Albertucci M. Nissen fundoplication for gastroesophageal reflux disease: evaluation of primary repair in 100 consecutive patients. Ann Surg. 1986;204:9–20.
29. Dallemagne b WJM. Jehaes C, et al. Surg Laparosc Endosc Percutan Tech. 1991;1:138–43.

Evaluation of GERD: Symptoms and Disease Classification

6

Amber Shada

Gastroesophageal reflux, or retrograde movement of gastric contents across the lower esophageal sphincter (LES), is relatively common, seen in almost two-thirds of adults in the United States [4]. It is physiologically normal and in fact occurs several times each day in normal healthy individuals. Whenever the pressure gradient between stomach and esophagus is high enough to overcome the LES pressure, retrograde movement of gastric contents will occur. Typically this occurs in the form of a transient lower esophageal sphincter relaxation (TLESR) [2]. This is caused by shortening of the LES during gastric distension, as commonly happens after meals [12]. In most individuals, TLESRs are often brief and asymptomatic. In some cases, TLESRs can be more frequent, longer lasting, or more acidic, allowing excessive exposure of the esophageal mucosa to gastric acid [8]. Over time, this can lead to failure of the LES and symptomatic gastroesophageal reflux. The esophagus, upon receipt of acidic refluxate, will attempt to clear contents back toward the stomach with peristaltic activity. However, the effectiveness of this is variable depending upon underlying esophageal function. Gastroesophageal reflux disease, over time, can cause ineffective motility of the esophagus, in turn worsening the effect of reflux on the esophageal mucosa.

The typical symptoms of gastroesophageal reflux are heartburn and regurgitation. Heartburn is defined as a burning sensation in the retrosternal area [11]. Heartburn is caused when acids enter the squamous epithelium of the distal esophagus and stimulate nerve endings, producing a sensation of pain. In comparison, the columnar epithelium of the stomach is impervious to damage by acid. Regurgitation is defined as the perception of flow of refluxed gastric content (including acid) into the mouth or hypopharynx [11]. This results from either TLESRs or permanent damage to the lower esophageal sphincter causing complete failure of the LES to

A. Shada
Department of Surgery, University of Wisconsin, Madison, WI, USA
e-mail: shada@surgery.wisc.edu

J. Grams et al. (eds.), *The SAGES Manual of Foregut Surgery*,
https://doi.org/10.1007/978-3-319-96122-4_6

close. Regurgitation can be severe, with full column regurgitation of acidic gastric content and/or food.

Reflux can be seen in the presence of a normal LES that has transient lower esophageal sphincter relaxations. If an increased number of episodes occur, TLESRs can lead to microscopic changes to the LES. This can lead to destruction of the LES and worsening reflux or GERD.

There are also a number of atypical reflux symptoms. These are often accompanied by typical symptoms of GERD but are sometimes isolated. These include pulmonary symptoms such as chronic sore throat, cough, hoarseness, and asthma [3]. Dysphagia can also be an atypical symptom of GERD but does need further workup because dysphagia suggests possible underlying esophageal motility disorder or cancer. Dental erosions have been found to be associated with GERD as well [7]. Many patients with atypical GERD present initially to otolaryngologists, dentists, and allergists and may not see a surgeon until their symptoms become quite severe. It is important to keep GERD in the differential for patients that present with these atypical symptoms.

Despite this, it is important to realize that GERD is not a typical sole cause of these diseases but rather is often found to exacerbate them [11]. Patients can have a constellation of typical and atypical reflux symptoms, with no appreciable esophageal damage present. Gastroesophageal reflux disease (GERD) is the term used for reflux symptoms causing esophageal damage [11]. GERD can also be used to classify symptoms severe enough to impact quality of life.

Disease Classification

There are two types of epithelium in the upper digestive tract: squamous epithelium of the esophagus and columnar or oxyntic epithelium of the stomach. The latter is not damaged by acidic gastric contents. The squamous epithelium of the esophagus is damaged when exposed to pathologically high levels of acid.

This damage can manifest in a variety of ways. One result of chronic acid exposure is esophagitis. Esophagitis can be diagnosed with EGD and biopsy, although the characteristic findings of esophagitis (widened intracellular spaces, basal cell hyperplasia, intraepithelial eosinophils) are not specific to reflux esophagitis. Furthermore, the absence of these histologic changes does not rule out the presence of GERD. Thus, the diagnosis of GERD must be made in concert with clinical symptoms.

Esophagitis is classified as either erosive esophagitis or nonerosive esophagitis. Erosive esophagitis causes significant full-thickness mucosal damage of the esophagus, which can lead to ulcer formation. Ulcerations are visible on EGD, and the Los Angeles classification system is useful to determine the severity of esophagitis. The healing of these ulcers can in turn lead to stricture formation in the distal esophagus.

Erosive esophagitis is the most common macroscopic abnormality seen during EGD in patients with GERD. Despite that, it is still only seen in a minority of patients. On EGD, it is seen as a break in the mucosa. This can be either superficial (erosions) or full thickness (ulcerations). When it is full-thickness damage to the mucosa, it leads to more complications (strictures and ulcers) and an increased likelihood of disease that is refractory to medical management. As these areas cyclically break down and heal, strictures often form in the distal esophagus. Erosions have been classified by the Los Angeles classification system into grades A–D of severity, based upon percentage of circumference affected and size of mucosal break [5]. Esophagitis can also be found histopathologically, but the specificity of this to diagnose GERD is less reliable.

The majority of patients suffering from GERD have nonerosive esophageal reflux disease or NERD. Nonerosive disease is defined as reflux-associated symptoms in the absence of mucosal breaks at endoscopy [11]. This is less likely than erosive disease to cause long-term structural damage to the esophagus. They also typically have fewer complications (strictures, etc.) than patients with erosive reflux disease. Patients with NERD can have excellent acid control on proton pump inhibitors (PPI). In fact, PPI use has been successful in moving patients from erosive to nonerosive reflux disease in large numbers. Histologically, biopsies of the esophagus of patients with NERD will have early signs of damage such as dilated intracellular spaces [9, 10]. These are visible early on only using electron microscopy and as damage progresses will become visible on light microscopy as well [10].

Another potential result of squamous epithelial cell exposure to acid is columnar metaplasia. Columnar metaplasia can occur early in the disease course and can be seen in the majority of patients with chronic GERD [1]. Gastric reflux can damage the squamous epithelium to the stem cell layer, which is significantly deep to alter the proliferation of the squamous epithelial cells, leading to columnar metaplasia [1, 6]. Columnar metaplasia, or Barrett's esophagus, begins in the distal-most esophagus but can extend proximally as damage continues, leading to visible metaplasia or columnar-lined esophagus. This can progress to dysplastic Barrett's esophagus and finally adenocarcinoma of the esophagus [1]. Long-segment Barrett's esophagus is one of the most reliable risk factors for development of esophageal adenocarcinoma [11].

A patient with reflux symptoms will often undergo upper endoscopy to evaluate the extent of damage from reflux. This will allow designation of erosive versus nonerosive disease. Additionally, tissue biopsies of the gastroesophageal junction can evaluate for signs of esophagitis as well as columnar metaplasia indicative of Barrett's esophagus.

Summary

Reflux symptoms are relatively common. Gastroesophageal reflux disease is the presence of esophageal damage accompanying reflux symptoms.

GERD can be characterized by erosive and nonerosive esophagitis.

Erosive esophagitis is more likely to lead to stricture, ulcers, and metaplasia in the distal esophagus, as a result of full-thickness mucosal injury.

References

1. Chandrasoma P, Wijetunge S, Demeester SR, Hagen J, Demeester TR. The histologic squamo-oxyntic gap: an accurate and reproducible diagnostic marker of gastroesophageal reflux disease. Am J Surg Pathol. 2010;34(11):1574–81. https://doi.org/10.1097/PAS.0b013e3181f06990.
2. Dent J, Dodds WJ, Friedman RH, Sekiguchi T, Hogan WJ, Arndorfer RC, Petrie DJ. Mechanism of gastroesophageal reflux in recumbent asymptomatic human subjects. J Clin Invest. 1980;65(2):256–67. https://doi.org/10.1172/jci109667.
3. el-Serag HB, Sonnenberg A. Comorbid occurrence of laryngeal or pulmonary disease with esophagitis in United States military veterans. Gastroenterology. 1997;113(3):755–60.
4. Everhart JE, Ruhl CE. Burden of digestive diseases in the United States part I: overall and upper gastrointestinal diseases. Gastroenterology. 2009;136(2):376–86. https://doi.org/10.1053/j.gastro.2008.12.015.
5. Genta RM, Spechler SJ, Kielhorn AF. The Los Angeles and Savary-Miller systems for grading esophagitis: utilization and correlation with histology. Dis Esophagus. 2011;24(1):10–7. https://doi.org/10.1111/j.1442-2050.2010.01092.x.
6. Karam SM. Lineage commitment and maturation of epithelial cells in the gut. Front Biosci. 1999;4:D286–98.
7. Munoz JV, Herreros B, Sanchiz V, Amoros C, Hernandez V, Pascual I, et al. Dental and periodontal lesions in patients with gastro-oesophageal reflux disease. Dig Liver Dis. 2003;35(7):461–7.
8. Schneider JH, Kuper MA, Konigsrainer A, Brucher BL. Transient lower esophageal sphincter relaxation and esophageal motor response. J Surg Res. 2010;159(2):714–9. https://doi.org/10.1016/j.jss.2009.02.021.
9. Solcia E, Villani L, Luinetti O, Trespi E, Strada E, Tinelli C, Fiocca R. Altered intercellular glycoconjugates and dilated intercellular spaces of esophageal epithelium in reflux disease. Virchows Arch. 2000;436(3):207–16.
10. Tobey NA, Hosseini SS, Argote CM, Dobrucali AM, Awayda MS, Orlando RC. Dilated intercellular spaces and shunt permeability in nonerosive acid-damaged esophageal epithelium. Am J Gastroenterol. 2004;99(1):13–22.
11. Vakil N, van Zanten SV, Kahrilas P, Dent J, Jones R. The Montreal definition and classification of gastroesophageal reflux disease: a global evidence-based consensus. Am J Gastroenterol. 2006;101(8):1900–20.; quiz 1943. https://doi.org/10.1111/j.1572-0241.2006.00630.x.
12. Wyman JB, Dent J, Heddle R, Dodds WJ, Toouli J, Downton J. Control of belching by the lower oesophageal sphincter. Gut. 1990;31(6):639–46.

Preoperative Workup of GERD

7

Amy Cha and Victoria M. Gershuni

Definition of Gastroesophageal Reflux Disease

The Montreal consensus definition of gastroesophageal reflux disease (GERD) is a condition that develops when the reflux of stomach contents causes troublesome symptoms and/or complications. Manifestations of GERD can be classified as esophageal or extraesophageal syndromes, with or without evidence of esophageal mucosal injury. This classification allows symptoms to define the disease but permits further characterization if mucosal injury is found on further study. Mucosal injury from GERD can progress to the well-recognized complications of esophagitis, stricture, intestinal metaplasia or Barrett's esophagus (BE), and adenocarcinoma [1].

Anatomy and Physiology of the Gastroesophageal Junction

The anatomical antireflux barrier at the gastroesophageal junction (GEJ) is created by the coordinated action of the lower esophageal sphincter (LES), diaphragmatic crura, segment of intra-abdominal esophagus, the angle of His, and peristaltic action propelling acid forward. At rest, the LES remains tonically contracted (10–30 mmHg) to create a zone of increased pressure compared to intraluminal gastric pressure (5 mmHg). The LES relaxes upon swallowing in advance of the peristaltic wave [2]. The crura of the diaphragm respond to changes in intra-abdominal pressure and can amplify LES contraction. Other components of acid clearance include saliva, gravity, and esophageal motility. Gastric dysmotility and delayed gastric emptying can likewise predispose to GERD. The symptoms and/or mucosal injury in GERD are attributed to increased esophageal exposure to gastric acid, often due

A. Cha (✉) · V. M. Gershuni
Department of Surgery, Hospital of the University of Pennsylvania, Philadelphia, PA, USA
e-mail: amycha@pennmedicine.upenn.edu

J. Grams et al. (eds.), *The SAGES Manual of Foregut Surgery*,
https://doi.org/10.1007/978-3-319-96122-4_7

to changes in the function of the LES. LES deterioration over time leads to decreased barrier of the esophagus from acid and bile exposure [2]. The disease includes both esophageal and extraesophageal syndromes and can progress from symptoms without esophageal injury (nonerosive) to complicated GERD. Up to 70% of patients who present with symptoms of GERD in the primary care setting do not have evidence of tissue injury [3].

Clinical Presentation

The Montreal classification divides GERD manifestations into esophageal and extraesophageal syndromes.

The esophageal syndromes include the typical reflux syndrome defined by the presence of troublesome heartburn and/or regurgitation. Heartburn and regurgitation can sometimes be accompanied by other symptoms such as epigastric pain or sleep disturbance due to nighttime heartburn. GERD can also cause episodes of chest pain that resemble ischemic cardiac chest pain, which is called reflux chest pain syndrome and considered an esophageal syndrome as well. Persistent or progressive dysphagia is a symptom of an esophageal syndrome with mucosal injury, as it is a warning symptom or alarm symptom for stricture or cancer of the esophagus which warrants investigation.

The extraesophageal syndromes include reflux-related cough, laryngitis, asthma syndromes, and associations with dental erosion, sinusitis, aspiration, pulmonary fibrosis, pharyngitis, hoarseness, globus sensation, or recurrent otitis media. It is important to remember that an association of these syndromes and GERD exists, but it is rare for extraesophageal syndromes to occur in isolation without concomitant manifestations of typical esophageal syndrome. These syndromes are usually multifactorial with GERD as only one of several potential triggers, and data showing a benefit of reflux treatments on these syndromes are weak.

Due to the wide range of presentation in GERD patients, it is important that other etiologies such as cardiopulmonary disease, other foregut disease, and motility disorders also be ruled out prior to surgical treatment of GERD. Although GERD is a common entity, the signs and symptoms are nonspecific. The presentation is heterogeneous and dependent on the patient's perception of symptoms, which can overlap the symptoms of other upper gastrointestinal disorders like achalasia, gastroparesis, and functional dyspepsia [3].

Epidemiology

Recent epidemiologic studies have reported the prevalence of GERD with at least one episode of heartburn and/or regurgitation weekly to be as high as 30% in Western countries, which is up from 20% in 2005 [4]. Evidence suggests disease burden may be increasing worldwide, even as the range of geographical areas studied has expanded considerably. Studies have demonstrated that as many as 7% of

Americans have daily episodes of heartburn and 42% of Americans suffer from at least one episode per month [5]. These data suggest that GERD is likely to remain a common reason for physician office visits, both primary and referral, around the world.

Treatment Options

The primary treatment options for GERD include medical therapy with proton pump inhibitors and/or H2 receptor antagonists or laparoscopic surgical reconstruction by fundoplication. Acid-suppressive therapies may reduce or eliminate the symptom of heartburn by increasing the pH of gastric secretions, but they do not address the anatomically defective antireflux barrier and esophageal exposure to any weakly acidic gastric contents that may continue to reflux in some patients. Despite adequate acid suppression, 32% of patients in randomized studies and 45% in observational studies were found to have persistent symptoms [5]. However, not all patients who fail to respond to medical therapy have GERD. It is important to study these patients to distinguish those with persistent symptoms due to GERD vs non-GERD causes. This is emphasized by the finding that nearly 30% of patients who present with a chief complaint of GERD do not end up having abnormal distal esophageal acid exposure and, thus, would not benefit from an antireflux operation [5].

When surgical treatment is considered, objective esophageal testing is imperative to document the presence of GERD. While symptoms are indicative of GERD, they are unreliable in establishing the diagnosis without additional esophageal function tests. The goal of preoperative testing is to establish the presence of abnormal esophageal acid exposure and correlate reflux events with symptoms. Laparoscopic fundoplication is highly effective in patients with documented abnormal esophageal acid exposure and typical GERD symptoms of heartburn and regurgitation. Proper patient selection by objective esophageal testing is critical to achieve excellent surgical outcomes.

Esophageal Testing

Upper endoscopy is important to assess for esophageal mucosal injury as a manifestation of GERD, namely, esophagitis and BE. The Los Angeles (LA) classification was introduced into practice to objectively describe the severity of esophagitis. LA grade A and mild B esophagitis can have wide inter-observer variability and be diagnostically nonspecific, so the Esophageal Diagnostic Advisory Panel recommends these patients require pH testing to document the presence of GERD. Patients with LA grade C or D esophagitis do not require pH testing, as long as achalasia and pill esophagitis have been excluded. BE is defined as columnar-lined segment of esophagus visible on endoscopy in conjunction with pathologic findings of intestinal metaplasia with presence of goblet cells; it represents an advanced form of

GERD. The Prague classification is an objective description for the endoscopic appearance of BE, but there is inter-observer variability particularly in short-segment lesions <1 cm, and only 50% of short-segment BE lesions were confirmed histologically. The Esophageal Diagnostic Advisory Panel makes a distinction between short-segment BE (<3 cm) requiring pH testing to document the presence of GERD before antireflux surgery [5]. Patients with long-segment BE (≥3 cm) do not require pH testing prior to antireflux surgery [5]. Endoscopic findings of BE or a stricture are the most sensitive indicators of short esophagus that will require Collis gastroplasty. Finally, upper endoscopy is useful in eliminating errors in pH testing such as misplaced pH probe or capsule, especially important in the diagnosis of patients who may have nonerosive reflux disease. This distinct subgroup of GERD patients has no mucosal injury on endoscopy but can be further subcategorized with careful pH testing. Patients with abnormal pH test but no mucosal injury are commonly encountered, requiring additional testing to document pathological GERD. Particular attention should be paid to obtaining thorough surgical history and history of other gastrointestinal symptoms in these patients to consider whether antireflux surgery may worsen the non-GERD symptoms. Patients with no mucosal injury and a normal pH test but with symptoms and reflux events that temporally correlate may have acid hypersensitivity. Patients with no mucosal injury with a normal pH test and no symptom correlation with reflux events by definition must have a non-GERD etiology for their symptoms. These two groups of patients with no mucosal injury and negative pH test might not be adequately treated with antireflux surgery, and in these patients surgery should be avoided [5].

All patients who are considered for antireflux surgery require barium esophagram. A barium esophagram provides the surgeon with useful anatomic and functional information. It will reveal the presence and size of hiatal hernia, diverticulum, stricture, esophageal length, and even gastroesophageal reflux events with provocative maneuvers. It is not, however, a reliable predictor of short esophagus as the endoscopic findings of stricture or BE are [5]. Barium esophagram can further differentiate between a type I sliding hiatal hernia and paraesophageal hernias (types II, III, IV). Paraesophageal hernias may be associated with increasing GERD symptoms and gastric volvulus may result in catastrophic complications. The workup may require barium esophagram, upper endoscopy, and manometry because an antireflux procedure is performed as an intergral part of the procedure. pH testing is not required in these patients.

Ambulatory pH testing is the gold standard for determining presence of pathological GERD. It is required for all patients being considered for antireflux surgery [6] with very few exceptions: type III paraesophageal hernia which must be repaired regardless of GERD, long-segment BE (≥3 cm), or LA grade C or D esophagitis if achalasia and pill esophagitis have been excluded. The Esophageal Diagnostic Advisory Panel consensus was that pH testing off acid suppression at least 7 days [6] should be performed in all patients with nonerosive GERD, those with LA grade A or mild B esophagitis, and those with short-segment BE (<3 cm). pH testing off acid suppression is an important measurement in the management of patients with GERD not responding to PPI therapy as well; those who have a normal pH study may then stop PPI therapy which is of no benefit to them [6]. pH testing can be performed by transnasal catheter for 24 h or wireless pH capsule for 48 h. An abnormal 24-h pH test in a PPI-dependent patient with typical symptoms predicts successful outcomes with antireflux surgery, whereas those with typical symptoms without abnormal pH test are less likely to have successful surgical outcomes. 48-h pH testing can increase detection accuracy and sensitivity for abnormal esophageal acid exposure by as much as 22% [5]. Multichannel intraluminal impedance (MII)-pH is a promising tool to detect any type of reflux event regardless of acid or nonacid pH, especially in patients refractory to PPI therapy. Additional studies are needed to clarify the value of 24-h MII-pH (on acid suppression) in predicting outcomes of antireflux surgery. The Esophageal Diagnostic Advisory Panel maintains that testing off acid suppression should be used to determine if there is pathologic GERD [5]. Finally, the symptom index (SI) and symptom association probability (SAP) are the symptom association values calculated by the analysis software to evaluate the temporal association between clinical symptoms and reflux events. The SI is a measure of the strength of the association between symptoms and reflux events; ≥50% is considered positive. The SAP determines whether this relationship could have occurred by chance; >95% is statistically significant. These calculated values have only been validated for acid-related heartburn, regurgitation, and chest pain, and not nonacid by MII-pH. The values are also highly dependent on the numbers of symptoms noted by patients during the testing period [5].

Manometry should also be performed in all patients being considered for antireflux surgery to exclude achalasia or other underlying esophageal motility disorder which may have been misdiagnosed as GERD. Sixty percent of GERD patients might have defective LES on manometry, and impaired esophageal motility is associated with the severity of esophagitis as well. Now, 32-channel high-resolution manometry is easier, faster, and more accurate. Manometry can be used to assess peristaltic coordination and contractile force of the esophageal body, which can guide the surgeon in choosing the type of antireflux procedure. Patients with frequent failed or weak peristalsis might have less dysphagia with partial fundoplication, but no controlled data support the practice of tailoring the degree of fundoplication to the preoperative esophageal motility. The precise location of the LES can be measured for accurate pH capsule or catheter placement. Nevertheless, manometry is also not a reliable predictor of the short esophagus as the upper endoscopic finding of BE or stricture [5].

Gastric emptying study should be obtained selectively. Delayed gastric emptying symptoms include bloating, abdominal distension, and nausea, but these are nonspecific and overlap with the symptoms of functional dyspepsia. Even 30% of patients with functional dyspepsia will have delayed gastric emptying, and the study does not distinguish gastroparesis from functional dyspepsia. Twenty percent of patients with GERD have delayed gastric emptying which improves with fundoplication, reducing the capacity of the fundus and the radius of the proximal stomach, generating a higher intraluminal pressure and promoting the passage of food bolus. Persistent delayed gastric emptying can worsen gas bloat after antireflux surgery, but 31% of patients were found to have delayed gastric emptying preoperatively that did not predict the outcome of fundoplication [5, 7]. Currently there are no established gastric emptying study values that predict the worsening of gas bloat postoperatively. It should be obtained selectively in patients with significant nausea, vomiting, and bloating or those with retained food on endoscopy [7].

Laryngopharyngeal reflux (LPR) symptoms may be a result of irritation of the hypopharynx by acid reflux, but other causative factors include tobacco, alcohol, allergies, postnasal drip, and chronic sinusitis to name a few. Empiric PPI therapy is usually recommended but demonstrates no therapeutic benefit in recent meta-analyses [1]. Outcomes of antireflux surgery performed for LPR symptoms are less favorable compared with those achieved in patients with typical GERD symptoms. In an attempt to measure LPR events from acid reflux, the oropharyngeal pH catheter and hypopharyngeal MII (HMII)-pH catheter have been introduced and investigated. There is a lack of data to support the use of oropharyngeal pH or HMII-pH testing for improving patient selection for antireflux surgery. For patients with LPR symptoms who undergo these tests, a positive pH test documenting pathologic acid exposure in the distal esophagus is still required to justify antireflux surgery.

Indications for Surgery

From a surgical perspective, GERD is a mechanical failure of the lower esophageal sphincter (LES), appropriate gastric emptying, and coordinated esophageal peristalsis. A single test cannot make the diagnosis alone; rather, the several diagnostic studies taken together provide a full picture of GERD to determine whether it is amenable to surgical treatment. Based on SAGES guidelines, objective evidence of esophageal reflux must be demonstrated prior to surgery. These include any mucosal break from adjacent normal-appearing esophageal mucosa in a symptomatic patient, peptic stricture in the absence of malignancy, biopsy-proven Barrett's esophagus (BE), or prolonged exposure to acidic pH as demonstrated by esophageal pH monitoring probe.

Only after successful objective identification of pathologic acid exposure should surgery be pursued in the following situations [7]:

1. Patients who have failed conservative therapy with lifestyle change and medical management as determined by inadequate symptom management, severe regurgitation despite acid suppression, or side effects secondary to acid-suppressing medications.
2. Patients who wish to pursue surgery for quality of life considerations (cost, need for lifelong medication use, etc.) despite adequate medical management.
3. Demonstration of GERD complications, including BE or peptic stricture.
4. Extra-intestinal manifestations of GERD: asthma, pulmonary fibrosis, throat clearing, aspiration, cough, etc.

References

1. Wayman J, Myers JC, Jamieson GG. Preoperative gastric emptying and patterns of reflux as predictors of outcome after laparoscopic fundoplication. Br J Surg. 2007;94:592–8.
2. Mikami DJ, Murayama KM. Physiology and Pathogenesis of Gastroesophageal Reflux Disease. Surg Clin N Am. 2015:515–25.
3. Vakil N, van Zanten SV, Kahrilas P, et al. The Montreal definition and classification of gastroesophageal reflux disease: a global evidence-based consensus. Am J Gastroenterol. 2006;101:1900–20.
4. El-Serag HB, Sweet S, Winchester CC, Dent J. Update on the epidemiology of gastro-oesophageal reflux disease: a systematic review. Gut. 2014;63(6):871–80.
5. Jobe BA, Richter JE, Hoppo T, et al. Preoperative diagnostic workup before antireflux surgery: an evidence and experience-based consensus of the esophageal diagnostic advisory panel. J Am Coll Surg. 2013;217(4):586–97.
6. Richter JE, Pandolfino JE, Vela MF, et al. Utilization of wireless pH monitoring technologies: a summary of the proceedings from the Esophageal Diagnostic Working Group. Dis Esophagus. 2012;26:755–65.
7. Stefanidis D, Hope WW, Kohn GP, et al. Guidelines for surgical treatment of gastroesophageal reflux disease. Surg Endosc. 2010;24:2647–69.

Identifying Patients with Eosinophilic Esophagitis

8

Rebecca L. Gunter and Luke M. Funk

Eosinophilic esophagitis (EoE) is a chronic immune/antigen-mediated esophageal disease that presents as esophageal dysfunction in the setting of localized eosinophilic predominant inflammation. The most recent practice guideline from the American College of Gastroenterology defines EoE by the following criteria: symptoms related to esophageal dysfunction and the presence of eosinophil-predominant inflammation isolated to the esophagus that persists after a trial of proton pump inhibitors (PPI) in the absence of a secondary cause of esophageal eosinophilia [1]. Its prevalence has been increasing, due in part to increased awareness of the condition and more frequent diagnosis, but also as a result of a true increase in the incidence of disease. The estimated prevalence of EoE in the United States between 2010 and 2015 was 30.0/100,000 for adults age 18–65 years and 12.8/100,000 for adults over the age of 65 [2].

Diagnosis

History and Physical Exam

The typical EoE patient is a young or middle-aged male with a history of atopy. Men outnumber women (3:1). The most common presenting symptom of EoE is dysphagia due to esophageal dysfunction or food impaction. These symptoms are more often experienced with solid foods than with liquids, and patients may have a history of avoiding high-consistency foods. Dysphagia in patients with EoE is a

R. L. Gunter
Department of Surgery, University of Wisconsin Hospital and Clinics, Madison, WI, USA

L. M. Funk (✉)
Division of Minimally Invasive, Foregut, and Bariatric Surgery; Department of Surgery, University of Wisconsin Hospital and Clinics, Madison, WI, USA
e-mail: funk@surgery.wisc.edu

J. Grams et al. (eds.), *The SAGES Manual of Foregut Surgery*,
https://doi.org/10.1007/978-3-319-96122-4_8

result of chronic inflammation, dysmotility, and fibrostenotic remodeling. Additional behavior modifications related to dysphagia are commonly reported, such as eating slowly or needing to swallow multiple times to fully clear the food bolus from the esophagus. Patients may also report heartburn or atypical chest pain.

EoE is increasingly recognized as a manifestation of a food sensitization or allergy. A history of atopy should alert the treating physician to the possibility of EoE. As many as 70% of children and adults with EoE have a history of asthma, allergic rhinitis, and/or atopic dermatitis [3].

The Eosinophilic Esophagitis Activity Index (EEsAI) is a validated, patient-reported survey instrument that characterizes symptom severity and may be used for ongoing evaluation during and after therapy [4]. This survey is based on seven items assessing the frequency and duration of dysphagia, the severity of dysphagia when eating foods of eight different consistencies, and behavioral changes (avoidance, modification, and slow eating of certain foods) as a result of their dysphagia. The EEsAI evaluates these items over the past 24 h, 7 days, and 30 days. The Dysphagia Symptom Questionnaire (DSQ) and the Mayo Dysphagia Questionnaire (MDQ) are alternative survey measures that are used to assess EoE severity, but they are less specific in regard to food consistency and behavioral modifications [5, 6]. While the EEsAI, DSQ, and MDQ are useful in following symptom evolution over time, they are not sufficient to indicate endoscopic or histologic severity or remission, as symptoms and objective findings are inconsistently correlated [7].

Physical examination is generally unremarkable in patients with EoE, though 10% of patients with EoE also have eczema [8]. Despite its relationship with other allergic conditions, allergy testing either by skin prick or serum tests for IgE is not useful and is generally not recommended [9].

Differential Diagnosis

Patients presenting with dysphagia or food impaction should be evaluated for mechanical causes of obstruction such as a neoplasm, esophageal stricture, or epiphrenic diverticula, as well as primary esophageal motility disorders such as achalasia or systemic sclerosis. A complete history and physical can help narrow the differential diagnosis, but additional diagnostic measures are often required to reach a final diagnosis, including upper endoscopy, esophageal biopsies, esophageal manometry, and barium esophagram. Elevated levels of eosinophils found in the esophageal epithelium, the hallmark of eosinophilic esophagitis, may be seen in a variety of other conditions. These include inflammatory bowel diseases, IgE-mediated food allergies, celiac disease, hypereosinophilic syndrome, GERD, infectious diseases, and toxic injury.

Upper Endoscopy

Endoscopy is used to diagnose EoE, monitor disease progression and remission, and guide therapy. EoE manifests a variety of endoscopic findings, including mucosal edema, esophageal rings (also known as trachealization or corrugation), furrows (also known as felinization), exudates or plaques, luminal narrowing, and mucosal fragility during endoscopic evaluation (Fig. 8.1) [1]. Due to the wide range of endoscopic features and the variability in endoscopists' evaluation and descriptive terminology, a classification and scoring system for EoE was developed and validated in 2013 [10, 11]. This score, known as the EoE Endoscopic Reference Score (EREFS) system, encompasses the five primary endoscopic findings of EoE: edema, rings, exudate, furrows, and strictures [12]. Each of these parameters is given a grade and used to generate a score (Table 8.1). A score of 2.0 or greater has an 88% sensitivity and 92% specificity for diagnosing EoE [13].

A history suggestive of EoE and supporting endoscopic findings must be confirmed by mucosal biopsies demonstrating eosinophil-predominant inflammation. Biopsies should be taken at the time of endoscopy from at least two different locations in the esophagus, usually in the proximal and distal halves of the esophagus. This point is especially important because while patients with GERD may have esophageal eosinophilia located in the distal esophagus, patients with EoE will have diffuse eosinophilia throughout the esophagus. It is recommended to obtain multiple biopsies due to the patchy and heterogeneous nature of EoE. Though the number of biopsies needed is debatable, diagnostic sensitivity can approach 100% with 6–9 biopsies [14, 15].

Other Imaging and Diagnostic Tools

Barium esophagram may be useful to detect esophageal narrowing not appreciated on endoscopy. Compared to barium esophagram, endoscopy has a sensitivity of only 14.7% and a specificity of 79.2% for detecting esophageal narrowing [16]. Its use may be reserved for patients presenting with persistent dysphagia and normal endoscopic findings. Endoscopic and endoluminal ultrasonography may detect esophageal mural thickening, though this has been used primarily in studies examining steroid effectiveness [17, 18].

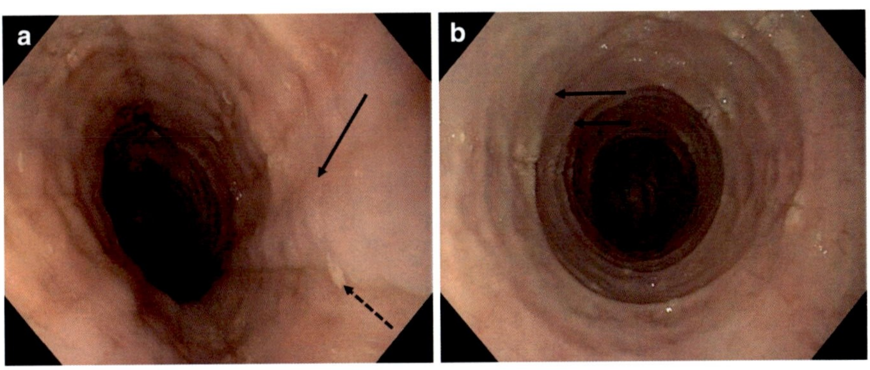

Fig. 8.1 (**a**) Longitudinal furrows *(arrow)* and exudates *(dashed arrow)* are visible throughout the esophagus; (**b**) fixed concentric rings *(arrows)* are seen down the length of the esophagus. (Images courtesy of Dr. Anurag Soni, Department of Medicine, Division of Gastroenterology and Hepatology, University of Wisconsin)

Table 8.1 Eosinophilic Esophagitis Endoscopic Reference Score (EREFS) grading system

Major features
Edema
Grade 0: absent (distinct vascularity present)
Grade 1: loss of clarity or absence of vascular markings
Fixed rings
Grade 0: none
Grade 1: mild (subtle circumferential ridges)
Grade 2: moderate (distinct rings that do not impair passage of a standard adult endoscope)
Grade 3: severe (distinct rings that do not permit passage of a standard adult endoscope)
Exudates
Grade 0: none
Grade 1: mild (lesions involving <10% of the esophageal surface area)
Grade 2: severe (lesions involving >10% of the esophageal surface area)
Furrows
Grade 0: none
Grade 1: present
Stricture
Grade 0: none
Grade 1: present
Minor features
Crepe paper esophagus (mucosal fragility or laceration upon simple passage of an endoscope)
Grade 0: absent
Grade 1: present
Narrow-caliber esophagus (reduced luminal diameter of the majority of the tubular esophagus)
Grade 0: absent
Grade 1: present

Patients with EoE may have decreased esophageal distensibility and abnormal motility, which can be detected with esophageal manometry or by using a functional luminal imaging probe (FLIP). Documented derangements of esophageal motility include hypertensive or weak peristaltic function and poor esophageal shortening upon swallowing [18]. Distensibility measured by FLIP is significantly decreased throughout the length of the esophagus and at the gastroesophageal junction in patients with EoE [19, 20].

Histology

The primary histologic finding of EoE on histology is an elevated number of intraepithelial eosinophils (Fig. 8.2). Most diagnostic criteria use a threshold of at least 15 eosinophils per high-powered field [1, 21]. Eosinophils may be clustered in microabscesses (aggregates of four or more eosinophils) and are often located at or near the epithelial surface, a phenomenon called "surface layering." The basal layer of the epithelium may be thickened to a significant degree, comprising nearly the entire epithelium. Intracellular edema can be significant, making intercellular bridges that are normally invisible to light microscopy readily apparent. The normally thin and loose connective tissue of the lamina propria can become thick and dense with collagen fibers. Eosinophils and other inflammatory cells may also

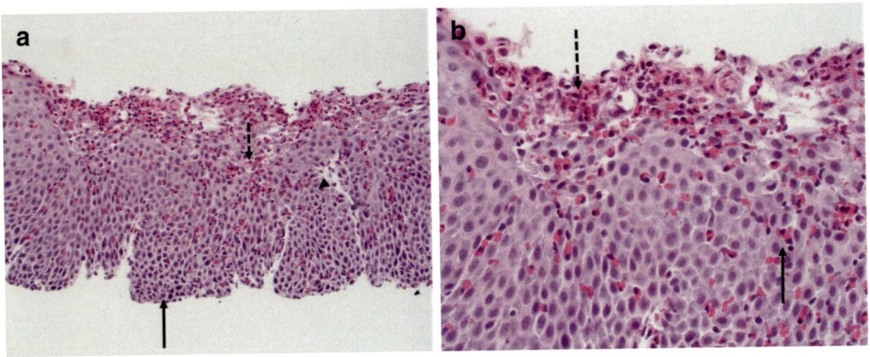

Fig. 8.2 (**a**) Esophageal biopsy showing basal cell hyperplasia *(solid arrow)*, intercellular edema or spongiosis *(arrowhead)*, and marked increase in intraepithelial eosinophils with eosinophilic microabscesses *(dashed arrow)*; (**b**) increased intraepithelial eosinophils *(solid arrow)* and eosinophilic microabscesses *(dashed arrow)* at greater magnification. (Images courtesy of Dr. Rao Watson, Department of Pathology and Laboratory Medicine, University of Wisconsin)

be seen in the lamina propria, though these do not contribute to the intraepithelial eosinophil count used to make the diagnosis of EoE [21].

Distinction from GERD

The presentation of EoE can be very similar to that of gastroesophageal reflux disease (GERD). EoE was initially believed to be a marker for GERD [22, 23]. Both can be characterized by heartburn, chest pain, or dysphagia. The most commonly reported symptom in EoE is dysphagia with food impaction, whereas patients with GERD more frequently complain of heartburn and regurgitation. It is important to differentiate EoE patients from patients with GERD because their treatments differ substantially.

Attwood et al. first described EoE as being separate from GERD in 1993 in a case series of patients who presented with dysphagia but whose endoscopic images and pH monitoring demonstrated no evidence of acid reflux. Esophageal biopsies of these patients showed elevated eosinophils in the esophageal epithelium compared to a control cohort of patients known to have GERD (56 eosinophils/HPF in patients with EoE vs. 3.3 eosinophils/HPF in patients with GERD) [24]. The following year, Straumann et al. termed this "idiopathic eosinophilic esophagitis" [25]. The endoscopic findings of EoE are typically evenly distributed across the esophagus and are characteristically different than those of GERD, which are localized to the distal esophagus.

Treatment

Treatment of EoE is directed at symptom reduction, remission of endoscopic and histologic disease manifestations, and prevention of long-term sequelae (e.g., strictures, luminal narrowing). Several therapeutic options are available, which may be used alone or in combination.

Diet Modification

Diet modification may be attempted to alleviate symptoms and reverse esophageal fibrostenosis. Accepted regimens include elemental diets, allergy testing-directed elimination diets, and empiric food elimination. Because elemental diets are poorly tolerated, and the predictive value of allergy testing is limited, empiric food elimination has become the preferred method. The most popular regimen is the six-food elimination diet, removing the six most common food allergens (milk protein, wheat, eggs, soy, peanuts/tree nuts, and seafood) for 6 weeks (the *induction* phase). Following this period, foods are sequentially reintroduced with repeated endoscopies to monitor for disease recurrence (the *reintroduction* phase). Once the food trigger is identified, patients are counseled to continue avoiding it in their diets (the *maintenance* phase).

Prospective randomized clinical trials have demonstrated that the six-food elimination diet decreases the level of eosinophilia in 65–75% of patients and decreases symptom scores by up to 94% [26, 27]. Milk protein and wheat are the most frequently identified food triggers. This approach is especially useful for patients seeking non-pharmacologic treatments, though the need for frequent endoscopies and their associated cost are notable drawbacks. Alternatives to the six-food elimination diet are the four-food elimination diet (eliminating milk protein, wheat, eggs, and soy) and empiric elimination of cow's milk alone. These have the advantage of being less restrictive, and they can identify the food trigger faster. Most patients who fail can be rescued with the full six-food elimination diet [28].

Medications

Swallowed topical steroids are used as first-line therapy. Budesonide and fluticasone are most commonly prescribed. In a prospective randomized controlled trial of 36 patients, treatment with a 15-day course of budesonide decreased eosinophilia (47.8–17.7 eosinophils/HPF), induced full histologic remission in 72%, and significantly decreased reported symptoms [29]. These results were durable out to 50 weeks, and long-term therapy showed a trend toward normalization of any evidence of esophageal remodeling prior to initiation [17]. Fluticasone has been shown to induce complete histologic remission in 65–68% of participants, but does not cause a significant reduction in reported symptoms [30, 31]. Cessation of either therapy results in relapse in nearly all patients, and thus patients should continue topical steroids as maintenance therapy. Esophageal candidiasis is a potential adverse outcome of topical steroids (found in up to 30% of patients), though this is often asymptomatic and detected on endoscopy alone. Because EoE is localized to the esophagus, systemic steroids are reserved for patients with severe symptoms and in need of rapid therapy [9].

Proton pump inhibitors were historically the first-line therapy for EoE. Initially, it was believed that patients who had symptom relief with PPI therapy had GERD and those who saw no benefit had true EoE. However, there is a growing awareness of a subset of patients with esophageal eosinophilia whose symptoms respond to PPI, but have no evidence of GERD. This condition has been termed PPI-responsive esophageal eosinophilia (PPI-REE) [32]. Three mechanisms of action for this effect have been proposed. The first is that PPIs themselves have anti-inflammatory properties and can reduce eosinophil migration into the esophageal epithelium [33]. The second is that patients with PPI-REE have improved epithelial barrier function after receiving PPI therapy, preventing potential food allergens from crossing the mucosal layer [34]. A final proposed mechanism is that some patients with EoE may also have a component of acid reflux that responds to PPI therapy. Regardless of mechanism, it is reasonable to initiate PPI therapy for patients with EoE as a first step, reserving topical steroid therapy for those who do not respond.

Endoscopic Therapy

In addition to its role in diagnosis and disease surveillance, endoscopy has important therapeutic uses. More than 70% of patients with EoE have evidence of decreased esophageal distensibility. Long-standing EoE can result in esophageal remodeling leading to strictures, [35] which are identified in 30–80% of adults with EoE. The risk of each of these changes increases with disease duration [18]. Endoscopic balloon dilation is an effective treatment of these complications and the resultant dysphagia. In a retrospective study of 10 patients with steroid-refractory EoE, all patients improved their dysphagia scores after 1–5 dilation sessions [36]. Another study of 207 patients found that esophageal dilation increased esophageal diameter between 5 and 7 mm. This correlated with a significant improvement in dysphagia symptoms in 93% of patients, with a median follow-up of 17 months [37]. More than half of patients require more than one dilation session to achieve success [38]. The best predictor of success is the esophageal caliber achieved at the end of dilation therapy. Despite initial safety concerns raised due to the mucosal fragility seen in EoE, complication rates are similar to those undergoing esophageal dilation for other causes [39].

A subset of patients with EoE have a diffusely stenotic, extremely narrow-caliber esophagus. These patients are typically older and have had a longer symptom duration. They are often resistant to steroid therapy and require multiple dilations to achieve symptom relief [40].

Conclusion

EoE is an increasingly common disease whose hallmark symptoms overlap with GERD. Surgeons who perform endoscopy may be involved in its diagnosis and endoscopic treatment of complications resulting from long-standing EoE. There is no role for surgical intervention in the management of EoE.

References

1. Dellon ES, Gonsalves N, Hirano I, Furuta GT, Liacouras CA, Katzka DA, et al. ACG clinical guideline: evidenced based approach to the diagnosis and management of esophageal eosinophilia and eosinophilic esophagitis (EoE). Am J Gastroenterol. 2013;108:679–92; quiz 693
2. Mansoor E, Cooper GS. The 2010-2015 prevalence of eosinophilic esophagitis in the USA: a population-based study. Dig Dis Sci. 2016;61:2928–34.
3. Hirano I. 2015 David Y. Graham lecture: the first two decades of eosinophilic esophagitis-from acid reflux to food allergy. Am J Gastroenterol. 2016;111:770–6.
4. Schoepfer AM, Straumann A, Panczak R, Coslovsky M, Kuehni CE, Maurer E, et al. Development and validation of a symptom-based activity index for adults with eosinophilic esophagitis. Gastroenterology. 2014;147:1255–66. e21
5. Dellon ES, Irani A-M, Hill MR, Hirano I. Development and field testing of a novel patient-reported outcome measure of dysphagia in patients with eosinophilic esophagitis. Aliment Pharmacol Ther. 2013;38:634–42.
6. Grudell ABM, Alexander JA, Enders FB, Pacifico R, Fredericksen M, Wise JL, et al. Validation of the Mayo dysphagia questionnaire. Dis Esophagus. 2007;20:202–5.
7. Safroneeva E, Straumann A, Coslovsky M, Zwahlen M, Kuehni CE, Panczak R, et al. Symptoms have modest accuracy in detecting endoscopic and histologic remission in adults with eosinophilic esophagitis. Gastroenterology. 2016;150:581–90. e4
8. Miehlke S. Clinical features of eosinophilic esophagitis. Dig Dis. 2014;32:61–7.
9. Richter JE. Current Management of Eosinophilic Esophagitis 2015. J Clin Gastroenterol. 2016;50:99–110.
10. Kim HP, Vance RB, Shaheen NJ, Dellon ES. The prevalence and diagnostic utility of endoscopic features of eosinophilic esophagitis: a meta-analysis. Clin Gastroenterol Hepatol. 2012;10:988–96. e5
11. Peery AF, Cao H, Dominik R, Shaheen NJ, Dellon ES. Variable reliability of endoscopic findings with white-light and narrow-band imaging for patients with suspected eosinophilic esophagitis. Clin Gastroenterol Hepatol. 2011;9:475–80.
12. Hirano I, Moy N, Heckman MG, Thomas CS, Gonsalves N, Achem SR. Endoscopic assessment of the oesophageal features of eosinophilic oesophagitis: validation of a novel classification and grading system. Gut. 2013;62:489–95.
13. Dellon ES, Cotton CC, Gebhart JH, Higgins LL, Beitia R, Woosley JT, et al. Accuracy of the eosinophilic esophagitis endoscopic reference score in diagnosis and determining response to treatment. Clin Gastroenterol Hepatol. 2016;14:31–9.
14. Saffari H, Peterson KA, Fang JC, Teman C, Gleich GJ, Pease LF. Patchy eosinophil distributions in an esophagectomy specimen from a patient with eosinophilic esophagitis: implications for endoscopic biopsy. J Allergy Clin Immunol. 2012;130:798–800.
15. Gonsalves N, Policarpio-Nicolas M, Zhang Q, Rao MS, Hirano I. Histopathologic variability and endoscopic correlates in adults with eosinophilic esophagitis. Gastrointest Endosc. 2006;64:313–9.
16. Gentile N, Katzka D, Ravi K, Trenkner S, Enders F, Killian J, et al. Oesophageal narrowing is common and frequently under-appreciated at endoscopy in patients with oesophageal eosinophilia. Aliment Pharmacol Ther. 2014;40:1333–40.
17. Straumann A, Conus S, Degen L, Frei C, Bussmann C, Beglinger C, et al. Long-term budesonide maintenance treatment is partially effective for patients with eosinophilic esophagitis. Clin Gastroenterol Hepatol. 2011;9:400–9. e1
18. Hirano I, Aceves SS. Clinical implications and pathogenesis of esophageal remodeling in eosinophilic esophagitis. Gastroenterol Clin N Am. 2014;43:297–316.
19. Kwiatek MA, Hirano I, Kahrilas PJ, Rothe J, Luger D, Pandolfino JE. Mechanical properties of the esophagus in eosinophilic esophagitis. Gastroenterology. 2011;140:82–90.

20. Nicodème F, Hirano I, Chen J, Robinson K, Lin Z, Xiao Y, et al. Esophageal distensibility as a measure of disease severity in patients with eosinophilic esophagitis. Clin Gastroenterol Hepatol. 2013;11:1101–7. e1
21. Collins MH. Histopathologic features of eosinophilic esophagitis. Gastrointest Endosc Clin N Am. 2008;18:59–71. viii – ix
22. Winter HS, Madara JL, Stafford RJ, Grand RJ, Quinlan JE, Goldman H. Intraepithelial eosinophils: a new diagnostic criterion for reflux esophagitis. Gastroenterology. 1982;83:818–23.
23. Brown LF, Goldman H, Antonioli DA. Intraepithelial eosinophils in endoscopic biopsies of adults with reflux esophagitis. Am J Surg Pathol. 1984;8:899–905.
24. Attwood SE, Smyrk TC, Demeester TR, Jones JB. Esophageal eosinophilia with dysphagia. A distinct clinicopathologic syndrome. Dig Dis Sci. 1993;38:109–16.
25. Straumann A, Spichtin HP, Bernoulli R, Loosli J, Vögtlin J. Idiopathic eosinophilic esophagitis: a frequently overlooked disease with typical clinical aspects and discrete endoscopic findings. Schweiz Med Wochenschr. 1994;124:1419–29.
26. Gonsalves N, Yang G-Y, Doerfler B, Ritz S, Ditto AM, Hirano I. Elimination diet effectively treats eosinophilic esophagitis in adults; food reintroduction identifies causative factors. Gastroenterology. 2012;142:1451–9.e1; quiz e14–5
27. Lucendo AJ, Arias Á, González-Cervera J, Yagüe-Compadre JL, Guagnozzi D, Angueira T, et al. Empiric 6-food elimination diet induced and maintained prolonged remission in patients with adult eosinophilic esophagitis: a prospective study on the food cause of the disease. J Allergy Clin Immunol. 2013;131:797–804.
28. Molina-Infante J, Arias A, Barrio J, Rodríguez-Sánchez J, Sanchez-Cazalilla M, Lucendo AJ. Four-food group elimination diet for adult eosinophilic esophagitis: a prospective multicenter study. J Allergy Clin Immunol. 2014;134:1093–9. e1
29. Straumann A, Conus S, Degen L, Felder S, Kummer M, Engel H, et al. Budesonide is effective in adolescent and adult patients with active eosinophilic esophagitis. Gastroenterology. 2010;139:1526–37, 1537.e1.
30. Butz BK, Wen T, Gleich GJ, Furuta GT, Spergel J, King E, et al. Efficacy, dose reduction, and resistance to high-dose fluticasone in patients with eosinophilic esophagitis. Gastroenterology. 2014;147:324–33. e5
31. Alexander JA, Jung KW, Arora AS, Enders F, Katzka DA, Kephardt GM, et al. Swallowed fluticasone improves histologic but not symptomatic response of adults with eosinophilic esophagitis. Clin Gastroenterol Hepatol. 2012;10:742–9. e1
32. Molina-Infante J, Ferrando-Lamana L, Ripoll C, Hernandez-Alonso M, Mateos JM, Fernandez-Bermejo M, et al. Esophageal eosinophilic infiltration responds to proton pump inhibition in most adults. Clin Gastroenterol Hepatol. 2011;9:110–7.
33. Cheng E, Zhang X, Huo X, Yu C, Zhang Q, Wang DH, et al. Omeprazole blocks eotaxin-3 expression by oesophageal squamous cells from patients with eosinophilic oesophagitis and GORD. Gut. 2013;62:824–32.
34. Van Rhijn BD, Weijenborg PW, Verheij J, van den Bergh Weerman MA, Verseijden C, van den Wijngaard RMJGJ, et al. Proton pump inhibitors partially restore mucosal integrity in patients with proton pump inhibitor-responsive esophageal eosinophilia but not eosinophilic esophagitis. Clin Gastroenterol Hepatol. 2014;12:1815–23.e2.
35. Dellon ES, Kim HP, Sperry SLW, Rybnicek DA, Woosley JT, Shaheen NJ. A phenotypic analysis shows that eosinophilic esophagitis is a progressive fibrostenotic disease. Gastrointest Endosc. 2014;79:577–85.e4.
36. Schoepfer AM, Gschossmann J, Scheurer U, Seibold F, Straumann A. Esophageal strictures in adult eosinophilic esophagitis: dilation is an effective and safe alternative after failure of topical corticosteroids. Endoscopy. 2008;40:161–4.
37. Schoepfer AM, Gonsalves N, Bussmann C, Conus S, Simon H-U, Straumann A, et al. Esophageal dilation in eosinophilic esophagitis: effectiveness, safety, and impact on the underlying inflammation. Am J Gastroenterol. 2010;105:1062–70.

38. Runge TM, Eluri S, Cotton CC, Burk CM, Woosley JT, Shaheen NJ, et al. Outcomes of esophageal dilation in eosinophilic esophagitis: safety, efficacy, and persistence of the Fibrostenotic phenotype. Am J Gastroenterol. 2016;111:206–13.
39. Jacobs JW, Spechler SJ. A systematic review of the risk of perforation during esophageal dilation for patients with eosinophilic esophagitis. Dig Dis Sci. 2010;55:1512–5.
40. Eluri S, Runge TM, Cotton CC, Burk CM, Wolf WA, Woosley JT, et al. The extremely narrow-caliber esophagus is a treatment-resistant subphenotype of eosinophilic esophagitis. Gastrointest Endosc. 2016;83:1142–8.

Laryngopharyngeal Reflux (LPR)

9

Krzysztof Nowak, Saurabh Sharma, and Subhash Kini

Introduction

Laryngopharyngeal reflux (LPR) can be defined as influx of stomach contents into the upper airway, especially the laryngopharynx and posterior nasopharynx. As a result, affected individuals complain of various laryngopharyngeal and respiratory symptoms caused by the damage to the upper airway epithelium.

LPR is primarily a clinical diagnosis, usually based on the presence of several symptoms, which most often include hoarseness, nonproductive throat clearing, sensation of having excess mucous in the throat, globus pharyngeus, difficulties swallowing, dry cough, and difficulties breathing. Multiple analyses and surveys show that heartburn complaints occur in no more than 40% of affected (LPR) patients.

Due to the variability of its clinical presentation, confusing sets of symptoms, and lack of reliable testing methods, there are no agreed upon diagnostic criteria for LPR. As a result, it is often underdiagnosed and undertreated in spite of being a very common condition. Reflecting this confusion is the use of many different synonyms such as extra-esophageal reflux (EER), reflux laryngitis, laryngeal reflux, gastropharyngeal reflux, pharyngoesophageal reflux, supraesophageal reflux, and silent or atypical reflux.

The aim of this chapter is to give a succinct overview of the current understanding of LPR.

K. Nowak
ENT and Allergy Associates, Yonkers, NY, USA

S. Sharma
Department of Bariatric and Robotic Surgery Fortis Hospital, Mohali, Punjab, India

S. Kini (✉)
Department of Surgery, Icahn School of Medicine at Mount Sinai St. Luke's, New York, NY, USA
e-mail: subhash.kini@mountsinai.org

J. Grams et al. (eds.), *The SAGES Manual of Foregut Surgery*,
https://doi.org/10.1007/978-3-319-96122-4_9

History

Reports of association between vocal cord granulomas and laryngopharyngeal reflux have been mentioned as early as in the late 1960s. In a breakthrough 1991 article, Dr. Koufman presented a detailed description of various aspects of reflux in the laryngopharyngeal region and provided important observations about the clinical presentation, diagnosis, and proposed management at that time [1]. In 2002, Koufman et al. published the official position statement of the American Academy of Otolaryngology and stressed that LPR is a distinct clinical entity separate from gastroesophageal reflux disease (GERD) [2]. Guidelines presented by the American Gastroenterological Association Institute in 2008 presented a different perspective describing GERD as having two different types of syndromes, esophageal, and extra-esophageal (pertaining to LPR).

In spite of growing number of publications, there is still little awareness and understanding of LPR in the medical community except for otolaryngologists, voice specialist, and foregut and esophageal specialists.

Epidemiology

Because of lack of diagnostic criteria, it is difficult to estimate the true incidence of LPR. There are no large population-based studies that have examined this carefully. Most recent estimates of GERD prevalence in North America are in the range of 18.1–27.8%. LPR can be considered as a subset of GERD, and clinical experience of many experts in the field points to this condition being very prevalent. Kaufmann reported an incidence of LPR to be 50% in patients with laryngeal and voice symptoms [3]. An analysis conducted at a large group specialty practice in the New York City area (ENT and Allergy Associates) in 2016 showed that 9.7% of all adult patients seen that year (29,473 out of 304,362) carried the diagnosis of GERD or LPR. It is estimated that the economic impact of diagnosing and treating LPR can be 5–6 times higher than that of GERD [4].

Pathophysiology

The pathophysiology of LPR is a complex interplay between abnormal function of esophageal sphincters, esophageal motility, and the efficacy of various defense mechanisms (presence of saliva, mucous barrier, and activity of carbonic anhydrase), which ultimately affect the extent and frequency of exposure to acid, bile, and pepsin on the laryngopharyngeal mucosa.

Lower esophageal sphincter dysfunction and esophageal dysmotility directly contribute to prolonged esophageal acid clearance in patients with LPR [5].

Abnormal upper esophageal sphincter (UES) function is another critical factor in LPR pathophysiology. Inappropriate premature relaxation of the UES during a reflux event leads to airway damage. It has been shown that prolonged mucosal damage is associated with laryngopharyngeal sensory deficits. Patients with GERD and cough have impaired laryngopharyngeal sensitivity, which in turn further diminishes UES function and leads to more reflux events.

Rarely, LPR may also be caused by presence of the so-called inlet patch, which is heterotopic acid-secreting gastric mucosa in the upper esophagus.

Acid

The larynx and hypopharynx have a neutral pH of 7.0 and are extremely sensitive to changes of pH caused by stomach acid and bile. In addition, the upper airway lining has no good mechanisms to protect itself from the effects of the contents of gastric reflux.

Any exposure of the laryngopharynx to stomach acid will initiate epithelial damage. This damage can be a result of direct acidification of the cellular microenvironment or augmentation of pepsin's enzymatic action. Highly acidic foods may themselves also contribute to this process. Even a mildly acidic pH of 6.5 can initiate the activity of pepsin and lead to epithelial damage.

Pepsin

As mentioned above, acid does not act alone in damaging the upper aerodigestive tract mucosa. Pepsin, a proteolytic enzyme secreted in the stomach, is considered to be one of the primary causes of mucosal damage in LPR. Pepsin has been found in higher concentrations in the laryngeal mucosa and respiratory secretions in LPR patients when compared with controls. Initially, pepsin has been thought to cause epithelial damage by its proteolytic activity in digesting the molecules that maintain cohesion between the cells. However, recent studies have shown that pepsin is also endocytosed by the airway and possibly esophageal epithelial cells. It is then retained in the intracellular vesicles of low pH, in which the enzyme's proteolytic activity is restored. It has been demonstrated that in such setting, pepsin causes mitochondrial damage, significant cell toxicity, and changes in the expression of several genes implicated in stress and toxicity [6].

It has been also suggested that exposure of the larynx and pharynx to pepsin causes damage to the mucosa through depletion of carbonic anhydrase III enzyme, which plays a key role in the regulation of pH and protection of tissues from the effects of acid [7]. A positive association between macroscopic findings of inflammation and damage in LPR and presence of pepsin in tracheal aspirates has been shown. There is growing evidence that the damaging effect of pepsin and lack of carbonic anhydrase activity may lead to carcinogenesis.

Bile Acids

Bile acids are also part of duodenal-gastric refluxate. Laryngopharyngeal mucosa is not adapted for bile exposure. Higher concentrations of bile acids in saliva have been found in LPR patients. Considering the neutral pH of laryngopharyngeal mucosa, the unconjugated bile acids like chenodeoxycholic acid may have a significant damaging effect [8].

Clinical Presentation

LPR is notoriously difficult to diagnose because most of the symptoms associated with it are not very specific, and its presentation is pleomorphic. Patients present with various combinations and severity of symptoms. Heartburn and other "typical" complaints of GERD are often absent. As mentioned before, a diagnostic gold standard for LPR has not been established.

The most common presenting symptoms of LPR are laryngeal in nature and include hoarseness, globus pharyngeus, perception of excess mucous in the throat accompanied by constant nonproductive throat clearing, dry or itchy throat, and chronic or recurrent dry cough. Many patients have stridor, which is mistaken for wheezing and therefore misdiagnosed as asthma. Reflux-induced chronic laryngitis has been associated with development of subglottic stenosis, laryngeal granulomas, contact ulcers, vocal nodules, and laryngeal carcinoma.

LPR is one of the most common causes of chronic cough. Cough in LPR is mostly nonproductive. Affected persons often experience fits of unstoppable cough to the point of tearing, loss of bladder control, and gagging. Cough often interferes with sleep. Complaints of shortness of breath are also very common and can be very distressing. Patients report inability to take a breath in (inspiratory dyspnea) and suffocating sensations that cause panic reactions, which prompt them to seek immediate help in the emergency rooms.

Other less frequently observed (or possibly less reported) symptoms associated with LPR include complaints of bad taste in the throat and mouth, water brash (regurgitation of excessive amounts of saliva), night sweats, sore throat on waking up, itchy ears, nasal congestion, and even tooth erosion. There are also reports of significant coexistence between LPR and obstructive sleep apnea. In addition, laryngopharyngeal reflux has been associated with chronic rhinosinusitis and chronic otitis media. Pepsin has been consistently detected in significant proportion of chronic middle ear effusions in children and has been associated with chronic otitis media.

Multiple authors have reported that LPR is responsible for causing bronchoconstriction and asthma symptoms, but careful review of medical literature does not provide a clear proof. Shortness of breath and complaints of wheezy respiratory noises should be attributed primarily to laryngospasms and resulting stridor, especially when pulmonary function tests are normal.

Because of the predominance of respiratory complaints and paucity of classical GERD symptoms, many patients present themselves first to their primary care physician, pulmonologist, allergy specialist, or otolaryngologist rather than to a gastroenterologist or a surgeon.

Diagnosis

The diagnosis of LPR is based on the combination of clinical suspicion, presenting symptoms, and exclusion of other conditions that may present with similar complaints. To clarify or facilitate the diagnosis, one can also use clinical diagnostic tools (questionnaires), perform endoscopic evaluations, pH probe tests, and check for presence of pepsin in the upper airway.

Role of Reflux Symptom Index (RSI)

One of the few validated clinical diagnostic tools used most frequently to facilitate the diagnosis of LPR is reflux symptom index (RSI), which consists of a set of nine questions addressing the most common symptoms and their severity. RSI is a useful tool but has significant limitations. It was developed as a severity assessment and outcomes instrument for patients already suspected and managed for LPR. RSI's validity and reliability was based on evaluation of only 25 patients already diagnosed with LPR and 25 controls [9]. In addition, some of the RSI questions do not appear to be well formulated (multiple symptoms lumped together) and miss some important symptoms or complaints helpful in the diagnosis of LPR (e.g., throat dryness or bad taste in the throat or mouth).

Laryngoscopy

Laryngoscopy (indirect laryngoscopy or fiber-optic nasolaryngoscopy) is an integral part of a patient's evaluation to rule out any other laryngeal disorders (including vocal cord nodules and carcinoma), which may cause hoarseness, dysphonia, and cough. It is important to stress that the laryngoscopic findings typical for LPR such as posterior laryngeal edema, true vocal fold edema, and pseudosulcus are not diagnostic by themselves. Studies show poor correlation between clinical symptoms and endoscopic findings of LPR.

The typical laryngoscopic changes associated with LPR include edema and erythema of the posterior commissure, which is referred to as posterior laryngitis. Additional reported changes are vocal cord edema, pseudosulcus vocalis (edema of the undersurface of the vocal fold), presence of thick endolaryngeal mucous, lymphoid hyperplasia of the posterior pharynx (cobblestoning), and much more rarely granuloma formation, contact ulcers, subglottic stenosis, posterior glottic stenosis, and strictures. To provide a more consistent way of reporting fiber-optic laryngoscopy findings, Belafsky et al. created a reflux finding score (RFS) in 2001 [10]. RFS, however, has not become a useful diagnostic tool because of poor correlation between its scores and the clinical symptoms, pH probe results, and response to therapy.

Chest Imaging and Pulmonary Function Tests

In cases of chronic cough, a careful history should be obtained to rule out chronic respiratory infections and other noninfectious chronic respiratory conditions. Imaging studies, such as a chest X-ray or chest CT and pulmonary function tests, have to be performed to help make the diagnosis.

Dual pH Probe with Impedance Monitoring

Classic esophageal pH probe studies have major diagnostic and practical limitations. A large international study performed in a primary care setting showed that standard pH probe testing failed to diagnose approximately one-third of patients with established acid reflux disease. Standard esophageal monitoring for LPR is not very sensitive.

Dual pH probe and impedance monitoring can be helpful in diagnosing LPR. The proximal probe is located near the upper esophageal sphincter. A major challenge with dual pH measurement is achieving the optimal location of the upper esophageal probe in relation to the upper esophageal sphincter (UES). If the placement is too low or too high in relation to the UES, the test may show falsely positive or negative results.

An alternative to esophageal pH probes is the pharyngeal pH probe test (Restech system), which measures acid exposure in mid-pharynx. This probe is easy to place, well-tolerated, and potentially more sensitive than traditional esophageal pH testing, capable of detecting liquid and aerosolized droplets. Studies with oropharyngeal pH probes are encouraging though more data in the form of randomized controlled studies are needed [11, 12].

The benefits of the oropharyngeal pH probe are relatively low cost, ease of placement, and minimal discomfort to the patient.

Esophagogastroduodenoscopy (EGD)

Even though EGD does not prove or disprove the diagnosis of LPR, it still plays an important role in patient's assessment and formulating a management plan.

EGD can show the presence of hiatal hernia, active esophagitis, strictures, Schatzki rings, Barrett's esophagus, and other less common esophageal disorders such as achalasia or eosinophilic esophagitis. It also helps to rule out malignancy. EGD is an important preoperative assessment tool in LPR patients who are appropriate candidates for surgical anti-reflux procedures. Some studies have shown that endoscopic symptoms of severe GERD increase the probability of LPR diagnosis.

Pepsin Detection

As we have already discussed, pepsin is not native to the oropharynx or esophagus. Detection of pepsin in the oropharynx is thus indicative of reflux. A recent systematic review reported that pepsin is a reliable marker for diagnosing LPR [13]. Pepsin can be found in trace amounts in the upper aerodigestive tract in healthy asymptomatic individuals but at much lower levels when compared with LPR patients.

A few years ago, a new diagnostic tool, Peptest, emerged which has been available in the UK and Europe and has just been approved by the FDA in the USA in 2017. Peptest is an in vitro lateral flow device that uses monoclonal antibodies to detect pepsin in samples of coughed up saliva/respiratory secretions. Peptest has been shown to be highly accurate and has validated performance measures in detection of GERD. Its sensitivity and specificity are reported to reach 87% [13, 14]. It has a positive predictive value of 85% and negative predictive value of 68% in a blinded study where GERD was confirmed using pH measurement and EGD [14].

Trial of Pharmacotherapy and Reflux Precautions

Good clinical response to empirical therapy with PPIs and H2 blockers can be used to help in the diagnosis of LPR. Good response to treatment may help in avoiding excessive testing and provide quick relief to the patient. Lack of convincing response to acid suppressants and reflux precautions within 4–8 weeks of treatment should prompt the physician to investigate further and clarify the diagnosis.

In spite of many conflicting studies regarding efficacy of these treatments, there is a general consensus to conduct an initial empirical treatment with proton pump inhibitors (PPIs) twice a day for 2–3 months. Good clinical response is considered to be a diagnostic confirmation. Medications, however, reduce only the production of acid in the stomach, but non-acid or weakly acidic reflux may still persist. This may explain the fact that multiple studies show that failure of treatment even with high-dose acid suppression (PPIs given twice a day) may reach up to 30% of cases.

Treatment

Lifestyle Modification

Lifestyle and dietary modifications can be of very significant help in many cases and should be strongly recommended to all patients. Cessation of smoking, stopping alcohol and coffee use, complete avoidance of carbonated drinks, weight loss, no eating before lying down, and elevation of the head of the bed by 4–6 inches are universal recommendations. Avoidance of reflux-triggering foods such as coffee, chocolate, vinegar, mint, fatty and spicy foods, citrus fruits, tomatoes and their products, fresh onions, and garlic can greatly reduce symptoms and significantly augment the effects of medical therapy. There are several books available for the general public that deal especially with the dietary recommendations for patients in GERD and LPR.

Medical Therapy

PPIs are the first-line treatment in pharmacological management of LPR. These medications can provide significant relief for many patients with LPR and have shown their superiority over lifestyle modification alone in alleviating symptoms in LPR patients. PPIs have been shown to improve the RSI scores in LPR patients compared to the placebo-treated group. This is supported by strong evidence both by randomized trials and meta-analyses. Response to treatment, however, has been variable [15–18].

There is still no agreement on what should be the recommended duration of the initial treatment with PPIs. Recommendations vary anywhere between 6 and 12 weeks based on improvement in symptoms and RSI scores. Many patients are unable to stop PPIs due to quick recurrence of symptoms.

Recently, there has been increasing concern regarding the adverse effects of PPIs. Reports of adverse outcomes with long-term PPIs include nephritis, osteoporosis with risk of bone fractures, dementia, increased risk of *C. difficile* infection, and premature death [19]. In light of these reports, the treatment duration of PPIs and risk benefit of long-term treatment should be carefully weighed.

H2 blockers and antacids are used as an adjunct therapy and have limited role as sole therapy in the management of LPR.

Prokinetic agents have also been studied in combination with PPIs in treatment of LPR. The data is not strong for recommendation of prokinetic agents in addition to PPIs.

Endoluminal Treatment

Various endoluminal devices have been approved by FDA for treatment of GERD. These include EsophyX® transoral incisionless fundoplication device, LINX® magnetic beads system, and Stretta® procedure.

EsophyX® is a transoral incisionless fundoplication (TIF) device. There is some data to support the effectiveness of EsophyX® in treating patients with LPR with subsequent improvement in RSI or atypical symptoms. TIF also lead to significant decrease in PPIs use in treated patients. Limited data is available on long-term durability of this treatment. Serious adverse outcome is reported anywhere between 0.14% and 4% [20, 21].

Stretta® procedure is an endoscopic therapy which delivers radiofrequency energy to the lower esophageal sphincter muscle. This causes remodeling of muscle fibers and improved LES function. There is paucity of literature regarding the Stretta® procedure for LPR. In one study, the Stretta® procedure has been shown to be equally effective in improving symptoms of LPR and decrease in use of PPIs [22].

Both abovementioned endoluminal therapies have not shown superiority when compared to 360 degree (Nissen) fundoplication. Some studies have shown inferior results when compared with Nissen fundoplication, whereas others have shown these to be equivalent to partial (Toupet and Dor) fundoplication.

More data on long-term follow-up of endoluminally treated patients is needed to decide the effectiveness of these treatment strategies.

Surgical Therapy

Fundoplication or Anti-Reflux Surgery

Anti-reflux surgery has been reserved as a treatment modality for medically refractory LPR, patients who do not want to take long-term PPI, and severe GERD associated with LPR.

Preoperative planning and workup is an essential prerequisite for anti-reflux surgery.

EGD is usually the initial step. A barium esophagogram helps in assessing the anatomical and, perhaps, functional aspect of the esophagus and helps in ruling out achalasia and large hiatal hernias. It serves as a good test for follow-up post anti-reflux surgery.

Esophageal manometry is important in determining presence of achalasia and other motility disorders of the esophagus. One should proceed to full fundoplication (Nissen) only if the motility is normal (>70% normal swallows). Otherwise, one should do a partial fundoplication (commonly Toupet).

Dual pH monitoring and impedance measurement with or without oropharyngeal pH monitoring support LPR diagnosis and are usually part of preoperative workup.

A laparoscopic Nissen fundoplication is a standard 2–3-cm-long, complete 360 degree loose gastric fundal wrap, whereas a Toupet fundoplication is a 270 degree partial wrap. Anti-reflux surgery has good outcomes in carefully selected LPR patients, but the results are slightly inferior when compared with GERD outcomes [23].

Cough has been shown to improve after anti-reflux surgery. The response rate is variable anywhere between 30% and 80% in literature. The difference between Nissen and Toupet in relieving cough symptom of LPR has been shown to be not significant in one study [24].

Hoarseness, one of the common symptoms of LPR, is also shown to improve after anti-reflux surgery. The data is limited, and no trials have been done to compare various surgical techniques.

The above statements are supported by Brown et al. in a large prospective study which reported significant improvement in atypical symptoms of GERD, cough, wheeze, and hoarseness, in patients undergoing anti-reflux surgery (Nissen) for GERD [25].

Zhang et al. reported improvement in RSI score in LPR patients after Nissen fundoplication when compared with PPI group. LPR was diagnosed using oropharyngeal pH monitoring and using high-resolution manometry and endoscopy for associated GERD [26]. At 2-year follow-up, independence from PPI was marked in surgery group, and overall satisfaction was better in surgery group.

Complaints of shortness of breath and difficulties with breathing (often associated with asthma) have also been shown to improve with surgery (Nissen fundoplication) when compared with medical treatment group [27], with a decrease in beta-agonist, and oral corticosteroid use in asthmatics has also been reported after Nissen fundoplication [28].

New Frontiers

Epidermal growth factor (EGF) is a cell growth-stimulating cytokine and plays a role in cell differentiation. It can be a potential marker for LPR diagnosis. Salivary EGF levels were found to be low in patients with reflux laryngitis (LPR) when compared with healthy controls. But there was no change in EGF level posttreatment [29].

The following biomarkers have been identified in medial arytenoid biopsy specimens of LPR patients: (1) mucosal defense markers MUC2, MUC5B, and CDH1, (2) squamous/columnar marker KRT14, and (3) inflammatory markers CD1d, CRNN, and TGFb-1. These biomarkers have promising potential in identification and probably in the diagnosis of LPR [30].

Conclusion

Despite having a significant disease burden, the awareness of LPR in the medical community remains low. As a result, it is underdiagnosed and undertreated. LPR requires a high degree of clinical suspicion and experience on behalf of the physician to diagnose and treat. For patients who do not respond to medical therapy, laparoscopic fundoplication offers great relief of symptoms.

References

1. Koufman JA. The otolaryngologic manifestations of gastroesophageal reflux disease (GERD): a clinical investigation of 225 patients using ambulatory 24-hour pH monitoring and an experimental investigation of the role of acid and pepsin in the development of laryngeal. Laryngoscope. 1991;101:1–78.
2. Koufman JA, Aviv JE, Casiano RR, Shaw GY. Laryngopharyngeal reflux: position statement of the committee on speech, voice, and swallowing disorders of the American Academy of Otolaryngology-Head and Neck Surgery. Otolaryngol Head Neck Surg. 2002;127:32–5.
3. Koufman J. Prevalence of reflux in 113 consecutive patients with laryngeal and voice disorders. Otolaryngol Head Neck Surg. 2000;123:385–8.

4. Francis DO, Rymer JA, Slaughter JC, et al. High economic burden of caring for patients with suspected Extraesophageal reflux. Am J Gastroenterol. 2013;108:905–11.
5. Peters JH, Demeester TR. Gastroesophageal barrier. 7th ed: Shackelford's Surg Aliment Tract; 2007. https://doi.org/10.1016/B978-1-4377-2206-2.00015-4.
6. Samuels TL, Johnston N. Pepsin as a causal agent of inflammation during nonacidic reflux. Otolaryngol Head Neck Surg. 2009;141:559–63.
7. Johnston N, Knight J, Dettmar PW, Lively MO, Koufman J. Pepsin and carbonic anhydrase Isoenzyme III as diagnostic markers for Laryngopharyngeal reflux disease. Laryngoscope. 2004;114:2129–34.
8. Sasaki CT, Marotta J, Chow J, Hundal J, Eisen RN. Bile-induced laryngitis: is there a basis in evidence? Ann Otol Rhinol Laryngol. 2005;114:192–7.
9. Belafsky PC, Postma GN, Koufman JA. Validity and reliability of the reflux symptom index (RSI). J Voice. 2002;16:274–7.
10. Belafsky PC, Postma GN, Koufman JA. The validity and reliability of the reflux finding score (RFS). Laryngoscope. 2001;111:1313–7.
11. Wiener GJ, Tsukashima R, Kelly C, Wolf E, Schmeltzer M, Bankert C, Fisk L, Vaezi M. Oropharyngeal pH monitoring for the detection of liquid and aerosolized supraesophageal gastric reflux. J Voice. 2009;23:498–504.
12. Desjardin M, Roman S, Des SB, Gourcerol G, Coffin B, Ropert A, Mion F, Zerbib F. Pharyngeal pH alone is not reliable for the detection of pharyngeal reflux events:a study with oesophageal and pharyngeal pH-impedance monitoring. United Eur Gastroenterol J. 2013;1:438–44.
13. Calvo-Henríquez C, Ruano-Ravina A, Vaamonde P, Martínez-Capoccioni G, et al. Is pepsin a reliable marker of Laryngopharyngeal reflux? A systematic review. Otolaryngol Neck Surg. 2017;19459981770943
14. Saritas Yuksel E, Hong SKS, Strugala V, Slaughter JC, Goutte M, Garrett CG, Dettmar PW, Vaezi MF. Rapid salivary pepsin test: blinded assessment of test performance in gastroesophageal reflux disease. Laryngoscope. 2012;122:1312–6.
15. Chappity P, Kumar R, Deka RC, Chokkalingam V, Saraya A, Sikka K. Proton pump inhibitors versus solitary lifestyle modification in Management of Laryngopharyngeal Reflux and Evaluating who is at risk: scenario in a developing country. Clin Med Insights Ear Nose Throat. 2014;7:1–5. https://doi.org/10.4137/CMENT.S13799.
16. Guo H, Ma H, Wang J. Proton pump inhibitor therapy for the treatment of laryngopharyngeal reflux. J Clin Gastroenterol. 2015;50:1–6.
17. Wei C. A meta-analysis for the role of proton pump inhibitor therapy in patients with laryngopharyngeal reflux. Eur Arch Otorhinolaryngol. 2016;273:3795–801.
18. Lam PKY, Ng ML, Cheung TK, Wong BYH, Tan VPY, Fong DYT, Wei WI, Wong BCY. Rabeprazole is effective in treating laryngopharyngeal reflux in a randomized placebo-controlled trial. Clin Gastroenterol Hepatol. 2010;8:770–6.
19. Xie Y, Bowe B, Li T, Xian H, Yan Y, Al-Aly Z. Risk of death among users of proton pump inhibitors: a longitudinal observational cohort study of United States veterans. BMJ Open. 2017;7:e015735.
20. Trad KS, Turgeon DG, Deljkich E. Long-term outcomes after transoral incisionless fundoplication in patients with GERD and LPR symptoms. Surg Endosc Other Interv Tech. 2012;26:650–60.
21. Testoni PA, Testoni S, Mazzoleni G, Vailati C, Passaretti S. Long-term efficacy of transoral incisionless fundoplication with Esophyx (Tif 2.0) and factors affecting outcomes in GERD patients followed for up to 6 years: a prospective single-center study. Surg Endosc Other Interv Tech. 2015;29:2770–80.
22. Yan C, Liang WT, Wang ZG, Hu ZW, Wu JM, Zhang C, Chen MP. Comparison of Stretta procedure and toupet fundoplication for gastroesophageal reflux disease-related extra-esophageal symptoms. World J Gastroenterol. 2015;21:12882–7.
23. Sidhwa F, Moore A, Alligood E, Fisichella PM. Diagnosis and treatment of the Extraesophageal manifestations of gastroesophageal reflux disease. Ann Surg. 2017;265:63–7.
24. Koch OO, Antoniou SA, Kaindlstorfer A, Asche KU, Granderath FA, Pointner R. Effectiveness of laparoscopic total and partial fundoplication on extraesophageal manifestations of gastro-

esophageal reflux disease: a randomized study. Surg Laparosc Endosc Percutaneous Tech. 2012;22:387–91.

25. Brown SR, Gyawali CP, Melman L, Jenkins ED, Bader J, Frisella MM, Brunt LM, Eagon JC, Matthews BD. Clinical outcomes of atypical extra-esophageal reflux symptoms following laparoscopic antireflux surgery. Surg Endosc Other Interv Tech. 2011;25:3852–8.
26. Zhang C, Hu Z-W, Yan C, Wu Q, Wu J-M, Du X, Liu D-G, Luo T, Li F, Wang Z-G. Nissen fundoplication *vs* proton pump inhibitors for laryngopharyngeal reflux based on pH-monitoring and symptom-scale. World J Gastroenterol. 2017;23:3546.
27. Sontag SJ, O'Connell S, Khandelwal S, Greenlee H, Schnell T, Nemchausky B, Chejfec G, Miller T, Seidel J, Sonnenberg A. Asthmatics with gastroesophageal reflux: long term results of a randomized trial of medical and surgical antireflux therapies. Am J Gastroenterol. 2003;98:987–99.
28. Da SAPC, Tercioti-Junior V, Lopes LR, Coelho-Neto JDS, Bertanha L, Rodrigues PRDF, Andreollo NA. Laparoscopic antireflux surgery in patients with extra esophageal symptoms related to asthma. Arq Bras Cir Dig. 2014;27:92–5.
29. Eckley CA, Sardinha LR, Rizzo LV. Salivary concentration of epidermal growth factor in adults with reflux laryngitis before and after treatment. Ann Otol Rhinol Laryngol. 2013;122:440–4.
30. Wood JM, Hussey DJ, Woods CM, Astill D, I Watson D, Lee B, Carney AS. Does gene expression in laryngeal subsites differ between patients with laryngopharyngeal reflux and controls? Clin Otolaryngol. 2018;43(1):158–63. https://doi.org/10.1111/coa.12918.

Management of Esophageal Peptic Stricture

10

Jeffrey W. Hazey and Mazen R. Al-Mansour

Introduction

Since the introduction of proton pump inhibitors, the incidence of esophageal peptic stricture (EPS) has declined significantly [1]. Nonetheless, EPS remains a common cause of dysphagia and is the most common cause of benign esophageal strictures. Up to 25% of benign esophageal strictures result from other causes including eosinophilic esophagitis, radiation, caustic ingestion, and iatrogenic (following creation of surgical anastomoses, sclerotherapy, mucosal ablation, and endoscopic resections). EPS is typically a manifestation of prolonged gastro-esophageal reflux disease (GERD). Chronic exposure of the distal esophagus to gastric acid results in erosive esophagitis with subsequent collagen deposition, fibrosis, and luminal narrowing. These strictures are usually located at the distal esophagus and are short in length. EPS affects only 10 percent of GERD patients presenting for medical treatment. The subset of patients with GERD that develop EPS tend to be older, have longer duration of symptoms, have higher incidence of esophageal dysmotility, and have lower esophageal sphincter pressures on manometry [2, 3]. This chapter focuses on the evaluation and different methods and equipment for the treatment of EPS.

J. W. Hazey (✉)
Division of General and Gastrointestinal Surgery, Department of Surgery, The Ohio State University, Wexner Medical Center, Columbus, OH, USA
e-mail: Jeffrey.hazey@memorialohio.com

M. R. Al-Mansour
Department of General and Gastrointestinal Surgery, The Ohio State University, Wexner Medical Center, Columbus, OH, USA

J. Grams et al. (eds.), *The SAGES Manual of Foregut Surgery*,
https://doi.org/10.1007/978-3-319-96122-4_10

Indications

Patients with EPS most often present with dysphagia. As the esophagus narrows, solid food dysphagia progresses over time to affect swallowing of liquids as well. Gastric acid suppression and esophageal dilation are the backbones of the treatment of benign esophageal stricture and have a long track record of efficacy and safety. The goals of treatment of EPS are to alleviate dysphagia, allow oral nutrition, prevent aspiration risk, and prevent stricture recurrence.

Esophageal dilation is contraindicated in the cace of significant coagulopathy and severe cardiopulmonary disease, in the case of malignant stricture, and in the setting of acute esophageal perforation.

Patient Evaluation Prior to Dilation

Evaluation of patients with suspected EPS usually includes contrast esophagogram and endoscopy. Barium esophagogram is often the first test obtained to evaluate dysphagia. It allows delineation of the esophagogastric anatomy and helps characterize the stricture (diameter, length, location, tortuosity, and number of strictures). In addition, it helps identify other anatomic abnormalities such as esophageal diverticula and hiatal hernias, findings that may influence treatment decisions.

Endoscopic evaluation of the stricture allows visual inspection of the mucosa along with determination of the diameter of the stricture. It also allows mucosal sampling, which is essential in ruling out malignancy and other benign etiologies of esophageal stricture such as eosinophilic esophagitis, which is associated with increased incidence of dilation-induced perforation.

Esophageal Dilation

The mainstay of the treatment of EPS is esophageal dilation and acid suppressive therapy. Mechanical esophageal dilation (bougienage) has been described for centuries. Carved whalebones were used for this purpose in the seventeenth century, and the initial reports of bougienage are traced back to the nineteenth century [4, 5].

Instruments

There are two main types of esophageal dilators. Table 10.1 provides a summary of those dilators:

A. *Mechanical dilators (bougie type)* are long tapered tubes that are pushed transorally down into the esophagus. Different types of mechanical dilators exist; the most common are:

– *Weighted dilators* (e.g., Maloney and Hurst dilators): these are flexible rubber weighted tubes that are passed blindly without the need for a guidewire. They were previously weighted with mercury, which is now substituted with tungsten due to concerns of leakage and mercury poisoning. They can have either a tapered tip (Maloney) or a rounded tip (Hurst) (Fig. 10.1).

Table 10.1 Types of esophageal dilators

Dilator	Description	Need for guidewire	Reusable
Mechanical (bougie) dilators			
Maloney	Tapered tip Flexible rubber weighted with mercury or tungsten	No	Yes
Hurst	Rounded tip Flexible rubber weighted with mercury or tungsten	No	Yes
Savary-Gilliard® (Wilson-Cook, Inc., Winston-Salem, NC)	Long tapered tip Polyvinyl Radiopaque marker at the base of taper identifying the point of maximum diameter	Yes	Yes
American Dilation System® (CR Bard, Inc., Billerica, MA)	Flexible, tapered short tip Polyvinyl Radiopaque throughout length of dilator	Yes	Yes
Eder-Puestow	Olive tip Metal	Yes	Yes
Balloon dilators			
TTS balloon	Passed via the working channel of the endoscope	Available in some models	No
OTW balloon	Passed over a guide wire	Yes	No

TTS through-the-scope, *OTW* over-the-wire

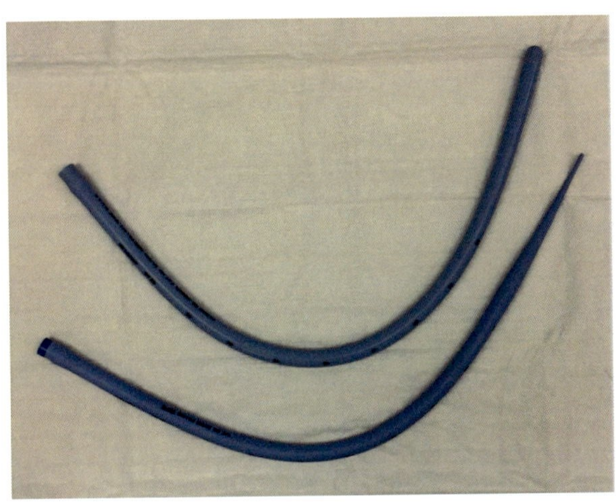

Fig. 10.1 Weighted mechanical dilators: Maloney dilator at the bottom, Hurst dilator at the top

- *Wire-guided dilators* (e.g., Savary-Gilliard dilator, American Dilation System): these dilators are made of polyvinyl chloride and are passed over a guidewire (Fig. 10.2).

Mechanical dilators come in multiple sizes (5–20 mm or 15–60 F). As they are pushed in, they incrementally exert both radial and longitudinal (shear) forces that are thought to disrupt the fibrous tissue causing the stricture to stretch. As the dilator is advanced, the stricture is stretched gradually starting at the proximal end.

B. *Balloon dilators* can be classified into two types:
- *Through-the-scope (TTS) balloon*
- *Over-the-wire (OTW) balloon*

Balloon dilators exert radial dilation force simultaneously across the length of the stricture which results in disruption of the fibrous tissue with subsequent relief of the stricture [6, 7]. The balloons are pressurized and come in different sizes (6–20 mm) that correspond to different preset pressures. Some TTS balloons come with a single size, and some can expand to three different sizes (with 1–1.5 mm increments) depending on the applied atmospheric pressure. The latter are often referred to as controlled radial expansion (CRE) balloons. CRE balloons allow serial dilations to be performed without exchanging the balloon (Fig. 10.3).

Technique

Stricture dilation is usually performed as an ambulatory procedure and is mostly performed in the endoscopy unit. The patient is instructed to avoid oral intake overnight. Anticoagulants and antiplatelet agents are held (if needed) in preparation for the procedure to minimize bleeding complications. Topical application of a local anesthetic to the throat may be used to minimize gagging. Moderate sedation, deep sedation, or general anesthesia can be used according to patient factors and endoscopist preferences. Antibiotic prophylaxis is not warranted even in patients with

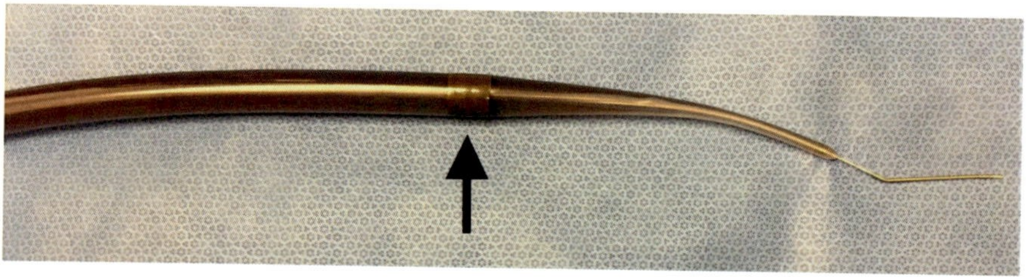

Fig. 10.2 Savary dilator, black arrow points to the radiopaque marker at the base of the taper marking the point of maximum diameter

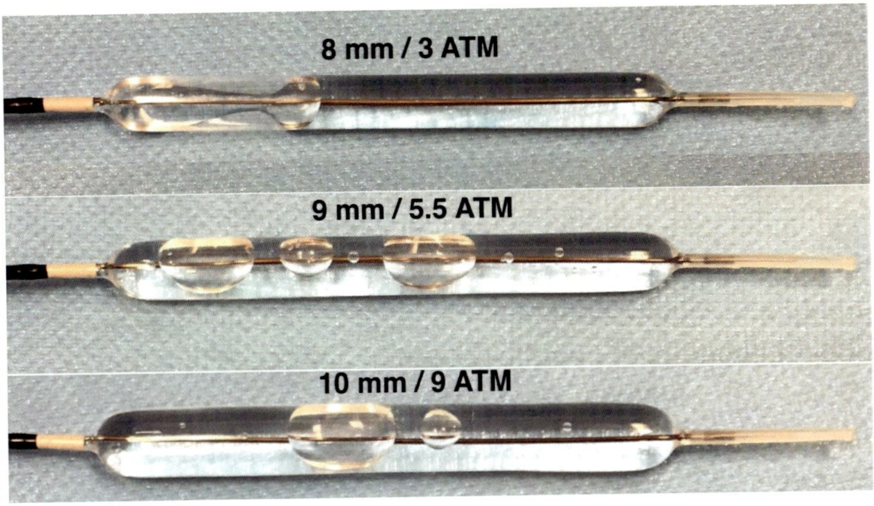

Fig. 10.3 Controlled radial expansion (CRE) through-the-scope (TTS) balloon

high risk for bacterial endocarditis according to the guidelines of the American Society for Gastrointestinal Endoscopy and the American Heart Association [8, 9]. The patient is positioned in the left lateral decubitus position with the head of the bed elevated, although supine placement in patients undergoing general anesthesia is an acceptable alternative. Weighted dilators can be passed in the upright sitting position. To obtain safe and adequate dilation of complex strictures, serial dilations over multiple sessions might be necessary.

Whether using a mechanical dilator or a balloon dilator, the diameter of the initial dilator should be the same as the diameter of the stricture itself. This could be estimated by radiological evaluation or by comparison to the diameter of the endoscope [5]. It is helpful to know that the diameters of the standard esophagogastroduodenoscopy scope and the nasopharyngeal (NP) scope are 8.8 mm and 5.9 mm, respectively.

Mechanical dilation When a Savary dilator is used, a guidewire is passed across the narrowed segment. This could be performed using endoscopic or fluoroscopic guidance. If the endoscope can traverse the stenosis, fluoroscopy is not necessary. The wire can be passed via the working channel of the endoscope into the stomach under direct visualization. However, the use of fluoroscopy is recommended when the endoscope cannot traverse the stenosis in order to confirm appropriate intraluminal placement.

Visualizing the wire below the diaphragm on fluoroscopy and the lack of resistance to wire advancement ensures appropriate intraluminal positioning of the wire. The scope is then withdrawn while keeping the wire in place. The dilator is lubricated generously and is then pushed over the wire while paying attention to the resistance met and observing the presence of blood when the dilator is withdrawn.

The lack of resistance and blood suggests that the dilator was too small and a larger diameter dilator should be used instead. If significant resistance is met, the operator should stop and downsize the dilator in order to avoid esophageal perforation. Maloney and Hurst dilators are utilized in a similar fashion, albeit without the need for wire guidance. Studies showed conflicting results regarding the utility of fluoroscopy in improving the outcomes of mechanical dilation [10–16].

It is imperative that the endoscopist ensures that the entire tapered portion of the dilator traverses the stricture. This ensures adequate dilation to the desired target diameter and also allows for accurate documentation of the diameter of the stricture. Wire-guided mechanical dilators have radiopaque portions that allow fluoroscopic confirmation of full dilation. When using weighted dilators, the endoscopist can use the measurement markings on the dilator itself. After determining the distances of the proximal and distal ends of the stricture from the incisors, the dilator is pushed until the base of the taper (point of maximum diameter) has passed through the distal end of the stricture. Maloney dilators have two sets of measurement markings that are often color-coded. The first set determines the distance from the tip of the dilator, and other set describes the distance from the base of the taper (point of maximum diameter). The endoscopist should ensure familiarity with the measurement markings prior to commencing the dilation process.

Through-the-scope (TTS) balloon dilation The balloon is passed via the working channel of the endoscope beyond the stricture. It is then pulled back so that the center of the balloon lies against the area of maximal luminal narrowing. The balloon is then inflated to its smaller diameter with the inflation maintained for 30–60 s. Using commercially available inflation devices, application of the appropriate level of atmospheric pressure can be ensured (Fig. 10.4). As with mechanical dilation, resistance to the inflation can be appreciated by the assistant while the balloon is being inflated and is used to judge the degree of inflation. If appropriate level of

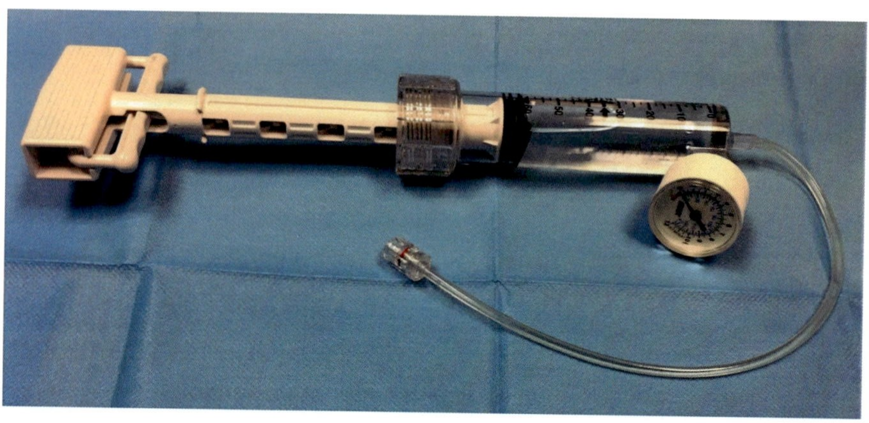

Fig. 10.4 Inflation pump. Allows accurate inflation of the balloon dilator to the appropriate diameter

resistance is noted, the balloon can be inflated to a larger diameter. It is necessary to maintain the position of the balloon by keeping it close to the tip of the endoscope and holding it in place as it enters the endoscope working channel to prevent antegrade or retrograde sliding (Fig. 10.5). If fluoroscopy is being used, the balloon can be filled with diluted water-soluble contrast. As the stricture is being dilated, the operator can observe the relief of the "balloon waist" indicating adequate stretching of the stricture. As is the case with wire-guided mechanical dilators, the TTS balloons can also be passed over a wire if the stricture is too narrow to allow the passage of the endoscope (Fig. 10.6).

Over-the-wire (OTW) balloon dilation After passing a guidewire through the narrowed segment as described above, the balloon is passed under fluoroscopic guidance over the wire across the stricture and then pulled back to lay inside the stricture. It is then inflated with dilute water-soluble contrast while watching the balloon waist develop and subsequently disappear by fluoroscopy. This, in addition to the free movement of the inflated balloon across the dilated stricture, confirms adequate dilation [17].

When using mechanical dilators, we recommend using a maximum of three serial mechanical dilations per session without exceeding 6 F (2 mm) increase in the stricture size. When using TTS balloons, our practice is to use three

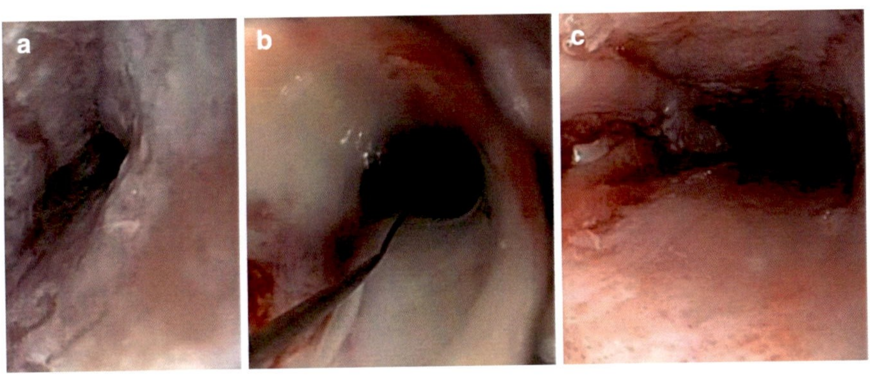

Fig. 10.5 Endoscopic view of balloon dilation. (**a**) Esophageal stricture before dilation. (**b**) Endoscopic view during balloon dilation: by pulling the balloon closer to the scope, the dilation process can be visualized endoscopically. (**c**) The appearance of the stricture following dilation demonstrating the larger luminal diameter

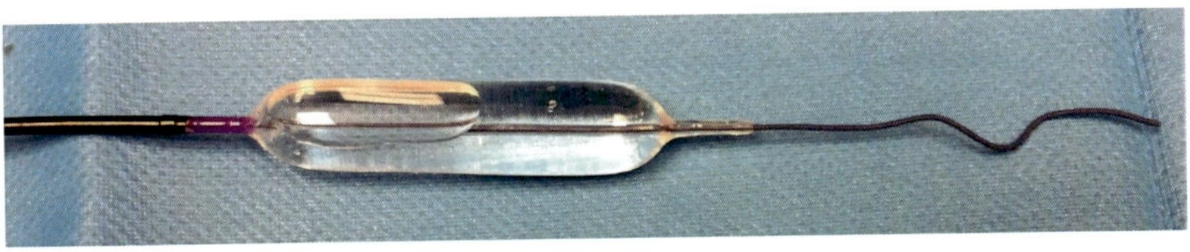

Fig. 10.6 Wire-guided through-the-scope (TTS) balloon

increments in size (e.g., 12, 13.5, 15 mm) during a single session. A more conservative approach may be used for tighter and longer strictures to minimize complication risks.

The number of sessions is guided by the response to dilation and the patient's symptoms. In many patients with simple strictures, adequate dilation could be achieved in a single session. Some patients undergoing initial dilation of tight strictures may require repeat dilations every 5–7 days. The frequency of dilations can be reduced subsequently and is tailored to the patient's symptoms. Generally, the largest dilator size used in the last session could be used as the first dilator size for the current session, keeping in mind that strictures tend to shrink. It is our practice to perform endoscopic assessment of the diameter of the stricture prior to repeat dilation. Other factors that may help determine the size of the subsequent dilators is the degree of resistance encountered during the previous dilation session and the patient's tolerance to the procedure. Generally speaking, dilation to 18 mm (54 F) allows intake of a regular diet. Patients tend to report solid food dysphagia with a 13 mm (39 F) esophageal diameter. These values provide a rough guide as to the end point of dilation. It is rarely necessary to dilate an esophageal stricture beyond 20 mm (60 F).

Outcomes Both mechanical and balloon dilators are highly effective in alleviating the symptoms of esophageal stricture [18]. Studies comparing the outcomes and complication rates of esophageal dilation using mechanical and balloon dilators showed variable results without clear advantage of one system over the other [19–22]. The choice of dilation system should be based on the experience of the endoscopist with the dilation device. Blind passage of Maloney dilator should be avoided in complex strictures and when other anastomotic factors (e.g., large hiatal hernia or esophageal diverticulum) are present due to the increased risk of perforation [23].

Complications Esophageal dilation inherently results in disruption of the esophageal wall at the site of the stricture. Minor bleeding resulting from mucosal tears at the time of the procedure is an expected finding when successful dilation is accomplished. Perforation is the most common major complication following esophageal dilation. The incidence of this complication is estimated to range between 0.1% and 0.8%. Risk factors for perforation include underlying inflammatory disorders (e.g., eosinophilic esophagitis, severe erosive esophagitis), a history of prior perforation, high inflation pressures, prior radiation exposure, endoscopist inexperience, a large hiatal hernia, and blind passage of dilators in complex strictures [23–26]. The risk of perforation seems to be more related to the pathology of the stricture rather than the method of dilation. This serious complication is associated with 20% risk of mortality [27]. Esophageal perforation should be suspected in patients who develop chest pain, abdominal pain, tachycardia, tachypnea, and/or fever after dilation. Early identification of esophageal perforation is paramount since delays in diagnosis and treatment can result in increased morbidity and mortality rates. The diagnosis can be confirmed by contrast esophagogram and/or chest CT scan. The details of management of esophageal perforation are beyond the scope of this chapter, but the treatment options can be generally classified into medical, endoscopic, or surgical treatments. Medical treatment includes avoidance of oral intake, nutritional support with parenteral nutrition, drainage of infected fluid collections, and broad-spectrum antibiotics. Endoscopic treatment usually includes the placement of a plastic or covered metallic stent across the perforation. Other endoscopic treatment options include using clips to close the defect and endoluminal vacuum therapy. Surgical treatment might be necessary particularly if the diagnosis is delayed and may include surgical repair, diversion, or esophagectomy. The choice of treatment is guided by clinical and radiological assessment.

Significant bleeding is uncommon after esophageal dilation. The incidence rate is estimated at 0.2% [24]. Unless coagulopathy is present, the bleeding is usually self-limited, and watchful waiting is often all that is needed. More significant bleeding requires endoscopic evaluation and treatment.

Chest pain can be observed in some patients even in the absence of perforation. It is usually a self-limited problem; however, esophageal perforation needs to be excluded in these patients.

Esophageal dilation is the endoscopic procedure with the highest risk of transient bacteremia. Bacteremia rates ranging from 22% to 72% were observed after esophageal dilation [28–30]. Complications resulting from bacteremia are infrequent; therefore, antibiotic prophylaxis for bacterial endocarditis is not recommended for these procedures [8, 9].

Management after dilation Gastric acid suppression is mandatory following dilation for EPS. Persistent exposure to gastric acid can result in recurrent strictures due to subsequent esophagitis and fibrosis. Studies of the natural history of EPS after dilation before the widespread use of proton pump inhibitors (PPIs) estimated a 50% rate of recurrence [31, 32]. PPIs have been shown to reduce the need for repeat dilations and improve dysphagia scores after EPS dilations. PPIs are more effective in preventing restenosis than H2 receptor blockers [33–36].

EPS is more likely to recur in patients who report persistent heartburn including those on PPIs [37]. These patients may benefit from antireflux surgery (fundoplication) after the stricture has been appropriately dilated.

Refractory Strictures

Some patients continue to have persistent symptoms despite aggressive dilation schedules and acid suppressive therapy. Self-dilation at home using Maloney dilators has been described [38, 39]. This requires a highly motivated patient, and many patients are not appropriate candidates. Therapeutic options for patients with recalcitrant EPS include intralesional corticosteroid injections, esophageal stent placement, endoscopic electroincision, topical application of Mitomycin C, and surgical treatment.

Intralesional corticosteroid injection has been employed to prevent restenosis following dilation [40–42]. While the exact mechanism is not well understood, it is thought that corticosteroids may impair collagen deposition and enhance local collagen breakdown and therefore prevent stricture recurrence [43]. A solution of triamcinolone acetonide (Kenalog) with a concentration of 10–40 mg/mL is injected at four quadrants at the narrowest portion of the stricture using a sclerotherapy needle just prior to dilation. A randomized sham-controlled trial has shown significant reduction in EPS recurrence after dilation (13% versus 60%) in patients who received the corticosteroid injection [44].

Esophageal stents have been used for the management of benign esophageal strictures including EPS. The stent applies radial pressure to the stricture and is ideally left in place for 6 weeks to allow tissue remodeling in order to prevent recurrence. Uncovered metal stents should *not* be used for benign esophageal strictures, since tissue ingrowth prevents stent removal and can lead to in-stent stenosis and fistula formation. Similarly, partially covered self-expanding metal stents (PCSEMS) may also get embedded at the ends making subsequent removal challenging. Fully covered self-expanding metal stents (FCSEMS) have a silicone or polyurethane cover that prevents tissue ingrowth and allows removability. Recent guidelines published by European Society of Gastrointestinal Endoscopy recommend using FCSEMS over PCSEMS for benign esophageal stricture [45, 46]. Nonmetal stents (including plastic and biodegradable stents) have also been used for this purpose.

Inconsistent outcomes and high rates of complications have limited the use of esophageal stents for management of esophageal strictures [47–51]. The most common problem is stent migration. A flared flanges (dog bone) design where the diameter of the stent at both ends is larger than the diameter at the middle seems to help minimize this problem (Fig. 10.7). Esophageal stents vary in length (5–15 cm), shaft diameter (12–23 mm), and flare diameter (20–30 mm). Other serious complications of esophageal stents including perforation, bleeding, and fistula formation have been reported. Stent intolerance in the form of chest pain is also another common problem. Patients frequently describe severe heartburn when the stent is placed across the lower esophageal sphincter. A meta-analysis of 18 studies

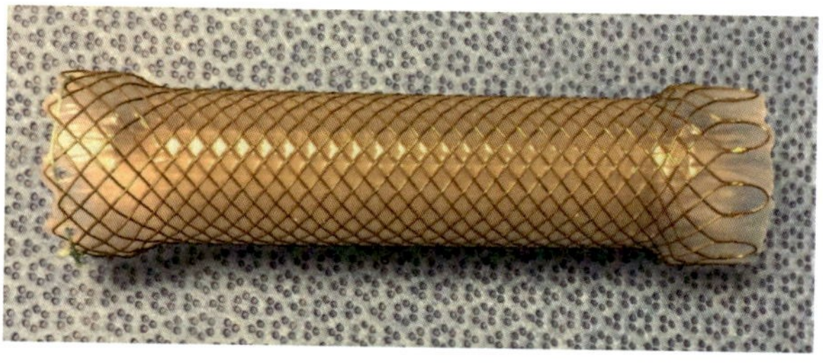

Fig. 10.7 Full covered self-expanding metal stent with flared flanges

and 444 patients who had esophageal stent placement for the management of benign esophageal strictures including EPS has shown 41 percent clinical success rate, with a migration rate of 29 percent and a 21 percent adverse event rate. No clinically significant difference in outcomes or complications was noted between SEPS, FCSEMS, and biodegradable stents [52]. Table 10.2 summarizes the types of stents used for the management of benign esophageal strictures.

Endoscopic incisional therapy has been described in the management of refractory esophageal stricture particularly anastomotic strictures and Schatzki's ring. An electrosurgical needle knife is used to create radial incisions at the stricture, which allows dilation to a larger diameter [53]. Its use in the treatment of EPS has not been adequately examined [54, 55].

Topical application of Mitomycin C (an anti-neoplastic agent with anti-fibroblastic effects) has been described in cases of recalcitrant strictures particularly in the pediatric population. These include strictures resulting from radiation, caustic ingestion, and postsurgical (tracheoesophageal fistula correction) and endoscopic mucosal resections. The effectiveness of Mitomycin C as an adjunct to dilation for EPS needs further investigation [56, 57].

Table 10.2 Types of esophageal stents used for benign esophageal strictures

Stent	Examples	Description	Removable
SEPS	Polyflex® (Rüsch, Kernen, Germany)	Polyester braid with full silicone covering	Yes
Biodegradable stent	SX-Ella BD® (Ella-CS, Hradec, Kralove, Czech Republic)	Made of dissolvable polymers or absorbable suture material (e.g., polydioxanone)	Not needed
FCSEMS	Alimaxx-ES® (Merit Medical Systems Inc., South Jordan, Utah, USA) Wallflex® (Boston Scientific Inc., Natick, MA) Bonastent® (EndoChoice Inc., Alpharetta, GA) Evolution® (Cook Medical Inc., Winston-Salem, NC)	Silicone, polyester, or polyurethane coated, with a scaffolding of Nitinol, stainless steel, or Elgiloy. Come in either straight design or with flared flange (dog bone) design	Yes
PCSEMS	Ultraflex® (Microvasive/Boston Scientific Corp, Natick, MA, USA)	Silicone, polyester, or polyurethane coated, with a scaffolding of Nitinol, stainless steel, or Eligiloy except at the ends	Yes but removal can be challenging

SEPS self-expanding plastic stent, *FCSEMS* fully covered self-expanding metal stent, *PCSEMS* partially covered self-expanding metal stents

While uncommon, some strictures are resistant to endoscopic therapy, and these patients should be considered for surgical therapy including esophagectomy with reconstruction using gastric, jejunal, or colonic conduits.

Conclusion

Esophageal peptic stricture is a manifestation of chronic gastroesophageal reflux disease characterized by fibrotic narrowing of the distal esophagus resulting in dysphagia. Gastric acid suppression and esophageal dilation are the mainstays of treatment. Mechanical dilation (bougienage) and balloon dilation are similarly efficacious and safe methods of esophageal stricture dilation. Esophageal perforation is the most common serious complication. Refractory strictures can be treated with endoscopic stenting or intralesional corticosteroid injection.

References

1. Ruigómez A, García Rodríguez LA, Wallander M-A, Johansson S, Eklund S. Esophageal stricture: incidence, treatment patterns, and recurrence rate. Am J Gastroenterol. 2006;101:2685–92.
2. Marks RD, Richter JE. Peptic strictures of the esophagus. Am J Gastroenterol. 1993;88:1160–73.
3. Ahtaridis G, Snape WJ, Cohen S. Clinical and manometric findings in benign peptic strictures of the esophagus. Dig Dis Sci. 1979;24:858–61.
4. Spiess AE, Kahrilas PJ. Treating achalasia: from whalebone to laparoscope. JAMA. 1998;280:638–42.
5. Ferguson DD. Evaluation and management of benign esophageal strictures. Dis Esophagus Off J Int Soc Dis Esophagus. 2005;18:359–64.
6. Abele JE. The physics of esophageal dilatation. Hepato-Gastroenterology. 1992;39:486–9.
7. McLean GK, LeVeen RF. Shear stress in the performance of esophageal dilation: comparison of balloon dilation and bougienage. Radiology. 1989;172:983–6.
8. Wilson W, Taubert KA, Gewitz M, Lockhart PB, Baddour LM, Levison M, Bolger A, Cabell CH, Takahashi M, Baltimore RS, Newburger JW, Strom BL, Tani LY, Gerber M, Bonow RO, Pallasch T, Shulman ST, Rowley AH, Burns JC, Ferrieri P, Gardner T, Goff D, Durack DT, American Heart Association Rheumatic Fever, Endocarditis, and Kawasaki Disease Committee, American Heart Association Council on Cardiovascular Disease in the Young, American Heart Association Council on Clinical Cardiology, American Heart Association Council on Cardiovascular Surgery and Anesthesia, Quality of Care and Outcomes Research Interdisciplinary Working Group. Prevention of infective endocarditis: guidelines from the American Heart Association: a guideline from the American Heart Association Rheumatic Fever, Endocarditis, and Kawasaki Disease Committee, Council on Cardiovascular Disease in the Young, and the Council on Clinical Cardiology, Council on Cardiovascular Surgery and Anesthesia, and the Quality of Care and Outcomes Research Interdisciplinary Working Group. Circulation. 2007;116:1736–54.
9. ASGE STANDARDS OF PRACTICE COMMITTEE, Banerjee S, Shen B, Baron TH, Nelson DB, Anderson MA, Cash BD, Dominitz JA, Gan SI, Harrison ME, Ikenberry SO, Jagannath SB, Lichtenstein D, Fanelli RD, Lee K, van Guilder T, Stewart LE. Antibiotic prophylaxis for GI endoscopy. Gastrointest Endosc. 2008;67:791–8.
10. Kozarek RA, Patterson DJ, Ball TJ, Gelfand MG, Jiranek GE, Bredfeldt JE, Brandabur JJ, Wolfsen HW, Raltz SL. Esophageal dilation can be done safely using selective fluoroscopy and single dilating sessions. J Clin Gastroenterol. 1995;20:184–8.
11. Ho SB, Cass O, Katsman RJ, Lipschultz EM, Metzger RJ, Onstad GR, Silvis SE. Fluoroscopy is not necessary for Maloney dilation of chronic esophageal strictures. Gastrointest Endosc. 1995;41:11–4.

12. McClave SA, Brady PG, Wright RA, Goldschmid S, Minocha A. Does fluoroscopic guidance for Maloney esophageal dilation impact on the clinical endpoint of therapy: relief of dysphagia and achievement of luminal patency. Gastrointest Endosc. 1996;43:93–7.
13. Tucker LE. The importance of fluoroscopic guidance for Maloney dilation. Am J Gastroenterol. 1992;87:1709–11.
14. Wang Y-G, Tio T-L, Soehendra N. Endoscopic dilation of esophageal stricture without fluoroscopy is safe and effective. World J Gastroenterol. 2002;8:766–8.
15. Raymondi R, Pereira-Lima JC, Valves A, Morales GF, Marques D, Lopes CV, Marroni CA. Endoscopic dilation of benign esophageal strictures without fluoroscopy: experience of 2750 procedures. Hepato-Gastroenterology. 2008;55:1342–8.
16. Kabbaj N, Salihoun M, Chaoui Z, Acharki M, Amrani N. Safety and outcome using endoscopic dilatation for benign esophageal stricture without fluoroscopy. World J Gastrointest Pharmacol Ther. 2011;2:46–9.
17. Saeed ZA. Balloon dilatation of benign esophageal stenoses. Hepato-Gastroenterology. 1992;39:490–3.
18. Riley SA, Attwood SEA. Guidelines on the use of oesophageal dilatation in clinical practice. Gut. 2004;53(Suppl 1):i1–6.
19. Scolapio JS, Pasha TM, Gostout CJ, Mahoney DW, Zinsmeister AR, Ott BJ, Lindor KD. A randomized prospective study comparing rigid to balloon dilators for benign esophageal strictures and rings. Gastrointest Endosc. 1999;50:13–7.
20. Shemesh E, Czerniak A. Comparison between Savary-Gilliard and balloon dilatation of benign esophageal strictures. World J Surg. 1990;14:518–21; discussion 521–522
21. Saeed ZA, Winchester CB, Ferro PS, Michaletz PA, Schwartz JT, Graham DY. Prospective randomized comparison of polyvinyl bougies and through-the-scope balloons for dilation of peptic strictures of the esophagus. Gastrointest Endosc. 1995;41:189–95.
22. Cox JG, Winter RK, Maslin SC, Dakkak M, Jones R, Buckton GK, Hoare RC, Dyet JF, Bennett JR. Balloon or bougie for dilatation of benign esophageal stricture? Dig Dis Sci. 1994;39:776–81.
23. Hernandez LV, Jacobson JW, Harris MS, Hernandez LJ. Comparison among the perforation rates of Maloney, balloon, and savary dilation of esophageal strictures. Gastrointest Endosc. 2000;51:460–2.
24. Mandelstam P, Sugawa C, Silvis SE, Nebel OT, Rogers BH. Complications associated with esophagogastroduodenoscopy and with esophageal dilation. Gastrointest Endosc. 1976;23:16–9.
25. Piotet E, Escher A, Monnier P. Esophageal and pharyngeal strictures: report on 1,862 endoscopic dilatations using the Savary-Gilliard technique. Eur Arch Otorhinolaryngol. 2008;265:357–64.
26. Silvis SE, Nebel O, Rogers G, Sugawa C, Mandelstam P. Endoscopic complications. Results of the 1974 American Society for Gastrointestinal Endoscopy Survey. JAMA. 1976;235:928–30.
27. Brinster CJ, Singhal S, Lee L, Marshall MB, Kaiser LR, Kucharczuk JC. Evolving options in the management of esophageal perforation. Ann Thorac Surg. 2004;77:1475–83.
28. Botoman VA, Surawicz CM. Bacteremia with gastrointestinal endoscopic procedures. Gastrointest Endosc. 1986;32:342–6.
29. Nelson DB, Sanderson SJ, Azar MM. Bacteremia with esophageal dilation. Gastrointest Endosc. 1998;48:563–7.
30. Bautista-Casasnovas A, Varela-Cives R, Estévez Martínez E, Jardón Bahía JA, Barca PR, Dargallo Carbonell T, Villanueva Jeremias A, Cadranel S, Tojo R. What is the infection risk of oesophageal dilatations? Eur J Pediatr. 1998;157:901–3.
31. Patterson DJ, Graham DY, Smith JL, Schwartz JT, Alpert E, Lanza FL, Cain GD. Natural history of benign esophageal stricture treated by dilatation. Gastroenterology. 1983;85:346–50.
32. Glick ME. Clinical course of esophageal stricture managed by bougienage. Dig Dis Sci. 1982;27:884–8.
33. Marks RD, Richter JE, Rizzo J, Koehler RE, Spenney JG, Mills TP, Champion G. Omeprazole versus H2-receptor antagonists in treating patients with peptic stricture and esophagitis. Gastroenterology. 1994;106:907–15.

34. Smith PM, Kerr GD, Cockel R, Ross BA, Bate CM, Brown P, Dronfield MW, Green JR, Hislop WS, Theodossi A. A comparison of omeprazole and ranitidine in the prevention of recurrence of benign esophageal stricture. Restore Investigator Group. Gastroenterology. 1994;107:1312–8.
35. Silvis SE, Farahmand M, Johnson JA, Ansel HJ, Ho SB. A randomized blinded comparison of omeprazole and ranitidine in the treatment of chronic esophageal stricture secondary to acid peptic esophagitis. Gastrointest Endosc. 1996;43:216–21.
36. Swarbrick ET, Gough AL, Foster CS, Christian J, Garrett AD, Langworthy CH. Prevention of recurrence of oesophageal stricture, a comparison of lansoprazole and high-dose ranitidine. Eur J Gastroenterol Hepatol. 1996;8:431–8.
37. Said A, Brust DJ, Gaumnitz EA, Reichelderfer M. Predictors of early recurrence of benign esophageal strictures. Am J Gastroenterol. 2003;98:1252–6.
38. Dzeletovic I, Fleischer DE, Crowell MD, Pannala R, Harris LA, Ramirez FC, Burdick GE, Rentz LA, Spratley RV, Helling SD, Alexander JA. Self-dilation as a treatment for resistant, benign esophageal strictures. Dig Dis Sci. 2013;58:3218–23.
39. Grobe JL, Kozarek RA, Sanowski RA. Self-bougienage in the treatment of benign esophageal stricture. J Clin Gastroenterol. 1984;6:109–12.
40. Orive-Calzada A, Bernal-Martinez A, Navajas-Laboa M, Torres-Burgos S, Aguirresarobe M, Lorenzo-Morote M, Arevalo-Serna JA, Cabriada-Nuño JL. Efficacy of intralesional corticosteroid injection in endoscopic treatment of esophageal strictures. Surg Laparosc Endosc Percutan Tech. 2012;22:518–22.
41. Kochhar R, Ray JD, Sriram PV, Kumar S, Singh K. Intralesional steroids augment the effects of endoscopic dilation in corrosive esophageal strictures. Gastrointest Endosc. 1999;49:509–13.
42. Kirsch M, Blue M, Desai RK, Sivak MV. Intralesional steroid injections for peptic esophageal strictures. Gastrointest Endosc. 1991;37:180–2.
43. Russell SB, Trupin JS, Myers JC, Broquist AH, Smith JC, Myles ME, Russell JD. Differential glucocorticoid regulation of collagen mRNAs in human dermal fibroblasts. Keloid-derived and fetal fibroblasts are refractory to down- regulation. J Biol Chem. 1989;264:13730–5.
44. Ramage JI, Rumalla A, Baron TH, Pochron NL, Zinsmeister AR, Murray JA, Norton ID, Diehl N, Romero Y. A prospective, randomized, double-blind, placebo- controlled trial of endoscopic steroid injection therapy for recalcitrant esophageal peptic strictures. Am J Gastroenterol. 2005;100:2419–25.
45. Spaander MCW, Baron TH, Siersema PD, Fuccio L, Schumacher B, Escorsell À, Garcia-Pagán J-C, Dumonceau J-M, Conio M, de Ceglie A, Skowronek J, Nordsmark M, Seufferlein T, Van Gossum A, Hassan C, Repici A, Bruno MJ. Esophageal stenting for benign and malignant disease: European Society of Gastrointestinal Endoscopy (ESGE) Clinical Guideline. Endoscopy. 2016;48:939–48.
46. Gangloff A, Lecleire S, Di Fiore A, Huet E, Iwanicki-Caron I, Antonietti M, Michel P. Fully versus partially covered self-expandable metal stents in benign esophageal strictures. Dis Esophagus. 2015;28:678–83.
47. Dua KS, Vleggaar FP, Santharam R, Siersema PD. Removable self- expanding plastic esophageal stent as a continuous, non-permanent dilator in treating refractory benign esophageal strictures: a prospective two-center study. Am J Gastroenterol. 2008;103:2988–94.
48. Holm AN, de la Mora Levy JG, Gostout CJ, Topazian MD, Baron TH. Self- expanding plastic stents in treatment of benign esophageal conditions. Gastrointest Endosc. 2008;67:20–5.
49. Evrard S, Le Moine O, Lazaraki G, Dormann A, El Nakadi I, Devière J. Self- expanding plastic stents for benign esophageal lesions. Gastrointest Endosc. 2004;60:894–900.
50. Repici A, Hassan C, Sharma P, Conio M, Siersema P. Systematic review: the role of self-expanding plastic stents for benign oesophageal strictures. Aliment Pharmacol Ther. 2010;31:1268–75.
51. Song HY, Jung HY, Park SI, Kim SB, Lee DH, Kang SG, Il Min Y. Covered retrievable expandable nitinol stents in patients with benign esophageal strictures: initial experience. Radiology. 2000;217:551–7.

52. Fuccio L, Hassan C, Frazzoni L, Miglio R, Repici A. Clinical outcomes following stent placement in refractory benign esophageal stricture: a systematic review and meta-analysis. Endoscopy. 2016;48:141–8.
53. Samanta J, Dhaka N, Sinha SK, Kochhar R. Endoscopic incisional therapy for benign esophageal strictures: technique and results. World J Gastrointest Endosc. 2015;7:1318–26.
54. Lee WK, Kim BS, Yang MA, Yun SH, Lee YJ, Kim JW, Cho JW. An intractable caustic esophageal stricture successfully managed with sequential treatment comprising incision with an insulated-tip knife, balloon dilation, and an oral steroid. Clin Endosc. 2016;49:560.
55. Simmons DT, Baron TH. Electroincision of refractory esophagogastric anastomotic strictures. Dis Esophagus. 2006;19:410–4.
56. Rosseneu S, Afzal N, Yerushalmi B, Ibarguen-Secchia E, Lewindon P, Cameron D, Mahler T, Schwagten K, Köhler H, Lindley KJ, Thomson M. Topical application of mitomycin-C in oesophageal strictures. J Pediatr Gastroenterol Nutr. 2007;44:336–41.
57. Deng H-Y, Wang W-P, Lin Y-D, Chen L-Q. Can mitomycin facilitate endoscopic dilatation treatment of benign oesophageal stricture? Interact Cardiovasc Thorac Surg. 2017;24(1):112–4.

Medical Management of GERD

11

Feng Li, Stephanie Denise Pointer, and Jon P. Walker

Introduction

Prior to considering surgical therapy for the management of GERD, one must consider the medical options, for which there are many. This chapter aims to give a broad overview of the medical options available to the treating physician. Prior to pursuing therapy, it is critical to make an assessment as to the etiology of the GERD symptoms. For example, the therapy for erosive esophagitis may differ from nonerosive reflux disease (NERD). It will also be very important to appreciate the therapeutic options for other conditions with similar symptoms, such as functional heartburn, hypersensitive esophagus, and non-acid reflux.

These therapies have several mechanisms, including decreasing intragastric pH, esophageal exposure to gastric contents, and sensitivity of the esophagus to any potential exposures.

Lifestyle and Dietary Interventions in the Management of GERD

The cornerstone of therapy for GERD, regardless of the etiology, is lifestyle and dietary modifications. These modifications include weight management, exercise, tobacco cessation, minimizing alcohol, and dietary modifications [1].

Weight loss is strongly recommended in patients with a BMI (body mass index) > 25 or patients with recent weight gain, in order to improve GERD

F. Li · S. D. Pointer · J. P. Walker (✉)
Division of Gastroenterology, Hepatology, and Nutrition, The Ohio State University Wexler Medical Center, Columbus, OH, USA
e-mail: Jon.walker@osumc.edu

J. Grams et al. (eds.), *The SAGES Manual of Foregut Surgery*,
https://doi.org/10.1007/978-3-319-96122-4_11

symptoms [2–4]. Obesity has been demonstrated to be an independent risk factor for GERD. The pathophysiological mechanisms for the increased risk include lower esophageal sphincter abnormalities, increased risk of hiatal hernia, and increased intragastric pressure [5]. One cross-sectional study demonstrated that obese participants were 2.5 times more likely to have reflux symptoms or esophageal erosions compared to participants with a normal (<25) BMI [6]. A similar study demonstrated that in patients with GERD, elevated BMI was associated with more severe and more frequent reflux symptoms and esophagitis [7].

Dietary modifications can be vital in the management of GERD and reflux symptoms. While the data supporting the recommendations is not particularly strong, selective elimination could be considered for patients who can correlate their symptoms with a particular food or beverage item. Food items that have historically been targeted for avoidance include chocolate, citrus, tomato-based products, peppermint, caffeine, spicy foods, carbonated beverages, and onion [1]. Other lifestyle modifications include avoiding large meals, decreased fat intake, and elevation of the head of the bed [8]. Most importantly, avoidance of recumbency within 2–3 h of meals has been shown to decrease nocturnal gastric acidity and nocturnal GERD symptoms [9, 10].

Tobacco cessation may result in improvement of GERD symptoms [11]. One recent study evaluated the effect of smoking cessation on GERD symptoms in patients who were treated with varenicline (a nicotinic receptor partial antagonist that is used to aid in smoking cessation) before and 1 year after smoking cessation. Patients who were treated with varenicline were asked to complete a self-reported questionnaire that detailed their smoking history and GERD symptoms. In the patients who were able to successfully achieve smoking cessation, 43.9% had improvement in their GERD symptoms compared to 18.2% in the patients who did not achieve smoking cessation.

A summary of the lifestyle and pharmacologic management of GERD is summarized in Table 11.1.

Medication Management of GERD

Medical management of GERD focuses on raising intragastric pH, promoting forward motility, and manipulating lower esophageal sphincter pressure [12]. Standard medical therapies for patients failing lifestyle modifications include antacids, sucralfate, H2 receptor antagonists, and proton pump inhibitors. Other options for GERD include prokinetics and baclofen.

Both step-up and step-down [13, 14] approaches to therapy have been proposed. The step-down approach initiates treatment with more potent antisecretory drugs and then de-escalates therapy as symptoms improve. Step-up therapy involves incrementally increasing potency of therapy until symptoms are controlled. Typically step-down therapy will result in more rapid improvement in symptoms,

Table 11.1 Lifestyle and pharmacologic management of GERD

Therapy	Pregnancy category	Use during lactation (Y/N)	Comments
Weight loss [7, 9]	–	–	Studies have shown improvement in GERD symptoms and esophageal pH
Elevation of head of bed [10–12]	–	–	Studies have shown improvement in GERD symptoms and esophageal pH
Avoidance of late night meals [13, 14]	–	–	Studies have shown improvement in nocturnal gastric acidity
Tobacco and alcohol cessation [17–19]	–	–	Studies have not shown improvement in GERD symptoms
Avoidance of chocolate, caffeine, spicy foods, citrus, carbonated beverages	–	–	No studies have been performed, but selective elimination could be considered for some patients if they can correlate improvement of their symptoms with elimination of selected food item
Antacids (calcium carbonate) [12]	Category C	Yes	–
Sucralfate	Category B	Yes	–
H2 receptor clocker: Cimetidine [12]	Category B	Yes	The American Academy of Pediatrics classified as compatible with breast feeding
H2 receptor blocker: Ranitidine [12]	Category B	Yes	–
H2 receptor blocker: Famotidine [12]	Category B	Yes	Lowest concentrations in breast milk of all H2 receptor blockers
Proton pump inhibitors (PPIs) [12]	Category B[a]	No	Studies have shown growth retardation in infant mice of lactating rats

[a]All PPIs, *except* omeprazole, are pregnancy category B. Omeprazole is pregnancy category C

whereas step-up therapy will reduce PPI use, resulting in lower costs and less adverse effects related to PPI therapy. Therefore, step-down therapy should be considered in patients with complications of GERD (such as esophagitis) or more frequent/severe symptoms.

Antacids

Antacids contain medications such as aluminum hydroxide or calcium carbonate that neutralize gastric pH. While they may provide rapid onset of relief of symptoms [15], antacids do not provide long-lasting symptom control and thus require frequent dosing. In addition, they are not effective in healing esophagitis [12]. Therefore, use of antacids is mainly limited to on-demand therapy for mild GERD symptoms.

Sucralfate

Sucralfate is a complex salt composed of sucrose sulfate and aluminum hydroxide. It inhibits the activity of the enzyme pepsin and protects against the formation of ulcers [16]. It is a topical agent that binds to the mucosal surface and promotes healing and protects from acid injury. It is very poorly absorbed from the GI tract thereby exerting its therapeutic effect through local mucosal protection [16].

Sucralfate has been shown to be, potentially, efficacious in improving reflux symptoms in patients with reflux esophagitis and nonerosive reflux disease (NERD) [17]. In a placebo-controlled trial, patients with reflux treated with sucralfate had significantly higher response compared to placebo (71% vs 29%, $p < 0.001$). However, sucralfate has a short duration of action and limited efficacy compared to PPI.

A study was performed comparing the effect of sucralfate gel versus placebo in patients with NERD [18]. A total of 141 patients with moderate to severe gastroesophageal reflux symptoms (without erosions or ulcers at endoscopy) were treated for 6 weeks in a randomized, double-blind, placebo-controlled study with either 1 g sucralfate gel BID or placebo [18]. In the sucralfate treatment group, 45% of patients reported a "good" or "excellent" overall response in their symptoms compared with 22% of patients in the placebo group [18]. This study concluded that sucralfate gel was superior in the treatment of NERD compared to placebo [18].

One randomized controlled trial compared sucralfate and ranitidine in reflux esophagitis to determine if sucralfate is an effective alternative in the treatment of reflux esophagitis [19]. A total of 49 patients with reflux esophagitis were treated for 8 weeks with either 1 g of sucralfate suspension four times daily or one 150 mg ranitidine film-coated tablet twice daily [19]. After 8 weeks of treatment, reflux esophagitis was healed in 14 (out of 22) patients in the sucralfate treatment group and 13 (out of 19) patients in the ranitidine treatment group [19]. Both forms of treatment were tolerated well and had similar positive effect on symptoms, and there were no differences in the endoscopic findings after treatment. This study concluded that sucralfate is an effective alternative treatment in the treatment of reflux esophagitis [19]. There are studies that also demonstrate that sucralfate may aid in mucosal repair and ulcer healing. Sucralfate is typically used in conjunction with other GERD medications. Because it is not teratogenic, it is also considered safe to be used in pregnancy and is classified as pregnancy category B.

H2 Receptor Antagonists

H2 receptor antagonists (H2RAs) reduce acid secretion by inhibiting the histamine-2 receptor on the gastric parietal cell, which regulates acid secretion. H2RAs provide longer duration of relief compared to antacids but have slower onset of action [20].

Proton Pump Inhibitors

Proton pump inhibitors (PPIs) are the most potent antisecretory therapy. They work by binding irreversibly to the hydrogen-potassium-ATPase pump on parietal cells, thus blocking acid secretion into the gastric lumen. In general, all PPIs should be dosed approximately 30–60 min before a meal for maximal effect and are most effective when taken at least 30 min before the first meal of the day because H-K-ATPase numbers are at their peak following a prolonged fast.

PPIs also have superior healing rates of erosive esophagitis compared to H2RAs (92.1% vs 69.9% at 8 weeks), and in a study comparing lansoprazole to ranitidine, patients on lansoprazole reported improved symptoms, including less daytime heartburn, burning in the upper abdomen, and gastroesophageal regurgitation at the end of the 8-week study period [21, 22].

Among patients with nonerosive reflux disease, a Cochrane review showed that PPI therapy is superior to both H2RAs and prokinetics for heartburn relief [23]. The relative risks for heartburn remission in placebo-controlled trials were 0.37 (95% CI 0.32–0.44) for PPI, 0.77 (95% CI 0.60–0.99) for H2RA, and 0.86 (95% CI 0.73–1.01) for prokinetics. Even among patients with typical heartburn symptoms but normal endoscopic findings, PPI remained superior to H2RA (heartburn remission RR 0.78, 95% CI 0.62–0.97), although the difference was smaller compared to patients treated empirically.

Furthermore, in patients with symptoms of GERD, but normal endoscopy findings (endoscopy-negative reflux disease/ENRD), a short course of antisecretory drugs is effective in controlling symptoms. In this group, PPIs were also superior to H2RAs (four trials), although the difference was smaller compared to studies of patients treated empirically. In the only trial comparing an antisecretory (omeprazole) with a prokinetic agent (cisapride), outcome was in favor of the PPI. No placebo-controlled trials on the efficacy of prokinetics for ENRD were identified.

In patients with erosive esophagitis, PPI therapy has superior rates of healing and decreased relapse compared to H2RA and placebo [24]. A large meta-analysis comparing PPI, H2RA, sucralfate, and placebo in erosive esophagitis confirmed superior healing with PPIs (84% +/− 11% PPI, 52% +/− 17% H2RA, 39% +/− 22% sucralfate, 28% +/− 16% placebo) [25].

There have been no significant differences in symptomatic relief among different PPIs [26]. In terms of mucosal healing of erosive esophagitis, esomeprazole demonstrated a slight increase in probability of healing erosive esophagitis (RR 1.05, 95% CI 1.02–1.08) [26]. The clinical significance of this is unclear, and typically PPIs can be used interchangeably.

The vast majority (~70–80%) of patients with GERD would be expected to respond completely to standard PPI therapy. One of the most common reasons for failure is poor compliance with dosage recommendations. It is highly recommended that providers first have a discussion with patients regarding the proper use and timing of PPI therapy before increasing dosing or considering it a treatment failure. Other risk factors for lack of symptom control despite medical therapy include longer duration of symptoms, presence of hiatal hernia, and extra-esophageal symptoms [27].

Patients with otherwise noncomplicated reflux can be managed with either on-demand or intermittent PPI therapy [13, 28]. Maintenance therapy should be considered for patients with refractory symptoms or complications such as erosive esophagitis due to the high rate of recurrence off PPI. For instance, among patients with LA grade B-C esophagitis, nearly all will relapse symptomatically by 6 months [27].

PPI therapy is highly effective, but patients should be counseled regarding potential adverse effects, which can include vitamin and mineral deficiencies, bone fractures, enteric infections, pneumonia, and cardiovascular risk with co-prescription with clopidogrel. In addition, more recent studies have shown an association between chronic PPI use and the development of dementia and chronic kidney disease.

It has been hypothesized that acid suppression therapy can reduce B12 levels. The first step in cobalamin absorption is dependent on acid and pepsin to release cobalamin from dietary proteins. Thus, reduction in intragastric acid can decrease bioavailability of B12 for absorption. However, two reviews did not show evidence of B12 deficiency in patients on chronic PPI [29, 30]. It should be noted that the elderly may be at increased risk of B12 deficiency and B12 deficiency should still be considered in this population.

Similarly, absorption of dietary iron also relies on gastric acid to dissociate iron salts from food. Conditions that decrease gastric acid such as atrophic gastritis and vagotomy have been associated with iron deficiency. However, normal subjects on PPI therapy have not been shown to develop iron deficiency [29].

Hypomagnesemia has been reported in association with PPI use [31]. Serious adverse effects of hypomagnesemia can include tetany, cardiac arrhythmias, and seizure. Based on multiple case reports, the FDA issued a warning in 2011 regarding long-term (greater than 1 year) PPI use and the risk of hypomagnesemia [32]. In about 25% of the cases of hypomagnesemia, oral magnesium supplementation was insufficient, requiring discontinuation of the PPI. Therefore, it is reasonable to monitor magnesium levels in patients expected to be on prolonged PPI or in patients who take PPI with other medications (diuretics) that lower magnesium.

Concerns have also been raised regarding risk of osteoporosis. Prior studies have shown conflicting results, but a recent prospective cohort study demonstrated that PPI use was significantly associated with a shorter time to first non-traumatic fracture (hazard ratio 1.75, 95% confidence interval 1.4–2.17) [33]. Given the significant morbidity associated with osteoporosis-related fractures, the risk of PPI use should be carefully considered in populations at risk for osteoporosis.

PPIs are also thought to be associated with increased risk of enteric infections. By decreasing gastric acidity, PPI therapy may promote growth of gut microflora. Systematic reviews have demonstrated increased risk of salmonella, campylobacter, and *C. difficile* infections for patients on PPI therapy [34]. The risks and benefits of PPI therapy should be considered carefully in patients at risk for enteric infections, especially those at risk for *C. difficile*.

The data regarding risk of pneumonia with PPI use is conflicting. A large review and meta-analysis demonstrated increased risk of pneumonia in patients using PPIs (adjusted OR 1.27, 95% CI 1.11–1.46) in the observational studies, but this relationship was not seen with the randomized studies [35]. On the other hand, a more recently published meta-analysis did demonstrate increased risk of community-acquired pneumonia among patients on PPI therapy (OR 1.36, 95% CI 1.12–1.65) [36]. Interestingly, on sub-group analysis, short duration of use was associated with increased risk of community-acquired pneumonia, while chronic use was not. This risk associated with short-term use has also been reported in other studies [37, 38]. The mechanism behind this is unclear. Further studies are needed to better delineate the risks of pneumonia associated with PPI therapy.

Clopidogrel is a commonly used antiplatelet medication. In 2009, the FDA issued a warning regarding the possibility of increased cardiovascular events among patients taking both clopidogrel and PPI therapy, as both medications are metabolized through the CYP 2C19 pathway. These recommendations were based on in vitro studies, which demonstrated decreased inhibition of platelet aggregation by clopidogrel in combination with PPI [39]. However, clinical data does not support any evidence of increased cardiovascular events with this medication combination. An analysis of well-controlled randomized trials concluded that there was no risk of adverse cardiac outcomes [40]. In fact, there may be increased risk of bleeding complications without PPI therapy in high-risk individuals on antiplatelet therapy.

Recent population database studies have raised the concern that long-term PPI use may be associated with dementia as well as chronic kidney disease. In a retrospective population cohort study, there was an association between the use of chronic PPIs and the development of chronic kidney disease (in analysis adjusted for demographic, socioeconomic, and clinical variables, HR, 1.50, 95% CI 1.14–1.96). In addition, there was a dose-dependent risk of CKD with PPI use, with twice-daily dosing being associated with increased risk. On the other hand, there was no increase in CKD risk with H2RA [41]. At this time, more studies are needed to confirm any causative relationship between PPI use and CKD development.

A large population database analysis demonstrated an association between regular PPI use and onset of dementia (HR 1.44; 95% CI, 1.36–1.52) [42]. In mouse models, PPI therapy with lansoprazole has been associated with increased deposition of beta-amyloid, which could be a mechanism for this association [43]. Similar to the study showing association with CKD, there was no clear demonstration of a causative relationship with dementia in this study.

In a recent review by the American Gastroenterological Association, it was determined that the use of long-term PPI therapy is effective and very safe. However, given these reports regarding rare but potentially serious complications from long-term PPI use, we recommend that PPIs be used judiciously and only when indicated.

The proposed risks of proton pump inhibitors and suggested practice recommendations are summarized in Table 11.2.

Table 11.2 Summary of proton pump inhibitor therapy risks and suggested practice recommendations

Risk	Summary	Practice recommendations
Nutritional		
B12 deficiency	Very rare. Elderly and malnourished at higher risk	No need for routine screening Could be considered in elderly or malnourished
Iron deficiency	Little data that PPI contributes to clinically significant iron deficiency	No need for routine screening
Hypomagnesemia	Rare, case reports published in literature	Be aware of risks of hypomagnesemia, hypokalemia, hypocalcemia. Consider checking levels in patients if there are cardiac risk factors
Fracture risk	Inconsistent studies, more recent studies do show association with fragility fractures	No recommendation for routine bone density screening
Infectious		
Enteric infections	Increased risk of salmonella, campylobacter, *C. difficile*	Consider risk/benefit especially in patients at risk for *C. difficile*
Pneumonia	Conflicting data Most associated with short-term use	PPI should not be withheld from patients when indicated
Medication interactions		
Clopidogrel	No evidence of increased cardiovascular risk	No limitations
Other complications		
Chronic kidney disease	Association between development of chronic kidney disease and PPI use in dose-dependent relationship	Discuss risks and benefits with patient. Use lowest possible PPI dose
Dementia	Association between development of dementia and chronic PPI use	Discuss risks and benefits with patient

Prokinetics

Prokinetic medications such as metoclopramide have been shown to increase lower esophageal sphincter pressure, increase esophageal peristalsis, and increase gastric emptying [44]. There is limited data showing clinical benefit of adding metoclopramide to PPI therapy. The combination of metoclopramide in addition to H2RA has not been shown to have any incremental benefit over either agent alone [45].

Unfortunately, the routine use of metoclopramide is limited by its central nervous system side effects, including drowsiness, agitation, dystonic reactions, and tardive dyskinesia [46]. The FDA has issued a black box warning regarding risk of tardive dyskinesia, an often irreversible movement disorder, with chronic use of metoclopramide [47].

An alternative to metoclopramide is domperidone, which currently requires an application for investigation drug usage permit from the FDA and is not currently approved for GERD. Although domperidone and metoclopramide have similar efficacy in gastroparesis, they have not been compared in GERD [48]. It is important to note that while on therapy, routine EKGs are needed to monitor for prolonged QT interval, which can cause ventricular arrhythmias and sudden cardiac death [49].

Macrolide antibiotics, such as azithromycin, have been shown to reduce acid reflux in addition to their prokinetic effect. However their use is limited by tachyphylaxis [50].

Baclofen

Baclofen is another alternative therapy for refractory GERD. Baclofen works through reducing transient LES relaxations, which are an important contributor to reflux [51, 52]. Baclofen has also been shown to decrease the amount of postprandial acid and non-acid reflux events [53], nocturnal reflux [54], and belching [55].

However, baclofen is not used more widely due to such side effects as drowsiness, nausea, headaches, asthenia, and tachyphylaxis. In addition, it is not currently approved by the FDA for treatment of GERD.

Management of Gastroesophageal Reflux Symptoms in Pregnancy and During Lactation

Gastroesophageal reflux symptoms are estimated to occur in up to 50% of pregnancies [56, 57]. These symptoms are typically due to the mechanical pressure that is placed on the stomach and bowel as the uterus enlarges. There is limited data to determine if there is a hormonal correlation with GERD symptoms in pregnancy. Symptoms typically manifest in the first trimester of pregnancy and resolve after delivery [58, 59].

Treatment of GERD symptoms in pregnancy typically follows a stepwise approach (Fig. 11.1). Lifestyle modifications are recommended as first-line therapy. If symptoms persist despite lifestyle modifications, calcium-containing antacids, sucralfate, and promotility drugs (i.e., metoclopramide (pregnancy category B)) are typically recommended, followed by H2 blockers (pregnancy category B) and proton pump inhibitors (pregnancy category C) [16].

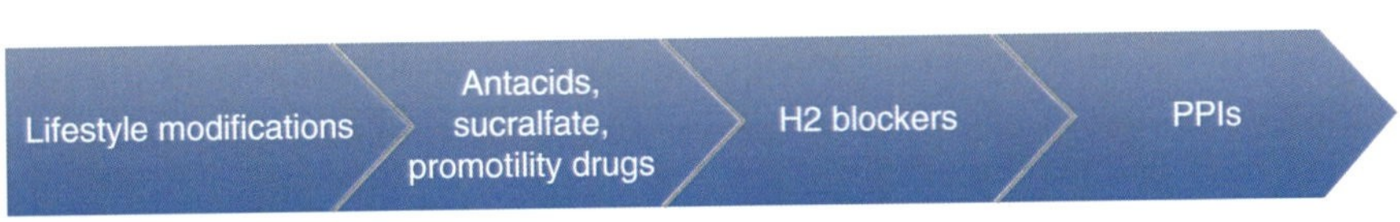

Fig. 11.1 Stepwise approach to management of GERD in pregnancy

All H2 receptor blockers are excreted in human breast milk, and the effects of these drugs are unknown on the nursing human infant [60]. One review examined available data regarding the levels of H2 receptor blockers in breast milk and found that ranitidine and famotidine are safest to use during lactation, with famotidine being preferred because of its lower concentration in human breast milk [16, 61–64]. There is no data available on the use of sucralfate during breastfeeding; however, because it is virtually unabsorbed enterally, it is considered acceptable to use while breastfeeding without precautions [16, 60, 65, 66]. Proton pump inhibitors (PPIs) are typically not recommended for use by lactating mothers. Women with severe GERD symptoms can either take PPIs and discontinue lactation or use a different class of reflux therapy [16].

NERD (Nonerosive Reflux Disease) and Non-acid Reflux Management

Nonerosive reflux disease is a subset of GERD that is characterized by symptoms of reflux without mucosal erosions on endoscopy, but with evidence of pathologic levels of reflux on pH or pH-impedance monitoring. The potential causes for symptoms in NERD are microscopic inflammation, visceral hypersensitivity, or sustained esophageal contractions [67].

PPIs have been shown to be effective in NERD. However, patients with NERD have been shown to be less responsive to PPIs than patients who have erosive esophagitis by approximately 20–40% after 4 weeks of treatment [68].

Non-acid reflux disease is a subset of GERD that is characterized by symptoms of reflux; however, there is minimal to no response to PPI treatment, nor is there evidence of pathologic acid reflux during pH testing. Therefore, acid reflux does not appear to be the underlying disorder [69]. Bile acid sequestrants and oatmeal have been used to treat reflux symptoms. However, there is little data to assess the efficacy of these modalities. Baclofen can also be an option in treating non-acid reflux [69–71].

Functional Heartburn Management

Functional heartburn is the term used to describe the symptoms of a select group of patients who have heartburn symptoms but have normal esophageal acid exposure and no correlation between rare reflux events and their symptoms [70].

Therapy for functional heartburn involves a stepwise approach to alleviating symptoms (Fig. 11.2). The first step is lifestyle modification that includes avoiding triggers and identifying psychosocial features associated with symptoms [70]. Close communication between the gastroenterologist/surgeon, primary care physician, and, sometimes, psychiatry/psychology plays an important role in this aspect of therapy. If lifestyle modifications fail to improve symptoms, patients can then be treated with acid suppression [70]. While there may be no evidence in the patients' history or objective testing for acid reflux, there is data to suggest that acid

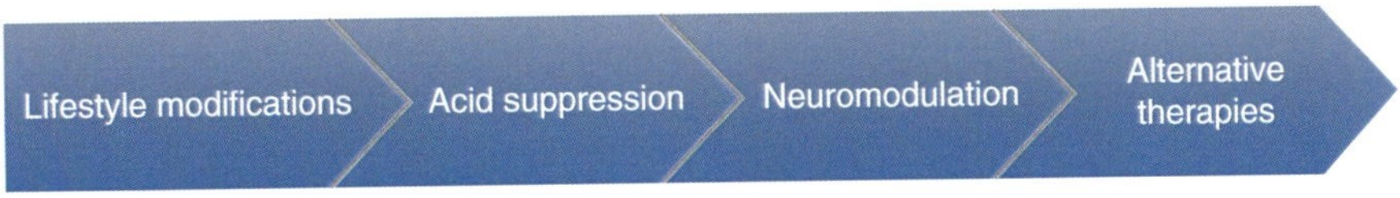

Fig. 11.2 Stepwise approach to management of functional heartburn

suppression can be beneficial in some patients with functional heartburn. This may represent the likely overlap between hypersensitive esophagus and functional heartburn [71, 72]. If acid suppression fails to improve symptoms, patients can then be treated with neuromodulatory medications that include tricyclic antidepressants (TCAs), selective serotonin reuptake inhibitors (SSRIs), and melatonin [70]. If neuromodulatory therapies fail to adequately improve symptoms, patients can be treated with alternative therapies which include biofeedback, acupuncture, and esophageal-directed hypnotherapy [70].

While there is limited data to assess the effectiveness of neuromodulatory medications, one study found that imipramine (tricyclic antidepressant) did improve quality of life in patients suffering from functional heartburn; however, it did not relieve symptoms more effectively than placebo [73]. In this study, patients with established diagnoses of esophageal hypersensitivity or functional heartburn were randomized to receive either 8 weeks of imipramine 25 mg once daily or placebo [73]. The primary outcome was relief of symptoms, and the secondary outcome was improvement in the quality of life [73]. Patients receiving imipramine did not have a higher rate of satisfactory improvement in symptoms compared to patients receiving placebo [73]. Nonetheless, other trials show that tricyclic antidepressants can control esophageal pain in both healthy subjects and those that have functional esophageal disorders [74]. Thus, neuromodulatory therapy has become an important treatment modality in functional heartburn.

References

1. Nwokediuko SC. Current trends in the management of gastroesophageal reflux disease: a review. ISRN Gastroenterol. 2012;2012:391631.
2. Jacobson BC, et al. Body-mass index and symptoms of gastroesophageal reflux in women. N Engl J Med. 2006;354(22):2340–8.
3. Fraser-Moodie CA, et al. Weight loss has an independent beneficial effect on symptoms of gastro-oesophageal reflux in patients who are overweight. Scand J Gastroenterol. 1999;34(4):337–40.
4. Mathus-Vliegen LM, Tytgat GN. Twenty-four-hour pH measurements in morbid obesity: effects of massive overweight, weight loss and gastric distension. Eur J Gastroenterol Hepatol. 1996;8(7):635–40.
5. Nam SY. Obesity-related digestive diseases and their pathophysiology. Gut Liver. 2016;11:323.
6. El-Serag HB, et al. Obesity is an independent risk factor for GERD symptoms and erosive esophagitis. Am J Gastroenterol. 2005;100(6):1243–50.
7. Nocon M, et al. Association of body mass index with heartburn, regurgitation and esophagitis: results of the Progression of Gastroesophageal Reflux Disease study. J Gastroenterol Hepatol. 2007;22(11):1728–31.

8. Harvey RF, et al. Effects of sleeping with the bed-head raised and of ranitidine in patients with severe peptic oesophagitis. Lancet. 1987;2(8569):1200–3.
9. Duroux P, et al. Early dinner reduces nocturnal gastric acidity. Gut. 1989;30(8):1063–7.
10. Orr WC, Harnish MJ. Sleep-related gastro-oesophageal reflux: provocation with a late evening meal and treatment with acid suppression. Aliment Pharmacol Ther. 1998;12(10):1033–8.
11. Kohata Y, et al. Long-term benefits of smoking cessation on gastroesophageal reflux disease and health-related quality of life. PLoS One. 2016;11(2):e0147860.
12. Hunt RH. Importance of pH control in the management of GERD. Arch Intern Med. 1999;159(7):649–57.
13. Inadomi JM, et al. Step-down management of gastroesophageal reflux disease. Gastroenterology. 2001;121(5):1095–100.
14. Inadomi JM, et al. Step-down from multiple-to single-dose proton pump inhibitors (PPIs): a prospective study of patients with heartburn or acid regurgitation completely relieved with PPIs. Am J Gastroenterol. 2003;98(9):1940–4.
15. Weberg R, Berstad A. Symptomatic effect of a low-dose antacid regimen in reflux oesophagitis. Scand J Gastroenterol. 1989;24(4):401–6.
16. Richter JE. Review article: the management of heartburn in pregnancy. Aliment Pharmacol Ther. 2005;22(9):749–57.
17. Wang YK, et al. Current pharmacological management of gastroesophageal reflux disease. Gastroenterol Res Pract. 2013;2013:983653.
18. Simon B, Ravelli GP, Goffin H. Sucralfate gel versus placebo in patients with non-erosive gastro-oesophageal reflux disease. Aliment Pharmacol Ther. 1996;10(3):441–6.
19. Simon B, Mueller P. Comparison of the effect of sucralfate and ranitidine in reflux esophagitis. Am J Med. 1987;83(3b):43–7.
20. Wolfe MM, Sachs G. Acid suppression: optimizing therapy for gastroduodenal ulcer healing, gastroesophageal reflux disease, and stress-related erosive syndrome. Gastroenterology. 2000;118(2 Suppl 1):S9–31.
21. Robinson M, et al. A comparison of lansoprazole and ranitidine in the treatment of erosive oesophagitis. Aliment Pharmacol Ther. 1995;9(1):25–31.
22. Vantrappen G, et al. Omeprazole (40 mg) is superior to ranitidine in short-term treatment of ulcerative reflux esophagitis. Dig Dis Sci. 1988;33(5):523–9.
23. Sigterman KE, et al. Short-term treatment with proton pump inhibitors, H2-receptor antagonists and prokinetics for gastro-oesophageal reflux disease-like symptoms and endoscopy negative reflux disease. Cochrane Database Syst Rev. 2013;(5):1–84.
24. Labenz J, Malfertheiner P. Treatment of uncomplicated reflux disease. World J Gastroenterol. 2005;11(28):4291–9.
25. Chiba N, et al. Speed of healing and symptom relief in grade II to IV gastroesophageal reflux disease: a meta-analysis. Gastroenterology. 1997;112(6):1798–810.
26. Gralnek IM, et al. Esomeprazole versus other proton pump inhibitors in erosive esophagitis: a meta-analysis of randomized clinical trials. Clin Gastroenterol Hepatol. 2006;4(12):1452–8.
27. Dickman R, et al. Comparison of clinical characteristics of patients with gastroesophageal reflux disease who failed proton pump inhibitor therapy versus those who fully responded. J Neurogastroenterol Motil. 2011;17:387.
28. Pace F, et al. Systematic review: maintenance treatment of gastro-oesophageal reflux disease with proton pump inhibitors taken 'on-demand'. Aliment Pharmacol Ther. 2007;26(2):195–204.
29. Sheen E, Triadafilopoulos G. Adverse effects of long-term proton pump inhibitor therapy. Dig Dis Sci. 2011;56(4):931–50.
30. Lodato F, et al. Adverse effects of proton pump inhibitors. Best Pract Res Clin Gastroenterol. 2010;24(2):193–201.
31. Hoorn EJ, et al. A case series of proton pump inhibitor-induced hypomagnesemia. Am J Kidney Dis. 2010;56(1):112–6.
32. FDA Drug Safety Communication: Low magnesium levels can be associated with long-term use of proton pump inhibitor drugs (PPIs). 2011 [cited 2016 November 29]; Available from: http://www.fda.gov/safety/medwatch/safetyinformation/ucm258810.htm.

33. Fraser LA, et al. The effect of proton pump inhibitors on fracture risk: report from the Canadian Multicenter Osteoporosis Study. Osteoporos Int. 2013;24(4):1161–8.
34. Bavishi C, Dupont H. Systematic review: the use of proton pump inhibitors and increased susceptibility to enteric infection. Aliment Pharmacol Ther. 2011;34(11–12):1269–81.
35. Eom C-S, et al. Use of acid-suppressive drugs and risk of pneumonia: a systematic review and meta-analysis. Can Med Assoc J. 2011;183(3):310–9.
36. Johnstone J, Nerenberg K, Loeb M. Meta-analysis: proton pump inhibitor use and the risk of community-acquired pneumonia. Aliment Pharmacol Ther. 2010;31(11):1165–77.
37. Giuliano C, Wilhelm SM, Kale-Pradhan PB. Are proton pump inhibitors associated with the development of community-acquired pneumonia? A meta-analysis. Expert Rev Clin Pharmacol. 2012;5(3):337–44.
38. Hermos JA, et al. Risk of community-acquired pneumonia in veteran patients to whom proton pump inhibitors were dispensed. Clin Infect Dis. 2011;54(1):33–42.
39. Sibbing D, et al. Impact of proton pump inhibitors on the antiplatelet effects of clopidogrel. Thromb Haemost. 2009;101(4):714–9.
40. Gerson LB, et al. Lack of significant interactions between clopidogrel and proton pump inhibitor therapy: meta-analysis of existing literature. Dig Dis Sci. 2012;57(5):1304–13.
41. Lazarus B, et al. Proton pump inhibitor use and the risk of chronic kidney disease. JAMA Intern Med. 2016;176(2):238–46.
42. Gomm W, et al. Association of proton pump inhibitors with risk of dementia: a pharmacoepidemiological claims data analysis. JAMA Neurol. 2016;73(4):410–6.
43. Badiola N, et al. The proton-pump inhibitor lansoprazole enhances amyloid beta production. PLoS One. 2013;8(3):e58837.
44. Champion M. Prokinetic therapy in gastroesophageal reflux disease. Can J Gastroenterol = J can gastroenterol. 1997;11:55B–65B.
45. Richter JE, et al. Omeprazole versus ranitidine or ranitidine/metoclopramide in poorly responsive symptomatic gastroesophageal reflux disease. Am J Gastroenterol. 1996;91(9):1766–72.
46. Rao A, Camilleri M. Review article: metoclopramide and tardive dyskinesia. Aliment Pharmacol Ther. 2010;31(1):11–9.
47. Reglan (metoclopramide) tablets, ODT (Orally Disintegrating Tablets), and injection. 2009 [cited 2016 November 29]; Available from: http://www.fda.gov/Safety/MedWatch/SafetyInformation/ucm170934.htm.
48. Maddern G, et al. Domperidone, metoclopramide, and placebo: all give symptomatic improvement in gastroesophageal reflux. J Clin Gastroenterol. 1986;8(2):135–40.
49. van Noord C, et al. Domperidone and ventricular arrhythmia or sudden cardiac death. Drug Saf. 2010;33(11):1003–14.
50. Rohof WO, et al. Effect of azithromycin on acid reflux, hiatus hernia and proximal acid pocket in the postprandial period. Gut. 2012;61(12):1670–7.
51. Koek G, et al. Effect of the GABAB agonist baclofen in patients with symptoms and duodeno-gastro-oesophageal reflux refractory to proton pump inhibitors. Gut. 2003;52(10):1397–402.
52. Grossi L, et al. Effect of baclofen on oesophageal motility and transient lower oesophageal sphincter relaxations in GORD patients: a 48-h manometric study. Neurogastroenterol Motil. 2008;20(7):760–6.
53. Vela M, et al. Baclofen decreases acid and non-acid post-prandial gastro-oesophageal reflux measured by combined multichannel intraluminal impedance and pH. Aliment Pharmacol Ther. 2003;17(2):243–51.
54. Orr W, et al. The effect of baclofen on nocturnal gastroesophageal reflux and measures of sleep quality: a randomized, cross-over trial. Neurogastroenterol Motil. 2012;24(6):553–e253.
55. Cange L, et al. Baclofen-mediated gastro-oesophageal acid reflux control in patients with established reflux disease. Aliment Pharmacol Ther. 2002;16(5):869–73.
56. Ronkainen J, et al. High prevalence of gastroesophageal reflux symptoms and esophagitis with or without symptoms in the general adult Swedish population: a Kalixanda study report. Scand J Gastroenterol. 2005;40(3):275–85.

57. Shaw MJ, et al. When does simple heartburn become a diseases? Gastroenterology. 1998;114:A284.
58. Charan M, Katz PO. Gastroesophageal reflux disease in pregnancy. Curr Treat Options Gastroenterol. 2001;4(1):73–81.
59. Anton CR, Anton E, Stanciu C. Gastroesophageal reflux disease in pregnancy. Rev Med Chir Soc Med Nat Iasi. 2001;105(1):43–7.
60. Broussard CN, Richter JE. Treating gastro-oesophageal reflux disease during pregnancy and lactation: what are the safest therapy options? Drug Saf. 1998;19(4):325–37.
61. Riley A, Crowley P, Harrison C. Transfer of ranitidine to biological fluids: milk and semen. In: The clinical use of ranitidine, Medicine Publishing Foundation Series, vol. 5. Oxford: Medicine Publishing Foundation; 1982. p. 77–86.
62. Kearns G, et al. Appearance of ranitidine in breast milk following multiple dosing. Clin Pharm. 1984;4(3):322–4.
63. Knigge UP. Histaminergic regulation of prolactin secretion. Dan Med Bull. 1990;37(2):109–24.
64. Perret G, et al. Effect of a short-term oral administration of cimetidine and ranitidine on the basal and thyrotropin-releasing hormone-stimulated serum concentrations of prolactin, thyrotropin and thyroid hormones in healthy volunteers. Pharmacology. 1986;32(2):101–8.
65. Lewis J, Weingold A. The use of gastrointestinal drugs during pregnancy and lactation. Am J Gastroenterol. 1985;80(11):912–23.
66. Hagemann TM. Gastrointestinal medications and breastfeeding. J Hum Lact. 1998;14(3):259–62.
67. Chen C-L, Hsu P-I. Current advances in the diagnosis and treatment of nonerosive reflux disease. Gastroenterol Res Pract. 2013;2013:653989.
68. Dean BB, et al. Effectiveness of proton pump inhibitors in nonerosive reflux disease. Clin Gastroenterol Hepatol. 2004;2(8):656–64.
69. Storr MA. What is nonacid reflux disease? Can J Gastroenterol. 2011;25(1):35–8.
70. Hachem C, Shaheen NJ. Diagnosis and Management of Functional Heartburn. Am J Gastroenterol. 2016;111(1):53–61; quiz 62.
71. Kavitt RT, et al. Symptom reports are not reliable during ambulatory reflux monitoring. Am J Gastroenterol. 2012;107(12):1826–32.
72. Rosen R, et al. Intraesophageal pressure recording improves the detection of cough during multichannel intraluminal impedance testing (pH-MII) in children. J Pediatr Gastroenterol Nutr. 2014;58(1):22.
73. Limsrivilai J, et al. Imipramine for treatment of esophageal hypersensitivity and functional heartburn: a randomized placebo-controlled trial. Am J Gastroenterol. 2016;111(2):217–24.
74. Prakash C, Clouse RE. Long-term outcome from tricyclic antidepressant treatment of functional chest pain. Dig Dis Sci. 1999;44(12):2373–9.

12 Laparoscopic Anti-reflux Surgery: Nissen and Partial Fundoplications

Gustavo Fernandez Ranvier, Daniela Guevara, and Barry Salky

Indications

Laparoscopic fundoplication is the gold standard surgical treatment of moderate to severe gastroesophageal reflux disease (GERD) [1].

Gastroesophageal reflux disease is common in the general population, and although it may present as acid reflux, heartburn, or chest pain, its symptomatology may be caused by a number of disease processes such as a hiatal hernia, achalasia, diffuse esophageal spasm, gastritis, gastric or duodenal ulcers, or coronary artery disease among others. Patients who suffer from GERD that has been severe and unresponsive to medical treatment (medications, lifestyle, and habit changes) associated with the following medical conditions may be candidates for an anti-reflux surgery:

- High volume reflux
- Erosive esophagitis
- Benign stricture secondary to GERD
- Barrett's columnar-lined epithelium (without high grade dysplasia or carcinoma) in conjunction with symptoms not improved with medical treatment
- Atypical or respiratory symptoms with a good response to medical treatment
- Failed optimal medical treatment
- Noncompliance with medical therapy
- Risk factors that predict a poor response to medical therapy:
  - Nocturnal reflux on 24-h esophageal PH study
  - Structurally deficient lower esophageal sphincter
  - Mixed reflux of gastric or duodenal juice
  - Mucosal injury at presentation

G. F. Ranvier (✉) · D. Guevara · B. Salky
Division of Metabolic, Endocrine and Minimally Invasive Surgery, Department of Surgery, Mount Sinai Hospital, Icahn School of Medicine at Mount Sinai, New York, NY, USA
e-mail: gustavo.fernandez-ranvier@mountsinai.org

J. Grams et al. (eds.), *The SAGES Manual of Foregut Surgery*,
https://doi.org/10.1007/978-3-319-96122-4_12

About one-third to half of patients with GERD may present with laryngopharyngeal reflux (LPR) and report upper respiratory symptoms including hoarseness, laryngitis, wheezing, nocturnal asthma, chronic coughing, aspiration, or dental erosion [2]. Relief of respiratory symptoms is usually achievable by fundoplication in patients who also have typical reflux symptoms; however, poorer outcomes may be expected in those patients with LPR in association with abnormalities of esophageal motility. As with GERD with classic symptoms of acid reflux or heartburn, the primary treatment of LPR is still medical, and these patients should be referred to gastroenterologists or ENT physicians who specialize in LPR before considering surgery. A common error is to define the presence of gastroesophageal reflux disease by endoscopic esophagitis. Limiting the diagnosis to patients with endoscopic esophagitis ignores a large population of patients without mucosal injury who may have severe symptoms of gastroesophageal reflux and could be considered for anti-reflux surgery.

Preoperative Workup: Defining Reflux Disease

The most precise approach to define gastroesophageal reflux disease is to measure the basic pathophysiologic abnormality of the disease [3]. The work up consists of:

- *Upper endoscopy:* A detailed esophageal and gastric endoscopy should be performed to assess the esophageal and gastric mucosa and presence or absence of a hiatal hernia and for further assessment of other pathologic findings such as malignancy prior to proceeding with a surgical anti-reflux procedure.
- *24-hour pH monitoring*: It is the gold standard to assess the degree and pattern of esophageal exposure to acid gastric juice. Although symptoms may differ from GERD, in those cases when laryngopharyngeal reflux disease is suspected (in general a flexible fiber-optic laryngoscopy will demonstrate erythema and inflammation of the vocal cords and pharynx), a dual pH sensor probe to measure acid exposure to the upper esophagus and larynx should be performed. The Bravo® reflux testing system measurements of acid exposure are adequate for GERD (heartburn), but cannot be used for diagnosis of LPR since the placement of the capsule high in the esophagus is not well tolerated by the patients.
- *High-resolution manometry (HRM) with esophageal pressure topography (EPT):* It is an important and essential tool for evaluation of the upper and lower esophageal sphincter and motor function of the body of the esophagus prior to any anti-reflux procedure. HRM is performed with catheters equipped with multiple sensors distributed longitudinally and radially in the esophagus allowing simultaneous pressure measurements in the sphincters and the esophagus. The EPT is represented by a three-dimensional plotting format for interpretation of the HRM. Esophageal pressure measurements are converted into a color scale using cold colors for interpretation of low pressures and hot color for interpretation of high pressures. This study may provide alternative diagnosis, such as scleroderma or achalasia, for which anti-reflux surgery may be contraindicated. In

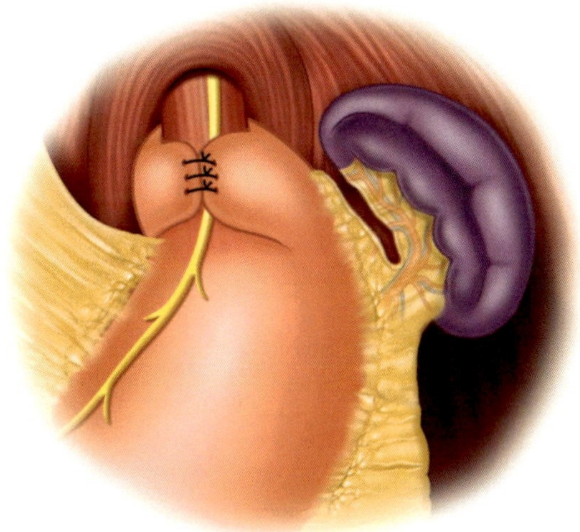

Fig. 12.1 Nissen fundoplication

addition this will help determine if there is sufficient motor power in the body of the esophagus to propel a bolus of food through a newly reconstructed valve. Patients with normal peristaltic contractions do well with a 360° Nissen fundoplication (Fig. 12.1). When peristalsis is decreased or severely disordered (greater than 30% simultaneous contractions or dropped waves) or the amplitude of the contraction in one or more of the lower esophageal segment is below 20 mmHg, a partial fundoplication is recommended, especially if the patient has clinical dysphagia.

- *Assessment of esophageal length:* This is done to exclude esophageal shortening. Repetitive injury causes scarring and fibrosis and ultimately results in anatomic shortening of the esophagus in a small group of patients. This compromises the ability to do an adequate tension-free repair without a potential breakdown or thoracic migration of the stomach. It is essential to identify these patients preoperatively.
- Esophageal length is best assessed using video roentgenographic contrast studies and endoscopic findings together. It has been our experience that when the gastroesophageal (GE) junction is above 30 cm from the incisors or there is a documented stricture, the probability of encountering a short esophagus increases considerably.

Choice of Operation

Selection of a partial versus complete fundoplication is based upon an assessment of the esophageal contractility and the clinical presence of dysphagia [4, 5]. The surgeon should be careful with performing a 360° fundoplication in those patients with clinical dysphagia. Those with weak esophageal contractions (amplitudes of contractions <30% simultaneous waves) may have increased outflow resistance associated with a complete fundoplication, which will dramatically increase the dysphagia postoperatively. If the esophagus is found to be short at surgery besides appropriate circumferential dissection in an attempt to bring the esophagus to the abdomen, a Collis gastroplasty may be necessary.

In those patients with normal esophageal length and motility, our operation of choice is a laparoscopic Nissen fundoplication, but we recognize that some surgeons perform a partial fundoplication even with normal motility.

In those patients with decreased motility and dysphagia, our preference is to perform a partial fundoplication. If the patient has decreased motility without dysphagia, a Nissen fundoplication is a reasonable option.

Surgical Techniques

A number of anti-reflux procedures have been described for the treatment of GERD. The most common procedures are Nissen fundoplication and a 270° partial fundoplication (Toupet). We recognize that other procedures exist, but we do not have any clinical experience with them (e.g., Hill procedure).

Patient Position and Room Setup

1. The patient may be positioned in a modified lithotomy position or with split legs depending on the surgeon's preference.
2. The surgeon stands between the legs and works with both hands with the monitor overlying the head of the patient. This allows the right- and left-handed instruments to approach the hiatus with appropriate angulation and exposure.
3. The patient is placed at 30–45° of reverse Trendelenburg position to allow displacement the transverse colon and small bowel inferiorly to keep them away from obstructing the surgical maneuvers and the view of the video camera.

Trocar Position and Principles of Exposure

1. Four 5-mm and one 10-mm port are utilized with a 0°-, 30°-, and/or 45°-angled laparoscope.
2. The abdominal cavity is accessed with a 5 mm direct viewing in the left upper abdominal quadrant (midclavicular line), 2–3″ below the costal margin (right operating port).
3. Place the left operating port in the right upper abdominal quadrant (midclavicular line), 2–3″ below the costal margin. This allows triangulation between the camera and the two instruments being in direct line with the camera.
4. Place one lateral retracting port below the costal margin in the lateral left upper quadrant (anterior axillary line).
5. Place the camera port (10-mm) above the umbilicus, one-third of the distance between the umbilicus and xiphoid process and 2–3″ to the left of the midline. In patients with large body habitus, this port may be needed to be placed half of the distance between the umbilicus and the xiphoid process.

6. A Nathanson retractor is carefully placed through an epigastric incision (and to the left of the falciform ligament) for anterior retraction of the liver and exposure of the esophageal hiatus. This maneuver exposes the esophageal hiatus. The stomach can subsequently be manipulated and retracted with an blunt grasper to expose and better visualize the hiatus. In the presence of a hiatal hernia, reduction of the hernia with the excision of the hernia sac and fixation will need to be accomplished.

I. *Nissen Procedure (Complete 360° Fundoplication)*

The critical elements of laparoscopic Nissen fundoplication are:

1. Crural dissection, identification, and preservation of both vagus nerves
2. Circumferential dissection of the esophagus
3. Fundus mobilization by division of short gastric vessels (a Nissen-Rossetti fundoplication is a variant of the Nissen procedure without division of the short gastric vessels)
4. Crural closure
5. Creation of a short, loose fundoplication by enveloping the anterior and posterior wall of the fundus around the lower esophagus

1. *Crural dissection* begins with identification of either the left or the right crus. Laparoscopic scissors, blunt graspers, or an energy device should be used for dissection.
   (a) Begin the dissection by incising the gastro-hepatic ligament. This will expose the lesser sac with the caudate lobe, the right crus, and the vena cava.
   (b) A replaced left hepatic artery arising from the left gastric artery will be present in up to 25% of patients. It should be identified and preserved.
   (c) After incising the gastro-hepatic ligament, the right crus is dissected from the anterior to posterior trying to preserve the covering muscular fascia of the crus intact.
   (d) With careful maneuvers and retracting the right crus laterally, the mediastinum just lateral and posterior to the esophagus should be dissected. The dissection continues into the mediastinum in order to separate the esophagus from its surrounding structures; this will be a critical step to allow proper mobilization of the esophagus into the abdominal cavity. The right, posterior vagus is in this area, and it must be identified. The junctions of the left and right crural fibers are identified just posterior to the esophagus from the right side.
   (e) Anterior dissection at the level of the phrenoesophageal ligament should be performed with care to prevent injury to the phrenic artery and vein as they course the anterior aspect of the hiatus. The left, anterior vagus nerve is just beneath the ligament and must be identified and preserved. The left crus is then dissected from anterior to posterior separating the esophagus from the left crus.
   (f) By retracting the esophagus anteriorly, the left and right crural junction can be then identified. A complete dissection of the lateral and inferior

aspect of the left crus and fundus of the stomach is the key maneuver allowing circumferential mobilization of the esophagus. By retracting the gastric fundus to the right, a better exposure of the left crus can be accomplished.

2. *Circumferential dissection of the esophagus* can be accomplished by careful dissection of the lateral, anterior, and posterior soft tissues within the hiatus with the purpose of bringing 3–4 cm of the esophagus into the abdomen without tension.
   (a) In the presence of severe esophagitis, transmural inflammation, esophageal shortening, and/or a large posterior fat pad, this dissection may be difficult. Alternatively, the hiatus can be approached from the left side after dividing the short gastric vessels.
   (b) After circumferential dissection of the hiatus, a Penrose drain can be passed around the esophagus and be used as an esophageal retractor to facilitate the procedure.
3. *Fundus mobilization:* Complete fundus mobilization allows construction of a tension-free fundoplication.
   (a) The gastrosplenic ligament is incised approximately one-third the distance down the greater curvature of the stomach with an energy device close to the stomach; graspers are used for lateral retraction to enter the lesser sac. Dissect and divide the short gastric vessels with the aid of an energy device. The dissection also includes posterior attachments of the upper stomach and continues until the right crus and caudate lobe can be seen from the left side (complete mobilization).
4. *Crural closure*: With or without a blunt-tipped 36 Fr. bougie (surgeon's preference).
   (a) Retracting the esophagus anterior and to the patient's left, identify the left and right crura for repair.
   (b) Using 0 weight interrupted nonabsorbable sutures on a non-cutting needle with pledgets, the crural defect is approximated in a U-shaped manner. The number of sutures will depend on the hiatal opening size. While intracorporeal knot tying can be performed, we prefer to use an extracorporeal knot here.
   (c) It is important not to narrow the hiatus during this part of the procedure.
5. Creation of a short, loose fundoplication.
   (a) Grasp the posterior fundus, and pass it to the right posterior to the esophagus, making sure that the proper portion of the fundus has been brought posterior. We confirm this by making a "shoe shine" maneuver with the stomach behind the esophagus.
   (b) Place two anchoring sutures of 2-0 silk between the stomach-esophagus-stomach, making sure the sutures don't take the anterior vagus nerve to complete the fundoplication. When finished, the fundoplication should be

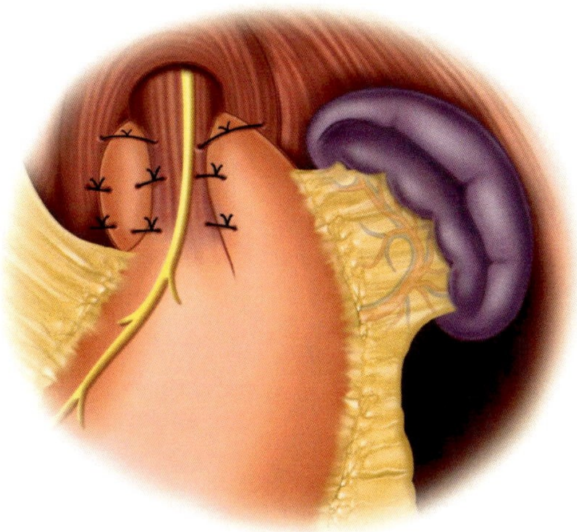

Fig. 12.2 Toupet fundoplication

loose and floppy. A 5-mm instrument should be able to be passed between the fundoplication and the esophagus easily. Although this step can be done without a calibrating bougie, most authors recommend the use of a 54–60 Fr. bougie.

(c) Assure hemostasis and port closure.

II. *Toupet Procedure (Partial 270° Fundoplication)*

Although the orientation of partial fundoplication may be either partial 180° anterior wrap (Dor), posterior, or lateral, we favor the laparoscopic Toupet procedure (270° posterior fundoplication) (Fig. 12.2).

1. All the mobilization steps of the Nissen are performed first. The short gastric vessels also need to be mobilized in a Toupet fundoplication. The Penrose drain is removed now.
2. The fundus is brought behind the esophagus so that the posterior portion of the fundus is visible. The blunt grasper from the left lateral 5 mm trocar is used to hold the fundus up for exposure to the left crus from the right side.
3. Three 2-0 silk sutures are used to fix the fundus to the left crus. It is important to place these sutures first, as once the fundoplication is constructed, the left crus will not be easily seen. Intracorporeal suturing and knot tying is preferred in this step.
4. Three 2-0 silk sutures are then placed on the posterior fundus to the right crus of the diaphragm. Intracorporeal suturing and knot tying is preferred in this step.
5. Once the posterior fixation is completed, the anterior sutures are placed, three on the right and three on the left, approximating the fundus to the esophagus, so that the fundoplication incorporates 270° of the esophagus. The top suture on each side incorporates the fundus with the diaphragmatic crural sutures to

make collar stiches. Care is taken to avoid the anterior vagus nerve during this portion of the procedure.

Postoperative Care

1. A nasogastric tube is not necessary.
2. Pain is managed with per oral narcotics or ketorolac for the first 24 h and oral hydrocodone or NSAIDS thereafter as necessary.
3. A barium esophagram is performed the morning after the surgery to confirm that the stomach is below the diaphragm. If this is confirmed, then room temperature or warm clear liquids are begun, and the patient is discharged. On the other hand, if the wrap has migrated cephalad into the mediastinum, the patient should be taken to the operative room for immediate revision of the fundoplication. We keep the patient on clear liquids for a few days, assuming the normal post op dysphagia is present. Otherwise the diet can be advanced to a puree diet.

Immediate Postoperative Symptom Management

It is common for patients to have a change in the swallowing mechanism after a fundoplication. The key is to explain this preoperatively to all patients, so that these symptoms are expected, and the patients understand what to expect.

1. Dysphagia: Postoperative dysphagia is a common symptom after fundoplication. It is our experience that a 360° wrap produces more dysphagia than a 270° wrap. The dysphagia can last up to 6 weeks. During this period, patients are placed on dietary modification. For the first 2–3 days, all patients are placed on a liquid only diet. If the dysphagia begins to dissipate rapidly (the norm), the diet is advanced to "smoothies" for 2–3 days. If the patients tolerate smoothies, then they are advanced to a solid diet. Patients are told to avoid bread, well-done meats, dry foods (white meat chicken or tuna), carbonated beverages, and cold liquids or food. This limitation is continued until the temporary dysphagia has resolved, usually a couple of months. If the dysphagia continues past 6 weeks, we study the patient with a barium esophagram. We have found this to generate more information than an EGD. Persistent dysphagia is usually secondary to a tight wrap. While we will perform endoscopic balloon dilation, these patients almost always need further surgery with loosening of the wrap or conversion to a partial fundoplication. It does take up to 2 months for all the swelling to go away from the fundoplication, so time should be allow for recovery with a need to study or instrument them before that time.
2. Gas-bloat syndrome: This is a poorly understood syndrome with a wide variety of presentations. By far, most of the symptoms are mild and tend to disappear as

the swelling around the fundoplication goes away. It is seen much less in partial fundoplication than complete fundoplication. Patients must be instructed to avoid carbonated beverages and sipping hot liquids through a straw. The most common presentation is epigastric distention and discomfort after eating. Persistence with severe symptoms is very unusual but, if present, requires surgery with take down of the wrap. "Gas pains" are part of this syndrome. It is secondary to the increase in swallowed air in the intestinal tract especially the splenic flexure area of the colon. It disappears over time, and it is associated with increased passage of flatus as well.

3. Hiccough: It is a very common symptom in the early postoperative course of fundoplication. It is seen more often in those with GERD and large hiatal hernias. It is unusual to last more than 2 weeks.
4. Shoulder pain: It is common to have referred pain from the phrenic nerve to the shoulders. C3 and C4 nerve root distribution of the phrenic nerve is in the neck and medial portion of the shoulder. It can be the most painful part of the surgery. It responds well to anti-inflammatory medication and an application of a local heating pad. It is unusual for this to last more than 2 weeks.

Postoperative Complications

The most common reasons for failure are disruption of the sutures in the diaphragm causing a recurrent hiatal hernia fundoplication with cephalad migration of the wrap into the chest. This may also be the consequence of an improperly mobilized esophagus. If there is no angulation of the stomach and the esophagus, this usually remains as an asymptomatic process. However, if angulation occurs, then dysphagia commonly occurs. It also can lead to disruption of the wrap and recurrence of the GERD. The primary treatment of recurrent reflux symptoms is medication. If medical treatment fails, revisional surgery may be needed.

In a study of 1751 patients that had a laparoscopic fundoplication for GERD, 109 patients underwent revisional surgery after a median postoperative time of 26 months after the primary procedure. The indications for revisional surgery were dysphagia in 52 patients (47.7%), reflux in 36 (33%), paraesophageal herniation in 16 (14.6%), and atypical symptoms in 5 patients (4.6%). However, the success rate for revisional surgery is lower than primary surgery with least success in those patients in whom indication for revisional surgery was dysphagia [6].

The safety of laparoscopic fundoplication has now been established. Mortality is rare following an elective anti-reflux procedure, whether open or laparoscopic. Complications associated with surgical techniques and postoperative recovery have improved. Laparoscopic fundoplication has decreased the incidence of splenic injury compared to open surgery. Intraoperative esophageal or gastric injury is rare, especially if a bougie is not utilized. Cumulative results suggest an incidence of pulmonary embolism of less than 0.5%.

Postoperative Outcomes

Several studies have compared outcomes between a laparoscopic Nissen and the laparoscopic Toupet fundoplication. In general, the prevalence of postoperative dysphagia, gas-bloat syndrome, inability to belch, and reoperation rates seems to be higher in those patients undergoing Nissen fundoplication. However, dysphagia in those patients undergoing Nissen fundoplication seems to be a self-limited problem in the majority of cases. While a shorter operative time and higher postoperative lower esophageal sphincter pressures are associated with the Nissen fundoplication, both procedures have demonstrated equivalent improvement in quality of life and long-term control of GERD.

References

1. Broeders JA, Mauritz FA, Ahmed Ali U, et al. Systematic review and meta-analysis of laparoscopic Nissen (posterior total) versus Toupet (posterior partial) fundoplication for gastro-oesophageal reflux disease. Br J Surg. 2010;97(9):1318–30.
2. Johnson WE, Hagen JA, DeMeester TR, et al. Outcome of respiratory symptoms after antireflux surgery on patients with gastroesophageal reflux disease. Arch Surg. 1996;131:489.
3. Singhal V, Khaitan L. Preoperative evaluation of gastroesophageal esophageal reflux disease. Surg Clin North Am. 2015;95:615.
4. Ludemann R, Watson DI, Jamieson GG, et al. Five-year follow up of a randomized clinical trial of laparoscopic total versus anterior 180 degrees fundoplication. Br J Surg. 2005;92:240.
5. Du X, Hu Z, Yan C, et al. A meta-analysis of long follow-up outcomes of laparoscopic Nissen (total) versus Toupet (270°) fundoplication for gastro-esophageal reflux disease based on randomized controlled trials in adults. BMC Gastroenterol. 2016;16(1):88.
6. Lamb PJ, Myers JC, Jamieson GG, Thompson SK, Devitt PG, Watson DI. Long-term outcomes of revisional surgery following laparoscopic fundoplication. Br J Surg. 2009;96(4):391–7.

Laparoscopic Antireflux Surgery: Magnetic GEJ Augmentation

13

Matias Mihura and Brian E. Louie

Introduction

Gastroesophageal reflux disease (GERD) is a common disease of the gastrointestinal tract, with an increasing incidence, especially among people in western countries. The dominant treatment for patients with uncomplicated GERD is medical therapy in the form empiric anti-secretory therapy particularly proton pump inhibitors (PPIs) combined with lifestyle modifications such as weight loss, elevation of the head of bed, smaller meal size, and avoidance of trigger foods. Despite this, almost 40% of patients have incomplete control of their symptoms despite high doses of medication [1, 2].

Until recently, the only alternative treatment was surgical reconstruction of the gastroesophageal junction with antireflux surgery, commonly Nissen fundoplication. Surgeons have used this operation for over 70 years since it was first published to control GERD [1]. Over the years, it has undergone various modifications but has remained essentially the same. Long-term outcomes of antireflux surgery show equivalent if not superior results to those on PPI therapy [2–4]. Despite these results, it is estimated that only 1% of patients with chronic GERD will be offered and undergo antireflux surgery [5, 6]. The reasons for this are multifaceted but are driven by patient and referring physician concerns about increased rates of flatulence, the inability to belch and vomit, and, most importantly, variance in efficacy and long-term satisfaction [2, 3].

Magnetic sphincter augmentation (MSA) was developed to address these issues while still providing long-term reflux control through a simple, standardized laparoscopic procedure. This chapter will review the development of the device, describe the current surgical technique for implantation, review the outcomes, and discuss the future directions of the device.

M. Mihura · B. E. Louie (✉)
Division of Thoracic Surgery, Swedish Cancer Institute, Seattle, WA, USA
e-mail: brian.louie@swedish.org

J. Grams et al. (eds.), *The SAGES Manual of Foregut Surgery*,
https://doi.org/10.1007/978-3-319-96122-4_13

Magnetic Sphincter Augmentation Device

The magnetic sphincter device consists of a series of magnets coated in parylene and hermetically sealed inside titanium cases. The beads are interlinked together with titanium wires forming a flexible ring that rests around the LES in a circular fashion [7]. The magnetic attraction of the beads provides a sustained force to augment the LES barrier. When closed, the beads rest on the titanium struts near to each other but not touching in a "Roman arch" configuration (Fig. 13.1). This allows the ring to rest on the outer surface of the esophagus without compressing the distal esophagus. The magnetic force of the MSA device is highest when the device is closed and opens in response to a bolus of food passing through the gastroesophageal junction (Fig. 13.2). The device is manufactured in different sizes, from 13 to 17 beads, and is capable of almost doubling its size when fully expanded.

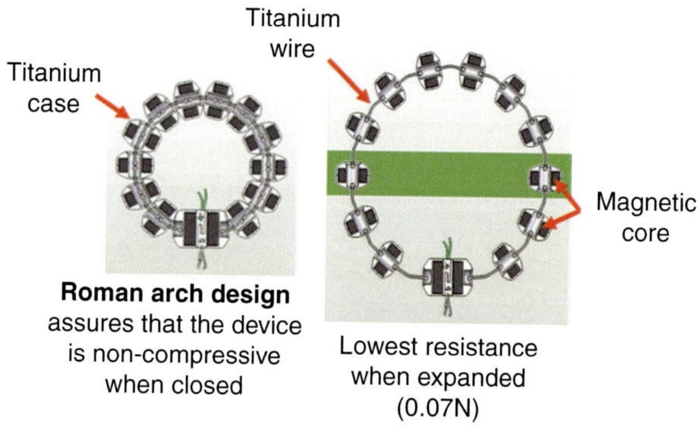

Fig. 13.1 Roman arch design of the magnetic sphincter device. (Image courtesy of Torax Medical Incorporated)

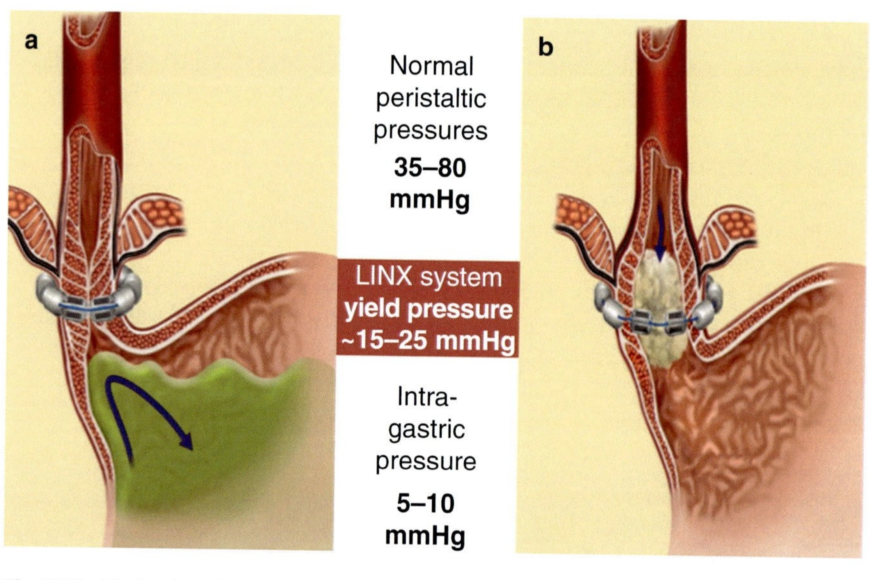

Fig. 13.2 Mechanism of action of the magnetic sphincter device. (**a**) MSA keeps LES closed. (**b**) MSA opens to food bolus. MSA magnetic sphincter augmentation, LES lower esophageal sphincter. (Image courtesy of Torax Medical Incorporated)

Toward Augmentation of the Lower Esophageal Sphincter

The concept of augmenting the lower esophageal sphincter (LES) was first described by Angelchik who developed an implantable silicone prosthesis that he proposed as a device to reduce hiatal hernias but was found to also control GERD [6]. In an attempt to provide an explanation for the effectiveness of this device, Samelson et al., using canine models, placed 3 mm wide rubber bands calibrated at a pressure of 25 mm Hg at the level of the gastroesophageal junction in order to simulate the prosthesis [7]. He determined that the ligatures raised the gastric pressure at which the sphincter opened. Without a ligature, the opening pressure of the LES occurred with an infused volume of 1250 cc and a gastric pressure of 7 mm Hg, whereas a 4 cm ligature around the GEJ allowed it to open 2250 cc and 18 mm Hg, respectively. In a similar fashion, the initial ex vivo studies of the MSA device were performed using a porcine stomach model with the pylorus ligated and a magnetic sphincter device placed around the LES with different magnetic forces. Water was perfused into the stomach through a posterior gastrotomy, and gastric yield pressures were found to correlate directly with magnetic forces as measured with a manometry catheter [5].

The subsequent in vivo animal studies were done in ten live male Sinclair pigs since porcine peristaltic pressures are similar to those in humans. All the animals underwent implantation of the device with different magnetic forces and were followed closely for 20–44 weeks. These studies confirmed normal eating patterns with no observed effects on eating behavior or weight gain in any of the animals; that the esophageal mucosa appeared normal at all endoscopies and no erosion or migration was observed at necropsy; that the devices were confined to the esophageal adventitia and encapsulated in fibrous tissue; that average LES pressure rose from 22.9 to 35.6 mmHg after surgery but, interestingly, did not correlate with the increasing magnetic forces; and that esophageal peristaltic pressures were adequate to open the augmented LES, without changes in eating behavior, even at the highest closed magnetic force tested [5].

Human trials with MSA began with 38 patients undergoing implantation between February 2007 and October 2008 at four different centers in the USA and Europe, and their results were reported in four separate papers representing results defined as short term, 1–2 years, 4 years, and 5 years of follow-up [8–11]. The results in these initial 38 patients demonstrated initial improvements in symptom control, improvements in measured distal esophageal acid exposure, and 80–85% of patients free from daily PPI use. These results were sustained at the 1–2-year, 4-year, and 5-year reports (Table 13.1).

With encouraging results from this initial trial, a larger multicenter trial began in January 2009 at 14 centers (13 in the USA and 1 in the Netherlands). The 3-year outcomes demonstrated that 64% of patients had achieved a reduction of 50% or more in the % time pH < 4 compared to baseline with a full 58% whose esophageal acid exposure normalized [12]. Additionally, a 50% reduction in the quality of life scores and a 50% reduction in the dose of PPIs were achieved in 92% and 93% of

Table 13.1 Results of the feasibility trial

Author	N	Follow-up	GERD-HRQL (Off PPIs)	PPI cessation % (n)	pH testing
Bonavina et al. [8]	38	Mean 209 days (12–434)	Median: decreased from 26 to 2.6 at 6 months $p < 0.005$	89% off PPIs at 3 months	Median total % time pH < 4: from 8.4% to 1.1% $p < 0.001$ Median DeMeester score: from 29.3 to 4.2[a] $p < 0.001$
Bonavina et al. [9]	44	Median 895 days (226–1144)	Mean: decreased by 85% at 1 year and 90% at 2 years $p < 0.0001$	90% at 1 year and 86% at 2 years off PPIs	Mean total % time pH < 4: from 11.9% to 3.1% at 1 year and 2.4 at 2 years. Both $p < 0.0001$ Mean DeMeester score: from 42.3 to 11.9 at 1 year and 9.4 at 2 years.[b] Both $p < 0.0001$
Lipham et al. [10]	44	Median 3.7 years (119–1827 days)	Mean: decreased from 25.7 ± 6.4 at baseline to 3.3 ± 3.7 $p < 0.001$	80% free from daily PPIs	Mean total % time pH < 4: from 11.9% to 3.8% $p < 0.001$ Mean DeMeester score: from 42.3 to 14.7[c] $p < 0.05$
Saino et al. [11]	44[d]	5 years	Mean: decreased from 25.7 to 2.9 $p < 0.01$ 93.9% with at least 50% reduction in total score	87.8% (29/33) were off medication 93.9% achieved a reduction of 50% or more in their daily dose	Mean total % time pH < 4 = from 11.9% to 4.6% $p < 0.01$ Mean DeMeester score: from 42.3 to 16.1 $p < 0.01$

[a]24/38 completed the esophageal pH testing
[b]40/44 completed their clinical and pH-metry assessment at either 1 or 2 years of follow-up
[c]20/44 completed esophageal pH testing at 3 years
[d]33/44 completed the 5-year follow-up and 20/44 patients completed esophageal pH testing at 5 years

patients, respectively. There was a significant improvement in the median DeMeester score from 36.6 to 13.5 at 1 year ($p < 0.001$). The 40% of patients identified with esophagitis at baseline decreased to 12% at year 1 and to 11% at year 2 ($p < 0.001$ for both comparisons). With these encouraging results, MSA with the LINX® Reflux Management System received FDA approval in 2012 as an alternative option in the treatment of GERD (Table 13.2).

Table 13.2 Results of the pivotal trial

Author	N	Follow-up	GERD-HRQL (Off PPIs)	PPI cessation % (n)	pH testing
Ganz et al. [12]	100	3 years[a]	Median: decreased from 27 at baseline to 2 at 3 years $p < 0.005$	87% (72/83) off PPIs at 3 years	Median total % time pH < 4: from 10.9% to 3.3% $p < 0.001$ Median DeMeester score: from 36.6 to 13.5[a] $p < 0.001$
Ganz et al. [16]	100[b]	5 years	Median: decreased from 27 at baseline to 4 at 5 years $p < 0.001$ 83% with at least 50% reduction in total score	75.3% were off PPIs at 5 years 89.4% achieved a reduction of 50% or more in their daily dose	No pH testing at 5 years

[a]98/100 completed follow-up at 1 year, 90/100 at 2 years, and 85/100 at 3 years. 96/100 completed esophageal pH testing at 1 year
[b]85/100 completed 5-year follow-up

Indications

The indications for implantation of a magnetic sphincter are the same as for any other established surgical treatment for GERD. These patients have chronic symptoms of GERD documented by objective testing, a clinical response to PPI therapy, and desire an alternative to medical therapy.

There are specific recommendations to guide patient selection for MSA that include:

- Age > 18
- Typical GERD symptoms, at least partially responsive to PPIs
- Los Angeles grade A or B esophagitis
- Hiatal hernia < 3 cm
- BMI < 35 kg/m^2
- Esophageal motility with >70% of effective swallows and distal wave amplitude > 35 mmHg

Furthermore, MSA is not recommended in the following situations:

- Large or paraesophageal hiatal hernias
- Los Angeles grade C or D esophagitis
- Barrett's esophagus
- Prior esophageal or gastric surgery
- Need for MRI > 1.5 Tesla
- History of dysphagia

The only known absolute contraindications to implantation are an allergy to titanium, stainless steel, nickel, or other ferrous materials and the presence of esophageal cancer.

Preoperative Evaluation

The preoperative evaluation of a potential patient for LINX implantation is the same as for any other antireflux procedure. It is recommended that patients undergo the standard tests of upper endoscopy, barium swallow, 24 or 48 h pH testing, and high-resolution manometry. Additional tests such as gastric emptying studies may be performed at the surgeon's discretion.

Surgical Technique

The surgical technique for implantation has evolved over the past 5 years since MSA was introduced in the USA. Initial implants were completed using a minimal dissection technique hoping to leave as much of the native structure of the reflux barrier intact. Over time it has been become recognized that some of the surgical principles of antireflux surgery must be maintained. Specifically, hiatal closure and restoration of intra-abdominal LES length are required so that the device is clearly secured around the distal esophagus just above the endoscopic gastroesophageal junction.

Patients are positioned in low lithotomy position under general anesthesia. Five ports are usually required positioned similarly to those used for fundoplication. We place a 11 mm camera port cephalad and to the left of the umbilicus, a 5 mm subxiphoid port for the Nathanson liver retractor, a 5 mm port at the left costal margin sited at edge of the greater curve, a 5 mm port at the left costal margin entering just above the left colon, and a 5 mm port in the right subcostal space (Fig. 13.3). The hiatus is probed carefully to assess for the presence of a hiatal hernia or diaphragmatic laxity (Fig. 13.4a small dimple and Fig. 13.4b – small HH).

We describe the original minimal dissection technique below. If used, it should only be used when patients with no hernia, a Hill grade 1 valve, and no laxity in the diaphragm at laparoscopy. At most centers performing MSA, a complete hiatal dissection has been adopted for all cases but especially if a hiatal hernia is detected and/or a Hill grade 2 or worse valve is encountered.

Minimal Dissection Technique

Dissection begins by dividing the gastro-hepatic ligament with the hook cautery above and below to the hepatic branch of the anterior vagus nerve, thereby preserving it. The peritoneum is incised along the right crus adjacent to the esophagus at the

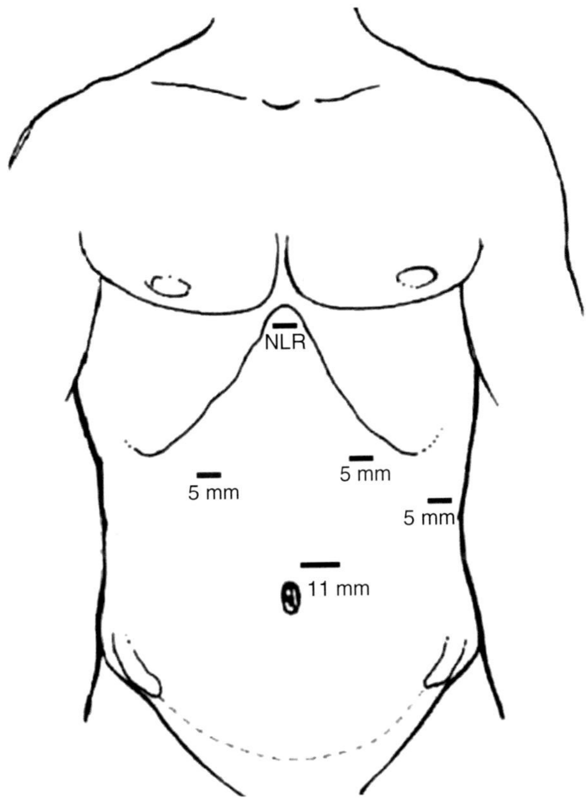

Fig. 13.3 Port placement. NLR Nathanson liver retractor

level of the hepatic vagal branch. Following the trajectory to the left side, the landing zone along the left crus is freed up by taking the attachments down staying along the crural muscle until the edge of the esophagus is identified. We then tunnel along the crural pillars toward the landing zone in the retroesophageal space to allow a Penrose drain to come through this window. The hiatus is inspected posteriorly to assess for the presence of any unsuspected hiatal hernia. If there is one, the placement of one or more posterior crural stitches is indicated. A tunnel is then created between the posterior vagus nerve and the esophageal wall, and the Penrose drain is passed through this tunnel to exclude the posterior vagal nerve.

The anterior and lateral attachments along the esophagus are dissected taking care not to injure the anterior vagal nerve but to expose the esophageal wall by bringing the fat pad onto the stomach. The MSA device sizing instrument is passed between the esophagus and the posterior vagus and wrapped around the esophagus at the level of the GEJ. Two measurements are taken to determine the size of device to be implanted. Finally the MSA device is placed through the opening between the vagus nerve and the esophagus and secured anteriorly with the anchoring clasp

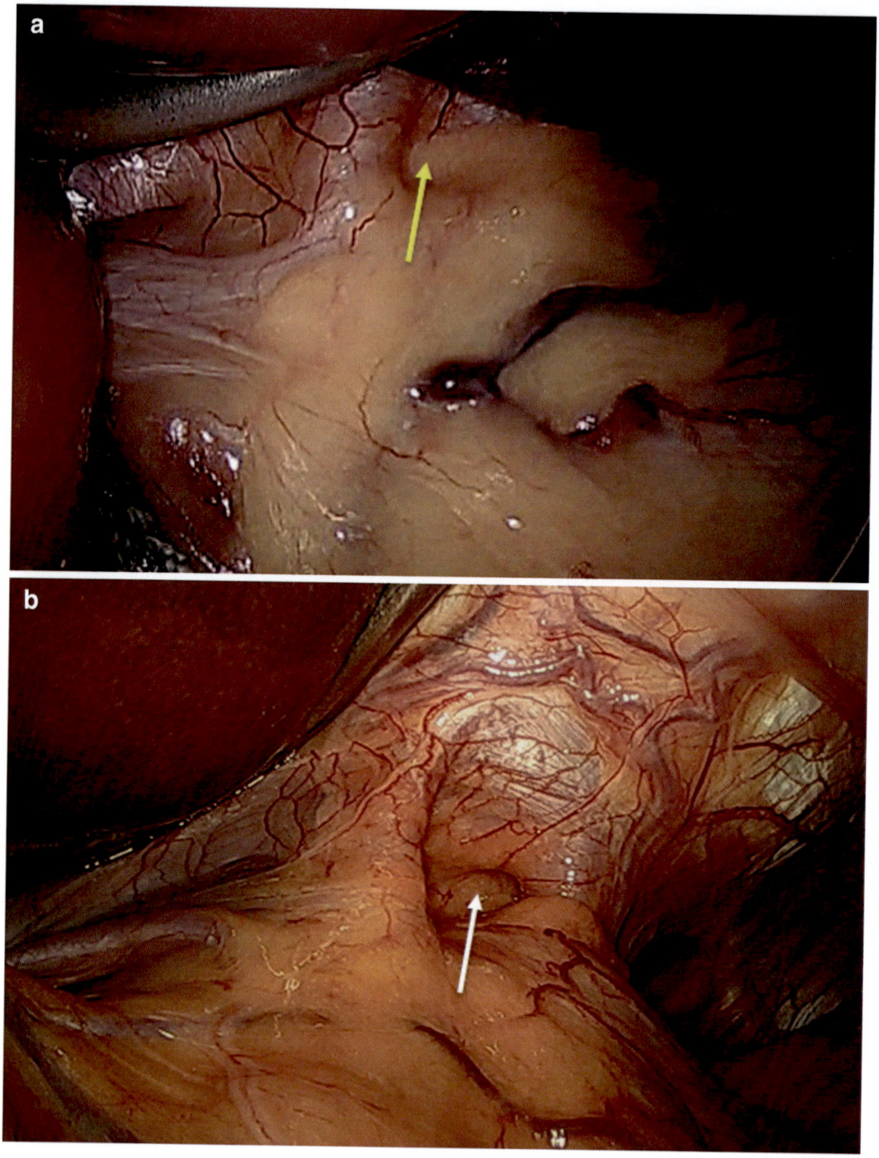

Fig. 13.4 Intraoperative assessment of the hiatus. (**a**): Hiatus with a small "dimple" or minimal hiatal hernia (yellow arrow). (**b**): Hiatus with a small hiatal hernia (white arrow)

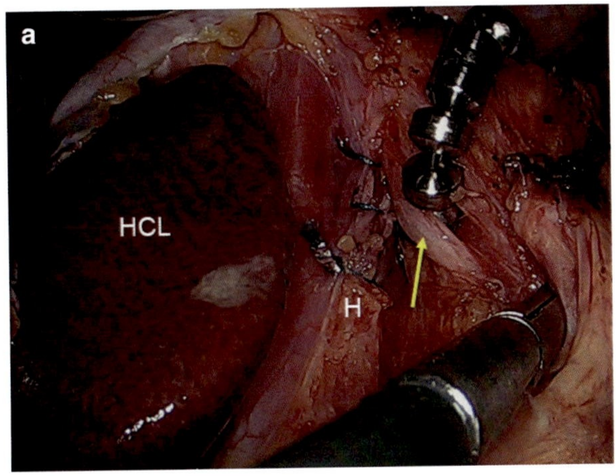

Fig. 13.5 Laparoscopic location of the magnetic sphincter after implantation. Yellow arrow marking posterior vagus nerve. HCL Hepatic caudate lobe, H Hiatus closed with three posterior stitches

(Fig. 13.5). A postoperative upper endoscopy is useful to confirm the correct placement of the device on the distal esophagus just above the rugal folds.

Complete Hiatal Dissection Technique

A complete hiatal dissection is undertaken to restore intra-abdominal length and is the same as the dissection used in preparation for a Nissen fundoplication. The hiatus is then closed primarily with sutures posteriorly until the opening matches the size of the esophagus. The posterior vagus is excluded, the esophagus sized, and the device implanted as described above.

Postoperative Management

Postoperatively, patients are started on liquids and oral pain medication the day of surgery. Our preference is to obtain a barium swallow after the procedure to confirm the position of the device and assess esophageal emptying. Once this is confirmed, a regular oral diet is instituted with instructions to eat five smaller meals and to take a small amount of solid food each waking hour to "exercise" or activate the device into the open and closed positions.

Eating recommendations are given to every patient before discharge. In our opinion, this is extremely important to decrease the rate of postoperative dysphagia. Patients are reminded that after the device is implanted, they need to eat slowly, avoiding large meals and the extremes of temperature. It's preferred to eat smaller amounts of food more frequently rather than a few large meals. PPIs are stopped the day of surgery though some suggest reducing their PPI medication immediately after surgery to a half dose or switching to ranitidine 300 mg/day for 2 weeks and then stopping [13].

Follow-up is done in a scheduled fashion. Patients are seen 2 weeks after surgery with a chest x-ray in order to assess the device position. They are then seen at 6 weeks, at 6 months, and at 12 months, then annually after the first year. We strongly recommend EGD, pH testing, and manometry 1 year after implantation. When the patient reports uncontrollable or new symptoms, evaluation is recommended and is tailored to the symptoms but often includes upper endoscopy to assess for erosion.

Complications

Complications after implantation of a MSA device are uncommon in clinical practice. In a safety analysis of the first 1000 device implantations and a follow-up of 6 years, the overall event rates were 0.1% for intra-/perioperative complications; 1.3% for readmissions, mainly in the early postoperative period; 5.6% for esophageal dilations required for dysphagia; 3.4% for reoperation for device removal with a median implant duration at time of device removal of 94 days (range 6–1302); and 0.1% for device erosion corresponding to 1 case in the late postoperative period [14].

The same trend followed a recent publication of more than 3200 devices implanted in the USA from 2012 to 2016 with a median implant duration of 1.4 years [15]. No perioperative deaths or life-threatening complications were reported. There were no device malfunctions or unanticipated events. The overall rate of device removal was 2.7% (89/3283) with dysphagia (52/89, 58.4%) and persistent reflux symptoms (19/89, 21.3%) being the most common causes of removal. The overall rate of device erosion was 0.15% (5/3283) and no migrations were reported.

Table 13.3 summarizes the complications reported in these two safety analyses of approximately 4000 patients implanted with MSA.

Dysphagia

The most common side effect described by patients after magnetic sphincter augmentation remains dysphagia, which occurs in two distinct patterns. The first is

Table 13.3 Overall complications after MSA implantation

Study	*N*	Perioperative complications % (*n*)	Readmission % (*n*)	Esophageal dilation % (*n*)	Device removal % (*n*)	Device erosion % (*n*)	Device migration %	Device malfunction %
Lipham et al. [14]	1048	0.1% (1)	1.3% (14)	5.6% (59)	3.4% (36)	0.1% (1)	0%	0%
Smith et al. [15]	3283	0%	–	–	2.7% (89)	0.15% (5)	0%	0%

during the immediate postoperative period and is fairly predictable in time course and resolution since it closely matches the time period of scarring and encapsulation of the device. Although this is universally well tolerated, there is some individual variability in regard to both duration and intensity. The biggest success factor in the management of this has been the clinician and patient understanding and pre-procedural expectation setting regarding this process. Encouraging patients to have frequent small meals and avoid a liquid-only diet has helped maintain the ability to tolerate a diet through this early period of dysphagia. It has been rare that a true intervention such as dilation has been required to address this dysphagia. Early in the clinical experience, there was a tendency to want to take action through dilation, which potentially could have extended and increased the inflammatory process. For patients whose dysphagia is not well managed through counseling and diet, current best practice is to consider a short course of steroids to reduce inflammation and swelling and allow for the natural healing process to run its course prior to the consideration of dilation [16].

The second pattern for dysphagia, which is much less common, does not appear to follow the expected time course described above. These patients have more significant symptoms that may include repeated vomiting, severe chest pain, and food impaction. In these uncommon instances, these patients may have developed secondary spastic motility disturbances leading to chest pain. Alternatively, albeit rare, they may develop pseudoachalasia or secondary motility disorder simply from implantation of the device (Fig. 13.6a, b). Manometry is often helpful in these situations. These situations have also been reported after fundoplication and lap band implantation. Lastly, the development of new-onset dysphagia or worsening dysphagia after a period of stability warrants further investigation particularly upper endoscopy and/or barium swallow to evaluate for the potential for erosion or migration.

Intra-/Perioperative Complications

Intraoperative and perioperative complications are reported to occur in 0.1% of cases [14]. The range of intraoperative complications is likely no different and probably less than Nissen fundoplication because of less dissection. Nevertheless, if they occur, they are generally related to performance of the laparoscopy. Similarly, perioperative complications are also likely related to the laparoscopy. Complications specific to MSA could include esophageal injury during the posterior dissection and exclusion of the posterior vagal nerve. In this situation, it is recommended to repair the injury using standard surgical principles and abort implantation of the device because of the potential risk for leakage and subsequent infection and erosion of the device.

Device Removal and Migration

Early in the MSA experience, the most common reason for device removal was dysphagia with a reported incidence of 1.6% (17/1048) [14]. However, with increasing

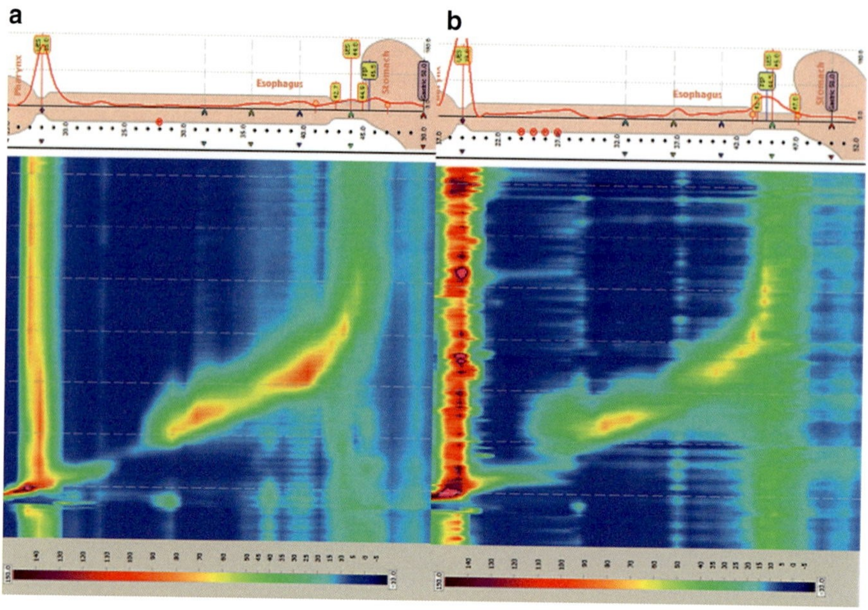

Fig. 13.6 High-resolution manometry of patient pre- and post-MSA demonstrating new dysmotility. (**a**): Pre-MSA manometry with almost normal motility. Esophageal body with 100% peristalsis, normal distal contractile integral (DCI) at 1553.5 mmHg-cm-s, and slightly elevated intrabolus pressure at 18.8 mmHg. Normal LES basal pressure at 8.5 mmHg (normal 4.8–32 mmHg) and normal integrated relaxing pressure (IRP) at 12 mmHg. (**b**): Post-MSA manometry 2 months after extraction with abnormal motility defined by esophageal body with 100% peristalsis and normal DCI, but with a notable compartmentalized esophageal pressurization. Increased IBP of 27.2 mmHg. Increased LES basal pressure at 33.4 mmHg with abnormal relaxation (IRP) of 21.1 mmHg

experience and better management, the rate of dysphagia has decreased, and the need to remove the devices is becoming less common. Still, dysphagia is the most likely reason for device removal. Device removals for MRI preparation have also become less common with the most recent version of the device, which is compatible with a 1.5 Tesla magnet. The term migration evokes the idea that the device has moved, but, in patients undergoing reoperation, the device is usually found at the gastroesophageal junction but that the junction has migrated through an unrecognized hiatal hernia. Verbal communication with other surgeons suggests that many are dissecting out the device, restoring esophageal length, and reclosing the crura to reconstruct the hiatus in order to preserve the device. Alternatively, the patient and surgeon may opt to remove the device and then re-site it or convert to a Nissen or Toupet fundoplication depending on the presence or absence of GERD symptoms.

Device Erosion

Device erosion remains a rare event. Updated data over and above the most recent safety analysis confirms 13 known cases of erosion with a rate of occurrence of less than 0.2% that is significantly lower than the larger devices of lap band or

Angelchik. Current understanding is that erosions generally occur around 24 months post implant. They are often detected by a change in status with the development of new-onset GERD or more commonly dysphagia. All device erosions have been successfully removed endoscopically [17] or laparoscopically [20]. Current best practice is to remove it endoscopically because it preserves the external planes intra-abdominally and allows for elective conversion to another antireflux procedure if the patient remains symptomatic after the esophageal wall has healed.

Several endoscopic options have been reported. First, an Olympus Endoloop Cutter (Olympus Medical Systems, Center Valley, PA, USA) (Fig. 13.7a, b) can be used to cut the titanium bar between the beads and gently extract it from the tunnel. Second, a newly developed DC Clip Cutter, which was made to remove the Over-the-Scope Clip (Ovesco Endoscopy AG, Tubingen, Germany), was used to cut the titanium bar [17]. This device is described as a bipolar grasping device that is connected to an electrical generator producing direct current impulses and

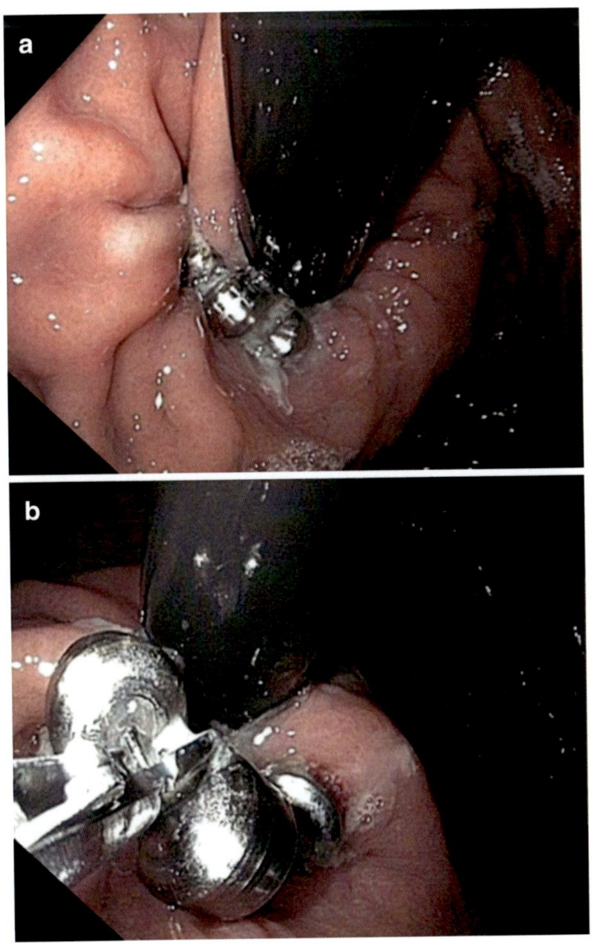

Fig. 13.7 (**a**): Endoscopic view of an eroded MSA device. (**b**): Undergoing removal with an endoloop cutter

fits via the 3.2 mm working channel of a therapeutic endoscope. Lastly, it's possible that using an endoscopic/ERCP mechanical lithotripter device (Olympus Medical Systems, Center Valley, PA, USA) will snap the titanium wire by looping a guide wire around the titanium bar and withdrawing both ends of wire. The wires are then threaded through the reusable outer sheath and into the handle, thereby allowing the loop of wire to tightened around the device using the wire to disrupt the device.

Gastroparesis

Anecdotal reports of gastroparesis developing after MSA implantation have been circulated though none have been reported in the published literature. The mechanism for this development remains unclear since this would require both vagal nerves to be divided. Even in patients who have experienced device erosion where the anterior vagal nerve is potentially in jeopardy, there have been no reported cases of gastroparesis. Standard treatment for the gastroparesis is recommended until further information is elucidated.

Outcomes of Magnetic Sphincter Augmentation

Observational Single-Arm Studies

At present, single-arm observational studies have reported both short- and long-term outcomes including the primary studies leading up to FDA approval [13, 16] (Tables 13.1, 13.2, and 13.4). Short-term outcomes have reported generally at 1 year of follow-up. These studies show consistent improvement in symptom control as evidenced by improvements in GERD-HRQL and freedom from PPIs ranging from 75% to 89%. Objective evidence of reflux assessed by pH probe analysis show a range of normalization from 50% to 85% including the MSA arm of the comparative trials. This has improved over time likely due to increasing experience.

At present, there is only limited long-term follow-up data. Ganz et al. reported on the long-term outcomes on 100 patients who formed the initial study cohort [18]. With an 85% (85/100 patients) of 5-year follow-up, 83% of patients achieved a 50% or greater reduction in GERD-HRQL scores, and median GERD-HRQL scores off PPIs decreased from 27 at baseline to 4 after 5 years of surgery ($p < 0.001$). Moreover, they obtained a decrease in patients who reported moderate to severe heartburn from 89% to 11.9% and regurgitation from 57% to 1.2% ($p < 0.001$ for all comparisons). When analyzing the use of PPIs, 75.3% of patients were off medication at 5 years, and 9.4% used them only as needed. Furthermore, this group reported endoscopic outcomes. Healing of esophagitis occurred in 26 of 34 patients at 5 years (76.5%), and in patients without it at baseline, 43 of 48 (90%) continued to have no esophagitis, whereas 4 patients developed grade A and 1 patient grade B

Table 13.4 Short- and medium-term outcomes

Author	N	Follow-up	GERD-HRQL (Off PPIs)	PPI cessation % (n)	pH testing
Bonavina et al. [13]	100[a]	Median of 3 years	Median: improved from 24 at baseline to 2 at last follow-up	85% off PPI at last follow-up	Median total % time pH < 4: from 8% to 3.2% $p < 0.001$ Median DeMeester score: from 30.1 to 11.2 $p < 0.001$
Czosnyka et al. [16]	102	Mean of 7.6 months	Median: improved from 27 at baseline to 5 at last follow-up ($p < 0.001$)	–	–

[a]95% with follow-up ≥1 year (1 year, $n = 42$; 2 years, $n = 8$; 3 years, $n = 15$; and 5 years, $n = 30$). Esophageal pH testing done on 30/100 patients with a mean follow-up for esophageal pH testing of 4.2 years

esophagitis. Similar results were reported by Saino et al. who reported on the first 44 patients undergoing MSA.

Comparative Outcomes with Fundoplication

Although there are no randomized clinical trials published comparing MSA vs standard antireflux operations, there have been several comparative studies.

There have been four predominantly single- or dual-center comparative studies comparing the outcomes of magnetic sphincter augmentation to Nissen fundoplication with follow-up limited to about 12 months [19–22]. These studies show that MSA results in similar improvements in GERD-HRQL when compared to Nissen fundoplication and similar rates of freedom from PPIs in the studies reporting that outcome. Only one study reported objective pH testing postoperatively and showed significant improvements from preoperatively but also significant differences favoring Nissen fundoplication [20]. One trial compared MSA to Toupet fundoplication with median follow-up of 45 months and showed equivalent improvements in GERD-HRQL and PPI utilization post procedure [23] (Table 13.5).

A large multi-institutional study of 354 patients with at least 12 months of follow-up compared MSA with Nissen fundoplication both overall and in a propensity-matched analysis [24]. This study showed that MSA in patients with uncomplicated GERD results in equivalent symptom control, improved quality of life with less adverse effects, but lower rate of freedom from PPI when compared to fundoplication. There was significant improvement in GERD-HRQL scores compared to baseline (from 21 to 3 for MSA and from 19 to 4 for LNF), with no significant differences between groups. Patients with MSA had a more physiologic sphincter based on the ability to belch and vomit (MSA 96% and 95% vs LNF 69% and 43% $p < 0.001$). After propensity matching, the MSA group still had significantly a lower freedom from PPI when compared to NF (76% vs 88%).

Table 13.5 Outcomes of studies comparing different types of fundoplication with MSA

Author	Procedure	N	Follow-up (months)	Median GERD-HRQL	PPI cessation % (n)	pH testing	Dysphagia/ dilation	Gas-related symptoms	Ability to belch and vomit % (n)	Reoperation (%)
Louie et al. [20]	MSA	34	6	5	100% (24/24)	DeMeester score: 14.2 % time <4: 4.6	40.2[a] Dilation: 4.2% (1/24)	1.32[b]	67% (16/24) $p = 0.0001$	0
	LNF	32	10	5.1 $p = 0.93$	96.9% (31/32)	DeMeester score: 5.1. $p = 0.0001$ % time <4: 1.1 $p = 0.0001$	36.9 Dilation: 0% $p = 0.24$	2.36 $p = 0.059$	0% (0/32)	0
Riegler et al. [21]	MSA	202	12	3	81.8%	–	7% Dilation: $p = \text{ns}$	10%	Belch: 98.4% Vomit: 91.3%	4%
	LNF/LTF	47	12	3.5 $p = 0.18$	63% $p = 0.009$	–	10.6% $p = 0.373$ Dilation: $p = \text{ns}$	31.9% $p < 0.001$	Belch: 88.9% $p = 0.007$ Vomit: 44.4% $p < 0.001$	6.4%
Sheu et al. [22]	MSA	12	7	–	–	–	83% Dilation: 50%	0%[c]	–	–
	LNF	12	7	–	–	–	58% $p = 0.37$ Dilation: 0% $p = 0.014$	33% $p = 0.21$	–	–

Reynolds et al. [19]	MSA	50	12	4.2	83% (39/47)	–	10.6% (5/47)[d] Dilation: 16% (8/50)	Overall: 27.7% (13/47) Severe: 0%	Belch: 91.5% (43/47) Vomit: 95.7% (45/47)	0
	LNF	50	12	4.3 $p = 0.88$	91.5% (43/47) $p = 0.355$	–	12.8% (6/47) $p = 0.766$ Dilation: 10% (5/50) $p = 0.554$	Overall: 38.3% (18/47) $p = 0.067$ Severe: 10.6% (5/47) $p = 0.022$	Belch: 74.5% (35/47) $p = 0.028$ Vomit: 78.7% (37/47) $p = 0.05$	0
Asti et al. [23]	MSA	135	44	0	$p =$ ns	–	$p =$ ns	$p =$ ns	–	$p =$ ns
	LTF	103	42	2 $p =$ ns		–			–	

Abbreviation: *LTF* laparoscopic Toupet fundoplication, *LNF* laparoscopic Nissen fundoplication, *MSA* magnetic sphincter augmentation, *NS* no statistical difference

[a]Measured by dysphagia score (ranges from 0 to 45, with 0 being the most severe dysphagia and 45 being no dysphagia)

[b]Values extrapolated from the GERD-HRQL scores. Lowest values indicate less symptoms

[c]Includes bloating, flatulence, and/or diarrhea

[d]Values in % (n). Corresponds to moderate/severe dysphagia: symptoms more than once a week, regurgitation of undigested food, vomiting, or requiring dietary modifications

Factors Influencing Outcomes of MSA

Despite fairly consistent results across multiple studies with symptomatic improvement in 80% and freedom from PPIs in 75%, there are still some patients who do not attain the benefits of MSA. It is not entirely clear why certain patients do not benefit from MSA, but several factors have been identified that are likely to influence the outcomes of MSA.

The first factor is the need to convert a defective lower esophageal sphincter into a competent sphincter since restoration of these characteristics is directly related to reflux control [25, 26]. In patients with a deficit in one or more of these components of the LES, resting pressure < 6 mmHg, total LES length < 2 cm, or intra-abdominal LES length < 1 cm, the ability of MSA to restore the LES to normal was 77% in patients with only one structural defect compared to 56% in patients with two or three defects [27]. Patients who converted to a normal sphincter had better reflux control and were less likely to be on PPIs compared to patients who remained with a defective sphincter.

The second factor is the patient's characteristics. A recent multivariable analysis of 170 patients implanted with a MSA device identified that excellent/good outcomes (defined by GERD-HRQL scores <15, no PPI use, and grade A or no esophagitis) were negatively impacted by BMI > 35 (OR = 0.9, p = 0.02), elevated preoperative LES residual pressure (OR = 0.92, p = 0.03), and structurally defective LES, while the presence of a Hill grade 2 valve trended toward significance [28]. The negative impact of BMI in the outcomes of MSA is understandable through several mechanisms that have been studied before: elevated BMI increases the pressure gradient between the abdominal cavity and the intrathoracic esophagus [29], higher BMI patients are associated with increased transient LES sphincter relaxations or shortenings that promote postprandial reflux events [30], and higher BMI patients are more likely to have a structurally defective sphincter and defective esophageal acid clearance [31, 32].

The fact that a defective valve affects outcome also makes sense since one of the key points in every antireflux procedure is restoring intra-abdominal esophageal length and, therefore, helping to restore the basal LES pressure. It is likely that the surgeon controls some of the ability to help restore a structurally defective LES by carefully assessing the hiatus and restoring intra-abdominal length and hiatal closure. There is likely some interplay between the Hill grade and how the surgeon assesses and repairs the hiatus. A Hill grade 4 valve is likely to undergo complete dissection and repair which will restore length and therefore pressure, whereas a Hill 2 valve may appear relatively normal at laparoscopy and not have as much length restored when a simple cruroplasty is performed rather than a complete dissection [28].

Potential Indications for MSA

Although the initial implantation criteria for MSA are restricted to patients with GERD symptoms with hiatal hernias less than 3 cm in size and normal motility, MSA, theoretically, can be used in almost any situation where augmentation of the

LES is required. It must be remembered that these extended indications are based on surgical judgment and not on the basis of any body of evidence or literature.

The most obvious consideration by foregut surgeons is to use MSA in hernias that are larger than 3 cm and might even be classified as paraesophageal hernias. Several centers are currently enrolling patients with sliding hiatal hernias that are 4–7 cm into a 5-year follow-up registry. Early results from 1 center have shown that it is feasible to implant the device in 52 patients with a hernia between 3 and 7 cm. At a median follow-up of 12 months, GERD-HRQL decreased from 20.5 to 3.6 and had lower PPI use compared to patients with hernias < 3 cm and similar rates of dysphagia [33]. There were no recurrences at this early follow-up. Additionally, 2 centers enrolled 200 patients with 78% of patients having hernias larger than 5 cm and/or a paraesophageal hernia. All hernias were primarily repaired with 83% having an absorbable mesh onlay followed by implantation of a magnetic sphincter device [34]. At a median follow-up of 8.6 months, 156 patients had improved GERD-HRQL scores and freedom from PPIs in 94%. Objective follow-up was completed in only 51 patients with 3 asymptomatic hernias (<3 cm) and 1 symptomatic hernia (8% recurrence 4/51) who underwent successful hernia repair without MSA manipulation.

One area of particular interest where MSA might play a key role is in the management of GERD in patients who are post sleeve gastrectomy. The LES is likely to be rendered weaker after a sleeve gastrectomy due to division of some of the collar sling fibers that enhance the angle of His. Loss of the angle reduced the intrinsic LES pressure significantly, thereby allowing easier egress of reflux into the esophagus [35, 36]. Augmentation of the weakened LES with a magnetic sphincter is an attractive option for these patients whose only alternative is conversion to a Roux-en-Y gastric bypass, an operation they often decline when discussing the options for weight loss surgery. A pilot study of seven patients undergoing MSA after sleeve gastrectomy confirmed feasibility of placement as well as improvement in their symptoms at very early follow-up of 4 weeks [37]. A larger trial is underway in Europe currently and planning for a US trial is also well underway.

Patients experiencing GERD after a Roux-en-Y gastric bypass for weight loss are much less common than patients post sleeve. The mechanism of action in this group is less clear though loss of the angle of His, a relatively large pouch, and some dilation of the distal esophagus likely contribute to the development of GERD. A single-case series of two patients is reported showing improvement in GERD-HRQL [38].

Conclusion

Magnetic sphincter augmentation with the LINX® Reflux Management System is a novel device made of an expansible bracelet of magnetic beads designed to be placed around the gastroesophageal junction with a standardized laparoscopic procedure. This device can augment the function of the lower esophageal sphincter by preventing premature opening of the sphincter, thereby preventing reflux of gastric contents into the lower esophagus, while maintaining the ability to permit the passage of the food bolus and to belch and vomit. Magnetic sphincter augmentation has demonstrated in multiple studies consistent improvements in patient symptoms as measured by the GERD-HRQL instrument, freedom from PPIs, and improving objective pH control. These outcomes confirm that MSA is an effective method of controlling troublesome GERD symptoms. Future studies are required to determine its role outside of the initial indications for its use.

References

1. Nissen R. Eine einfache Operation zur Beeinflussung der Refluxoesophagitis. Schweiz Med Wochenschr. 1956;86:590–2.
2. Lundell L, Miettinen P, Myrvold H, Pedersen S, Liedman B, Hatlebakk J, et al. Continued (5-year) followup of a randomized clinical study comparing antireflux surgery and omeprazole in gastroesophageal reflux disease. Am Coll Surg [Internet]. 2001;192(2):172–9. Available from: http://www.sciencedirect.com/science/article/pii/S1072751500007973.
3. Lundell L, Miettinen P, Myrvold HE, Hatlebakk JG, Wallin L, Engström C, et al. Comparison of outcomes twelve years after antireflux surgery or omeprazole maintenance therapy for reflux esophagitis. Clin Gastroenterol Hepatol [Internet]. 2009;7(12):1292–8. Available from: https://doi.org/10.1016/j.cgh.2009.05.021.
4. Galmiche J-P, Hatlebakk J, Attwood S, Ell C, Fiocca R, Eklund S, et al. Laparoscopic antireflux surgery vs esomeprazole treatment for chronic GERD. JAMA [Internet]. 2011;305(19):1969–77. Available from: http://jama.jamanetwork.com/article.aspx?doi=10.1001/jama.2011.626.
5. Angelchik JP, Cohen R. A new surgical procedure for the treatment of gastroesophageal reflux and hiatal hernia. Surg Gynecol Obstet [Internet]. 1979;148(2):246–8. Available from: http://www.ncbi.nlm.nih.gov/pubmed/154176.
6. Samelson SL, Weiser HF, Bombeck CT, Siewert JR, Ludtke FE, Hoelscher AH, et al. A new concept in the surgical treatment of gastroesophageal reflux. Ann Surg [Internet]. 1983;197(3):254–9. Available from: http://www.pubmedcentral.nih.gov/articlerender.fcgi?artid=1352726&tool=pmcentrez&rendertype=abstract.
7. Ganz RA, Gostout CJ, Grudem J, Swanson W, Berg T, DeMeester TR. Use of a magnetic sphincter for the treatment of GERD: a feasibility study. Gastrointest Endosc. 2008;67(2):287–94.
8. Bonavina L, Saino GI, Bona D, Lipham J, Ganz RA, Dunn D, et al. Magnetic augmentation of the lower esophageal sphincter: results of a feasibility clinical trial. J Gastrointest Surg. 2008;12(12):2133–40.
9. Bonavina L, DeMeester T, Fockens P, Dunn D, Saino G, Bona D, et al. Laparoscopic sphincter augmentation device eliminates reflux symptoms and normalizes esophageal acid exposure. Ann Surg. 2010;252(5):857–62.
10. Lipham JC, DeMeester TR, Ganz RA, Bonavina L, Saino G, Dunn DH, et al. The LINX® reflux management system: confirmed safety and efficacy now at 4 years. Surg Endosc Other Interv Tech. 2012;26(10):2944–9.
11. Saino G, Bonavina L, Lipham JC, Dunn D, Ganz RA. Magnetic sphincter augmentation for gastroesophageal reflux at 5 years: final results of a pilot study show long-term acid reduction and symptom improvement. J Laparoendosc Adv Surg Tech A [Internet]. 2015;25(10):787–92. Available from: http://www.scopus.com/inward/record.url?eid=2-s2.0-84945588819&partnerID=tZOtx3y1.
12. Ganz RA, Peters JH, Horgan S, et al. Esophageal sphincter device for gastroesophageal reflux disease. N Engl J Med. 2013;368(8):719–27. http://www.ncbi.nlm.nih.gov/pubmed/23425164
13. Bonavina L, Saino G, Bona D, Sironi A, Lazzari V. One hundred consecutive patients treated with magnetic sphincter augmentation for gastroesophageal reflux disease: 6 years of clinical experience from a single center. J Am Coll Surg [Internet]. 2013;217(4):577–85. Available from: https://doi.org/10.1016/j.jamcollsurg.2013.04.039.

14. Lipham JC, Taiganides PA, Louie BE, Ganz RA, Demeester TR. Safety analysis of first 1000 patients treated with magnetic sphincter augmentation for gastroesophageal reflux disease. Dis Esophagus. 2015;28(4):305–11.
15. Smith CD, Ganz RA, Lipham JC, Bell RC, Rattner DW. Lower esophageal sphincter augmentation for gastroesophageal reflux disease: the safety of a modern implant. J Laparoendosc Adv Surg Tech [Internet]. 2017;27(6):lap.2017.0025. Available from: http://online.liebertpub.com/doi/10.1089/lap.2017.0025.
16. Czosnyka NM, Buckley FP, Doggett SL, Vassaur H, Connolly EE, Borgert AJ, et al. Outcomes of magnetic sphincter augmentation – a community hospital perspective. Am J Surg. 2016;213:1019.
17. Bauer M, Meining A, Kranzfelder M, Jell A, Schirren R, Wilhelm D, et al. Endoluminal perforation of a magnetic antireflux device. Surg Endosc Other Interv Tech [Internet]. 2015;29(12):3806–10. Available from: https://doi.org/10.1007/s00464-015-4145-6.
18. Ganz RA, Edmundowicz SA, Taiganides PA, Lipham JC, Smith CD, DeVault KR, et al. Long-term outcomes of patients receiving a magnetic sphincter augmentation device for gastroesophageal reflux. Clin Gastroenterol Hepatol [Internet]. 2016;14(5):671–7. Available from: https://doi.org/10.1016/j.cgh.2015.05.028.
19. Reynolds JL, Zehetner J, Wu P, Shah S, Bildzukewicz N, Lipham JC. Laparoscopic magnetic sphincter augmentation vs laparoscopic nissen fundoplication: a matched-pair analysis of 100 patients. J Am Coll Surg [Internet]. 2015;221(1):123–8. Available from: https://doi.org/10.1016/j.jamcollsurg.2015.02.025.
20. Louie BE, Farivar AS, Shultz D, Brennan C, Vallières E, Aye RW. Short-term outcomes using magnetic sphincter augmentation versus nissen fundoplication for medically resistant gastroesophageal reflux disease. Ann Thorac Surg. 2014;98(2):498–505.
21. Riegler M, Schoppman SF, Bonavina L, Ashton D, Horbach T, Kemen M. Magnetic sphincter augmentation and fundoplication for GERD in clinical practice: one-year results of a multicenter, prospective observational study. Surg Endosc. 2015;29:1123–9.
22. Sheu EG, Nau P, Nath B, Kuo B, Rattner DW. A comparative trial of laparoscopic magnetic sphincter augmentation and Nissen fundoplication. Surg Endosc. 2015;29(3):505–9.
23. Asti E, Bonitta G, Lovece A, Lazzari V, Bonavina L. Longitudinal comparison of quality of life in patients undergoing laparoscopic Toupet fundoplication versus magnetic sphincter augmentation: observational cohort study with propensity score analysis. Medicine (Baltimore). 2016;95(30):e4366.
24. Warren HF, Reynolds JL, Lipham JC, Zehetner J, Bildzukewicz NA, Taiganides PA, et al. Multi-institutional outcomes using magnetic sphincter augmentation versus Nissen fundoplication for chronic gastroesophageal reflux disease. Surg Endosc Other Interv Tech. 2016;30(8):3289–96.
25. Lord RVN, Demeester SR, Peters JH, Hagen JA, Elyssnia D, Sheth CT, et al. Hiatal hernia, lower esophageal sphincter incompetence, and effectiveness of nissen fundoplication in the spectrum of gastroesophageal reflux disease. J Gastrointest Surg. 2009;13(4):602–10.
26. Crookes PF, Ritter MP, Johnson WE, Bremner CG, Peters JH, DeMeester TR. Static and dynamic function of the lower esophageal sphincter before and after laparoscopic Nissen fundoplication. J Gastrointest Surg. 1997;1(6):499–504.
27. Warren HF, Louie BE, Farivar AS, Wilshire C, Aye RW. Manometric changes to the lower esophageal sphincter after magnetic sphincter augmentation in patients with chronic gastroesophageal reflux disease. Ann Surg [Internet]. 2016;266(1):99. Available from: http://content.wkhealth.com/linkback/openurl?sid=WKPTLP:landingpage&an=00000658-900000000-96487.
28. Warren HF, Brown LM, Mihura M, Farivar AS, Aye RW, Louie BE. Factors influencing the outcome of magnetic sphincter augmentation for chronic gastroesophageal reflux disease. Surg Endosc. 2018;32(1):405–12.
29. Wu JC-Y, Mui L-M, Cheung CM-Y, Chan Y, Sung JJ-Y. Obesity is associated with increased transient lower esophageal sphincter relaxation. Gastroenterology. 2007;132(3):883–9.
30. El-Serag HB, Ergun GA, Pandolfino J, Fitzgerald S, Tran T, Kramer JR. Obesity increases oesophageal acid exposure. Gut. 2007;56(6):749–55.

31. Ayazi S, Hagen JA, Zehetner J, Ross O, Wu C, Oezcelik A, et al. The value of high-resolution manometry in the assessment of the resting characteristics of the lower esophageal sphincter. J Gastrointest Surg. 2009;13(12):2113–20.
32. Quiroga E, Cuenca-Abente F, Flum D, Dellinger EP, Oelschlager BK. Impaired esophageal function in morbidly obese patients with gastroesophageal reflux disease: evaluation with multichannel intraluminal impedance. Surg Endosc Other Interv Tech. 2006;20(5):739–43.
33. Rona KA, Reynolds J, Schwameis K, Zehetner J, Samakar K, Oh P, et al. Efficacy of magnetic sphincter augmentation in patients with large hiatal hernias. Surg Endosc Other Interv Tech. 2016;31(5):1–7.
34. Bell RCW, Buckely FP III, Freeman K, Doggett S, Heidrick R. Favorable results from a prospective evaluation of 200 patients with large hiatal hernias undergoing LINX magnetic sphincter augmentation. Surg Endosc. 2017;32:1762.
35. Thor KB, Hill LD, Mercer DD, Kozarek RD. Reappraisal of the flap valve mechanism in the gastroesophageal junction. A study of a new valvuloplasty procedure in cadavers. Acta Chir Scand. 1987;153(1):25–8.
36. Marchand P. The gastro-oesophageal "sphincter" and the mechanism of regurgitation. Br J Surg. 1955;42:504–13.
37. Desart K, Rossidis G, Michel M, Lux T, Ben-David K. Gastroesophageal reflux management with the LINX® system for gastroesophageal reflux disease following laparoscopic sleeve gastrectomy. J Gastrointest Surg. 2015;19(10):1782–6.
38. Muñoz-Largacha JA, Hess DT, Litle VR, Fernando HC. Lower esophageal magnetic sphincter augmentation for persistent reflux after Roux-en-Y gastric bypass. Obes Surg. 2016;26(2):464–6.

Laparoscopic Anti-reflux Surgery: Laparoscopic Roux-en-Y Gastric Bypass

14

Matthew Dong and Daniel M. Herron

Indications

Initially described by Mason in 1966, the Roux-en-Y gastric bypass (RYGB) became one of the most effective operative strategies for the management of morbid obesity. Many feel that it remains the gold standard treatment of morbid obesity, particularly with associated diabetes. In this population, RYGB has been demonstrated to result in a reduction in comorbid conditions and gastroesophageal reflux disease (GERD) in particular. The mechanisms for this are likely multifold: (1) reduction in the high gastroesophageal pressure gradient due to weight loss, (2) decreased acid exposure of the lower esophagus due to the separation of the antrum from the gastric pouch, and (3) improved clearance of gastric secretions and reflux from the distal esophagus due to improved drainage via the gastrojejunostomy.

As it treats both morbid obesity and weight-related medical comorbidities, RYGB should be offered as a first-line intervention for GERD in patients whose BMI is 35 kg/m^2 or greater. A recent study demonstrated a greater than 70% reduction in acid-reducing medication use in morbidly obese patients with GERD following RYGB after 1 year [1]. Because of the risks associated with RYGB, including dumping syndrome, marginal ulceration, and internal hernia formation, it should not be considered as a primary therapy for GERD in patients with a lower BMI. Patients who have had a previous anti-reflux surgery who demonstrated recurrence of their GERD symptoms require a complete preoperative evaluation to confirm the diagnosis of true recurrent reflux. This includes upper endoscopy, upper GI series, and 24-h pH monitoring. In cases where esophageal dysmotility is suspected, preoperative manometry is mandatory, as this is a contraindication to 360° fundoplication and is a relative contraindication to partial fundoplication. Discovery of a malpositioned fundoplication or paraesophageal hernia can be addressed with

M. Dong · D. M. Herron (✉)
Department of Surgery, Icahn School of Medicine at Mount Sinai, New York, NY, USA
e-mail: Daniel.Herron@mountsinai.org

J. Grams et al. (eds.), *The SAGES Manual of Foregut Surgery*,
https://doi.org/10.1007/978-3-319-96122-4_14

revision of the wrap. In cases of true recurrent GERD and no anatomic alterations of an appropriately placed fundoplication, RYGB remains an excellent secondary option for patients who have failed fundoplication or lower esophageal sphincter augmentation.

Patient Positioning and Room Setup

The patient is prepared in the perioperative area in the usual fashion. Perioperative antibiotics to cover skin flora and DVT chemoprophylaxis are administered prior to incision. Pneumatic sequential compression stockings are placed. Following the induction of general anesthesia, the patient is placed in the supine, split leg position, with the arms extended. Alternatively, the patient may be positioned supine, with a foot board. Placement of a Foley catheter is not necessary except in cases where a particularly long or difficult dissection is expected.

Operative Technique

Establishment of Pneumoperitoneum

Intra-abdominal access may be obtained using a 5 mm optical trocar, most commonly in the left upper quadrant. Alternatives include Veress needle or Hasson cut-down techniques. The abdomen is insufflated to 15 mmHg, and remaining trocars are placed under laparoscopic vision.

Trocar Placement

A 12 mm trocar is placed to the right of midline approximately two handbreadths below the xiphoid, with additional 5 mm trocars to the left of center at the same level as the 12 mm trocar and in the right upper quadrant at the midclavicular line, to create a lazy-U configuration. It is important that trocars not be placed too low in the abdomen such that they may restrict access during the dissection of the fundus and that they be placed widely enough to not interfere with one another while working from distance. A 30° laparoscope generally provides adequate visualization, but a 45° laparoscope may be employed as well.

Liver Retraction

A Nathanson liver retractor is placed via a subxiphoid incision. Access to the abdomen may be obtained using either a 5 mm trocar obturator or with a Tonsil clamp. The liver should be retracted to expose the angle of His and the gastrohepatic ligament.

Creation of the Gastric Pouch

The angle of His is mobilized away from the diaphragm. A window is then made in the gastrohepatic ligament just medial to the gastric wall using an advanced bipolar sealing and cutting device, approximately 5 cm distal to the gastroesophageal junction. Dissection is then performed bluntly into the retrogastric space. This preserves function of the vagus nerve. Alternatively, the dissection may be initiated by dividing the Pars flaccida to gain access to the lesser sac.

The stomach is then sequentially divided using a linear GIA stapler. The initial staple firing is made perpendicular to the lesser curve of the stomach, 5 cm below the gastroesophageal junction. The line of division is then carried superiorly toward the angle of His and just lateral to the anterior fat pad to create an approximately 15–20 cc pouch.

Gastrojejunostomy

There are three common techniques for creating the gastrojejunostomy: linear stapler, EEA stapler, and hand-sewn. Each technique has numerous sub-variants. Here, we describe our techniques for each.

Linear Stapler

A gastrotomy is created with either a monopolar hook or ultrasonic shears, posterior to the inferior portion of the staple line. Use of a bougie for counterpressure may be useful. The transverse mesocolon is elevated, and the ligament of Treitz is identified. The small bowel is run 50 cm, and an enterotomy is made. Utilizing a 45 mm gastric load linear stapler, a gastrojejunostomy is created. The goal anastomotic size is approximately 26–27 mm, to reduce the chance of stricture. The common enterotomy is closed with running 3-0 Vicryl suture in two layers. The small bowel is then divided with a bowel load GIA stapler. Alternatively, the small bowel may be divided prior to formation of the anastomosis.

EEA

In similar fashion, the small bowel is divided 50 cm distal to the ligament of Treitz. The staple line is removed from what will eventually become the Roux limb. An anvil attached to a delivery tube is introduced transorally and passed through the esophagus until the axle passes through a small gastrotomy. The delivery tube is removed when the anvil is in appropriate position in the gastric pouch. A lateral trocar site is dilated, and a 25 mm EEA is used to create the anastomosis. The cut end of the small bowel is closed and then removed by dividing with a GIA stapler.

Hand-Sewn

The gastrojejunostomy can also be performed with a hand-sewn technique. This can be performed on the anterior or posterior surface of the gastric pouch. A posterior outer layer with permanent or absorbable suture is created, and a linear gastrostomy and enterotomy are created approximately 25 mm in length. The anastomosis is then completed with running absorbable sutures for the inner layer followed by an anterior outer layer.

Jejunojejunostomy

With the small bowel previously divided 50 cm from the ligament of Treitz, a small enterotomy is made on the antimesenteric portion of the small bowel just proximal to the staple line. It is not necessary to notch the small bowel mesentery using this technique. The Roux limb is then run to the desired length, generally 100–150 cm. An antimesenteric enterotomy is then made in the Roux limb, and a generous anastomosis is made with a 60 mm bowel load GIA stapler. The common enterotomy is then closed either with 2-0 absorbable suture or may be approximated with interrupted sutures and then closed with an additional firing of the GIA stapler. If the latter technique is used, an anti-obstruction stitch between the Roux limb and the stapled end of the biliopancreatic limb is recommended.

Closure of Defects

In order to reduce the risk of internal hernia, the jejunojejunostomy mesenteric defect is closed using a running 3-0 silk suture. This suture line can be continued to create a second layer closure of the jejunojejunostomy. The space posterior to the Roux limb (the so-called pseudo-Petersen's space) is closed in a similar fashion. Trocar sites larger than 10 mm are closed with an absorbable suture utilizing a suture passer.

Leak Test

Prior to the conclusion of the operation, an intraoperative endoscopy is performed. This grants an opportunity to assess the patency of the gastrojejunostomy, to assess for anastomotic site hemorrhage, and to perform a leak test. The Roux limb is clamped with a bowel grasper and the gastric pouch insufflated with the pouch submerged in saline to assess for air leak. If present, this can typically be addressed using interrupted sutures.

Drains

Placement of closed suction drains is generally unnecessary but may be considered in cases with particularly difficult dissections or if there is concern with the gastrojejunostomy. If there is significant concern regarding the gastrojejunostomy, placement of a feeding remnant gastrostomy may be appropriate as well.

Special Considerations

Hiatal Hernia

A small hiatal or paraesophageal hernia is not a contraindication to Roux-en-Y gastric bypass for GERD, and it may be addressed at the time of surgery. After completely dissecting the hernia sac, the hiatus should be closed with permanent sutures. Placement of reinforcing mesh is not recommended. As the pouch will not accommodate a fundoplication, multiple pexy sutures may be placed between the pouch and diaphragm and the distal esophagus and diaphragm to keep the pouch within the abdomen. As in standard hiatal hernia repair, generous mobilization of the distal esophagus is critical to ensure a tension-free repair. A postoperative upper gastrointestinal series is recommended. Early postoperative recurrence should be treated with revision. Asymptomatic late recurrence does not require further intervention.

Previous Fundoplication

Revisional foregut surgery is challenging, as normal anatomic tissue planes may be obscured by scarring and postoperative anatomy can be quite variable. The liver is frequently scarred to the anterior wall of the stomach, and the dissection of this plane is often the first step in adequately visualizing and assessing the patient's anatomy. In taking down any previous fundoplication or other lower esophageal sphincter bolstering surgery, it is necessary to identify key structures. Intraoperative endoscopy can be helpful in multiple regards: identifying anatomy, inspecting an anastomosis, or performing a leak test. An upper gastrointestinal series on postoperative day 1 is recommended in any case of revisional foregut surgery.

Postoperative Management

Patients are transferred to the postanesthesia recovery unit. In the absence of contraindications, postoperative use of ketorolac and/or IV acetaminophen is routinely employed. Pain is initially managed with these agents and IV narcotics as needed. Patient-controlled analgesia (PCA) is generally unnecessary but is a reasonable option if these measures are insufficient. Patients are also initiated on an anti-nausea regimen, including scheduled ondansetron, scopolamine patch, and as needed trimethobenzamide.

Most patients can be transferred to a regular nursing floor, but step-down with continuous pulse oximetry may be necessary dependent upon the patient's medical comorbidities. Bariatric phase I diet is initiated either on the day of surgery or on the morning of the first postoperative day, and the patient is initiated on oral pain medications. Patients may be discharged home on the afternoon of postoperative day 1 if they are able to tolerate their diet and their pain is adequately controlled.

Postoperative Complications and Management

Bowel Obstruction

Small bowel obstruction or acute-onset abdominal pain in a patient with a known history of Roux-en-Y gastric bypass should always raise concern for the possibility of internal hernia. Although CT scan may be diagnostic and assist in cases with an equivocal history or exam, a negative CT scan does not rule out the possibility of internal hernia. The presence of a mesenteric swirl on CT is very specific but often not present. If internal hernia is suspected, a diagnostic laparoscopy is warranted since failure to promptly identify this complication can be catastrophic. Internal hernia may present at any point following gastric bypass, not only in the early postoperative period.

Other causes of gastrointestinal obstruction following gastric bypass include adhesions and kinking at the jejunojejunostomy. Symptoms frequently usually include pain, with nausea and vomiting less common. Diagnostic uncertainty often results from the fact that obstruction of the biliopancreatic limb may not result in nausea or emesis.

Internal hernia is treated with reduction of the hernia and closure of the defect with a running permanent suture. An adhesive obstruction is managed with adhesiolysis, and obstruction at the jejunojejunostomy may be due to stricture or intussusception and is variously treated with bypass of the affected area, reconfiguration of the anastomosis, or resection and reconstruction of the anastomosis.

In all cases of small bowel obstruction after gastric bypass, the small bowel must be run in its entirety and the patient's anatomy confirmed prior to any intervention.

Anastomotic Leak

Leak is a rare but potentially devastating early complication of gastric bypass. Although routine upper gastrointestinal series imaging is not required for primary Roux-en-Y gastric bypass, a low threshold for a contrast study is prudent. In patients with unexplained, persistent tachycardia or epigastric symptoms, an upper GI series should be obtained. If demonstrating a leak or if suspicion is high, a diagnostic laparoscopy is appropriate management.

During reoperation, an intraoperative leak test should be performed by instillation of air or blue dye into the gastric pouch. If an area of leak is identified, a primary repair and omental patch should be performed. A closed suction drain should also be placed. If no leak is identified after adequate investigation, placing a closed suction drain and observing the patient are appropriate.

In cases where severe inflammation is present and tissues are unable to be reapproximated, an omental patch and remnant gastrostomy tube placement is appropriate.

A delayed presentation leak is often amenable to CT-guided drainage and non-operative management with NPO, antibiotics, and TPN. In these cases, a negative upper GI should be obtained before initiation of oral feeding.

Bleeding

Acute postoperative bleeding (within the last 72 h) may initially present with unexplained, persistent tachycardia, shortness of breath, or vague upper gastrointestinal symptoms, creating diagnostic uncertainty as symptoms can mimic leak or DVT/PE, and these other complications should be ruled out in the absence of obvious gastrointestinal bleeding. Management varies depending upon the suspected location of the bleeding and the stability of the patient. The most common site of bleeding is from the cut edges of the stable lines.

Most commonly, non-operative management is sufficient, with fluid resuscitation, blood transfusion, and close observation alone. If significant endoluminal bleeding from the gastrojejunostomy is suspected, endoscopic intervention with endoscopically placed clips may be adequate. If these measures fail, operative intervention is warranted.

Marginal Ulcer

Perianastomotic ulceration is relatively uncommon following Roux-en-Y gastric bypass, but it can be a chronic and frustrating problem to manage when it does occur. Ulcers tend to form in the small bowel just distal to the gastrojejunostomy and are associated with chronic NSAID and tobacco use.

A thorough history and physical is mandatory in patients in whom the diagnosis is being considered. Patients may present with chronic burning epigastric pain, nausea, or other upper gastrointestinal symptoms, generally exacerbated by oral intake. Upper endoscopy is the confirmatory test of choice. Treatment consists of removal of the inciting stimulus, be it tobacco, use of NSAIDs, or occasionally reaction to suture material at the anastomosis. In the latter case, the foreign body can typically be easily removed endoscopically. Additionally, acid reduction with proton pump inhibitors and treatment with sucralfate or bismuth subsalicylate promote healing of the ulcer. *H. pylori* if present should be eradicated; typical regimens include proton pump inhibitors, clarithromycin, and amoxicillin, with or without metronidazole, or quadruple therapy with bismuth subsalicylate, metronidazole, tetracycline, and a PPI. Eradication should be ensured with urea nitrogen breath test, stool antigen test, and/or endoscopic biopsy where clinically appropriate. Finally, an interval endoscopy 4–6 weeks after definitive treatment of the underlying etiology should be performed to confirm resolution.

Patients without an obvious etiology for marginal ulcer or with ulcers refractory to the above measures should be investigated for gastro-gastric fistula with an upper GI series.

Stricture

Anastomotic stricture is a late complication following Roux-en-Y gastric bypass. It may occur in isolation, likely secondary to ischemia or technical error, or secondary to another condition, such as marginal ulcer. A careful history should be obtained, as symptoms may mimic normal postoperative changes. Postprandial epigastric or substernal pain, particularly with solid foods, despite appropriate measures of using small bites and thorough chewing of food boluses, is classic.

Diagnosis is confirmed with EGD, which also affords an opportunity to treat during the same procedure. Esophageal balloon dilators may be employed and are generally effective. Progressive dilation to a stomal diameter of 15–20 mm is appropriate. Perforation is rare and if small can generally be managed conservatively. Surgical revision is rarely required for anastomotic stricture but is indicated in cases where endoscopic dilation is not technically feasible or if the stricture recurs after multiple interventions.

Reference

1. Barr AC, et al. GERD and acid reduction medication use following gastric bypass and sleeve gastrectomy. Surg Endosc. 2017;31:410–5.

15 Endoscopic Reflux Treatments

Jeffrey D. E. Hawel and James C. Ellsmere

Introduction

The prevalence of gastroesophageal reflux disease (GERD) in Western countries ranges from 10% to 20% of the population [1]. Of those who suffer from GERD, as many as 40% will not respond to medical treatment [2]. Furthermore, the adverse effects of long-term proton pump inhibitor (PPI) use are not insignificant. Laparoscopic fundoplication offers improvement in control of symptoms and quality of life but comes with need for general anesthesia, surgical incisions, and risks inherent to any laparoscopic procedure. Symptom recurrence postlaparoscopic fundoplication can occur. Typically this requires reintroduction of PPI or sometimes revisional surgery. There is emerging data that endoscopic solutions can provide less invasive alternative therapies to treat GERD.

Endoscopic devices developed to treat GERD have been used since 2001 [3]. Several different approaches have been employed that alter the gastroesophageal junction to decrease reflux, namely, (i) implantation of prostheses to narrow the lumen, (ii) radiofrequency (RF) energy to induce remodeling, and (iii) sutured fundoplication. Devices designed to implant prostheses at the GEJ are no longer on the market largely because of rare but serious complications. Three endoscopic devices currently have FDA approval – Stretta®, EsophyX™, and MUSE™ – and are discussed below in further detail. A summary of these devices and their predecessors is outlined in Table 15.1.

J. D. E. Hawel · J. C. Ellsmere (✉)
Department of General Surgery, Dalhousie University, Halifax, NS, Canada
e-mail: jellsmer@dal.ca

J. Grams et al. (eds.), *The SAGES Manual of Foregut Surgery*,
https://doi.org/10.1007/978-3-319-96122-4_15

Table 15.1 Summary of endoscopic devices for the treatment of reflux disease

Device	Company	Method of action
FDA approved		
Stretta®	Mederi Therapeutics	RF delivery to the LES to promote remodeling and hypertrophy of the muscle
EsophyX™	EndoGastric Solutions	Transoral incisionless fundoplication using full-thickness polypropylene H-fasteners
MUSE™ system	Medigus Ltd.	Transoral incisionless fundoplication using a full-thickness stapling device under EUS guidance
No longer available		
EndoCinch	Bard	Partial-thickness sutured gastroplication
Enteryx	Boston Scientific	Injectable biocompatible polymer implant at the LES
Gatekeeper	Medtronic	LES submucosal implantation of hydrogel prosthesis
NDO Plicator	NDO	Full-thickness plication of the GEJ

Stretta® (Mederi Therapeutics)

The Stretta® procedure delivers radiofrequency (RF) energy to the lower esophageal sphincter (LES). Reflux is felt to be improved as a result of subsequent remodeling and thickening of the LES, leading to a reduction in compliance and an increase in basal pressure.

Stretta® can be safely used in patients with large hiatal hernias (>3 cm), short segment Barrett's esophagus, or even prior fundoplications [4, 5]. Erosive esophagitis should be treated medically until healed prior to performing Stretta.

The procedure begins with upper endoscopy to identify the location of the gastroesophageal junction. The RF delivery catheter, composed of four nickel-titanium treatment elements distributed radially around a balloon, is then delivered and positioned 2 cm proximal to the squamocolumnar junction. After insufflation of the balloon, the treatment elements are deployed 1–2 mm into the LES muscle to deliver the thermal treatments (Fig. 15.1). Temperature and impedance are measured along each treatment element by a RF generator system, and chilled water from the catheter irrigates the esophageal mucosa to prevent injury. Additional treatment sets are performed by rotating the catheter 45° and varying its linear position. A total of 15–25 treatment sets are created in most patients [4, 5].

A systematic review and meta-analysis published in 2012 by Perry et al. showed that RF treatment resulted in statistically significant improvement in heartburn scores, quality of life as measured by GERD-health-related quality of life (HRQL) scale, and reflux and dyspepsia scores. LES average pressure increased from 16.5 mmHg to 20.2 mmHg following Stretta, while esophageal acid exposure decreased from a pre-procedure DeMeester score of 44.4–28.5 post-procedure [6].

In line with these findings, the Stretta® procedure received strong recommendation in guidelines from SAGES, who considered it "appropriate therapy for patients being treated for GERD who are 18 years of age or older, who have had symptoms of heartburn, regurgitation, or both for 6 months or more, who have been partially or completely responsive to antisecretory pharmacologic therapy, and who have declined laparoscopic fundoplication" [7].

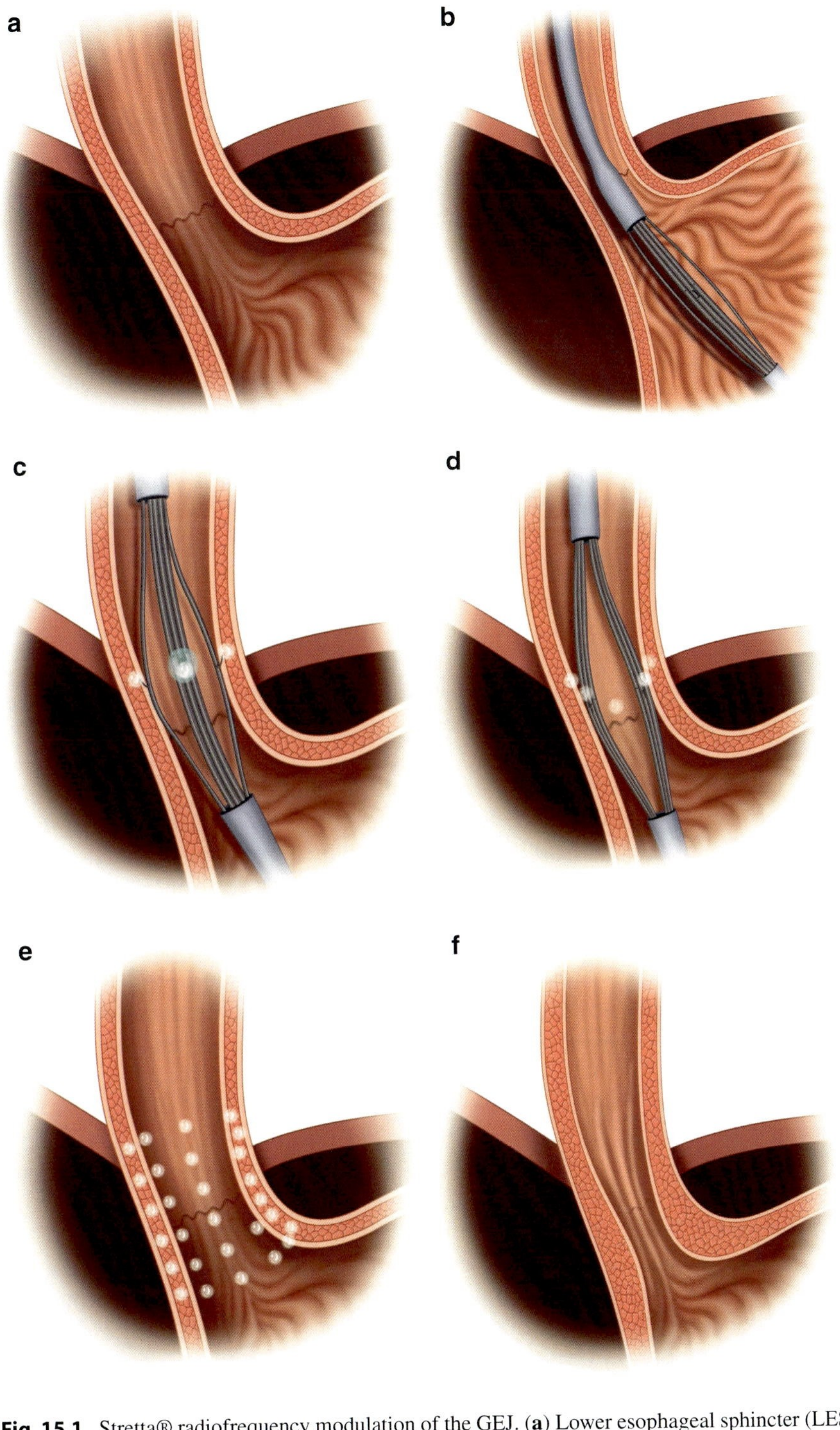

Fig. 15.1 Stretta® radiofrequency modulation of the GEJ. (**a**) Lower esophageal sphincter (LES) zone pretreatment. (**b**) Catheter insertion. (**c**) Initial axial burn. (**d**) Second axial burn; 45 °C burn. (**e**) Completion of RF treatments (eight per axial level) above/below gastroesophageal junction (GEJ). (**f**) LES zone posttreatment

However, the conclusions drawn by prior reviews were criticized for methodological error. This led to a subsequent rigorous systematic review and meta-analysis by Lipka et al. [8]. In this study, the outcomes assessed included: time the pH < 4 over 24 hours, lower esophageal sphincter pressure, ability to stop PPIs and HRQL. The pooled results of this study showed no difference when comparing Stretta to either sham or management with PPIs in patients with GERD.

An important consideration in reflux treatments, and indeed where many endoscopic therapies lack evidence, is long-term outcomes. Noar et al. recently published their 10-year data on 99 patients. Included in the trial were patients with previous fundoplication or large (>3 cm) hiatal hernias. Stretta showed durability and safety, with 72% of patients achieving normalization of GERD-HRQL scores. At 10 years, 23% of patients eliminated medical treatment entirely, and 41% of patients were off PPIs and taking no regular medical therapy. There were no major complications. Patients who initially partially respond are able to safely undergo repeat procedures to achieve maximal response, as was seen in 11 patients in the study [5].

Described serious adverse events associated with Stretta® in the US FDA maintained database are rare but include pneumonia, gastroparesis, esophageal perforation, cardiac arrest, and death [8]. Up to 50% of patients, however, have minor transient side effects following the procedure, the most common of which are chest discomfort and dyspepsia.

EsophyX™ (EndoGastric Solutions)

The EsophyX™ device was designed to create a full-thickness gastroesophageal valve, via transoral incisionless fundoplication (TIF). The initial TIF 1.0 technique created a 270°, 3 cm gastro-gastric plication centrally on the greater curvature at the squamocolumnar junction of the esophagus and the fundus. The TIF 2.0 creates a physiological valve via esophagogastric plication on the far posterior and anterior sides of the lesser curvature.

The technique is performed under general anesthesia with the patient in the left lateral decubitus position and can be completed in under an hour. Two endoscopists are required – one operates the device, while the other operates the endoscope to ensure proper exposure and continuous visualization throughout the entire procedure. The EsophyX™ device fits over a standard endoscope and is passed through the esophagus into the stomach. A helical screw is deployed and anchored into the fundus and used to draw gastric tissue into the device. Proprietary polypropylene H-fasteners are then delivered across the esophagus and gastric fundus to augment the valve (Fig. 15.2). Following completion of the procedure, the device is withdrawn, and endoscopy is repeated to evaluate the length and circumference of the newly created valve. Patients are usually admitted overnight for monitoring and discharged the following day [9].

The initial description of EsophyX™ (TIF 1.0) was published in 2008 by Cadiere et al. [9], and subsequent studies were small and observational in nature. However,

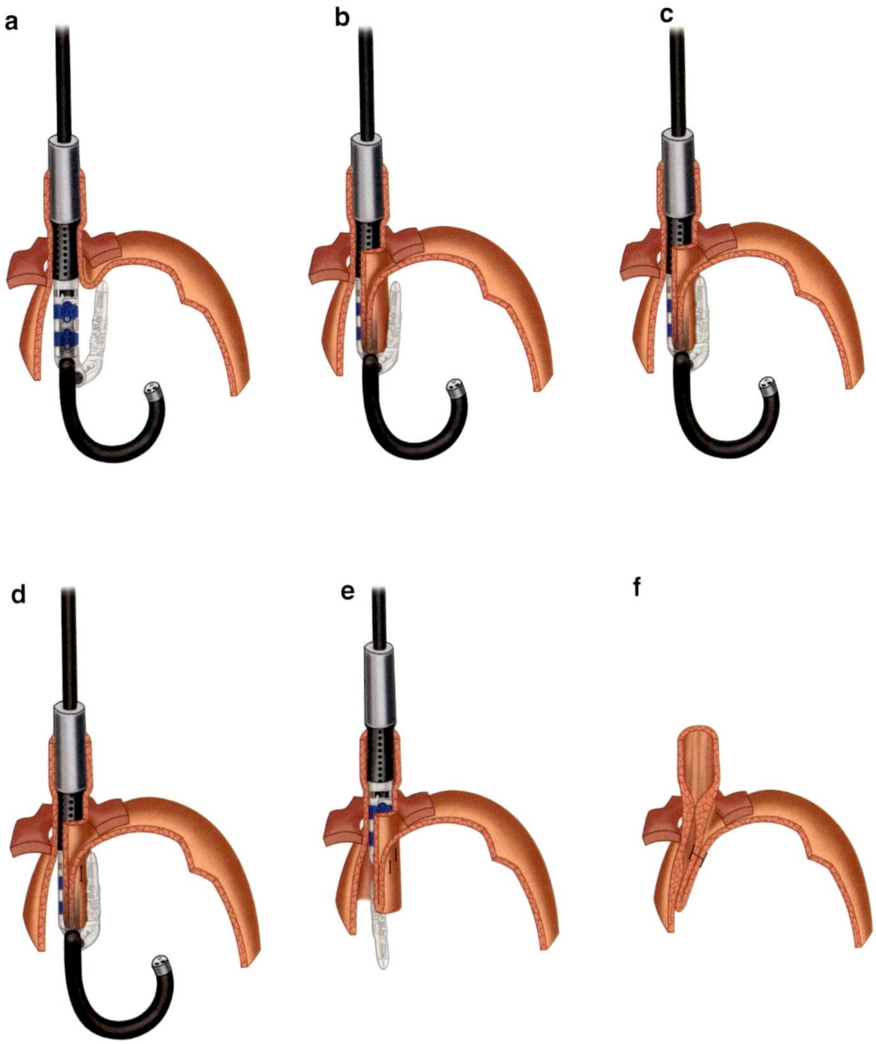

Fig. 15.2 EsophyX™ device for the creation of a transoral incisionless fundoplication. (**a**) Helix retractor engages fundus. (**b**) Fundus retracted. (**c**) Valve molded. (**d**) H-fasteners deployed. (**e**) Device retrieval. (**f**) Valve with serosa-to-serosa approximation below Z-line

five randomized control trials (RCTs) were published between 2014 and 2015, all of which studied the TIF 2.0 device. In 2016, Huang et al. summarized the available literature for EsophyX™ in their systematic review and meta-analysis. In their analysis of available RCTs, TIF was comparable with PPI therapy and showed improvement over sham groups with respect to esophageal acid exposure time. A significant reduction in total number of reflux episodes was seen following TIF in comparison to groups who did not undergo fundoplication. There was no significant difference in the incidence of acid reflux episodes compared to patients taking PPIs. In the observational studies, most patients eventually resumed PPIs in long-term follow-up; however, dosages generally were reduced. Weighted average rate of satisfaction with the procedure was 69.15% [10].

In this same systematic review, severe adverse events were seen in 2.4% of patients – 19 events in a total of 781 patients who underwent TIF. Severe adverse events included seven perforations, five cases of post-TIF bleeding, four cases of pneumothorax, one requiring intravenous antibiotics, and one involving severe epigastric pain. One death was reported 20 months after TIF [10].

MUSE™ System (Medigus Ltd.)

The Medigus Ultrasonic Surgical Endostapler (MUSE™) system combines a flexible video gastroscope with ultrasonography and a stapler mechanism. Similar to EsophyX™, it aims to create an endoscopic fundoplication, although a few key differences are present. First, ultrasound visualization ensures proper alignment of the anvil at the tip of the stapler cartridge on the shaft before firing. Second, staples are utilized rather than sutures, with the idea of creating a more permanent, true fundoplication.

The operator inserts the endoscope and retroflexes in the stomach. The top of the fundus is engaged with the tip of the endoscope and brought against the shaft of the endoscope, where the stapler cartridge is located (Fig. 15.3). The anvil and cartridge are aligned and locked by means of two pins that penetrate across the walls of the stomach and esophagus. A series of five staples arranged horizontally are fired. The staples are the same as those used for surgical gastrointestinal anastomoses. The scope is then rotated and the procedure repeated, thus creating a fundoplication of the anterior wall of the stomach [11].

Long-term clinical outcomes of 37 patients who underwent endoscopic fundoplication with the MUSE™ device were analyzed at baseline, 6 months, and 4 years post-procedure. At 6 months post-procedure, 83.8% remained off of PPIs. This dropped to 69.4% at 4 years. GERD-HRQL scores (off PPI) were significantly decreased. Significant reductions in the PPI dose required for patients who had resumed PPIs were also noted and were preserved at 4 years. Larger studies with sham control groups are awaited [12].

The most common adverse events reported were chest pain in 22% and sore throat in 21% of patients in the series from Zacherl et al. There were two severe adverse events in the series. The first presented with empyema and pneumothorax 3 days post-procedure and was managed with chest tube and antibiotic therapy. The second patient presented with an upper gastrointestinal hemorrhage 8 days post-procedure, requiring two-unit blood transfusion. Endoscopy did not reveal the source of the bleeding [13].

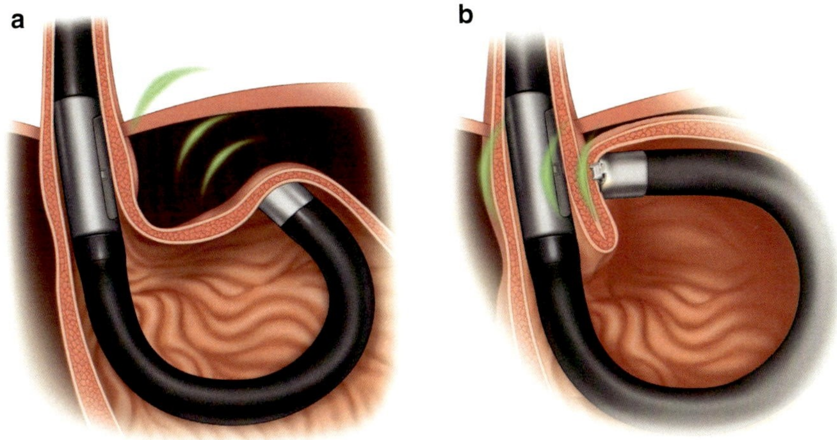

Fig. 15.3 MUSE™ System for the creation of an ultrasound-guided stapled fundoplication

Summary

Endoscopic therapies for GERD continue to evolve to meet patient needs. The goal is an effective mechanical solution that can be delivered with minimal morbidity and excellent long-term durability. There has been much progress over the last decade. Currently available devices – Stretta®, EsophyX™, and MUSE™ – have been shown to be safe and effective in improving symptom control and quality of life and offer a well-established alternative to laparoscopic interventions.

References

1. Dent J, El-Serag HB, Wallander MA, Johansson S. Epidemiology of gastro-oesophageal reflux disease: a systematic review. Gut. 2005;54:710–7.
2. El-Serag H, Becher A, Jones R. Systematic review: persistent reflux symptoms on proton pump inhibitor therapy in primary care and community studies. Aliment Pharmacol Ther. 2010;32(6):720–37.
3. Filipi CJ, Lehman GA, Rothstein RI, Raijman I, Stiegmann GV, Waring JP, Hunter JG, Gostout CJ, Edmundowicz SA, Dunne DP, Watson PA, Cornet DA. Transoral, flexible endoscopic suturing for treatment of GERD: a multicenter trial. Gastrointest Endosc. 2001;53(4):416–22.
4. Triadafilopoulos G, DiBaise JK, Nostrant TT, Stollman NH. The Stretta procedure for the treatment of GERD: 6 and 12 month follow-up of the US open label trial. Gastrointest Endosc. 2002;55(2):149–56.
5. Noar M, Squires P, Noar E, Lee M. Long-term maintenance effect of radiofrequency energy delivery for refractory GERD: a decade later. Surg Endosc. 2014;28:2323–33.
6. Perry KA, Banerjee A, Melvin WS. Radiofrequency energy delivery to the lower esophageal sphincter reduces esophageal acid exposure and improves GERD symptoms: a systematic review and meta-analysis. Surg Laparosc Endosc Percutan Tech. 2012;22(4):283–8.

7. Auyang ED, Carter P, Rauth T, et al. SAGES clinical spotlight review: endoluminal treatments for gastroesophageal reflux disease (GERD). Surg Endosc. 2013;27:2658–72.
8. Lipka S, Kumar A, Richter JE. No evidence for efficacy of radiofrequency ablation for treatment of gastroesophageal reflux disease: a systematic review and meta-analysis. Clin Gastroenterol Hepatol. 2015;13(6):1058–1067.e1.
9. Cadiere GB, Rajan A, Germay O, Himpens J. Endoluminal fundoplication by a transoral device for the treatment of GERD: a feasibility study. Surg Endosc. 2008;22:333–42.
10. Huang X, Chen S, Zhao H, Zeng X, Lian J, Tseng Y, Chen J. Efficacy of transoral incisionless fundoplication (TIF) for the treatment of GERD: a systematic review with meta-analysis. Surg Endosc. 2016;31:1032. [Epub ahead of print].
11. Kauer WK, Roy-Shapira A, Watson D, Sonnenschein M, Sonnenschein E, Unger J, Voget M, Stein HJ. Preclinical trial of a modified gastroscope that performs a true anterior fundoplication for the endoluminal treatment of gastroesophageal reflux disease. Surg Endosc. 2009;23(12):2728–31.
12. Kim HJ, Kwon CI, Kessler WR, Selzer DJ, McNulty G, Bapaye A, Bonavina L, Lehman GA. Long-term follow-up results of endoscopic treatment of gastroesophageal reflux disease with the MUSE™ endoscopic stapling device. Surg Endosc. 2016;30(8):3402–8.
13. Zacherl J, Roy-Shapira A, Bonavina L, Bapaye A, Kiesslich R, Schoppmann SF, Kessler WR, Selzer DJ, Broderick RC, Lehman GA, Horgan S. Endoscopic anterior fundoplication with the Medigus Ultrasonic Surgical Endostapler (MUSE™) for gastroesophageal reflux disease: 6-month results from a multi-center prospective trial. Surg Endosc. 2015;29(1):220–9.

Expert Commentary: Endoluminal Treatment for Gastroesophageal Reflux Disease

16

W. Scott Melvin

Gastroesophageal reflux disease (GERD) is a common disease affecting millions of patients throughout the world. Primary treatment has always relied on lifestyle adaptations with specific recommendations for losing weight, eliminating smoking, alcohol, and dietary changes. Other treatment options include acid control using proton pump inhibitors and histamine blockers. While many of these therapies are effective in reducing acid, most patient surveys demonstrate poor symptom control and significant deviations from high quality of life secondary to the symptoms of GERD.

Since the 1960s, surgical intervention in the form of a gastroesophageal fundoplication was reserved as the only interventional therapy for patients with severe symptoms, side effects, or extra-esophageal manifestations of their gastroesophageal reflux disease. Using traditional surgical techniques, there was significant morbidity and mortality associated with large operation, and so routine surgical interventions were not recommended. In the early 1990s, laparoscopic techniques were developed which allowed refinement and improvement and improved outcomes as laparoscopy was applied to gastroesophageal fundoplication. The evolution of instrumentation for the treatment of gastroesophageal reflux disease led to a significant expansion of the indications for anti-reflux surgery. The years following this growth allowed careful analysis and study of the appropriate indications and the outcomes associated with surgical intervention. However, the increased scrutiny associated with increased surgical volume did demonstrate some suboptimal outcomes. They were probably secondary to decrease in durability and variability in the surgical techniques during the course of the operations. Many physicians continued to have well-founded skepticism and were reluctant to recommend surgical intervention for most patients. This skepticism remains today and allows for hesitation in referring patients to surgery. Secondary to this, and during the time period, a

W. S. Melvin
Montefiore Medical Center, Albert Einstein College of Medicine, Bronx, NY, USA
e-mail: wsmelvin@montefiore.org

J. Grams et al. (eds.), *The SAGES Manual of Foregut Surgery*,
https://doi.org/10.1007/978-3-319-96122-4_16

variety of technological advances combined with talented investigators and innovators interested in decreasing the morbidity associated with even a laparoscopic surgery for the treatment of reflux disease, led to the advent of endoluminal options for therapy for GERD.

The indications for intervention remain somewhat controversial; however, most physicians recognize that acid exposure in the distal esophagus, as an objective measurement, is an indication for a procedure when the symptoms become persistent. Many patients additionally do not wish to maintain lifelong medical therapy, and so the desire to be off medicine is also a recommendation. Troublesome regurgitation and extra-esophageal manifestations including respiratory symptoms are a strong indication for patients with continued symptomatic reflux disease despite medical therapy. Endoluminal therapy can address the physiologic failure of the gastroesophageal sphincter, but not the significant anatomic derangements. Large hiatal hernias are seen in many patients with gastroesophageal reflux disease. Significant hiatal hernias have not been addressed using endoluminal techniques.

The initial forays utilizing the technology of the distal esophageal sphincter followed several pathways. These can broadly be divided into developing esophageal bulking agents; attempting to create bulk at the distal esophagus that decreases mechanical reflux, physiological manipulation, and/or manipulation of the lower esophageal sphincter; and providing a mechanical barrier in the form of an esophageal, gastric, or esophagogastric fundoplication or plication.

Attempts to develop a bulking agent that can be injected into the distal esophagus that was tunable and individualized seemed initially promising. Several devices and materials were widely tested and approved for use in a variety of countries. One product became FDA approved in the USA after extensive testing and was released into the market. However, post-approval market surveillance revealed difficulty in managing an intramural injection, including managing to keep the injectable material within the wall of the esophagus especially in the submucosal space. Some of these complications were associated with intra-arterial injections of foreign material, and the thought of continuing to use injectable bulking agents into the wall of the esophagus was largely abandoned.

Peripheral nerve ablation using radiofrequency energy was made available for a variety of applications throughout the body. This was applied to the lower esophageal sphincter, and it was largely due to the improvement and increased availability of the technology to adequately modulate and monitor the energy delivery in real time. The Stretta device was developed as a device to deliver a network of radiofrequency ablation nodes within the muscular wall of the esophagus. This network of heat created "nodes" delivered not only a small physiologic barrier but probably decreased compliance in the lower esophageal sphincter. A variety of data was accumulated over more than a decade, and this continues to demonstrate a reduction in symptoms and in some patients a decrease of distal esophageal acid exposure. The side effects remain quite minimal, and the safety profile is excellent. However, despite the encouraging data, and the widespread availability of the device, its use is somewhat still limited. One of the concerns remains is that the mechanism of action remains incompletely clear. It may represent a combination of decreased compliance in the distal esophagus, some mechanical scar in the distal esophageal wall, and more significantly it may disturb the vagal innervation of the distal esophagus completely eliminating transient lower esophageal sphincter relaxation in a patient with normal anatomy, especially those with daytime reflux.

A variety of mechanical "suturing" or stapling mechanical devices were developed in the field to gather tissue at the distal esophagus, at the proximal stomach, or at the GE junction to increase a mechanical barrier to prevent reflux or recreate the angle of His. The culmination of the work seems to conclude that full-thickness plication of the gastric and esophageal wall is important to provide durability and significant effect rather than just mucosal gathering. Two devices eventually emerged that currently are approved for use in the USA and have significant data surrounding them. The EsophyX device applies full-thickness "H"-type fasteners between the esophagus and the stomach creating a partial fundoplication. Multiple fasteners can be placed along the proximal stomach with an articulated arm that is placed over the scope in a device that can be used to tailor a less than circumferential wrap, and it is associated with an articulated tissue grasper that helps invaginate tissue into the jaws. Medigus has been less well-studied. This also provides a full-thickness fastening between the esophagus and the stomach using mechanical metal staples. The staples are loaded into the intraesophageal portion of the device and delivered against an anvil that is attached to the shaft of the orally placed scope. The device uses ultrasound guidance to prevent trapping of extra-esophageal tissue as well as locating the device anvil as well. The use of the transoral fundoplication is now widely accepted as a technique. It has received a reimbursement code from the federal government in the USA, and the data continues to be accumulated on the efficacy of this device and the appropriateness of the devices in a variety of patients with symptomatic reflux disease.

Conclusions

Currently, there are three endoluminal devices approved for use in the USA. These are Stretta, EsophyX, and Medigus. Both Stretta and EsophyX are widely available and have had extensive clinical evaluation throughout the world.

Stretta is unique in that it has a very good safety profile accomplished with few side effects. It can be accomplished in about 30 minutes in a gastroenterology suite or an operating room. It can be given with sedation or general anesthesia. Patients can be active and have little postoperative discomfort for symptomatology. It was approved by the Federal Drug and Food Administration in the year 2000, and it received a CPT code in 2004 (43257). Currently, the body of data suggests that 55–80% of people have significant or complete resolution of symptoms as well as data that demonstrates an improved quality of life in relation to gastroesophageal reflux symptomatology.

EsophyX was first approved by the US Federal Drug Administration in 2007 as an over-the-scope endoluminal fundoplication device. Multiple case series have been reported as well as several sham-controlled trials that demonstrate efficacy in treating reflux including respiratory symptoms associated with gastroesophageal reflux. Most of the collected data has demonstrated significant ability to reduce symptoms in patients with normal anatomy. More recently, data has been accumulated in case series that demonstrates the ability to perform a partial fundoplication with the device at the time of laparoscopy to repair a hiatal hernia. This indication was recently approved by the FDA and added to the material information. The durability of the device remains of some concern and has not been completely well-described. The device and procedure do have their own CPT code that was approved in 2016 and are available throughout the USA.

In order to provide the best individualized care for patients with troublesome gastroesophageal reflux disease, a full "tool box" is helpful. This tool box should include endoluminal therapy for patients who meet the strict criteria of having relatively normal anatomy or desire interventional therapy to reduce their need for medications. Indications for therapy are somewhat controversial still but clearly for patients with documented gastroesophageal acid reflux, normal motility, and relatively normal anatomy. Patients who continue to have significant symptoms on medication or patients who desire to terminate their medical therapy may benefit from a minimally invasive or endoluminal procedure. Both of these techniques are relatively safe and well-tolerated. The durability of each of the techniques continues to be studied, and further data is being accumulated as we go forward. At the current time, it seems reasonable to offer endoluminal therapy as a first step or as a rescue therapy for patients who have mechanical abilities to be treated this way.

Major surgical societies and scientific boards have taken the task of evaluating different endoluminal therapies for reflux. The only significant review and guidelines have been published by The Society of American Gastrointestinal and Endoscopic Surgeons. In May of 2017, a clinical spotlight review, Endoluminal Treatments for Gastroesophageal Reflux Disease, was released after approval by the board of directors of SAGES. This included a systemic review and had various recommendations. The final recommendations included conclusions on transoral incisionless fundoplication as well as radiofrequency ablation of the lower esophageal sphincter.

The final recommendations for Stretta are "Based on existing evidence, Stretta significantly improves health-related quality of life score, heartburn scores, the incidence of esophagitis and esophageal acid exposure in patients with GERD, but does not increase lower esophageal sphincter basal pressure. In addition, it decreases the use of PPIs by approximately 50%. The effectiveness of the procedure diminishes somewhat over time, but persistent effects have been described up to 10 years after the procedure in appropriately selected patients with GERD. Stretta is more effective than medical therapy, but less so than fundoplication. Stretta is safe in adults and has a short learning curve" [1].

The recommendation for EsophyX is "Based on existing evidence, Esophyx can be performed with an acceptable safety risk in appropriately selected patients. The procedure leads to a better control of GERD symptoms compared with medical therapy in the short term (six months), but appears to lose effectiveness during long-term follow up, and is associated with moderate patient satisfaction scores. Objective reflux measures improve similarly after the procedure compared with medical therapy. No comparative controlled trials exist between transoral fundoplication and surgical fundoplication, but preliminary evidence suggests that the latter can be used safely after transoral failure." [1]

The final determination for treatment should be individualized for each patient based on objective data and symptom complex and rendered by an experienced clinician with adequate knowledge of the disease process and treatment options.

Reference

1. www.sages.org/publications/guidelines/endoluminal-treatments-for-gastroesophageal-reflux-disease-gerd.

17 Laparoscopic Antireflux Surgery: Reoperations at the Hiatus

Abhishek D. Parmar and Kyle A. Perry

Introduction and Epidemiology

Laparoscopic Nissen fundoplication is regarded as the gold standard operation for medically intractable gastroesophageal reflux disease. As surgeons have increasingly performed this operation over time, complications and the need for reoperation are also becoming increasingly common. While several studies have established the long-term efficacy of fundoplication for improving symptoms of reflux disease, it is still an operation that carries a significant risk for reoperation [1].

Rates of reoperation after initial antireflux surgery in the literature have been widely reported, from greater than 10% in the era of early adoption of laparoscopic fundoplication in the 1990s to as low as less than 3% in one systematic review [2]. Population-based studies estimate a reoperation rate of approximately 5%, usually within 1–2 years after fundoplication. In a nationwide Danish study of 2465 patients, 5% of patients required reoperation, with the risk highest in the first 2 years postoperatively [3]. Similarly, a population-based study of 13,000 Californians with uncomplicated GERD who underwent fundoplication from 1995 to 2010 identified a reoperation rate of 6.9% at 10 years [4]. In this study, younger, female patients were more likely to undergo reoperation, also more likely in the first 2 years postoperatively.

Causes for reoperation are most often due to recurrent reflux symptoms or dysphagia. Anatomic causes of fundoplication failure include transmediastinal

A. D. Parmar (✉)
Division of Gastrointestinal Surgery, Department of Surgery, University of Alabama School of Medicine, Birmingham, AL, USA
e-mail: aparmar@uabmc.edu

K. A. Perry
Division of General and Gastrointestinal Surgery, The Ohio State University, Columbus, OH, USA
e-mail: kyle.perry@osumc.edu

J. Grams et al. (eds.), *The SAGES Manual of Foregut Surgery*,
https://doi.org/10.1007/978-3-319-96122-4_17

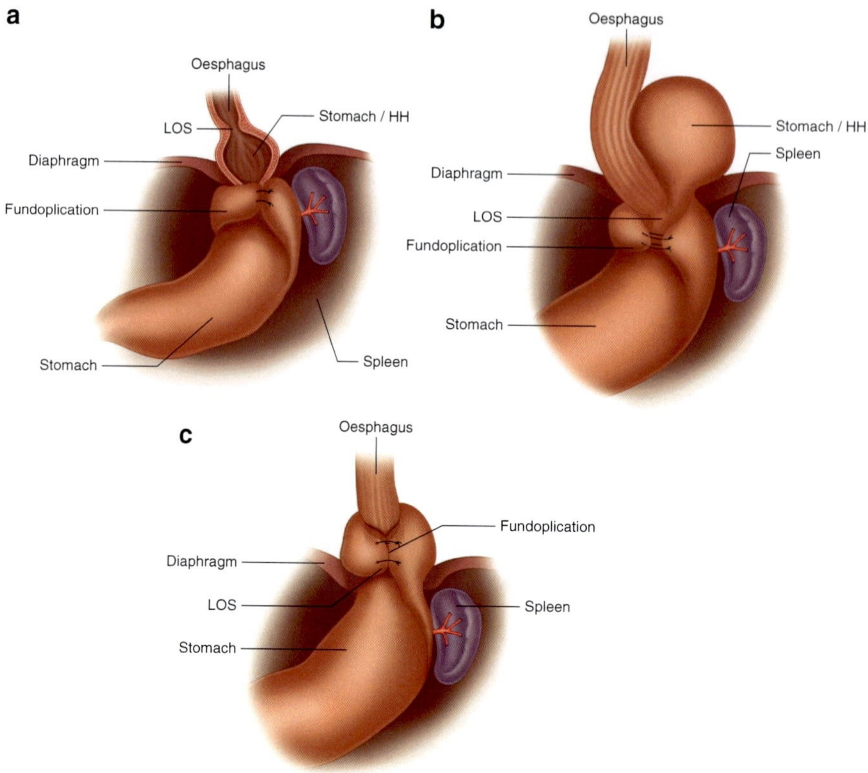

Fig. 17.1 Patterns of failure. (Suppiah et al. [9])

migration, fundoplication issues (tight wrap, slipped wrap), unrecognized shortened esophagus, or previously undiagnosed esophageal dysmotility, with transmediastinal migration being the most common [5–8]. An alternate classification has been proposed by Suppiah et al., in which (1) the wrap may have either "telescoped" or slipped, (2) a paraesophageal hernia may have developed, or (3) crural failure occurred with wrap herniation into the chest [9] (Fig. 17.1). Indications for surgery and etiologies of wrap failure as observed from the most recent systematic review of 930 redo antireflux operations by Symons et al. in 2011 are depicted in Table 17.1 [10].

Clinical Evaluation and Management

When considering reoperative surgery of the hiatus, it is essential to distinguish between radiographic recurrence and symptomatic recurrence. Studies have demonstrated that while radiographic hiatal hernia recurrence after Nissen fundoplication may be common, this may or may not be clinically relevant in the absence of

Table 17.1 Indications for reoperation and etiology of wrap failure after primary antireflux surgery

Indications for reoperation			Etiology of wrap failure		
Primary indication for reoperation	Number	Percentage	Etiology of wrap failure	Number	Percentage
Recurrent GERD	377	59.4	Hiatal hernia	336	44.1
Dysphagia	194	30.6	Disrupted	120	15.8
Gas bloat	29	4.6	Slipped	89	11.7
Hiatal hernia	14	2.2	Twisted	43	5.6
Other	21	3.2	Misplaced	30	3.9
			Other	144	19

Adapted from van Beek et al. [6]
GERD gastroesophageal reflux disease

significant symptoms that warrant repair. Oelschlager et al. [11] reviewed their experience in a multi-institutional cohort of 60 patients who underwent laparoscopic repair of large hiatal hernias. At a median of 58 months postoperatively, the group identified a radiographic recurrence on upper gastrointestinal series in 34 patients (57%). However, there was no difference in quality of life scores between patients with or without radiographic recurrence. As such, experts in foregut surgery recommend reoperation only be undertaken in the context of foregut symptomatology (recurrent or new reflux and/or dysphagia) *with* anatomic/radiographic findings that may be correctable surgically [7].

History and Physical Exam

A careful assessment of symptom severity and detail should be obtained prior to any intervention. Multiple standardized scoring systems are available, with the Visick score, dysphagia severity score, and GERD health-related quality of life surveys being developed specifically for symptoms of reflux [12, 13]. The patient's symptomatology should be used as a key determinant to guide preoperative testing and evaluation. Patient symptoms are generally classified into two groups: recurrent reflux-type symptoms and dysphagia. Eliciting the specific conditions in which these symptoms occur (solid versus liquid oral intake, presence and timing of regurgitation) can help differentiate primary or secondary esophageal dysmotility from an anatomic obstruction at a tight or herniated wrap. In addition, a focused assessment to identify symptoms of delayed gastric emptying would warrant additional imaging [14]. Care should be taken to ensure that patient symptoms are not expected side effects of fundoplication such as mild, early postoperative dysphagia, gas bloating, or an inability to belch. In this setting, dysphagia symptoms can often be successfully managed by endoscopic balloon dilation. Symptoms that persist beyond 6 months after surgery warrant evaluation and consideration for reoperation.

Finally, as with any reoperation, a thorough review of the patient's prior operative note and/or discussion with the operating surgeon should be undertaken to identify specific operative details that might affect reoperation. These details might include technical details that could contribute to failure, such as failure to reduce and excise a hernia sac, inability to achieve adequate intra-abdominal length (and reasons for this), failure to adequately transect the short gastric vessels for an adequate distance, anatomic aberrations (such as a replaced or accessory left hepatic artery), or any other specific issues that may affect operative approach.

Surgeons undertaking redo fundoplications should take care to counsel patients about these risks and reasonable expectations for success and complications following surgery. Once reoperation is considered, rates of success are diminished, while rates of perioperative complications are increased compared to primary antireflux surgery [5, 6, 10]. Several systematic reviews have established that success, as defined by symptom improvement or resolution, is generally achieved in only 70–84% of patients following reoperative antireflux surgery, and this decreases with each successive reoperation [7]. In addition, the risk for complications can range from 14 to 21%, with most series citing gastrointestinal perforation as the most common complication. Finally, since rates of success diminish considerably with each successive reoperation, surgeons must balance the likelihood of success with repeat fundoplication with the benefit of conversion to Roux-en-Y gastric bypass as a definitive antireflux operation, particularly for obese patients.

Imaging and Interventions

Standard imaging and interventions prior to considering reoperative surgery of the hiatus include a repeat of the tests ordered prior to the primary antireflux operation. The evidence-based standards for preoperative imaging testing include an upper endoscopy, pH study with or without multichannel intraluminal impedance, barium upper gastrointestinal series, and esophageal manometry [15]. Upper endoscopy is an essential component to the evaluation in these patients to rule out pre-existing Barrett's dysplasia or underlying invasive malignancy as a potential cause for dysphagia. pH study is necessary to assess the presence or absence of objective reflux as a cause for patient symptoms, and correlation should be made with patient's symptoms as well as previous pH study. Barium esophagram demonstrates the patient's foregut anatomy and can help identify a herniated, slipped, or tight fundoplication as a cause of prolonged postoperative dysphagia. Finally, manometry will determine if the patient's cause for dysphagia may be due to underlying primary or secondary esophageal dysmotility. In addition, patients with severe dysmotility or esophageal aperistalsis might benefit from a partial redo fundoplication to reduce the risk of postoperative dysphagia. Patients with symptoms of delayed gastric emptying or with a history of known bilateral vagotomy during index operation should also undergo a technetium-labeled gastric emptying study. Objective evidence for delayed gastric emptying might prompt consideration for a gastric emptying procedure (i.e., pyloroplasty or pyloromyotomy) at the time of reoperation or prior to consideration of hiatal reconstruction.

Technical Details

The choice of operative approach—open laparotomy, thoracotomy/thoracoscopy, or laparoscopy—should be left to the skill set of the surgeon. However, because the complication profile of reoperative laparoscopic surgery is improved compared to open surgery, and has documented safety and efficacy in the reoperative setting, we prefer the laparoscopic approach (Fig. 17.2) [1, 16].

While the technical components of laparoscopic reoperations of the hiatus are difficult to standardize given the variable patient presentations, there are several key steps during the dissection that are worth noting. The first is that adhesiolysis should be expected and should dictate peritoneal entry. The avoidance of prior open or laparoscopic incisions is essential to prevent iatrogenic injury. Intraperitoneal access can be achieved using open or closed approaches. Also, surgeons should be willing to place additional ports or modify port placement as needed if significant adhesions are present [16].

The next consideration is the approach to the initial hiatal dissection. Due to the extensive adhesions around the hiatus and the risk for iatrogenic esophageal or gastric injury, it is important to consider multiple possible approaches to the hiatus. One approach is to begin the dissection along the liver capsule in the region of the Pars flaccida (Fig. 17.2a). In this manner, the stomach can be mobilized to expose the caudate lobe of the liver and facilitate visualization of the right crus of the diaphragm (Fig. 17.2b). Alternatively, the lesser sac can be entered along the greater curvature of the stomach to expose the left diaphragmatic crus. Once the medial border of the crus can be clearly identified, careful sharp dissection can be used to achieve a circumferential dissection of the hiatus and the reduction of any herniated stomach and allow placement of a Penrose drain around the distal esophagus prior to beginning the mediastinal dissection (Fig. 17.2c).

Mediastinal dissection should proceed with caution as with any primary antireflux surgery, with care taken to avoid iatrogenic injury to the esophagus, vagus nerves, and stomach and to preserve the peritoneal lining of the crura if possible [8]. The gastroesophageal fat pat should be removed, and endoscopy may be utilized to accurately identify the gastroesophageal junction. Because the most common cause of failure is due to herniation of the wrap into the chest, care must be taken to first ensure adequate intra-abdominal esophageal length of at least 3 cm and then to perform adequate hiatal closure, which has been observed as a central cause for herniation (Fig. 17.2d) [16]. Calibrating the hiatal closure over a 44F Maloney dilator or bougie can assist in optimal hiatal closure, as can reducing the pneumoperitoneum setting to 8 mmHg. Finally, if hiatal closure proves difficult, a right-sided relaxing incision may also be performed [17], although this does have the theoretical risk for herniation. Consideration should also be given to reinforcing the hiatal closure with mesh, which likely reduces the risk of early hiatal hernia recurrence but with the potential for mesh-related complication and questionable long-term benefit [18, 19]. If intra-abdominal length cannot be obtained due to extensive mediastinal scarring or adhesions, an esophageal lengthening procedure should be performed. We prefer the wedge fundectomy approach as this can achieve adequate esophageal length using a totally laparoscopic approach (Fig. 17.2e, f) [20].

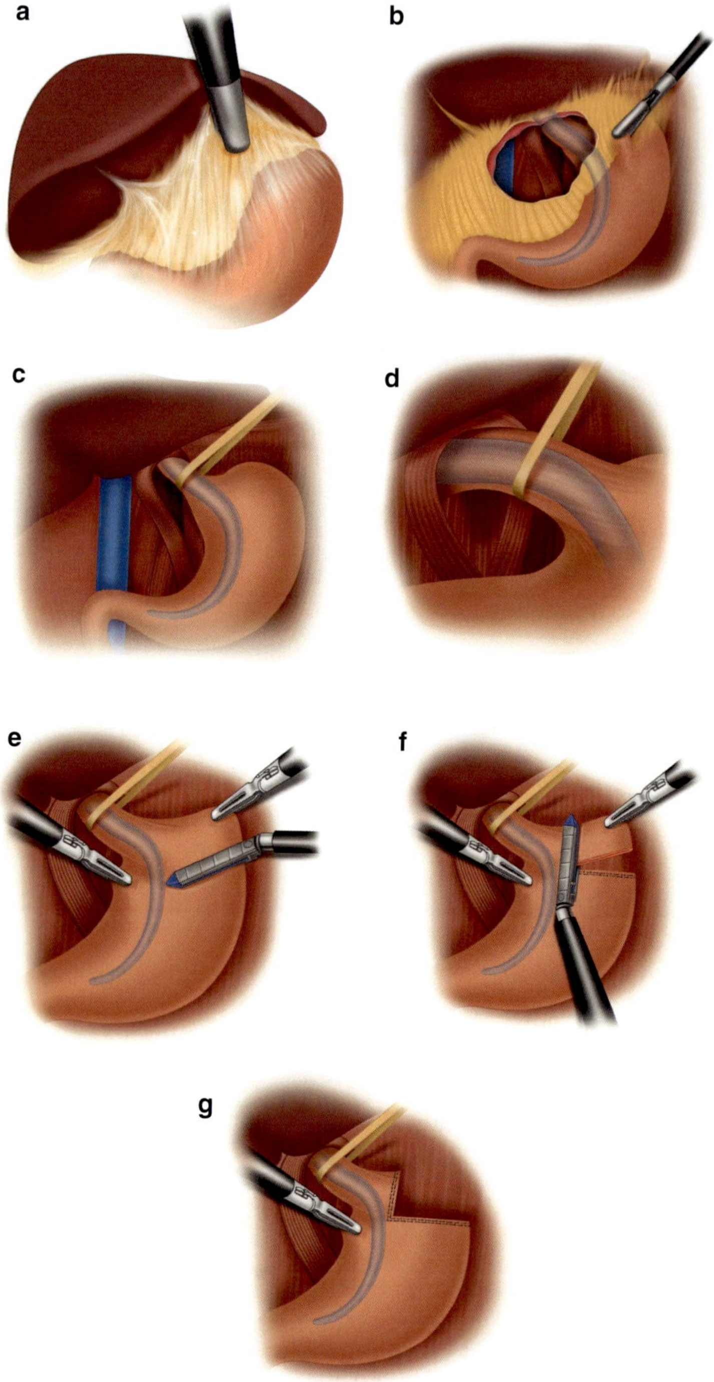
a
b
c
d
e
f
g

Finally, the previous fundoplication should be completely taken down, the stomach placed in the in situ position, and the wrap redone regardless of the gross appearance intraoperatively or on prior imaging tests (Fig. 17.2g). Techniques to perform wrap takedown can include the use of sharp dissection, energy devices, or a stapler at the fundoplication. A partial fundoplication should be considered in lieu of a floppy Nissen fundoplication in cases of severe dysphagia or established esophageal dysmotility on preoperative manometry. Key pitfalls and technical conduct of fundoplication creation have been discussed previously [21].

Repeat Reoperations of the Hiatus

Success rates are known to decrease with each successive reoperation, so we need to consider the approach to the patient with failure after a reoperation of the hiatus. These patients represent a complex group, and particular attention must be focused on the details of their symptoms in concert with repeat imaging and physiologic studies. Smith et al. published their experience in over 300 patients undergoing reoperative surgery [7]. The indications for redo-redo surgery in these patients were more likely to be due to wrap herniation and dysphagia than an inadequate wrap or recurrent reflux. In their high-volume experience, failure rates increased with successive repeat operation, from less than 3% after initial operation to over 7% with each successive procedure. In addition, they observed no increase in operative complications including gastric or esophageal perforation between a single reoperation and multiple reoperations. Despite lower success rates, the overwhelming majority of patients reported that they would recommend reoperation as a means to improve their quality of life, a finding that has been reproduced at other high-volume centers [22].

While these reports are reassuring, these reoperations were performed by experienced surgeons at high-volume centers for foregut surgery, and the outcomes may not be generalizable to all surgeons or practice models. Wilshire et al. published their experience with reoperative hiatal surgery in 2016 [23] and reported that patients who had undergone more than one reoperation had a significantly increased risk for intraoperative complications compared to a single reoperation (36% vs. 23%, $p = 0.002$) with worse quality of life outcomes. As historical failure rates may exceed 50% with a third reoperation [24], consideration in these cases should be made to convert the fundoplication to a Roux-en-Y gastric bypass, particularly for patients who are morbidly obese [25, 26].

Fig. 17.2 Technical details of operation. (**a**): Wrap/stomach is densely adhered to liver capsule, with Pars flaccida obliterated, (**b**): Wrap mobilized free from liver capsule, right crus, and IVC in view, (**c**): Penrose utilized for retraction and mediastinal mobilization, (**d**): Esophagus mobilized to obtain three centimeters of intra-abdominal length, (**e**): Wedge fundectomy, (**f**): Wedge fundectomy, (**g**): Fundoplication taken down

Key Points

- Reoperative antireflux surgery is a complex undertaking and should only be performed by experienced surgeons with specific expertise and/or training in foregut surgery.
- Laparoscopy has become the standard of care for reoperations of the hiatus and should be attempted initially.
- Optimal preoperative evaluation, including thorough history taking and testing, is essential in the selection of patients who would benefit from reoperative antireflux surgery.
- Preoperative testing should include at minimum upper endoscopy, pH study with or without multichannel intraluminal impedance, barium upper gastrointestinal series, and esophageal manometry.
- Technical points of the operation include safe peritoneal entry, use of the caudate lobe to guide initial hiatal dissection, obtaining adequate intra-abdominal esophageal length, and re-performance of the fundoplication.
- Multiple reoperations at the hiatus should be approached with caution, and strong consideration should be given to conversion to Roux-en-Y gastric bypass.

Summary

Reoperative antireflux surgery is a complex undertaking, with significant risk for complications and failure. Careful selection of patients who might benefit from reoperation, through informed history taking and preoperative evaluation, are vital components in the care of these patients. Reoperation should only be undertaken by surgeons with significant technical expertise in advanced laparoscopy and with an understanding of several key technical points. Finally, avoidance of multiple reoperations should be balanced with the risk for complications in conversion to Roux-en-Y gastric bypass. Only while employing all these considerations can outcomes be fully optimized for this patient population.

References

1. Oor JE, Roks DJ, Broeders JA, Hazebroek EJ, Gooszen HG. Seventeen-year outcome of a randomized clinical trial comparing laparoscopic and conventional Nissen fundoplication: a plea for patient counseling and clarification. Ann Surg. 2017;266(1):23–8.
2. Carlson MA, Frantzides CT. Complications and results of primary minimally invasive antireflux procedures: a review of 10,735 reported cases. J Am Coll Surg. 2001;193(4):428–39.
3. Funch-Jensen P, Bendixen A, Iversen MG, Kehlet H. Complications and frequency of redo antireflux surgery in Denmark: a nationwide study, 1997-2005. Surg Endosc. Mar 2008;22(3):627–30.
4. Zhou T, Harnsberger C, Broderick R, et al. Reoperation rates after laparoscopic fundoplication. Surg Endosc. 2015;29(3):510–4.
5. Furnée EJ, Draaisma WA, Broeders IA, Gooszen HG. Surgical reintervention after failed antireflux surgery: a systematic review of the literature. J Gastrointest Surg. 2009;13(8):1539–49.

6. van Beek DB, Auyang ED, Soper NJ. A comprehensive review of laparoscopic redo fundoplication. Surg Endosc. 2011;25(3):706–12.
7. Smith CD, McClusky DA, Rajad MA, Lederman AB, Hunter JG. When fundoplication fails: redo? Ann Surg. 2005;241(6):861–9; discussion 869–871.
8. Awais O, Luketich JD, Schuchert MJ, et al. Reoperative antireflux surgery for failed fundoplication: an analysis of outcomes in 275 patients. Ann Thorac Surg. 2011;92(3):1083–9; discussion 1089–1090.
9. Suppiah A, Sirimanna P, Vivian SJ, O'Donnell H, Lee G, Falk GL. Temporal patterns of hiatus hernia recurrence and hiatal failure: quality of life and recurrence after revision surgery. Dis Esophagus. 2017;30(4):1–8.
10. Symons NR, Purkayastha S, Dillemans B, et al. Laparoscopic revision of failed antireflux surgery: a systematic review. Am J Surg. 2011;202(3):336–43.
11. Oelschlager BK, Petersen RP, Brunt LM, Soper NJ, Sheppard BC, Mitsumori L, Rohrmann C, Swanstrom LL, Pellegrini CA. Laparoscopic paraesophageal hernia repair: defining long-term clinical and anatomic outcomes. J Gastrointest Surg. 2012;16:453–9.
12. VISICK AH. A study of the failures after gastrectomy. Ann R Coll Surg Engl. 1948;3(5):266–84.
13. Velanovich V, Vallance SR, Gusz JR, Tapia FV, Harkabus MA. Quality of life scale for gastroesophageal reflux disease. J Am Coll Surg. 1996;183(3):217–24.
14. Hamrick MC, Davis SS, Chiruvella A, et al. Incidence of delayed gastric emptying associated with revisional laparoscopic paraesophageal hernia repair. J Gastrointest Surg. 2013;17(2):213–7.
15. Jobe BA, Richter JE, Hoppo T, et al. Preoperative diagnostic workup before antireflux surgery: an evidence and experience-based consensus of the esophageal diagnostic advisory panel. J Am Coll Surg. 2013;217(4):586–97.
16. Horgan S, Pohl D, Bogetti D, Eubanks T, Pellegrini C. Failed antireflux surgery: what have we learned from reoperations? Arch Surg. 1999;134(8):809–15; discussion 815–807.
17. Cohn TD, Soper NJ. Paraesophageal hernia repair: techniques for success. J Laparoendosc Adv Surg Tech A. 2017;27(1):19–23.
18. Oelschlager BK, Pellegrini CA, Hunter J, et al. Biologic prosthesis reduces recurrence after laparoscopic paraesophageal hernia repair: a multicenter, prospective, randomized trial. Ann Surg. 2006;244(4):481–90.
19. Stadlhuber RJ, Sherif AE, Mittal SK, et al. Mesh complications after prosthetic reinforcement of hiatal closure: a 28-case series. Surg Endosc. 2009;23(6):1219–26.
20. Zehetner J, DeMeester SR, Ayazi S, Kilday P, Alicuben ET, DeMeester TR. Laparoscopic wedge fundectomy for collis gastroplasty creation in patients with a foreshortened esophagus. Ann Surg. 2014;260(6):1030–3.
21. Peters JH, DeMeester TR, Crookes P, et al. The treatment of gastroesophageal reflux disease with laparoscopic Nissen fundoplication: prospective evaluation of 100 patients with "typical" symptoms. Ann Surg. 1998;228(1):40–50.
22. Del Campo SEM, Mansfield SA, Suzo AJ, Hazey JW, Perry KA. Laparoscopic redo fundoplication improves disease-specific and global quality of life following failed laparoscopic or open fundoplication. Surg Endosc. 2017;31(11):4649–55.
23. Wilshire CL, Louie BE, Shultz D, Jutric Z, Farivar AS, Aye RW. Clinical outcomes of reoperation for failed antireflux operations. Ann Thorac Surg. 2016;101(4):1290–6.
24. Little AG, Ferguson MK, Skinner DB. Reoperation for failed antireflux operations. J Thorac Cardiovasc Surg. 1986;91(4):511–7.
25. Grover BT, Kothari SN. Reoperative antireflux surgery. Surg Clin North Am. 2015;95(3):629–40.
26. Frezza EE, Ikramuddin S, Gourash W, et al. Symptomatic improvement in gastroesophageal reflux disease (GERD) following laparoscopic Roux-en-Y gastric bypass. Surg Endosc. 2002;16(7):1027–31.

Classification and Evaluation of Diaphragmatic Hernias

18

Adham R. Saad and Britney L. Corey

Introduction

Patients with diaphragmatic hernias are referred to surgeons to determine the necessity for intervention. Often these hernias are incidental findings from diagnostic evaluations for reflux or ulcer disease, but they can also present in dire need of urgent surgery. Understanding the evaluation and treatment of diaphragmatic hernias is essential to determining the appropriate treatment. It is important to know the classification of the different types of diaphragmatic hernias and how to adequately evaluate them so that patients get proper treatment with the appropriate urgency. The large majority of these cases are not emergencies, and it is imperative that the patient gets a complete workup prior to surgical intervention to prevent debilitating postoperative complications. Through a discussion of the anatomy of the diaphragm and the esophageal hiatus, the pathophysiology of these hernias is more clear. In addition, the different types of hernias, their classification, and their appropriate evaluation will be discussed.

A. R. Saad
Minimally Invasive GI Surgery, Department of Surgery, University of Alabama at Birmingham, Birmingham, AL, USA

B. L. Corey (✉)
Department of Surgery, University of Alabama at Birmingham, Birmingham Veteran's Affairs Medical Center, Birmingham, AL, USA
e-mail: blprince@uabmc.edu

J. Grams et al. (eds.), *The SAGES Manual of Foregut Surgery*,
https://doi.org/10.1007/978-3-319-96122-4_18

Anatomic Considerations

Embryology

The diaphragm develops between the 3rd and 10th weeks of gestation and is derived from four precursors: (1) the septum transversum, (2) two pleuroperitoneal folds, (3) cervical myotomes, and (4) the dorsal mesentery [1] (Fig. 18.1). The septum tranversum forms the central tendon, and the two pleuroperitoneal folds grow medially to join this tendon. The posteromedial portion is formed from the dorsal mesentery which contains the aorta, inferior vena cava, and esophagus. The crura are created from migration of myoblasts to this dorsal mesentery. The third, fourth, and fifth cervical myotomes provide the diaphragmatic musculature [2]. Congenital defects occur with failure of the pleuroperitoneal folds to develop, as there is no scaffolding for the musculature to develop upon [1].

Diaphragm

The diaphragm has three muscle groups: sternal, costal, and lumbar, which all join at the central tendon and create a dome-shaped membrane separating the thoracic and abdominal cavities [2]. There are three distinct foramina: aortic, esophageal, and caval. The aortic hiatus at T12 is the most posterior and contains the aorta, the thoracic duct, and azygous veins. It is bordered posteriorly by the vertebral bodies, anteriorly by the median arcuate ligament, and laterally by the crural origins.

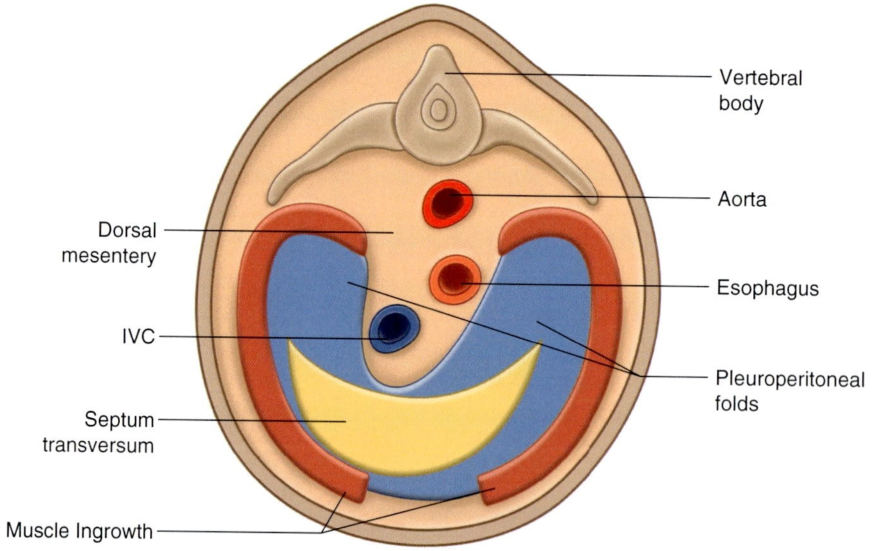

Fig. 18.1 Embryology of the diaphragm

At T10, the esophageal hiatus is the only foramen surrounded completely by muscle. The caval opening is the most anterior lying between T8 and T9 [1] and is completely surrounded by the central tendon of the diaphragm.

Blood is supplied by the right and left phrenic arteries, the intercostal arteries, and musculophrenic branches of the internal thoracic arteries [1]. Muscular and sensory innervation is provided by the left and right phrenic nerves which arise from the C3, C4, and C5 rami [2].

Hiatal Anatomy

The majority of diaphragmatic hernias occur through the esophageal hiatus, therefore it is essential to understand this anatomy (Fig. 18.2). The right and left diaphragmatic crus are muscular fibers that arise from the anterior longitudinal ligaments and are anchored at the lumbar vertebrae. As the right crus emerges from the anterior longitudinal ligament, it splits into two arms, one coursing medially and wrapping posterior to the esophagus and the other wrapping anteriorly. These arms decussate anterior to the esophagus where, along with the left crus, they attach at the central tendon of the diaphragm [3].

The esophagus is anchored to the crus by the phrenoesophageal membrane, which is formed from fused endothoracic and endoabdominal fascias. Additional posterior support is provided by the vagus nerves and radicles of the left gastric artery and vein. The phrenoesophageal membrane is attached circumferentially on the esophagus at the squamocolumnar junction. An intact membrane prevents herniation through the hiatus [4].

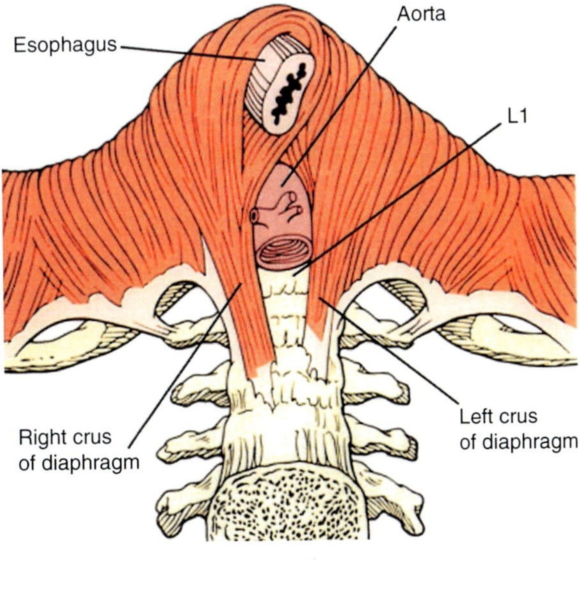

Fig. 18.2 Anatomy of the hiatus. (From Kahrilas et al. [4])

Esophagogastric Junction

The esophagogastric junction can be difficult to clinically define because of its intrinsic mobility (Fig. 18.3). Defining a true hiatal hernia depends on the relative positioning of the esophagus, the stomach, and the hiatus which is constantly variable [3]. Esophageal shortening occurs with contraction of the longitudinal muscles which elevates the distal esophagus [5]. With lifting of the distal esophagus, the esophagogastric junction is elevated above the hiatus, and there is physiological herniation [6]. It is known that this normal herniation occurs during primary and secondary peristalsis, esophageal distension, and transient relaxations of the lower esophageal sphincter [7]. Once the inciting stimulus for physiologic herniation ceases, the intrinsic elastic recoil of the phrenoesophageal membrane returns the

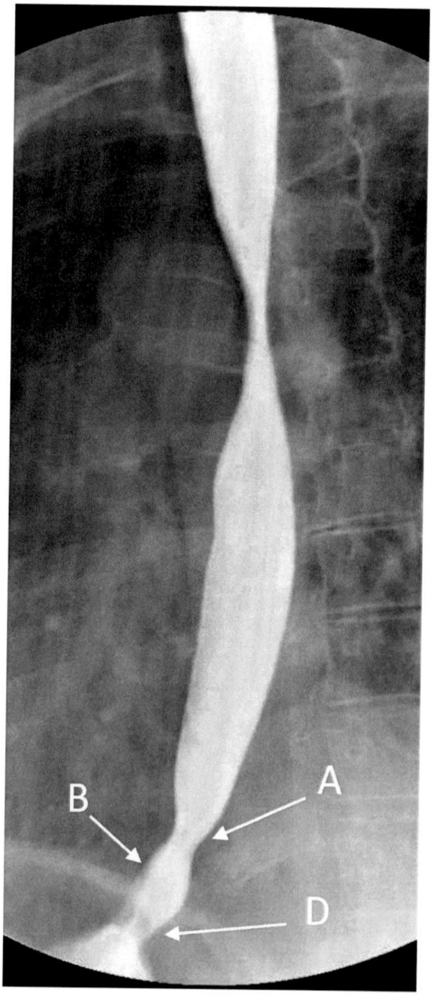

Fig. 18.3 Normal barium swallow. (A) "A" ring, (B) "B" ring or Z-line, and (D) diaphragmatic impression

esophagogastric junction to the abdomen [3]. This variability in relative anatomy at the hiatus creates unique challenges in the diagnosis and treatment of hiatal hernias. It is helpful to localize the esophagogastric junction with endoscopy although it can be difficult to get an accurate picture of its location relative to other relevant structures.

Pathophysiology

Risk Factors

Obesity causes gradual increases in intra-abdominal pressure which creates forces that encourage hiatal herniation [8]. Body mass index (BMI) has a direct relationship with increasing risk of hiatal hernia [9]. Clinically, many surgeons hesitate to offer hiatal hernia repair for patients with elevated body mass index because of increased risk of re-herniation. There is some controversy as to whether obesity increases the likelihood of recurrence after surgery at the hiatus. In a study comparing antireflux surgery outcomes in obese patients (BMI > 30), overweight patients (BMI 25–29.9), and nonobese (BMI < 25), obese patients had significantly higher recurrence rates (31%) versus the overweight (8%) and the nonobese (4.5%) [10]. More recent studies make the case that obesity has no effect on outcomes after antireflux surgery with or without concurrent hiatal hernia repair. Winslow et al. [11] showed that although surgery in the obese population is more difficult with significantly greater operative times, there was no difference in recurrence rates, symptoms, and patient satisfaction. In a prospective analysis of both clinical and objective outcomes, there were no differences in quality of life measures and recurrence rates between the obese and nonobese groups [12]. This controversy supports a frank discussion between obese patients and physicians as to the ideal timing for repair.

Age is also associated with increased risk for hiatal herniation. As the elasticity and recoil of the phrenoesophageal membrane decrease with age, the risk of herniation increases [9]. This is discussed in more detail in the pathophysiology section.

Previous surgery at the hiatus is another known risk factor for hiatal herniation. In a prospective study, radiologic recurrence after hiatal hernia repair has been reported as 57% (median follow-up = 58 months), although the majority of these were not clinically relevant and only 3% required reoperation [13]. Another study showed a radiologic recurrence rate of 27% at 1 year follow-up with no clinically relevant recurrences and no identifiable risk factors for recurrence [14]. It is assumed that each subsequent repair would have an increased likelihood of recurrence.

Other known risk factors include thoracoabdominal trauma most commonly from motor vehicle collisions [15]. Skeletal deformities such as scoliosis that change the anatomy of the diaphragm also increase risk [16]. Finally, congenital deformities are the most common cause of diaphragmatic hernia in children [17].

Causal Theories

As was well described in a review article by Weber et al., there are three theories of causation of hiatal hernia: (1) increased intra-abdominal pressure forcing the gastroesophageal junction into the chest, (2) displacement of the gastroesophageal junction into the chest due to esophageal shortening from fibrosis or excess vagal stimulation, and (3) gastroesophageal junction migration due to enlargement of the hiatus from congenital defects or acquired molecular/cellular changes. Through their review, they conclude that none of these theories are definitive and that causation is likely multifactorial [18].

Increased Intra-Abdominal Pressure

As previously discussed, obesity is a known risk factor for development of hiatal hernia which supports this causal theory. It has been shown that with increases of BMI of one point, intragastric pressure increases by 0.3 mmHg and intraesophageal pressure rose by 0.17 mmHg; waist circumference increases of 1 cm increased intragastric and intraesophageal pressures by 0.16 mmHg and 0.1 mmHg, respectively [6]. These gradients would theoretically transfer forces leading to hiatal herniation.

Esophageal Shortening/Vagal Stimulation

With contraction of the longitudinal muscles of the esophagus, physiological herniation is proposed to occur during swallowing [6]. It has been shown that with inhibitory vagal innervation anterior to the stomach cardia, this physiological herniation is not allowed to occur. Therefore, it is theorized that damage to the vagal nerve at the esophagogastric junction can cause either a decrease in this inhibitory function or an increase in stimulation of the longitudinal muscles resulting in chronic herniation over time [19].

Hiatal Enlargement

Through a combination of changes in the molecular makeup of the tissues that create the hiatus, progressive weakening can lead to physical weakening that can allow herniation. On analysis of the phrenoesophageal, gastrohepatic, and gastrophrenic ligaments at the time of fundoplication for gastroesophageal reflux disease, those patients with concurrent hiatal hernia were found to have 50% less elastin than those without hiatal hernias [20]. Impairments in collagen have been shown in both inguinal and incisional hernias, which would beg the question as to collagen involvement in hiatal hernia [21, 22]. Although this question is yet to be answered, it is not unreasonable to theorize that collagen also plays a role at the hiatus. Crural muscle fibers also seem to be involved in weakening of the hiatus. At the microscopic level, when comparing crural muscle in patients with and without hiatal hernia, there appears to be degradation of the myofibrils and degeneration of the muscular architecture in the patients with hiatal hernia [23]. Therefore, hiatal enlargement through a combination of tissue factors at the supportive ligaments and impairments of crural muscle is highly supported.

Types of Diaphragmatic Hernias

Hiatal Hernias

Hiatal hernias are categorized into sliding or paraesophageal hernias with four recognized types (Fig. 18.4).

Type I Hiatal Hernia

Type I hiatal hernia is commonly described as a sliding hiatal hernia and occurs when the esophageal hiatus is dilated enough to allow herniation of the gastric cardia and bringing the gastroesophageal junction above the diaphragm. While they are the most common of the diaphragmatic hernias, they are also the most difficult to

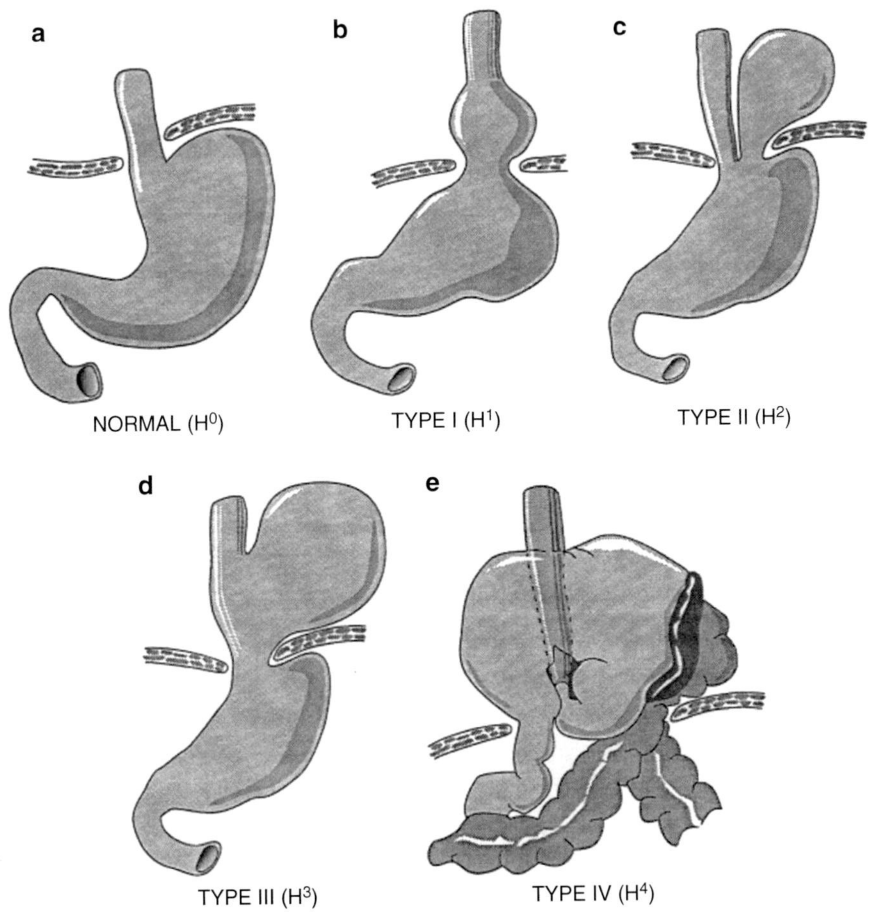

Fig. 18.4 (**a**) Normal hiatus, (**b**) Type I sliding hernia, (**c**) Type II paraesophageal, (**d**) Type III paraesophageal, and (**e**) Type IV. (From Zaman and Lidor [14])

define [3] because of the previously described phenomenon of "physiologic herniation" [6]. With these hernias, the phrenoesophageal ligament is weakened and thinned but remains intact. Therefore, there is a widening of the hiatus that allows the gastric cardia to herniate into the mediastinum. These hernias become clinically significant because of their association with gastroesophageal reflux [3]. This is likely due to the significantly larger cross-sectional opening at the esophagogastric junction in patients with hiatal hernias versus patients without hiatal hernia at different intragastric pressures, as was eloquently described in a study by Pandolfino et al. [24]. The hiatus becomes circular in dimension as opposed to elliptical [24].

Paraesophageal

These hernias are less common than the sliding type hiatal hernia and correspond to approximately 5–15% of all hiatal hernias [25]. Although these hernias are also associated with gastroesophageal reflux, their clinical significance is rooted in the mechanical complications [3] to include obstruction, dysphagia, and organ strangulation.

Type II

These hernias result when there is an actual defect in the phrenoesophageal membrane that allows herniation of the gastric fundus while the gastroesophageal junction remains tethered at the hiatus [26].

Type III

Type III hernias are viewed as a progression of a Type I or II hiatal hernia (Fig. 18.5). As the Type II hernia enlarges, there is continued weakening of the phrenoesophageal membrane that allows the gastroesophageal junction to slide into the mediastinum [3]. Therefore, the Type III hernia is by definition a combination of the Type I and Type II hiatal hernias.

Type IV

These are large hernias where the hiatus has enlarged enough to accommodate herniation of other organs in addition to the stomach. These can be associated with a large variety of symptom profiles.

Congenital

Morgagni

This hernia was first described by anatomist Giovanni Morgagni in 1769 as an "anterior retrosternal diaphragmatic defect that occurs between the xiphoid process of the sternum and costochondral attachments of the diaphragm" [2] (Fig. 18.6). These hernias result from a failure of the complete migration of muscle fibers to cover a triangular space between the sternum and bilateral costal margins, and herniation of abdominal contents usually results from trauma, obesity, or pregnancy [27]. Although these hernias are congenital, they are often not diagnosed until adulthood when they become symptomatic or as an incidental finding [28]. These hernias should always be

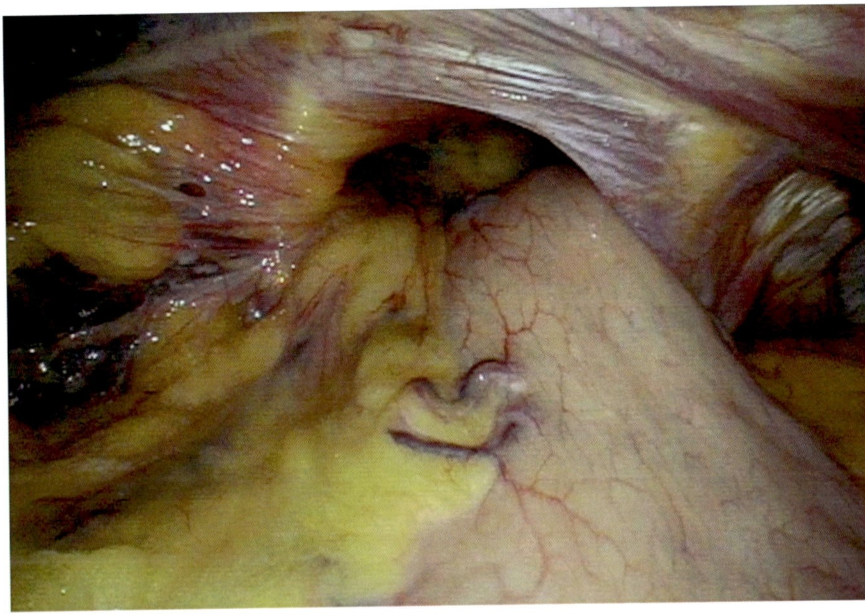

Fig. 18.5 Intraoperative view of sliding hiatal hernia with cardia and gastroesophageal junction above the diaphragm

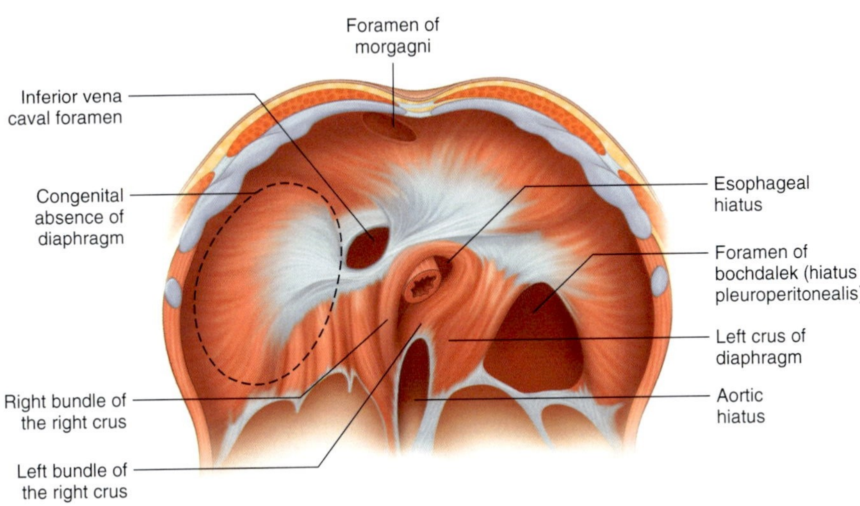

Fig. 18.6 Anatomy of Morgagni and Bochdalek hernias. (From http://www.continentalhospitals.com/blog/diaphragmatic-hernia/)

repaired upon diagnosis for fear of complications of obstruction or strangulation. Repair is usually completed transabdominally, although a transthoracic approach may be required for herniation above the carina with the use of mesh for larger defects [2]. Minimally invasive techniques have been an accepted approach for many years [27].

Bochdalek

Bochdalek hernias comprise 90% of congenital diaphragmatic hernias [29]. The diagnosis is often made with antenatal scans or at the time of delivery with respiratory distress [29]. As first described by anatomist Vincenz Bochdalek, these are congenital diaphragmatic hernias that occur during early embryologic development (Fig. 18.6). During this phase of development, the gastrointestinal tract is formed, and due to abnormal development of the pleuroperitoneal canal, the viscera become contained in the chest which prevents normal development of the lung [2]. Therefore, this pulmonary hypoplasia as well as associated vascular and cardiac abnormalities can result in a neonatal mortality of almost 50% [29]. For these patients, intensive cardiac and respiratory support are required for whatever period is necessary to obtain clinical stability with surgical intervention as a secondary goal [29]. Primary repair is often achievable, although more complex repairs may require a patch for a large defect and/or silo placement to allow return of the viscera to the abdomen [2].

Evaluation

Clinical Presentation

Chronic Symptoms

Most chronic symptoms result from the anatomic changes at the esophagogastric junction [30]. Most commonly patients will complain of reflux symptoms to include both heartburn and regurgitation. The hernia causes separation of the lower esophageal sphincter from the diaphragmatic crus which leads to acid exposure at the esophagus [25]. Concurrently, once this acid refluxes into the esophagus, the hiatal hernia compounds the exposure by also preventing acid clearance [31]. Increased intragastric pressures caused by the hernia also impair gastric emptying which complicates the reflux mechanism further [30].

Dysphagia may be the presenting symptom when the herniated portion compresses the distal esophagus. Stasis within the herniated stomach can also lead to symptoms of dysphagia [25]. Simple discoordination at the distal esophagus caused by the separation of the lower esophageal sphincter and the crura is often experienced as dysphagia by the patient [25].

Bleeding or anemia can be the presenting sign in patients with Cameron lesions, although other sites of gastrointestinal hemorrhage must be excluded [30]. Chest pain is a non-specific symptom associated with hiatal hernia, although, again, cardiopulmonary etiologies must be ruled out. Progressive dyspnea can be a presenting symptom that is often assigned to a cardiopulmonary or age-related source [32]. If hiatal hernia is identified as the source of dyspnea, repair can result in improvements in pulmonary function which correlate to the size of the hernia [33].

Acute Symptoms

Symptoms in the acute setting are primarily associated with paraesophageal hernias and are related to obstruction, ischemia, or volvulus [25]. Patients who present with obstruction usually have non-distended abdomens, can usually be managed with nasogastric decompression, and often resolve spontaneously [30]. For those who are unable to be managed nonoperatively due to a deteriorating clinical picture, the concern is strangulation and eventual necrosis of the stomach. Although necrosis is rare, it is the leading cause of mortality from hiatal hernia [34]. Patients in whom necrosis is possible, emergency diagnostic upper endoscopy or surgical intervention are essential.

Radiography

The primary role of both chest radiography and computed tomography is initial identification of the hernia either incidentally or in the acute setting. For adequate radiologic evaluation of a hiatal hernia, the primary study is a barium swallow because it identifies the anatomy of the hernia, the relative orientation of the hernia contents, and localizes the gastroesophageal junction (Fig. 18.7). In addition, this

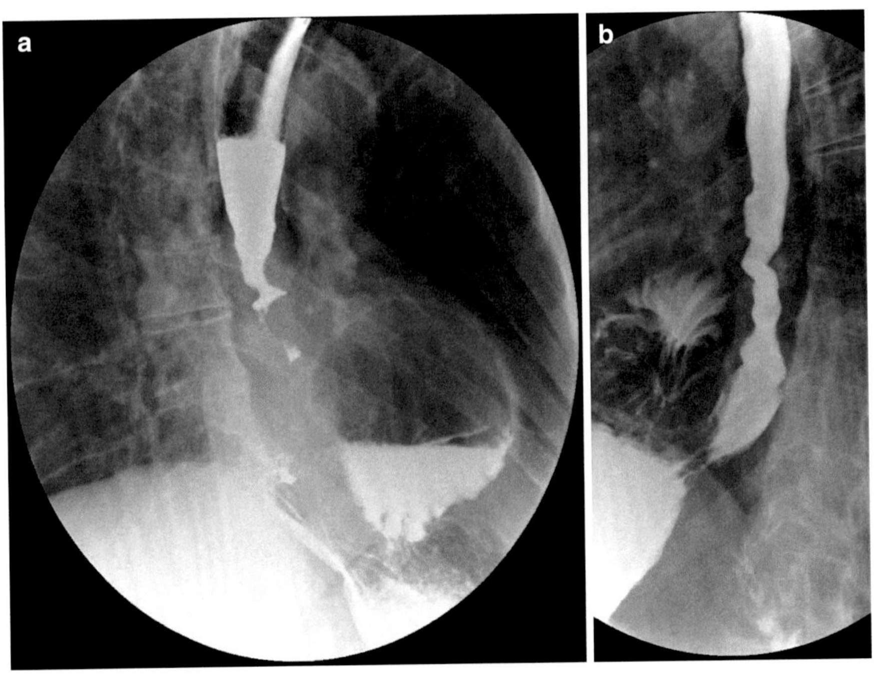

Fig. 18.7 Barium swallow. (**a**) Type III paraesophageal hernia depicting herniation of the gastric cardia and fundus above the diaphragmatic hiatus. (**b**) Type II paraesophageal hernia with herniation of the gastric fundus adjacent to esophagus with the esophagogastric junction still tethered at the hiatus

study is conducted in real time, so it allows the radiographer to identify the anatomy as it relates to other key structures and how these essential elements interact. For paraesophageal hernias, the imaging and diagnosis is fairly straightforward, whereas the diagnosis of Type I hiatal hernias can be more difficult.

Because of variations in protocol and radiographic criteria for defining hiatal hernias, there can be significant differences in interpretations of barium swallows. In order to visualize the key structures, they have to be distended, which intrinsically changes their relative positions. This distension causes shortening of the esophagus and displacement of the esophagogastric junction which is the basis of the 2 cm rule [3]. The 2 cm rule states that there must be more than 2 cm between the diaphragmatic hiatus and the squamocolumnar junction (or B ring) for diagnosis of a Type I hiatal hernia [35]. Without visualization of the B ring, three rugal folds above the diaphragm are necessary for diagnosis. Additionally, the timing of measurements during the peristaltic sequence can have significant effects on the results. If measurements are taken early in the peristaltic sequence, the size of the hernia will appear significantly larger than if the measurements are taken at the end of the sequence [3]. These variations can make the sizing and identification of small sliding hernias especially difficult and intrinsically erratic. Barium swallow can also help identify issues with esophageal motility which can be further elucidated with high-resolution manometry.

Endoscopy

Upper endoscopy is an important part of the evaluation of hiatal hernias. It allows for accurate diagnosis of hiatal herniation and is important in evaluating potential complications such as bleeding and dysphagia (Fig. 18.8). A Type I hiatal hernia is defined on endoscopy as a 2 cm separation of the squamocolumnar junction and the

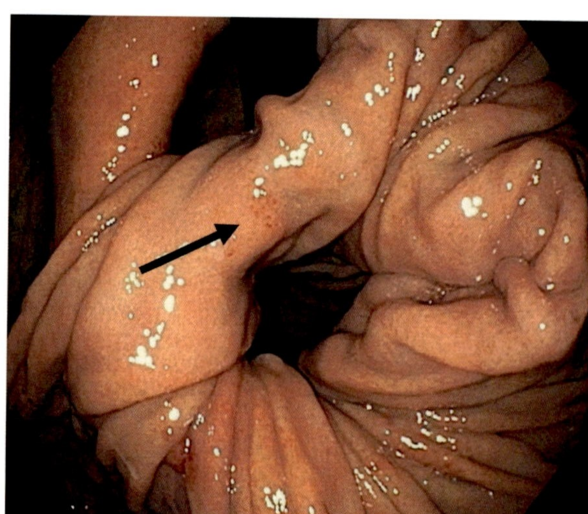

Fig. 18.8 Retroflexed endoscopic view of paraesophageal hernia. Arrow indicates early Cameron lesions which are a common etiology of anemia in patients with hiatal hernia

diaphragmatic pinch as the stomach encounters the crura. This diagnostic criterion can be limited in settings such as Barrett's metaplasia or esophagitis where the squamocolumnar junction is obscured. The mobile nature of the esophagogastric junction can also make measurements quite difficult. Paraesophageal hernias are a more straightforward diagnosis although endoscopy can be difficult due to the tortuous path.

Just as with barium swallow, there can be significant variations between endoscopic technique and interpretation. Bytzer showed that patient history alone can bias interpretation of endoscopic images where only 23% of endoscopists showing the same video case interpreted the same diagnosis [36]. This inherent variability in endoscopy and its interpretation can limit the value of information drawn from endoscopy, especially in hiatal hernias less than 3 cm in size [3]. Retrograde view can provide some extra information about the integrity of the hiatus and displacement of the squamocolumnar junction relative to the hiatus. Additionally, variations in the extent of gastric distention with insufflation may cause an inherent 2 cm error in size measurement [3].

Manometry

The esophagogastric junction can be identified with high-resolution manometry because of three physiologic phenomenon: (1) intragastric pressure is greater than intraesophageal pressure, most notably during inspiration, (2_ the pressure wave seen at the esophagogastric junction has both tonic (representing the lower esophageal sphincter) and phasic (representing the crura) elements, and (3) there is relative movement and intraluminal pressure changes at the esophagogastric junction during respiration [3]. High-resolution manometry with pressure plotting helps locate the upper esophageal sphincter, lower esophageal sphincter, and crural diaphragm in real time as the three high-pressure zones. A separation of greater than 2 cm between the lower esophageal sphincter and crural diaphragm is defined as a hiatal hernia [25]. There can be great variation in how well defined these high-pressure zones are in individuals which can create some interpretive variability in diagnosis [3]. Even with this variability, high-resolution manometry has dramatically improved diagnostic capabilities because of its ability to localize the lower esophageal sphincter and crural diaphragm in real time without swallow or distension-related distortions seen in barium swallow and endoscopy [3].

Diagnostic Summary

Although all the diagnostic modalities are plagued with some inadequacies, it is important for the clinician to take all the information provided to formulate a reasonable approach to the care of the patient. It is important for the gastroenterologists, surgeons, and radiologists to discuss the more complex cases where the diagnosis is not so apparent. It is imperative for each institution to create protocols and diagnostic standardization to promote consistency between different practitioners. Precise discussion of patient-specific symptoms can provide invaluable clues as to the diagnosis and predict which symptoms can be alleviated with surgical intervention to maintain patient satisfaction.

References

1. Bryant AS, Cerfolio RJ. Chapter 42. Diaphragmatic procedures. In: Souba WW, editor. ACS Surgery: Principles & Practice. New York: WebMD; 2007. p. 464.
2. Maish MS. The diaphragm. Surg Clin North Am. 2010;90(5):955–68.
3. Kahrilas PJ, Kim HC, Pandolfino JE. Approaches to the diagnosis and grading of hiatal hernia. Best Pract Res Clin Gastroenterol. 2008;22(4):601–16.
4. Kahrilas PJ, Lin S, Chen J, et al. The effect of hiatus hernia on the gastro-oesophageal junction pressure. Gut. 1999;44(4):476–82.
5. Pouderoux P, Lin S, Kahrilas PJ. Timing, propagation, coordination, and effect of esophageal shortening during peristalsis. Gastroenterology. 1997;112(4):1147–54.
6. Pandolfino JE, Zhang QG, Ghosh SK, et al. Transient lower esophageal sphincter relaxations and reflux: mechanistic analysis using concurrent fluoroscopy and high-resolution manometry. Gastroenterology. 2006;131(6):1725–33.
7. Shi G, Pandolfino JE, Joehl RJ, et al. Distinct patterns of oesophageal shortening during primary peristalsis, secondary peristalsis, and transient lower oesophageal sphincter relaxation. Neurogastroenterology Motil. 2002;14(5):505–12.
8. Pandolfino JE, El-Seraq HB, Zhang Q, et al. Obesity: a challenge to esophagogastric junction integrity. Gastroenterology. 2006;130(3):639–49.
9. Menon S, Trudgill N. Risk factors in the aetiology of hiatus hernia: a meta-analysis. Eur J of Gastroenterol Hepatol. 2011;23(2):133–8.
10. Perez AR, Moncure AC, Rattner DW. Obesity adversely affects the outcome of antireflux operations. Surg Endosc. 2001;15(9):986–9.
11. Winslow ER, Frisella MM, Soper NJ, et al. Obesity does not adversely affect the outcome of laparoscopic antireflux surgery (LARS). Surg Endosc. 2003;17(12):2003–11.
12. Luketina RR, Koch OO, Köhler G, et al. Obesity does not affect the outcome of laparoscopic antireflux surgery. Surg Endosc. 2015;29(6):1327–33.
13. Oelschlager BK, Petersen RP, Brunt LM, et al. Laparoscopic paraesophageal hernia repair: defining long-term clinical and anatomic outcomes. J Gastrointest Surg. 2012;16:453–9.
14. Zaman JA, Lidor AO. The optimal approach to symptomatic paraesophageal hernia repair: important technical considerations. Curr Gastroenterol Rep. 2016;18(10):53.
15. Eren S, Ciris F. Diaphragmatic hernia: diagnostic approaches with review of the literature. Eur J Radiol. 2005;54(3):448–59.
16. Schuchert MJ, Adusumilli PS, Cook CC, et al. The impact of scoliosis among patients with giant paraesophageal hernia. J Gastrointest Surg. 2011;15(1):23–8.
17. Karpelowsky JS, Wieselthaler N, Rode H. Primary paraesophageal hernia in children. J Pediatr Surg. 2006;41(9):1588–93.
18. Weber C, Davis CS, Shankaran V, et al. Hiatal hernias: a review of the pathophysiologic theories and implication for research. Surg Endosc. 2011;25(10):3149–53.
19. Christensen J, Miftakhov R. Hiatus hernia: a review of evidence for its origin in esophageal longitudinal muscle dysfunction. Am J Med. 2000;108(Suppl 4a):3S–7S.
20. Curci JA, Melman LM, Thompson RW, et al. Elastic fiber depletion in the supporting ligaments of the gastroesophageal junction: a structural basis for the development of hiatal hernia. J Am Coll Surg. 2008;207(2):191–6.
21. Rosch R, Klinge U, Si Z, et al. A role for the collagen I/III and MMP-1/−13 genes in primary inguinal hernia. BMC Med Genet. 2002;3:2.

22. Si Z, Bhardwai R, Rosch R, et al. Impaired balance of type I and type III procollagen mRNA in cultured fibroblasts of patients with incisional hernia. Surgery. 2002;131(3):324–31.
23. Fei L, del Genio G, Rossetti G, et al. Hiatal hernia recurrence: surgical complication or disease? Electron microscope findings of the diaphragmatic pillars. J Gastrointest Surg. 2009;13(3):459–64.
24. Pandolfino JE, Shi G, Trueworthy B, et al. Esophagogastric junction opening during relaxation distinguishes nonhernia reflux patients, hernia patients, and normal subjects. Gastroenterology. 2003;125(4):1018–24.
25. Roman S, Kahrilas PJ. The diagnosis and management of hiatus hernia. BMJ. 2014;349:g1654.
26. Skinner DB. Chapter 53. Hernias. In: Berk JE, editor. Gastroenterology. Philadelphia: W.B. Saunders; 1985. p. 705.
27. Minneci PC, Deans KJ, Kim P, et al. Foramen of Morgagni hernia: changes in diagnosis and treatment. Ann Thorac Surg. 2004;77(6):1956–9.
28. Nasr A, Fecteau A. Foramen of Morgagni hernia: presentation and treatment. Thorac Surg Clin. 2009;19(4):463–8.
29. McHoney M. Congenital diaphragmatic hernia, management in newborn. Pediatr Surg Int. 2015;31(11):1005–13.
30. Collet D, Luc G, Chiche L. Management of large Para-esophageal hiatal hernias. J Visc Surg. 2013;150(6):395–402.
31. Jones MP, Sloan SS, Jovanovic B, et al. Impaired egress rather than increased access: an important independent predictor of erosive oesophagitis. Neurogastroenterol Motil. 2002;14(6):625–31.
32. Khanna A, Finch G. Paraesophageal herniation: a review. Surgeon. 2011;9(2):104–11.
33. Low DE, Simchuk EJ. Effect of paraesophageal hernia repair on pulmonary function. Ann Thorac Surg. 2002;74(2):333–7.
34. Bawahab M, Mitchell P, Church N, et al. Management of acute paraesophageal hernia. Surg Endosc. 2009;23(2):255–9.
35. Ott DJ, Gelfand DW, Chen YM, et al. Predictive relationship of hiatal hernia to reflux esophagitis. Gastrointest Radiol. 1985;10(4):317–20.
36. Bytzer P. Information bias in endoscopic assessment. Am J Gastroenterol. 2007;102(8):1585–7.

Laparoscopic Hiatal Hernia Repair

19

Andrew M. Ibrahim and Dana A. Telem

Introduction

An estimated 75% of hiatal hernias are now being repaired through a laparoscopic approach [1]. This chapter will briefly outline the indications, technique, and perioperative considerations for the laparoscopic repair of hiatal hernias. The previous chapter (Chap. 18) discusses the classification and evaluation of diaphragmatic hernias including presentation and workup approach. The following chapter (Chap. 20) within this manual describes the transthoracic approach as an alternative to laparoscopic repair.

Indications

Preoperative Indications

Indications for electively operating on hiatal hernias should take into account the type of hernia, the associated symptoms, and patient's comorbidities. The presentation of a hiatal hernia can range from asymptomatic to life threatening (Table 19.1). Many hiatal hernias are discovered incidentally and have no symptoms. Alternatively, hiatal hernias may present with mild symptoms including epigastric pain, dysphagia, reflux symptoms, or early satiety. Finally, patients with hiatal hernia can present acutely when their stomach or other abdominal contents become strangulated.

A. M. Ibrahim (✉)
Robertwood Johnson Clinical Scholar, Department of Surgery, University of Michigan, Ann Arbor, MI, USA
e-mail: iandrew@umich.edu

D. A. Telem
Michigan Comprehensive Hernia Program, Department of Surgery, University of Michigan, Ann Arbor, MI, USA

J. Grams et al. (eds.), *The SAGES Manual of Foregut Surgery*,
https://doi.org/10.1007/978-3-319-96122-4_19

Table 19.1 Presentation of hiatal hernias

No symptoms
Often discovered incidentally on imaging obtained for another purpose
Mild symptoms
Epigastric pain, dysphagia, early satiety, reflux
Life threatening
When a hiatal hernia has led to strangulation of abdominal contents

In 2013, the SAGES Board of Governors approved the following guidelines for hiatal hernia repair that take into account type of hernia, presentation, and the patient's comorbidities [2]:

1. Repair of a Type I hernia in the absence of reflux disease is not necessary.
2. All symptomatic paraesophageal hiatal hernias should be repaired, particularly those with acute obstructive symptoms or which have undergone volvulus.
3. Routine elective repair of completely asymptomatic paraesophageal hernias may not always be indicated. Consideration for surgery should include the patient's age and comorbidities.
4. Acute gastric volvulus requires reduction of the stomach with limited resection if needed.

Consistent with these guidelines, the authors prefer a "watchful waiting" approach for asymptomatic patients as well as those with mild symptoms and significant comorbid conditions.

(Note, a discussion of indications and approach and an acute gastric volvulus hernia are discussed in Chap. 22).

Intraoperative Indications

Hiatal hernias may be discovered incidentally during another abdominal operation. For example, a review of 35,947 Roux-en-Y gastric bypass procedures found that 2233 (~6%) had an incidental hiatal hernia [3]. Subsequent studies noted that patients undergoing bariatric procedures who had their hiatal hernias repaired at the same time reported lower rates of reflux symptoms [4–6]. For this reason, most surgeons now routinely repair hiatal hernias discovered during bariatric operations.

Technique

Below we describe our approach to a laparoscopic hiatal hernia repair. We include "key steps" that have broad consensus from minimally invasive surgeons, as well as "additional considerations" where there is some debate and conflicting evidence.

Key Steps Key steps to repair of the hiatal hernia include:

- Reducing the hernia contents
- Mobilization of the hernia sac
- Mobilizing the esophagus
- Closure of the cura
- Anti-reflux procedure (fundoplication, gastroplasty)

Reducing Hernia Sac Contents The hernia sac often extends well into the thoracic cavity and may include abdominal contents such as the stomach, small bowel, or colon. These should be reduced with atraumatic graspers and returned into the abdominal cavity. In some cases, taking some of the short gastric vessels may be necessary to reduce the contents.

Mobilization of the Hernia Sac After reducing the hernia contents, the sac should be mobilized away from mediastinal structures. Because the sac forms an avascular plane, it should be bluntly dissected away from intrathoracic structures with minimal bleeding. A critical step in this portion of the operation is to identify and preserve the vagal nerves that run along the esophagus. If there is a concern of encountering a replaced left hepatic artery while dissecting the sac, the vessel should be clamped and the liver observed.

Mobilization of the Esophagus Because the hernia contents invariably travel along the esophagus, it is common for the esophagus to be partially displaced into the thoracic cavity. To avoid recurrence, the esophagus should be mobilized and distal end restored to its intraabdominal location (Fig. 19.1). Generally, at least 3 centimeters of the esophagus should sit comfortably below the diaphragm. If this

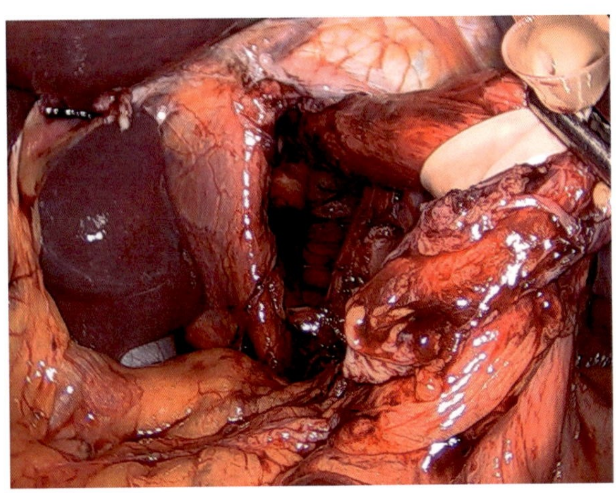

Fig. 19.1 Mobilization of the esophagus. Because the hernia contents invariably travel along the esophagus, it is common for the esophagus to be partially displaced into the thoracic cavity. To avoid recurrence, the esophagus should be mobilized and distal end restored to its intraabdominal location

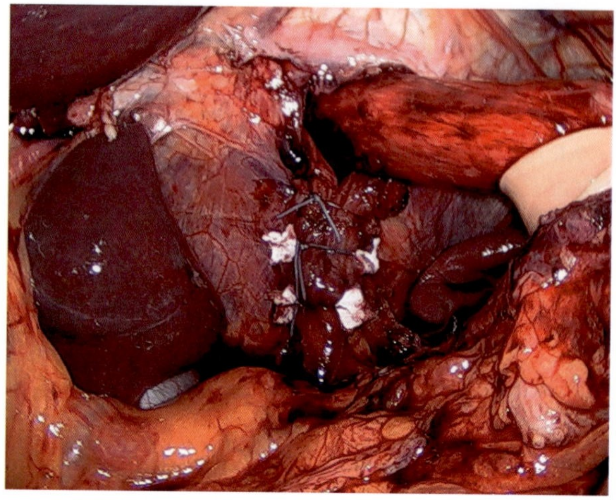

Fig. 19.2 Closure of the cura. After the esophagus has been mobilized, the hernia defect around the cura should be closed. This should be a tension-free repair with horizontal interrupted sutures placed posterior to the esophagus

is not possible, an esophageal lengthening procedure (e.g., Collis gastroplasty) should be performed. (See Chap. 21 for a full discussion of esophagus lengthening procedures.)

Closure of the Cura After the esophagus has been mobilized, the hernia defect around the cura should be closed (Fig. 19.2). This should be a tension-free repair with horizontal interrupted sutures placed posterior to the esophagus. For larger defects, relaxing incisions along the lateral diaphragm can be made to facilitate approximating the cura. Mesh reinforcement has been a matter of debate and discussed in detail in Chap. 24.

Anti-reflux Procedures There is increasing consensus among surgeons that an anti-reflux procedure should be performed on patients undergoing hiatal hernia repair. This is because the hiatal repair disrupts the phrenoesophageal ligament and predisposes patients to reflux symptoms. Anti-reflux fundoplication options include a partial wrap (e.g., Toupet) or a full wrap (e.g., Nissen). Preoperative motility studies and description of patient symptoms help inform which wrap is most appropriate.

Additional Steps to Consider

In contrast to the broad agreement about the key steps listed above, there is variability in the use of gastropexy, hernia sac excision, and robotics for hiatal hernia repair. We discuss each of them here.

Gastropexy To help prevent recurrence, some surgeons also perform an anterior gastropexy. This is typically done by securing the anterior stomach to the anterior abdominal wall with two nonabsorbable stitches. The rationale for this approach is supported by two early, short-term studies that found gastropexy to be associated with decreased recurrence [7, 8]. A subsequent study, however, with longer-term follow-up found no difference in rates of recurrence between patients receiving gastropexy and no gastropexy [9].

Hernia Sac Excision There is debate about whether or not the hernia sac should be excised. Advocates for sac excision point toward studies suggesting that this reduces hernia recurrence [10, 11]. Those who do not perform sac excision point out that these studies are underpowered and that dissection alone is sufficient [12]. The current SAGES guidelines consider both sides by recommending that the hiatal hernia sac should be dissected (strong recommendation) and preferably excised (weak recommendation) [2].

Robotics Compared to open abdominal surgery, the laparoscopic approach for hiatal hernia repair has been associated with decreased morbidity and shorter length of stay [13, 14], making it the preferred approach [15]. The role of robot-assisted minimally invasive surgery is less defined. On one hand, the robot may be helpful in operating in tight spaces with improved dexterity around the hiatus. However, the lack of haptic feedback may threaten the quality of suture tying around the cura that is key to the operation. At present, there does not appear to be a clear advantage to make the robot a preferred approach over standard laparoscopy [16, 17].

Challenges encouraged during laparoscopic hiatal hernia repair and potential solutions are reviewed in Table 19.2.

Post-operative Management

Diet Early post-operative dysphagia rates have been reported as high as 50%. We recommend patients to begin with a clear liquid diet and advance as tolerated. Ice and cold liquids should be avoided as they can cause irritation and are poorly tolerated.

Table 19.2 Challenges encountered during hiatal hernia repair

Challenge	Potential solution
Short esophagus	Collis gastroplasty
Diaphragm tension during defect closure	Lateral relaxing incisions
Enter pleural cavity during dissection	Close defect OR use red rubber catheter during operation, then ask anesthesia to hyper-inflate to remove CO_2 OR leave alone
Concern for replaced left hepatic artery during dissection	Clamp vessel, observe liver perfusion before taking vessel

Antiemetics Antiemetic medications also have an important role in the immediate post-operative period. Early gagging, belching, and retching are thought to predispose patients to early failure of their hiatal hernia repair and anti-reflux procedure [18]. For this reason, many surgeons schedule antiemetics in the immediate post-operative period with low threshold for subsequent as needed doses.

Imaging Signs and symptoms concerning for a hernia recurrence or leak are indications for contrast imaging. In asymptomatic patients, contrast imaging is not routinely performed. Some surgeons, however, do obtain post-operative contrast imaging to confirm new anatomy, particularly in challenging cases.

Post–operative Complications

Post-operative complications can be classified into early and late complications.

Early Complications

The most frequent complication observed in the immediate post-operative period occurs due to iatrogenic injury to structures surrounding the hiatus. Injury to the pleural cavity can result in a pneumothorax. Missed bowel injury (often from traction) can manifest as a delayed perforation that requires reoperation. And although quite rare, the dreaded complication of an early recurrence of the hiatal hernia has been described. This latter complication underscores the motivation behind aggressive antiemetic medications in the immediate post-operative period.

Unrelated to the iatrogenic injury, patients undergoing hiatal hernia repair are also at notable risk for post-operative myocardial infarction, pneumonia, and respiratory distress. The incidence of these complications likely reflects the older age demographic that develop hiatal hernias and undergo surgery. This set of complications supports the position of many surgeons to not operate on asymptomatic hiatal hernias in older patients with significant comorbidities.

Late Complications

Complications have also been described well after the immediate post-operative period. Delayed gastric emptying can occur as a result of irritation or injury to the vagus nerve during the operation. Dysphagia has also been observed, particularly with patients who underwent a full Nissen fundoplication. Because of this observation, some surgeons favor only a partial wrap in patients who have any evidence of esophageal dysmotility preoperatively.

Post-operative Outcomes

Post-operative outcomes after hiatal hernia repair include rate of recurrence and improvement in preoperative symptoms.

Recurrences detected by endoscopy or contrast studies range from 4 to 42% [19–23]. Larger hernias appear to have higher rates of recurrence. Nearly all studies have consistently reported that radiographic recurrences are often associated with no new symptoms. As such, many people also consider following symptoms and quality of life scores.

Multiple studies demonstrate that patients do have a significant improvement in symptoms related to their hiatal hernia. For example, a review of 111 patients undergoing hiatal hernia repair observed their symptoms scores decreased significantly at 1- and 3-year follow-up compared to their preoperative baseline [24]. Consistent with the data on radiologic recurrence and symptoms, many patients who experience a small recurrence appear to still report improved quality of life after hiatal hernia repair [25].

References

1. Nguyen NT, Christie C, Masoomi H, Matin T, Laugenour K, Hohmann S. Utilization and outcomes of laparoscopic versus open paraesophageal hernia repair. Am Surg. 2011;77(10):1353–7.
2. Kohn GP, Price RR, DeMeester SR, et al. Guidelines for the management of hiatal hernia. Surgical Endoscopy and Other Interventional Techniques. 2013;27(12):4409–28.
3. Kothari V, Shaligram A, Reynoso J, Schmidt E, McBride CL, Oleynikov D. Impact on perioperative outcomes of concomitant hiatal hernia repair with laparoscopic gastric bypass. Obes Surg. 2012;22(10):1607–10.
4. Flanagin BA, Mitchell MT, Thistlethwaite WA, Alverdy JC. Diagnosis and treatment of atypical presentations of hiatal hernia following bariatric surgery. Obes Surg. 2010;20(3):386–92.
5. Merchant AM, Cook MW, Srinivasan J, Davis SS, Sweeney JF, Lin E. Comparison between laparoscopic paraesophageal hernia repair with sleeve gastrectomy and paraesophageal hernia repair alone in morbidly obese patients. Am Surg. 2009;75(7):620–5.
6. Salvador-Sanchis JL, Martinez-Ramos D, Herfarth A, Rivadulla-Serrano I, Ibanez-Belenguer M, Hoashi JS. Treatment of morbid obesity and hiatal paraesophageal hernia by laparoscopic roux-en-Y gastric bypass. Obes Surg. 2010;20(6):801–3.
7. Poncet G, Robert M, Roman S, Boulez JC. Laparoscopic repair of large hiatal hernia without prosthetic reinforcement: late results and relevance of anterior gastropexy. Journal of gastrointestinal surgery : official journal of the Society for Surgery of the Alimentary Tract. 2010;14(12):1910–6.
8. Ponsky J, Rosen M, Fanning A, Malm J. Anterior gastropexy may reduce the recurrence rate after laparoscopic paraesophageal hernia repair. Surg Endosc. 2003;17(7):1036–41.
9. Diaz S, Brunt LM, Klingensmith ME, Frisella PM, Soper NJ. Laparoscopic paraesophageal hernia repair, a challenging operation: medium-term outcome of 116 patients. Journal of Gastrointestinal Surgery: Official Journal of the Society for Surgery of the Alimentary Tract. 2003;7(1):59–66. discussion 66-57.
10. Edye M, Salky B, Posner A, Fierer A. Sac excision is essential to adequate laparoscopic repair of paraesophageal hernia. Surg Endosc. 1998;12(10):1259–63.
11. Leeder PC, Smith G, Dehn TC. Laparoscopic management of large paraesophageal hiatal hernia. Surg Endosc. 2003;17(9):1372–5.

12. Watson DI, Davies N, Devitt PG, Jamieson GG. Importance of dissection of the hernial sac in laparoscopic surgery for large hiatal hernias. Arch Surg. 1999;134(10):1069–73.
13. Oelschlager BK, Pellegrini CA. Paraesophageal hernias: open, laparoscopic, or thoracic repair? Chest Surg Clin N Am. 2001;11(3):589–603.
14. Zehetner J, Demeester SR, Ayazi S, et al. Laparoscopic versus open repair of paraesophageal hernia: the second decade. J Am Coll Surg. 2011;212(5):813–20.
15. Oleynikov D, Jolley JM. Paraesophageal hernia. Surg Clin North Am. 2015;95(3):555–65.
16. Galvani CA, Loebl H, Osuchukwu O, Samame J, Apel ME, Ghaderi I. Robotic-assisted Paraesophageal hernia repair: initial experience at a single institution. J Laparoendoscop Advanc Surg Tech Part A. 2016;26(4):290–5.
17. Gehrig T, Mehrabi A, Fischer L, et al. Robotic-assisted paraesophageal hernia repair--a case-control study. Langenbeck's Archives of Surgery/Deutsche Gesellschaft fur Chirurgie. 2013;398(5):691–6.
18. Iqbal A, Kakarlapudi GV, Awad ZT, et al. Assessment of diaphragmatic stressors as risk factors for symptomatic failure of laparoscopic nissen fundoplication. J Gastrointestinal Surgery: Official Journal of the Society for Surgery of the Alimentary Tract. 2006;10(1):12–21.
19. Alicuben ET, Worrell SG, DeMeester SR. Impact of crural relaxing incisions, Collis gastroplasty, and non-cross-linked human dermal mesh crural reinforcement on early hiatal hernia recurrence rates. J Am Coll Surg. 2014;219(5):988–92.
20. Antoniou SA, Antoniou GA, Koch OO, Pointner R, Granderath FA. Lower recurrence rates after mesh-reinforced versus simple hiatal hernia repair: a meta-analysis of randomized trials. Surg Laparosc Endosc Percutan Tech. 2012;22(6):498–502.
21. Antoniou SA, Koch OO, Antoniou GA, Pointner R, Granderath FA. Mesh-reinforced hiatal hernia repair: a review on the effect on postoperative dysphagia and recurrence. Langenbeck's Archives of Surgery/Deutsche Gesellschaft fur Chirurgie. 2012;397(1):19–27.
22. Falk GL. Early hiatal hernia recurrence rates. J Am Coll Surg. 2015;220(5):968.
23. Hashemi M, Peters JH, DeMeester TR, et al. Laparoscopic repair of large type III hiatal hernia: objective followup reveals high recurrence rate. J Am Coll Surg. 2000;190(5):553–60. discussion 560-551.
24. Lidor AO, Steele KE, Stem M, Fleming RM, Schweitzer MA, Marohn MR. Long-term quality of life and risk factors for recurrence after laparoscopic repair of paraesophageal hernia. JAMA Surg. 2015;150(5):424–31.
25. Lidor AO, Kawaji Q, Stem M, et al. Defining recurrence after paraesophageal hernia repair: correlating symptoms and radiographic findings. Surgery. 2013;154(2):171–8.

Transthoracic Hiatal Hernia Repair

20

Paul Linsky and Benjamin Wei

With the widespread acceptance of and access to laparoscopy, the use of a transthoracic approach for repairing a hiatal hernia has become a rare event. Laparoscopic hiatal hernia repair, typically paired with a fundoplication and/or gastropexy, has become the most common method of dealing with this pathology. A NSQIP database retrospective review examined over 8000 patients who had paraesophageal hernia repair from 2005 to 2011; only 2.4% underwent transthoracic repair [1]. However, in certain situations, such as in a patient who has had multiple transabdominal repairs or otherwise has a hostile abdomen, transthoracic hiatal hernia can be an important alternative.

Indications

Any patient with a hiatal hernia or paraesophageal hernia is a candidate for this procedure. A laparoscopic or robotic transabdominal approach, however, is generally the first choice for a first-time or initial reoperative approach given its benefits in terms of recovery time, postoperative pain, and decreased respiratory complications. A transthoracic approach is particularly beneficial for a few subsets of patients. An obvious advantage is seen in the rare case of a patient also requiring treatment of disease of the left chest, whether it involves the lung, esophagus, or chest wall, in which simultaneous transthoracic hiatal hernia repair makes sense. A more common scenario involves a patient who has undergone multiple previous transabdominal

P. Linsky
Department of Surgery, Division of Cardiothoracic Surgery, University of Alabama Birmingham, Birmingham, AL, USA

B. Wei (✉)
Department of Surgery, University of Alabama-Birmingham Medical Center, Birmingham, AL, USA
e-mail: bwei@uab.edu

J. Grams et al. (eds.), *The SAGES Manual of Foregut Surgery*,
https://doi.org/10.1007/978-3-319-96122-4_20

hernia repair operations or multiple abdominal operations. Operating in a virgin field may reduce the chance of intraoperative complications related to accessing the abdominal cavity and the hernia itself. Prior transthoracic hiatal hernia repair also may predispose a patient to requiring a repeat transthoracic approach; that said, we often approach these patients through the abdomen and employ VATS or thoracotomy only if intrathoracic adhesions prevent the hernia from being reduced.

The answer to the question of whether to operate on all large paraesophageal hernias remains elusive. Conventional thinking dictates repair for any patient found to have one in order to eliminate the risk of strangulation. Others believe that the risk of needing emergency surgery for a paraesophageal hernia is low, at closer to 10–15% over a patient's lifetime, or around 1.1% per year [2, 3]. Therefore, some feel that asymptomatic patients can be managed conservatively, especially patients at higher operative risk. Generally speaking, however, paraesophageal hernia repair should be offered to *symptomatic* patients if their operative risk is acceptable. Symptoms of paraesophageal hernia include postprandial abdominal or chest pain, dysphagia, dyspnea, regurgitation, postprandial vomiting, GERD, and early satiety.

Preoperative Evaluation

As for any operation, a complete history and focused physical exam should be performed on all patients. Patients should be asked about the symptoms noted above. Anemia can also be a manifestation of paraesophageal hernia, as it can arise from the chronic low-grade loss of blood from gastric ulcers/erosions and gastritis in the incarcerated stomach. On the other hand, the clinician should not always assume that respiratory and gastrointestinal issues are automatically related to the hernia. A thorough assessment of the patient's cardiopulmonary and gastrointestinal issues with any relevant testing should be done. Specifically, the preoperative evaluation for a transthoracic hiatal hernia is the same as for a transabdominal approach. It consists of obtaining a barium or gastrografin swallow study to assess anatomy. Upper endoscopy can be employed but more often is performed on the day of surgery to detect the rare concomitant esophageal or gastric pathology that would dictate a different strategy. Manometry can be attempted but is often unsuccessful for patients with large paraesophageal hernias. Similarly, pH study is often difficult due to technical reasons. In addition, the conduct of the operation in our experience is unlikely to change based on results from this testing. A CT scan of the chest and abdomen is not mandatory but helpful for determining what organs are herniated into the chest and revealing any other intra-abdominal or intrathoracic abnormality that needs to be considered. Infrequently, a patient with an elevated hemidiaphragm due to eventration or paralysis can be confused with a large paraesophageal hernia; generally, however, the history of the patient can reveal the culprit injury in cases of diaphragmatic paralysis. Fluoroscopy with the patient sniffing or inspiring should detect paradoxical motion of the hemidiaphragm in these cases. In addition, close attention to the CT scan should be paid; a thin section of diaphragm may be visible and allow for differentiation between a massive paraesophageal hernia and elevated hemidiaphragm.

Pulmonary function should be assessed; many patients will describe dyspnea as a symptom of their hernia, and it is helpful to know how impaired their lungs are and if they have any coexisting pulmonary disease that would make recovery from a thoracotomy more difficult. This also serves as a baseline to which postoperative values can be compared. Consideration to having a workup for myocardial ischemia in higher-risk patients should be given.

Technique

The technique described is for the open transthoracic hiatal hernia repair. Few case reports of completely thoracoscopic hiatal hernia repair exist [4, 5]. A double-lumen endotracheal tube is placed at the time of intubation. An esophagoscope can be inserted in order to act as a stent preventing the hiatal repair from being too tight, although the surgeon should recognize that an adult endoscope is equivalent only to an approximately 36 Fr bougie (standard bougie size for this purpose is 51–54 Fr). The patient is positioned in right lateral decubitus. A left posterolateral thoracotomy is performed. The chest is typically entered through the sixth or seventh interspace. The left lung must be mobilized superiorly to provide adequate exposure to the hiatus. Therefore, the inferior pulmonary ligament is incised to the level of the inferior pulmonary vein. Next, the mediastinal pleura is incised and the pleura overlying the esophagus is opened. Adequate mobilization is then performed by mobilizing the esophagus from the carina to the diaphragm. The hernia sac is then dissected off the esophagus and mobilized so that it can be reduced through hiatal defect. This generally requires circumferential freeing of the sac from the edge of the hiatal defect. Occasionally short gastric vessels require division in order to fully reduce the stomach. The diaphragmatic hiatus can be purposefully enlarged during the process of mobilizing and reducing the hernia to facilitate this process. The fundus of the stomach is restored to its normal anatomic position; the crural approximation sutures are placed, but not tied. During mobilization of the anterior esophageal fat pad, the vagus nerves need to be identified and protected. Mobilization of the fat pad enables identification of GEJ to determine if there is appropriate intra-abdominal esophageal length. Additionally, the dissection not only allows for identification of the anterior vagus but also creates better adhesion of the stomach to the future fundoplication. If the patient has a shortened esophagus, a Collis gastroplasty can be performed at this time. If performing this, consideration should be given to replacing the esophagoscope with a 54 Fr bougie to avoid narrowing. Gastroplasty is accomplished by using a GIA stapler and stapling into the stomach, parallel to the esophagus near the cardia of the stomach.

After this is completed, both crura are identified. It is critical to identify clearly the right crus of the diaphragm, which can be difficult to see as it is located at the bottom of the surgical field; a Babcock or Allis clamp can be used to grasp the crus and ensure that solid tissue is available for suturing. Once all of the anatomy is delineated, the crural sutures may be placed. Crural sutures are usually needed both posterior and anterior to the esophagus and left untied for now. The use of laparotomy pads or surgical towels to keep the abdominal contents in place during this part of the operation can be helpful. Sutures to reapproximate the cut edges of any diaphragm that was divided to help reduce the hernia can be placed and tied.

We typically perform a Belsey Mark IV fundoplication [6]. This fundoplication is a partial wrap of 270 degrees made with two rows of three horizontal mattressed, 2–0 or 3–0 braided polyester or silk sutures (Fig. 20.1). The sutures should be placed in the seromuscular layer (or to be accurate, in the adventitial and muscular layers of the esophagus and seromuscular layer of the stomach), but deep enough to bring the fundus to the esophagus without tension or tearing. If a staple line is present from the gastroplasty, the middle suture of each row should straddle it. The other sutures of each row are therefore 135 degrees left and right of the middle suture. The

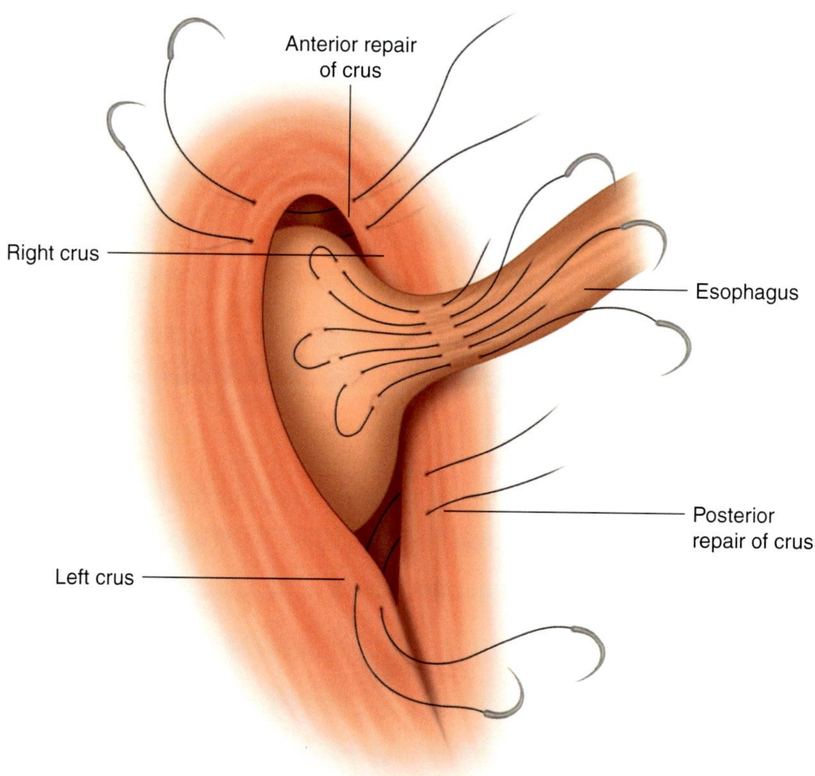

Fig. 20.1 (**a**) First row of horizontal mattress sutures for Belsey Mark IV fundoplication during transthoracic hiatal hernia repair. (**b**) Second row of horizontal mattress sutures (transdiaphragmatic) for Belsey Mark IV fundoplication

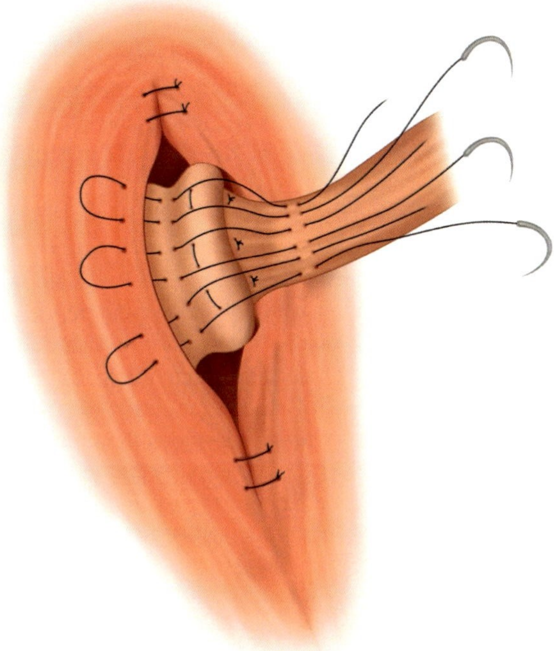

Fig. 20.1 (continued)

next row is spaced 1–1.5 cm from the fold created by tying down the sutures in the previous row. This row of sutures is placed into the diaphragm as well, to secure the repair to it. After the esophageal and gastric "bites" are taken, the needle is then passed through the diaphragm about 1 centimeter from the edge, from inferior to the diaphragm to superior so that the knot is tied on the thoracic side of the repair. These should follow in the orientation of the previous rows and respect the 270-degree spacing of the fundoplication. The GEJ and the fundoplication are translocated into the abdomen when these sutures are tied.

A Nissen fundoplication can be performed through a thoracotomy as well; for obvious reasons, this requires somewhat greater mobilization of the fundus than a Belsey fundoplication.

At this point, the crural sutures are then tied, reapproximating the hiatus. When tied, the reconstructed hiatus should open enough to slide a finger next to and past the esophagus.

A chest tube should be placed in the left chest and the thoracotomy closed in the usual fashion.

Postoperative Care

Immediately postoperatively, two key patient factors must be assessed and controlled. These are patient nausea and gastric distension. Both directly affect the tension and stress placed on the newly reconstructed hiatus and constructed fundoplication. Scheduled antiemetics should be considered given the recent gastric surgery and possible emetogenic effects of anesthetics and analgesics. We do not routinely place a nasogastric tube. However, if significant distention is visible on postoperative radiograph, placement can be considered.

Pain control is critical following thoracotomy. Modalities to control pain should be escalated if necessary. Patient-controlled intravenous analgesia is often, but not always, necessary. Certain institutions may prefer preoperative placement of an epidural catheter, paravertebral catheter or nerve block, or long-acting liposomal bupivacaine nerve block. Non-narcotic measures such as nonsteroidal anti-inflammatory drugs, acetaminophen, lidocaine patches, and muscle relaxants should also be utilized in order to decrease the amount of narcotic required and thereby reduce the adverse side effects of their administration. Intravenous fluids should be minimized given that they appear to increase the risk of pulmonary complications. Any of these outcomes could prolong recovery. The head of the patient's bed is best to be elevated to 30 degrees. This should assist in reducing edema, helping pulmonary function, and draining any fluid in the chest. Chest tube management can be left to the surgeon's preference, but we recommend obtaining a chest x-ray to ensure proper re-expansion of the lung and proper position of the chest tube and nasogastric tube, if employed. Patients can take sips of liquid the afternoon/evening of surgery but should be instructed to seek assistance if there is any urge to retch or vomit.

On postoperative day 1, the patient should be instructed and encouraged to be out of bed and ambulate as much as he or she can tolerate. An esophagram is generally obtained to both check for perforation and to establish a baseline with regard to the radiographic appearance of the esophagogastric junction and wrap. Some postoperative edema, manifested by slow transit of contrast through the fundoplication, is to be expected. If it had been placed, the nasogastric tube can usually be removed. Chest tube removal should follow usual parameters in terms of absence of air leak and reasonable daily output (up to 400–500 cc per day) and full re-expansion of the lung with minimal to no pneumothorax. Deep vein thrombosis prophylaxis should be used (and should have been initiated prior to general anesthesia).

The appropriate progression of the diet is always a question following any alimentary surgery, and the transthoracic hiatal hernia repair is no different. Delayed gastric emptying should always be on the mind of the surgeon. Even the patient tolerating clear liquids may not be able to advance to regular or soft diet quickly. A postoperative ileus is not uncommon following transthoracic hiatal hernia repair. Conservative management would wait for the patient to have evidence of return of bowel function in the form of flatus prior to advancing past clears. This pace may be too slow for some. Each surgeon should prepare their own algorithm to advance the patient's diet. We generally only advance to a soft diet while in the hospital. Patients may be discharged when the chest tube has been removed, tolerating a reasonable diet, and pain control managed with oral medications alone. Proton-pump inhibitors or other GERD medications are generally continued in the acute setting and may be discontinued later if the patient is able.

At discharge, instructions to the patient include remaining on a soft diet for 2–3 weeks and to chew food very thoroughly prior to swallowing. As with any post-operative patients, activity and weight lifting restrictions do apply. An increase in intra-abdominal pressure could result in injury to the repair and recurrence, as well as pose a risk of incisional hernia and bowel obstruction. Follow-up is scheduled within 2–4 weeks. A repeat esophagram at that visit is unnecessary.

Postoperative Complications

The complications of this operation are a combination of the typical complications seen in hiatal and paraesophageal surgery and thoracic surgery. The use of a thoracotomy does cause increased pain, especially in comparison with laparoscopic approaches. Atrial fibrillation is a risk following thoracotomy but is controlled with rate and/or rhythm control and is usually self-limited. Pneumonia can occur; post-operative pulmonary toilet and early ambulation are used to prevent this complication, which is managed with antibiotics. If significant adhesions between the hernia and the lung were lysed, an air leak may be present; this typically resolves with observation alone. Chest tube output tends to be higher following thoracotomy than VATS. Bleeding requiring transfusion and/or reoperation is, and should be, quite rare. Short gastric arteries can be susceptible to delayed bleeding. Additionally, Belsey described the presence of a communicating artery that connects the inferior phrenic artery to the left gastric artery. It is typically in a thick tissue band that must be divided to properly mobilize the stomach from the hiatus. As with any surgery, scrupulous detail to hemostasis must be performed. Additionally, Orringer reported bleeding from shallow ulcers after this operation [7]. These were formed proximal to strictures and resulted from erosive esophagitis. Management, as with any upper gastrointestinal bleeds, involves endoscopy to assess and possibly control the bleeding, blood transfusion if the patient is unstable, and intravenous antacid therapy. In Orringer's series, no surgery was required, and only PPI or H2 blockers were needed [7].

Dysphagia is the most common complication in both immediate and delayed postoperative period. Initially, this is due to edema at the surgical site and resolves with time and patience. Prolonged dysphagia is often due to stricture of the distal esophagus. This stricture is often present at the time of the operation and can be the result of overtightening of the hiatus. Often, a single dilation with a balloon or bougie is all that is necessary to improve the patient's swallowing. In a few patients, repeated dilatations may be needed.

Leak can occur either in the esophagus or the stomach. For the esophagus and sometimes the proximal esophagus, a contrast exam is helpful. An uncontained leak in the esophagus may benefit from stent placement, while a contained leak typically can be managed without it. The leak should be reassessed in 3–4 weeks; if healed, oral nutrition should be initiated. Reoperative thoracotomy should be considered if stenting is unsuccessful. If a gastroplasty is performed or if considerable amount of tension is placed on the repair due to inadequate mobilization or retching or gastric distension, the stomach can leak. With a stapled gastroplasty, inadequate tissue compression or overdistension prior to healing can be the cause. Any patient with unexplained tachycardia or signs of sepsis should be evaluated for a leak. Many patients can be treated nonoperatively by making the patient NPO and starting intravenous antibiotics. Some form of nutrition should be instituted, whether enterally via a feeding tube of some kind or parenterally. Clinical deterioration or peritonitis should provide the impetus for operative reexploration and repair, typically through a transabdominal route in cases of suspected gastric perforation. Alternatively, the hiatal hernia repair can be taken down and the stomach examined through the chest.

With mobilization of the esophagus from the arch to the diaphragm and dissection at the gastroesophageal junction, permanent or temporary injury to one or both vagus nerves can result in delayed gastric emptying, or gastroparesis. This is manifested by nausea/vomiting and inability to tolerate oral intake after surgery, sometimes accompanied by bloating and/or abdominal pain. A distinction should be drawn between stricture and gastroparesis given their differing treatments; esophagram and gastric emptying study can be helpful for diagnosis. As transthoracic hiatal hernia repair often tends to be performed in the context of prior operations on the esophagogastric junction, delayed gastric emptying is not uncommon. If delayed gastric emptying is suspected in the preoperative setting, a gastric emptying study should be performed in order to confirm that this is a pre-existing problem. Promotility agents often relieve the symptoms of gastroparesis. Placement of gastric pacemakers and pyloroplasty are more extreme options for gastroparesis not responding to medical therapy.

Recurrence of the hernia after repair, whether transthoracic or otherwise, can occur. A distinction, however, should be drawn between recurrences that are clinically relevant and warrant reoperation and recurrences that are only radiologic in nature and asymptomatic or minimally symptomatic. Patients do not tolerate well a fundoplication that has herniated into the chest but remains intact. If significant dysphagia, regurgitation, or vomiting occurs, reoperative repair should be contemplated. Early dehiscence of the repair and recurrence of the hernia can occur acutely in the setting of postoperative retching/vomiting; reoperation should be offered in this situation.

Postoperative Outcomes

Few large series of transthoracic hiatal hernia repairs exist. The transthoracic approach comprised only 2.4% of all repairs performed from 2005 to 2011 in the NSQIP database [1]. The vast majority of patients in that review underwent laparoscopic repair (78.4%). The open transabdominal approach was less prevalent but still almost ten times more common than the transthoracic approach (19.2%). In that study, the mortality of the transthoracic approach was more than laparoscopic, 1.5% vs. 0.5%, but less than the open transabdominal approach (2.6%). Length of stay was twice as long compared to the laparoscopic approach. However, patients were sicker and more likely to have CHF and COPD. After adjustment for age, ASA, emergency cases, functional status, and steroid use, the transthoracic approach still had increased odds of overall and serious morbidity compared to laparoscopic repair (OR 2.73 and OR 2.49 respectively, $p < 0.001$).

Long-term outcomes over a 20-year period were reported from Emory University in 1997 [8]. They reported 276 patients that underwent the Belsey Mark IV fundoplication. It should be noted that only 9.7% of these patients were noted to have a paraesophageal hernia. The overall perioperative morbidity and mortality rates were low, at 10.1% and 0.4%, respectively. Early reoperation (0.7%), leak (0.7%), stricture (0.4%), and other major complications were all rare. Late reoperations occurred in eight patients. Dysphagia was absent or only occasional in 79%; 6% required intervention for dysphagia. GERD symptoms were absent or occasional in 84% of patients.

In 2004, the University of Michigan published their 25-year experience of 240 patients undergoing transthoracic repair for paraesophageal hiatal hernia [9]. Of these, 96% underwent a combined Collis-Nissen operation in 96%, Nissen fundoplication in 3%, and a Belsey Mark IV in 1 patient. The investigators reported a 1.7% perioperative death rate, median length of hospital stay of 7 days, and early reoperation in 5% of patients. Median follow-up was 27.8 months, and "satisfactory" results by patient report were achieved in 85%. Of 153 patients who underwent routine pre-discharge postoperative esophagram, 77% had satisfactory postoperative appearance, with 17% having delayed esophageal emptying and 5% with esophageal dysmotility. Four patients had early anatomic recurrences that were all reoperated on. A liberal policy of dilational therapy led to 31% undergoing dilation for dysphagia after surgery, but only 8% received more than one dilation. Late postoperatively, only six patients required further surgery (four for recurrent herniation, two for esophagectomy due to stenosis at the GE junction). Of 45 patients who had both preoperative and postoperative pH testing, 88% had preoperative abnormal reflux compared to 4% postoperatively. Dysmotility also decreased postoperatively, from 27% preoperative to 7% postoperative.

Taylor et al. have demonstrated that reoperative transthoracic hiatal hernia repair can also be done safely [10]. Major postoperative complications occurred in only 12% of their overall group of 65 patients (42 patients in initial group, 23 patients in reoperative group). In-hospital mortality occurred in only one patient (initial repair). Reoperative transthoracic hiatal hernia repair was associated with higher postoperative symptomatic bloating and dysphagia scores and less improvement in GERD-related quality of life scores compared to initial repair. Overall quality of life scores, however, were similar.

Conclusion

Although a minimally invasive transabdominal approach is now the preferred initial approach to paraesophageal hernia due to decreased perioperative morbidity, transthoracic hiatal hernia repair is a useful operation for certain patients. The few reports that exist come from large, specialized centers but demonstrate very good short-term results and long-term freedom from reoperation, reflux, and dysphagia.

References

1. Mungo B, Molena D, Stem M, et al. Thirty-day outcomes of paraesophageal hernia repair using the NSQIP database: should laparoscopy be the standard of care? J Am Coll Surg. 2014;219:229–36.
2. Stylopoulos N, Gazelle GS, Rattner DW. Paraesophageal hernias: operation or observations? Ann Surg. 2002;236:492–501.
3. Sihvo EI, Salo JA, Rasanene JV, Rantanen TK. Fatal complications of adult paraesophageal hernia: a population-based study. J Thorac Cardiovasc Surg. 2009;137:419–24.
4. Hurley JP, McCarthy JF, Wood AE. Thoracoscopic assisted paraesophageal hernia repair. Scand J Thorac Cardiovasc Surg. 1994;28:94–6.
5. Sartotelli KH, Rothenberg SS, Karrer FM, Lilly JR. Thoracoscopic repair of hiatal hernia following fundoplication: a new approach to an old problem. J Laparoendosc Surg. 1996;6 Suppl 1:S91–3.
6. Belsey R. Mark IV repair of hiatal hernia by the transthoracic approach. World J Surg. 1977;1:475–81.
7. Orringer MB, Sloan H. Complications and failings of the combined Collis-Belsey operation. J Thorac Cardiovasc Surg. 1977;74:726–35.
8. Fenton KN, Miller JI, Lee RB, Mansour KA. Belsey Mark IV antireflux procedure for complicated gastroesophageal reflux disease. Ann Thorac Surg. 1997;64:790–4.
9. Patel HJ, Tan BB, Yee J, et al. A 25-year experience with open primary transthoracic repair of paraesophageal hiatal hernia. J Thorac Cardiovasc Surg. 2004;127:843–9.
10. Taylor MD, Nagji AS, Kozower BD, et al. Quality of life following primary vs. redo transthoracic paraesophageal hernia repairs. Int Cardiovasc Thorac Surg. 2007;7:71–4.

21 Esophageal Lengthening Procedures

Monisha Sudarshan and Shanda Haley Blackmon

The concept of acquired short esophagus is possibly one of the most controversial aspects in surgery for benign esophageal disease. Many experienced surgeons challenge the existence of this condition [1, 2], whereas others attest to the importance of its recognition and treatment to optimize surgical outcomes. Regardless, esophageal lengthening procedures are useful techniques in the armamentarium of an upper GI surgeon and are the focus of this chapter.

Incidence and Pathophysiology

The incidence of shortened esophagus is challenging to ascertain due to a lack of uniform definition with a wide variation in the surgical literature. Recent studies at high-volume centers identify rates between 0% and 18% [3–5] depending on the need for extensive mediastinal dissection and Collis gastroplasty. Pathophysiology of a foreshortened esophagus is multifactorial and attributed to chronic inflammation in the setting of GERD. A lax lower esophageal sphincter results in refluxed gastric juices with edema and inflammation seeping from the mucosa into the esophageal wall. Chronicity of this insult causes transmural inflammation and longitudinal fibrosis and is presumed to be the cause of a shorter esophagus [6, 7].

Treating a short esophagus or intra-abdominal esophageal length of <2.5 cm is imperative to ensure decreased tension of the wrap, prevent wrap failure, and avoid recurrence. Of particular importance is the higher failure rates noted for giant para-esophageal hernias where a lengthening procedure will be of benefit [8].

M. Sudarshan · S. H. Blackmon (✉)
Department of Thoracic Surgery, Mayo Clinic, Rochester, MN, USA
e-mail: Blackmon.shanda@mayo.edu

J. Grams et al. (eds.), *The SAGES Manual of Foregut Surgery*,
https://doi.org/10.1007/978-3-319-96122-4_21

Preoperative Prediction of the Short Esophagus

No single preoperative test is adequate to predict the need for esophageal lengthening maneuvers, although a patient with a giant paraesophageal hernia that has been present for more than 30 years with severe reflux is certainly a warning sign. The usual battery of preoperative tests for GERD patients includes upper endoscopy, pH study, manometry, and an upper GI contrast esophagogram (Fig. 21.1). Some studies suggested that presence of long segment (>5 cm) nonreducible type I hernia or a type III hernia on esophagogram were predictive of a short esophagus [9]; however other investigations have yielded a positive predictive value of only 50% for barium esophagograms [6]. Esophageal length on manometry is useful if found to be below

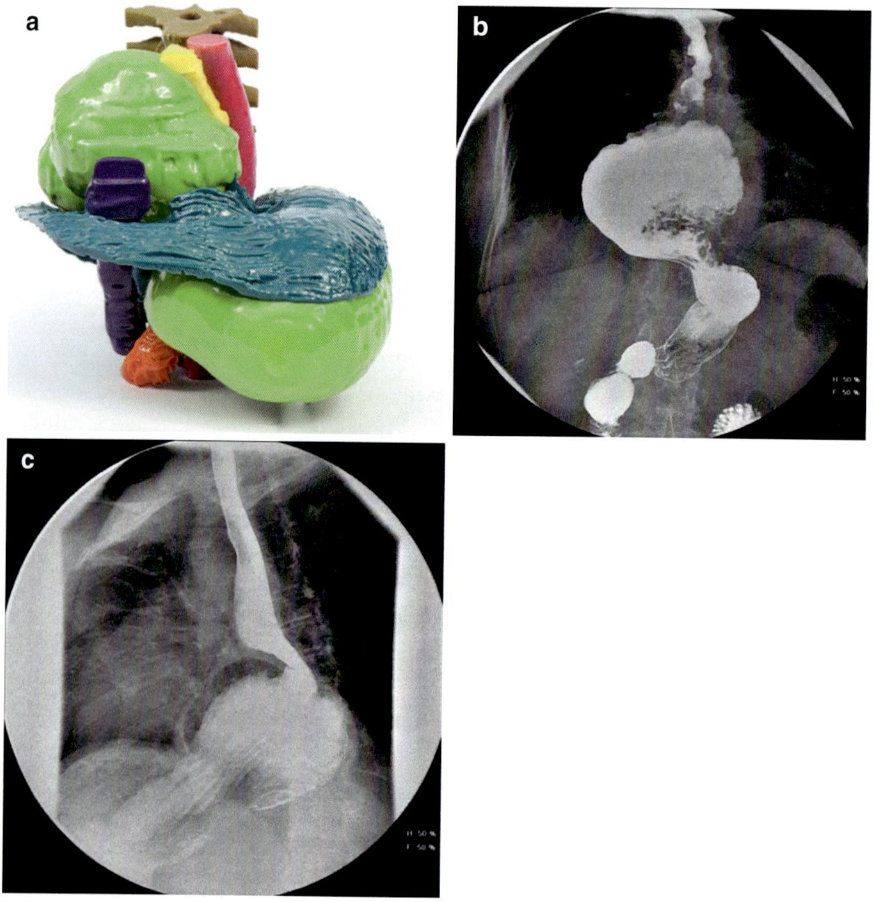

Fig. 21.1 (**a**) 3-D model of a giant paraesophageal hernia. (**b**, **c**) Preoperative esophagograms demonstrating giant paraesophageal hernias in patients with long-standing reflux. Both patients required a modified Collis wedge gastroplasty

Table 21.1 Predictive factors for an esophageal lengthening procedure

Long history of GERD (>30 years)
Failed reflux operation
Presence of a stricture >1 cm
Type III and IV hernia
Esophageal length < 5th percentile on manometry
Esophageal length index <19.5 on endoscopy

Esophageal length index: esophageal length (cm)/patients' height (meters)
GERD gastroesophageal reflux disease

the 5th percentile, but absolute values are difficult to interpret due to variation according to body habitus [10].

Endoscopic measurements of esophageal length, when corrected for height, have been used for prediction. The esophageal length index (ELI) is the ratio of esophageal length (cm) to the patient's height (meters) with an ELI of 19.5 or less having a positive predictive value of 81% and a negative predictive value of 83% [11]. The use of information from all tests conducted preoperatively will aid in prognostication of a lengthening procedure; however definite assessment takes place intraoperatively (Table 21.1).

Intraoperative Evaluation for Conducting a Lengthening Procedure

Prior to determining esophageal length, any intrathoracic stomach must be completely reduced along with removal of the hernia sac. Classification of circumferential mediastinal mobilization of the esophagus is labeled as type I if the length is less than 5 cm and type II when it is between 5 and 10 cm [6]. The vagus nerves must be identified and preserved during this mobilization in order to prevent delayed gastric emptying postoperatively. After a type I mobilization is completed, the gastroesophageal fat pad is dissected medially, and any tubes in the esophagus are withdrawn. Starting from the left side of the patient, the gastroesophageal fat pad is removed sparing the vagus to reveal the esophagogastric junction. The very best way to identify this is in conjunction with intraoperative endoscopy and transillumination of the esophagogastric junction (top of the rugal folds). One must be aware not to merely identify the squamocolumnar junction, as many of these patients may have Barrett's esophagus, and this line may be falsely high above the esophagogastric junction. Intra-abdominal esophageal length can be estimated by measuring the distance from the hiatus to the gastroesophageal junction without utilizing any instruments to pull down on the esophagus during the measurement with an aim of 2.5 cm to ensure minimal tension on the fundoplication. If the intra-abdominal length is suboptimal, further mediastinal dissection of up to 10 cm (type II mobilization) should be completed for mobilization. Some authors have identified the carina [12] or the inferior pulmonary veins [13] as their upper limit. Extensive mediastinal dissection

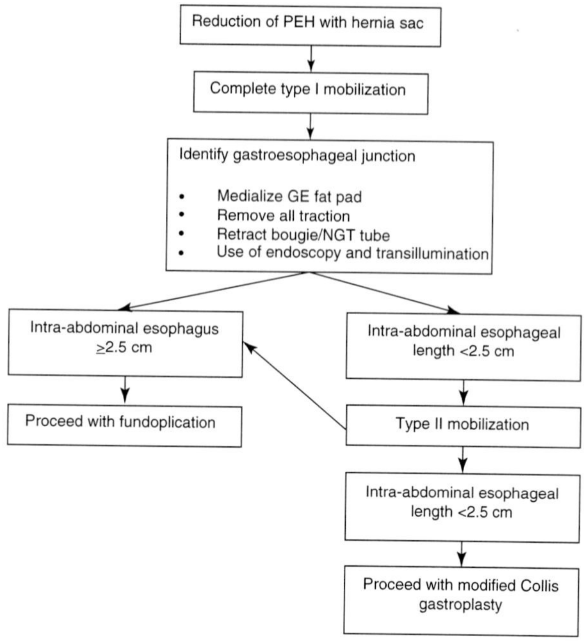

Fig. 21.2 Intraoperative decision-making algorithm

generally yields an adequate intra-abdominal length [14]; however, if this is still insufficient, modified Collis gastroplasty techniques will be required to decrease tension (Fig. 21.2) and reduce recurrence.

Techniques for Esophageal Lengthening

The original Collis gastroplasty described in 1957 was performed through a thoracoabdominal incision [15]. With the progress of minimally invasive techniques, currently the modified Collis wedge gastroplasty is completed laparoscopically, often using the same port placement required for the fundoplication. Our standard port placement is a 5 mm epigastric port for a Nathanson liver retractor, two surgeon ports in the right midclavicular (5 mm) and left subcostal (10 mm) region, a supra-umbilical camera port (10 mm), and a midaxillary assistant port (5 mm).

The left subcostal operator port is upsized to a 12 mm port and a 50F bougie is inserted. The surgeon retracts the stomach just beyond the angle of His using the right operator port, and the assistant applies downward traction near the first short gastric artery in order to fan out the stomach in preparation for a wedge gastroplasty. A reticulating endoscopic stapler is introduced through the left subcostal port and fired at a 45-degree angle aiming for 3 cm below the GEJ and abutting the bougie. Usually two to three firings of the linear stapler may be required (Fig. 21.3). Then, a vertical firing of the staple parallel to the bougie results in completion of the

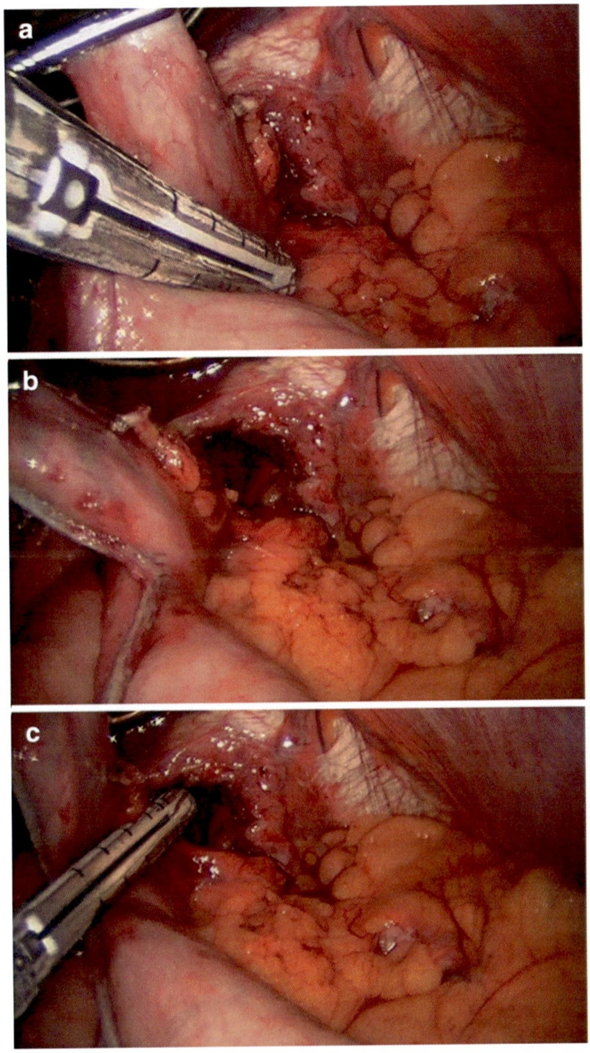

Fig. 21.3 Construction of the modified Collis wedge gastroplasty. (**a**) First staple fire at 45 degrees with bougie in place. (**b**) and (**c**) Second staple fire parallel to the esophagus completing the wedge gastroplasty

wedge. A fundoplication can be completed in the usual manner for a wrap fashioned around this neo-esophagus with the bougie still in place. The wrap should ideally cover the staple line, and it is not typically necessary to oversew the staple line. Of note, performing a lengthening procedure on a stomach with ischemic changes such as patients with volvulus is highly discouraged due to increased risk of leak.

Important aspects to consider when performing the wedge gastroplasty include avoiding a 90-degree angle with the stapler which inadvertently removes a larger portion of the fundus, leaving the same length gained on the esophagus but a smaller portion of fundus to perform the wrap. The use of a bougie is imperative to avoid stenosis of the neo-esophagus.

A modified Collis gastroplasty can be performed with a Nissen and Toupet [16] and less often with a Dor [17] fundoplication. Type of fundoplication will be dictated by the preoperative esophageal motility studies and factors including scleroderma, diffuse esophageal spasm, and achalasia.

Slight variations to the modified Collis gastroplasty are published in the current literature with good outcomes. Wilson and colleagues [18] describe their approach consisting of a single fire of the endoscopic stapler parallel to the bougie through a single left anterior axillary line intercostal space incision after completing all the usual steps laparoscopically. The group describes obviating the need for a wedge fundectomy and crossing staple lines with this technique.

Postoperative Management

A nasogastric tube is inserted intraoperatively, and postoperative nausea is carefully controlled to avoid retching or vomiting which strains the wrap. We selectively perform barium swallow on postoperative day 1, and if no leak is confirmed, the nasogastric tube is removed, and the patient resumes a clear fluid diet. Gradual progression to a soft fundoplication diet is advised and discharged is planned typically on POD 1. Occasionally esophagograms performed after Collis gastroplasty may be misinterpreted as recurrence due to the presence of rugal folds above the wrap, and caution must be exercised when reading these images.

Review of Outcomes

Prevention of staple line leak is a foremost priority after a modified Collis procedure. In recent series, the incidence for wedge gastroplasty does not demonstrate any significant increased leak risk in comparison with a fundoplication-only cohort [19, 20].

Furthermore, since the neo-esophagus lacks motility, worsened dysphagia is another concern for these patients. Studies have demonstrated a slightly higher rate of dysphagia in comparison with fundoplication-only patients; however these have not been statistically significant. Furthermore, when comparing pre- and postoperative dysphagia symptoms, consistent improvement in the modified Collis cohort has been noted [19].

Due to an aperistaltic segment and wrap around the mucosa that can still produce acid, increased reflux is another postoperative issue to consider. Studies have confirmed a longer acid clearance time in patient with a Collis gastroplasty in comparison with a fundoplication-only group [21]. However, reflux symptoms and use of anti-reflux medication have demonstrated to be comparable in the two groups [19].

Recurrence rates or wrap failure after a Collis gastroplasty ranges between 0% and 18% in a recent review of current literature [22]. It is difficult to compare recurrence rates as patients are not followed routinely with imaging, and the definition of recurrence differs among studies (radiologic vs. clinical). In a few studies, wrap failure and recurrence for giant paraesophageal hernias (where a Collis gastroplasty is now often employed) who received only a fundoplication were between 32% and 42% [23–25]. Therefore, this suggests a trend of improved outcomes with the modified Collis procedure.

Summary

A key to the success of the reflux operation and paraesophageal hernia repair is a tension-free intra-abdominal wrap. Esophageal lengthening procedures are required when there is a less than 2.5 cm of intra-abdominal esophagus. Conditions often associated with this include chronic GERD, giant hernia, and presence of a stricture; however, ultimately the need for a Collis gastroplasty can only be determined intraoperatively. Type II mobilization of the esophagus is critical to gaining length in addition to careful determination of the gastroesophageal junction. The modified Collis gastroplasty holds the potential to decrease recurrence and wrap failure in the properly selected patient population. It is associated with minimal morbidity with most studies demonstrating equivalent quality of life outcomes in comparison with fundoplication-only cohorts.

References

1. Madan AK, Frantzides CT, Patsavas KL. The myth of the short esophagus. Surg Endosc. 2004;18(1):31–4.
2. Korn O, Csendes A, Burdiles P, Braghetto I, Sagastume H, Biagini L. Length of the esophagus in patients with gastroesophageal reflux disease and Barrett's esophagus compared to controls. Surgery. 2003;133(4):358–63.
3. Swanstrom LL, Marcus DR, Galloway GQ. Laparoscopic Collis gastroplasty is the treatment of choice for the shortened esophagus. Am J Surg. 1996;171(5):477–81.
4. Awad ZT, Mittal SK, Roth TA, Anderson PI, Wilfley WA Jr, Filipi CJ. Esophageal shortening during the era of laparoscopic surgery. World J Surg. 2001;25(5):558–61.
5. O'Rourke RW, Khajanchee YS, Urbach DR, Lee NN, Lockhart B, Hansen PD, Swanstrom LL. Extended transmediastinal dissection: an alternative to gastroplasty for short esophagus. Arch Surg. 2003;138(7):735–40.
6. Horvath KD, Swanstrom LL, Jobe BA. The short esophagus: pathophysiology, incidence, presentation, and treatment in the era of laparoscopic antireflux surgery. Ann Surg. 2000;232(5):630–40.
7. Gozzetti G, Pilotti V, Spangaro M, Bassi F, Grigioni W, Carulli N, Loria P, Felice V, Lerro F, Mattioli S. Pathophysiology and natural history of acquired short esophagus. Surgery. 1987;102(3):507–14.
8. Terry ML, Vernon A, Hunter JG. Stapled-wedge Collis gastroplasty for the shortened esophagus. Am J Surg. 2004;188(2):195–9.
9. Bremner RM, Bremner CG, Peters JH. Fundamentals of antireflux surgery. In: Peters JH, DeMeester TR, editors. Minimally invasive surgery of the foregut. 1st ed. St Louis: Quality Medical Publishing; 1994. p. 119–243.
10. Gastal OL, Hagen JA, Peters JH, Campos GM, Hashemi M, Theisen J, Bremner CG, DeMeester TR. Short esophagus: analysis of predictors and clinical implications. Arch Surg. 1999;134(6):633–6.

11. Yano F, Stadlhuber RJ, Tsuboi K, Garg N, Filipi CJ, Mittal SK. Preoperative predictability of the short esophagus: endoscopic criteria. Surg Endosc. 2009;23(6):1308–12.
12. Swanstrom LL, Hansen P. Laparoscopic total esophagectomy. Arch Surg. 1997;132(9): 943–7.
13. DeMeester SR. Laparoscopic paraesophageal hernia repair: critical steps and adjunct techniques to minimize recurrence. Surg Laparosc Endosc Percutan Tech. 2013;23(5): 429–35.
14. Bochkarev V, Lee YK, Vitamvas M, Oleynikov D. Short esophagus: how much length can we get? Surg Endosc. 2008;22(10):2123–7.
15. Collis JL. An operation for hiatus hernia with short oesophagus. Thorax. 1957;12(3): 181–8.
16. J Z, DeMeester SR, Ayazi S, Kilday P, Alicuben ET, DeMeester TR. Laparoscopic wedge fundectomy for collis gastroplasty creation in patients with a foreshortened esophagus. Ann Surg. 2014;260(6):1030–3.
17. Latzko M, Borao F, Squillaro A, Mansson J, Barker W, Baker T. Laparoscopic repair of paraesophageal hernias. JSLS. 2014;18(3):e2014.00009.
18. Wilson JL, Bradley DD, Louie BE, Aye RW, Vallières E, Farivar AS. Laparoscopy with left chest collis gastroplasty: a simplified technique for shortened esophagus. Ann Thorac Surg. 2014;98(5):1860–2.
19. Nason KS, Luketich JD, Awais O, Abbas G, Pennathur A, Landreneau RJ, Schuchert MJ. Quality of life after collis gastroplasty for short esophagus in patients with paraesophageal hernia. Ann Thorac Surg. 2011;92(5):1854–60.
20. Houghton SG, Deschamps C, Cassivi SD, Allen MS, Nichols FC 3rd, Barnes SA, Pairolero PC. Combined transabdominal gastroplasty and fundoplication for shortened esophagus: impact on reflux-related and overall quality of life. Ann Thorac Surg. 2008;85(6): 1947–52.
21. Mor A, Lutfi R, Torquati A. Esophageal acid-clearance physiology is altered after Nissen-Collis gastroplasty. Surg Endosc. 2013;27(4):1334–8.
22. Kunio NR, Dolan JP, Hunter JG. Short esophagus. Surg Clin North Am. 2015;95(3): 641–52.
23. Hashemi M, Peters JH, DeMeester TR, Huprich JE, Quek M, Hagen JA, Crookes PF, Theisen J, DeMeester SR, Sillin LF, Bremner CG. Laparoscopic repair of large type III hiatal hernia: objective followup reveals high recurrence rate. J Am Coll Surg. 2000;190(5):553–60.
24. Khaitan L, Houston H, Sharp K, Holzman M, Richards W. Laparoscopic paraesophageal hernia repair has an acceptable recurrence rate. Am Surg. 2002;68(6):546–51.
25. Jobe BA, Aye RW, Deveney CW, Domreis JS, Hill LD. Laparoscopic management of giant type III hiatal hernia and short esophagus. Objective follow-up at three years. J Gastrointest Surg. 2002;6(2):181–8; discussion 188.

Management of Acute Gastric Volvulus

22

Kathleen Simon and Jon Gould

Introduction

Acute gastric volvulus is a surgical emergency defined as rotation of the stomach greater than 180 degrees, causing foregut luminal obstruction and compromising blood flow to the stomach. Mortality of acute gastric volvulus has historically been as high as 60% with complicated volvulus; however with advances in diagnosis and management to include laparoscopic and endoscopic intervention, the mortality has declined to 15–20% [1, 2]. A high index of suspicion is necessary to ensure a prompt work-up and intervention as the cohort of patients likely to be affected by this phenomenon are elderly patients with concomitant comorbid conditions.

Pathophysiology

Gastric volvulus shows no predilection for gender or race. It is most common in the sixth decade of life although 20–30% occur in children less than 1 year of age. The stomach is held in position by four ligaments: the gastrocolic, gastrohepatic, gastrophrenic, and gastrosplenic ligaments. These ligaments along with the pylorus and gastroesophageal junction aid in fixing the stomach in position that naturally prevents rotation. Primary gastric volvulus is idiopathic abnormal rotation of the stomach greater than 180° and occurs in approximately 30% of individuals to present with volvulus. Primary gastric volvulus includes abnormalities in these fixation points and may occur due to an inherent anatomic characteristic such as congenital abnormalities in fixation [3, 4]. Secondary gastric volvulus is more common, occurring in 60–70% of patients [5]. In this case gastric volvulus may be associated with

K. Simon · J. Gould (✉)
Department of Surgery, Medical College of Wisconsin, Milwaukee, WI, USA
e-mail: jgould@mcw.edu

J. Grams et al. (eds.), *The SAGES Manual of Foregut Surgery*,
https://doi.org/10.1007/978-3-319-96122-4_22

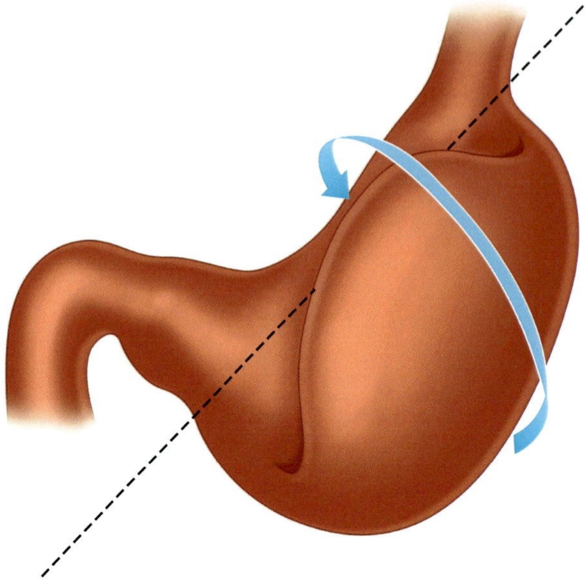

Fig. 22.1 Organoaxial volvulus of the stomach. There is rotation along the long axis of the stomach from the hiatus to the pylorus

disorders of the spleen or diaphragm, including hernias or eventration. A common association is that with paraesophageal hernia [6].

Abnormal rotation of the stomach is described by three different classifications and around two axes of rotation. Organoaxial rotation is that along the axis running from the gastroesophageal junction to the pylorus causing rotation of the greater curve of the stomach superior-medially to the lesser curve (Fig. 22.1). This is the most common axis of rotation and makes up approximately 60% of cases. This type of gastric volvulus is associated with paraesophageal hernias or diaphragmatic abnormalities. Mesenteroaxial volvulus is that within the transverse or short axis of the stomach, where the pylorus is rotated anterior and superior to the gastroesophageal junction (Fig. 22.2). This occurs in approximately 30% of cases. A combination of these two classifications makes up the third and rarest type of gastric volvulus [4, 7, 8]. Differentiating between these types of gastric volvulus may be achieved on preoperative imaging. Mesenteroaxial rotation on abdominal x-ray imaging would appear as an inverted stomach [6].

Acute versus chronic gastric volvulus is a pivotal differentiation as the need and urgency of repair and mortality associated with nonoperative management are vastly different. Acute gastric volvulus is a surgical emergency as ischemia may develop in the gastric wall leading to perforation with or without cardiorespiratory compromise if a hiatal hernia is concurrently present.

Presentation

Patients presenting with gastric volvulus most commonly present with clinical findings secondary to foregut luminal obstruction. Symptoms may be acute or chronic in nature, constant or intermittent. The classic description of a patient with acute

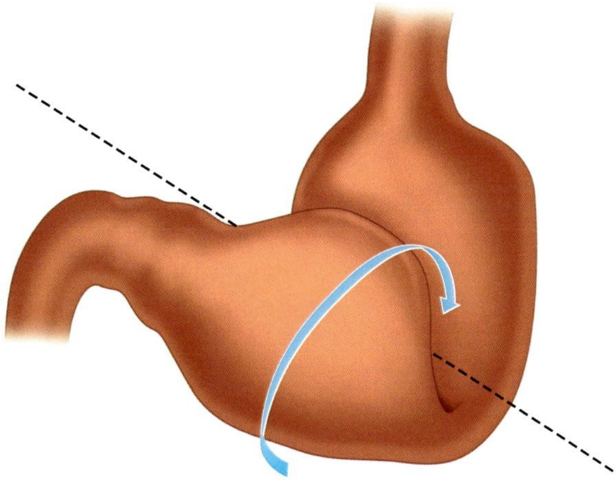

Fig. 22.2 Mesenteroaxial volvulus. There is rotation along the short axis of the stomach transecting the lesser and greater curves

gastric volvulus is described by the eponym Borchardt's triad—epigastric abdominal pain, retching, and inability to pass a nasogastric tube. Less commonly patients may present with hematemesis secondary to gastric ischemia, mucosal sloughing, mucosal tear, or peptic ulcer disease.

Patients in extremis with clinical features consistent with shock may harbor gastric ischemia or perforation. Acute gastric volvulus in conjunction with a paraesophageal hernia is of particular urgency due to its intrathoracic position and risk of cardiopulmonary compromise [7]. Case reports have documented the effects of acute gastric volvulus within the chest leading to cardiac tamponade, respiratory compromise, or mediastinitis with resulting risk of mortality [8].

In contrast, patients with a chronic relapsing gastric volvulus may present with non-specific gastrointestinal symptoms such as nausea and abdominal pain, postprandial bloating, or early satiety [9].

Diagnosis

Several imaging studies can assist in confirming at diagnosis of acute gastric volvulus and assist with operative planning.

A plain film x-ray of the chest may demonstrate a retro-cardiac mass with an air-fluid level. Additional studies to investigate these findings may include an upper endoscopy, upper gastrointestinal (UGI) fluoroscopic exam, or computed tomography (CT) scan.

When patients present with hematemesis, an upper endoscopy is often performed. It has been demonstrated in the literature that endoscopy can be helpful in making the diagnosis of acute gastric volvulus in two thirds of patients and is diagnostic itself in one third of patients [3]. There are several findings on endoscopy that may lead to the diagnosis of acute gastric volvulus including mucosal edema, erosions or ulcerations, and inability to pass through the pylorus. These findings may increase the index of suspicion for acute gastric volvulus and prompt further imaging [5].

A CT scan of the chest and abdomen can be helpful in several ways. Not only does a CT scan provide a confirmation of a diagnosis of gastric volvulus but it also assists in operative planning. Presence of a hiatal hernia or defect in the diaphragm can be evaluated ahead of time as well as the integrity of the gastric wall and presence or absence of threatened or ischemic bowel. Providing a 3D reconstructed view of the gastric vasculature with a CT angiogram can further describe the degree of ischemia and definitively describe the volvulus as acute or chronic [5].

A definitive diagnosis can be achieved by obtaining an UGI. This may demonstrate the site of obstruction, the orientation of the stomach, as well as a pointed or downturned pylorus [10]. In a single institution review of cases, it has been demonstrated that barium studies have been the most helpful in achieving a diagnosis of gastric volvulus [11]. Out of 25 studies performed during their institutional review, 14 were diagnostic of gastric volvulus. Of the remaining 11 studies performed, 7 were suggestive of the diagnosis. This study more than any other imaging study, x-ray, CT scan, or endoscopy, was most beneficial in making the diagnosis.

Management Strategies

Management of an acute gastric volvulus is traditionally a surgical emergency due to the risk of ischemia with resulting increased morbidity and mortality. Prompt initiation of therapy should include decompression of the stomach with a nasogastric tube versus endoscopic decompression. The original description of definitive surgical management of gastric volvulus was described by Tanner et al. in 1964. The methods described follow two main principles: repair any precipitating condition and prevent recurrence [6]. Surgical intervention includes reduction of the volvulized stomach, resection of gastric necrosis if present, and gastropexy.

The procedures described in the early literature for gastric volvulus were performed for both chronic and acute presentations, and all were performed with an open midline laparotomy. Due to the increased prevalence of gastric volvulus in the elderly population, the pendulum had swung to a more conservative approach, especially in those whom the volvulus is suspected to be chronic [12].

Approaching acute gastric volvulus laparoscopically has been demonstrated to be safe and effective, with shorter hospital length of stay compared to those approached open [2, 11]. Standard treatment components include reduction of the volvulized stomach with gastropexy [2]. In patients with gastric volvulus associated with a paraesophageal hernia, the treatment algorithm includes reduction of the hernia, hiatal hernia repair, and fundoplication with or without gastropexy. In high-risk patients with significant comorbidities, operating time can be minimized by limiting the operation to reduction of the volvulus and gastropexy alone. Long-term studies are limited as to the outcome of these patients and recurrence rates without diaphragmatic repair. Likewise, in patients with a high operative risk, authors have described placement of a percutaneous endoscopic gastrostomy tube (PEG) as a means of gastropexy in cases of chronic gastric volvulus although long-term outcomes have not been reported [11, 13]. There have been cases reported in the pediatric literature of recurrent gastric volvulus after gastropexy alone suggesting this may not be a definitive solution [14].

Endoscopic reduction of gastric volvulus has been described most commonly for chronic gastric volvulus although multiple case series have been published suggesting possible utility in acute gastric volvulus as well [15–17]. Endoscopic detorsion is a method used for reduction in order to bridge the patient for an elective repair as it offers no definitive prevention of recurrence. The technique is described as an "alpha loop technique" in which the scope is introduced into the stomach, retroflexed to create an alpha loop, and then by torqueing the endoscope clockwise, the volvulized stomach is reduced [15]. Omata et al. described a case of acute mesenteroaxial gastric volvulus successfully reduced endoscopically allowing the patient to be discharged and undergo a laparoscopic gastropexy in an elective setting [16]. This technique was able to be performed as the patient did not exhibit signs of bowel ischemia which would warrant immediate operative intervention. Endoscopic decompression has also been used as an alternative to surgical intervention on patients determined to be at prohibitively high risk.

Conclusions

Acute gastric volvulus is a rare, life-threatening condition which demands a high index of suspicion for expeditious work-up and intervention. Diagnosis is made most commonly with barium upper GI studies and CT imaging with or without upper endoscopy. Treatment is initiated with gastric decompression with a nasogastric tube or endoscopic decompression. Definitive surgical management includes reduction of the volvulized stomach, resection of gastric necrosis if present, and gastropexy. Precipitating conditions should be addressed concurrently including repair of diaphragmatic hernia and fundoplication as indicated. Endoscopic techniques for gastric decompression as a bridge to definitive management are recently being described. Use of PEG tubes as definitive management may be indicated in high-risk patients without signs of ischemia in order to avoid high-risk surgery although long-term data regarding recurrence rates are limited.

References

1. Haas O, Rat P, Christophe M, Friedman S, Favre JP. Surgical results of intrathoracic gastric volvulus complicating hiatal hernia. Br J Surg. 1990;77(12):1379–81.
2. Palanivelu C, Rangarajan M, Shetty AR, Senthilkumar R. Laparoscopic suture gastropexy for gastric volvulus: a report of 14 cases. Surg Endosc. 2007;21(6):863–6.
3. Gourgiotis S, Vougas V, Germanos S, Baratsis S. Acute gastric volvulus: diagnosis and management over 10 years. Dig Surg. 2006;23(3):169–72.
4. McElreath DP, Olden KW, Aduli F. Hiccups: a subtle sign in the clinical diagnosis of gastric volvulus and a review of the literature. Dig Dis Sci. 2008;53(11):3033–6.
5. Larssen KS, Stimec B, Takvam JA, Ignjatovic D. Role of imaging in gastric volvulus: stepwise approach in three cases. Turk J Gastroenterol. 2012;23(4):390–3.
6. Tanner NC. Chronic and recurrent volvulus of the stomach with late results of "colonic displacement". Am J Surg. 1968;115(4):505–15.

7. Rashid F, Thangarajah T, Mulvey D, Larvin M, Iftikhar SY. A review article on gastric volvulus: a challenge to diagnosis and management. Int J Surg. 2010;8(1):18–24.
8. Williamson JM, Dalton RS, Mahon D. Acute giant gastric volvulus causing cardiac tamponade. J Gastrointest Surg. 2010;14(7):1199–200.
9. Shivanand G, Seema S, Srivastava DN, Pande GK, Sahni P, Prasad R, et al. Gastric volvulus: acute and chronic presentation. Clin Imaging. 2003;27(4):265–8.
10. Al-Balas H, Hani MB, Omari HZ. Radiological features of acute gastric volvulus in adult patients. Clin Imaging. 2010;34(5):344–7.
11. Teague WJ, Ackroyd R, Watson DI, Devitt PG. Changing patterns in the management of gastric volvulus over 14 years. Br J Surg. 2000;87(3):358–61.
12. Katkhouda N, Mavor E, Achanta K, Friedlander MH, Grant SW, Essani R, et al. Laparoscopic repair of chronic intrathoracic gastric volvulus. Surgery. 2000;128(5):784–90.
13. Kawai M, Hiramatsu M, Lee SW, Tokuhara T, Fujita Y, Nomura E, et al. Endoscopy-assisted percutaneous anterior gastropexy for gastric volvulus: a minimally invasive technique using a special instrument. Endoscopy. 2013;45(Suppl 2 UCTN):E151–2.
14. Colijn AW, Kneepkens CM, Taets van Amerongen A, Ekkelkamp S. Gastric volvulus after anterior gastropexy. J Pediatr Gastroenterol Nutr. 1993;17(1):105–7.
15. Wolfgang R, Lee JG. Endoscopic treatment of acute gastric volvulus causing cardiac tamponade. J Clin Gastroenterol. 2001;32(4):336–9.
16. Omata J, Utsunomiya K, Kajiwara Y, Takahata R, Miyasaka N, Sugasawa H, et al. Acute gastric volvulus associated with wandering spleen in an adult treated laparoscopically after endoscopic reduction: a case report. Surg Case Rep. 2016;2(1):47. 47,016-0175-0. Epub 2016 May 24.
17. Kilincalp S, Akinci H, Coban S. Successful treatment of acute gastric volvulus by emergency endoscopic reduction in a patient with cerebral palsy. Endoscopy. 2014;46(Suppl 1 UCTN):E375–6.

Surgical Management: Other Diaphragmatic Hernias in Adults

23

Taher Gulamhusein, Nabeel R. Obeid, and Aurora D. Pryor

The Diaphragm: Embryology, Anatomy, and Physiology

Embryology

The diaphragm begins to form during the fourth week of gestation from the fusion of four embryonic precursors: the septum transversum anteriorly, the pleuroperitoneal folds dorsolaterally, the crura from the esophageal mesentery dorsally, and the body wall mesoderm posteriorly.

The septum transversum is the precursor to the central tendon, arises from the ventral body wall, and initiates the developmental process. It encircles the esophagus and great vessels and fuses with the foregut mesentery to separate the pleural and peritoneal cavities posteromedially.

The dorsal mesentery of the esophagus ultimately becomes the diaphragmatic crura and attaches the foregut to the dorsal body wall [1, 2]. The lateral margins of the diaphragm then develop from muscles of the thoracic wall and the pleuroperitoneal folds. Neuromuscularization of the diaphragm proceeds in conjunction with the events above and completes the maturation of the primitive structure. The right pleuroperitoneal membrane typically closes before the left. Formation of the primitive diaphragm is generally completed by the eighth week of gestation [3].

T. Gulamhusein · A. D. Pryor (✉)
Department of Surgery, Stony Brook Medicine, Stony Brook University Hospital, Stony Brook, NY, USA
e-mail: aurora.pryor@stonybrookmedicine.edu

N. R. Obeid
Department of Surgery, Stony Brook Medicine, Stony Brook, NY, USA

J. Grams et al. (eds.), *The SAGES Manual of Foregut Surgery*,
https://doi.org/10.1007/978-3-319-96122-4_23

Anatomy

The diaphragm has three muscular components which radiate outward and are attached to a large central tendon. They are separated from each other by intervening nonmuscular areas and are named the (1) pars lumbaris, (2) pars costalis, and (3) pars sternalis. The muscles of the diaphragm are continuous with the transversus abdominis muscle of the inner abdominal wall. The costal (pars costalis and sternalis) and crural (pars lumbaris) components of the muscular diaphragm have distinct embryologic precursors, neurologic innervations, and functional properties.

Muscular Portion of the Diaphragm

The pars sternalis is the smallest muscular component and originates from the posterior layer of the rectus sheath. It inserts onto the central tendon of the diaphragm. There are narrow gaps on both sides of the pars sternalis (the sternocostal triangles) which separate it from the pars costalis. In the normal diaphragm, these gaps are made of connective tissue which contains the internal thoracic/superior epigastric vessels. The right sternocostal triangle is also known as the triangle of Morgagni and the left, the triangle of Larrey [2, 4].

The pars costalis arises from upper margins of the lower 6 ribs (ribs 7 through 12). The lumbocostal triangles, also known as Bochdalek's gaps, separate the pars costalis from the pars lumbaris. They are covered by fascia, peritoneum, and pleura.

The pars lumbaris, the most powerful part of the diaphragm, lies bilaterally to the spine and forms the right and left crura. The crura originate from the anterior surface of the lumbar vertebrae, the intervertebral disks, and the anterior longitudinal ligament [5]. The right crus, the larger of the two, extends toward the middle part of the central tendon superiorly and eventually splits to form the esophageal hiatus, where it is the sole contributor to the esophageal hiatus in 60% of individuals. The remaining 40% of individuals have contributions from both crura. The split fibers meet again to form the anterior aspect of the aortic hiatus. It should be noted that while the esophageal crura contains muscular and tendinous components, only the tendinous component has enough strength to hold sutures over time. The right crus forms the ligament of Treitz inferiorly. The left crus runs upward to the left of the esophageal hiatus, runs behind the right crus, and inserts onto the central tendon [2].

The Tendinous Portion of the Diaphragm

The central tendon is the thickest and highest part of the diaphragm. It is described as having a cloverleaf shape, with one anterior and two lateral leaflets. It is not centrally located, nor is it symmetric—it lies more anteriorly than posteriorly, and the right leaf of the tendon is the largest of all three.

The superior surface of the central tendon is attached to the pericardium. The downward pressure from the heart centrally and the upward pressure from the liver laterally give the diaphragm a saddlelike appearance on a chest radiograph. At rest, the right dome lies at the fourth intercostal space and the left at the fifth to sixth intercostal space [5]. Inspiration promotes descent of both domes to two intercostal levels lower than their resting positions [2].

Blood Supply and Lymphatic Drainage of the Diaphragm

The diaphragm has a rich blood supply that is derived from four groups of arteries: (1) the pericardiophrenic arteries, (2) the musculophrenic arteries, (3) the superior and inferior phrenic arteries, and (4) the intercostal arteries.

The internal thoracic arteries, which arise from the proximal subclavian arteries, give off the pericardiophrenic arteries which travel with the phrenic nerves from the chest to the thoracic side of the diaphragm. They ultimately anastomose with the musculophrenic and superior phrenic arteries. As the internal thoracic artery continues its course through the chest, it gives off the musculophrenic artery just before entering the Morgagni's space (on the right) and the Larrey's space (on the left), after which it becomes the superior epigastric artery. The superior phrenic arteries arise directly from the thoracic aorta and provide blood supply to the thoracic side of the diaphragm.

The inferior phrenic arteries, which come off the abdominal aorta, provide the majority of the blood supply to the diaphragm. The right inferior phrenic artery rarely arises from the right renal artery. Each inferior phrenic artery splits into medial and lateral branches which collateralize with the musculophrenic, pericardiophrenic, and intercostal arteries. The intercostal arteries supply the peripheral parts of the costal diaphragm.

The thoracic diaphragm drains into the azygous and hemiazygous veins, and the abdominal side of the diaphragm drains into the inferior vena cava via the inferior phrenic veins.

The lymphatic drainage of the diaphragm plays a pivotal role in draining the peritoneal cavity. It consists of three sets of lymphatic systems, (1) the anterior system, (2) the lateral system, and (3) the posterior system [2, 4].

Neural Innervation of the Diaphragm

The diaphragm is innervated primarily by the phrenic nerves, which provide motor and sensory fibers. The costal part of the diaphragm also receives some contribution from the intercostal nerves.

The phrenic nerves mainly originate from the fourth nerve roots but receive contributions from the third and fifth roots as well. They course craniocaudally anterior to the hilum of the lungs and lie on the lateral surface of the pericardium along with the pericardiophrenic vessels [2, 4].

Openings of the Diaphragm

The diaphragm has three major anatomic openings to allow structures to pass between the abdominal and thoracic cavities: (1) the aortic, (2) the esophageal, and (3) the inferior vena cava orifices.

The aortic hiatus is located anterior to T12. Its borders are the vertebral body posteriorly, the crural diaphragm bilaterally, and the median arcuate ligament anteriorly. The aorta, aortic plexus, thoracic duct, and azygous vein pass through the aortic hiatus. The median arcuate ligament forms an arch anterior to the hiatus at the level of the celiac trunk and connects the two crura of the diaphragm [6].

The esophageal hiatus is located slightly to the left of midline at the level of T10 and is anterior to the aortic hiatus. It is formed by the median arcuate ligament posteriorly. Anterolaterally it is normally formed by the diaphragmatic crura and by splitting of the medial fibers of the right crus. There are many anatomic variations of the relative contributions of the right and left crural fibers to the esophageal hiatus [4]. The esophageal hiatus permits the passage of the esophagus, the anterior and posterior vagal trunks, and the phrenicoabdominal branch of the left phrenic nerve, which supplies sensory fibers to the pancreas and peritoneum.

The phrenoesophageal ligament, which is an extension of the inferior diaphragmatic fascia, attaches the esophagus to the diaphragm. It is responsible for preventing upward displacement of the esophagus.

The foramen vena cava is located at the right portion of the central tendon at the level of T8 and T9. It allows for passage of the vena cava and the right phrenic nerve. It is located completely within the central tendon and therefore does not have any muscular borders.

Larrey's and Morgagni's gaps, the left and right sternocostal triangles, respectively, allow for the internal mammary vessels to descend into the anterior abdominal wall, where they are known as the superior epigastric arteries. The lumbocostal triangles, located posteriorly, only contain a few muscle fibers and do not contain major anatomical structures.

Physiology

The major functions of the diaphragm are involved in supporting various respiratory and gastrointestinal processes.

The Respiratory Functions of the Diaphragm

The foremost function of the diaphragm is to contribute to the mechanics of the respiratory cycle. It is the muscle which is responsible for the majority of the work of breathing in normal individuals and in those with lung diseases. Paralysis of the non-diaphragmatic respiratory muscles does not lead to respiratory distress, but paralysis of both domes of the diaphragm will result in hypercarbia and respiratory failure [2].

With inspiration, muscle fiber contraction initially pulls the central tendon, which has an effect of expanding the thoracic volume. Secondly, the two domes of the diaphragm flatten to some extent, which pushes the intra-abdominal organs down and increases the intra-abdominal pressure. This increased intra-abdominal pressure is transmitted onto the zone of apposition, which results in an outward expansion of the rib cage. Thirdly, during deeper inspiration, the peripheral parts of the diaphragm unravel from the lateral walls of the chest, and this permits a widening of the costodiaphragmatic recesses. The net effect of the opposing forces of the contracting and descending diaphragm to the abdominal contents has a net effect on forcing the ribs upward and outward [2, 5].

Expiration is primarily driven by diaphragmatic relaxation and the elastic recoil forces of the lungs and thoracic wall. The elastic recoil allows for air to be drawn out passively from the lungs. The abdominal muscles contribute to some degree, as they push back displaced components of the intra-abdominal cavity [7].

The Gastroesophageal Functions of the Diaphragm

The contributions of the diaphragm to gastroesophageal function often get overshadowed by its obvious role in the pulmonary system. The crural part of the diaphragm plays important roles in swallowing, vomiting, and preventing gastroesophageal reflux. The gastroesophageal roles of the diaphragm are discussed in other chapters of this text.

Congenital Diaphragmatic Hernias

Bochdalek Hernias

Pathophysiology

Bochdalek hernia (BH), also known as posterolateral diaphragmatic hernia, is a congenital diaphragmatic hernia. Its development can be traced to failure of fusion or closure of the posterolateral components of the diaphragm during development. The frequency in neonates is about 1 per 7000, and the male/female ratio ranges from 3:2 to 2:1, depending on the series [8, 9]. In 78–90% of cases, it is located on the left diaphragmatic side, theorized to be due to fusion of the pleuroperitoneal folds on the right side first, which occurs around the eighth week of embryologic development. Furthermore, it is thought that left-sided hernias are more common because of the coverage provided by the liver on the right side [10]. The presence of a hernia sac depends on when the fusion takes place, as it is absent in over 85% of cases in some series [11]. The most common organs herniated through a BH are colon (70%), stomach (43%), spleen (28%), duodenopancreatic complex (11%), liver (7%), omentum (6%), kidney (4%), and retroperitoneal fat (3%) [12]. In 26% of cases, BH is associated with congenital anomalies, including pulmonary hypoplasia, hydrocephaly, and Arnold-Chiari malformation [13].

Clinical Presentation

Typically, Bochdalek hernias manifest at an early age with respiratory distress. This is thought to be due to compression of the gastrointestinal tract leading to pulmonary hypoplasia from lack of maturation of the parenchyma. Neonates may develop cyanosis and dyspnea and may be found to have cardiac deviation to the contralateral hemithorax.

Rarely, these hernias may present in the adult patient, with an incidence of 0.17% based on radiographic literature [14, 15]. Adult-onset presentation may range from mild shortness of breath to gastric volvulus. Bochdalek hernias can also be incidental findings on imaging done for other reasons. An extensive meta-analysis revealed the average age of presentation for adult Bochdalek hernias was 40 years, with no significant gender predilection; some reports have suggested they may present even earlier, at an average age of 28 years [10, 16]. It is consistently found that Bochdalek hernias are diagnosed at a much earlier age than Morgagni hernias, discussed below.

Left-sided hernias were encountered in 78–90% of the cases reported, with the size of the defect being independent of laterality. Generally, symptomatic adults with Bochdalek hernias typically present with GI symptoms, including vague abdominal pain and/or distension, with pain being the most common complaint (69%) and pregnancy the most common precipitating factor due to increased intra-abdominal pressure [10, 17]. The nonspecific nature of these symptoms contributes to the difficulty in diagnosis. Complications of Bochdalek hernias include gastric volvulus, incarceration, obstruction, strangulation, pulmonary symptoms, dysphagia, GERD, and hemorrhage.

Work-Up and Evaluation

As previously mentioned, making the correct diagnosis can be quite challenging. Physical examination is often nonspecific, although diminished breath sounds and presence of bowel sounds may provide a clinical clue. Radiographic investigation is the mainstay. Routine imaging such as chest X-ray (CXR) may reveal diagnostic clues like an elevated hemidiaphragm (Fig. 23.1) or air meniscus sign, but many times these studies are found to be unremarkable. Therefore, a negative CXR does not rule out the diagnosis of a diaphragmatic hernia.

Generally, barium contrast studies are used to confirm clinical suspicion in the pediatric population, showing abdominal contents displaced into the chest or an "upside down stomach" (Fig. 23.2). In the adult patient, the most definitive study is a computerized tomography (CT) scan (Fig. 23.3), which has been shown to have the most sensitivity and specificity [18, 19]. An MRI with three-dimensional reconstruction can also aid in differentiating the soft tissue planes.

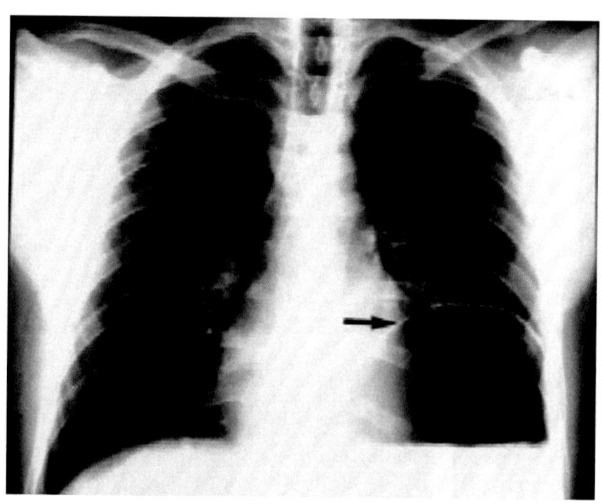

Fig. 23.1 Chest X-ray revealing an elevated left hemidiaphragm (arrow), an early but nonspecific radiographic finding of diaphragmatic hernia. (Used with permission from Wolters Kluwer Health, Inc.; Bujanda et al. [17])

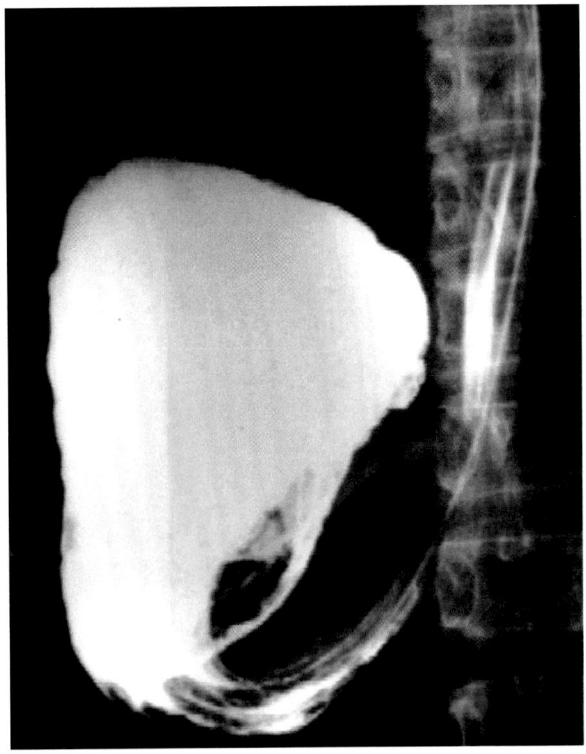

Fig. 23.2 Contrast radiograph revealing gastric herniation with "upside-down stomach" sign. (Used with permission from Wolters Kluwer Health, Inc.; Bujanda et al. [17])

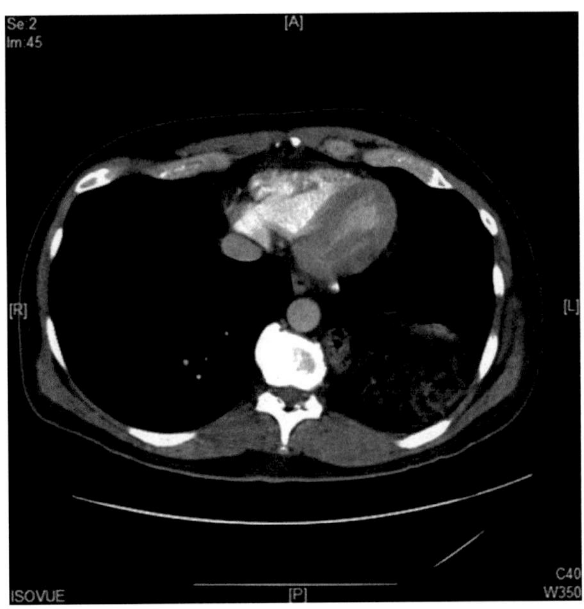

Fig. 23.3 CT scan showing evidence of left posterolateral diaphragmatic hernia with the colon and omentum. (Used with permission from Springer-Verlag; Brown et al. [10])

Indications for Repair

Given the relative rarity of Bochdalek hernias, and therefore only scattered case reports or series in the literature, there are no well-established guidelines for operative intervention. It is generally recommended that patients undergo repair if deemed to be an appropriate surgical candidate. This is true regardless of symptomatology or the incidental nature of the diagnosis. Certainly, symptoms attributed to the presence of a BH or complications of the hernia, such as obstruction, are indications for repair.

Technique for Repair

Surgical repair of the defect can be performed transabdominally or with a thoracic approach, and in both cases can be done open or with minimally invasive techniques [20]. The first reported laparoscopic repair was in 1998, and the minimally invasive approach has been gaining popularity ever since [21]. In a comprehensive meta-analysis from 2011, most Bochdalek hernia repairs were performed via laparotomy (38%), as opposed to 12% laparoscopically, with other approaches including thoracotomy, thoracoscopic, or combined [10]. Of those that were emergent, 42% were done with laparotomy vs. 19% via laparoscopy. Primary repair was achieved in 95% of open cases and in 53% of laparoscopic cases.

For the laparoscopic repair, patients are positioned in the lateral decubitus with reverse Trendelenburg position to maximize exposure. Four to five trocars can be used to triangulate the target of the left upper quadrant (assuming a left-sided hernia defect). The operation begins with reduction of hernia contents with or without excision of the hernia sac (if present) in order to clearly define the defect. For smaller defects, leaving the sac in place may facilitate the repair. If incarcerated, the diaphragm may need to be incised radially to effectively reduce hernia contents. In some instances, in order to gain full exposure and to assess the extent of the defect, one may need to mobilize the spleen as well as the left lateral liver by incising the triangular ligament.

At this time, attention then turns to repair of the defect, which is closed in a transverse fashion, from medial to lateral. This is performed with permanent suture, taking large bites of tissue in order to avoid tearing the muscle.

Chest tubes are placed routinely by some, while others use a red rubber suction catheter to evacuate the pleural cavity prior to transabdominal closure. With CO_2 pneumoperitoneum, evacuation may not be necessary unless ventilation is compromised. Due to the lack of peritoneal hernia sac in most cases, there is a risk for transient pneumothorax from direct communication of peritoneal and pleural spaces during laparoscopic insufflation. Unilateral lung ventilation or a thoracoscopic port may help to both assess the repair as well as to allow reinflation of the ipsilateral lung, followed by drainage of the pleural space.

The concept of primary vs. mesh repair is relevant to Bochdalek hernia, although there is a relative paucity of data on this compared to other hernia repairs. Primary repair of the diaphragm is achieved after successful reduction of contents with the determination that the repair will be under minimal to no tension and is often straightforward with smaller defect sizes due to redundancy of the

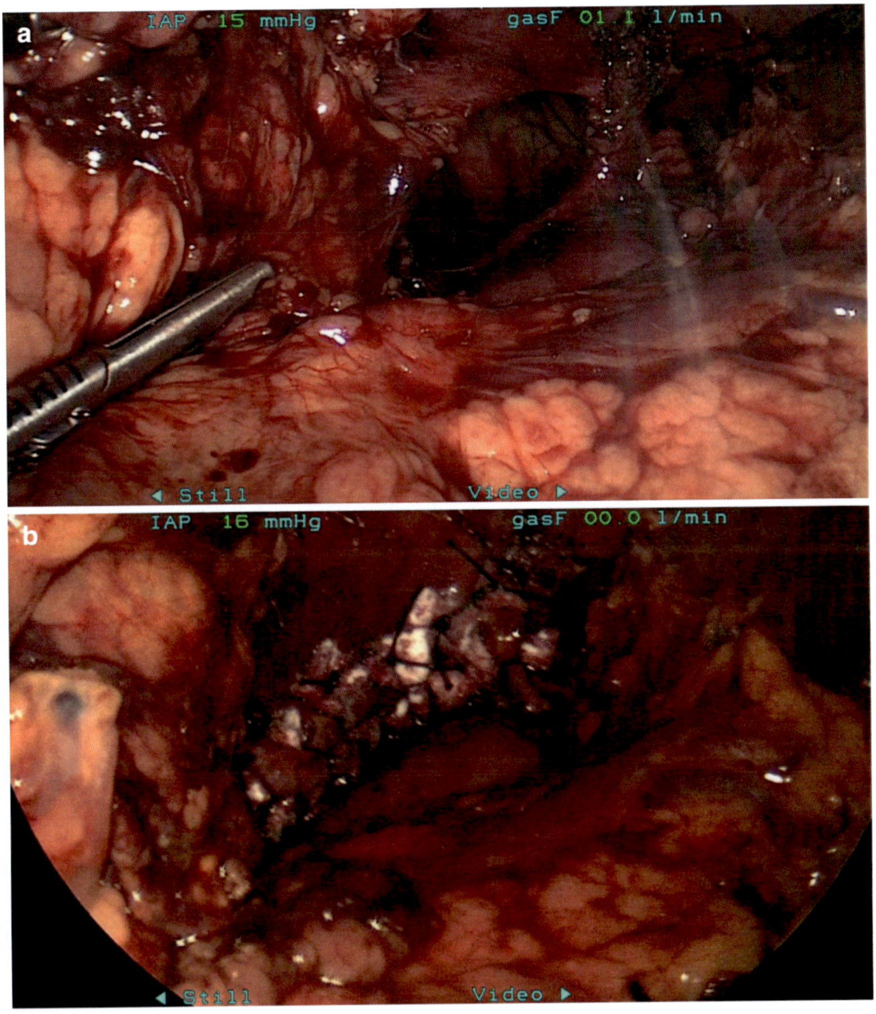

Fig. 23.4 (**a**, **b**) Intraoperative images depicting a Bochdalek hernia (**a**) before repair and (**b**) after primary repair with pledgets

diaphragm (Fig. 23.4). There have been case series with positive results using this technique [20].

Most surgeons recommend mesh in the setting of a large defect or significant tension on primary repair. Some recommend using mesh when defect size is greater than 8 cm in diameter [22]. Mesh is used more commonly in laparoscopic repair compared to open (60% vs. 7%) [10]. Dual-layer mesh appears to be most common, as it allows for visceral contact. The use of synthetic mesh such as Gore-Tex Dual-Mesh (Gore Medical, Flagstaff, AZ) with approximately 5 cm margins circumferentially with nonabsorbable tackers has been reported. Other case reports have used Dacron, Parietex (Sofradim, Trevoux, France), Marlex, and Surgisis (Cook

Urological, Fort Worth, TX). We suggest a nonporous permanent mesh if a bridging mesh is used. Mesh fixation should be performed with great caution, to avoid the potentially fatal complication of cardiac injury resulting in tamponade, especially with left-sided repairs. For this reason, suture fixation or glue adjuncts may be preferred. A survey by the Society of American Gastrointestinal and Endoscopic Surgeons (SAGES) found that most surgeons use sutures for hiatal hernia fixation, followed by tacking in 24% [23].

Postoperative Management

Again, no standard protocol is in place given the infrequency of these operations. The diet can be started immediately postoperatively and advanced as tolerated. Patients should be cared for based on the operative approach. For laparoscopic repairs of small hernias, the patients can be managed in an ambulatory setting. If there is a high risk for cardiopulmonary event, the patient may need monitoring. If a chest tube was placed, the patient may need admission for tube management and removal when the output is low. Most surgeons will repeat imaging in 3–6 months to evaluate the repair.

Postoperative Complications

Overall, the morbidity after diaphragmatic repair of a Bochdalek hernia is related to the surgical technique. Laparoscopic repair has a lower morbidity than laparotomy (6% vs. 18%) [10]. Complications include infection, hemorrhage, respiratory failure, ileus, gastroesophageal reflux, chronic pain, hernia recurrence, and cardiac injury/tamponade.

Outcomes

In the neonatal population, prognosis is poor despite urgent surgical treatment. In adults, the mortality rate for elective surgery is less than 3% but rises to 32% when its diagnosis is delayed or complications develop [12]. Thirty-day mortality is low, ranging from 0 to 2% based on approach, and laparoscopy results in the shortest length of stay (4 days vs. 10–20 days for laparotomy or thoracotomy) [10]. Recurrence appears to be negligible in most series as well, with mean follow-up of 11–21 months.

Morgagni Hernias

Pathophysiology

Morgagni hernias (MH) are substernal diaphragmatic hernias originally described by Giovanni-Batista Morgagni in 1769 after autopsy examinations on an Italian stonecutter. In 1828, Larrey, Napoleon's surgeon, described a surgical approach to the pericardial cavity through an anterior diaphragmatic defect for the treatment of pericardial tamponade [24]. They both described a triangular space between the muscle fibers of the anterior diaphragm, caused by the passage of the superior epigastric vessels. Waelli made the first radiologic diagnosis of MH in 1911.

A failure of fusion of the pleuroperitoneal membranes, the septum transversum, and the dorsal mesentery results in a defect in this space [25]. During embryological development, there are multiple interrelated processes during diaphragmatic formation. The anterior aspect of the diaphragm is the last to form. This process is temporally related to the fusion of the sternum and to the period of embryologic development when there is a rapid increase in intra-abdominal contents. Errors in the coordination of these three processes lead to congenital weaknesses in the anterior aspect of the diaphragm, which predisposes to subsequent hernia formation [26].

When a hernia occurs on the left side of the sternum, it is named a Morgagni hernia; and when it occurs on the right, it is known as a Larrey hernia (LH). When a hernia is large enough so as to occupy both spaces, it is appropriately termed a Morgagni-Larrey hernia (MLH) [27]. Morgagni hernias are rare, with an occurrence of 1 in every 4800 live-born infants. They occur for 2–6% of all congenital diaphragmatic hernias and 2–4% of non-traumatic diaphragmatic hernias in adults [3, 28].

Hernias occur more often on the right (91%); it is theorized that this is due to the barrier effect of the heart, which prevents helps to prevent herniation on the left side [26]. The most commonly herniated contents include the omentum (65%), transverse colon (62%), stomach (8%), and liver (8%) [16, 27]. MH is associated with other abnormalities such as congenital heart diseases and Down syndrome [27]. Morgagni hernias generally contain a hernia sac.

Clinical Presentation

Of the two congenital diaphragmatic hernias, MH is more likely than BH to remain asymptomatic and evade diagnosis into adulthood. However, the literature also suggests that patients may be symptomatic up to 72% of the time with vague pain and pulmonary complaints and that MH simply goes overlooked given its relative rarity. As such, it may very well be a misconception that MH is an asymptomatic entity [26]. Oftentimes diagnosis is incidental; a Morgagni hernia may be discovered when imaging done for other reasons is suggestive or diagnostic [27]. MH may also be an incidental finding at laparoscopy. In a retrospective single-institution review at Massachusetts General Hospital, it was found that the average age at diagnosis of MH was 42 years [24].

When patients are symptomatic, MH present with primarily digestive and respiratory complaints due to the compression of intrathoracic organs by a hollow viscus. Unsurprisingly, shortness of breath (35%) and abdominal pain (31%) are usually the primary presenting symptoms. Whereas Bochdalek hernias may present with strangulated or gangrenous viscera, the Morgagni hernia generally presents with viable contents that are likely to be easily reduced from the hernia sac. Therefore, MH has a lower incidence of presenting with incarceration or strangulation [16].

Work-Up and Evaluation

Morgagni hernia is an elusive diagnosis which requires a high index of suspicion since it presents with nonspecific symptoms. In large hernias, a physical exam may demonstrate diminished breath and bowel sounds. Fortunately, Morgagni hernias may be diagnosed by one of several radiologic methods. In a retrospective review published in 2008, the most common diagnostic modality was chest radiography (93%), followed by computed tomography (CT) scan (47%), contrast enema (24%), and upper gastrointestinal study (23%) [26]. A chest X-ray may show an air-filled mass in the chest which would suggest a congenital diaphragmatic hernia. Contrast enemas may demonstrate colonic herniation into the chest. In more modern times, these modalities have largely been replaced by CT scans.

The advent of the CT scan has improved preoperative diagnostic ability for the diagnosis of Morgagni hernia. CT scans allow for the characterization of anterior mediastinal masses found on chest X-ray; a MH would present with a large paracardiac fat density with linear serpiginous densities consistent with omental blood vessels and an abnormally high-riding transverse colon. Differential diagnosis of such imaging findings would include a pericardial cyst, large fat pad, or a solid tumor. It should be noted that the presence of gas in the lesion is merely suggestive of herniation of hollow viscous, but does not confirm it; there have been case reports of gas containing lesions on chest X-ray which were not present on subsequent CT scans. This has been found to be secondary to intermittent spontaneous reduction of hernia contents [29].

Indications for Repair

Generally, after a Morgagni hernia has been diagnosed, the treatment is to proceed with surgical correction if the patient is deemed to be a good candidate for surgery. This is irrespective of symptoms and is done to prevent future potential complications of incarceration and strangulation.

Techniques for Repair

Much like for Bochdalek hernias, repair of Morgagni hernia has been reported via laparotomy, thoracotomy, thoracoscopy, and laparoscopy. Each of the four approaches has its risks and benefits. The abdominal approach allows for easier reduction of hernia contents and more thorough evaluation of the diaphragm for additional defects and concomitant repair. The primary advantage of the thoracic approach is that it provides easier dissection of the hernia sac off the mediastinal and pleural structures. Given the increasingly widespread use of laparoscopy and the relative ease of reducibility of the Morgagni hernia, the laparoscopic approach has been gaining in popularity. However, a review of the literature by Horton et al. in 2008 demonstrated that thoracotomy was still the most widely utilized approach (49%), with the likely reason being that it facilitated better sac excision. There have been only two documented cases of the thoracoscopic repair [26].

The first laparoscopic repair of MH was reported by Kuster et al. in 1992; a suturing technique was employed incorporating the abdominal fascia in the repair and securing the knots outside of the abdomen [30]. For various reasons, it appears that Morgagni hernia, as compared to Bochdalek hernia, is more amenable to laparoscopic repair. Firstly, patients with MH are more likely to present electively;

patients with Bochdalek hernia more often present with a clinical picture with elements of shock, which is worrisome for incarceration or strangulation. Secondly, the anterior location of the foramina of Morgagni and Larrey can be more easily approached laparoscopically, whereas the posterolateral location of the foramen of Bochdalek renders it more difficult to approach. Thirdly, the presence of a peritoneal sac in Morgagni hernias facilitates the reduction of intra-abdominal contents, whereas the lack of such a lining in Bochdalek hernias increases the risk of adhesions to intrathoracic structures [16]. Lastly, MH are oftentimes diagnosed at the time of laparoscopy being done for other reasons. MH repair has been conducted simultaneously with cholecystectomy, Nissen fundoplication, paraesophageal hernia repair, gastric bypass, gastrectomy, abdominal aortic aneurysm repair, and coronary artery bypass graft and even during pregnancy. As such, surgeons may be more willing to repair this hernia with minimally invasive techniques because the diagnosis is being made during laparoscopy [16, 26]. There is a case report of proceeding with laparoscopic repair while employing an abdominal wall lifting technique so as to avoid the consequences of pneumoperitoneum [31].

The decision to excise the hernia sac remains a point of contention. Those who abide by traditional surgical principles of sac excision claim that it increases the chance of obliteration of the hernia cavity and prefer to not leave behind a mesothelial-lined cavity in the chest [32]. Others believe that it is more prudent to leave the hernia sac in place to avoid injury to intrathoracic structures (i.e., the pleural lining and the pericardium) [16]. The natural history of an unexcised sac has not been studied, but Ramachandran and Arora reported complete resolution of a sac by CT scan 1 month postoperatively [33]. Some advocate for placement of a drain within the sac to prevent cyst formation [28].

Closure of the hernia defect is by means of primary repair or coverage of the defect with mesh. This is primarily dictated by the size of the defect and the ability to achieve a tension-free repair. Thoman et al. has suggested that defects greater than 20–30 cm^2 should be closed with prosthetic repair to avoid tension [34]. Given the rarity of this diagnosis, there is no clear consensus on which prosthesis is best for repair. At the time of writing, Swain et al. reported that 62% of Morgagni hernia repairs utilized a mesh-based repair [16]. Similar to Bochdalek hernias, there have been case reports utilizing many different prostheses with variable outcomes and long-term follow-up. Gore-Tex dual mesh (Gore Medical, Flagstaff, AZ), Dacron, Parietex (Sofradim, Trevoux, France), Marlex, polyvinylidene fluoride (PVDF, Dynamesh, IPOM), artificial pericardium patch, and bovine pericardium (Tutopatch, Tutogen Medical, Neunkirchen, Bavaria, DE) have been used [27, 35–37]. Mesh can be fixed in place using sutures or staples, taking great attention to avoid injury to nearby structures. As with Bochdalek hernia, if the mesh is used to bridge a gap in the diaphragm, we suggest a permanent nonporous mesh.

The technique for laparoscopic repair is similar to a typical setup for a laparoscopic Nissen fundoplication with the patient positioned supine +/– lithotomy position. The patient is placed in reverse Trendelenburg and three to five ports are placed with care not to place the ports near the costal margin. After insufflation of the abdomen and introduction of a supraumbilical laparoscope, the hernia is identified and the contents are reduced and assessed for viability.

After successful reduction, the sac may or may not be excised. If the decision is made to proceed with sac excision, thoracoscopy may be a helpful adjunct for larger defects. Thereafter, attention is turned to closure of the diaphragmatic defect. Size of the defect, tissue quality, and surgeon experience dictate how closure will proceed. We typically used permanent sutures placed with a suture passer. When utilizing mesh, most authors advocate for at least 1.5–2.5 cm overlap [25–27, 38]. We suggest at least 3 cm to allow for postoperative mesh shrinkage. Dual-sided synthetics offer the advantage of visceral contact and have therefore gained popularity. Many authors who utilize polypropylene mesh cover the mesh with omentum, peritoneal flap, or the falciform ligament to prevent adhesions with intra-abdominal organs [28].

Postoperative Management

There is no unified consensus for the postoperative management of patients who undergo repair of a Morgagni hernia; management parallels that reported for Bochdalek hernia, above. Patients are generally placed in a postoperative setting which allows for cardiopulmonary monitoring as needed. They are started on a diet and advanced as tolerated. Patients are discharged when they are able to tolerate a diet, have achieved adequate pain control, and are able to ambulate without issue. This ranges from ambulatory to 8 days [38].

Long-term follow-up varies, but short-term follow-up is usually within the 3–6-month period. The patient may or may not have a barium enema or CT completed to confirm infradiaphragmatic positioning of the transverse colon [25].

Postoperative Complications

Overall, the morbidity and mortality after repair of Morgagni hernia are related to the surgical technique. Minimally invasive techniques have fewer complications and lower morbidity. Laparotomy has a reported 17% complication rate compared to 5% for laparoscopy; however, patients undergoing laparotomy more often undergo emergency surgery and may be more predisposed to developing postoperative complications [26]. Complications include infection, hemorrhage, respiratory failure, ileus, gastroesophageal reflux, chronic pain, hernia recurrence, and cardiac injury/tamponade.

Outcomes

Outcomes after Morgagni hernia repair demonstrate negligible rates of recurrence with variable follow-up ranging from anywhere between 1 month to 7 years. As would be expected, the average hospital length of stay is greatest for open thoracic (14 days) and abdominal (11 days) approaches; laparoscopy has an average length of stay of only 3 days. Thirty-day mortality is highest for patients undergoing laparotomy (4%), but as stated above, this may reflect the poorer health status of patients who require emergent surgery [26, 38].

Acquired Diaphragmatic Hernias

Traumatic Diaphragmatic Hernias

Historical Background

Traumatic diaphragmatic hernias were first reported by Sennertus in 1541, who reported a delayed herniation of abdominal viscera through an injured diaphragm. Ambroise Pare reported a case of traumatic diaphragmatic rupture at autopsy in 1579 in a patient who was a captain in the French military and died 8 months after sustaining a gunshot wound to the abdomen. Autopsy results showed strangulation of the colon through a small diaphragmatic defect which could only admit the tip of the small finger. Bowditch made the first antemortem diagnosis of traumatic diaphragmatic rupture in 1853, and the first successful repair was performed by Riolfi in 1886 [39].

Incidence, Etiology, and Pathophysiology

Diaphragmatic injuries are frequently missed or may present in a delayed fashion, and as such the actual incidence of injuries may be higher than what is reported in the literature. Rubikas reported a 2.1% incidence of diaphragmatic injury in patients with blunt trauma and a 3.5% incidence after penetrating trauma [40]. However, there have been rates of traumatic diaphragmatic injuries as high as 5% for patients who have been hospitalized after motor vehicle accidents and as high as 15% for patients who sustained penetrating injuries to the lower chest and upper abdomen [41].

In a large review of traumatic diaphragmatic injuries, Shah et al. reports that three-quarters of traumatic diaphragmatic injuries are due to blunt trauma, whereas the remaining are due to penetrating trauma [39]. However, there may be variations in the incidence and etiology of diaphragmatic injuries which is reflected by the demographic of the population served. Multiple single-institution reviews of traumatic diaphragmatic injuries from Quebec, Senegal, and Turkey revealed a penetrating etiology in 60–70% of patients treated for traumatic diaphragmatic injury [42–44].

It is important to distinguish between an isolated diaphragmatic injury and the occurrence of a diaphragmatic hernia secondary to this injury. Despite having a higher incidence of penetrating diaphragmatic injury, Hanna et al. showed that diaphragmatic hernia occurred more frequently when the diaphragmatic injury was secondary to blunt trauma. The size of the diaphragmatic defect was also significantly larger in blunt trauma patients, likely associated with the increased pressure gradient across the diaphragm that is associated with blunt injury [42]. Approximately 88% of blunt diaphragmatic injuries reported in the literature were the result of motor vehicle collisions [45]. Penetrating injuries are usually the result from stabs or gunshots. Penetrating injury could potentially be more dangerous, as the smaller defects would increase the risk of strangulation of herniated contents.

The diaphragm may sustain injury by multiple mechanisms. Impact to the chest wall may cause avulsion of the diaphragm from its points of attachment or cause shearing injury to the dome. Injury may also be caused by a sudden increase in transdiaphragmatic pressure which is transmitted to the diaphragm by the abdominal viscera [39, 46]. The weakest point of the diaphragm during its embryological development is the posterolateral portion which arises from the pleuroperitoneal membrane. The pressure gradient generated across this point during a high-impact traumatic event (such as a motor vehicle collision or a fall) is usually the inciting event that leads to traumatic diaphragmatic rupture in blunt trauma. Blunt traumatic injury generally results in an injury pattern of large 5–15 cm radial tears in the posterolateral aspect of the diaphragm. Herniation of intra-abdominal contents is promoted by the pressure gradient between the abdominal and thoracic cavities.

The effects of a ruptured diaphragm are primarily on circulation and respiration. Diaphragmatic action accounts for 66% of the tidal volume when lying supine; functional loss of one hemidiaphragm may result in a 25% to 50% decrease in pulmonary function [39]. Herniated viscera may cause compression of the lungs or displacement of the mediastinum with resultant impaired venous return to the heart. This may be further complicated by incarceration and strangulation.

It has consistently been shown that most traumatic ruptures occur on the left side of the diaphragm [44]. The right hemidiaphragm is stronger than the left and is also afforded protection by the liver. This accounts for nearly a three to nine times more frequency of injuries to the left side [46, 47]. The liver helps in dissipating the increased intra-abdominal pressure over a larger area. It is likely that right-sided injuries may also be underreported given the diagnostic difficulty of uncovering injuries on that side. We recently managed a right-sided diaphragmatic hernia which presented 2 weeks after the index traumatic event. The hernia was repaired thoracoscopically due to the presence of significant intrathoracic adhesions (Fig. 23.5).

Traumatic injuries to the diaphragm may also be iatrogenic. We have managed pericardial defects after pericardial windows and accidental chest tube placement through the diaphragm.

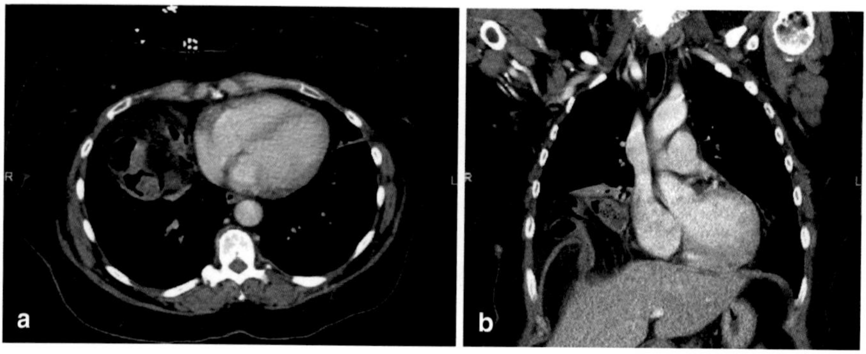

Fig. 23.5 (**a**, **b**) Representative (**a**) axial and (**b**) coronal CT scan images from the case of a 61-year-old female from our institution who presented with a traumatic right-sided diaphragmatic hernia 2 weeks after motor vehicle collision. Herniated contents included the omentum and colon. She underwent thoracoscopic hernia repair using interrupted #0 Surgidac sutures (Covidien, Dublin, Republic of Ireland)

Clinical Presentation

Grimes described the natural history of traumatic diaphragmatic rupture in three phases: the acute phase, the latent phase, and the obstructive phase.

The acute phase begins from the time of trauma to the apparent recovery from primary injuries. Abdominal pain, respiratory distress, and cardiac dysfunction characterize this phase. However, the associated injuries from trauma overwhelmingly influence the acute phase. In the setting of penetrating injury, when the injury was in the abdomen, there is up to an 83.3% rate of associated intra-abdominal organ injury requiring surgical attention. When the penetrating wound is in the chest, associated organ injury has been reported to be 54.8% [42]. Given that various studies have found a significantly increased injury severity score in patients with blunt diaphragmatic injury as compared to those without blunt diaphragmatic injury [45], it should come as no surprise that the diagnosis of a ruptured diaphragm is frequently missed in the acute phase as attention is directed toward stabilization of shock, respiratory insufficiency, coma, and other visceral injuries. Anywhere between 33% and 66% of traumatic diaphragmatic ruptures are missed during this period [39, 48].

The latent phase begins when the intra-abdominal viscera begin to occupy the diaphragmatic defect and herniate into the thoracic cavity. This is accompanied with upper gastrointestinal complaints as well as pain in the left shoulder, chest, or upper quadrant. Dyspnea or orthopnea may be present. Physical exam may reveal diminished breath sounds.

Lastly, the obstructive phase begins. It manifests as signs of visceral obstruction or ischemia of strangulated contents. Presenting symptoms include nausea, vomiting, severe abdominal pain, and significant respiratory distress. Case series have shown that the majority (85%) of strangulation occurs within 3 years of trauma and that 90% of strangulated diaphragmatic hernias are of traumatic origin [39].

Work-Up and Evaluation

Radiographic Imaging

Traumatic diaphragmatic rupture may be associated with high morbidity and mortality due to a difficulty in making the diagnosis and the high number of associated injuries. The rate of missing a diaphragmatic injury is upward of 66% [46, 49]. Diagnosis requires a high index of suspicion.

Most frequently, a supine chest radiograph is the first imaging study conducted to evaluate for thoracic and intra-abdominal trauma. The diagnostic sensitivity of a plain chest radiograph for the diagnosis of diaphragmatic rupture ranges from 27 to 60% for left-sided hernias and 17 to 33% for right-sided hernias. Placement of a nasogastric tube prior to obtaining the chest radiographic may aid in diagnosis; identification of the tube above the level of the left hemidiaphragm would be suggestive of diaphragmatic rupture. Other features on radiograph include obliteration of the diaphragmatic contour, mediastinal shift to the contralateral side, or an ipsilateral pleural effusion [46].

Computed tomographic images are the gold standard imaging modality for diagnosing acute traumatic diaphragmatic rupture, but they are far from perfect. Murray et al. concluded in 1996 that CT imaging has a 66% specificity in diagnosing acute diaphragmatic ruptures after blunt trauma. Earlier reports found that the diagnostic accuracy of CT for diaphragmatic rupture has a sensitivity ranging from 14 to 71% and specificity of 76% to 99%, with an increased sensitivity and specificity for left-sided injuries [50, 51]. However, recent improvements in CT technology, particularly multi-slice CT, may allow for increased sensitivity, specificity, and accuracy of diagnosis by dramatically reducing motion and beam hardening artifacts and improving spatial resolution. Sarita et al. found that the sensitivity, specificity, and accuracy of multidetector computed tomogram (MDCT) scan were 100%, 93%, and 95%, respectively. MDCT may reveal diaphragmatic discontinuity, thickening of the diaphragm, a collar sign, visceral herniation, or a dependent viscera sign [49].

Role of Laparoscopy

The use of minimally invasive techniques to diagnose diaphragmatic injuries was initially described in the 1970s when thoracoscopy was first utilized to diagnose acute diaphragmatic lacerations from penetrating trauma to the left chest [41]. There have been a few studies conducted which demonstrate the utility of diagnostic laparoscopy to identify suspected acute diaphragmatic rupture and herniation, especially given the variable diagnostic accuracy of radiography in detecting these injuries. Murray et al. found a 24% incidence of occult diaphragmatic injury in the setting of penetrating trauma to the left lower chest in patients who lacked other clinical or radiographic findings to suggest such injury [52].

However, laparoscopic assessment should be used with caution; it is unadvisable in the treatment of patients who are likely to have associated injuries. There is up to a 41% rate of missing associated hollow viscus and solid organ injuries with the use of laparoscopy in the acute trauma setting [40]. As such, it is reasonable to proceed with a diagnostic laparoscopy when traumatic injury to the diaphragm is suspected in the absence of concomitant injuries or for subacute or chronic presentation.

Indications for Repair

The treatment for traumatic diaphragmatic rupture and hernia is operative intervention given the high morbidity and mortality associated with such injury. Defects in the diaphragm, no matter how small, will not heal spontaneously [53]. This is in part due to the thoracoabdominal pressure gradient, which will naturally favor enlargement of the defect with herniation of abdominal contents [46].

Techniques for Repair

The operative approach to the repair diaphragmatic injuries is dependent on multiple factors. Consideration is given to the presence of other intra-abdominal injuries, patient stability, the technical ability of the surgeon, and the chronicity, location, and the size of the diaphragmatic injury.

Laparotomy is utilized in the acute setting when there is a high likelihood of associated intra-abdominal injuries or the patient is unstable and not deemed to be a candidate for laparoscopy. The standard open repair of a diaphragmatic hernia utilizes simple, figure-of-eight, or horizontal mattress sutures using nonabsorbable material [41]. A thoracotomy may also be included to facilitate the reduction of hernia contents in the event they cannot be reduced successfully via laparotomy alone. The thoracic approach is particularly helpful for right-sided defects, as the location of the liver can make abdominal access difficult. A mesh may also be required, although there are many case reports which indicate that small defects are amenable to primary repair without any untoward consequences. Mihos et al. described the repair of 65 patients with traumatic diaphragmatic rupture (of which eight patients had herniation) via a combination of laparotomy and thoracotomy. Most patients had an injury severity score (ISS) reflective of major polytrauma. Repairs were conducted primarily using interrupted and running nonabsorbable suture. Postoperative complications were related to the injury burden and not necessarily to the method of repair [24]. Failure to reapproximate diaphragmatic gaps in the acute setting may be amenable to a delayed bridging mesh repair [54].

Some authors advocate for an open approach for defects greater than 10 centimeters [41]. Dirican et al. reviewed the repair of 48 diaphragmatic hernias; the eight patients who underwent a polypropylene mesh repair had a mean defect size of 7.87 centimeters, whereas the patients who underwent primary repair had a mean rupture size of 4.35 centimeters. There were no complications in the postoperative follow-up periods of the patients in the study. Early postoperative deaths were found to be a result of associated injuries, and not the diaphragmatic injury itself. The six early mortalities in the study were a result of irreversible hemorrhagic shock [44].

Hernia location also dictates operative approach. Right-sided hernias are better suited for open or thoracoscopic repair because of the spatial and visual constraints of the right upper quadrant of the abdomen, particularly for defects obscured by the liver. Laparoscopy is also more difficult with hernias anterior to the esophageal hiatus and adjacent to the pericardium. The diaphragm is thin, taut, immobile, and very close to the pericardium in the area just anterior to the esophagus. Improper suture placement in this area may injure the pericardium, and sutures placed too superficially for fear of such injury increase the risk of recurrence [55]. Additionally, chronic traumatic diaphragmatic hernias located in the central portion of the diaphragm may be difficult to repair because of significant tension on the closure. The edges of chronic diaphragmatic hernias become fibrotic with time and, as such, are better suited for a mesh-based repair. Large, chronic hernias may benefit from a thoracic approach to facilitate adhesiolysis [41, 56].

Reina et al. published a case report and literature review on traumatic intrapericardial diaphragmatic hernias – a rare entity for which there were only 82 documented cases published at the time [57]. These hernias occur with rupture of the central portion of the diaphragm, and most cases involved herniation of the transverse colon, stomach, or greater omentum. These types of hernias may also be iatrogenic. Authors advocated for an open repair via an abdominal or thoracic approach, depending on acute or chronic period of presentation, respectively. Amazingly, just 8 years after that literature review, McCutcheon et al. reported the first case of a completely laparoscopic repair of a patient who presented 4 months

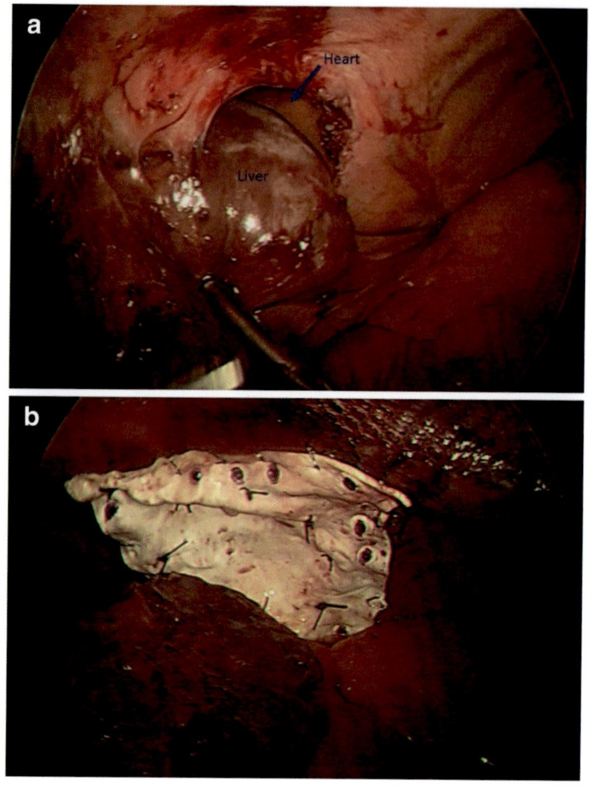

Fig. 23.6 (**a**, **b**) Intraoperative images from the case of a 63-year-old female with prior pericardial window complicated by a large diaphragmatic hernia (**a**) with the left lobe of the liver herniated into the pericardium, (**b**) repaired using a 10 × 10 cm nonporous mesh (Gore Medical, Flagstaff, AZ)

after the inciting traumatic incident. Exploration revealed a 6 × 5 cm defect in the central tendon with herniation of incarcerated transverse colon and omentum in the pericardial sac which was repaired using a simple expanded polytetrafluoroethylene (ePTFE) soft tissue patch. The patient did well and was discharged postoperative day 5, with no signs of recurrence at 6-month follow-up [58]. We presented a similar case in 2011 of a patient with pericardial hernia following pericardial window. Recently, we had a similar case in 2016 which involved herniation of the liver after a pericardial window; nonporous mesh was successfully used to repair the hernia defect (Fig. 23.6).

Frantzides and Carlson described the first laparoscopic repair of a penetrating diaphragmatic injury in 1994 [59]. An acute traumatic diaphragmatic hernia which would be a straightforward candidate for laparoscopic repair would need to be of small size, located in the left hemidiaphragm, and be an isolated injury. Such injuries are generally a result of penetrating mechanisms. However, case reports of laparoscopic repair with onlay polypropylene mesh have demonstrated successful repair of traumatic diaphragmatic hernias up to a size of 10 centimeters in patients with high injury severity scores who sustained blunt trauma, suggesting that appropriate patient selection and surgeon skill may allow for successful laparoscopic repair [53].

A laparoscopic approach is not necessarily contraindicated for a chronic diaphragmatic hernia, which has traditionally been addressed with a thoracic approach. Rather, thoracoscopy has the disadvantages of requiring lateral positioning of the patient and single-lung ventilation which could be avoided by using laparoscopy. Chronic hernias may also be repaired laparoscopically if the patient has favorable factors (i.e., location and size of hernia as well as burden of adhesions) and if surgeon experience permits such repair [55]. Matthews et al. showed successful laparoscopic repair of chronic diaphragmatic hernias of various sizes, preferring to use a mesh-based repair for defects larger than 3 × 6 centimeters with no documented recurrences at a mean follow-up period of 8 months [41]. With advancements in laparoscopic surgery and surgeon expertise, it is even possible to repair chronic recurrent traumatic hernias, such as was described by Frantzides et al., who successfully repaired a 8 × 10 centimeter recurrent chronic traumatic diaphragmatic hernia using a 15 × 22 centimeter PTFE mesh [60].

The application of mesh in diaphragmatic injuries secondary to high-velocity trauma may be contraindicated in the setting of solid or hollow viscous injuries given the risk of mesh infection. Biological mesh has been recommended as an alternative to synthetic mesh in hostile environments with high risk of mesh infection. Biological mesh has the ability to incorporate into the surrounding tissues with decreased risks of infection, adhesion, erosion, extrusion, and rejection compared with a synthetic mesh, but there is limited evidence to support its widespread use [53, 61, 62]. We caution against using it as a bridge repair due to remodeling over time.

Postoperative Management, Complications, and Outcomes

Postoperative Management

Postoperative management of patients who sustain diaphragmatic injuries is often complicated due to the injury burden from acute trauma. Fluid management, monitoring of electrolytes, and respiratory support are the cornerstones of management. For open repairs in the acute setting, the mean duration of mechanical respiratory support can be last over a week, and many patients may require tracheostomy to facilitate weaning of ventilator support [63].

The postoperative management of chronic diaphragmatic hernias is much less involved given that they are discovered remote from the initial trauma. Unsurprisingly, a laparoscopic approach is associated with a decreased hospital length of stay when compared with open surgery; the average difference in length of stay may be as upward as 10 days in favor of the laparoscopic group [64].

Complications

Pulmonary complications predominate postoperatively in the acute setting, with atelectasis being the most frequent complication reported. There is also a high incidence of prolonged respiratory failure, with an associated 45% mortality rate. Postoperative sepsis is most often secondary to wound infection and pneumonia [63, 65].

Outcomes from acute traumatic diaphragmatic hernia repair are primarily related to the burden of traumatic injury sustained to the patient. Mortality rates vary from 1% to 28% in the literature [39]. In a case series of 105 patients with traumatic diaphragmatic injury, Hanna et al. found an overall mortality rate of 18.1%, with no significant difference between mechanisms of injury. All of the mortalities had associated injuries requiring operative intervention. Predictors of death for blunt traumatic injury were traumatic brain injury and ISS greater than 15; for penetrating injury, only ISS was found to be a predictor of mortality [42].

Outcomes

Outcomes of traumatic diaphragmatic hernia are difficult to assess owing to poor long-term follow-up of the patient population. Hanna et al. were only able to successfully follow up 13 patients out of 76 patients who were alive at discharge. Two patients were found to have recurrence, and this was attributed to the use of absorbable suture [42].

The literature shows that laparoscopic repairs have a low rate of perioperative complications. At this time, the literature shows that only two studies have reported complications – one of trocar site herniation and the other of pleural effusion [66, 67]. Postoperative follow-up across the literature ranges from 1 week to 42 months with acceptably low recurrence rates, suggesting that the laparoscopic approach is safe and feasible for the repair of traumatic diaphragmatic hernias [64, 68].

Conclusions

Diaphragmatic hernias are rare and due to both congenital and traumatic causes, although the tenets of repair and postoperative management are relatively universal. Most of these hernias can be addressed laparoscopically, but thoracoscopic and open approaches may be needed. Much like in abdominal wall hernia, tissue repair is optimal if it can be accomplished in a tension-free manner, but mesh may be required for larger defects. Outcomes are generally good and recovery based on the operative approach.

References

1. Ashcraft KW, Holcomb GW, Murphy JP, Ostlie DJ, editors. Ashcraft's pediatric surgery. 6th ed. London/New York: Saunders/Elsevier; 2014.
2. Anraku M, Shargall Y. Surgical conditions of the diaphragm: anatomy and physiology. Thorac Surg Clin. 2009;19(4):419–29. https://doi.org/10.1016/j.thorsurg.2009.08.002.
3. Eren S, Çiriş F. Diaphragmatic hernia: diagnostic approaches with review of the literature. Eur J Radiol. 2005;54(3):448–59. https://doi.org/10.1016/j.ejrad.2004.09.008.
4. Downey R. Anatomy of the normal diaphragm. Thorac Surg Clin. 2011;21(2):273–9. https://doi.org/10.1016/j.thorsurg.2011.01.001.
5. Schumpelick V, Steinau G, Schlüper I, Prescher A. Surgical embryology and anatomy of the diaphragm with surgical applications. Surg Clin North Am. 2000;80(1):213–39.
6. Nason LK, Walker CM, McNeeley MF, Burivong W, Fligner CL, Godwin JD. Imaging of the diaphragm: anatomy and function. Radiographics. 2012;32(2):E51–70.

7. Maish MS. The diaphragm. Surg Clin North Am. 2010;90(5):955–68. https://doi.org/10.1016/j.suc.2010.07.005.
8. Perez Cabanas I, de Miguel Velasco M, Rodriguez Garrido J. Perez_Necrosis gastrica total por hernia de Bochdalek.pdf. Necrosis Gástrica Total Por Hernia Bochdalek Estrangulada En El Adulto. 1991;5:385–7.
9. Ferrer A. Alternativas a la polisomnografía convencional en el diagnóstico y tratamiento del síndrome de apneas durante el sueño. Arch Bronconeumol. 1995;31:259–63.
10. Brown SR, Horton JD, Trivette E, Hofmann LJ, Johnson JM. Bochdalek hernia in the adult: demographics, presentation, and surgical management. Hernia. 2011;15(1):23–30. https://doi.org/10.1007/s10029-010-0699-3.
11. Thomas S, Kapur B. Adult Bochdalek hernia—clinical features, management and results of treatment. Jpn J Surg. 1991;21(1):114–9.
12. Fingerhut A, Purcher J, Pelletier J. Deux Obs Hernia Diaphragmatique Postero-Laterale Congenitale Dite Bochdalek Revel L'age. Adulte Par Complicat Sev. 1978;115:135–43.
13. Alfonso L, Centeno C, Alvarez F. Severas malformaciones asociadas a hernia diafragmática congénita: factores condicionantes de mortalidad. An Esp Pedr. 1993;1:22–4.
14. Mullins ME, Saini S. Imaging of incidental Bochdalek hernia. Semin Ultrasound CT MRI. 2005;26(1):28–36. https://doi.org/10.1053/j.sult.2004.10.006.
15. Mullins ME, Stein J, Saini SS, Mueller PR. Prevalence of incidental Bochdalek's hernia in a large adult population. Am J Roentgenol. 2001;177(2):363–6.
16. Swain JM, Klaus A, Achem SR, Hinder RA. Congenital diaphragmatic hernia in adults. Surg Innov. 2001;8(4):246–55.
17. Bujanda L, Larrucea I, Ramos F, Muñoz C, Sánchez A, Fernández I. Bochdalek's hernia in adults. J Clin Gastroenterol. 2001;32(2):155–7.
18. Tokumoto N, Tanabe K, Yamamoto H, Suzuki T, Miyata Y, Ohdan H. Thoracoscopic-assisted repair of a bochdalek hernia in an adult: a case report. J Med Case Rep. 2010;4(1):1.
19. Yamana D, Ohba S. Three-dimensional image of Bochdalek diaphragmatic hernia; a case report. Radiat Med. 1994;12:39–41.
20. Thanakumar J, Krishnan A, John P. Reduced port laparoscopic repair of Bochdalek hernia in an adult: a first report. J Minimal Access Surg. 2012;8(4):158. https://doi.org/10.4103/0972-9941.103131.
21. Al-Emadi M, Helmy I, Abu Nada M, Hamad A-J. Al_Emadi_Laparoscopic repair of Bochdalek Hernia in an Adult.pdf. Surg Laparosc Endosc Percutan Tech. 1999;9(6):423–5.
22. Slesser AA, Ribbans H, Blunt D, Stanbridge R, Buchanan GN. A spontaneous adult right-sided Bochdalek hernia containing perforated colon. JRSM Short Rep. 2011;2(7):54. https://doi.org/10.1258/shorts.2011.011056.
23. Frantzides CT, Carlson MA, Loizides S, et al. Hiatal hernia repair with mesh: a survey of SAGES members. Surg Endosc. 2010;24(5):1017–24. https://doi.org/10.1007/s00464-009-0718-6.
24. Minneci PC, Deans KJ, Kim P, Mathisen DJ. Foramen of Morgagni hernia: changes in diagnosis and treatment. Ann Thorac Surg. 2004;77(6):1956–9. https://doi.org/10.1016/j.athoracsur.2003.12.028.
25. Marin-Blazquez AA, Candel MF, Parra PA, et al. Morgagni hernia: repair with a mesh using laparoscopic surgery. Hernia. 2004;8(1):70–2. https://doi.org/10.1007/s10029-003-0145-x.
26. Horton JD, Hofmann LJ, Hetz SP. Presentation and management of Morgagni hernias in adults: a review of 298 cases. Surg Endosc. 2008;22(6):1413–20. https://doi.org/10.1007/s00464-008-9754-x.
27. Yavuz N, Yigitbasi R, Sunamak O, As A, Oral C, Erguney S. Laparoscopic repair of Morgagni hernia. Surg Laparosc Endosc Percutan Tech. 2006;16(3):173–6.
28. Bortul M, Calligaris L, Gheller P. Laparoscopic repair of a Morgagni-Larrey hernia. J Laparoendosc Adv Surg Tech Part A. 1998;8(5):309–13.
29. Fagelman D, Caridi J. Fagelman_CT diagnosis of hernia of morgagni.pdf. Gastrointest Radiol. 1984;9(1):153–5. https://doi.org/10.1007/BF01887823.
30. Kuster GG, Kline LE, Garzo G. Diaphragmatic hernia through the foramen of Morgagni: laparoscopic repair case report. J Laparoendosc Surg. 1992;2(2):93–100.

31. Orita M, Okino M, Yamashita K, Morita N, Esato K. Laparoscopic repair of a diaphragmatic hernia through the foramen of Morgagni. Surg Endosc. 1997;11(6):668–70.
32. Ackroyd R, Watson D. Ackroyd_Laparoscopic repair of a hernia of Morgagni using a suture technique.pdf. J R Coll Surg Edinb. 2000;45(6):400–2.
33. Ramachandran M, Dip M, Arora V. Ramchandran_Laparoscopic transabdominal repair of hernia of Morgagni-Larrey.pdf. Surg Laparosc Endoscpy Percutaneous Tech. 1999;9(5):358–61.
34. Thoman DS, Hui T, Phillips EH. Laparoscopic diaphragmatic hernia repair. Surg Endosc Interv Tech. 2002;16(9):1345–9.
35. Nguyen T, Eubanks PJ, Nguyen D, Klein SR. The laparoscopic approach for repair of Morgagni hernias. JSLS. 1998;2(1):85–8.
36. Godazandeh G, Mortazian M. Laparoscopic repair of Morgagni hernia using polyvinylidene fluoride (PVDF) mesh. Middle East J Dig Dis MEJDD. 2012;4(4):232–5.
37. Li S, Liu X, Shen Y, Wang H, Feng M, Tan L. Laparoscopic repair of Morgagni hernia by artificial pericardium patch in an adult obese patient. J Thorac Dis. 2015;7(4):754.
38. Percivale A, Stella M, Durante V, et al. Laparoscopic treatment of Morgagni-Larrey hernia: technical details and report of a series. J Laparoendosc Adv Surg Tech. 2005;15(3):303–7.
39. Shah R, Sabanathan S, Mearns A, Choudhury A. Traumatic rupture of diaphragm. Ann Thorac Surg. 1995;60(5):1444–9. https://doi.org/10.1016/0003-4975(95)00629-Y.
40. Rubikas R. Diaphragmatic injuries. Eur J Cardiothorac Surg. 2001;20(1):53–7.
41. Matthews BD, Bui H, Harold KL, et al. Laparoscopic repair of traumatic diaphragmatic injuries. Surg Endosc. 2003;17(2):254–8. https://doi.org/10.1007/s00464-002-8831-9.
42. Hanna WC, Ferri LE, Fata P, Razek T, Mulder DS. The current status of traumatic diaphragmatic injury: lessons learned from 105 patients over 13 years. Ann Thorac Surg. 2008;85(3):1044–8. https://doi.org/10.1016/j.athoracsur.2007.10.084.
43. Thiam O, Konate I, Gueye ML, et al. Traumatic diaphragmatic injuries: epidemiological, diagnostic and therapeutic aspects. Springerplus. 2016;5(1) https://doi.org/10.1186/s40064-016-3291-1.
44. Dirican A, Yilmaz M, Unal B, Piskin T, Ersan V, Yilmaz S. Acute traumatic diaphragmatic ruptures: a retrospective study of 48 cases. Surg Today. 2011;41(10):1352–6. https://doi.org/10.1007/s00595-010-4518-3.
45. Ali S, PS MHK, Lins M. Update on managing diaphragmatic rupture in blunt trauma: a review of 208 consecutive cases. Can J Surg. 2009;52(3):177.
46. Sangster G, Ventura VP, Carbo A, Gates T, Garayburu J, D'Agostino H. Diaphragmatic rupture: a frequently missed injury in blunt thoracoabdominal trauma patients. Emerg Radiol. 2007;13(5):225–30. https://doi.org/10.1007/s10140-006-0548-y.
47. Shapiro M, Heiberg E, Durham R, Luchtefeld W, Mazuski J. The unreliability of CT scans and initial chest radiographs in evaluating blunt trauma induced diaphragmatic rupture. Clin Radiol. 1995;51:27–30.
48. Mihos P, Potaris K, Gakidis J, et al. Traumatic rupture of the diaphragm: experience with 65 patients. Injury. 2003;34(3):169–72.
49. Magu S, Agarwal S, Singla S. Computed tomography in the evaluation of diaphragmatic hernia following blunt trauma. Indian J Surg. 2012;74(4):288–93. https://doi.org/10.1007/s12262-011-0390-7.
50. Murray JG, Caoili E, Gruden JF, Evans SJ, Halvorsen RA Jr, Mackersie RC. Acute rupture of the diaphragm due to blunt trauma: diagnostic sensitivity and specificity of CT. AJR Am J Roentgenol. 1996;166(5):1035–9.
51. Peer SM, Devaraddeppa PM, Buggi S. Traumatic diaphragmatic hernia-our experience. Int J Surg. 2009;7(6):547–9. https://doi.org/10.1016/j.ijsu.2009.09.003.
52. Murray JA, Demetriades D, Asensio JA, et al. Occult injuries to the diaphragm: prospective evaluation of laparoscopy in penetrating injuries to the left lower chest. J Am Coll Surg. 1998;187(6):626–30.
53. Siow SL, Wong CM, Hardin M, Sohail M. Successful laparoscopic management of combined traumatic diaphragmatic rupture and abdominal wall hernia: a case report. J Med Case Rep. 2016;10(1) https://doi.org/10.1186/s13256-015-0780-8.

54. Kishore GSB, Gupta V, Doley RP, et al. Traumatic diaphragmatic hernia: tertiary centre experience. Hernia. 2010;14(2):159–64. https://doi.org/10.1007/s10029-009-0579-x.
55. Zerey M, Heniford BT, Sing RF. Laparoscopic repair of traumatic diaphragmatic hernia. Oper Tech Gen Surg. 2006;8(1):27–33. https://doi.org/10.1053/j.optechgensurg.2006.04.006.
56. Simpson J, Lobo DN, Shah AB, Rowlands BJ. Traumatic diaphragmatic rupture: associated injuries and outcome. Ann R Coll Surg Engl. 2000;82(2):97.
57. Reina A, Vidana E, Soriano P, et al. Traumatic intrapericardial diaphragmatic hernia: case report and literature review. Injury. 2001;32(2):153–6.
58. McCutcheon BL, Chin UY, Hogan GJ, Todd JC, Johnson RB, Grimm CP. Laparoscopic repair of traumatic intrapericardial diaphragmatic hernia. Hernia. 2010;14(6):647–9. https://doi.org/10.1007/s10029-009-0596-9.
59. Carlson MA. Brief clinical report laparoscopic repair of a penetrating injury to the diaphragm: a case report. J Laparoendosc Surg 1994;4(2):153–6.
60. Frantzides C, Madan A, O'Leary P, Losurdo J. Frantzides Laparoscopic repair of a recurrent chronic traumatic diaphragmatic hernia.pdf. February 2003.
61. Zhong T, Janis JE, Ahmad J, Hofer SOP. Outcomes after abdominal wall reconstruction using acellular dermal matrix: a systematic review. J Plast Reconstr Aesthet Surg. 2011;64(12):1562–71. https://doi.org/10.1016/j.bjps.2011.04.035.
62. Garvey PB, Martinez RA, Baumann DP, Liu J, Butler CE. Outcomes of Abdominal Wall reconstruction with acellular dermal matrix are not affected by wound contamination. J Am Coll Surg. 2014;219(5):853–64. https://doi.org/10.1016/j.jamcollsurg.2014.06.021.
63. Rodriguez-Morales G, Rodriguez A, Shatney C. Acute rupture of the diaphragm in blunt trauma: analysis of 60 patients. J Trauma. 1986;26(5):438–44.
64. Liao C-H, Chu C-H, Wu Y-T, et al. The feasibility and efficacy of laparoscopic repair for chronic traumatic diaphragmatic herniation: introduction of a novel technique with literature review. Hernia. 2016;20(2):303–9. https://doi.org/10.1007/s10029-015-1405-2.
65. Sharma O. Sharma_Traumatic diaphragmatic rupture_not an uncommon entity.pdf. J Trauma. 1989;29(5):678–82.
66. Matz A, Alis M, Charuzi I, Kyzer S. The role of laparoscopy in the diagnosis and treatment of missed diaphragmatic rupture. Surg Endosc. 2000;14(6):537–9. https://doi.org/10.1007/s004640000112.
67. Schneider C, Tamme C, Scheidbach H, Delker-Wegener S, Köckerling F. Laparoscopic management of traumatic ruptures of the diaphragm. Langenbeck's Arch Surg. 2000;385(2):118–23.
68. Meyer G, Hüttl TP, Hatz RA, Schildberg FW. Laparoscopic repair of traumatic diaphragmatic hernias. Surg Endosc. 2000;14(11):1010–4. https://doi.org/10.1007/s004640000206.

Expert Commentary: Mesh Reinforcement of Hiatal Closure

24

Mohammed Al Mahroos, Carmen L Mueller, and Gerald M. Fried

Introduction

Laparoscopic paraesophageal hernia (PEH) repair has posed a challenge to surgeons ever since Cuschieri reported the first case in 1992 [1]. To this day, it remains a technically demanding procedure that requires advanced training and expertise [2].

The principles of PEH repair, whether laparoscopic or open, involve primary closure of the hiatus around the esophagus after complete reduction of the hernia sac. However, this repair is associated with a high failure rate, which has led surgeons to use prosthetic graft materials to reinforce the hiatal closure. This approach was extrapolated from success with tension-free mesh repairs of other types of hernias, such as abdominal wall defects. Multiple variations to the traditional PEH repair have been tried, with a view to refine the technique and reduce the risk of recurrence.

Attempts at crural reinforcement date back almost 100 years. Hedblom et al. first used autologous fascia lata in 1925 to buttress the crural closure [3, 4]. Later, prosthetic materials such as tantalum [5], polyvinyl formaldehyde sponge [6], and polytetrafluoroethylene (PTFE) [7] were introduced as reinforcement materials for use at the hiatus. Currently, several different types of prosthetics, in a wide range of materials and sizes, are available for this purpose. Regardless of approach, however, the recurrence rate remains between 20–59% at 5 years [8–12]. For the purpose of this report, we will use the term "mesh" to describe these materials used to support

M. Al Mahroos · C. L. Mueller
Department of General Surgery, McGill University, Montreal, QC, Canada

G. M. Fried (✉)
Department of Surgery, McGill University Health Centre, Montreal, QC, Canada
e-mail: gerald.fried@mcgill.ca

J. Grams et al. (eds.), *The SAGES Manual of Foregut Surgery*,
https://doi.org/10.1007/978-3-319-96122-4_24

the hiatal closure, although some of these products are solid sheets of material with various surfaces designed to promote or discourage ingrowth, while others are truly mesh with various weights and pore sizes.

Despite the high recurrence rate, most recurrences are asymptomatic and infrequently require a repeat operation [13–15]. Moreover, reported sequelae of the use of synthetic materials near the esophagus are not inconsequential and include erosion, perforation, obstruction, and increased risk of major complications at revisional surgery. Bioabsorbable and bioprosthetic meshes seem to be safer than synthetic meshes at the hiatus, but are considerably more costly and may be associated with a higher risk for delayed recurrences.

In this chapter, we will review the literature comparing outcomes of hiatal mesh reinforcement to simple closure during laparoscopic paraesophageal hernia repair.

Synthetic (Nonabsorbable) Mesh

Types

Polypropylene, polytetrafluoroethylene (PTFE), and polypropylene with covalently bonded titanized surface (Timesh ®) are types of synthetic mesh that are commonly used for this purpose.

Impact on Recurrence

Synthetic mesh reinforcement seems to reduce at least short-term recurrences of PEH compared to primary closure alone.

During the 1990s, multiple small series were published regarding the use of synthetic mesh reinforcement during paraesophageal hernia repair [16–19]. These reports were quite heterogeneous, with each group reporting a different technique for reinforcing the hiatus with mesh and each using different materials. These were small case series ($n = 1$–5), and follow-up was limited to 3–6 months. There were no mesh-related complications reported, possibly due to the small number of patients and short follow-up.

Carlson MA et al. [20] reported the very first randomized controlled trial (RCT) of laparoscopic paraesophageal hernia repair with prosthetic reinforcement [20]. These authors randomized 31 patients to posterior cruroplasty vs cruroplasty with mesh reinforcement using polytetrafluoroethylene (PTFE). The mesh was used as onlay reinforcement in a keyhole fashion to accommodate the esophagus. All patients underwent an esophagogastroduodenoscopy (EGD) and esophagogram at 3 months after surgery and every 6 months thereafter, with a median follow-up ranging between 12 and 36 months. No recurrences were reported in the mesh group; three recurrences (18.8%) were reported in the cruroplasty-alone group. Of these, two underwent repeat operative repair for symptoms. Unfortunately, perioperative symptoms and quality of life were not reported in either group, and the definition of "recurrence" was not described.

Since this study, there have been multiple RCTs comparing laparoscopic hiatal hernia repair with mesh to simple closure of the hiatus (Table 24.1). Many of these reported reduced recurrence rates with synthetic mesh and an increased need for reoperation for symptomatic recurrence in patients repaired without mesh [18, 21]. The follow-up intervals in these studies ranges from 6 to 36 months.

Cost

While very few trials report cost of repair with synthetic mesh versus primary closure, use of mesh is logically more costly than primary closure alone. The mesh itself has an inherent cost, and the additional operating room time needed to place the mesh after primary crural closure must be factored in as well. In one study, an additional cost of $1050 USD was estimated with the use of PTFE when compared to primary closure [20]. Another report found use of PTFE for hiatal reinforcement increased case costs by $960+/−70 USD [22]. The additional cost for the mesh techniques needs to be balanced against the substantial cost of reoperation for a symptomatic recurrence. These data are not available.

Synthetic Nonabsorbable Mesh-Related Complications

Several types of complications have been described following crural reinforcement with synthetic mesh during paraesophageal hernia repair. Bleeding, stricture, and erosion of mesh into the stomach or esophagus (Figs. 24.1 and 24.2) are the most commonly reported [21, 23, 24].

Esophageal stenosis causing dysphagia is an oft-described sequela of using synthetic nonabsorbable mesh at the hiatus. These cases frequently require either operative or endoscopic intervention to treat the dysphagia. If the mesh can be removed endoscopically, the resulting stricture may be dilated, potentially avoiding operative intervention. If reoperation is necessary, however, the risk of partial esophagectomy or gastrectomy is high [16, 25–31]. One publication reported 20 cases of mesh-related complications after laparoscopic paraesophageal hernia repair, 8 involving polypropylene and 12 involving PTFE. The complications included mesh erosion in 12 patients and dense fibrosis around the esophagus in the remaining 8, all causing significant dysphagia. Only two of these patients were managed non-operatively [32]. The remaining patients required operations ranging from laparoscopic retrieval of mesh to esophagectomy.

All available RCTs comparing permanent synthetic hiatal mesh to absorbable mesh or no mesh have had short follow-up durations (12–36 months), which may explain the low rate of reported mesh-related complications in these trials. In a recent survey of European surgeons using synthetic mesh for hiatal reinforcement, 523 respondents reported encountering mesh complications at least once in their

Table 24.1 Randomized controlled trials, systematic reviews, and meta-analyses comparing paraesophageal hernia repair with mesh to simple closure of the hiatus

Authors	Year	Type	Inclusion criteria	Exclusion criteria	Mesh used	N	Follow-up	QoL/need for reoperation	Recurrence detection method	Outcomes
Carlson et al.	1999	RCT	Defects >8 cm. Lap PEH with mesh vs no mesh	Defects <8 cm	PTFE	31	12–36 m	NR.	EGD. Esophagogram.	Decreased recurrence with mesh. No mesh-related complication.
Frantzides et al.	2002	RCT	Lap PEH with mesh vs no mesh		PTFE	72	12 m	QoL = NR. Reoperation: 5/8 patients (no mesh group).	EGD. Esophagogram.	Decreased recurrence with mesh. No mesh-related complications.
Graderath et al.	2005	RCT	Lap PEH with mesh vs no mesh	Poor esophageal motility	Polypropylene	100	12 m	QoL = NR. Reoperation: 4/4 (no mesh group).	EGD. Barium swallow.	Decreased recurrence with mesh. More dysphagia with mesh at 1 week,6 weeks, and 3 months.
Oelschlager et al.	2006	RCT	Lap PEH repair with biologic mesh vs no mesh	Recurrence, previous gastric surgery, emergency surgery	Surgisis	108	6 m	QoL = both significantly improved (mesh>none mesh). Reoperation:NA.	UGI series.	Decreased short-term recurrence with mesh. No mesh-related complications.
Oelschlager et al.	2011	RCT-FU	5 years F/u on RCT from 2006		Surgisis	72	5 ys	QoL = no difference. Reoperation: 2/20 no mesh group & 0/14 mesh group.	UGI series.	No difference. No difference in complications.
Antoniou et al.	2012	MA	RCT mesh vs no mesh	None	Variety	267(3 RCTs)	6–12 m	NR.	EGD. Barium swallow.	Decreased recurrence with mesh. Possible more dysphagia with mesh repair.

Furnee et al.	2013	SR	Lap PEH repair with mesh	Studies with <10 pt., emergency surgery	Biomesh and polypropylene	924 (26 study)	25 m	NR.	N/a.	Decreased in short term. Similar long-term recurrence. 0.2% esophageal erosion and 0.5% extensive mesh-related fibrosis.
Watson et al.	2014	RCT	Cruroplasty vs absorbable vs nonabsorbable mesh		Surgisis and Timesh	126	12 m	QoL = NR. Reopration = 0/5.	EGD. Barium swallow.	No difference in recurrence. No difference in complications.
Antoniou et al.	2015	MA	Biologic mesh vs cruroplasty	If no specific f/u modality	Biologic	295(5 studies)	12–36 m	NR.	EGD. Barium swallow.	Decreased short-term recurrence with mesh. No difference in long-term recurrence. Complications not reported.
Koetji et al.	2015	RCT	Cruroplasty vs absorbable vs nonabsorbable		Surgisis and Timesh	126	24 m	QoL = no difference. Reoperation: NR.	EGD. Barium swallow.	No difference in QoL or recurrence. Complications not reported.
Memon et al.	2016	MA	RCTs only, LAP PEH repair with mesh and no mesh	Non randomized reports and emergency cases	Variety	406(4 studies)	6 m	QoL = NR. Reoperation: (OR 3.73) in favor of mesh group	EGD. Barium swallow.	No difference in short-term complications.
Tam et al.	2016	MA	Large PEH repair with mesh vs no mesh	Studies not reporting recurrence	Variety	13 study	6 m–5y	QoL = no difference. Reoperation = no difference.		Available evidence is weak. Cannot routinely recommend mesh.

RCT randomized controlled trials, *SR* systematic review, *MA* meta-analysis

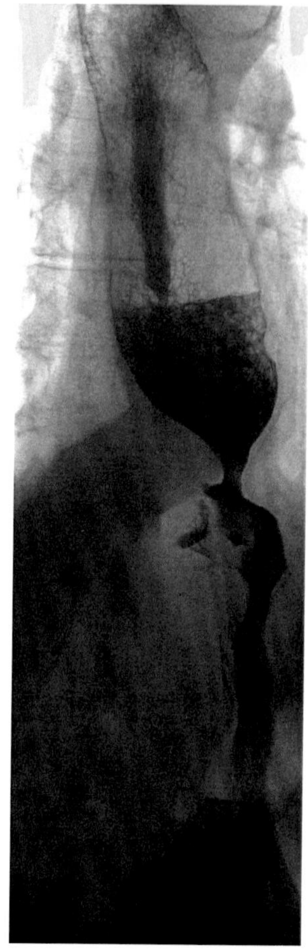

Fig. 24.1 Upper GI study showing severe esophageal stricture caused by synthetic (permanent) mesh used to reinforce the hiatus during HH repair and sleeve gastrectomy

careers. These complications included mesh erosion (21%), esophageal stenosis (25%), mesh infection (7%), and cardiac tamponade (7%) [33]. The respondents to this survey highlight the very real, and often delayed, risk of serious complications of synthetic mesh for paraesophageal hernia repair.

The use of Teflon pledgets has also been associated with complications. In one retrospective review of 1175 cases of laparoscopic paraesophageal hernia repair, 11 patients developed symptoms from Teflon pledgets erosion that occurred more than 2 months after surgery [34]. These patients presented with dysphagia, recurrent symptoms of reflux, and melena.

Absorbable Mesh

Types

Surgisis®, Strattice ™, Alloderm®, and Gore's BioA® are the more commonly reported absorbable products used for hiatal hernia repair.

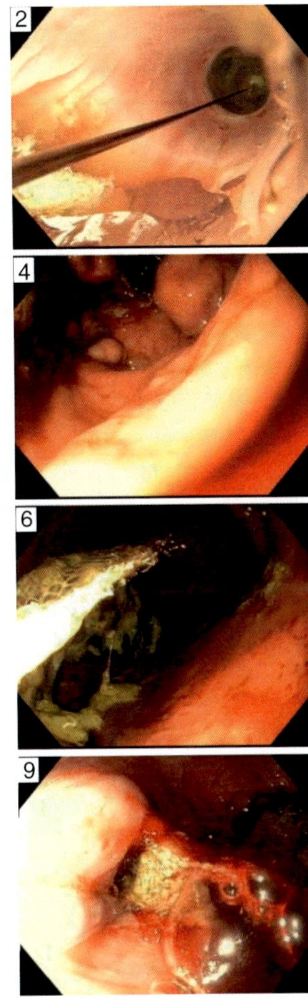

Fig. 24.2 Gastroscopy showing synthetic mesh erosion into the esophagus causing significant stricture. The patient presented with severe dysphagia several years after PEH repair. Multiple endoscopic dilatations were required. The mesh was retrieved endoscopically

Impact on Recurrence

Similarly to synthetic nonabsorbable mesh, multiple RCTs and systematic reviews have been conducted comparing absorbable or biologic mesh to simple closure of the hiatus. The well-known RCT by Oelschlager et al., in 2006 [35], compared Surgisis® to simple closure of the diaphragmatic pillars. In the Surgisis® group, a piece of Surgisis® was prepared and cut in a U configuration. The mesh was then placed with the base of the U overlying the posterior hiatal closure and sutured in place with interrupted sutures. A total of 108 patients were randomized and followed for 6 months. Recurrence was defined as a hiatal hernia >2 cm diagnosed on upper gastrointestinal imaging or the need for reoperation secondary due to wrap disruption, migration, or herniation at any time during the study period. Initial results showed a significantly lower recurrence rate in the mesh group versus the simple closure group (9 vs 24%, $p = 0.04$). Based on these early results, the authors concluded that hiatal reinforcement with Surgisis® resulted in fewer recurrences when compared to simple closure of the hiatus [35]. This trial stimulated enthusiasm for the use of biologic material to supplement crural closure. However, a follow-up study of these same patients examining recurrence rates at 5 years showed no difference between groups [10].

Two RCTs compared synthetic mesh, biologic mesh, and simple closure after PEH repair. These studies found no difference in recurrence rates among all three groups at 12 months [36] and 24 months [11], with recurrence rates ranging from 12% to 30%.

No reports could be found specifically examining the efficacy of bioprosthetic absorbable mesh for crural reinforcement. A retrospective review of a single institution database found no significant difference in hernia recurrence rates or complications with BioA® and biologic meshes [37]. Another retrospective series of 114 patients undergoing both sliding and PEH repair with BioA® mesh reported a recurrence rate of 0.9% with a median follow-up of 1 year. While this low recurrence rate is highly encouraging, this study has several significant limitations, including its retrospective nature, lack of long-term follow-up, and inclusion of small (sliding) hiatal hernias [38]. No mesh-related complications were reported in either series. As prospective data are lacking, no meaningful conclusions can be drawn regarding the efficacy of bioprosthetic mesh for prevention of hiatal hernia recurrence.

Cost

No trials have directly compared cost differences between various mesh repairs versus primary closure alone. However, use of these meshes is clearly more costly than simple primary closure. While costs of materials vary somewhat by region, biologic meshes have been reported to cost up to $1202 USD per case and other materials up to $483 USD [39].

Absorbable Mesh-Related Complications

Mesh-related complications are in general far less common or devastating for absorbable meshes compared to permanent synthetic crural reinforcements. Fibrosis and dysphagia seem to be the most common sequelae of absorbable mesh placed next to the esophagus. One series described four patients who developed dysphagia and pain after paraesophageal hernia repair with absorbable mesh reinforcement. Of these, one required reoperation to remove the mesh as it was determined to be the cause of his dysphagia, and another required multiple endoscopic dilatations [34]. Another series described 6 patients who developed dysphagia due to extensive fibrosis around the gastroesophageal junction after absorbable mesh use [32].

As with randomized controlled trials of permanent mesh for hiatal reinforcement, most RCTs examining outcomes with absorbable mesh report only short-term outcomes. In the Oelschlager 5-year follow-up study of 108 patients randomized to no mesh versus Surgisis reinforcement, no significant mesh-related complications were reported [10]. In general, it seems complications of absorbable mesh occur less frequently, and are less devastating, than those encountered when permanent mesh is used at the hiatus.

Meta-analyses of Randomized Controlled Trials

Since the results of individual RCTs regarding the value of mesh reinforcement at the hiatus have been conflicting, numerous systematic reviews and meta-analyses (SR&MAs) have been conducted [2, 9, 40–43]. Most of these grouped synthetic and biologic meshes together in their analysis of outcomes, and the majority have concluded there is insufficient evidence to support routine mesh reinforcement of any type at the hiatus.

In 2016 alone, there were two such systematic reviews and meta-analyses published [2, 9]. Memon et al. reviewed four randomized controlled trials (406 patients) comparing mesh repair to simple closure during laparoscopic hernia repair [9]. The median follow-up was 6 months. They concluded that all included RCTs suffered from poor methodological quality and that there is presently no evidence to support the routine use of mesh. The report by Tam et al. (2016) analyzed 26 studies comparing mesh repair to simple closure in laparoscopic paraesophageal hernia repair with recurrence as the primary outcome [2]. They found the odds of hernia recurrence in the mesh repair group were 49% less (OR 0.51, 95% CI 0.30 to 0.87; $p = 0.014$) relative to the baseline group of simple repair. However, there was no significant difference in the need for reoperation between mesh and non-mesh groups (odds ratio 0.42, 95% CI 0.13 to 1.37; $p = 0.149$). Furthermore, the included studies were highly variable with respect to type of mesh used, definition of recurrence, and time to objective follow-up, which ranged between 6 and 117 months, such that a favorable conclusion toward mesh repair could not be made. Of the studies included in the same meta-analysis, three studies reported six mesh-related complications including five mesh erosion into the esophagus and one unspecified complication requiring mesh removal [2].

Significance of Hiatal Hernia Recurrence After Paraesophageal Hernia Repair

Recurrence has classically been used as a metric of quality after paraesophageal hernia repair. As such, the goal of paraesophageal hernia repair historically has been to avoid recurrences of any size, even small type I hernias. As described above, the majority of RCTs and other studies examining mesh reinforcement after hiatal closure report follow-up of only ~6–24 months; few of these report on pre- vs postoperative quality of life or symptoms (Table 24.1). The one trial which did report on these outcomes at 5 years in patients receiving biologic vs no mesh found no differences in symptoms, quality of life, or need for reoperation between groups, regardless of hernia recurrence [10].

In the absence of direct data, need for reoperation may be used as a surrogate for poor quality of life or intolerable symptoms. In large series reporting on 5–10 years of follow-up, the rate of reoperation appears to be quite low (0–4.8%) [8, 10]. Furthermore, in studies that have reported long-term quality of life and symptoms scores, these appear to improve and remain stable over time irrespective of hernia recurrence [8, 44–46]. In light of these results, it seems that anatomical recurrence alone is not a sufficient indicator of operative "failure" after PEH repair.

Summary

Despite numerous RCTs and other clinical reports, the available data do not presently support the routine use of mesh for crural reinforcement over primary cruroplasty alone. While synthetic nonabsorbable mesh use has been shown to result in lower anatomic recurrence rates, most recurrences are of little clinical significance and do not warrant the risk of catastrophic complications from permanent mesh placed at the hiatus. Absorbable materials might lessen the risk of serious complications but result in similar long-term recurrence rates to primary closure with considerable additional cost.

As such, it is our opinion, based on the available evidence at this time, that routine mesh reinforcement after primary hiatal hernia repair is of little clinical value and associated with elevated risk of complications and cost. We recommend against the use of permanent mesh entirely and suggest that bioabsorbable meshes be used only selectively.

References

1. Cuschieri A, Shimi S, Nathanson LK. Laparoscopic reduction, crural repair, and fundoplication of large hiatal hernia. Am J Surg. 1992;163(4):425–30.
2. Tam V, Winger DG, Nason KS. A systematic review and meta-analysis of mesh vs suture cruroplasty in laparoscopic large hiatal hernia repair. Am J Surg. 2016;211(1):226–38.
3. Hedblom CA. The selective surgical treatment of diaphragmatic hernia. Ann Surg. 1931;94(4):776–85.
4. Hedblom CA. Diaphragmatic hernia: a study of three hundred and seventy eight cases in which operation was performed. JAMA. 1925;85:947.
5. Fusco EM. The repair of hiatus hernia with tantalum mesh. Mil Med. 1960;125:189–90.
6. Friedman MH, Mackenzie WC. The clinical use of polyvinyl sponge (ivalon) in the repair of oesophageal hiatus hernia. Can J Surg. 1961;4:176–82.
7. Merendino KA, Dillard DH. Permanent fixation by teflon mesh of the size of the esophageal diaphragmatic aperture in hiatus herniplasty; a concept in repair. Am J Surg. 1965;110:416–20.
8. Le Page PA, et al. Durability of giant hiatus hernia repair in 455 patients over 20 years. Ann R Coll Surg Engl. 2015;97(3):188–93.
9. Memon MA, et al. Suture cruroplasty versus prosthetic hiatal herniorrhaphy for large hiatal hernia: a meta-analysis and systematic review of randomized controlled trials. Ann Surg. 2016;263(2):258–66.

10. Oelschlager BK, et al. Biologic prosthesis to prevent recurrence after laparoscopic paraesophageal hernia repair: long-term follow-up from a multicenter, prospective, randomized trial. J Am Coll Surg. 2011;213(4):461–8.
11. Koetje JH, et al. Quality of life following repair of large hiatal hernia is improved but not influenced by use of mesh: results from a randomized controlled trial. World J Surg. 2015;39(6):1465–73.
12. Mattar SG, et al. Long-term outcome of laparoscopic repair of paraesophageal hernia. Surg Endosc. 2002;16(5):745–9.
13. Allison PR. Hiatus hernia: (a 20-year retrospective survey). Ann Surg. 1973;178(3):273–6.
14. Lebenthal A, Waterford SD, Fisichella PM. Treatment and controversies in paraesophageal hernia repair. Front Surg. 2015;2:13.
15. Smith GS, et al. Symptomatic and radiological follow-up after para-esophageal hernia repair. Dis Esophagus. 2004;17(4):279–84.
16. Edelman DS. Laparoscopic paraesophageal hernia repair with mesh. Surg Laparosc Endosc. 1995;5(1):32–7.
17. Paul MG, et al. Laparoscopic tension-free repair of large paraesophageal hernias. Surg Endosc. 1997;11(3):303–7.
18. Frantzides CT, Carlson MA. Prosthetic reinforcement of posterior cruroplasty during laparoscopic hiatal herniorrhaphy. Surg Endosc. 1997;11(7):769–71.
19. Watanabe G, et al. Laparoscopic repair of a paraesophageal hiatus hernia without fundoplication. Surg Today. 1997;27(11):1093–6.
20. Carlson MA, Richards CG, Frantzides CT. Laparoscopic prosthetic reinforcement of hiatal herniorrhaphy. Dig Surg. 1999;16(5):407–10.
21. Granderath FA, et al. Impact of laparoscopic nissen fundoplication with prosthetic hiatal closure on esophageal body motility: results of a prospective randomized trial. Arch Surg. 2006;141(7):625–32.
22. Frantzides CT, et al. A prospective, randomized trial of laparoscopic polytetrafluoroethylene (PTFE) patch repair vs simple cruroplasty for large hiatal hernia. Arch Surg. 2002;137(6):649–52.
23. Arendt T, et al. Dysphagia due to transmural migration of surgical material into the esophagus nine years after Nissen fundoplication. Gastrointest Endosc. 2000;51(5):607–10.
24. Trus TL, et al. Complications of laparoscopic paraesophageal hernia repair. J Gastrointest Surg. 1997;1(3):221–7. discussion 228
25. Carlson MA, et al. Management of intrathoracic stomach with polypropylene mesh prosthesis reinforced transabdominal hiatus hernia repair. J Am Coll Surg. 1998;187(3):227–30.
26. Schauer PR, et al. Comparison of laparoscopic versus open repair of paraesophageal hernia. Am J Surg. 1998;176(6):659–65.
27. Coluccio G, et al. Dislocation into the cardial lumen of a PTFE prosthesis used in the treatment of voluminous hiatal sliding hernia, a case report. Minerva Chir. 2000;55(5):341–5.
28. van der Peet DL, et al. Laparoscopic treatment of large paraesophageal hernias: both excision of the sac and gastropexy are imperative for adequate surgical treatment. Surg Endosc. 2000;14(11):1015–8.
29. Rumstadt B, et al. Gastric mesh erosion after hiatoplasty for recurrent paraesophageal hernia. Endoscopy. 2008;40(Suppl 2):E70.
30. Griffith PS, et al. Rejection of goretex mesh used in prosthetic cruroplasty: a case series. Int J Surg. 2008;6(2):106–9.
31. Tatum RP, et al. Complications of PTFE mesh at the diaphragmatic hiatus. J Gastrointest Surg. 2008;12(5):953–7.
32. Stadlhuber RJ, et al. Mesh complications after prosthetic reinforcement of hiatal closure: a 28-case series. Surg Endosc. 2009;23(6):1219–26.
33. Huddy JR, et al. Laparoscopic repair of hiatus hernia: does mesh type influence outcome? A meta-analysis and European survey study. Surg Endosc. 2016;30(12):5209–21.
34. Antonakis F, Kockerling F, Kallinowski F. Functional results after repair of large hiatal hernia by use of a biologic mesh. Front Surg. 2016;3:16.

35. Oelschlager BK, et al. Biologic prosthesis reduces recurrence after laparoscopic paraesophageal hernia repair: a multicenter, prospective, randomized trial. Ann Surg. 2006;244(4):481–90.
36. Watson DI, et al. Laparoscopic repair of very large hiatus hernia with sutures versus absorbable mesh versus nonabsorbable mesh: a randomized controlled trial. Ann Surg. 2015;261(2):282–9.
37. Jones R, et al. Long-term outcomes of radiologic recurrence after paraesophageal hernia repair with mesh. Surg Endosc. 2015;29(2):425–30.
38. Alicuben ET, Worrell SG, DeMeester SR. Resorbable biosynthetic mesh for crural reinforcement during hiatal hernia repair. Am Surg. 2014;80(10):1030–3.
39. Chiruvella A, Lomelin D, Oleynikov D. A cost-comparison of mesh usage in laparoscopic paraesophageal hernia repair. In: Sages. Boston: Sages Archives; 2016.
40. Antoniou SA, et al. Lower recurrence rates after mesh-reinforced versus simple hiatal hernia repair: a meta-analysis of randomized trials. Surg Laparosc Endosc Percutan Tech. 2012;22(6):498–502.
41. Antoniou SA, et al. Laparoscopic augmentation of the diaphragmatic hiatus with biologic mesh versus suture repair: a systematic review and meta-analysis. Langenbeck's Arch Surg. 2015;400(5):577–83.
42. Rathore MA, et al. Metaanalysis of recurrence after laparoscopic repair of paraesophageal hernia. JSLS. 2007;11(4):456–60.
43. Furnee E, Hazebroek E. Mesh in laparoscopic large hiatal hernia repair: a systematic review of the literature. Surg Endosc. 2013;27(11):3998–4008.
44. Lidor AO, et al. Long-term quality of life and risk factors for recurrence after laparoscopic repair of paraesophageal hernia. JAMA Surg. 2015;150(5):424–31.
45. Targarona EM, et al. Long-term outcome and quality of life after laparoscopic treatment of large paraesophageal hernia. World J Surg. 2013;37(8):1878–82.
46. Mittal SK, et al. Outcomes after repair of the intrathoracic stomach: objective follow-up of up to 5 years. Surg Endosc. 2011;25(2):556–66.

Historical Perspective: Evolution of the Diagnosis and Management of Barrett's Esophagus

25

Reginald C. W. Bell

Introduction

The history of Barrett's esophagus provides insight into current understanding not only of esophageal cancer but also of the anatomy and physiology of hiatal hernia and GERD.

A current definition of Barrett's esophagus is "the condition in which metaplastic columnar epithelium replaces the stratified squamous epithelium that normally lines the distal esophagus and predisposes to cancer development" [36, 39, 43, 48, 49]. Although straightforward, the definition of and ability to precisely identify the esophagogastric junction and agreement on what constitutes metaplastic epithelium that predispose to cancer development remain problematic.

When Norman Barrett first described esophageal ulcers associated with reflux esophagitis, he believed that the esophagus ended at the squamocolumnar junction (SCJ, the top of the columnar epithelium) and that the segment we now call "Barrett's esophagus" was an axially herniated, acid-secreting gastric tube with normal gastric mucosa. There was no mention of extension of columnar epithelium up the esophagus nor of it being metaplastic or predisposing to cancer risk.

Reviewing the history of Barrett's esophagus provides a framework for our current understanding of and confusion about what constitutes Barrett's esophagus. Issues that have arisen during this history include:

1. Whether columnar lining in a tubular section of the foregut represented a tubularized stomach or changes in the esophagus.
2. If the columnar lining was indeed a change in the esophagus, did it represent congenital heterotopic glands or metaplastic change?

R. C. W. Bell
Institute of Esophageal and Reflux Surgery, 499 E Hampden Ave., Suite 400, Englewood 80113, CO, USA
e-mail: reg@iersurgery.com

J. Grams et al. (eds.), *The SAGES Manual of Foregut Surgery*,
https://doi.org/10.1007/978-3-319-96122-4_25

3. If metaplastic change, what was the cause?
4. Whether some extent of columnar mucous but not acid-secreting lining was normal and protective against acid, or whether this cardiac mucosa was a pathologic finding.
5. Whether intestinal metaplasia found on esophageal biopsy is required for the diagnosis of Barrett's.
6. What extent of columnar lined esophagus is required for a diagnosis of Barrett's.
7. Whether cardiac mucosa represents the early stage in the development of Barrett's esophagus.
8. Whether there is a point at which cardiac mucosa will go on to metaplastic, precancerous Barrett's or "regress" to oxyntocardiac mucosa that lacks malignant potential.

Barrett's esophagus is characterized by a metaplastic epithelium in the distal esophagus which may (or may not) be visualized as columnar epithelium during flexible endoscopy. To understand the history, definition, and current controversies surrounding Barrett's esophagus requires an understanding of what defines the gastroesophageal junction and the various histologies present in this region.

Anatomy of the Gastroesophageal Junction

(a) The term "gastroesophageal junction" (GEJ), as it lacks modifiers, implies that there is just one junction. However, the GEJ can be visualized histologically, anatomically, endoscopically, and by manometry. Unfortunately not all these visions coincide and have been one source of confusion.

(b) Anatomic: Most would agree that the anatomic GEJ is where the tubular esophagus ends and the billowing of the proximal stomach starts when examining an ex vivo esophagus and stomach. It is assumed that the transition from two layers of muscularis propria to three layers coincides with the finding of peritoneal lining. In a normal person this would be an oblique junction starting at the angle of His (typically fairly clearly seen) and extending medially and inferiorly toward the lesser curve (where peritoneal lining is used to define the transition). Visualization of the squamocolumnar junction on retroflex view of the distal esophagus is a normal finding indicating the anatomic/endoscopic GEJ. If the squamocolumnar junction is not visualized on retroflexion, this can indicate a fixed hiatal hernia or a condition in which rugal folds extend up the distal esophagus.

(c) Endoscopic: The most commonly used definition of the GEJ is the proximal limit of the rugal folds seen during sedated endoscopy with minimal esophageal distention. McClave in 1987 described a normal SCJ as proximal to within 2 cm of the rugal folds, including in a patient with hiatal hernia [21]. Eventually clinicians decided that the proximal limit of gastric rugal folds reliably coincided with muscular GEJ. The latter is not true.

Using the proximal limit of the rugal folds is recognized as problematic because it will vary with the amount of esophageal distention, the normal slippage of mucosa over the muscularis propria, the presence of a hiatal hernia, and a more recent recognition that rugal folds may be present in a dilated distal esophagus due to longstanding GERD.

The surgeon who performs esophageal surgery is actually fairly well equipped to discern the relation of the start of the rugal folds and the anatomic GEJ by performing flexible endoscopy after division of the phrenoesophageal membrane: with the stomach distended, the endoscope is drawn back until the billowing ends and a tube begins. This almost always corresponds to the angle of His. If rugal folds extend proximally into the tube, this represents development of rugal folds within the distal esophagus (a dilated distal esophagus). Without this maneuver, i.e., during normal endoscopic examination, the uppermost limit of the rugal folds would mistakenly be diagnosed as the GEJ.

(d) Manometric: Esophageal manometry characterizes a high-pressure zone in the distal esophagus which consists of the lower esophageal sphincter and the crural diaphragm. In the absence of a hiatal hernia, the lower end of the high-pressure zone corresponds to the anatomic GEJ. Paull was the first to use manometry to localize esophageal biopsies and in so doing described fundic-type epithelium in the distal esophagus (what is now called oxyntocardiac mucosa). Multiple studies have found a correlation between the length of Barrett' s esophagus and shortening of the lower esophageal sphincter [10, 28].

(e) Histologic: Allison in 1957 argued that columnar lining in the tubular area, which Barrett had thought gastric, was indeed esophageal due to the presence of submucosal glands in this mucus-secreting epithelium. He also found anatomic evidence to support this conclusion.

1. Histology of the Gastroesophageal Junction
   (a) Stratified squamous epithelium: This is a normal epithelium found only in the esophagus. It may have mucosal and submucosal glands. The presence of glands has helped define the anatomic esophagus even when the more superficial region has been superseded by metaplastic epithelium, but may not be seen on routine endoscopic biopsies.
   (b) Oxyntic mucosa: This is a normal columnar epithelium which is composed of parietal and chief, parietal, and mucous cells. The surface and foveolar layers consist of mucous cells; parietal and chief cells are found in straight tubular glands.
   (c) Cardiac mucosa: Once thought a normal finding in the distal esophagus, it is becoming accepted that this is an abnormal, metaplastic epithelium. It is composed of mucous cells (no parietal, chief, or goblet cells). Also called junctional mucosa or mucous-cell-only mucosa, it is seen in the esophagus.
   (d) Oxyntocardiac mucosa, also called fundic-type epithelium: This is an abnormal mucosa comprised of parietal cells and mucous cells. Initially described by Paull in 1976 [29]. It can resemble gastric oxyntic mucosa if there are numerous parietal cells and few mucous cells, in which case the finding of mucous cells mixed with parietal cells within the glands establishes it as oxyntocardiac. The term oxyntocardiac was introduced

in 2000 by Chandrasoma to clarify that this mucosa is only seen in the esophagus proper, and not in the gastric fundus [11].

(e) Esophageal intestinal metaplasia: Often considered the *sine qua non* of Barrett's esophagus, intestinal metaplasia (IM) is characterized by the finding of goblet cells. Goblet cells secrete acid mucin, which distends the lateral borders of the cell creating a goblet appearance. These cells stain with Alcian blue and are also recognized during fluorescein dye infusion using confocal laser endomicroscopy [22, 25]. Early reports recognized this type of epithelium as predisposed to malignancy; by reverse logic it is often seen as necessary finding to diagnose Barrett's esophagus (if Barrett's esophagus is taken to mean any condition in the esophagus that predisposes to malignancy). As we will see, more recent research indicates that cardiac mucosa also predisposes to malignancy [9].

(f) Atrophic oxyntic mucosa, also called atrophic gastritis: This is an abnormal, mucous-cell-only epithelium with loss of parietal cells, and so may resemble cardiac mucosa, which is also a mucous-cell-only epithelium. Atrophic gastritis has a flat surface and involves large areas of the stomach, compared to cardiac mucosa, which is hyperplastic, often inflammatory, and limited to the distal esophagus and 3 cm distal to the currently defined esophagogastric junction. Atrophic gastritis can be a result of *H. pylori* infection or autoimmune gastritis.

(g) Gastric intestinal metaplasia: Consisting of goblet cells in oxyntic mucosa. It is typically seen in severe cases of atrophic gastritis where there is parietal cell loss. When parietal cells are seen, the diagnosis is clear; otherwise the distinction from esophageal intestinal metaplasia (Barrett's esophagus) can be difficult [10] (Table 25.1).

Table 25.1 Table of epithelial types in the region of the GEJ

Cell type	Defining cell type	Location	Additional characteristics	
Squamous epithelium	Squamous	Esophagus	Submucosal glands	Ki67 only in suprabasal region
Intestinal metaplasia	Goblet cells	Esophageal	Within cardiac mucosa	
		Gastric	Within (atrophic) oxyntic mucosa	
Cardiac	Mucous cells, no parietal or goblet cells	Esophagus	Carditis – inflammatory cells	
Oxyntocardiac	Mucous and parietal cells, no chief cells	Esophagus	Paull: atrophic epithelium	
Oxyntic	Parietal and chief cells	Gastric		
Atrophic oxyntic	Oxyntic but with some or complete loss of parietal cells, may have only mucous cells or goblet cells (IM)	Gastric		Associated with *H. pylori*

Synopsis of Errors Along the Way

1. Barrett thinks that the esophagus ends at the squamocolumnar junction.
   (a) Barrett corrects that idea and agrees peritoneal lining is good definition.
2. Barrett and Allison think that this columnar epithelium in the distal esophagus is gastric (acid-secreting) in nature.
3. Barrett and Allison among others believe the columnar epithelium to be congenital.
4. The terms gastric and fundic mucosa become used indiscriminately, with varied interpretations.
5. Hayward advocates that up to 2 cm of mucus-secreting epithelium in the distal esophagus is normal, protecting proximal squamous epithelium from gastric acid. Thus mucus-secreting epithelium without parietal cells (now called cardiac mucosa) is largely ignored.
6. A research criterion – 3 cm of columnar lined esophagus – becomes a de facto requirement for Barrett's esophagus. Along with Hayward's position that up to 2 cm of columnar lined esophagus is normal, columnar lined esophagus of <3 cm is largely ignored.
7. Although the association of Barrett's esophagus with severe reflux disease was correct, many incorrectly assumed that Barrett's would only be seen in patients with severe reflux disease.
8. Intestinal metaplasia (presence of goblet cells) transitioned from being the most common and easiest to identify criterion for Barrett's esophagus to being the *sine qua non* and became required for the diagnosis of Barrett's. (Correctly, intestinal metaplasia does seem to have the highest risk of developing cancer.)

Preview of Key Insights

1. Barrett recognizes that there is something different about the lining below certain types of mid-esophageal ulcers.
2. Allison posits that the peritoneal reflection defines gastroesophageal junction and finds that columnar epithelium extends proximal to the gastroesophageal junction. Barrett agrees.
3. Hayward posits correctly that columnar epithelium in the esophagus is metaplastic.
4. Paull confirms that junctional mucosa (now called cardiac mucosa) and gastric fundic-type mucosa (now called oxyntocardiac mucosa) are present in the manometrically defined lower esophagus. When present, IM was always above junctional mucosa which when present was always above gastric fundic-type mucosa.
5. Spechler et al. find that intestinal metaplasia is present in patients with <3 cm of columnar lined esophagus, including those without severe reflux disease.
6. Chandrasoma argues that cardiac mucosa results from injury to the esophagus. The histologic criterion for the esophagogastric junction, which was only described previously (and incorrectly) by Norman Barrett as the end of

squamous epithelium, is now reversed: the EGJ is defined as the start of gastric epithelium defined by the presence of parietal (oxyntic) cells. Anything above this is acquired due to reflux damage and has the potential for increasing the risk of adenocarcinoma.

Norman Barrett's Personal Life

Norman Barrett was a pioneer in thoracic surgery whose contributions extended well beyond the condition that bears his name. Born in Australia in 1903, he received his medical training in England and the USA. In 1948 he founded the first thoracic surgery department at St. Thomas Hospital in London. He was the first editor of the journal *Thorax* and remained so for 25 years. Many of the early articles pertinent to the history of Barrett's esophagus were published in *Thorax*. His contributions to thoracic surgery included a technique for enucleation of pulmonary hydatid cysts, known as "the Barrett technique." He performed the first successful repair of a Boerhaave's perforation of the distal esophagus. Barrett was instrumental in the acceptance of Heller's myotomy over esophagogastrostomy for achalasia [20].

A General History of Barrett's Esophagus

Norman Barrett's first description of reflux-induced change in the esophagus was not that of columnar lining, but of peptic ulcer. Antedating Barrett's pivotal 1950 description, Albers in 1839 described peptic ulcer of the esophagus [3], and Tileston described 3 cases of peptic ulcer of the esophagus associated with gastric-type epithelium and thought the ulceration is due to incompetence of the cardia, i.e., to GERD [47].

Allison in 1948 described various types of hiatal hernia and also heterotopic (not metaplastic) gastric mucosa [1]. Allison believed that a short esophagus was not congenital but secondary to acquired sliding hernia leading to peptic injury with associated contraction. He refuted the current concept that these ulcers were due to congenital shortening of the esophagus leading to gastric reflux. He proposed instead that acquired hiatal hernia led to incompetence of the cardia and gastric reflux.

Norman Barrett in 1950 described ulcers associated with reflux esophagitis with resultant circumferential and longitudinal stricture, pulling the stomach up above the hiatus resulting in a tubularized stomach covered by peritoneum [3]. He defined the esophagus as that portion of foregut lined by squamous epithelium that was distal to cricopharyngeus. As the descriptions entailed patients with peptic ulcers or strictures, the gastric-type epithelium in this gastric tube was, not illogically, considered to be acid-secreting gastric mucosa.

Allison and Johnstone 1953 in an article titled "The Oesophagus Lined with Gastric Mucous Membrane" described a segment of columnar lined esophagus (CLE) interposed between the squamocolumnar junction and the stomach [2]. Their criteria for considering this columnar lining to be esophagus included (1) a lack of peritoneal lining, (2) the presence of longitudinal and circular musculature of normal esophagus, (3) findings of islands of squamous epithelium in this area, (4) a lack of oxyntic cells, and (5) the presence of typical esophageal mucous glands in the submucosa. This gastric-type lining of the esophagus (though lacking oxyntic cells) was considered at the time most often congenital and not acquired. The ulcerations were always associated with hiatal hernia, and so it was also not clear to what extent the gastric-type lining or the hernia contributed to the ulcers. This was also called "gastric mucosa of the cardiac type" and was considered to be in the esophagus. Though gastric mucosa in the esophagus was recognized as heterotopic and not normal, it was not yet understood to be acquired or metaplastic. The article discusses whether peptic ulcer healing in an acid environment would be with gastric or squamous epithelium, and if the former, then gastric mucosa in the esophagus could be an acquired condition and "calls for further investigation." The term "Barrett's ulcers" is introduced in reference to chronic esophageal ulcers occurring in the gastric lined portion of the esophagus. Unlike peptic ulcers of the esophagus, Barrett's ulcers were more likely to bleed or perforate. One patient developed cancer – called a gastric cancer – in this paper. The paper contains pathologic descriptions of seven patients and refers to cardiac mucosa without oxyntic glands, sometimes with goblet cells.

Barrett's 1957 paper "The Lower Esophagus Lined by Columnar Epithelium" recognized Allison and Johnson's research. Barrett reversed his earlier belief that the gastric lined tube was the stomach and agreed that it indeed was a portion of the esophagus. He suggested the term "columnar epithelium" as it was descriptive and without an etiologic implication [4]. Barrett thought the best etiologic explanation was congenital, "the result of a failure of the embryonic lining of the gullet to achieve normal maturity." He discusses but ultimately rejects the idea that damage to the esophagus could result in replacement of squamous epithelium by the more quickly growing columnar epithelium. Thus "Barrett's ulcer" became "Barrett's esophagus" denoting columnar lining of the lower esophagus. Both Allison and Barrett recognized the possibility that columnar epithelium was acquired and due to reflux, but still felt it was congenital. By the 1960s columnar epithelium was recognized to be an acquired condition due to reflux injury with subsequent healing with a mucous lined epithelium that was protective against further peptic injury.

Hayward, in 1961, in an editorial that was conceptual rather than based in science, described columnar transformation of the esophagus as a sequence related to peptic injury and was the first to argue that this was "metaplastic" [17]. Important aspects of this paper are as follows: (1) He defines EGJ anatomically, not related to mucosa changes, as end of the tube. (2) He advocates getting rid of the term "cardia" as it is a vague anatomic entity. (3) He recognizes that mucosa slides up and down up to 2 cm in normal swallowing. (4) He proposes that it is normal for there to be a section of columnar epithelium interposed between squamous and oxyntic mucosa, composed of mucous cells without oxyntic cells. Columnar epithelium is a normal and necessary protective boundary between acid-producing gastric mucosa and acid-sensitive squamous epithelium. This portion of the esophagus would typically be lined by what he terms "junctional" epithelium (mucus-secreting epithelium, devoid of oxyntic cells; mention is not yet made of goblet cells). As peptic injury progresses up the esophagus, healing occurs in a metaplastic fashion, and this junctional mucosa extends ever proximally. Hayward thought this approach had the following implications: (1) Carcinoma of the cardia should be regarded as a variant of esophageal cancer. (2) Reflux injury leads to proximal extension of the junctional epithelium. It is not congenital ectopic tissue. (3) Were it congenital ectopic tissue, then any treatment of complications (ulcer or stricture) should involve resection of this tissue on the other hand, if it is acquired, then surgery to correct reflux might be more appropriate, and might lead to regression of junctional epithelium. In retrospect, the introduction of the concept of "junctional" epithelium still left confusion on whether even a small amount of mucus but non-acid-producing epithelium just below squamous epithelium was normal (implication, congenital) or acquired (metaplastic) (Fig. 25.1).

Actual proof that columnar lined esophagus could be acquired awaited the work of Cedric Bremner, who induced columnar lined epithelium in dogs by surgically creating an incompetent sphincter and reflux [8].

With evolving recognition that a segment of columnar lined esophagus (CLE) was present in some patients – typically those with hiatal hernia and reflux – a better understanding of the cell types comprising this segment evolved. Barrett and Allison both had considered this segment to be acid-secreting gastric epithelium, though possibly producing more mucus and less acid than typical gastric epithelium. Bosher and Taylor in 1951 were the first to describe goblet cells in columnar lined esophagus [6]. Morson and Belcher in 1952 described an esophageal adenocarcinoma surrounded by intestinal-type epithelium with goblet cells [23]. Hayward in his 1961 editorial describes junctional mucosa as comprised of mucus-secreting cells, devoid of acid-secreting oxyntic cells, but does not mention goblet cells.

Paull in 1976 was the first to report findings in biopsies of patients with Barrett's esophagus in which the biopsies were guided specifically by esophageal manometry. The paper describes the following types of mucosa present in or above the manometrically determined lower esophageal sphincter:

- Distinctive specialized columnar epithelium with a villiform surface, mucous glands, Alcian blue-staining intestinal-type goblet cells, and no parietal or chief cells.
- Cardiac mucosa (Hayward's junctional type) composed only of mucus cells. No oxyntic (parietal, acid-secreting) cells.
- Gastric fundic-type epithelium with parietal cells and mucus. This is currently also called oxyntocardiac mucosa. In areas where parietal cells were present, the epithelium was markedly atrophic, and so not the same as true normal gastric fundic epithelium.

When present, specialized columnar epithelium was always the most proximal, and gastric fundic epithelium the most distal epithelium in Paull's description. Junctional (aka cardiac) epithelium was interposed between gastric fundic and specialized columnar or squamous epithelium [29]. Although this may seem straightforward, gastric fundic epithelium has oxyntic and mucus cells and when atrophic can have goblet cells. Junctional epithelium could only be distinguished from atrophic gastric epithelium if no oxyntic cells were seen on biopsy. At this point the concept of carditis – that junctional epithelium was inflammatory and so abnormal and metaplastic – had not been introduced.

As endoscopy became more prevalent, the need arose to define Barrett's esophagus based on endoscopic rather than surgical resection or autopsy findings. Biopsies of mucosa alone could not – at this time – distinguish normal gastric mucosa from metaplastic esophageal epithelium unless goblet cells were seen. Routine endoscopic biopsies do not extend deeply enough to pick up what are considered to be reliably defining characteristics of the esophagus – submucosal glands, circular and longitudinal muscularis, much less peritoneum or lack thereof (thank goodness!). An unreliable and variable endoscopic landmark – the start of the rugal folds – became the de facto definition of the gastroesophageal junction. Issues with using endoscopic landmarks include variability of the proximal extent of rugal folds with varying esophageal distention and mucosal slippage over the

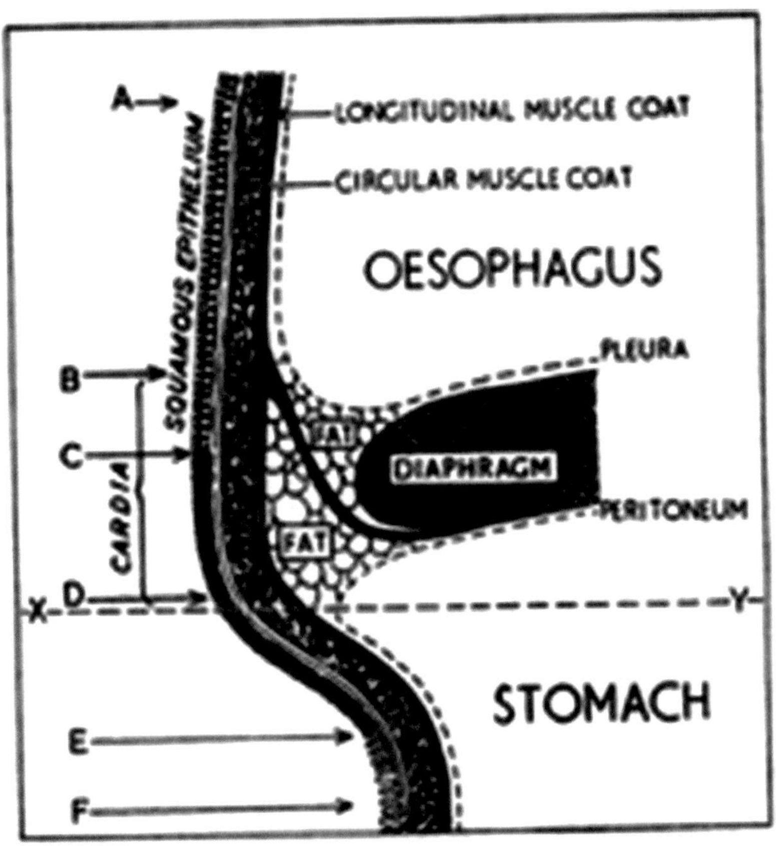

Fig. 25.1 Hayward's conception of junctional epithelium [17]

muscularis during swallowing. Hayward's influence had led to the belief that 2 cm of junctional mucosa was normal. Recognizing the inherent limitations in endoscopic biopsies and wishing to avoid confounding factors including false-positive biopsies of goblet cell gastric mucosa, researchers required a minimum of 3 cm of columnar lined esophagus to include a patient in studies of Barrett's esophagus [41]. By the early 1990s, this minimum of 3 cm of columnar lined esophagus evolved from a research criterion to a clinical definition of Barrett's [30]. Endoscopists tended to ignore and not biopsy columnar epithelium of less than 3 cm. As Barrett's esophagus had been associated with severe GERD, patients with minimal GERD symptoms were also ignored.

In 1994 Spechler et al. challenged the concept of the 3 cm rule by performing routine biopsies of patients (not just those with severe GERD) with less than 3 cm of columnar lined epithelium and found intestinal metaplasia in 18% [44]. This somewhat unexpected finding, present even in patients with no signs or symptoms of GERD, was subsequently confirmed by other investigators [31, 32, 50]. The concept and terminology of short-segment Barrett's esophagus (SSBE) (< 3 cm of IM) emerged, and IM of ≥ 3 cm termed long-segment Barrett's esophagus (LSBE). The association of Barrett's esophagus of any length with increased esophageal acid exposure (81% in SSBE, 100% in LSBE) and decreased LES competency led to Barrett's esophagus being diagnostic of GERD and an indication for treatment outside of pH testing [12].

Nandurkar in 1997, using Alcian blue staining as the standard to identify goblet cells, found that 50% of Barrett's would be missed by H&E staining alone [25]. Alcian blue staining replaced H&E staining as the criterion for goblet cells.

Since the clinical importance of Barrett's esophagus was related to its precancerous condition, and goblet cells were the hallmark of Barrett's esophagus, clinicians tended to regard any biopsy of the distal esophagus showing goblet cells "Barrett's," regardless of its visible extent. To help eliminate false-positive biopsies of gastric epithelium, some investigators wished to maintain a minimum of 1 cm of columnar lined esophagus. To a certain extent, this concern about the potential for false-positive biopsies holds true today in the recommendaton advanced by some GI societies not to biopsy a normal-appearing SCJ [38].

Should any finding of goblet cells in biopsies of the EGJ should be considered Barrett's esophagus and not gastric IM due to atrophic gastritis? As adenocarcinoma has developed in patients with goblet cells found on routine biopsies of the EGJ, consensus has developed that goblet cell metaplasia should be considered Barrett's esophagus regardless of length. Should cardiac mucosa be considered metaplastic and having premalignant potential? Work by Chandrasoma and others has demonstrated that cardiac mucosa is indeed metaplastic. Hence the current definition of Barrett's esophagus as "the condition in which any extent of metaplastic columnar epithelium that predisposes to cancer development replaces the stratified squamous epithelium that normally lines the distal esophagus" [43].

Early investigators postulated that gastric-type epithelium migrated proximally onto GERD-damaged epithelium [2]. The current hypothesis is that GERD damages the squamous epithelium resulting in the exposure of multipotential stem cells in the basal layer to refluxed gastric juice, triggering abnormal, metaplastic differentiation [18, 35].

It is interesting that, in an era of DNA analysis, the most specific diagnostic criterion for Barrett's esophagus is still the finding of goblet cells on biopsy, a concept introduced in 1951. This is true not only in the clinical setting but in the research setting, where various markers such as p53 have proved neither more specific nor predictive of the risk of developing Barrett's, nor of it progressing to dysplasia [42].

IM, Barrett's, and Risk of Adenocarcinoma

Small case series such as those of Barrett and Allison in the 1950s included patients with adenocarcinoma within a segment of columnar lined esophagus, but the cancers were thought to be gastric in origin based on the belief that columnar lined esophagus was congenital gastric-type mucosa. Morson and Belcher in 1952 may have been the first to describe an esophageal adenocarcinoma arising in the presence of goblet cells [23]. Barrett in 1957 posited that adenocarcinomas arising in columnar lined epithelium above the GEJ were not due to upward growth of a gastric cancer, but arose *de novo* in columnar lined esophagus. He based this concept on his finding adenocarcinomas in the proximal region of columnar lined esophagus that did not extend down to the GEJ, and were amenable to resection [4].

During the 1970s case reports of finding dysplasia or esophageal adenocarcinoma in Barrett's epithelium emerged [5, 16, 29]. By the 1980s it was fairly widely accepted that esophageal adenocarcinoma was found in the presence of surrounding IM, that the IM often exhibited dysplasia, and that therefore IM was the precursor of esophageal adenocarcinoma. IM became the *sine qua non* of clinically significant BE. Goblet cells in IM were easily identifiable. As there was no known role for cardiac or fundic-type epithelium in the course of esophageal injury, these epithelial types were largely ignored by clinicians and researchers.

Gastric cardia adenocarcinomas had been considered gastric in origin, even though they typically involved the distal esophagus. Clark in 1994 reported findings of IM in 42% of cardiac cancers and 79% of esophageal cancers, but only 5% of subcardiac carcinomas [13]. Subsequent confirmatory studies led to the reclassification of cardiac cancers from being of gastric to esophageal in origin, and to an understanding of GERD as the etiology of these cancers [45].

After Spechler's finding of intestinal metaplasia in patients with minimal visible columnar epithelium, short-segment Barrett's esophagus (SSBE) also came to be regarded as a premalignant condition. Weston in 1997 found dysplasia at presentation in 8% of SSBE *v* 24% of LSBE, though only the LSBE went on to develop HGD or adenocarcinoma [51]. Sharma found a similar prevalence of dysplasia in SSBE, an incidence of 5.7%/year, and progression to HGD and adenocarcinoma. The need for surveillance in SSBE, as was being done for LSBE, was established [40].

Barrett's esophagus circa 2,000 was defined as the presence of intestinal metaplasia in any visible area of columnar epithelium that was present above the GEJ, the GEJ understood to be the proximal limits of the rugal folds at endoscopy.

Three questions arise from this definition that persist today regarding the risk of cancer: (1) What is the risk of intestinal metaplasia progressing to cancer if the biopsy is taken from an endoscopically normal esophagus without visible columnar lined esophagus? If present, how should this be followed or treated? (2) If there is visible columnar lined esophagus without IM on biopsy, is this still a condition that predisposes to cancer and so falls under the clinical definition of Barrett's? (3) Are there other cellular and epithelial findings that predispose toward the development of adenocarcinoma?

(1) The malignant potential of intestinal metaplasia on a biopsy of a normal-appearing SCJ remains enigmatic. From a scientific point of view, it would make sense to biopsy patients with a normal SCJ and follow them to see if those with IM have any increased risk of malignancy. Perhaps because of increased sampling error, perhaps because of economic/cost issues of surveillance in this patient population, scientific rigor has been overruled in clinical practice. Consider the 2011 American Gastroenterological Association's technical review on the management of Barrett's esophagus: "The inclusion of patients with cardia-type epithelium under the rubric of 'Barrett's esophagus' would substantially increase the number of patients with that disorder, which would substantially increase treatment costs. The benefits of surveillance and treatment programs for Barrett's esophagus are debated, even for patients with intestinal metaplasia, whose cancer risk is far better defined. The likelihood of finding intestinal-type epithelium in Barrett's esophagus varies directly with the extent of the esophageal columnar lining, and the issue of whether to consider cardia-type epithelium a marker for Barrett's esophagus usually concerns only patients with short segments of esophageal columnar epithelium (generally segments considerably less than 3 cm in extent). The clinical benefit of biopsy sampling for patients with such short segments of esophageal columnar epithelium has not been established [43]." The British Society of Gastroenterology recommends that even an irregular Z-line with tongues less than 1 cm should not be biopsied because the clinical significance of IM in this region is unclear. "Surveillance is generally not recommended in patients with IM at the cardia or in those with an irregular Z-line regardless of the presence of IM (Recommendation grade C)" [14].

(2) Lack of IM on biopsies of visible columnar lined esophagus probably indicates a sampling error. When followed, most patients will demonstrate IM on subsequent biopsies [14]. When IM is not present in these biopsies, cardiac mucosa is typically found.

(3) There is increasing evidence that cardiac mucosa, once considered a normal finding, is not only pathologic but predisposes to malignancy. In the earliest part of disease, injured esophageal squamous epithelium heals as cardiac mucosa, with inflammatory cells seen deeper in the epithelium. Histochemical and genetic studies of cardia-type epithelium have revealed DNA and other abnormalities (villin, CDX2) similar to those found in specialized intestinal metaplasia, abnormalities that may predispose to cancer development [15, 19]. Clinical evidence that cardiac mucosa may have by itself an increased risk of malignancy was found by

Takubo. Of 141 patients with minute (mucosal) Barrett's Epithelium, more than 70% of primary small adenocarcinomas (<2 cm) of the esophagus were adjacent to cardiac/fundic-type rather than intestinal-type mucosa. Moreover, intestinal metaplasia was not observed in any areas of the endoscopic mucosal resection specimens in 64 (56.6%) of the 113 cases [46]. Not all studies have confirmed this [24].

Development of Treatment of Barrett's Esophagus

In the 1950s the only treatment for Barrett's ulcers and strictures refractory to dilation was esophagectomy. Columnar lined epithelium per se needed no treatment. Recognition that Barrett's was an acquired condition and not congenital led to the concept that it might be prevented or at least treated by methods other than resection.

As acid-suppressive medications became more common, the severe ulcers and strictures requiring resection seen in the 1950s became less common, and are rarely seen today.

As recognition of the malignant potential of Barrett's esophagus increased and as flexible endoscopy became more widespread, surveillance programs were developed including the Seattle Protocol.

The question then emerged regarding when dysplastic Barrett's merited esophagectomy as opposed to continued surveillance. Findings on esophagectomy specimens performed for HGD demonstrated invasive adenocarcinoma in 50% of cases, and surgeons argued that esophagectomy was the appropriate treatment for HGD [26].

If Barrett's esophagus and subsequent dysplasia resulted from damaged squamous epithelium exposed to uncontrolled exposure to gastric contents, then it was not illogical to think that re-injury to the Barrett's esophagus in the setting of controlled exposure to gastric contents (typically PPI therapy) might allow the esophagus to heal with more normal, neo-squamous epithelium with elimination of or prevention of dysplasia. In the early 1990s, endoscopic laser therapy was the first energy source to be reported effective in ablating Barrett's esophagus [7, 34]. Sampliner reported ablation of Barrett's and subsequent healing with normal squamous epithelium using multipolar electrical cautery in 1996 [33].

The use of laser or multipolar cautery was tedious as it applied pin-point energy to a broad area. The earliest broad-based energy source employed visible light to a broad area of Barrett's esophagus that had been subjected to a cytotoxic photosensitizing agent. These cytotoxic photosensitizers such as porfimer sodium were selectively retained by neoplastic tissue, enabling somewhat selective killing of neoplastic cells. However, the photosensitizing agents remained in the skin for extended periods (up to a month with porfimer), making patients sensitive to ambient sunlight or even strong indoor light. Additionally, depth of injury was not predictable, and strictures occurred in up to 30% of patients so treated [27].

Ablation of defined yet broad areas of Barrett's became facile with endoscopically guided catheters consisting of evenly spaced radial electrodes that delivered radiofrequency energy along the length of the electrodes (up to 3 cm). Barrx RFA provided a controlled depth of burn, with a stricture rate of 8% or less. Multiple studies have demonstrated its efficacy in treating high-grade dysplasia, low-grade dysplasia, and even non-dysplastic Barrett's [37].

The development of techniques to resect larger areas of esophageal mucosa (endoscopic mucosal resection, EMR) has enabled both tissue diagnosis and the ability to remove nodular lesions not amenable to ablation techniques. A combination of EMR and ablation can provide the most comprehensive method to deal with Barrett's esophagus, and both techniques will be discussed in another chapter.

Summary

One cannot appreciate the history of Barrett's esophagus without some understanding of histology. Current controversies regarding the diagnosis and management of Barrett's, and regarding the malignant potential of reflux-induced injury to the esophagus, become more clear with a historical perspective.

The history of Barrett's esophagus has propelled us from a belief that columnar lined epithelium around certain ulcers was congenital, anatomically stomach, and of gastric cell type, to a knowledge that it is acquired, anatomically esophagus, and comprised of metaplastic esophageal epithelium. Cardiac epithelium was considered to be a normal, protective barrier; now it is being recognized as abnormal and likely having malignant potential. Early researchers defined columnar lined esophagus as the end of squamous epithelium and ignored when it ended; current research is focused on when metaplastic changes start distally at the junction with gastric oxyntic mucosa. We have probably gone backward in other ways: Early anatomic descriptions wherein all layers of the esophagus were analyzed to determine the GEJ have given way to less precise, unreliable endoscopic finding based on mucosal folds. We have also probably gone backward in basing our current understanding and tenets about a "normal squamocolumnar junction" and its potential to be considered Barrett's esophagus not upon routine scientific studies, but upon society recommendations that certain areas not be routinely studied.

Looking ahead, the concept, championed by Chandrasoma and others, that cardiac mucosa is due to reflux injury, is metaplastic, and predisposes to cancer seems to be gaining acceptance and will likely change the definition of Barrett's once again. The search for molecular markers will hopefully supplant the stalwart goblet cell as the defining characteristic of this entity which still bears Norman Barrett's name (Figs. 25.2, 25.3, 25.4, and 25.5).

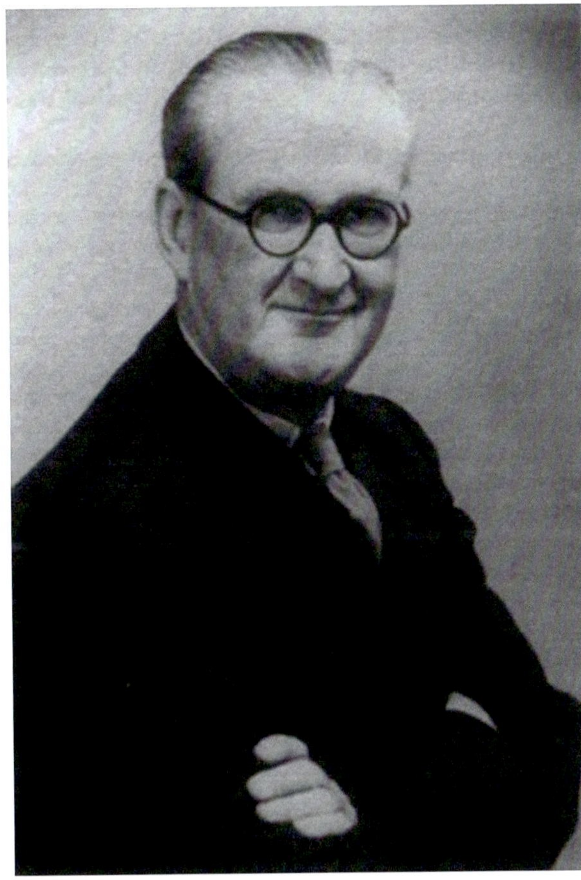

Fig. 25.2 Norman Barrett in 1958, age about 55 [20]

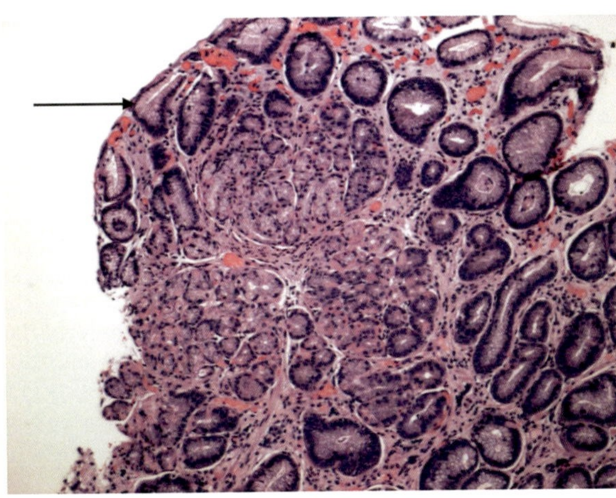

Fig. 25.3 Oxyntocardiac mucosa

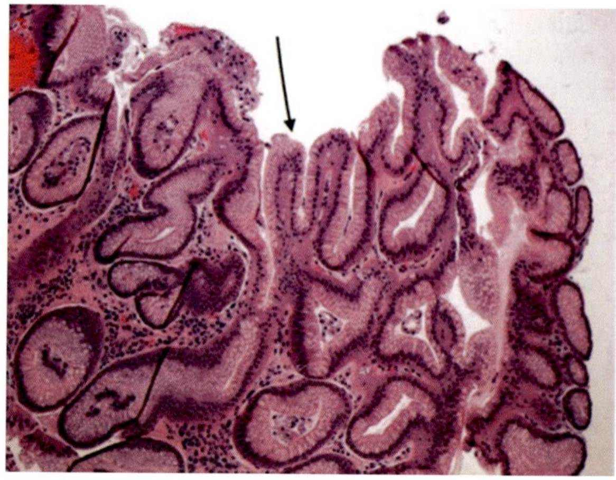

Fig. 25.4 Cardiac mucosa. Palisding rows of mucus-secreting cells illustrated by arrow

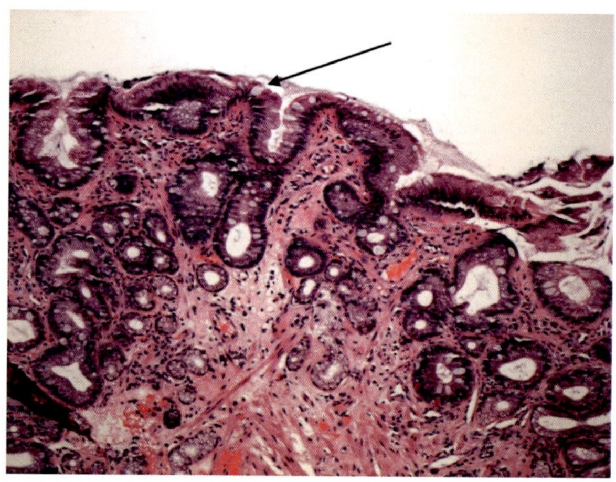

Fig. 25.5 Intestinal metaplasia. Goblet cell is illustrated by arrow

References

1. Allison PR. Peptic ulcer of the oesophagus. Thorax. 1948;3:20–42.
2. Allison PR, Johnstone AS. The oesophagus lined with gastric mucous membrane. Thorax. 1953;8:87–101.
3. Barrett NR. Chronic peptic ulcer of the oesophagus and 'oesophagitis'. Br J Surg. 1950;38:175–82.
4. Barrett NR. The lower esophagus lined by columnar epithelium. Surgery. 1957;41:881–94.
5. Belladonna JA, Hajdu SI, Bains MS, Winawer SJ. Adenocarcinoma in situ of Barrett's esophagus diagnosed by endoscopic cytology. N Engl J Med. 1974;291:895–6.
6. Bosher LH, Taylor FH. Heterotopic gastric mucosa in the esophagus with ulceration and stricture formation. J Thorac Surg. 1951;21:306–12.
7. Brandt LJ, Kauvar DR. Laser-induced transient regression of Barrett's epithelium. Gastrointest Endosc. 1992;38:619–22.
8. Bremner CG, Lynch VP, Ellis FH Jr. Barrett's esophagus: congenital or acquired? An experimental study of esophageal mucosal regeneration in the dog. Surgery. 1970;68:209–16.

9. Chandrasoma P. Pathophysiology of Barrett's esophagus. Semin Thorac Cardiovasc Surg. 1997;9:270–8.
10. Chandrasoma PD, Demeester TR. GERD: Reflux to Adenocarcinoma. Amsterdam: Elsevier; 2006.
11. Chandrasoma PT, Lokuhetty DM, Demeester TR, Bremmer CG, Peters JH, Oberg S, Groshen S. Definition of histopathologic changes in gastroesophageal reflux disease. Am J Surg Pathol. 2000;24:344–51.
12. Clark GW, Ireland AP, Peters JH, Chandrasoma P, Demeester TR, Bremner CG. Short-segment Barrett's esophagus: a prevalent complication of gastroesophageal reflux disease with malignant potential. J Gastrointest Surg. 1997;1:113–22.
13. Clark GW, Smyrk TC, Burdiles P, Hoeft SF, Peters JH, Kiyabu M, Hinder RA, Bremner CG, Demeester TR. Is Barrett's metaplasia the source of adenocarcinomas of the cardia? Arch Surg. 1994;129:609–14.
14. Fitzgerald RC, di Pietro M, Ragunath K, Ang Y, Kang JY, Watson P, Trudgill N, Patel P, Kaye PV, Sanders S, O'donovan M, Bird-Lieberman E, Bhandari P, Jankowski JA, Attwood S, Parsons SL, Loft D, Lagergren J, Moayyedi P, Lyratzopoulos G, de Caestecker J, British Society of Gastroenterology. British Society of Gastroenterology guidelines on the diagnosis and management of Barrett's oesophagus. Gut. 2014;63:7–42.
15. Hahn HP, Blount PL, Ayub K, Das KM, Souza R, Spechler S, Odze RD. Intestinal differentiation in metaplastic, nongoblet columnar epithelium in the esophagus. Am J Surg Pathol. 2009;33:1006–15.
16. Hankins JR, Cole FN, Attar S, Frost JL, McLaughlin JS. Adenocarcinoma involving the esophagus. J Thorac Cardiovasc Surg. 1974;68:148–58.
17. Hayward J. The lower end of the oesophagus. Thorax. 1961;16:36–41.
18. Jankowski JA, Wright NA, Meltzer SJ, Triadafilopoulos G, Geboes K, Casson AG, Kerr D, Young LS. Molecular evolution of the metaplasia-dysplasia-adenocarcinoma sequence in the esophagus. Am J Pathol. 1999;154:965–73.
19. Liu W, Hahn H, Odze RD, Goyal RK. Metaplastic esophageal columnar epithelium without goblet cells shows DNA content abnormalities similar to goblet cell-containing epithelium. Am J Gastroenterol. 2009;104:816–24.
20. Lord RV. Norman Barrett, "doyen of esophageal surgery". Ann Surg. 1999;229:428–39.
21. McClave SA, Boyce HW Jr, Gottfried MR. Early diagnosis of columnar-lined esophagus: a new endoscopic diagnostic criterion. Gastrointest Endosc. 1987;33:413–6.
22. Miehlke S, Morgner A, Aust D, Madisch A, Vieth M, Baretton G. Combined use of narrow-band imaging magnification endoscopy and miniprobe confocal laser microscopy in neoplastic Barrett's esophagus. Endoscopy. 2007;39(Suppl 1):E316.
23. Morson BC, Belcher JR. Adenocarcinoma of the oesophagus and ectopic gastric mucosa. Br J Cancer. 1952;6:127–30.
24. Murphy SJ, Johnston BT, Murray LJ. British Society of Gastroenterology guidelines for the diagnosis of Barrett's oesophagus: are we casting the net too wide? Gut. 2006;55:1821–2.
25. Nandurkar S, Talley NJ, Martin CJ, Ng TH, Adams S. Short segment Barrett's oesophagus: prevalence, diagnosis and associations. Gut. 1997;40:710–5.
26. Oberg S, Clark GW, Demeester TR. Barrett's esophagus. Update of pathophysiology and management. Hepato-Gastroenterology. 1998;45:1348–56.
27. Overholt BF, Wang KK, Burdick JS, Lightdale CJ, Kimmey M, Nava HR, Sivak MV Jr, Nishioka N, Barr H, Marcon N, Pedrosa M, Bronner MP, Grace M, Depot M, International Photodynamic Group for High-Grade Dysplasia In Barrett's Esophagus. Five-year efficacy and safety of photodynamic therapy with Photofrin in Barrett's high-grade dysplasia. Gastrointest Endosc. 2007;66:460–8.
28. Owen DA. Stomach. In: Sternberg SS, editor. Histology for pathologists. 2nd ed. Philadelphia: Lippincott-Raven Publishers; 1997.
29. Paull A, Trier JS, Dalton MD, Camp RC, Loeb P, Goyal RK. The histologic spectrum of Barrett's esophagus. N Engl J Med. 1976;295:476–80.
30. Reid BJ. Barrett's esophagus and esophageal adenocarcinoma. Gastroenterol Clin N Am. 1991;20:817–34.

31. Rex DK, Cummings OW, Shaw M, Cumings MD, Wong RK, Vasudeva RS, Dunne D, Rahmani EY, Helper DJ. Screening for Barrett's esophagus in colonoscopy patients with and without heartburn. Gastroenterology. 2003;125:1670–7.
32. Ronkainen J, Aro P, Storskrubb T, Johansson SE, Lind T, Bolling-Sternevald E, Vieth M, Stolte M, Talley NJ, Agreus L. Prevalence of Barrett's esophagus in the general population: an endoscopic study. Gastroenterology. 2005;129:1825–31.
33. Sampliner RE, Fennerty B, Garewal HS. Reversal of Barrett's esophagus with acid suppression and multipolar electrocoagulation: preliminary results. Gastrointest Endosc. 1996;44:532–5.
34. Sampliner RE, Hixson LJ, Fennerty MB, Garewal HS. Regression of Barrett's esophagus by laser ablation in an anacid environment. Dig Dis Sci. 1993;38:365–8.
35. Seery JP. Stem cells of the oesophageal epithelium. J Cell Sci. 2002;115:1783–9.
36. Shaheen NJ, Richter JE. Barrett's oesophagus. Lancet. 2009;373:850–61.
37. Shaheen NJ, Sharma P, Overholt BF, Wolfsen HC, Sampliner RE, Wang KK, Galanko JA, Bronner MP, Goldblum JR, Bennett AE, Jobe BA, Eisen GM, Fennerty MB, Hunter JG, Fleischer DE, Sharma VK, Hawes RH, Hoffman BJ, Rothstein RI, Gordon SR, Mashimo H, Chang KJ, Muthusamy VR, Edmundowicz SA, Spechler SJ, Siddiqui AA, Souza RF, Infantolino A, Falk GW, Kimmey MB, Madanick RD, Chak A, Lightdale CJ. Radiofrequency ablation in Barrett's esophagus with dysplasia. N Engl J Med. 2009;360:2277–88.
38. Sharma P. Recent advances in Barrett's esophagus: short-segment Barrett's esophagus and cardia intestinal metaplasia. Semin Gastrointest Dis. 1999;10:93–102.
39. Sharma P, McQuaid K, Dent J, Fennerty MB, Sampliner R, Spechler S, Cameron A, Corley D, Falk G, Goldblum J, Hunter J, Jankowski J, Lundell L, Reid B, Shaheen NJ, Sonnenberg A, Wang K, Weinstein W, AGA Chicago Workshop. A critical review of the diagnosis and management of Barrett's esophagus: the AGA Chicago Workshop. Gastroenterology. 2004;127:310–30.
40. Sharma P, Morales TG, Bhattacharyya A, Garewal HS, Sampliner RE. Dysplasia in short-segment Barrett's esophagus: a prospective 3-year follow-up. Am J Gastroenterol. 1997;92:2012–6.
41. Skinner DB, Walther BC, Riddell RH, Schmidt H, Iascone C, Demeester TR. Barrett's esophagus. Comparison of benign and malignant cases. Ann Surg. 1983;198:554–65.
42. Spechler SJ, Fitzgerald RC, Prasad GA, Wang KK. History, molecular mechanisms, and endoscopic treatment of Barrett's esophagus. Gastroenterology. 2010;138:854–69.
43. Spechler SJ, Sharma P, Souza RF, Inadomi JM, Shaheen NJ, American Gastroenterological, Association. American Gastroenterological Association technical review on the management of Barrett's esophagus. Gastroenterology. 2011;140:e18–52; quiz e13.
44. Spechler SJ, Zeroogian JM, Antonioli DA, Wang HH, Goyal RK. Prevalence of metaplasia at the gastro-oesophageal junction. Lancet. 1994;344:1533–6.
45. Stein HJ, von Rahden BH, Hofler H, Siewert JR. Carcinoma of the oesophagogastric junction and Barrett's esophagus: an almost clear oncologic model? Chirurg. 2003;74:703–8.
46. Takubo K, Aida J, Naomoto Y, Sawabe M, Arai T, Shiraishi H, Matsuura M, Ell C, May A, Pech O, Stolte M, Vieth M. Cardiac rather than intestinal-type background in endoscopic resection specimens of minute Barrett adenocarcinoma. Hum Pathol. 2009;40:65–74.
47. Tileston W. Peptic ulcer of the oesophagus. Am J Med Sci. 1906;132:240–65.
48. Vakil N, van Zanten SV, Kahrilas P, Dent J, Jones R, Global Consensus Group. The Montreal definition and classification of gastroesophageal reflux disease: a global evidence-based consensus. Am J Gastroenterol. 2006;101:1900–20; quiz 1943
49. Wang KK, Sampliner RE, Practice Parameters Committee of the American College of Gastroenterology. Updated guidelines 2008 for the diagnosis, surveillance and therapy of Barrett's esophagus. Am J Gastroenterol. 2008;103:788–97.
50. Weston AP, Krmpotich P, Makdisi WF, Cherian R, Dixon A, McGregor DH, Banerjee SK. Short segment Barrett's esophagus: clinical and histological features, associated endoscopic findings, and association with gastric intestinal metaplasia. Am J Gastroenterol. 1996;91:981–6.
51. Weston AP, Krmpotich PT, Cherian R, Dixon A, Topalosvki M. Prospective long-term endoscopic and histological follow-up of short segment Barrett's esophagus: comparison with traditional long segment Barrett's esophagus. Am J Gastroenterol. 1997;92:407–13.

Epidemiology of Barrett's Esophagus and Esophageal Cancer

26

Kunal Jajoo and Lawrence F. Borges

Epidemiology of Barrett's Esophagus

Introduction

Barrett's esophagus (BE) is a condition in which the normal stratified squamous epithelium of the distal esophagus is replaced by simple columnar epithelium that more closely resembles the lining of the small intestine. It arises as a consequence of repeated tissue injury in the distal esophagus, most commonly due to gastroesophageal reflux (GERD). BE is known to be a precursor lesion to the development of esophageal adenocarcinoma (EAC); however, optimal strategies for diagnosis and management are debated. BE is most commonly detected during upper endoscopy, where it appears as patches or tongues of salmon-colored mucosa rising into the tubular esophagus. Biopsies are necessary to confirm the diagnosis. As of 2016, the American College of Gastroenterology recommends that a diagnosis of BE should only be made if biopsies demonstrate specialized intestinal metaplasia (IM) with goblet cells [41], as this finding predicts a higher risk of malignant transformation. In contrast, the British Society of Gastroenterology recommends that IM should not be a prerequisite for diagnosis, but should be accounted for when making management and surveillance decisions [17].

Regional Prevalence

The estimated prevalence of BE among patients reporting symptomatic reflux or dyspepsia in the United States ranges from 6% to 20% [12, 48]. Interestingly,

K. Jajoo (✉) · L. F. Borges
Department of Medicine, Division of Gastroenterology, Brigham and Women's Hospital, Boston, MA, USA
e-mail: kjajoo@bwh.harvard.edu

J. Grams et al. (eds.), *The SAGES Manual of Foregut Surgery*,
https://doi.org/10.1007/978-3-319-96122-4_26

reported prevalence estimates among asymptomatic patients undergoing upper endoscopy in the United States are similar [19, 22, 48]. The majority of BE cases – from 6% to 17% – are so-called short-segment Barrett's esophagus (SSBE), in which the tongues of salmon-colored mucosa seen on endoscopy extend less than 3 cm into the esophagus. The minority – from 1.6% to 7% – are lesions that extend 3 cm or longer into the esophagus and are called long-segment Barrett's esophagus (LSBE). However, even in asymptomatic subjects, endoscopy-based studies may overestimate the true population prevalence. Autopsy data from the general population suggests that the prevalence of true BE is much lower, as only 11% of people had intestinal metaplasia found at the GE junction and only about 1% had BE found in the tubular esophagus [32].

In general, international prevalence estimates for BE are lower than in the United States. BE has been reported in only 1.6% of the general population in Sweden [38]. However, it was suggested that different thresholds for endoscopic suspicion of BE may account for some of this difference [37]. The reported prevalence of BE in most Asian countries is also lower than in the United States, estimated from 0.06% to 6% [9, 31]. Cultural and lifestyle factors may determine some of this difference. In addition, many Asian studies do not utilize the standard four-quadrant biopsy approach that is used in the United States, and a resulting decrease in sensitivity for detecting BE may also affect prevalence estimates. Notably, the reported prevalence rates of BE in Japan are often higher than other Asian countries (up to 19.9%). In Japan, many studies use the lower-esophageal palisade vessels as a landmark to identify the GEJ, despite demonstrated poor interobserver reliability [1]. When compared with the more widely accepted practice of using the longitudinal gastric folds to identify the GEJ, this difference in approach may explain some of the higher prevalence observed in Japanese studies [9].

Demographic and Clinical Risk Factors

BE is commonly considered to be a condition of older, Caucasian men. The incidence of BE rises with age, with the rate of new cases significantly increasing over the age of 50 [16]. Studies estimate that men have a 1.5–2-fold increased risk of developing Barrett's esophagus when compared to women [16, 48]. Men are also almost four times more likely than women to develop LSBE, which is likely related to a higher rate of severe reflux esophagitis in men [16, 18]. In a large study of over 20,000 patients presenting for endoscopy, Barrett's esophagus was also found more commonly in white Caucasian patients than in patients of either South Asian or Afro-Caribbean descent [18].

Obesity in the form of a larger waist circumference has been associated with an increased risk of developing BE. Reflux esophagitis is thought to play a role in these patients, as increased central adiposity has been correlated with more frequent reflux. Importantly, however, the association between larger waist circumference and BE remains significant after controlling for BMI and reflux symptoms, suggesting that other mechanisms may also play a role [14, 30]. Most traditional epidemiologic studies have failed to find a significant link between BMI and BE. This may be because a high BMI alone does not imply central obesity. Nevertheless, most clinicians will counsel their overweight patients with BE to lose weight. The presence of overt reflux symptoms is also a strong predictive factor. Subjects with symptomatic reflux were over ten times as likely to have BE compared with asymptomatic controls in a large Swedish case-control study [29].

Cigarette smoking has been associated with a multitude of malignant and premalignant conditions, and BE is no exception. A large meta-analysis, including 39 studies and over 7000 patients with BE, found that a history of ever smoking was associated with an over 40% increased risk of developing BE when compared to population-based controls. The association was weaker but still present when comparing BE cases with GERD controls [3]. Smoking intensity and duration are important, as there is a positive dose-dependent relationship between pack-years smoked and risk of BE, with the increase in risk for heavy smokers appearing to plateau after 20 pack-years. There also appears to be a synergistic effect between smoking and symptomatic reflux, as this combination of risk factors appears to account for almost 40% of the BE burden in these patients [13].

The majority of newly diagnosed cases of BE and associated esophageal cancer are sporadic. However, multiple familial case clusters have been reported in the literature raising suspicion for the presence of genetic susceptibility gene(s) in addition to shared environmental risk factors. In a modest-sized case-control study, after adjusting for age, sex, and a history of obesity, a positive family history was found to be an independent risk factor for BE, EAC, and EGJ adenocarcinoma [6]. Another large retrospective study that investigated the family histories of over 400 probands with BE or esophageal adenocarcinoma found evidence to suggest a genetic predisposition to the development of BE in 7% of cases [7].

Epidemiology of Esophageal Cancer

Introduction

Primary esophageal cancers include esophageal adenocarcinoma (EAC) and esophageal squamous cell (ESCC). Taken together, esophageal cancers represent the 8th most common type of cancer diagnosed worldwide, with over 450,000 new cases estimated annually. Esophageal cancer is also the 6th most common cause of cancer death. Approximately 400,000 deaths are attributed to esophageal cancer each year, accounting for nearly 5% of worldwide cancer mortality [20].

Regional Prevalence

The majority of esophageal cancer cases worldwide – about 80% – occur in less developed regions, with the highest rates found in Asia and Eastern Africa (see Fig. 26.1). Not surprisingly, mortality rates from esophageal cancer are also highest in these areas [2]. Esophageal cancer is relatively less prevalent in the United States, but still poses a significant burden. The American Cancer Society estimates that almost 17,000 new cases of esophageal cancer will be diagnosed in the United States in 2016 and that esophageal cancer will be responsible for almost 16,000 deaths [2].

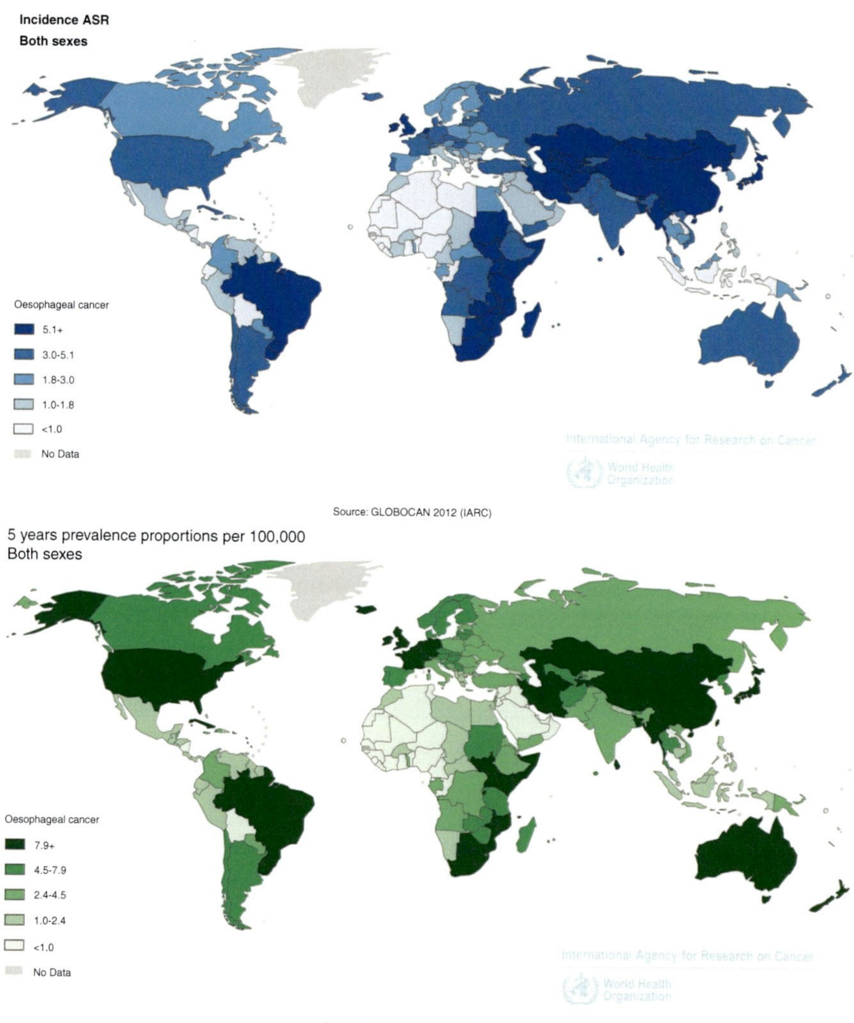

Fig. 26.1 World Health Organization maps showing the estimated worldwide incidence (above), and prevalence (below), of esophageal cancer, as of 2012

Most esophageal cancer diagnosed worldwide is ESCC, although the relative prevalence of ESCC and EAC varies by region [44]. ESCC is the most common form of esophageal cancer found in developing countries in Asia and the Middle East, including within the so-called esophageal cancer "belt" that extends from north-central China to parts of Iran. In contrast, the prevalence of EAC has risen steadily in many Western countries, and EAC is now the most common type of esophageal cancer seen in North America, Australia, and Europe.

Clinical Presentation

Early esophageal cancer is generally asymptomatic which makes early detection difficult. Dysphagia is the primary presenting symptom in over 70% of patients, and just over half will report weight loss as well [15]. Odynophagia and reflux may also be presenting symptoms but are less commonly reported. Laboratory evaluation may reveal anemia from slow but chronic blood loss at the tumor site. Specific findings on physical exam are uncommon but may include pleural effusion, lymphadenopathy, or dyspnea in cases of advanced disease.

Prognosis for patients with esophageal cancer depends primarily on stage at diagnosis. As of 2016, the American Cancer Society reports that 5-year survival for localized esophageal cancer – meaning no lymph node involvement or distant metastases – can be as high as 40% [2]. Long-term survival in these cases hinges on complete surgical resection. The 5-year survival rate for patients presenting with lymph node involvement drops quickly to 20%, and esophageal cancer with distant metastasis has the worst prognosis with a 5-year survival of less than 5%. Prognosis is generally similar between the two types of esophageal cancer, but there is some evidence that esophageal adenocarcinoma may respond more favorably to certain treatments [10].

Esophageal Adenocarcinoma

Demographic and Clinical Risk Factors

Barrett's esophagus is the single most important known risk factor for the development of EAC. A nationwide, population-based cohort study in Denmark found that patients with BE were 11 times more likely to develop EAC when compared to the general population. This translated to a 0.12% annual risk [24]. A large meta-analysis looking at 51 studies from the United States, Europe, and Australia found that the incidence of developing esophageal adenocarcinoma in patients with Barrett's esophagus was 6.3 per 1000 person-years, corresponding to an annual risk of 0.6%. This risk rose even further to 1% annually in the subgroup of patients who had BE with histological evidence of high-grade dysplasia [43].

Among patients with known BE, male gender confers a three-times increased risk of developing EAC. The risk of EAC also increases steadily with age. Patients with BE over the age of 70 are at more than threefold increased risk of developing

EAC compared to BE patients under age 50 and greater than 20-fold increased risk as compared to the general population [24]. Obesity is also a risk factor for EAC. Pooled data from 12 epidemiologic studies representing nearly 2000 cases of esophageal adenocarcinoma found a positive linear relationship between increasing BMI and risk of cancer [23]. Another study looking at genetic determinants of obesity estimates a 16% increased risk of EAC for each 1 kg/m^2 increase in BMI [45].

Certain lifestyle habits are also thought to pose an increased risk of EAC. There is strong evidence that cigarette smoking raises EAC risk in a dose-dependent relationship. A meta-analysis of over 30 studies showed that the relative risk of developing EAC or esophagogastric junction (EGJ) adenocarcinoma was increased 2.32 times overall for current smokers when compared to never smokers and the highest risks were seen in subjects who smoked over 2 packs per day or who had smoked for greater than 40 years. Interestingly, the risk was found to be lower but still significantly elevated in former smokers (RR 1.62), suggesting that any amount of cigarette exposure may have negative implications [46]. Alcohol, on the other hand, does not appear to increase risk of EAC. A nationwide, case-control study of esophageal cancer from Australia failed to observe any significant association between drinking alcohol and the risk of developing EAC [33]. With regard to diet, a 2013 meta-analysis, which included studies from both the United States and abroad, found a slightly higher risk of EAC in subjects who reported an increased consumption of red and processed meat [11].

Esophageal Squamous Cell Carcinoma

Demographic and Clinical Risk Factors

Risk factors for ESCC include some of the known EAC risk factors, as well as others that are unique to the squamous cell subtype (see Table 26.1). Patients with ESCC commonly have a history of tobacco and alcohol use. Regular tobacco smoking has been associated with a greater than threefold increased risk of developing ESCC compared with never use, and the risk of ESCC appears to increase with the number of cigarettes smoked per day and the use of unfiltered tobacco, such as pipe smoking [40]. Exposure to secondhand smoke alone also appears to

Table 26.1 Risk factors for esophageal cancer

Esophageal adenocarcinoma	Esophageal squamous cell carcinoma
Barrett's esophagus	Smoking tobacco
Gastroesophageal reflux	Alcohol
Obesity	High consumption of hot beverages
Smoking tobacco	Red and processed meats
Red and processed meats	Thoracic radiation
Family history	Family history
	Caustic injury
	Achalasia
	Human papillomavirus

pose some increased risk of ESCC [36]. Similar to tobacco, regular alcohol use raises the risk of ESCC in a dose-dependent manner. In a large meta-analysis of over 50 studies, moderate-to-heavy drinkers (> 12.5 grams of alcohol/day) were at least twice as likely to develop ESCC as nondrinkers [25], and this risk appears to increase with increased consumption [28, 33]. Smoking and drinking simultaneously appears to have a synergistic effect as the highest rates of ESCC are seen in these patients [33, 34].

Certain dietary habits are also thought to raise the risk of ESCC. A meta-analysis of over 20 studies looking at diet found that patients who reported a greater consumption of hot beverages were over twice as likely to develop ESCC, even after controlling for alcohol and tobacco use [4]. Repetitive, low-grade thermal injury to the esophageal lining may explain this association. Increased consumption of so-called pro-inflammatory foods, such as red and processed meats, is also thought to be a risk factor [35, 42]. In contrast, increased consumption of foods, such as olive oil, fish, whole grains, fruits, and vegetables, may be protective [27].

Prior medical history is also important in determining a patient's risk of ESCC. A preexisting diagnosis of achalasia is reported to raise the risk of ESCC by more than 16-fold, according to a large population-based study from Sweden; however, the mechanism behind this association is not known [39]. Patients with a history of thoracic radiation following mastectomy are also at increased risk, as their chances of developing ESCC are more than double of those without a history of thoracic radiation, starting just 5 years after radiation exposure [49]. ESCC is most common in the upper and middle thirds of the esophagus in these patients. There does not appear to be any increased risk of EAC in this population, perhaps because the lower esophagus is spared from radiation exposure. Caustic ingestion injury to the esophagus may also predispose to esophageal cancer, as reports estimate that it is a risk factor in 1–4% of all cases of esophageal carcinoma [5, 26]. The large majority of these are ESCC arising in the mid-esophagus, and the time between ingestion and presentation with cancer ranges considerably from 10 to 70 years. It is thus important to inquire about accidental ingestions during childhood, even in adult patients.

Given the well-known association between the human papillomavirus (HPV) and squamous cell cancers of the oropharynx, there has been much speculation about a link between HPV infection and esophageal cancer. Currently, the available evidence supports an association between HPV subtypes 16 and 18 and ESCC [47]. However, it remains unclear as to whether the presence of HPV in ESCC tumor cells has implications for prognosis or treatment [21]. This is an area of ongoing research that is sure to yield new insights in the near future.

While environmental and medical risk factors appear to be most important in the development of ESCC, there is likely some genetic component as well. For instance, light alcohol consumption (0–12.5 gms/day) has been associated with ESCC mainly in Asian studies. This suggests a lower threshold for ESCC development driven by genetic susceptibility in certain Asian populations [25]. The results from one Chinese case-control study appear to support this notion, as the authors report a twofold increased risk of developing ESCC for subjects with a family history of ESCC in a first-degree relative [8].

References

1. Amano Y, Ishimura N, Furuta K, Takahashi Y, Chinuki D, Mishima Y, Moriyama I, Fukuhara H, Ishihara S, Adachi K, Kinoshita Y. Which landmark results in a more consistent diagnosis of Barrett's esophagus, the gastric folds or the palisade vessels? Gastrointest Endosc. 2006;64(2):206–11. https://doi.org/10.1016/j.gie.2006.04.029.
2. American Cancer Society. Cancer facts & figures 2016; 2016.
3. Andrici J, Cox MR, Eslick GD. Cigarette smoking and the risk of Barrett's esophagus: a systematic review and meta-analysis. J Gastroenterol Hepatol. 2013;28(8):1258–73. https://doi.org/10.1111/jgh.12230.
4. Andrici J, Eslick GD. Hot food and beverage consumption and the risk of esophageal Cancer. Am J Prev Med. 2015;49(6):952–60. https://doi.org/10.1016/j.amepre.2015.07.023.
5. Appelqvist P, Salmo M. Lye corrosion carcinoma of the esophagus: a review of 63 cases. Cancer. 1980;45(10):2655–8. Retrieved from http://www.ncbi.nlm.nih.gov/pubmed/7378999.
6. Chak A, Lee T, Kinnard MF, Brock W, Faulx A, Willis J, Cooper GS, Sivak MV Jr, Goddard KAB. Familial aggregation of Barrett's oesophagus, oesophageal adenocarcinoma, and oesophagogastric junctional adenocarcinoma in caucasian adults. Gfut. 2002;51(3):323–8. Retrieved from http://www.ncbi.nlm.nih.gov/pubmed/12171951.
7. Chak A, Ochs-Balcom H, Falk G, Grady WM, Kinnard M, Willis JE, Elston R, Eng C. Familiarity in Barrett's esophagus, adenocarcinoma of the esophagus, and adenocarcinoma of the gastroesophageal junction. Cancer Epidemiol Biomark Prev. 2006;15(9):1668–73. https://doi.org/10.1158/1055-9965.EPI-06-0293.
8. Chang-Claude J, Becher H, Blettner M, Qiu S, Yang G, Wahrendorf J. Familial aggregation of oesophageal cancer in a high incidence area in China. Int J Epidemiol. 1997;26(6):1159–65. Retrieved from http://www.ncbi.nlm.nih.gov/pubmed/9447394.
9. Chang C-Y, Cook MB, Lee Y-C, Lin J-T, Ando T, Bhatia S, Chow WH, El-Omar EM, Goto H, Li YQ, McColl K, Rhee P-L, Sharma P, Sung JJ-Y, Wong JY-Y, Wu JC-Y, Ho K-Y. Current status of Barrett's esophagus research in Asia. J Gastroenterol Hepatol. 2011;26(2):240–6. https://doi.org/10.1111/j.1440-1746.2010.06529.x.
10. Chang DT, Chapman C, Shen J, Su Z, Koong AC. Treatment of esophageal cancer based on histology. Am J Clin Oncol. 2009;32(4):405–10. https://doi.org/10.1097/COC.0b013e3181917158.
11. Choi Y, Song S, Song Y, Lee JE. Consumption of red and processed meat and esophageal cancer risk: meta-analysis. World J Gastroenterol. 2013;19(7):1020. https://doi.org/10.3748/wjg.v19.i7.1020.
12. Connor MJ, Weston AP, Mayo MS, Sharma P. The prevalence of Barrett's esophagus and erosive esophagitis in patients undergoing upper endoscopy for dyspepsia in a VA population. Dig Dis Sci. 2004;49(6):920–4. Retrieved from http://www.ncbi.nlm.nih.gov/pubmed/15309878.
13. Cook MB, Shaheen NJ, Anderson LA, Giffen C, Chow W-H, Vaughan TL, Whiteman DC, Corley DA. Cigarette smoking increases risk of Barrett's esophagus: an analysis of the Barrett's and esophageal adenocarcinoma consortium. Gastroenterology. 2012;142(4):744–53. https://doi.org/10.1053/j.gastro.2011.12.049.
14. Corley DA, Kubo A, Levin TR, Block G, Habel L, Zhao W, Leighton P, Quesenberry C, Rumore GJ, Buffler PA. Abdominal obesity and body mass index as risk factors for Barrett's esophagus. Gastroenterology. 2007;133(1):34–41. https://doi.org/10.1053/j.gastro.2007.04.046.
15. Daly JM, Fry WA, Little AG, Winchester DP, McKee RF, Stewart AK, Fremgen AM. Esophageal cancer: results of an American College of Surgeons patient care evaluation study. J Am Coll Surg. 2000;190(5):562–72. Retrieved from http://www.ncbi.nlm.nih.gov/pubmed/10801023.
16. Edelstein ZR, Bronner MP, Rosen SN, Vaughan TL. Risk factors for Barrett's esophagus among patients with gastroesophageal reflux disease: a community clinic-based case–control study. Am J Gastroenterol. 2009;104(4):834–42. https://doi.org/10.1038/ajg.2009.137.
17. Fitzgerald RC, di Pietro M, Ragunath K, Ang Y, Kang J-Y, Watson P, Trudgill N, Patel P, Kaye PV, Sanders S, O'Donovan M, Bird-Lieberman E, Bhandari P, Jankowski JA, Attwood S, Parsons SL, Loft D, Lagergren J, Moayyedi P, Lyratzopoulos G, de Caestecker J, British

Society of Gastroenterology. British Society of Gastroenterology guidelines on the diagnosis and management of Barrett's oesophagus. Gut. 2014;63(1):7–42. https://doi.org/10.1136/gutjnl-2013-305372.

18. Ford AC, Forman D, Reynolds PD, Cooper BT, Moayyedi P. Ethnicity, gender, and socioeconomic status as risk factors for esophagitis and Barrett's esophagus. Am J Epidemiol. 2005;162(5):454–60. https://doi.org/10.1093/aje/kwi218.
19. Gerson LB, Shetler K, Triadafilopoulos G. Prevalence of Barrett's esophagus in asymptomatic individuals. Gastroenterology. 2002;123(2):461–7. https://doi.org/10.1053/gast.2002.34748.
20. Globocan. Fact Sheets by Cancer. Retrieved from http://globocan.iarc.fr/Pages/fact_sheets_cancer.aspx; 2012.
21. Guo L, Liu S, Zhang S, Chen Q, Zhang M, Quan P, Sun X-B. Human papillomavirus-related esophageal cancer survival. Medicine. 2016;95(46):e5318. https://doi.org/10.1097/MD.0000000000005318.
22. Hirota WK, Loughney TM, Lazas DJ, Maydonovitch CL, Rholl V, Wong RK. Specialized intestinal metaplasia, dysplasia, and cancer of the esophagus and esophagogastric junction: prevalence and clinical data. Gastroenterology. 1999;116(2):277–85. Retrieved from http://www.ncbi.nlm.nih.gov/pubmed/9922307.
23. Hoyo C, Cook MB, Kamangar F, Freedman ND, Whiteman DC, Bernstein L, Brown LM, Risch HA, Ye W, Sharp L, Wu AH, Ward MH, Casson AG, Murray LJ, Corley DA, Nyrén O, Pandeya N, Vaughan TL, Chow WH, Gammon MD. Body mass index in relation to oesophageal and oesophagogastric junction adenocarcinomas: a pooled analysis from the international BEACON consortium. Int J Epidemiol. 2012;41(6):1706–18. https://doi.org/10.1093/ije/dys176.
24. Hvid-Jensen F, Pedersen L, Drewes AM, Sørensen HT, Funch-Jensen P. Incidence of adenocarcinoma among patients with Barrett's esophagus. N Engl J Med. 2011;365(15):1375–83. https://doi.org/10.1056/NEJMoa1103042.
25. Islami F, Fedirko V, Tramacere I, Bagnardi V, Jenab M, Scotti L, Rota M, Corrao G, Garavello W, Schüz J, Straif K, Negri E, Boffetta P, La Vecchia C. Alcohol drinking and esophageal squamous cell carcinoma with focus on light-drinkers and never-smokers: a systematic review and meta-analysis. Int J Cancer. 2011;129(10):2473–84. https://doi.org/10.1002/ijc.25885.
26. Isolauri J, Markkula H. Lye ingestion and carcinoma of the esophagus. Acta Chir Scand. n.d.;155(4–5):269–71. Retrieved from http://www.ncbi.nlm.nih.gov/pubmed/2800875.
27. Jessri M, Rashidkhani B, Hajizadeh B, Jacques PF. Adherence to mediterranean-style dietary pattern and risk of esophageal squamous cell carcinoma: a case-control study in Iran. J Am Coll Nutr. 2012;31(5):338–51. Retrieved from http://www.ncbi.nlm.nih.gov/pubmed/23529991.
28. Ji J, Sundquist J, Sundquist K. Associations of alcohol use disorders with esophageal and gastric cancers. Eur J Cancer Prev. 2016;1 https://doi.org/10.1097/CEJ.0000000000000227.
29. Johansson J, Håkansson H-O, Mellblom L, Kempas A, Johansson K-E, Granath F, Nyrén O. Risk factors for Barrett's oesophagus: a population-based approach. Scand J Gastroenterol. 2007;42(2):148–56. https://doi.org/10.1080/00365520600881037.
30. Kubo A, Cook MB, Shaheen NJ, Vaughan TL, Whiteman DC, Murray L, Corley DA. Sex-specific associations between body mass index, waist circumference and the risk of Barrett's oesophagus: a pooled analysis from the international BEACON consortium. Gut. 2013;62(12):1684–91. https://doi.org/10.1136/gutjnl-2012-303753.
31. Lee HS, Jeon SW. Barrett esophagus in Asia: same disease with different pattern. Clin Endosc. 2014;47(1):15–22. https://doi.org/10.5946/ce.2014.47.1.15.
32. Ormsby AH, Kilgore SP, Goldblum JR, Richter JE, Rice TW, Gramlich TL. The location and frequency of intestinal metaplasia at the Esophagogastric junction in 223 consecutive autopsies: implications for patient treatment and preventive strategies in Barrett's esophagus. Mod Pathol. 2000;13(6):614–20. https://doi.org/10.1038/modpathol.3880106.
33. Pandeya N, Williams G, Green AC, Webb PM, Whiteman DC, Australian Cancer Study. Alcohol consumption and the risks of adenocarcinoma and squamous cell carcinoma of the esophagus. Gastroenterology. 2009;136(4):1215–24. https://doi.org/10.1053/j.gastro.2008.12.052.

34. Prabhu A, Obi KO, Rubenstein JH. The synergistic effects of alcohol and tobacco consumption on the risk of esophageal squamous cell carcinoma: a meta-analysis. Am J Gastroenterol. 2014;109(6):822–7. https://doi.org/10.1038/ajg.2014.71.
35. Qu X, Ben Q, Jiang Y. Consumption of red and processed meat and risk for esophageal squamous cell carcinoma based on a meta-analysis. Ann Epidemiol. 2013;23(12):762–70. https://doi.org/10.1016/j.annepidem.2013.09.003.
36. Rafiq R, Shah IA, Bhat GA, Lone MM, Islami F, Boffetta P, Dar NA. Secondhand smoking and the risk of esophageal squamous cell carcinoma in a high incidence region, Kashmir, India. Medicine. 2016;95(1):e2340. https://doi.org/10.1097/MD.0000000000002340.
37. Rex DK, Shaw M, Wong R. Prevalence of Barrett's esophagus. Gastroenterology. 2006;130:1373. https://doi.org/10.1053/j.gastro.2006.02.046.
38. Ronkainen J, Aro P, Storskrubb T, Johansson S, Lind T, Bolling–Sternevald E, Vieth M, Stolte M, Talley NJ, Agréus L. Prevalence of Barrett's esophagus in the general population: an endoscopic study. Gastroenterology. 2005;129(6):1825–31. https://doi.org/10.1053/j.gastro.2005.08.053.
39. Sandler RS, Nyrén O, Ekbom A, Eisen GM, Yuen J, Josefsson S. The risk of esophageal cancer in patients with achalasia. A population-based study. JAMA. 1995;274(17):1359–62. Retrieved from http://www.ncbi.nlm.nih.gov/pubmed/7563560.
40. Sewram V, Sitas F, O'Connell D, Myers J. Tobacco and alcohol as risk factors for oesophageal cancer in a high incidence area in South Africa. Cancer Epidemiol. 2016;41:113–21. https://doi.org/10.1016/j.canep.2016.02.001.
41. Shaheen NJ, Falk GW, Iyer PG, Gerson LB. ACG clinical guideline: diagnosis and Management of Barrett's esophagus. Am J Gastroenterol. 2016;111(1):30–50. https://doi.org/10.1038/ajg.2015.322.
42. Shivappa N, Zucchetto A, Serraino D, Rossi M, La Vecchia C, Hébert JR. Dietary inflammatory index and risk of esophageal squamous cell cancer in a case–control study from Italy. Cancer Causes Control. 2015;26(10):1439–47. https://doi.org/10.1007/s10552-015-0636-y.
43. Sikkema M, de Jonge PJF, Steyerberg EW, Kuipers EJ. Risk of esophageal adenocarcinoma and mortality in patients with Barrett's esophagus: a systematic review and meta-analysis. Clin Gastroenterol Hepatol. 2010;8(3):235–44. https://doi.org/10.1016/j.cgh.2009.10.010.
44. Thrift AP. The epidemic of oesophageal carcinoma: where are we now? Cancer Epidemiol. 2016;41:88–95. https://doi.org/10.1016/j.canep.2016.01.013.
45. Thrift AP, Shaheen NJ, Gammon MD, Bernstein L, Reid BJ, Onstad L, Risch HA, Liu G, Bird NC, Wu AH, Corley DA, Romero Y, Chanock SJ, Chow WH, Casson AG, Levine DM, Zhang R, Ek WE, MacGregor S, Ye W, Hardie LJ, Vaughan TL, Whiteman DC. Obesity and risk of esophageal adenocarcinoma and Barrett's esophagus: a Mendelian randomization study. JNCI. 2014;106(11) https://doi.org/10.1093/jnci/dju252. dju252–dju252.
46. Tramacere I, La Vecchia C, Negri E. Tobacco smoking and esophageal and gastric cardia adenocarcinoma. Epidemiology. 2011;22(3):344–9. https://doi.org/10.1097/EDE.0b013e31821092cd.
47. Wang J, Zhao L, Yan H, Che J, Huihui L, Jun W, Liu B, Cao B, Quan P. A meta-analysis and systematic review on the association between human papillomavirus (types 16 and 18) infection and esophageal cancer worldwide. PLoS One. 2016;11(7):e0159140. https://doi.org/10.1371/journal.pone.0159140.
48. Ward EM, Wolfsen HC, Achem SR, Loeb DS, Krishna M, Hemminger LL, DeVault KR. Barrett's esophagus is common in older men and women undergoing screening colonoscopy regardless of reflux symptoms. Am J Gastroenterol. 2006;101(1):12–7. https://doi.org/10.1111/j.1572-0241.2006.00379.x.
49. Zablotska LB, Chak A, Das A, Neugut AI. Increased risk of squamous cell esophageal cancer after adjuvant radiation therapy for primary breast cancer. Am J Epidemiol. 2005;161(4):330–7. https://doi.org/10.1093/aje/kwi050.

Diagnosis and Surveillance of Barrett's Esophagus

27

Oliver A. Varban

Introduction

Norman Barrett (1903–1979), a pioneering British thoracic surgeon, is widely recognized for his contributions to understanding gastroesophageal reflux and for describing the abnormal presence of columnar-lined esophagus in the presence of esophagitis [1]. Although coined Barrett's esophagus (BE), Barrett did not claim to be the first to describe the esophageal pathology and believed initially that the stomach was being drawn up by contractions of the esophagus rather than herniating through the hiatus. Later, he corrected his observations and recognized the importance of the sliding hiatus hernia and its effect on esophagitis [2]. He also made the original observation that the severity of the symptoms, such as pain, was not always proportional to the extent of esophageal inflammation [3].

Today, Barrett's esophagus is considered the most important risk factor for developing esophageal adenocarcinoma (EA), which has increased in incidence since the 1970s [4, 5]. The rationale for screening and surveillance of BE is to improve survival of EA through early detection of cancer. Guidelines on management are based on making an accurate histopathologic diagnosis of BE, which is obtained by performing a biopsy of the distal esophagus endoscopically. The relative risk of cancer is dependent on the histopathologic tissue types identified (i.e., nondysplastic vs low- or high-grade dysplasia) as well as the length of the segment of BE noted endoscopically. It is important to recognize that endoscopic surveillance has the potential for sampling error and the distribution of dysplasia and cancer can be highly variable. Moreover, surveillance programs can be expensive and time consuming. Understanding risk factors for BE, progression to EA, diagnostic criteria, and

O. A. Varban
Department of General Surgery, Michigan Medicine, University Hospital, University of Michigan, Ann Arbor, MI, USA
e-mail: ovarban@med.umich.edu

J. Grams et al. (eds.), *The SAGES Manual of Foregut Surgery*,
https://doi.org/10.1007/978-3-319-96122-4_27

histopathology is important in order to optimize resource utilization for screening and surveillance.

Risk Factors

Barrett's esophagus has been identified in approximately 1–2% of the population and in 15% of patients with chronic gastroesophageal reflux disease (GERD) [6–8]. Patients with GERD symptoms present for greater than 5 years have a higher likelihood of having BE (odds ratio (OR) 3.0, 95% confidence interval (CI) 1.2–8.0), and the likelihood increases with symptoms that are present for greater than 10 years (OR 6.4, 95% CI 2.4–17/1) [9]. Likewise, patients with early onset of GERD symptoms (i.e., weekly symptoms before the age of 30 years) have a higher likelihood of BE when compared to those that did not (OR 31.4, 95% CI 13.0–75.8) [9]. Presence of a hiatal hernia can also increase the risk of BE (OR 3.94, 95% CI 3.02–5.13) [10]. Male gender has been identified as a risk factor for BE, and a meta-analysis demonstrated that the overall pooled male/female ratio among patients with BE was 1.96:1 (95% confidence interval (CI) 1.77, 2.17/1) [11]. Compared to Caucasians, African Americans have a lower likelihood of BE (OR 0.34, 95% CI 0.12–0.97), indicating that Caucasian race is also a strong risk factor for BE [12]. Central obesity can contribute to an increased risk for BE when compared with patients with a normal body habitus (OR 2.0, CI 1.5–2.6), and this relationship persists after adjusting for BMI and GERD and is also consistent in both men and women [13, 14]. BE is more common in first- or second-degree relatives of patients with BE when compared to controls (24% vs 5% $p < 0.005$), and the association remains strong after adjusting for age, gender, and body mass index (OR 12, 95% CI 3.3–44.8) [15]. Although smoking is associated with a greater risk for BE compared with non-smokers (OR 1.44, 95% CI 1.20–1.74), alcohol use has not been demonstrated to be a significant risk factor for BE [16, 17]. Risk factors for BE have been summarized in Table 27.1.

Risk factors associated with the presence of dysplasia or EA in patients with BE include older age and length of BE segment. There is a reported 3.3% increase in dysplasia per year in patients diagnosed with BE [18]. Furthermore, in patients with a BE segment length of over 3 cm, there is a 14% risk of dysplasia for each additional centimeter of BE present. Other risk factors for developing neoplasia in the

Table 27.1 Risk factors for Barrett's esophagus

Risk factors
1. GERD
2. Age
3. Hiatal hernia
4. Male gender
5. Caucasian race
6. Family history of BE (first- or second-degree relatives)
7. Smoking

GERD gastroesophageal reflux disease, *BE* Barrett's esophagus presence of BE include central obesity and tobacco usage. It is important to note that there are certain medications that have been associated with reducing the risk of progression of BE to dysplasia including proton-pump inhibitors (PPIs), aspirin, nonsteroidal anti-inflammatory agents, and statins [19–21].

Diagnosis

Barrett's esophagus is diagnosed by identifying the presence of columnar-lined intestinal metaplasia (IM) in the distal esophagus, which is normally lined by stratified squamous epithelium (Fig. 27.1). The diagnosis is achieved by performing upper endoscopy and obtaining biopsies of salmon-colored mucosa that extends greater than 1 cm proximal to the gastroesophageal junction (GEJ). In patients with long segments (>2 cm) of suspected BE, eight random biopsies should be obtained.

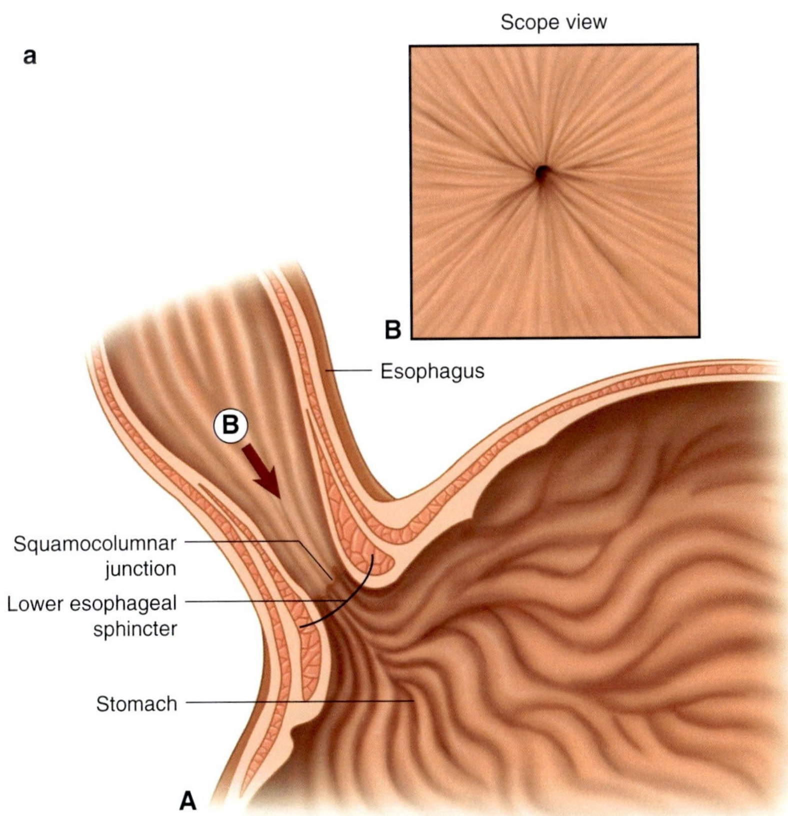

Fig. 27.1 (**a**) Endoscopic view of the gastroesophageal junction with a normal Z-line (squamocolumnar junction). (**b**) Endoscopic view of the gastroesophageal junction with Barrett's esophagus

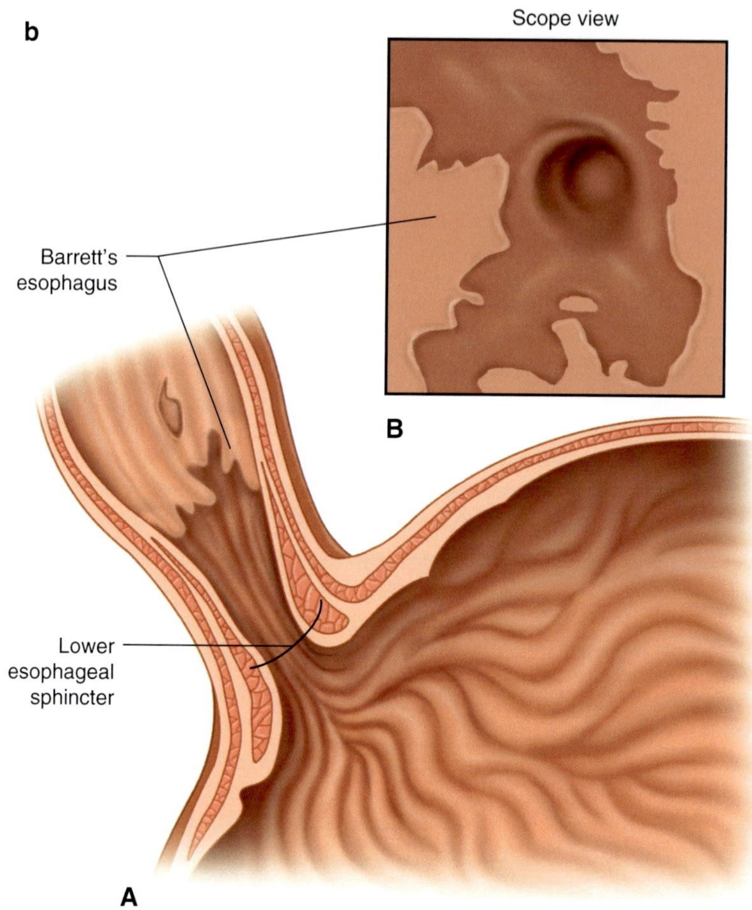

Fig. 27.1 (continued)

In patients with short segments (1–2 cm) of suspected BE, eight biopsies may not be possible, and so at least four biopsies per centimeter of circumferential BE and one biopsy per centimeter in tongues of BE should be obtained [18]. The location of the diaphragmatic hiatus, GEJ, and squamocolumnar junction (Z-line) should be reported by the endoscopist. In the presence of BE, the endoscopist should also describe the extent of metaplastic change using the Prague classification (Fig. 27.2) [22]. Assessment of the extent of BE on endoscopy is clinically important because more extensive disease is associated with a higher risk of dysplasia and EA.

High-definition, high-resolution white light endoscopy is the most common modality used for diagnosis. Alternatively, transnasal endoscopy is considered as an alternative to conventional upper endoscopy for BE screening [23, 24]. A wide variety of image enhancement techniques have been studied, such as methylene blue staining, acetic acid staining, indigo carmine staining, autofluorescence endoscopy,

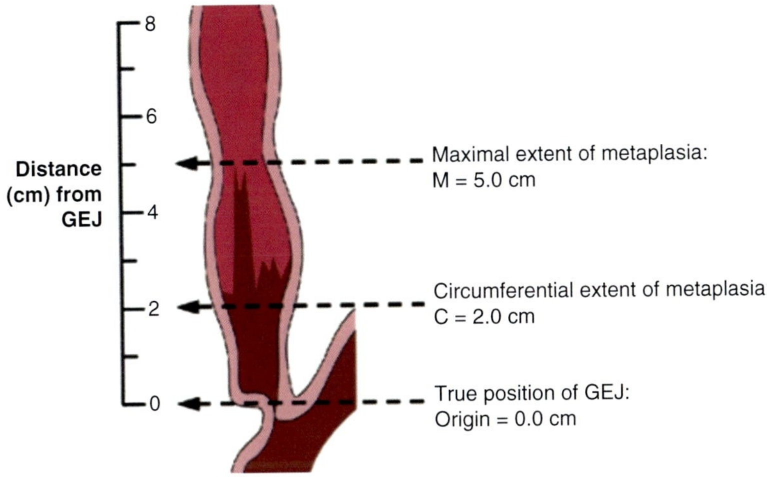

Fig. 27.2 Illustration of the Prague classification for Barrett's esophagus. (Adapted from Sharma et al. [22]). C, extent of circumferential metaplasia; M, maximal extent of metaplasia including the gastroesophageal junction (GEJ). The area of Barrett's esophagus is classified as C2M5

confocal laser endomicroscopy, volumetric laser endomicroscopy, spectroscopy, and molecular imaging. However, none of these methods have been determined to be superior. Electronic chromoendoscopy with either narrow-band imaging (NBI) or post-processing software systems allows for detailed imaging of the mucosal and vascular surface patterns in BE without the need for dye. When compared to high-definition white light endoscopy, NBI demonstrated no difference in the number of patients detected with dysplasia or neoplasia; however, fewer biopsies were required for NBI [25]. A meta-analysis evaluating the utility of electronic chromoendoscopy also suggested that this technology may increase the detection of dysplasia [26].

Histopathology

Barrett's esophagus is defined by the presence of intestinal metaplasia within visible columnar epithelium within the esophagus. Intestinal metaplasia refers to the transformation of squamous epithelium into columnar-lined epithelium consisting of goblet cells, which are recognized by a large cytoplasmic vacuole filled with blue-tinted mucin [27]. Alcian blue staining should be applied when there is doubt about the nature of goblet-shaped cells. Distended gastric foveolar cells may appear to be goblet cells ("pseudogoblet" cells), but they do not contain acid mucin and are therefore Alcian blue negative [28]. Additionally, IM identified below the GEJ should not be diagnosed as BE, since the changes are often secondary to *Helicobacter pylori* infection and its significance as a risk factor for EA is not well established [29]. Thus, it is important to obtain biopsies of BE that extends proximally 1 cm or greater from the GEJ and not in the presence of a normal Z-line or a Z-line with less than 1 cm of variability [18].

Neoplastic progression of BE is initiated by gastroesophageal reflux resulting in esophagitis, which in turn causes a subset of patients with IM to develop dysplasia, a precursor to EA. Histologically confirmed dysplasia is associated with a significant increased risk of EA; thus, understanding the degree of dysplasia is of clinical importance. During carcinogenesis, there is a spectrum of morphologic changes that are subdivided into four clinically significant groups: negative for dysplasia, low-grade dysplasia, high-grade dysplasia, and adenocarcinoma. These groups can be differentiated based on cytology, architecture, and degree of surface maturation among cells. Cytologic evaluation involves describing nuclear and cytoplasmic features such as size of nuclei, nuclear polarity, mitotic activity, and pleomorphism. Loss of nuclear polarity is an important feature that distinguishes high-grade dysplasia from low-grade dysplasia. It is evident when the nucleus is tilted, rounded, or horizontal to the basement membrane. Cellular architecture refers to the relationship of glands and lamina propria, which are well-spaced normally and demonstrate mild to marked distortion with crowded glands with dysplasia. Finally, normal cells demonstrate complete maturation, whereas dysplastic cells demonstrate minimal to no maturation. Biopsies with evidence of high-grade dysplasia should be evaluated for co-existing EA, which involves invasion into the lamina propria or muscularis mucosa. Other signs suggestive of EA include single cells in the lamina propria, desmoplasia, cribriform or solid tubular architecture, dilated tubules filled with necrotic debris, extensive neutrophilic infiltrate within the epithelium, ulcerated high-grade dysplasia, and neoplastic tubules incorporated into the overlying squamous epithelium [30]. Table 27.2 summarizes the histopathology of BE.

Although the presence of dysplasia is an important marker of cancer risk, considerable interobserver variability in the histopathologic interpretation of different degrees of dysplasia exists [31]. Current evidence supports confirmation of dysplasia by a second pathologist with extensive experience in BE interpretation [18]. In some cases biopsies may be indefinite for dysplasia. In these cases, there is pronounced inflammation or loss of surface epithelium along with cytologic atypia characterized by hyperchromasia, overlapping nuclei, irregular nuclear borders, and nuclear stratification. In addition, the cellular architecture is normal with some minimal gland crowding, and surface maturation is present. Given that the changes cannot be definitively described as reactive or neoplastic, repeat endoscopy within 6 months is recommended [27].

Since grading the degree of dysplasia accurately is important, biomarkers have been investigated in order to improve risk stratification of patients with BE. Specific immunohistochemical stains such as alpha-methylacyl CoA racemase (AMCAR), beta-catenin, cyclin DI, and p53 have shown some promise for differentiating neoplastic progression from reactive changes [32, 33]. Biomarkers that detect aneuploidy, increased tetraploidy, and loss of heterozygosity for chromosome 12p demonstrate some predictive value for neoplastic progression in patients with no dysplasia or low-grade dysplasia on biopsy, but have little utility in patients with high-grade dysplasia [34, 35]. Finally biomarker panels, which include detection of chromosomal abnormalities or tumor-suppressor gene-methylation patterns, have even identified patients with BE who progress to high-grade dysplasia 2 years

Table 27.2 Histopathology of Barrett's and risk of progression to esophageal adenocarcinoma

Histology	Hematoxylin and eosin stain (200×)	Risk of cancer progression
Negative for dysplasia	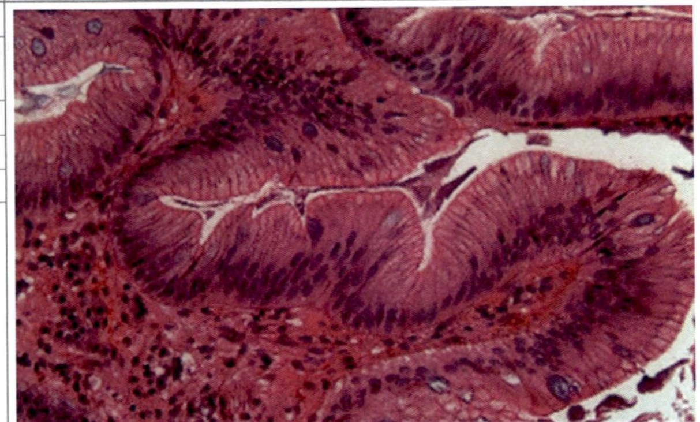	0.2–0.5% per year
Columnar cell metaplasia with mucin-filled, blue-tinted goblet cells		
Normal well-spaced glands		
Regular nuclei		
Smooth membranes		
Complete maturation		
Low-grade dysplasia	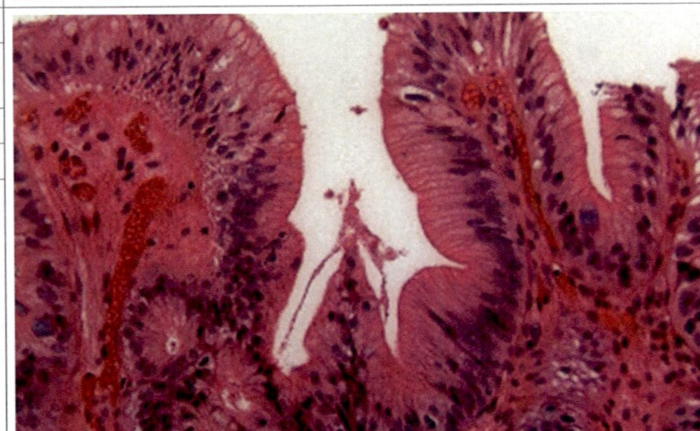	0.7% per year
Increased cellular atypia, hyperchromasia, pleomorphisms, and mitoses		
Gland crowding		
Maintained polarity		
Minimal maturation		

(continued)

Table 27.2 (continued)

Histology	Hematoxylin and eosin stain (200×)	Risk of cancer progression
High-grade dysplasia	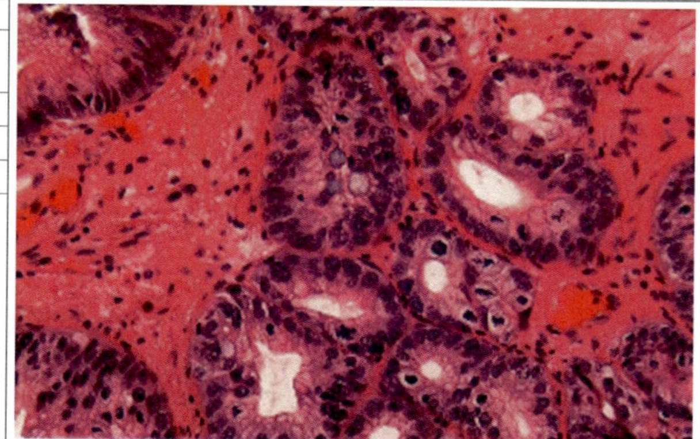	7% per year
Nuclear enlargement, prominent pleomorphism, atypical mitoses		
Crowded glands		
Cribriform or budding glands		
Loss of polarity		
No maturation		

Adapted from Shaheen et al. and Booth et al. [18, 27]

before histologic changes were detectable [36]. Despite its promise, biomarkers have yet to be validated in prospective controlled trials, and routine use is not advocated at this time.

Screening and Surveillance

Although Barrett's esophagus is a common condition and considered a precursor to esophageal adenocarcinoma, screening of the general population is not recommended by the American College of Gastroenterology [18]. In a meta-analysis reviewing the risk of EA and mortality in patients with BE, the data suggests that most patients with BE die of causes other than EA, indicating that patients should be counseled appropriately with regard to surveillance and therapeutic options [37]. Screening may be considered in high-risk patients such as men with chronic and/or frequent symptoms of gastroesophageal reflux and two or more risk factors for BE. In females, screening is not recommended but may be considered in individual cases if multiple risk factors for BE or EA are present [18].

After initial diagnosis of BE, management and surveillance should be performed depending on the degree of dysplasia. In patients with suspected BE and a lack of IM on histology, a repeat endoscopy should be performed in 1–2 years' time. For patients with BE without dysplasia, endoscopic surveillance should be performed every 3–5 years. In patents with BE and indefinite dysplasia, a repeat endoscopy should be performed in 3–6 months after the patient has been placed on acid-suppressive therapy. Patients with low-grade dysplasia may undergo endoscopic therapy or surveillance every 12 months. If endoscopic therapy has been performed, surveillance is recommended every 6 months in the first year following complete elimination of IM followed by yearly endoscopic surveillance thereafter. Meanwhile, patients with high-grade dysplasia should be managed with endoscopic therapy followed by endoscopic surveillance every 3 months for the first year following complete elimination of IM, every 6 months in the second year, and yearly thereafter. Figure 27.3 summarizes surveillance recommendations. Endoscopic surveillance should be performed by obtaining four-quadrant biopsies at 2 cm intervals without dysplasia and 1 cm intervals in patients with prior dysplasia [18].

A variety of endoscopic ablative therapies have been reported to eradicate IM in patients with BE. Radiofrequency ablation can be performed in the setting of low-grade and high-grade dysplasia and is currently the modality of choice [38]. Photodynamic therapy can be performed in patients with BE with high-grade dysplasia only but has a higher cost and side-effect profile [39]. Endoscopic mucosal resection (EMR) is performed when mucosal nodularity or ulcerations are detected. If low- or high-grade dysplasia is discovered, ablative therapy can be performed followed by surveillance. In the case of EA, lesions confined to the mucosa have a low rate of lymphatic involvement, and thus mucosal resection followed by ablative therapy to eradicate the remaining BE is considered acceptable treatment [18]. Otherwise, esophagectomy is the treatment of choice for candidates with T1a or T1b EA with poor differentiation and/or lymphovascular invasion. Antireflux surgery has

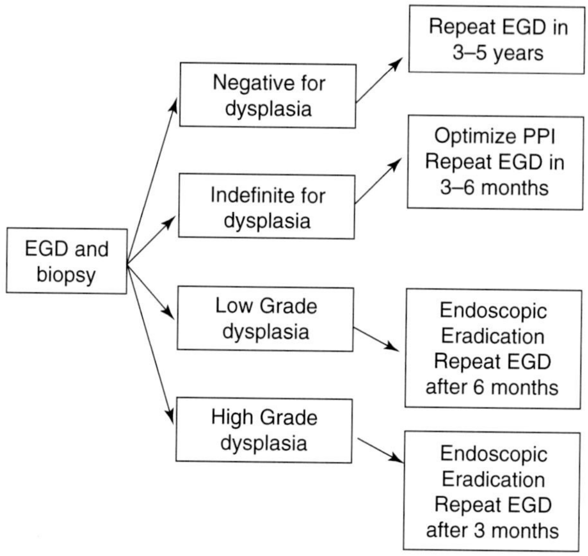

Fig. 27.3 Endoscopic surveillance of Barrett's esophagus according to histopathologic diagnosis. **EGD* esophagogastroduodenoscopy, *PPI* proton-pump inhibitor

demonstrated complete or partial regression of Barrett's mucosa with dysplasia regressing in nearly half of the patients at 5 years [40, 41]. However, the ACG does not consider antireflux surgery as an antineoplastic measure and only recommends surgery in patients with BE and GERD symptoms who are not well controlled by medical therapy [18]. To date, there has been no evidence to demonstrate the effectiveness of BE regression with magnetic sphincter augmentation devices. However, such prosthetic devices appear to result in pH normalization, cessation of PPI use, and improved quality of life in studies with 5-year follow-up [42].

Summary

Barrett's esophagus is a common condition that increases the likelihood for esophageal adenocarcinoma. Routine screening is not recommended for the general public but should be considered in patients with known risk factors. High-definition, high-resolution white light endoscopy with biopsy remains the gold standard for diagnosis, and the degree of dysplasia noted on histology dictates management.

References

1. Barrett NR. Chronic peptic ulcer of the oesophagus and 'oesophagitis'. Br J Surg. 1950;38:175–82.
2. Lord RV. Norman Barrett, "doyen of esophageal surgery". Ann Surg. 1999;229:428–39.

3. Barrett NR. Hiatus hernia: a review of some controversial points. Br J Surg. 1954;42:231–43.
4. Hur C, Miller M, Kong CY, et al. Trends in esophageal adenocarcinoma incidence and mortality. Cancer. 2013;119:1149–58.
5. Graham D, Lipman G, Sehgal V, Lovat LB. Monitoring the premalignant potential of Barrett's oesophagus'. Frontline Gastroenterol. 2016;7:316–22.
6. Johansson J, Håkansson HO, Mellblom L, et al. Prevalence of precancerous and other metaplasia in the distal oesophagus and gastro-oesophageal junction. Scand J Gastroenterol. 2005;40:893–902.
7. Ronkainen J, Aro P, Storskrubb T, et al. Prevalence of Barrett's esophagus in the general population: an endoscopic study. Gastroenterology. 2005;129:1825–31.
8. Zagari RM, Fuccio L, Wallander MA, et al. Gastro-oesophageal reflux symptoms, oesophagitis and Barrett's oesophagus in the general population: the Loiano-Monghidoro study. Gut. 2008;57:1354–9.
9. Lieberman DA, Oehlke M, Helfand M. Risk factors for Barrett's esophagus in community-based practice. GORGE consortium. Gastroenterology Outcomes Research Group in Endoscopy. Am J Gastroenterol. 1997;92:1293–7.
10. Andrici J, Tio M, Cox MR, Eslick GD. Hiatal hernia and the risk of Barrett's esophagus. J Gastroenterol Hepatol. 2013;28:415–31.
11. Cook MB, Wild CP, Forman D. A systematic review and meta-analysis of the sex ratio for Barrett's esophagus, erosive reflux disease, and nonerosive reflux disease. Am J Epidemiol. 2005;162:1050–61.
12. Abrams JA, Fields S, Lightdale CJ, Neugut AI. Racial and ethnic disparities in the prevalence of Barrett's esophagus among patients who undergo upper endoscopy. Clin Gastroenterol Hepatol. 2008;6:30–4.
13. Kubo A, Cook MB, Shaheen NJ, et al. Sex-specific associations between body mass index, waist circumference and the risk of Barrett's oesophagus: a pooled analysis from the international BEACON consortium. Gut. 2013;62:1684–91.
14. Thrift AP, Kramer JR, Alsarraj A, El-Serag HB. Fat mass by bioelectrical impedance analysis is not associated with increased risk of Barrett esophagus. J Clin Gastroenterol. 2014;48:218–23.
15. Chak A, Lee T, Kinnard MF, et al. Familial aggregation of Barrett's oesophagus, oesophageal adenocarcinoma, and oesophagogastric junctional adenocarcinoma in Caucasian adults. Gut. 2002;51:323–8.
16. Anderson LA, Cantwell MM, Watson RG, et al. The association between alcohol and reflux esophagitis, Barrett's esophagus, and esophageal adenocarcinoma. Gastroenterology. 2009;136:799–805.
17. Andrici J, Cox MR, Eslick GD. Cigarette smoking and the risk of Barrett's esophagus: a systematic review and meta-analysis. J Gastroenterol Hepatol. 2013;28:1258–73.
18. Shaheen NJ, Falk GW, Iyer PG, Gerson LB, American COG. ACG clinical guideline: diagnosis and management of Barrett's esophagus. Am J Gastroenterol. 2016;111:30–50; quiz 51
19. Singh S, Singh AG, Singh PP, Murad MH, Iyer PG. Statins are associated with reduced risk of esophageal cancer, particularly in patients with Barrett's esophagus: a systematic review and meta-analysis. Clin Gastroenterol Hepatol. 2013;11:620–9.
20. Singh S, Garg SK, Singh PP, Iyer PG, El-Serag HB. Acid-suppressive medications and risk of oesophageal adenocarcinoma in patients with Barrett's oesophagus: a systematic review and meta-analysis. Gut. 2014;63:1229–37.
21. Zhang S, Zhang XQ, Ding XW, et al. Cyclooxygenase inhibitors use is associated with reduced risk of esophageal adenocarcinoma in patients with Barrett's esophagus: a meta-analysis. Br J Cancer. 2014;110:2378–88.
22. Sharma P, Dent J, Armstrong D, et al. The development and validation of an endoscopic grading system for Barrett's esophagus: the Prague C & M criteria. Gastroenterology. 2006;131:1392–9.
23. Peery AF, Hoppo T, Garman KS, et al. Feasibility, safety, acceptability, and yield of office-based, screening transnasal esophagoscopy (with video). Gastrointest Endosc. 2012;75:945–953.e2.

24. Shariff MK, Bird-Lieberman EL, O'Donovan M, et al. Randomized crossover study comparing efficacy of transnasal endoscopy with that of standard endoscopy to detect Barrett's esophagus. Gastrointest Endosc. 2012;75:954–61.
25. Sharma P, Hawes RH, Bansal A, et al. Standard endoscopy with random biopsies versus narrow band imaging targeted biopsies in Barrett's oesophagus: a prospective, international, randomised controlled trial. Gut. 2013;62:15–21.
26. Qumseya BJ, Wang H, Badie N, et al. Advanced imaging technologies increase detection of dysplasia and neoplasia in patients with Barrett's esophagus: a meta-analysis and systematic review. Clin Gastroenterol Hepatol. 2013;11:1562–70.e1.
27. Booth CL, Thompson KS. Barrett's esophagus: a review of diagnostic criteria, clinical surveillance practices and new developments. J Gastrointest Oncol. 2012;3:232–42.
28. Spechler SJ, Goyal RK. The columnar-lined esophagus, intestinal metaplasia, and Norman Barrett. Gastroenterology. 1996;110:614–21.
29. Goldblum JR. The significance and etiology of intestinal metaplasia of the esophagogastric junction. Ann Diagn Pathol. 2002;6:67–73.
30. Zhu W, Appelman HD, Greenson JK, et al. A histologically defined subset of high-grade dysplasia in Barrett mucosa is predictive of associated carcinoma. Am J Clin Pathol. 2009;132:94–100.
31. Montgomery E, Bronner MP, Goldblum JR, et al. Reproducibility of the diagnosis of dysplasia in Barrett esophagus: a reaffirmation. Hum Pathol. 2001;32:368–78.
32. Shi XY, Bhagwandeen B, Leong AS. p16, cyclin D1, Ki-67, and AMACR as markers for dysplasia in Barrett esophagus. Appl Immunohistochem Mol Morphol. 2008;16:447–52.
33. van Dekken H, Hop WC, Tilanus HW, et al. Immunohistochemical evaluation of a panel of tumor cell markers during malignant progression in Barrett esophagus. Am J Clin Pathol. 2008;130:745–53.
34. Rabinovitch PS, Longton G, Blount PL, Levine DS, Reid BJ. Predictors of progression in Barrett's esophagus III: baseline flow cytometric variables. Am J Gastroenterol. 2001;96:3071–83.
35. Reid BJ, Levine DS, Longton G, Blount PL, Rabinovitch PS. Predictors of progression to cancer in Barrett's esophagus: baseline histology and flow cytometry identify low- and high-risk patient subsets. Am J Gastroenterol. 2000;95:1669–76.
36. Schulmann K, Sterian A, Berki A, et al. Inactivation of p16, RUNX3, and HPP1 occurs early in Barrett's-associated neoplastic progression and predicts progression risk. Oncogene. 2005;24:4138–48.
37. Sikkema M, de Jonge PJ, Steyerberg EW, Kuipers EJ. Risk of esophageal adenocarcinoma and mortality in patients with Barrett's esophagus: a systematic review and meta-analysis. Clin Gastroenterol Hepatol. 2010;8:235–44; quiz e32
38. Shaheen NJ, Sharma P, Overholt BF, et al. Radiofrequency ablation in Barrett's esophagus with dysplasia. N Engl J Med. 2009;360:2277–88.
39. Overholt BF, Lightdale CJ, Wang KK, et al. Photodynamic therapy with porfimer sodium for ablation of high-grade dysplasia in Barrett's esophagus: international, partially blinded, randomized phase III trial. Gastrointest Endosc. 2005;62:488–98.
40. Bamehriz F, Dutta S, Pottruff CG, Allen CJ, Anvari M. Does laparoscopic Nissen fundoplication prevent the progression of Barrett's oesophagus? Is the length of Barrett's a factor. J Minim Access Surg. 2005;1:21–8.
41. Hofstetter WL, Peters JH, DeMeester TR, et al. Long-term outcome of antireflux surgery in patients with Barrett's esophagus. Ann Surg. 2001;234:532–8; discussion 538
42. Ganz RA, Edmundowicz SA, Taiganides PA, et al. Long-term outcomes of patients receiving a magnetic sphincter augmentation device for gastroesophageal reflux. Clin Gastroenterol Hepatol. 2016;14:671–7.

28 Radiofrequency Ablation for Dysplastic Barrett's Esophagus

Yalini Vigneswaran and Michael B. Ujiki

Abbreviations

HGD	High-grade dysplasia
LGD	Low-grade dysplasia
PDT	Photodynamic therapy
RFA	Radiofrequency ablation

Indications

When Barrett's esophagus progresses to have abnormal histologic features, this can be classified as low-grade or high-grade dysplasia. Although most cases of Barrett's esophagus do not progress to dysplastic changes, when high-grade dysplasia is present, these lesions have a significant risk of progression to esophageal adenocarcinoma, reported as high as 20% per year [1–3]. Throughout the years, controversy has existed as to how to treat Barrett's esophagus and dysplasia in the setting of Barrett's esophagus. Radiofrequency ablative (RFA) therapy has now become the standard of care for high-grade dysplasia as opposed to observation alone, esophagectomy, or photodynamic therapy [1–7]. Ablation in these patients has demonstrated a high rate of complete eradication of dysplasia and decreased disease progression. It is important, however, that the endoscopist recognize and look for nodular disease prior to ablation. Any visible raised lesion must be addressed with endoscopic mucosal resection (EMR) prior to ablation in order to ensure that the ablation reaches the muscularis mucosae. In addition, sampling error can lead to

Y. Vigneswaran · M. B. Ujiki (✉)
Department of Surgery, NorthShore University Health System, University of Chicago Medical Center, Chicago, IL, USA
e-mail: mujiki@northshore.org

J. Grams et al. (eds.), *The SAGES Manual of Foregut Surgery*,
https://doi.org/10.1007/978-3-319-96122-4_28

under-staging in raised lesions, and EMR allows for a more accurate diagnosis which could lead to a treatment alternative more appropriate than ablation. We recommend that patients have two endoscopies in high definition with biopsies and within 2 months prior to undergoing ablation. Furthermore, it is recommended that the biopsies be reviewed by a pathologist specialized in Barrett's esophagus.

Ablation for patients with low-grade dysplasia as opposed to surveillance alone may still be considered controversial which will be discussed in more detail in Chap. 31. Suffice it to say, recent randomized controlled data has shown that ablation of low-grade dysplasia results in successful eradication and significantly lower progression rates when compared to surveillance alone [8, 9].

Device Technology

RFA therapy employs the principle of high power energy over a short period of time delivered to the superficial tissue of the esophagus. The ablation technique is applied by using either balloon-based bipolar radiofrequency electrodes or endoscope-mounted articulating bipolar electrodes for focal ablation (Fig. 28.1). The balloon-based bipolar radiofrequency electrode has an array of electrodes circumferentially along the surface of the balloon. The radiofrequency generator (Barrx FLEX energy generator) delivers a standardized amount of energy that is distributed over the surface area of the balloon, which then ablates the superficial tissue without injury to the submucosa below.

Endoscope-mounted bipolar electrodes come in different sizes and allow for focal ablation (Table 28.1). The electrodes articulate (up, down, left, right) which allow for optimal and focal tissue contact. Each of the different sizes fits on the end of a standard endoscope (8.6–9.8 mm diameter scope) and uses the same Barrx FLEX generator. The newest addition, the Channel RFA device, is a through-the-scope catheter and fits through the working channel of a standard endoscope.

Surgical Technique

Standard setup and procedure are followed as in routine endoscopy. Monitored anesthesia care is preferred but not mandatory. Initially the esophagus is sprayed with acetylcysteine 1% and subsequently flushed with water to clean away mucous and prepare it for good contact during ablation. If circumferential ablation is to be performed, the next step requires sizing the esophageal diameter. A sizing catheter is passed over a guidewire inserted endoscopically. This catheter has a small balloon (autosizing balloon) at the tip that inflates and, with the energy generator feedback, calculates the diameter of the esophagus to insure a good fit for contact without excess pressure on the wall during ablation. The sizing balloon is typically placed 6 cm above the proximal extent of the Barrett's esophagus and advanced 1 cm based on markings on the catheter. Advancement every 1 cm is continued after each size is recorded until the catheter is in the stomach. The appropriate treatment balloon

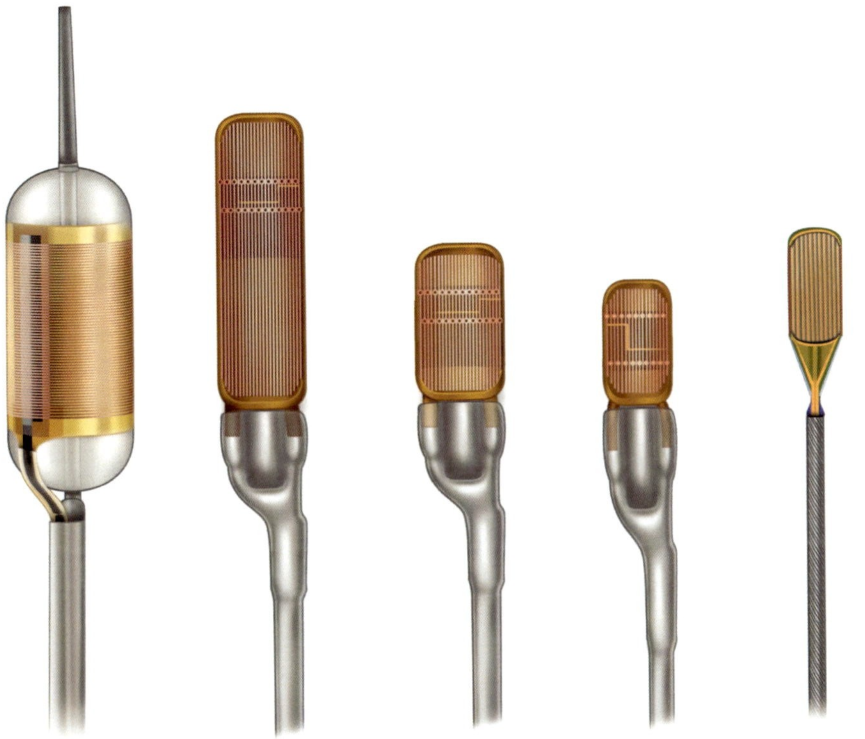

Fig. 28.1 Depiction of the various catheters used for radiofrequency ablation, including the balloon-based bipolar radiofrequency catheter for circumferential ablation as well as the various focal articulating bipolar electrodes

Table 28.1 Focal ablation catheters

Catheter	Size (length × width)
Barrx90 Ultra	40 mm × 13 mm
Barrx90	20.6 mm × 13.2 mm
Barrx60	15 mm × 10 mm
Channel RFA	15.7 mm × 7.5 mm

These catheters fit on the end of a standard endoscope (8.6–9.8 mm diameter scope) and are used with the Barrx FLEX generator. The newest addition, Channel RFA, fits through the working channel of a standard endoscope

catheter is then chosen based on this sizing. The outer diameter of the inflated ablation balloon should be smaller than the narrowest measured esophageal diameter. For example, if the smallest esophageal diameter measured is 29 mm, a 28 mm balloon should be chosen. Available balloon sizes are 18, 22, 25, 28, and 31 mm. One exception would be if a patient underwent prior EMR or ESD. In this case, the next smaller-size balloon should be chosen (i.e., 25 mm) in order to lower the risk of perforation.

The circumferential treatment balloon has electrodes 3 cm in length and covered with closely spaced radiofrequency electrodes as described above. After the sizing balloon is removed, the treatment balloon is placed over the guidewire, and the endoscope then follows the balloon for direct visualization. Treatment is started 1 cm proximal to the margin of visualized Barrett's esophagus. Approximately 10–12 J of energy is delivered in a circumferential manner to the tissue, and the treatment lasts for about 1–2 s. The circumferential balloon treatment is continued distally, with only small overlap between treatment areas to minimize regions at risk for stricture. Once the entire length of Barrett's is treated, the endoscope, balloon, and wire are removed. The balloon is gently inflated and cleaned outside of the patient. A soft cap is then placed on the tip of the endoscope, and the endoscope returned to the esophagus. The coagulum of the treated tissue is then gently scraped in a proximal to distal direction and the area forcefully rinsed with saline. The guidewire is then replaced, the endoscope removed, and the balloon catheter replaced over the guidewire. The endoscope is again introduced behind the balloon for direct visualization, and a second application of energy is delivered to all of the involved tissues in the same manner as the first application.

If focal ablation is performed with a mounted catheter (rather than the channel catheter), the electrode should be oriented to the 12 o'clock position on the video image. The endoscope and loaded catheter is then passed gently into the esophagus. The electrode is placed directly onto the involved mucosa and activated twice at 12–15 J. After all Barrett's tissue has been ablated, the electrode is used to push the coagulum off and the scope then removed to clean the electrode surface. The endoscope is then reinserted and the ablated areas treated again with a double application of 12–15 J.

Postoperative Management

After RFA is completed, maximal acid suppression is important in order to allow for the best chance at complete eradication of Barrett's esophagus. We prescribe either Nexium 40 mg twice daily or ask the patient to take a double dose of their proton-pump inhibitor twice daily for 2 weeks. In addition, we prescribe ranitidine 300 mg at bedtime for 2 weeks. Lastly, we prescribe sucralfate suspension, 1 g, four times daily for 2 weeks. After 2 weeks, these medications are discontinued with the exception of the proton-pump inhibitor.

It is recommended that patients be on a full (or nourishing) liquid diet for the first 24 h and then advance to a soft and general diet as tolerated. Patients should expect some throat and chest discomfort, but most are able to control this pain with liquid acetaminophen and/or ibuprofen. A minority of patients will require narcotic elixir.

For patients with high-grade dysplasia, after complete eradication, we recommend follow-up every 3 months for 1 year, every 6 months for the next year, and then yearly. Patients with low-grade dysplasia should be followed every 6 months for 1 year, then again after 1 year, and then once every 1–5 years. As follow-up studies are published and show long-term success, these follow-up periods may become more spaced out; however, currently there is not enough data to guide longer follow-up periods, and there is still risk of recurrent disease [10]. At these sessions, any residual Barrett's should be ablated. Most patients will require more than one session of ablation until there is complete eradication. If there appears to be complete eradication, biopsies every 1 cm in all four quadrants of the original length of Barrett's mucosa should be performed. If persistent Barrett's is noted after three or four separate ablations, we recommend that biopsies per the Seattle protocol be repeated prior to continuing with ablation in order to confirm that there has been no progression.

Complications

Radiofrequency ablation is very well tolerated. The most common side effect is postoperative chest pain. However this pain can often be managed with oral pain medications, viscous xylocaine or antacids. Risk of stricture post-RFA is a feared complication. Strictures after this treatment has been reported anywhere from 0% to 8% of cases [1, 5–7, 11]. However even when present, these strictures appear to be relatively easy to manage with dilation as compared to strictures that develop after photodynamic therapy [12]. Other complications such as bleeding and perforation are rare and infrequently reported.

Outcomes

The most common outcome of interest is eradication of dysplasia and reversion to squamous epithelium. Table 28.2 demonstrates various groups' outcomes after treating dysplasia with RFA. A recent meta-analysis reported complete eradication of dysplasia in 91% (95% CI, 87–95%) and complete eradication of intestinal metaplasia in 78% (95% CI, 70–86%). Furthermore after eradication, intestinal metaplasia recurred in only 13% of cases (95% CI, 9–18%) [4].

Table 28.2 Review of published outcomes after radiofrequency ablation for dysplasia

			Follow-up	Outcome		Stricture
	Study Size	Dysplasia types	(months)	CR-D	CR-IM	
Ganz et al. [5]	142	HGD	12	80.4%	54.3%	1 (0.7%)
Shaheen et al. [11]	106	LGD /HGD (51%)	24	95%	93%	8 (7.6%)
Velanovich [7]	66	LGD/HGD (18%)	12	100%	93%	4 (6.1%)
Sharma et al. [6]	63	LGD/HGD (38%)	24	89%	79%	1 (1.6%)

In comparison to other treatment modalities, RFA has the ability to treat long segments of disease with high rates of reversion to squamous epithelium. Randomized control trials have demonstrated the superior outcomes of RFA over surveillance alone for dysplasia [1, 9]. Although older treatment modalities such as multipolar electrocoagulation and argon plasma coagulation can lead to reversion to squamous epithelium, unlike RFA, these therapies treat small surface areas at each application; thus, treating long segments of disease became both difficult and time-consuming via these modalities. Photodynamic therapy (PDT) is a comparable therapy to RFA given the ability to treat long segments of disease easily; however, this therapy leads to lower rates of reversion. Additionally stricture rates after PDT are reported as high as 36% and result in densely fibrotic strictures that are highly resistant to dilation [2]. Lastly, RFA therapy has a reduced associated cost as compared to PDT.

Reports for longer follow-up are still required to understand the long-term efficacy of RFA treatment, and close surveillance is required to monitor for recurrent disease. However with these advances in RFA therapy, we have come a long way from morbid operations such as esophagectomy for high-grade dysplasia to relatively low-morbidity techniques which appear to effectively eradicate the disease.

Conclusions

RFA is a safe and efficacious treatment for high-grade dysplasia in the setting of Barrett's esophagus. This treatment has a low side effect and complication profile and can result in a high incidence of complete eradication of dysplasia and intestinal metaplasia.

References

1. Shaheen NJ, Sharma P, Overholt BF, Wolfsen HC, Sampliner RE, Wang KK, Galanko JA, Bronner MP, Goldblum JR, Bennett AE, Jobe BA, Eisen GM, Fennerty MB, Hunter JG, Fleischer DE, Sharma VK, Hawes RH, Hoffman BJ, Rothstein RI, Gordon SR, Mashimo H, Chang KJ, Muthusamy VR, Edmundowicz SA, Spechler SJ, Siddiqui AA, Souza RF, Infantolino A, Falk GW, Kimmey MB, Madanick RD, Chak A, Lightdale CJ. Radiofrequency ablation in Barrett's esophagus with dysplasia. N Engl J Med. 2009;360(22):2277–88.
2. Overholt BF, Lightdale CJ, Wang KK, Canto MI, Burdick S, Haggitt RC, Bronner MP, Taylor SL, Grace MG, Depot M, Esophagus IPGfH-GDiBs. Photodynamic therapy with porfimer sodium for ablation of high-grade dysplasia in Barrett's esophagus: international, partially blinded, randomized phase III trial. Gastrointest Endosc. 2005;62(4):488–98.
3. Overholt BF, Wang KK, Burdick JS, Lightdale CJ, Kimmey M, Nava HR, Sivak MV, Nishioka N, Barr H, Marcon N, Pedrosa M, Bronner MP, Grace M, Depot M, Esophagus IPGfH-GDiBs. Five-year efficacy and safety of photodynamic therapy with Photofrin in Barrett's high-grade dysplasia. Gastrointest Endosc. 2007;66(3):460–8.
4. Orman ES, Li N, Shaheen NJ. Efficacy and durability of radiofrequency ablation for Barrett's esophagus: systematic review and meta-analysis. Clin Gastroenterol Hepatol. 2013;11(10):1245–55.
5. Ganz RA, Overholt BF, Sharma VK, Fleischer DE, Shaheen NJ, Lightdale CJ, Freeman SR, Pruitt RE, Urayama SM, Gress F, Pavey DA, Branch MS, Savides TJ, Chang KJ, Muthusamy

VR, Bohorfoush AG, Pace SC, DeMeester SR, Eysselein VE, Panjehpour M, Triadafilopoulos G, Registry USM. Circumferential ablation of Barrett's esophagus that contains high-grade dysplasia: a U.S. multicenter registry. Gastrointest Endosc. 2008;68(1):35–40.

6. Sharma VK, Jae Kim H, Das A, Wells CD, Nguyen CC, Fleischer DE. Circumferential and focal ablation of Barrett's esophagus containing dysplasia. Am J Gastroenterol. 2009;104(2):310–7.
7. Velanovich V. Endoscopic endoluminal radiofrequency ablation of Barrett's esophagus: initial results and lessons learned. Surg Endosc. 2009;23(10):2175–80.
8. Small AJ, Araujo JL, Leggett CL, Mendelson AH, Agarwalla A, Abrams JA, Lightdale CJ, Wang TC, Iyer PG, Wang KK, Rustgi AK, Ginsberg GG, Forde KA, Gimotty PA, Lewis JD, Falk GW, Bewtra M. Radiofrequency ablation is associated with decreased neoplastic progression in patients with Barrett's esophagus and confirmed low-grade dysplasia. Gastroenterology. 2015;149(3):567–576.e563; quiz e513–564.
9. Phoa KN, van Vilsteren FG, Weusten BL, Bisschops R, Schoon EJ, Ragunath K, Fullarton G, Di Pietro M, Ravi N, Visser M, Offerhaus GJ, Seldenrijk CA, Meijer SL, ten Kate FJ, Tijssen JG, Bergman JJ. Radiofrequency ablation vs endoscopic surveillance for patients with Barrett esophagus and low-grade dysplasia: a randomized clinical trial. JAMA. 2014;311(12):1209–17.
10. Krishnamoorthi R, Singh S, Ragunathan K, A Katzka D, K Wang K, G Iyer P. Risk of recurrence of Barrett's esophagus after successful endoscopic therapy. Gastrointest Endosc. 2016;83(6):1090–1106.e1093.
11. Shaheen NJ, Overholt BF, Sampliner RE, Wolfsen HC, Wang KK, Fleischer DE, Sharma VK, Eisen GM, Fennerty MB, Hunter JG, Bronner MP, Goldblum JR, Bennett AE, Mashimo H, Rothstein RI, Gordon SR, Edmundowicz SA, Madanick RD, Peery AF, Muthusamy VR, Chang KJ, Kimmey MB, Spechler SJ, Siddiqui AA, Souza RF, Infantolino A, Dumot JA, Falk GW, Galanko JA, Jobe BA, Hawes RH, Hoffman BJ, Sharma P, Chak A, Lightdale CJ. Durability of radiofrequency ablation in Barrett's esophagus with dysplasia. Gastroenterology. 2011;141(2):460–8.
12. Shaheen NJ, Frantz DJ. When to consider endoscopic ablation therapy for Barrett's esophagus. Curr Opin Gastroenterol. 2010;26(4):361–6.

Endoscopic Mucosal Resection for Barrett's-Related Neoplasia

29

Kumar Krishnan and Srinadh Komanduri

Indication

Barrett's esophagus is a condition whereby the normal squamous epithelium is replaced by specialized intestine like mucosa. This process occurs in response to repetitive injury from reflux of gastroduodenal contents. The primary concern of this metaplastic process is the low but finite risk of malignant transformation. This process is thought to occur through a stepwise mechanism of cumulative genetic injury that results in dysplasia and subsequently malignancy [1]. Endoscopic therapy has largely replaced surgery for flat neoplastic disease within Barrett's esophagus. Radiofrequency ablation has demonstrated excellent efficacy and safety profile in multiple studies [2–4]. The primary limitation of mucosal ablative therapies for Barrett's esophagus is the inability to retain histology and provide detailed staging information on the neoplastic tissue. Further, lesions that may harbor disease deeper in the mucosa or submucosa should not undergo ablation due to the risk of inadequate treatment and subsequent risk of lymph node metastasis. This was highlighted by several surgical studies for suspected HGD which revealed that lymph node metastases were uncommon in patients with HGD or intramucosal carcinoma [5, 6]. However, lesions that involved the submucosa harbored lymph node metastasis at a rate of 20–25%. As such, accurate T staging is critical in managing patients with early esophageal neoplasia. While endoscopic ultrasound can be helpful, it is limited in distinguishing T1a from T1b lesion [7, 8]. Several studies have highlighted the importance of identifying such lesions, as ablation over such nodules

K. Krishnan (✉)
Division of Gastroenterology, Underwood Center for Digestive Disorders, Houston Methodist Hospital, Weill Cornell Medical College, Houston, TX, USA
e-mail: kkrishnan@mgh.harvard.edu

S. Komanduri
Department of Internal Medicine, Division of Gastroenterology, Northwestern University, Feinberg School of Medicine, Chicago, IL, USA

J. Grams et al. (eds.), *The SAGES Manual of Foregut Surgery*,
https://doi.org/10.1007/978-3-319-96122-4_29

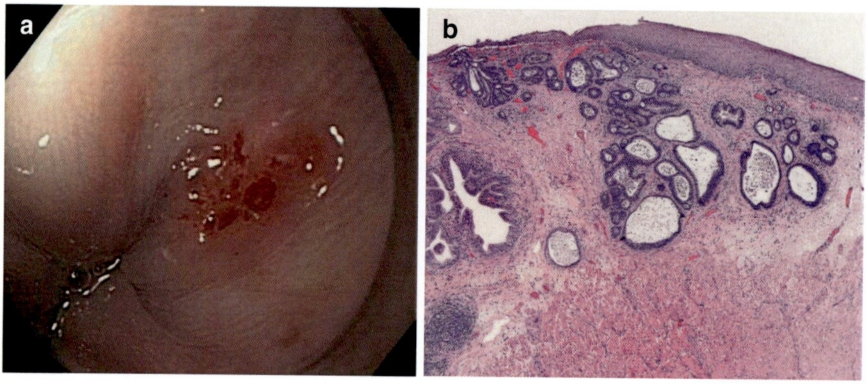

Fig. 29.1 (**a**) Squamous overgrowth. Endoscopic appearance of partial squamous overgrowth. (**b**) After endoscopic mucosal resection, histology reveals stratified squamous esophageal mucosa overlying deeper dysplastic glands

can result in squamous overgrowth of cancer (Fig. 29.1a, b) or inadequate treatment of esophageal cancer. For this reason, such lesions are best treated by endoscopic mucosal resection (EMR). EMR has the advantage of providing highly accurate T staging and can identify lesions that may require lymph node dissection. In addition to staging, EMR has been demonstrated to be highly effective for eradicating early mucosal adenocarcinoma of the esophagus [9] . One study also demonstrated that in 30% of cases, EMR specimens resulted in a change from initial diagnosis [10]. It is a useful adjunct to thermal ablative techniques, and the combination of both EMR with radiofrequency ablation is exceptionally effective in the management of dysplastic Barrett's esophagus with eradication rates for neoplastic Barrett's >90% [11].

Technique

Endoscopic resection for nodular Barrett's begins with appropriate identification of nodular disease. This requires a careful and comprehensive evaluation of the involved segment of Barrett's esophagus. This can be challenging due to peristalsis, secretion, and the mucous layer in the esophagus. As such, it is recommended to irrigate the distal esophagus with N-acetylcysteine to remove the layer of mucous on the surface of the esophagus, to better appreciate subtle changes within the mucosa. Optical enhancement is helpful, and this can take the form of either chemical chromoendoscopy (e.g., methylene blue) or optical chromoendoscopy (e.g., NBI). Recently, a validated NBI imaging criteria have been developed. These criteria focus on mucosal and vascular surface pattern irregularities to help identify areas of neoplastic Barrett's esophagus. Using these criteria, dysplastic areas can be assessed with 85% accuracy [12]. Once these areas have been identified, it is frequently helpful to apply cautery markings around the periphery of the lesion in order to ensure complete resection. This can be done with the tip of the snare using coagulation settings.

All endoscopic mucosal resection techniques involve the process of capturing mucosal tissue into a pseudopolyp configuration and subsequently using a standard snare to remove the pseudopolyp. The goal is to trap mucosal and some submucosal tissue while leaving the muscularis propria intact. The two primary techniques are referred to as band-assisted EMR and cap-assisted EMR. Both have demonstrated equal efficacy and safety. Cap-assisted EMR has the advantage of capturing slightly larger circumference of tissue, whereas band-assisted EMR has the advantage of easily developing multiple pseudopolyps for resection.

Cap-Assisted Endoscopic Mucosal Resection EMR

Cap EMR kits are commercially available from Olympus™ (Center Valley, PA). They consist of a translucent cap that fits on a standard gastroscope. The cap accommodates a snare which fits within a small groove within the distal end of the cap. Once the lesion of interest is targeted, a small submucosal injection is performed to slightly raise the lesion. The lesion is then targeted within the cap and suction is applied to bring the lesion into the cap. Once an adequate amount of tissue is captured within the cap, the assistant gently closes the snare (Fig. 29.2), and the pseudopolyp is carefully examined. Gentle shaking of the snare can help determine if muscle is trapped within the pseudopolyp. At this point, the pseudopolyp is resected using electrocautery. Either primary coagulation or a blended cutting current can be used. The base of the resection is carefully examined to assess for perforation. It is frequently helpful to use blue dye (indigo carmine or methylene blue) in the submucosal injection. This can help determine whether a deep resection has been performed. If the resection base is stained uniformly blue, then it is clear that only mucosa and submucosa has been resected. If there are areas of white or yellow surrounded by blue submucosa, this can indicate a deeper resection (e.g., target sign), and care should be made to assess for a perforation.

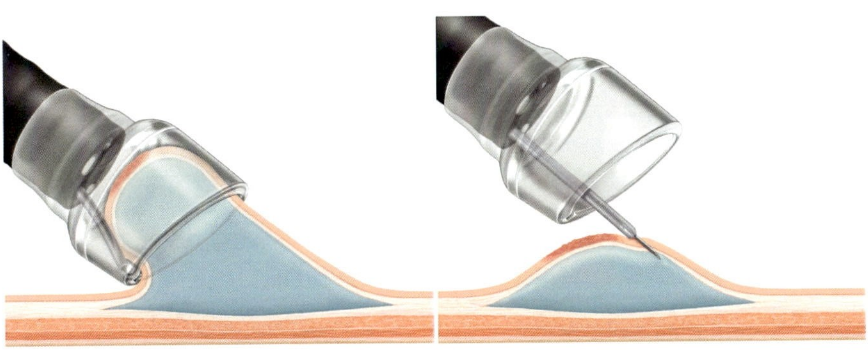

Fig. 29.2 Cap-assisted EMR. After submucosal injection, the cap is centered around the lesion of interest. It is suctioned into the cap and a snare is used to capture the lesion

Subsequently, the specimen should be retrieved, and additional resections can be performed if desired. It is important to note that the provided snare in some of the commercial cap EMR kits are single use, and additional resections may require a separate snare.

Band-Assisted EMR

Band-assisted EMR has largely replaced cap-assisted EMR as the primary EMR technique. There are two commercially available band-assisted EMR devices: the Duette© kit from Cook Medical (Bloomington, IN) and the Captivator© device from Boston Scientific (Marlborough, MA). Both devices function in a similar manner. Band-assisted EMR kits have a very similar installation to standard variceal banding kits. They consist of six rubber bands attached to a translucent cap. The rubber bands contain a tripwire/string that is passed through the working channel and connected to a knob at the insertion of the working channel. Similar to variceal band ligation, each band can be deployed by turning the knob at the working channel insertion.

The technique of band-assisted EMR is similar to cap EMR. The lesion of interest is targeted using the cap. Unlike cap-assisted EMR, submucosal injection is not required. Once the lesion of interest is targeted, it is centered within the cap and suction is applied. It is important to ensure the entire lesion is suctioned into the cap. The band is then deployed, thus creating a pseudopolyp. At this point, a snare is advanced through the working channel and positioned around the polyp. The snare can be placed either above or below the band; however, a slightly larger area will be obtained by placing the snare below the band (Fig. 29.3). Again, standard cautery (either coagulation or blended cut settings) is utilized, and the lesion is removed. Additional areas can then be resected to ensure wide margin resection. Further, a broader resection can be performed by deploying a second band adjacent to a resection base, thus creating a large resection area. Areas that do not adequately lift into the resection cap or appear ulcerated are indicative of extensive submucosal fibrosis or a lesion with infiltration into the muscular area. These lesions should not be treated with EMR and may require surgical resection.

Postoperative Management

Postoperative management of patients after endoscopic mucosal resection includes control of symptoms and prevention of complications. The most common symptom to be encountered is chest pain. This is a result of the iatrogenic ulcer that is created from the resection base. This is typically self-limited. We place all patients on a liquid diet for 24 h, followed by a soft diet for 1 week. Acid suppression is critical, with all patients placed on double-dose, proton-pump inhibitors. Sucralfate suspension is given for 1 week, and acetaminophen with codeine as an elixir is given on an as-needed basis for pain. As with all luminal resection, nonsteroidal

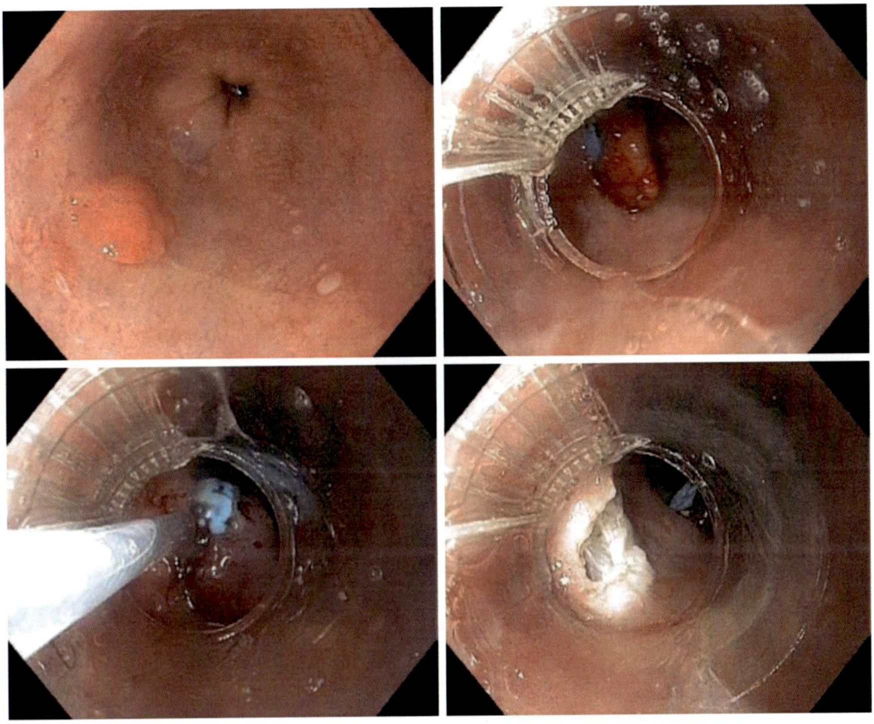

Fig. 29.3 Band-assisted EMR. A nodular lesion is noted in an area of flat Barrett's esophagus. Using the band-assisted device, the lesion is targeted. The lesion is suctioned in the cap and a band is deployed. The snare is placed below the band, and the lesion is removed en bloc

anti-inflammatory medications are avoided. We typically hold antiplatelet agents for 48 h after resection before carefully resuming.

Patients will require follow-up endoscopy in 2 months. At this point, additional endoscopic mucosal resection can be performed. If there are no areas of nodular disease, ablative techniques can be utilized.

Postoperative Complications

Endoscopic mucosal resection techniques have demonstrated relative safety. Major complications remain uncommon. Complications can be either early or late. The most common early complications are bleeding and perforation. A recent pooled systematic review noted the risk of bleeding to be 1.1% and perforation rates of 0.2% [11]. Immediate bleeding is the result of injury to penetrating submucosal vessels. This can be easily treated by centering the bleeding lesion with the cap and utilizing hemostatic forceps to coagulate the bleeding vessel. This is preferred over other thermal therapies that require coaptation of the vessel, which could lead to deep injury and perforation.

Perforation is a rare but severe complication of EMR. Full-thickness perforation of the esophagus can result in mediastinitis, pneumomediastinum, and rapid decompensation. Utilization of carbon dioxide for insufflation can prevent major respiratory issues from a perforation. Small perforations, when identified, may be able to be closed using hemostatic clips. Occasionally, tissue apposition is not amenable to closure using hemostatic clips. In this circumstance, alternatives include over the scope clip devices such as the OVESCO clip (OTSC, Carey, NC) or endoscopic suturing devices. In the absence of these devices and in the presence of a large perforation, a fully covered esophageal stent can be placed.

The most common late complication is the development of stricture. This has been noted in up to 10% of cases. Stricture rates correlate with the extent of resection, as those patients who undergo >50% circumferential EMR will almost uniformly develop esophageal stricture. Most strictures are amenable to endoscopic dilation techniques. Studies have demonstrated efficacy and safety of radical EMR with extensive mucosal resection; however, the stricture rates approach 50% in this patient population.

Postoperative Outcomes

Endoscopic mucosal resection is ideally utilized to treat visible lesions in the context of Barrett's neoplasia. As a monotherapy, however, two studies reveal that EMR can lead to complete eradication rates for Barrett's esophagus of 90–97% [13, 14]. More commonly, EMR is used as an adjunct in the comprehensive management of Barrett's esophagus, with an ablative technique used for flat Barrett's esophagus. Utilizing this approach eradication rates for Barrett's-associated neoplasia has been reported to be between 90% and 97% [15, 16]. This approach has resulted in far fewer strictures than with EMR alone and, as such, is the preferred treatment strategy for patients with Barrett's esophagus.

There is a paucity of data comparing cap-assisted vs band-assisted endoscopic mucosal resection in the context of neoplastic Barrett's esophagus. The advantages of each were discussed above. There does exist one randomized control trial comparing both approaches. This one study demonstrated the band-assisted EMR was faster and cheaper *compared* to cap EMR. There was no difference in perforation or bleeding risk. The size of each specimen was slightly larger in the cap EMR group, but the clinical relevance of this was not clear [17].

There is a growing interest in endoscopic submucosal dissection (ESD) as an alternative plan to EMR. This technique involves submucosal injection followed by dissection of the submucosal plane until complete en bloc resection has occurred. It is substantially more technically challenging compared to the EMR techniques and has not gained widespread acceptance in the United States. The largest multicenter study in the United States reveal that ESD performed at expert centers can be safely performed. En bloc resection rates were 96%. Strictures, however, were commonly encountered but managed endoscopically [18]. It is unclear, at present, the exact role of ESD in the management of Barrett's-associated neoplasia, and more data will be required before widespread use.

Conclusion

Endoscopic eradication therapy remains the primary treatment approach for neoplastic Barrett's esophagus. Visible lesions can frequently indicate more advanced disease and, as such, should be removed en bloc for accurate histologic analysis and staging. There are two primary techniques for endoscopic resection. Both are effective and have relative advantages. It is critical for endoscopists who perform endoscopic therapy for Barrett's esophagus to be proficient in EMR. Currently, many mechanisms exist for endoscopists to obtain proper training for all aspects of endoscopic eradication therapy. Successful outcomes including durable eradication of intestinal metaplasia, accurate staging, and avoidance of occult malignancy rely on successful endoscopic mucosal resection techniques.

References

1. Spechler SJ, Souza RF. Barrett's esophagus. N Engl J Med. 2014;371:836–45.
2. Shaheen NJ, Sharma P, Overholt BF, et al. Radiofrequency ablation in Barrett's esophagus with dysplasia. N Engl J Med. 2009;360:2277–88.
3. Phoa KN, van Vilsteren FG, Weusten BL, et al. Radiofrequency ablation vs endoscopic surveillance for patients with Barrett esophagus and low-grade dysplasia: a randomized clinical trial. JAMA. 2014;311:1209–17.
4. Shaheen NJ, Overholt BF, Sampliner RE, et al. Durability of radiofrequency ablation in Barrett's esophagus with dysplasia. Gastroenterology. 2011;141:460–8.
5. Rice TW, Zuccaro G Jr, Adelstein DJ, et al. Esophageal carcinoma: depth of tumor invasion is predictive of regional lymph node status. Ann Thorac Surg. 1998;65:787–92.
6. Stein HJ, Feith M, Bruecher BL, et al. Early esophageal cancer: pattern of lymphatic spread and prognostic factors for long-term survival after surgical resection. Ann Surg. 2005;242:566–73; discussion 573–5.
7. Falk GW. Endoscopic ultrasound in the evaluation of Barrett's esophagus: a preliminary report. Am J Gastroenterol. 1995;90:1187.
8. Spechler SJ, Sharma P, Souza RF, et al. American gastroenterological association technical review on the management of Barrett's esophagus. Gastroenterology. 2011;140:e18–52; quiz e13.
9. Pech O, May A, Manner H, et al. Long-term efficacy and safety of endoscopic resection for patients with mucosal adenocarcinoma of the esophagus. Gastroenterology. 2014;146:652–660.e1.
10. Wani S, Abrams J, Edmundowicz SA, et al. Endoscopic mucosal resection results in change of histologic diagnosis in Barrett's esophagus patients with visible and flat neoplasia: a multicenter cohort study. Dig Dis Sci. 2013;58:1703–9.
11. Desai M, Saligram S, Gupta N, et al. Efficacy and safety outcomes of multimodal endoscopic eradication therapy in Barrett's esophagus-related neoplasia: a systematic review and pooled analysis. Gastrointest Endosc. 2016;85(3):482–495.e4.
12. Sharma P, Bergman JJ, Goda K, et al. Development and validation of a classification system to identify high-grade dysplasia and esophageal adenocarcinoma in Barrett's esophagus using narrow-band imaging. Gastroenterology. 2016;150:591–8.
13. Anders M, Bahr C, El-Masry MA, et al. Long-term recurrence of neoplasia and Barrett's epithelium after complete endoscopic resection. Gut. 2014;63:1535–43.
14. Chennat J, Konda VJ, Ross AS, et al. Complete Barrett's eradication endoscopic mucosal resection: an effective treatment modality for high-grade dysplasia and intramucosal carcinoma–an American single-center experience. Am J Gastroenterol. 2009;104:2684–92.

15. Li N, Pasricha S, Bulsiewicz WJ, et al. Effects of preceding endoscopic mucosal resection on the efficacy and safety of radiofrequency ablation for treatment of Barrett's esophagus: results from the United States radiofrequency ablation registry. Dis Esophagus. 2016;29:537–43.
16. Phoa KN, Pouw RE, Bisschops R, et al. Multimodality endoscopic eradication for neoplastic Barrett oesophagus: results of an European multicentre study (EURO-II). Gut. 2016;65:555–62.
17. Pouw RE, van Vilsteren FG, Peters FP, et al. Randomized trial on endoscopic resection-cap versus multiband mucosectomy for piecemeal endoscopic resection of early Barrett's neoplasia. Gastrointest Endosc. 2011;74:35–43.
18. Yang D, Coman RM, Kahaleh M, et al. Endoscopic submucosal dissection for Barrett's early neoplasia: a multicenter study in the United States. Gastrointest Endosc. 2016;86(4):600–7.

The Role of Photodynamic Therapy and Cryotherapy for the Management of Barrett's Esophagus

30

Hope T. Jackson and Andrew S. Wright

Introduction

Gastroesophageal reflux can cause injury to the normal stratified squamous epithelium of the esophagus. This injury may lead to replacement of the normal esophageal lining by a metaplastic columnar intestinal-like epithelium known as Barrett's esophagus (BE). The clinical relevance of BE lies in its sequential progression from intestinal metaplasia (IM) to low-grade dysplasia (LGD), high-grade dysplasia (HGD), and, finally, invasive adenocarcinoma [1]. In the absence of dysplasia, BE is associated with a low annual incidence of progression to adenocarcinoma (less than 0.5), but the incidence of progression to adenocarcinoma is up to five times as high when dysplasia is present [2–6]. The management of BE with dysplasia and early cancer has shifted over the years, moving away from surgical resection (esophagectomy) to diagnostic and therapeutic endoscopy. Endoscopic therapy aims to remove the metaplastic or dysplastic tissue to a depth that destroys all the BE but minimizes damage to the submucosal layer of the esophagus to avoid stricture formation and transmural injury [7]. Several treatment options—endoscopic mucosal resection (EMR) and tissue ablative therapies such as radiofrequency ablation (RFA), photodynamic therapy (PDT), and cryotherapy (CT)—have been recognized as safe and effective therapies to accomplish this and are now the standard of care in many expert centers [8]. This chapter will focus on the role of photodynamic therapy and cryotherapy in the management of BE.

H. T. Jackson
University of Maryland School of Medicine, Baltimore, MD, USA
e-mail: hjackson@som.umaryland.edu

A. S. Wright (✉)
University of Washington Medical School, Seattle, WA, USA
e-mail: awright2@uw.edu

J. Grams et al. (eds.), *The SAGES Manual of Foregut Surgery*,
https://doi.org/10.1007/978-3-319-96122-4_30

Photodynamic Therapy

Technique

Photodynamic therapy (PDT) combines laser light and a photosensitizing agent that work together to cause selective tissue destruction. Sodium porfimer (Photofrin) is the only photosensitizing agent that is FDA approved in the United States and is given intravenously, while 5-aminolevulinic acid (5-ALA) is an oral agent approved for use in Europe. These agents are given 48–72 h before endoscopy and are absorbed preferentially by tissue with abnormal (hypermetabolic) activity. After the agent is fully absorbed by the target tissue, endoscopy is performed, and a laser light of appropriate power and wavelength is delivered to the affected area, activating the photosensitizing agent. The agent then reacts with oxygen causing free radicals that induce cell membrane damage and apoptosis [9].

Efficacy

Sodium porfimer (SP) is the photosensitizing agent approved in the United States for treatment of BE and HGD based on several studies. The first study came from Overholt and colleagues. This was a cohort study of 100 patients who had BE with dysplasia (HGD and LGD) who were treated with photodynamic therapy and followed for an average of 51 months [10]. These patients had a mean reduction in the length of Barrett's mucosa by 7 cm. Fifty-four percent of the patients had complete elimination of BE. Ninety-three percent of patients with LGD had complete remission, 78% of patients with HGD had complete remission, and 48% of those with early cancer had complete remission. Small areas of residual or nonresponding areas of BE were treated with a Nd:YAG laser with subsequent eradication. The study concluded that PDT alone or in combination with Nd:YAG laser thermal ablation provides effective endoscopic therapy for BE with dysplasia and can reduce the extent of and in some cases eliminate BE [10].

A larger multicenter, partially blinded, randomized clinical trial also conducted by Overholt et al. looked at a different cohort of patients with BE who had HGD [11]. Patients (208) were randomized to compare SP-PDT plus omeprazole therapy (138) versus omeprazole therapy alone (70). The study found that patients with SP-PDT with omeprazole had a significantly higher incidence of complete ablation of HGD than those in the omeprazole alone group (77% vs 39%). They concluded that SP-PDT was an effective therapy for ablating HGD in patients with BE and reducing the incidence of esophageal adenocarcinoma. This response was still present at a 5-year follow-up study [9]. Other centers have reported results of SP-PDT with similar outcomes [12–14].

5-Aminolevulinic acid (5-ALA) is an oral agent that is commonly chosen as the photosensitizing agent of choice in Europe. A study by Gossner et al. looked at 32 patients with BE (10) or superficial mucosal cancer (22) who underwent 5-ALA PDT [15]. The patients were maintained on omeprazole therapy, and the mean follow-up was 10 months. HGD was eradicated in all patients. Another study by Ackroyd et al. randomly assigned 36 patients to 5-ALA PDT or placebo followed by laser treatment [16]. Of the 18 patients given PDT, 89% showed macroscopic evidence of BE regression, and all had complete clearance of dysplasia. The area of BE was reduced by 30% in these patients. Only 11% of patients in the placebo group had a reduction in the area of BE, and only 33% of the placebo group had clearance of dysplasia. In terms of long-term outcomes, Pech et al. studied 66 BE patients with HGD (35) and adenocarcinoma (31) who were treated with 5-ALA PDT between 1996 and 2002 [17]. A complete response was observed in 97 and 100% in the two groups, respectively, at 37 months. Local recurrence was 3% (1) in those with HGD and 32% in those with adenocarcinoma during the entire study period.

Reported advantages of 5-ALA compared with SP are oral administration, shorter duration of skin photosensitivity (24–48 h versus 30 days), and preferential accumulation in the mucosa (SP also accumulates in the submucosa) which may limit tissue injury and, thus, complications such as stricture and perforation [15, 18, 19].

A single-center, randomized controlled trial by Dunn et al. compared SP-PDT and 5-ALA PDT. Sixty-four patients were randomized, 34 to 5-ALA and 30 to SP-PDT [20]. The median follow-up was 23 months. Strictures and skin photosensitivity were significantly more common with SP-PDT than 5ALA-PDT (33% vs 9% and 43% vs 6%, respectively). For BE less than 6 cm, complete regression of HGD was more likely with 5-ALA than SP. For BE greater than 6 cm, there was no significant difference in outcome between the PDT photosensitizers.

Complications

Several of the studies previously discussed describe complications associated with both SP and 5-ALA PDT. The SP-PDT multicenter trial by Overholt et al. reported patients experienced photosensitivity (69%), esophageal strictures (36%), and vomiting (32%) as the top 3 complications [11]. Odynophagia and fever were less commonly reported. The stricture rate was similar in Overholt's prior cohort study (34%) [10]. Elevated liver enzymes, chest pain, and neuropathy have been reported with the use of 5-ALA PDT [15–19]. Only Dunn et al. reported an incidence of strictures with 5-ALA use (9%) [20].

"Buried" Barrett's esophagus, residual BE that can become hidden under the neosquamous epithelium that forms following PDT, has also been reported as a potential complication. This can occur if PDT does not destroy all of the metaplastic epithelium. The partially treated mucosa may then heal with an overlying layer of neosquamous epithelium that then buries metaplastic glands where they can be missed on follow-up endoscopy [21]. This buried metaplasia may have malignant potential [22]. A systematic review by Gray and colleagues that included 22 studies of PDT for Barrett's esophagus with 953 patients found "buried metaplasia" in 14% (135) of patients [21]. The rate of buried glands has been shown to be significantly higher post-PDT (48%) than pre-PDT (20%), irrespective of the photosensitizing agent used [20]. The clinical relevance of buried Barrett's however is still controversial as it can be found in the absence of PDT, most commonly at the Z-line (squamocolumnar junction) [21].

Summary

PDT has been shown to be an effective minimally invasive alternative treatment to surgical resection for Barrett's esophagus with high-grade dysplasia. The side effect profile has limited its use as other endoscopic therapies have emerged. Future advances in PDT aim to focus on the development of photosensitizers with more favorable characteristics, non-laser methods of activating photosensitizers, and approaches that combine photodynamic therapy with other techniques.

Cryotherapy

Technique

The goal of cryotherapy is to create mucosal cellular destruction using freeze-thaw cycles. The therapy is performed by delivering low-pressure liquid nitrogen or carbon dioxide to the dysplastic area via a spray catheter. The treatment is applied for a total of 40s (two 20s applications or four 10s applications) and produces a 2 mm depth of injury [24]. The mechanism of injury to the mucosa involves cycles of rapid freezing and slow thawing that leads to the formation of extracellular and intracellular ice. This process disrupts cell membranes and causes tissue ischemia/destruction through vascular stasis from decreased blood flow, endothelial damage, and vascular thrombosis [25].

Efficacy

Johnston et al. reported the first study on the efficacy of cryotherapy for the treatment of BE [26]. This was a prospective single-center study of 11 patients with BE ranging from no dysplasia to HGD. Nine patients completed the study protocol, and 78% (7) of patients had complete eradication of BE at 6 months. Two patients were found to have buried BE. There were no reported complications at 12 months. Greenwald et al. published a similar prospective cohort study that found a 94% eradication rate for HGD with complications that included chest pain, dysphagia, and one gastric perforation [27].

Shaheen et al. subsequently published a multicenter retrospective study evaluating liquid nitrogen spray cryotherapy in patients with BE with HGD [28]. Ninety-eight patients were included, but only 58 patients completed treatment, comprising the efficacy cohort. The mean follow-up was 10.5 months. In the subset of patients completing therapy, complete eradication of HGD was seen in 97% of patients. Eighty-seven percent had complete eradication of all dysplasia with persistent non-dysplastic BE, and 57% had complete eradication of all BE. There were no esophageal perforations and strictures developed in three patients (5%) who were treated successfully with dilation. Two patients (3%) reported severe chest pain managed with oral narcotics. Buried BE was found in two subjects (3%).

Long-term efficacy studies are limited. Gosain et al. performed a retrospective study of 32 patients with BE with HGD [29]. Patients were treated with liquid nitrogen cryotherapy every 8 weeks (median treatment number was 4) until complete eradication of HGD and BE was confirmed by endoscopic biopsy. The median follow-up was 37 months. At the 2-year follow-up, complete eradication of HGD was found in all 32 patients and complete eradication of BE in 27 patients (84%). At the last follow-up of the study period, complete eradication of HGD was found in 31 patients (97%) and complete eradication of BE in 26 patients (81%). Recurrent HGD was found in six patients (18%), with complete eradication of HGD in five patients after repeat treatment. One patient progressed to adenocarcinoma and was subsequently downgraded to HGD after repeat cryotherapy. BE segment length greater than 3 cm was associated with a higher recurrence of BE but not HGD. Stricture was seen in three patients (9%) and all were successfully dilated.

Studies on the use of carbon dioxide cryotherapy for BE with dysplasia are also limited. Canto et al. reported, in abstract form only, on 44 patients with a median follow-up of 12 months [30]. Seven patients had failed prior treatment with photodynamic therapy or radiofrequency ablation. Treatment was completed in 23 patients, with complete eradication of HGD and BE seen in 21 (91%) and 22 patients (96%), respectively. Only two patients reported mild chest discomfort.

Xue et al. has the only published study on CO_2 cryotherapy [31]. This prospective, single-center study looked at 20 patients who were treated with CO_2 cryotherapy for BE. Ninety percent of patients had complete eradication of BE. At 6 months, one patient developed recurrent BE with no dysplasia and two patients had buried BE. Two patients developed mild chest discomfort which did not require treatment, and three patients developed esophagitis that was successfully treated with daily omeprazole. There were no reports of bleeding or perforation in this study, and the mean follow-up was 10 months.

There are no studies in the current literature that examine the efficacy of cryotherapy in combination with other endoscopic therapies, but the study by Canto and colleagues suggests there may be a role for cryotherapy when other therapies such as RFA and PDT fail. The most commonly reported side effects of this therapy are self-limited chest pain and dysphagia. Stricture, esophagitis, and perforation were less commonly reported.

Summary

Cryotherapy has been shown to be safe and efficacious in the treatment of BE with dysplasia. The low side effect profile, relatively simple technique, and high efficacy make it an attractive therapy of choice. Further long-term studies are needed, however, prior to recommending widespread use.

Comparisons to Other Endoscopic Therapies

Other endoscopic therapies such as radiofrequency ablation (RFA) (discussed in Chap. 28) and endomucosal resection (EMR, Chap. 29) are alternative endoscopic treatments for BE. There are no randomized comparative therapy studies in the current literature. One retrospective study does compare outcomes between PDT and RFA. Ertan et al. performed a single-institution retrospective analysis of patients who received PDT (33) and RFA (53) for BE with dysplasia [23]. Complete resolution of Barrett's occurred in 18 patients (54.5%) who received PDT and 47 patients (88.7%) who received RFA. In the PDT cohort, two patients reported photosensitivity reactions, nine (28%) developed strictures that required serial endoscopic dilations, and one patient developed an esophageal perforation that was managed nonoperatively. In the RFA cohort, two patients (4%) developed a stricture managed with dilation. No perforation was reported. Buried Barrett's was seen in four (12.5%) PDT patients and four (6%) RFA patients. According to the study's institution cost analysis, PDT was five times costlier than RFA. The authors concluded that RFA was more cost-effective than PDT and had a higher rate of resolution of BE without serious adverse events.

Conclusion

Endoscopic therapies to manage Barrett's esophagus continue to evolve. PDT and cryotherapy are safe and efficacious endoscopic therapies for the management of BE with dysplasia. Limited data exist to guide the choice between different endoscopic modalities for BE (RFA, cryotherapy, or PDT). Side effect profiles and the lack of long-term studies have limited the widespread adaptation of these techniques. Looking forward, long-term efficacy studies and technology advances are needed to further advance the endoscopic management of BE.

References

1. Pellegrini CA, Pohl D. High-grade dysplasia in Barrett's esophagus: surveillance or operation? J Gastrointest Surg. 2000;4(2):131–4.
2. Hvid-Jensen F, et al. Incidence of adenocarcinoma among patients with Barrett's esophagus. N Engl J Med. 2011;365(15):1375–83.
3. Rastogi A, et al. Incidence of esophageal adenocarcinoma in patients with Barrett's esophagus and high-grade dysplasia: a meta-analysis. Gastrointest Endosc. 2008;67(3):394–8.
4. Sharma P, et al. Dysplasia and cancer in a large multicenter cohort of patients with Barrett's esophagus. Clin Gastroenterol Hepatol. 2006;4(5):566–72.
5. Desai TK, et al. The incidence of oesophageal adenocarcinoma in non-dysplastic Barrett's oesophagus: a meta-analysis. Gut. 2012;61(7):970–6.

6. Shakhatreh MH, et al. The incidence of esophageal adenocarcinoma in a national veterans cohort with Barrett's esophagus. Am J Gastroenterol. 2014;109(12):1862–8. quiz 1861, 1869.
7. Dunkin BL, Lyons C. Endoscopic therapies for Barrett's esophagus. In: Swanstrom LL, Soper NJ, editors. Mastery of endoscopic and laparoscopic surgery. Philadelphia: Lippincott Williams & Wilkins; 2014.
8. Sappati Biyyani RS, Chak A. Barrett's esophagus: review of diagnosis and treatment. Gastroenterol Rep (Oxf). 2013;1(1):9–18.
9. Overholt BF, et al. Five-year efficacy and safety of photodynamic therapy with Photofrin in Barrett's high-grade dysplasia. Gastrointest Endosc. 2007;66(3):460–8.
10. Overholt BF, Panjehpour M, Haydek JM. Photodynamic therapy for Barrett's esophagus: follow-up in 100 patients. Gastrointest Endosc. 1999;49(1):1–7.
11. Overholt BF, et al. Photodynamic therapy with porfimer sodium for ablation of high-grade dysplasia in Barrett's esophagus: international, partially blinded, randomized phase III trial. Gastrointest Endosc. 2005;62(4):488–98.
12. Wang KK, Kim JY. Photodynamic therapy in Barrett's esophagus. Gastrointest Endosc Clin N Am. 2003;13(3):483–9. vii
13. Wolfsen HC, et al. Clinical experience of patients undergoing photodynamic therapy for Barrett's dysplasia or cancer. Aliment Pharmacol Ther. 2004;20(10):1125–31.
14. Wolfsen HC, Woodward TA, Raimondo M. Photodynamic therapy for dysplastic Barrett esophagus and early esophageal adenocarcinoma. Mayo Clin Proc. 2002;77(11):1176–81.
15. Gossner L, et al. Photodynamic ablation of high-grade dysplasia and early cancer in Barrett's esophagus by means of 5-aminolevulinic acid. Gastroenterology. 1998;114(3):448–55.
16. Ackroyd R, et al. Photodynamic therapy for dysplastic Barrett's oesophagus: a prospective, double blind, randomised, placebo controlled trial. Gut. 2000;47(5):612–7.
17. Pech O, et al. Long-term results of photodynamic therapy with 5-aminolevulinic acid for superficial Barrett's cancer and high-grade intraepithelial neoplasia. Gastrointest Endosc. 2005;62(1):24–30.
18. Barr H, et al. Eradication of high-grade dysplasia in columnar-lined (Barrett's) oesophagus by photodynamic therapy with endogenously generated protoporphyrin IX. Lancet. 1996;348(9027):584–5.
19. Ackroyd R, et al. 5-Aminolevulinic acid photosensitization of dysplastic Barrett's esophagus: a pharmacokinetic study. Photochem Photobiol. 1999;70(4):656–62.
20. Dunn JM, et al. A randomised controlled trial of ALA vs. Photofrin photodynamic therapy for high-grade dysplasia arising in Barrett's oesophagus. Lasers Med Sci. 2013;28(3):707–15.
21. Gray NA, Odze RD, Spechler SJ. Buried metaplasia after endoscopic ablation of Barrett's esophagus: a systematic review. Am J Gastroenterol. 2011;106(11):1899–908. quiz 1909.
22. Van Laethem JL, et al. Intramucosal adenocarcinoma arising under squamous re-epithelialisation of Barrett's oesophagus. Gut. 2000;46(4):574–7.
23. Ertan A, et al. Photodynamic therapy vs radiofrequency ablation for Barrett's dysplasia: efficacy, safety and cost-comparison. World J Gastroenterol. 2013;19(41):7106–13.
24. Azarm A, et al. Endoscopic management of Barrett's esophagus: advances in endoscopic techniques. Dig Dis Sci. 2012;57(12):3055–64.
25. Greenwald BD, Dumot JA. Cryotherapy for Barrett's esophagus and esophageal cancer. Curr Opin Gastroenterol. 2011;27(4):363–7.
26. Johnston MH, et al. Cryoablation of Barrett's esophagus: a pilot study. Gastrointest Endosc. 2005;62(6):842–8.
27. Greenwald BD, et al. Safety, tolerability, and efficacy of endoscopic low-pressure liquid nitrogen spray cryotherapy in the esophagus. Dis Esophagus. 2010;23(1):13–9.
28. Shaheen NJ, et al. Safety and efficacy of endoscopic spray cryotherapy for Barrett's esophagus with high-grade dysplasia. Gastrointest Endosc. 2010;71(4):680–5.
29. Gosain S, et al. Liquid nitrogen spray cryotherapy in Barrett's esophagus with high-grade dysplasia: long-term results. Gastrointest Endosc. 2013;78(2):260–5.

30. Canto MI. Carbon dioxide (CO2) cryotherapy is a safe and effective treatment of Barrett's esophagus (BE) with HGD/Intramucosal carcinoma. Gastrointest Endosc. 2009;69(5):AB341–AB341.
31. Xue HB, et al. A pilot study of endoscopic spray cryotherapy by pressurized carbon dioxide gas for Barrett's esophagus. Endoscopy. 2011;43(5):379–85.

31 Expert Commentary: Surveillance Versus Ablation for Patients with Low-Grade Dysplasia

John G. Hunter and Joseph M. Drosdeck

An estimated 25–40% of patients with Barrett's esophagus (BE) will be diagnosed with low-grade dysplasia (LGD) at some point in their lifetime [1]. Progression to high-grade dysplasia (HGD) or esophageal adenocarcinoma (EAC) is difficult to quantify but may occur at a rate of up to 13.4% per person-year [2]. Identifying those at risk for malignant transformation is challenging, partly because the diagnosis of LGD is difficult. A high degree of interobserver variability exists between pathologists [3], which has significant clinical implications. One report revealed that 85% of patients previously diagnosed with LGD were downgraded to non-dysplastic BE after evaluation by an expert gastrointestinal pathologist [2]. This underscores the importance of expert consultation to establish a firm diagnosis before proceeding with treatment.

Prior to the development of ablation therapy, patients and physicians lacked suitable treatment options for LGD and therefore adhered to a strict regimen of endoscopic surveillance [4]. Although this remains a viable option, endoscopic ablation technology has expanded the management of LGD by allowing for eradication of dysplastic mucosa, thereby minimizing the chances of carcinogenesis. Of the various ablation techniques available, radiofrequency ablation (RFA) has emerged as the most common and best-studied modality. A growing body of evidence supports RFA as a safe, effective, and durable treatment for LGD.

Among the most compelling evidence for RFA in patients with LGD is the AIM Dysplasia trial – a multicenter, randomized, sham-controlled trial that compared RFA plus endoscopic surveillance to endoscopic surveillance alone in patients with dysplastic BE. At 12 months, 90.5% of RFA-treated patients had complete eradication of LGD, compared to 22.7% of controls ($p < 0.001$). Patients who received

J. G. Hunter
Department of Surgery, OHSU, Portland, OR, USA

J. M. Drosdeck (✉)
Department of General Surgery, The Everett Clinic, Everett, WA, USA
e-mail: jdrosdeck@everettclinic.com

J. Grams et al. (eds.), *The SAGES Manual of Foregut Surgery*,
https://doi.org/10.1007/978-3-319-96122-4_31

ablation also had significantly less disease progression (3.6% vs. 16.3%, $p = 0.03$). Few serious adverse effects were noted, but RFA was associated with a significant increase in chest pain and a 6% stricture rate; all strictures were successfully managed with endoscopic dilation [5]. The 2- and 3-year results of the trial revealed a durable effect of RFA with a low rate of disease progression. Complete eradication of LGD and IM was observed in 98% of patients at 2 years. Follow-up at 3 years revealed complete eradication of dysplasia in 98% and complete eradication of intestinal metaplasia (IM) in 91% of patients. Predictors of complete response were sought, but none were statistically significant [6].

A recent randomized controlled trial published by Phoa et al. corroborated these findings. They compared RFA to endoscopic surveillance for patients with LGD and found that RFA significantly reduced the rate of progression to HGD and EAC over a 3-year follow-up period. Radiofrequency ablation reduced progression to HGD or EAC by 25% and reduced progression to EAC by 7.4%. Complete eradication of dysplasia was observed in 92.6% of patients after RFA. Treatment-related adverse events occurred in 19.1% of patients who received ablation. Stricture was the most common adverse event (11.8%) and was all treated successfully with endoscopic dilation. The data and safety monitoring board terminated the trial early due to superiority of ablation [7].

Radiofrequency ablation is a safe and effective treatment for LGD with a risk profile appropriately matched to the natural course of the disease. However, it does not provide indefinite eradication in all patients, and therefore, post-ablation surveillance is required [5–9]. With regard to cost-effectiveness, some evidence suggests RFA may be a cost-effective treatment for LGD, but a better understanding of its long-term efficacy is needed before drawing firm conclusions [10]. From a patient perspective, RFA improves disease-specific health-related quality of life secondary to a perceived decrease in the risk of cancer development [11]. Because patients face a diagnosis with an uncertain course, quality of life and psychological stress may play a significant part in their management decisions. Fortunately, endoscopic ablation technology has allowed the field to evolve past mere surveillance. In today's era, RFA should be discussed with, and considered in, all patients with LGD given its safety, efficacy, and durability.

References

1. Vieth M. Low-grade dysplasia in Barrett's esophagus – an innocent bystander? Contra. Endoscopy. 2007;39:647–9.
2. Curvers WL, ten Kate FJ, Krishnadath KK, et al. Low-grade dysplasia in Barrett's esophagus: overdiagnosed and underestimated. Am J Gastroenterol. 2010;105:1523–30.
3. Kerkhof M, van Dekken H, Steyerberg EW, et al. Grading of dysplasia in Barrett's oesophagus: substantial interobserver variation between general and gastrointestinal pathologists. Histopathology. 2007;50:920–7.
4. Shaheen NJ, Falk GW, Iyer PG, Gerson LB, American college of G. ACG clinical guideline: diagnosis and management of Barrett's esophagus. Am J Gastroenterol. 2016;111:30–50; quiz 1.

5. Shaheen NJ, Sharma P, Overholt BF, et al. Radiofrequency ablation in Barrett's esophagus with dysplasia. N Engl J Med. 2009;360:2277–88.
6. Shaheen NJ, Overholt BF, Sampliner RE, et al. Durability of radiofrequency ablation in Barrett's esophagus with dysplasia. Gastroenterology. 2011;141:460–8.
7. Phoa KN, van Vilsteren FG, Weusten BL, et al. Radiofrequency ablation vs endoscopic surveillance for patients with Barrett esophagus and low-grade dysplasia: a randomized clinical trial. JAMA. 2014;311:1209–17.
8. Orman ES, Kim HP, Bulsiewicz WJ, et al. Intestinal metaplasia recurs infrequently in patients successfully treated for Barrett's esophagus with radiofrequency ablation. Am J Gastroenterol. 2013;108:187–95; quiz 96.
9. Orman ES, Li N, Shaheen NJ. Efficacy and durability of radiofrequency ablation for Barrett's esophagus: systematic review and meta-analysis. Clin Gastroenterol Hepatol. 2013;11:1245–55.
10. Hur C, Choi SE, Rubenstein JH, et al. The cost effectiveness of radiofrequency ablation for Barrett's esophagus. Gastroenterology. 2012;143:567–75.
11. Shaheen NJ, Peery AF, Hawes RH, et al. Quality of life following radiofrequency ablation of dysplastic Barrett's esophagus. Endoscopy. 2010;42:790–9.

Historical Perspective: History of the Surgical Management of Achalasia

32

Julia Park and David W. Rattner

Introduction

Achalasia is a primary motility disorder of the esophagus with an incidence of 1 in 100,000 annually. It is best characterized by the existence of both: absence of esophageal peristalsis and failure of relaxation of the lower esophageal sphincter (LES). This is a progressive disease that if left untreated can evolve to a completely nonfunctional megaesophagus. The condition was first described in 1674 by Sir Thomas Willis in connection with a patient who used a cork-tipped whale bone to push food down after each meal. The pathophysiology of the disease remained undefined until 1891 when Mikulicz noted that esophageal obstruction was caused by a physiologic rather than anatomic defect and coined the term "cardiospasm." Over the past century, the development of fluoroscopy, flexible endoscopy, and more recently high-resolution manometry have transformed our understanding of achalasia. Furthermore, physiologic data now supplements anatomic information to guide therapeutic decision-making. Since defective esophageal peristalsis cannot be corrected, all surgical and endoscopic therapies for achalasia target the non-relaxing lower esophageal sphincter (LES). The introduction of minimally invasive surgery for achalasia in 1991 and the recent introduction of POEM (Per Oral Endoscopic Myotomy) in 2009 have revolutionized the treatment of achalasia and are now the most commonly utilized therapeutic modalities. Furthermore, in the digital era, patients with rare diseases commonly seek information about their condition and direct their own care. Therefore, patients, who in the past might have been told to have pneumatic dilations instead of invasive abdominal or thoracic surgery, now actively seek – often by Internet searches – minimally invasive surgical or endoscopic treatment for their disease.

J. Park · D. W. Rattner (✉)
Deptartment of Surgery, Massachussetts General Hospital, Harvard Medical School, Boston, MA, USA
e-mail: drattner@mgh.harvard.edu

J. Grams et al. (eds.), *The SAGES Manual of Foregut Surgery*,
https://doi.org/10.1007/978-3-319-96122-4_32

Treatment: Historical Perspective

Examining the evolution of the surgical management of achalasia dates back to a century ago and allows us to appreciate the evidence and observation-based deductions of many masters of surgery. The methods used during those times are still used as a foundation for current therapy of achalasia. Although there are reports of dilations dating as far back as 1674 and the 1800s, the actual pathophysiology of the disease was not known at that time. The term "cardiospasm" was adopted to describe this condition in 1891 by Mikulicz, reflecting the observation that a true stricture or anatomic obstruction was never seen. Throughout the nineteenth century into the early twentieth century, treatment consisted of dilations, reportedly using something as crude as a whale bone. Advancement of this technique over the years, best characterized by the experience at the Mayo Clinic, gave way to the development of a nonrigid bougie with a hydrostatic dilator mounted on it, which was used in over 800 patients up to early 1932. Complete relief was reported in 70%. At this time, there was very little understanding of the etiology of the disease, but what was for certain was the relief of symptoms (albeit temporary) that was seen in the afflicted [1–5]. This age-old technique, although modernized and perhaps more sophisticated technologically, is still utilized today.

The first surgical techniques were introduced by Mikulicz and involved performing a laparotomy, where gastrostomy was performed and the cardia was dilated with a clamp (Mikulicz operation) or even with digits on the hand (Schloffer and others). Recurrence was noted across the board, but temporary symptom relief was noted and enabled patients to eat. Complications included, but were not limited to, esophageal rupture and death. Reported in 1914, Dr. Arthur Hertz was the first to provide an alternative etiology and coined the term "achalasia" (Greek for "failure to relax"). After performing postmortems on patients with known cardiospasm, he was surprised to find that none revealed sphincter hypertrophy and proposed that, if in fact spasm of the muscle was the cause, there would be hypertrophy. He also proposed that serial rigid dilations would not be possible if spasm was present [1–4].

With x-ray imaging of these symptomatic patients, a hugely dilated megaesophagus was often seen. In order to address this particular aspect (which we now know as end-stage achalasia), multiple surgical treatments were designed to address the "common objective of straightening out the oesophagus" [6]. One such surgical technique included invagination or intussusception of the dilated esophagus onto itself (held together by interrupted sutures) via a neck incision (Freeman). The patient remained clinically well for years while he was being followed [6]. Herovsky first reported the use of an esophagogastrostomy from an abdominal incision by pulling down redundant esophagus and anastomosing it to the stomach. A number of others performed this operation (as well as modifications of it, i.e., anastomosing to first part of small bowel) in the following years, including Maingot, DeBakey, and Ochsner. Although immediate relief of symptoms was seen, patients were plagued by severe regurgitation and reflux [1, 4, 6]. Esophageal plication was also undertaken in order to address the megaesophagus. Esophageal plication, first reported by Reisinger in 1907 but modified and performed by many others, involved exposure of the esophagus through the posterior mediastinum or transpleurally and then excision of a vertical strip of the dilated esophagus 2–3 cm wide, with the subsequent esophageal re-approximation. Modifications include plication only without excision as well. Results were not favorable as this procedure did not address the cause of the problem [1, 4].

Establishment of the Myotomy and Fundoplication

In 1910, the first "cardioplasty" was performed by Wendel. It is reported that an anterior vertical incision was made on the cardia of the stomach and subsequently sutured transversely with excellent clinical outcome. A few years later in 1914, Heller described a more extensive cardioplasty, in which both an anterior and posterior extramucosal cardioplasty was performed transabdominally by dividing the peritoneum at the hiatus and pulling down the esophagus into the abdomen for exposure. This operation was well-accepted in Europe at the time. Other surgeons were performing this procedure and modifying it as well [1, 4, 7, 8]. Heller's operation was endorsed by many, and the general opinion on the matter is well-characterized in Maingot's words: "Oesophagocardiomyotomy is, in my opinion, worthy of a more general adoption, as it is a simple and safe operation, the technique is readily mastered, and the immediate and late results are most gratifying. Furthermore, these statements are confirmed by the excellent results obtained" [7]. This operation, revolutionary at the time, remains the foundation for what has become the gold standard for surgical treatment of achalasia today. The most common modifications included performing either a posterior or anterior myotomy (not both), with excellent symptom relief for both methods.

Although this procedure was quite successful in the treatment of achalasia over the next few decades, there was one resulting side effect: reflux esophagitis. In 1956, Rudolph Nissen described a fundoplication for the treatment of reflux, and in 1962, Dor proposed an operation that essentially addressed both achalasia and the resulting reflux esophagitis that would be encountered after surgical treatment of achalasia. It was a hybrid of the Heller myotomy and Nissen fundoplication and is commonly known as the anterior fundoplication. A transabdominal approach was undertaken, and an anterior myotomy 10 cm in length, which extended 5 cm onto the anterior wall of the stomach, was performed. The Dor fundoplication consisted of suturing the left side of the myotomy to the anterior wall of the stomach, and then the stomach was folded over to the right side of the myotomy and secured with sutures [9]. The Toupet fundoplication was also first reported around the same time but was not readily implemented until many years later [1]. The question of whether or not a fundoplication is required is a controversy that would be carried on for many years. This, of course, was followed by the next considerable discussion: which fundoplication is best?

The Heller myotomy with Dor fundoplication was widely accepted as the standard of care for achalasia. The first large case series (100 patients) reporting on long-term results of this surgical treatment (mean follow-up of almost 7 years) was published in 1988 by Csendes et al. and revealed good to excellent clinical outcomes in over 95% and objective reflux in 19% of patients. Csendes et al. performed an anterior myotomy 6 cm in length, with only 5–10 mm extension onto the stomach [10]. In 1992, Bonavina et al. published their results (median follow-up, 5.3 years) on over 200 patients in which a 10 cm long anterior myotomy (8 cm on esophagus, 2 cm onto the stomach) plus Dor fundoplication was performed. Ninety-four percent had good to excellent clinical outcomes reported, and 9% had abnormal acid exposure as determined by esophageal pH monitoring [11]. The difference in the length of the myotomy and how much is extended onto the stomach as portrayed between these two studies represents the beginning of a long-standing discussion in attempts to standardize the surgical technique. Further complicating this discussion was the fact that the majority of achalasia patients were treated surgically by thoracic surgeons who performed transthoracic rather than transabdominal myotomies. Addressing the question of whether a fundoplication is needed or not, a literature review of just over 5000 patients was analyzed by Andreollo et al., which concluded that a fundoplication was not necessary when Heller myotomy was performed through the chest vs. the abdomen [12]. This group postulated that the abdominal approach (including both open and laparoscopic) required mobilizing the phrenoesophageal ligament, which in turn disrupted the normal anti-reflux mechanism of the GE junction, thereby increasing postoperative reflux.

In the early 1990s, minimally invasive techniques were gaining acceptance in the surgical treatment of foregut disease. Cuschieri was the first to perform a laparoscopic Heller myotomy (LHM) in 1991 [13]. In the United States, Pellegrini performed the first laparoscopic myotomies, which were actually reoperations for insufficient thoracoscopic myotomies [14].

Comparison of the thoracoscopic vs. laparoscopic technique for Heller myotomy (no anti-reflux procedure for thoracoscopic, Dor fundoplication for laparoscopic) revealed faster recovery for patients in the laparoscopic group due to obvious drawbacks of entering the thoracic cavity for surgery, and a higher percentage of patients with abnormal acid exposure when objectively measured was seen in the thoracoscopic group [15]. Bonavina et al. was the first to report the feasibility and safety of laparoscopic Heller myotomy plus Dor fundoplication in 1995 [16], and by the end of the 1990s, the laparoscopic technique for the treatment of achalasia was the new gold standard.

As alluded to before, controversy remained about the length of myotomy required for adequate symptom relief. Patients who underwent standard Heller (1–2 cm extension of myotomy onto gastric wall) with Dor fundoplication and those that underwent "extended" myotomy (defined as 3 cm onto the stomach) with Toupet were compared, and relief from dysphagia was more prominent in the extended myotomy group [17]. This study and others have established the current practice today to ensure extension of the anterior myotomy well past the gastroesophageal junction.

Furthermore, most Heller myotomies today are combined with an anti-reflux procedure. A randomized control trial comparing Heller with and without Dor fundoplication found that the incidence of postoperative reflux measured by 24-h pH monitoring was 9% vs. 48% in those with and without fundoplication, respectively [18]. A meta-analysis by Campos et al. (2009) looking at all publications that reported postoperative 24-h pH monitoring confirms the higher rate of distal esophageal reflux (41.5%) without fundoplication as compared with 14.5% with fundoplication. As expected, incidence of postoperative reflux symptoms was observed in 31.5% after LHM without partial fundoplication vs. 9% in those with fundoplication [19–51]. Rawlings et al. compared Dor and Toupet after myotomy in a multicenter randomized control trial and found no significant difference in postoperative reflux and relief from dysphagia [52]. When confronted with a sigmoid-type esophagus and presumed nonexistent esophageal peristalsis in late- to end-stage achalasia, a fundoplication may be omitted as even a partial wrap can exacerbate dysphagia despite myotomy. A full Nissen fundoplication has been abandoned as the appropriate anti-reflux procedure as the incidence of dysphagia with Nissen proves to be unacceptably high vs. a partial wrap [53, 54].

Laparoscopic Heller Myotomy Outcomes

Clinical outcomes of laparoscopic Heller myotomy (LHM) with partial fundoplication have withstood the test of time. Success has been measured by both subjective resolution of symptoms using validated metrics [i.e., Eckardt score, Quality of Life in Reflux and Dyspepsia (QOLRAD), and Gastroesophageal Reflux Disease-Health-Related Quality of Life (GERD-HRQL), among others] and objective measurement utilizing manometry, pH monitoring, and upper endoscopy. Significant palliation of dysphagia was recorded in 89% (79–100%). Improvement of dysphagia remained the same between those with and without an anti-reflux procedure. In a meta-analysis encompassing over 3000 patients by Campos et al., rate of any complication was 6% and mortality was 0.1% (3 patients). Specifically, rate of mucosal perforation is 6.9%, but the clinical significance of perforation is 0.7% as most are recognized intraoperatively and immediately closed without any postoperative ramifications [19–51, 54, 55]. In those studies where postoperative 24-h pH monitoring was performed, 14.5% (0–44%) showed evidence of distal esophageal reflux. Those with symptomatic reflux represented a smaller percentage at 8.8% in those with a fundoplication [19–51].

Role of Robotic Surgery in the Treatment of Achalasia

Robotic surgery has been evaluated for nearly all aspects of gastrointestinal surgery. The robotic platform has been shown to be safe in patients undergoing Heller myotomy in multiple studies. The enhanced 3D view has been attributed to decreased incidence of intraoperative perforations of the esophagus, although the clinical outcomes are largely the same as compared with laparoscopic surgery. The significant cost, longer operating times, and limited availability are still barriers to widespread acceptance of the robotic platform for the surgical treatment of achalasia [56–63];

furthermore, perforations are in fact extremely uncommon with conventional laparoscopic Heller myotomy when performed by specialist surgeons [64].

Per Oral Endoscopic Myotomy (POEM)

In the continual pursuit for less invasive means of intervention, Inoue developed the POEM procedure and was the first to perform the endoscopic myotomy in patients with achalasia. This innovative endoscopic technique is outlined in detail by Inoue et al. [65], but in brief, it involves creation of a submucosal tunnel, dissection of the circular muscle fibers starting at 3 cm distal to the mucosal entry and 7 cm proximal to the gastroesophageal junction (GEJ) and extending to 2 cm past the GEJ, and closure of the mucosal entry site. In his first publication reporting the initial results, the patients had excellent clinical outcomes (improved dysphagia in 100%) and a significant reduction in LES pressure, with no serious complications recorded [65]. Since the introduction of the POEM procedure, it has been performed with increasing frequency. Subsequent studies have confirmed successful clinical outcomes using subjective metrics and range from 89% to 100% [55, 66–70]. Furthermore, this success rate remains high at 3-year follow-up, which is the longest reported to date [67]. Comparison with LHM reveals that clinical outcomes are similar between the two procedures at 6-month follow-up.

As there is no anti-reflux procedure performed with POEM, postoperative reflux has been a major concern. Esophagitis seen on postoperative endoscopy has been reported to occur in the range of 46–64.7% in short-term follow-up [55, 66–70]. Symptomatic reflux symptoms were seen in 21% at 3 year follow-up [67].

Conclusion

Advances in endoscopic and diagnostic techniques greatly enhanced the understanding of achalasia during the past century. Concurrently, new surgical modalities such as laparoscopic and endoluminal myotomies were developed that revolutionized the treatment of achalasia. Laparoscopic Heller myotomy and POEM are highly effective and have a lower perforation rates than the prior therapies such as pneumatic dilation that dominated in the twentieth century. Internet-savvy patients currently seek the least invasive methods for treatment in order to minimize pain and recovery time. Time will tell if the long-term results of POEM are equivalent to LHM and clarify the significance (if any) of increased esophageal acid exposure that has been observed in POEM patients.

References

1. Fisichella PM, Patti MG. From Heller to POEM (1914–2014): a 100-year history of surgery for achalasia. J Gastrointest Surg. 2014;18:1870–5.
2. Weber FP. Spasmodic stricture of the oesophagus (Cardiospasm), with fusiform dilatation above it. Proc R Soc Med. 1914;7(Clin Sect):147–51.

3. Hertz AF. Achalasia of the cardia (so-called cardio-spasm). Proc R Soc Med. 1915;8(Clin Sect):22–5.
4. Watts SH. Cardioplasty for Cardiospasm. Ann Surg. 1923;78(2):164–72.
5. Moersch HJ. Cardiospasm: diagnosis and treatment. Ann Surg. 1933;98(2):232–8.
6. Freeman L. An operation for the relief of cardiospasm associated with dilatation and tortuosity of the oesophagus. Ann Surg. 1923;78(2):173–5.
7. Maingot R. Extramucous oesophagocardiomyotomy in cardiospasm. Postgrad Med J. 1944;20(227):278–82.
8. Heller E. Extramukose Kardioplastik beim chronishen Kardiospasmus mit Dilatation des Oesophagus. Mitt Grenzgeb Med Chir. 1914;27:141–9.
9. Dor J, Humbert P, Dor V, et al. L'interet de la technique de Nissen modifiee dans la prevention de reflux après cardiomyotomie extramuqueuse de Heller. Meme Acad Chir (Paris). 1962;88:877–83.
10. Csendes A, Braghetto I, Mascaro J, et al. Late subjective and objective evaluation of the results of esophagomyotomy in 100 patients with achalasia of the esophagus. Surgery. 1988;104:469–75.
11. Bonavina L, Nosadini A, Bardini R, et al. Primary treatment of esophageal achalasia. Long-term resilts of myotomy and Dor fundoplication. Arch Surg. 1992;127(2):222–6.
12. Andreollo NA, Earlam RJ. Heller's myotomy for achalasia: is an added anti-reflux procedure necessary. Br J Surg. 1987;74:765–9.
13. Shimi S, Nathanson LK, Cuschieri A. Laparoscopic cardiomyotomy for achalasia. J R Coll Surg Edinb. 1991;36(3):152–4.
14. Pellegrini C, Wetter LA, Patti M, et al. Thoracoscopic esophagomyotomy. Initial experience with a new approach for the treatment of achalasia. Ann Surg. 1992;216(3):291–6.
15. Patti MG, Arcerito M, De Pinto M, et al. Comparison of thoracoscopic and laparoscopic Heller myotomy for achalasia. J Gastrointest Surg. 1998;2(6):561–6.
16. Bonavina L, Rosati R, Segalin A, et al. Laparoscopic Heller-Dor operation for the treatment of oesophageal achalasia: technique and early results. Ann Chir Gynaecol. 1995;84(2):165–8.
17. Wright AS, Williams CW, Pellegrini CA, et al. Long-term outcomes confirm superior efficacy of extended Heller myotomy with Toupet fundoplication for achalasia. Surg Endosc. 2007;21(5):713–8.
18. Richards WO, Torquati A, Holzman MD, et al. Heller myotomy versus Heller myotomy with Dor fundoplication for achalasia: a prospective randomized double-blind clinical trial. Ann Surg. 2004;240(3):405–12.
19. Campos GM, Vittinghoff E, Rabl C, et al. Endoscopic and surgical treatments for achalasia: a systematic review and meta-analysis. Ann Surg. 2009;249:45–57.
20. Delgado F, Bolufer JM, Martinez-Abad M, et al. Laparoscopic treatment of esophageal achalasia. Surg Laparosc Endosc. 1996;6:83–90.
21. Raiser F, Perdikis G, Hinder RA, et al. Heller myotomy via minimal-access surgery. An evaluation of antireflux procedures Arch Surg. 1996;131:593–7.
22. Anselmino M, Zaninotto G, Costantini M, et al. One-year follow-up after laparoscopic Heller-Dor operation for esophageal achalasia. Surg Endosc. 1997;11:3–7.
23. Vogt D, Curet M, Pitcher D, et al. Successful treatment of esophageal achalasia with laparoscopic Heller myotomy and Toupet fundoplication. Am J Surg. 1997;174:709–14.
24. Richards WO, Clements RH, Wang PC, et al. Prevalence of gastroesophageal reflux after laparoscopic Heller myotomy. Surg Endosc. 1999;13:1010–4.
25. Yamamura MS, Gilster JC, Myers BS, et al. Laparoscopic Heller myotomy and anterior fundoplication for achalasia results in a high degree of patient satisfaction. Arch Surg. 2000;135:902–6.
26. Zaninotto G, Costantini M, Molena D, et al. Treatment of esophageal achalasia with laparoscopic Heller myotomy and Dor partial anterior fundoplication: prospective evaluation of 100 consecutive patients. J Gastrointest Surg. 2000;4:282–9.
27. Ackroyd R, Watson DI, Devitt PG, et al. Laparoscopic cardiomyotomy and anterior partial fundoplication for achalasia. Surg Endosc. 2001;15:683–6.

28. Wills VL, Hunt DR. Functional outcome after Heller myotomy and fundoplication for achalasia. J Gastrointest Surg. 2001;5:408–13.
29. Pechlivanides G, Chrysos E, Athanasakis E, et al. Laparoscopic Heller cardiomyotomy and Dor fundoplication for esophageal achalasia: possible factors predicting outcome. Arch Surg. 2001;136:1240–3.
30. Donahue PE, Horgan S, Liu KJ, et al. Floppy Dor fundoplication after esophagocardiomyotomy for achalasia. Surgery. 2002;132:716–22.
31. Oelschlarger BK, Chang L, Pellegrini CA. Improved outcome after extended gastric myotomy for achalasia. Arch Surg. 2003;138:490–5.
32. Arain MA, Peters JH, Tamhankar AP, et al. Preoperative lower esophageal sphincter pressure affects outcome of laparoscopic esophageal myotomy for achalasia. J Gastrointest Surg. 2004;8:328–34.
33. Perrone JM, Frisella MM, Desai KM, et al. Results of laparoscopic Heller-Toupet operation for achalasia. Surg Endosc. 2004;18:1565–71.
34. Frantzides CT, Moore RE, Carlson MA, et al. Minimally invasive surgery for achalasia: a 10-year experience. J Gastrointest Surg. 2004;8:18–23.
35. Dempsey DT, Delano M, Bradley K, et al. Laparoscopic esophagomyotomy for achalasia; does anterior hemifundoplication affect clinical outcome? Ann Surg. 2004;239:779–85.
36. Avtan L, Avci C, Guvenc H, et al. Laparoscopic myotomy for oesophageal achalasia-adding an antireflux procedure is not always necessary. Int J Clin Pract. 2005;59:35–8.
37. Ramacciato G, D'Angelo FA, Aurello P, et al. Laparoscopic Heller myotomy with or without partial fundoplication: a matter of debate. World J Gastroenterol. 2005;11:1558–61.
38. Rossetti G, Brusciano L, Amato G, et al. A total fundoplication is not an obstacle to esophageal emptying after Heller myotomy for achalasia: results of a long-term follow up. Ann Surg. 2005;241:614–21.
39. Bonatti H, Hinder RA, Klocker J, et al. Long-term results of laparoscopic Heller myotomy with partial fundoplication for the treatment of achalasia. Am J Surg. 2005;190:874–8.
40. Rosemurgy A, Villadolid D, Thometz D, et al. Laparoscopic Heller myotomy provides durable relief from achalasia and savages failures after botox or dilation. Ann Surg. 2005;241:725–33.
41. Deb S, Deschamps C, Allen MS, et al. Laparoscopic esophageal myotomy for achalasia: factors affecting functional results. Ann Thorac Surg. 2005;80:1191–4.
42. Khajanchee YS, Kanneganti S, Leatherwood AE, et al. Laparoscopic Heller myotomy with Toupet fundoplication: outcomes predictors in 121 consecutive patients. Arch Surg. 2005;140:827–33.
43. Burpee SE, Mamazza J, Schlachta CM, et al. Objective analysis of gastroesophageal reflux after laparoscopic Heller myotomy: an anti-reflux procedure is required. Surg Endosc. 2005;19:9–14.
44. Katada N, Sakuramoto S, Kobayashi N, et al. Laparoscopic Heller myotomy with Toupet fundoplication for achalasia straightens the esophagus and relieves dysphagia. Am J Surg. 2006;192:1–8.
45. Torquati A, Richards WO, Holzman MD, et al. Laparoscopic myotomy for achalasia: predictors of successful outcome after 200 cases. Ann Surg. 2006;243:587–91.
46. Morino M, Rebecchi F, Festa V, et al. Preoperative pneumatic dilatation represents a risk factor for laparoscopic Heller myotomy. Surg Endosc. 1997;11:359–61.
47. Portale G, Costantini M, Rizzetto C, et al. Long-term outcomes of laparoscopic Heller-Dor surgery for esophageal achalasia: possible detrimental role of previous endoscopic treatment. J Gastrointest Surg. 2005;9:1332–9.
48. Smith CD, Stival A, Howell DL, et al. Endoscopic therapy for achalasia before Heller myotomy results in worse outcomes than Heller myotomy alone. Ann Surg. 2006;243:579–84.
49. Hunter JG, Trus TL, Branum GD, et al. Laparoscopic Heller myotomy and fundoplication for achalasia. Ann Surg. 1997;225:655–64.
50. Patti MG, Pellegrini CA, Horgan S, et al. Minimally invasive surgery for esophageal achalasia: an 8-year experience with 168 patients. Ann Surg. 1999;230:587–93.
51. Cade R. Heller's myotomy: thoracoscopic or laparoscopic? Dis Esophagus. 2000;13:279–81.

52. Rawlings A, Soper N, Oelschlager B, et al. Laparoscopic Dor versus Toupet fundoplication following Heller myotomy for achalasia: results of a multicenter, prospective randomized-controlled Trial. Surg Endosc. 2012;26(1):18–26.
53. Rebecchi F, Giaccone C, Farinella E, et al. Randomized controlled trial of laparoscopic Heller myotomy plus Dor fundoplication versus Nissen fundoplication for achalasia: long-term results. Ann Surg. 2008;248(6):1023–30.
54. Stefanidis D, Richardson W, Farrell TM, et al. Society of American gastrointestinal and endoscopic surgeons. SAGES guidelines for the surgical treatment of esophageal achalasia. Surg Endosc. 2012;26(2):296–311.
55. Moonen A, Boeckxstaens G. Current diagnosis and management of achalasia. J Clin Gastroenterol. 2014;48:484–90.
56. Afaneh C, Finnerty B, Abelson JS, et al. Robotic-assisted Heller myotomy: a modern technique and review of outcomes. J Robot Surg. 2015;9(2):101–8.
57. Talamini M, Campbell K, Stanfield C. Robotic gastrointestinal surgery: early experience and system description. J Laparoendosc Adv Surg Tech A. 2002;12(4):225–32.
58. Melvin WS, Dundon JM, Talamini M, et al. Computer-enhanced robotic telesurgery minimizes esophageal perforation during Heller myotomy. Surgery. 2005;138(4):553–8.
59. Horgan S, Galvani C, Gorodner MV, et al. Robotic-assisted Heller myotomy versus laparoscopic Heller myotomy for the treatment of esophageal achalasia: multicenter study. J Gastrointest Surg. 2005;9(8):1020–9.
60. Galvani C, Gorodner MV, Moser F, et al. Laparoscopic Heller myotomy for achalasia facilitated by robotic assistance. Surg Endosc. 2006;20(7):1105–12.
61. Huffmanm LC, Pandalai PK, Boulton BJ, et al. Robotic Heller myotomy: a safe operation with higher postoperative quality-of-life indices. Surgery. 2007;142(4):613–8.
62. Shaligram A, Unnirevi J, Simorov A, et al. How does the robot affect outcomes? A retrospective review of open, laparoscopic, and robotic Heller myotomy for achalasia. Surg Endosc. 2012;26(4):1047–50.
63. Perry KA, Kanji A, Drosdeck JM, et al. Efficacy and durability of robotic Heller myotomy for achalasia: patient symptoms and satisfaction at long-term follow-up. Surg Endosc. 2014;28(11):3162–7.
64. Nau P, Rattner D. Laparoscopic Heller myotomy as the gold standard for treatment of achalasia. J Gastrointest Surg. 2014;18(12):2201–7.
65. Inoue H, Minami H, Kobayashi Y, et al. Peroral endoscopic myotomy (POEM) for esophageal achalasia. Endoscopy. 2010;42(4):265–71.
66. Swanstrom LL, Kurian A, Dunst CM, et al. Long-term outcomes of an endoscopic myotomy for achalasia: the POEM procedure. Ann Surg. 2012;256:659–67.
67. Inoue H, Sato H, Ikeda H, et al. Per-oral endoscopic Myotomy: a series of 500 patients. J Am Coll Surg. 2015;221(2):256–64.
68. Schneider AM, Louie BE, Warren HF, et al. A matched comparison of per oral endoscopic myotomy to laparoscopic Heller myotomy in the treatment of achalasia. J Gastrointest Surg. 2016;20:1789–96.
69. Stavropoulos SN, Modayil RJ, Freidel D, et al. The international per oral endoscopic myotomy survey (IPOEMS): a snapshot of the global POEM experience. Surg Endosc. 2013;27:3322–38.
70. Hungness ES, Teitelbaum EN, Santos BF, et al. Comparisons of perioperative outcomes between peroral esophageal myotomy (POEM) and laparoscopic Heller myotomy. J Gastrointest Surg. 2013;17:228–35.

Epidemiology, Evaluation, and Classification of Achalasia and Other Esophageal Motility Disorders

33

Wayne S. Lee, Ali Rezaie, and Miguel A. Burch

Introduction

With a patient population of increasingly advanced age, dysphagia is a commonly encountered symptom. Of all motor dysfunctions of the esophagus, achalasia is the best defined in the literature and will be the primary subject of this chapter. However, the workup for dysphagia is based upon wide differential diagnoses; thus a thorough understanding of other esophageal dysmotility disorders is crucial. The prevalence of swallowing difficulty in the community-dwelling elderly ranges from 5% to 72% with a mean of 15%, with risk factors being advanced age, history of clinical disease, and physical frailty [1]. Although the majority of these will be secondary to oropharyngeal dysfunction, it is important for the discerning surgeon to identify and treat esophageal motility disorders.

Epidemiology

Historically the incidence of achalasia is 0.5–1.5 new cases per 100,000 in North America and Europe [2–5]. As achalasia is an incurable disorder, its prevalence is much greater than its incidence at 8–10 per 100,000 [5, 6]. Interestingly in regions with more widespread use of high-resolution manometry (HRM), the incidence and prevalence have increased by two- to threefold compared to values prior to its prevalent use in mid-2000s [7]. Hospitalizations for achalasia have remained stable for

W. S. Lee · M. A. Burch (✉)
Department of Minimally Invasive Surgery, Cedars-Sinai Medical Center, Los Angeles, CA, USA
e-mail: Miguel.burch@cshs.edu

A. Rezaie
Department of Medicine, GI Motility Program, Cedars-Sinai Medical Center, Los Angeles, CA, USA

J. Grams et al. (eds.), *The SAGES Manual of Foregut Surgery*,
https://doi.org/10.1007/978-3-319-96122-4_33

the past few decades; however, there is an age-related increase in incidence in patients older than 50 with peak between 65 and 84. Achalasia affects all ethnicities and genders equally [8, 9]; however, other studies have demonstrated a slight male predominance [10].

Although the vast majority of achalasia seems to be sporadic de novo diagnoses, genetic predispositions have also been described. Allgrove syndrome, characterized by 3 A's (alacrima, adrenal insufficiency, and achalasia), is a rare disorder in which defect in the AAAS gene leads to a defective ALADIN protein [11]. Familial clustering has also been described in an autosomal dominant inheritance pattern [12, 13]. Associations between achalasia and both Parkinson's disease and Down syndrome have been described as well [14–17].

Other esophageal motility disorders are less well characterized from a population standpoint. However the relative incidences may be estimated from studies in comparison to achalasia. In an Irish study of 5184 consecutive patients undergoing manometry studies referred for reflux-related symptoms over a 10-year period, 4% had achalasia, 1.4% had nutcracker esophagus, 1.0% had hypertensive lower esophageal sphincter, 0.2% had diffuse esophageal spasm (DES), and 0.2% had scleroderma [18]. Approximately 20–50% of gastroesophageal reflux disease (GERD) patients have ineffective esophageal motility (IEM) [19]. It can also be seen in up to 30% of patients with nonobstructive dysphagia that is unrelated to GERD [20].

Pathophysiology

Failure of lower esophageal sphincter relaxation with aperistalsis is pathognomonic for achalasia. Although the root cause for achalasia seems to be multifactorial, the common end result is characterized by progressive degeneration of nitric oxide producing inhibitory neurons in the mid and distal esophagus. Inflammation and fibrosis of the myenteric (Auerbach's) plexus is seen in pathologic specimens. Replacement of the nerves with collagen and hypertrophy of the muscularis propria has also been found [21, 22]. The selective loss of inhibitory innervation leads functionally to lack of deglutitive relaxation of the esophagogastric junction (EGJ) and inability of the esophageal body to contract in a peristaltic fashion. As excitatory postganglionic neurons are spared, cholinergic stimulation leads to unopposed high lower esophageal sphincter pressure at rest. The unremitting lower esophageal sphincter contraction creates an impediment for bolus passage into the stomach, leading to a gradual dilation of the esophageal body. The natural history of untreated achalasia was described by Ellis in 1960, dividing the clinical features into three chronologic stages: onset, silent period, and progressive deterioration [23]. Ultimately, severe achalasia is characterized by massive esophageal dilation, acting as a reservoir of fermented undigested food. This end-stage achalasia is referred to as sigmoid esophagus as it is characterized by dilatation and nondependent curvature shape.

Several mechanisms for the etiology of achalasia have been proposed, including infectious, immunologic, and genetic causes. The basis for infectious and autoimmune causes is derived from studies that demonstrate higher antibody titers for

Varicella zoster virus in patients with achalasia. Varicella zoster virus DNA have also been found in esophageal myenteric plexus in achalasia patients [24]. The theory of viral infection triggering neuronal degeneration is strengthened by an association between achalasia and antecedent viral infection. Higher rates of allergic and autoimmune disorders were also found in achalasia patients and their first-degree relatives [25]. Secondary achalasia caused by *Trypanosoma cruzi* infection (Chagas disease) is also well established to be pathophysiologically indistinguishable from idiopathic achalasia [26]. In addition to familial clustering and gene defects, Allgrove syndrome, the genetic implications for achalasia include polymorphisms found in nitric oxide synthase and vasoactive intestinal peptide receptor 1 proteins [27, 28].

The pathophysiology of other esophageal motility disorders is not as well described in the literature. DES is characterized by dysfunction in the intrinsic neural regulation in esophageal smooth muscle, as normal striated muscle peristalsis is usually intact in the upper third [29]. Endoscopic sonographic evaluation has demonstrated increased esophageal muscle mass in patients with DES and high amplitude esophageal contraction [30]. However dissimilar to achalasia, pathologic specimens of patients with DES and nutcracker esophagus demonstrate the presence of ganglia [31]. Thus, muscular hypertrophy may be secondary to increased bolus resistance through the esophagus and EGJ, rather than a primary cause of DES [29]. Nitric oxide seems to be an important mediator in DES [32]. A similar mechanism seems to be implicated in jackhammer esophagus and hypertensive lower esophageal sphincter, as phosphodiesterase-5 inhibitors such as sildenafil seem to ameliorate symptoms of both. This mechanism is through an increase in intracellular cyclic-GMP, which enhances nitric oxide-induced smooth muscle relaxation [33]. Clinically, jackhammer esophagus patients with impaired EGJ relaxation have been found to be prone to developing peristaltic dysfunction and achalasia [34]. IEM seems to be due to decreased cholinergic stimulation throughout the esophageal body. Potential causes include impaired neuromuscular control, muscular hypertrophy, extensive fibrosis, and inflammatory mediators.

Evaluation

Due to a broad differential diagnosis, the workup for esophageal motility disorders should begin with detailed history taking (Table 33.1). Meticulous symptom recognition should lead to the referral of appropriate diagnostic testing. Dysphagia is the most common symptom in achalasia, occurring in more than 90% [35]. Dysphagia is usually gradual starting initially with "chest fullness" and progressing to "sticking sensation." However, symptoms may be severe at the time of diagnosis, with dysphagia to both liquids and solids. Oropharyngeal dysphagia should be distinguished from esophageal dysphagia by inquiring about immediate regurgitation and aspiration with drinking thin liquids. It can also be associated with nasopharyngeal regurgitation, drooling, and concurrent or underlying neurologic or muscular diseases [35]. Common neuromuscular pathologies associated with oropharyngeal

Table 33.1 Differential diagnosis of esophageal dysmotility

Primary
Achalasia
Diffuse esophageal spasm
Hypertensive lower esophageal sphincter
Hypercontractile (jackhammer) esophagus
Weak peristalsis/ineffective esophageal motility
Hypotensive lower esophageal sphincter
Secondary
Malignancy/pseudoachalasia (primary esophageal, metastatic)
Rheumatologic (scleroderma, systemic lupus erythematosus, Raynaud's phenomenon, Sjögren's syndrome)
Infectious (Chagas disease, candida, cytomegalovirus, herpes simplex virus, human immunodeficiency virus)
Infiltrative (eosinophilic esophagitis, amyloidosis, sarcoidosis)
Iatrogenic (post gastric banding, post vagotomy)
Medications

dysfunction include stroke, traumatic brain injury, myasthenia gravis, and amyotrophic lateral sclerosis; anatomic conditions include cricopharyngeal bar and Zenker's diverticulum. Cervical dysphagia should be worked up to rule out distal esophageal obstruction, as the location of obstruction may be subjective. In general, esophageal motility disorders can cause dysphagia to both liquid and solids, and mechanical obstructions cause dysphagia to solids more so than liquids; however, mechanical obstructions may cause functional esophageal dysmotility, which may cause dysphagia to liquids as well.

Heartburn (75%) and regurgitation (45%) are also common in achalasia, which may initially be misdiagnosed as GERD [35]. Regurgitation of bland undigested food and saliva may occur at night, causing patients to wake up choking and coughing. The severity of regurgitation may be progressive as the esophagus dilates. Belching and halitosis can also occur from undigested food in the esophagus. The reservoir of stagnant food particles may undergo fermentation, leading to heartburn. Surgical treatment of heartburn symptoms such as GERD with fundoplication without additional workup to rule out achalasia or other esophageal motility disorders may be disastrous.

Noncardiac chest pain (20%), epigastric pain (15%), and odynophagia (<5%) may also be present [35]. Although symptoms of dysphagia and regurgitation may be ameliorated with pneumatic dilation or surgical myotomy, relief of chest pain is usually less consistent. Achalasia-related chest pain is more common in younger patients; a majority will have improvement of chest pain with advancing age, though only a minority will have complete resolution of pain [36]. Studies have demonstrated patients with noncardiac chest pain to have lower thresholds for pain in response to esophageal distension due to hypersensitization [37]. There is a broad overlap of sensory experience to different esophageal stimuli (mechanical distension, thermal, and electrical), which suggests polymodal sensory signaling to the brain, which are nonspecific. Esophageal exposure to acid also evokes hypersensitivity to pain [38].

Respiratory symptoms occur in achalasia patients approximately 20–40% of the time, including cough, asthma, and sore throat, likely caused by chronic aspiration [35, 39]. The symptoms may be more common at night due to recumbent position.

Weight loss may be a late finding, as most patients will resort to dietary modification to ameliorate their dysphagia. Rapid weight loss should heighten clinical suspicion of pseudoachalasia, the incidence of which may be as high as 2–4%. These patients usually present as an older population, with a shorter history of dysphagia [40].

The Eckardt score is a standardized scoring system for achalasia based on clinical symptoms to provide an objective quantitative measure of clinical severity [41]. It was initially developed to assess clinical improvement after pneumatic dilation. Depending on the frequency of esophageal symptoms (dysphagia, regurgitation, retrosternal pressure sensation), individual scores between 0 and 3 (never, occasionally, daily, with each meal) are added up. Additional scores of 0–3 for weight loss (none, <5 kg; 5–10, >10) are added as well, for a total maximum score of 12. Clinical stages were defined based on the score: stage 0, 0–1; stage 1, 2–3; stage 2, 4–6; and stage 3, >6. The scoring system has been validated to assess posttreatment symptoms [42]. A score of 0–1 suggested successful treatment and remission; failure is defined as stage 2 and 3. The pre-treatment Eckardt score of ≥9 has also been found to be associated with primary failure after peroral endoscopic myotomy as well as recurrence [43].

Diagnostic Studies

Barium Swallow

The barium swallow study is the best initial diagnostic study to assess esophageal structure and function, with the benefit of being low cost and widely available. High-quality visualization of the mucosa may be accomplished with the addition of effervescent solution to provide both air and liquid contrast. Esophageal motility can also be assessed by obtaining single swallows of contrast from the cervical esophagus to emptying through the EGJ. Timed spot films can also be taken at 1, 2, and 5 min after swallowing a set volume of barium. This timed barium swallow allows for assessment of delayed esophageal emptying, which in normal individuals should occur in less than 1 min. The addition of a solid phase such as bread to the standard liquid barium swallow may increase the overall yield, especially in those with symptoms of solid food dysphagia.

Tapered narrowing at the EGJ or the classic bird's beak appearance may be seen in achalasia along with a dilated esophageal body (Fig. 33.1). Due to the outlet obstruction, a constant column of air fluid level may be seen, as hydrostatic pressure drives emptying of barium through the narrowed EGJ. This height is usually proportional to the severity of achalasia. Whereas primary and secondary peristalses are initiated by deglutition and focal distension of the esophageal body, respectively, tertiary contractions are nonpropulsive events and may be seen on barium swallow

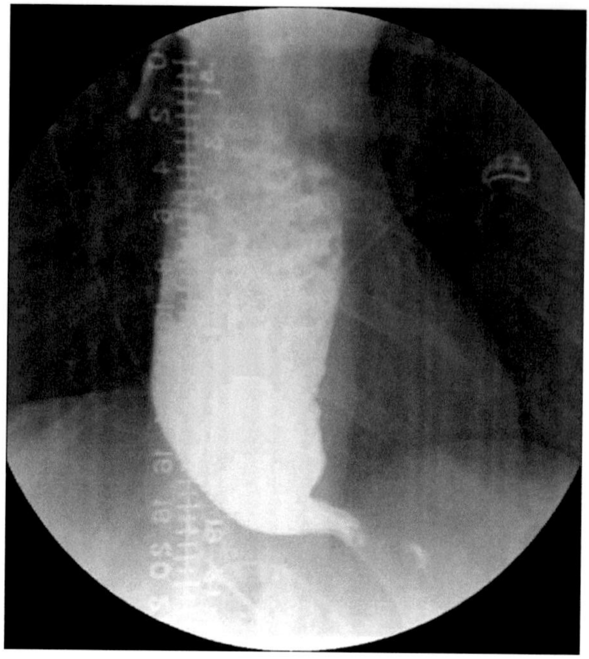

Fig. 33.1 Barium esophagram of a patient with achalasia with bird's beak appearance

in vigorous achalasia and presbyesophagus. Epiphrenic diverticulum can also sometimes be seen.

The severity of achalasia can be graded based on esophageal diameter on radiologic findings: early achalasia (<4 cm), moderate achalasia (4–6 cm), and severe achalasia (>6 cm) [44]. This third and final stage of achalasia as described by Ellis is characterized by progressive deterioration including malnutrition, severe weight loss, and respiratory complications [23]. On barium swallow this is typified by massive dilation, elongation, and tortuosity as a sigmoid esophagus.

Sensitivity for diagnosing DES on barium swallow is lower than achalasia as the condition is usually intermittent. Classic findings include corkscrew or rosary-bead appearance; however, nonspecific findings of delayed esophageal emptying may be more commonly seen.

Nutcracker/jackhammer esophagus is characterized by high-amplitude, but otherwise normal, peristalsis and will have normal barium swallow findings.

Endoscopy

Esophagogastroduodenoscopy with biopsies should be performed in patients with dysphagia to rule out pseudoachalasia/malignancy, esophagitis secondary to GERD, hiatal hernia, and eosinophilic esophagitis. Other mechanical obstructive lesions, such as esophageal strictures, webs, and rings, may be identified and potentially amenable to concurrent endoscopic dilation. Endoscopic ultrasound may be beneficial in select cases with high suspicion of pseudoachalasia.

Depending on severity, patients with achalasia will have findings of esophageal dilation, liquid pooling with undigested food/pills, and difficulty traversing across the EGJ. Tortuosity and epiphrenic diverticula may also be seen in advanced stages.

pH Study

In patients with dysphagia and heartburn, pH studies may sometimes be obtained demonstrating acid exposure of the distal esophagus. It is important to distinguish between lower pH environments due to GERD versus fermentation from esophageal stasis secondary to achalasia. In the classic acid reflux, several sharp spikes will be seen on the pH tracing associated with episodes of reflux. In fermentation secondary to stasis from achalasia, a slow, gradual drop in pH may sometimes be seen following a meal (Fig. 33.2).

Computed Tomography

Computed tomography of the chest and abdomen may be useful in the evaluation for extrinsic compression or with clinical suspicion of pseudoachalasia.

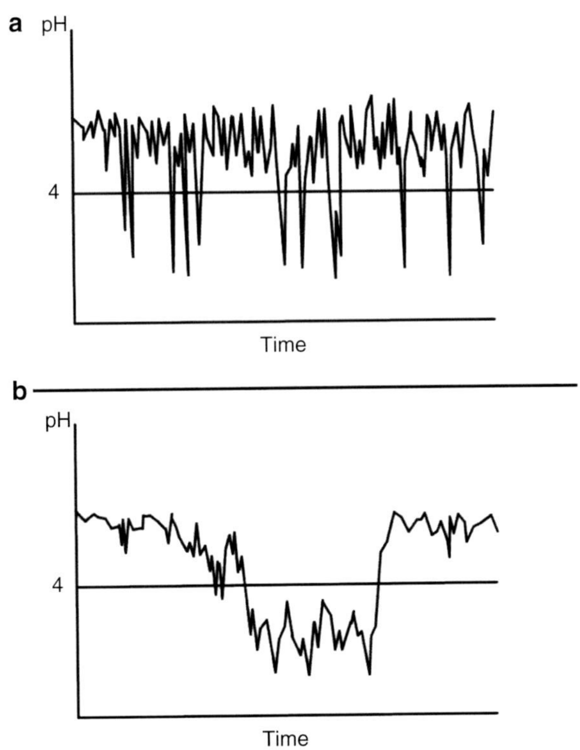

Fig. 33.2 Typical pH study tracing patterns in GERD and achalasia. (**a**) Gastroesophageal reflux disease characterized by multiple sharp spikes. (**b**) Achalasia with slow gradual decline in pH due to acidic fermentation after a meal due to stasis

Manometry

Esophageal manometry is a functional study by positioning intraluminal pressure sensors throughout the entire length of the esophagus. Conventional manometry is comprised of multiple water-perfused sensors placed 3–5 cm apart and performed in the supine position to avoid confounding factors of gravity and hydrostatic pressure. Impedance testing can be done concurrently to detect bolus passage by measuring the different resistance of air, liquid, and esophageal mucosa.

High-resolution manometry has largely replaced conventional manometry as it provides a continuum of intraluminal pressure monitoring using 36 solid-state sensors. Additionally, the study may be performed in the upright position, which is more physiologic to assess deglutition. The results are intuitively depicted as an esophageal pressure topography (EPT) that plots the length of the esophagus over time, with pressure color coded to provide isobaric contour data. In a randomized controlled trial comparing conventional and HRM, a diagnosis was more frequently established with HRM, with a higher sensitivity for diagnosing achalasia [45].

To accurately interpret findings on HRM, it is necessary to be familiar with some of the key features on the EPT plot. In a normal plot, there are two constant high-pressure zones at rest that designate the upper and lower esophageal sphincters (LES). There are also two troughs in a normal peristaltic wave, one proximal and one distal. There is an inflection point in the peristaltic wave where deglutition slows down (within 3 cm of the EGJ) that is represented by the contractile deceleration point (CDP) (Fig. 33.3).

Main findings regarding the EGJ on HRM are the EGJ morphology and the integrated relaxation pressure (IRP). The imprinted pressures from the LES and diaphragmatic hiatus (visible with respiration) determine the EGJ. Hiatal hernia is present when the diaphragmatic pinch of the hiatus and LES pressure zones are separated by more than 2 cm. The IRP is measured as the mean of the 4 s of the maximal LES relaxation within the 10-s relaxation window after swallow is initiated. Normal IRP is less than 15 mmHg, whereas consistently high IRPs with multiple swallows indicate failure of LES relaxation [46].

Characteristics of the esophageal body on HRM include peristaltic integrity, distal latency (DL), and distal contractile integral (DCI). Peristaltic integrity may be described as an intact peristalsis or fragmented (<5 cm break) based on breaks seen in the 20 mmHg isobaric contour. DL is the period of quiescence between the initiation of deglutition at the upper esophageal sphincter and the CDP. A shortened DL (<4.5 s) is indicative of premature contraction. A standardized measurement of the contractile vigor is the DCI, which is measured as the product of length, time, and amplitude above 20 mmHg between the proximal and distal troughs. Normal values are spread over a wide range – from 450 to 8000 mmHg-s-cm. Elevated values indicate hypercontractile esophagus [46] (Table 33.2).

High-resolution manometry has significantly improved diagnosis of achalasia by providing a detailed functional assessment of the esophagus, specifically EGJ relaxation and IRP. Using an IRP above 15 mmHg to detect achalasia, HRM had a sensitivity and specificity of 98% and 96%, respectively [47]. In 2008, Pandolfino et al. published a classification system for achalasia based on HRM findings, subdividing

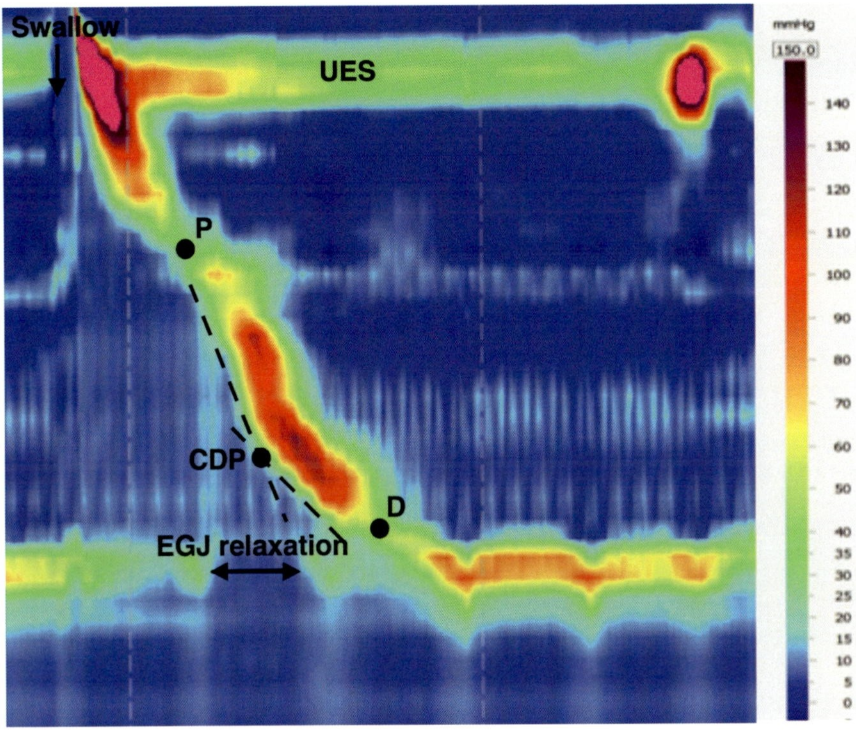

Fig. 33.3 Esophageal pressure topography of a normal swallow. Two high-pressure zones characterized by the upper esophageal sphincter (UES) and the esophagogastric junction (EGJ). Two troughs are visualized, one proximal (P) and one distal (D). The contractile deceleration point (CDP) is marked by the inflection point between the initial and terminal portions of the swallow. The EGJ relaxation window is a 10-s time-period, which occurs after deglutition

patients into three categories [48] (Fig. 33.4). Type I (classic) achalasia is characterized by no distal esophageal pressurization in at least eight swallows out of ten. In type II achalasia, there is panesophageal pressurization greater than 30 mmHg in two or more swallows. Type III (spastic) achalasia has two or more spastic contractions without evidence of peristalsis. These spastic contractions are distinguished from type II pressurization by rapid contractions and shortened DL. Chest pain was more common in type II and III compared to type I. The subclassification had prognostic value to treatment modalities, with type II being most responsive to myotomy and dilation. Type I patients had better outcomes with myotomy as initial treatment compared to endoscopic therapy. Type III had the worst outcomes regardless of treatment with Botox injection, endoscopic dilation, or surgical myotomy [48]. In 2010, these results were externally validated in patients who underwent Heller myotomy with Dor fundoplication as primary treatment. The study demonstrated that higher failure rates were seen in type III achalasia patients, as well as in those with LES resting pressure >30 mmHg [49]. HRM can also be used to evaluate secondary achalasia (Fig. 33.5), as well as provide detailed information after treatment (Fig. 33.6).

Table 33.2 Abnormal esophageal contractile patterns

Contraction vigor
Failed: DCI <100 mmHg-s-cm
Weak: DCI between 100 and 450 mmHg-s-cm
Hypercontractile: DCI ≥8000 mmHg-s-cm
Contractile pattern
Premature: DL <4.5 s and DCI >450 mmHg-s-cm
Fragmented: large break (>5 cm) in 20 mmHg isobaric contour with DCI >450 mmHg-s-cm

Modified from Chicago Classification, v.3 [46]

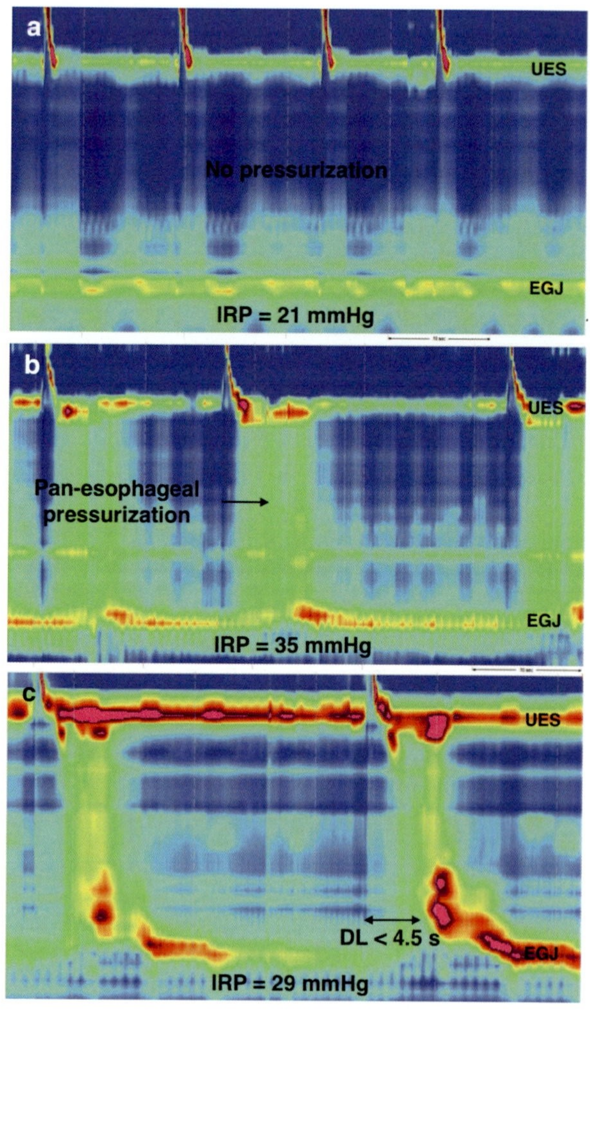

Fig. 33.4 High-resolution manometry of achalasia subtypes. In all cases there is failure of relaxation of the esophagogastric junction (EGJ) (IRP > 15 mmHg) and aperistalsis. (**a**) In type 1, there is absence of pressurization with wet swallows. (**b**) In type 2, there is panesophageal pressurization caused by intrabolus pressure. (**c**) Type 3 achalasia is characterized by premature spastic contractions, defined as distal latency less than 4.5 s. *EGJ* esophagogastric junction, *DL* distal latency, *IRP* integrated relaxation pressure, *UES* upper esophageal sphincter

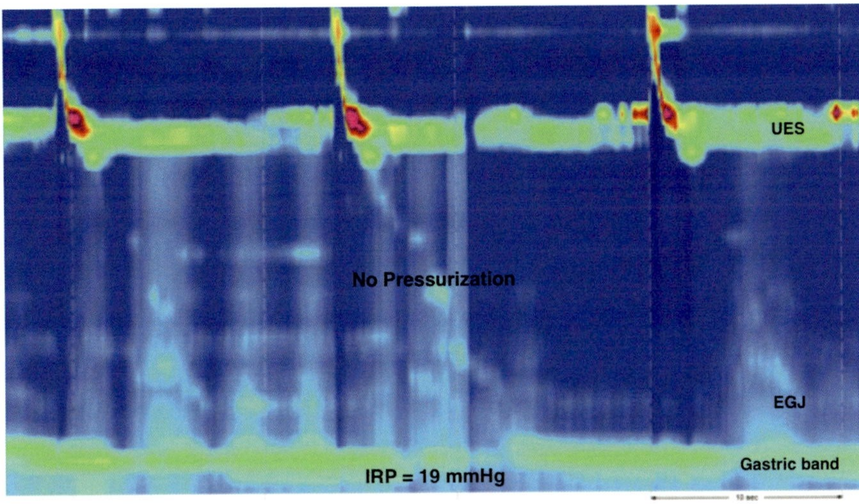

Fig. 33.5 Esophageal pressure topography in a patient with a long-standing history of gastric band presenting with dysphagia and demonstrating aperistalsis and no pressurization. *EGJ* esophagogastric junction, *IRP* integrated relaxation pressure, *UES* upper esophageal sphincter

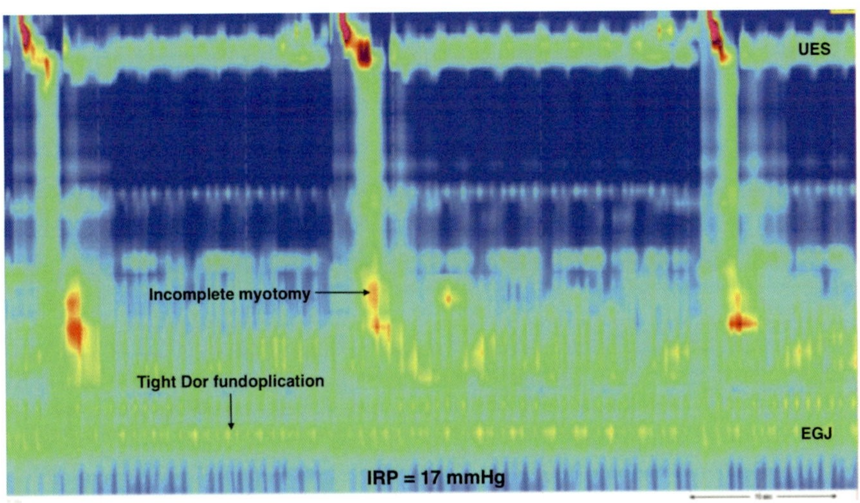

Fig. 33.6 Esophageal pressure topography in a type 3 achalasia patient after incomplete myotomy and a tight Dor fundoplication, characterized by residual spastic contractions above the level of the myotomy and an elevated IRP. *EGJ* esophagogastric junction, *IRP* integrated relaxation pressure, *UES* upper esophageal sphincter

Table 33.3 The Chicago classification hierarchical analysis

1. IRP ≥15 mmHg and 100% failed peristalsis or spasm (disorder of EGJ outflow obstruction)
(a) Achalasia
(i) Type I: no contractility
(ii) Type II: ≥20% panesophageal pressurization
(iii) Type III: ≥20% spasm (DL <4.5 s)
2. IRP ≥15 mmHg, some intact/weak peristalsis (disorder of EGJ outflow obstruction)
(a) EGJ outflow obstruction
(i) Incompletely expressed achalasia
(ii) Mechanical obstruction
3. IRP normal and short DL or high DCI or aperistalsis (other major disorders of peristalsis)
(a) Diffuse esophageal spasm: ≥20% premature (DL <4.5 s)
(b) Jackhammer esophagus: ≥20% DCI >8000 mmHg-s-cm
(c) Absent contractility (100% failed peristalsis): consider achalasia
4. IRP normal and ≥ 50% ineffective swallows (minor disorders of peristalsis)
(a) Ineffective motility (IEM)
(b) Fragmented peristalsis: ≥50% fragmented swallows and not effective
5. IRP normal and > 50% effective swallows (normal)

Modified from Chicago Classification, v.3 [46]

In an effort to characterize other esophageal motility disorders based on HRM findings, the International High-Resolution Manometry Working Group developed the Chicago classification (Table 33.3). It was initially published in 2012 [50], with the most recent revision (version 3.0) in 2015 [46]. It utilizes a hierarchal approach to sequentially evaluate for outflow disorders of the EGJ and other major and minor disorders of peristalsis. The algorithm is primarily based on the IRP, peristaltic integrity, and contractility patterns. Elevated IRP ≥15 mmHg with aperistalsis is diagnostic of achalasia, while partial peristaltic function raises suspicion for EGJ outflow obstruction such as mechanical obstruction or incompletely expressed achalasia. Other disorders of peristalsis that do not fall into the above categories are further stratified. DES is defined by at least 2 of 10 swallows demonstrating shortened distal latency of less than 4.5 s. Jackhammer esophagus is characterized by extreme contraction vigor with DCI >8000 mmHg-s-cm in at least two of ten swallows and is pathologically associated with dysphagia and noncardiac chest pain. Previous DCI values that were used to define nutcracker esophagus are now known to be within the limits of normal values in asymptomatic individuals (450–8000 mmHg-s-cm); thus this condition of hypertensive peristalsis is of unknown clinical significance and has been omitted in the most recent version of Chicago classification. Other miscellaneous disorders of peristalsis include absent contractility, ineffective motility, and fragmented peristalsis.

References

1. Madhavan A, LaGorio LA, Crary MA, Dahl WJ, Carnaby GD. Prevalence of and risk factors for dysphagia in the community dwelling elderly: a systematic review. J Nutr Health Aging. 2016;20(8):806–15.
2. Mayberry JF, Atkinson M. Studies of incidence and prevalence of achalasia in the Nottingham area. Q J Med. 1985;56(220):451–6.
3. Mayberry JF, Atkinson M. Variations in the prevalence of achalasia in Great Britain and Ireland: an epidemiological study based on hospital admissions. Q J Med. 1987;62(237):67–74.
4. Howard PJ, Maher L, Pryde A, Cameron EW, Heading RC. Five year prospective study of the incidence, clinical features, and diagnosis of achalasia in Edinburgh. Gut. 1992;33(8):1011–5.
5. Sadowski DC, Ackah F, Jiang B, Svenson LW. Achalasia: incidence, prevalence and survival. A population-based study. Neurogastroenterol Motil. 2010;22(9):e256–61.
6. Mayberry JF. Epidemiology and demographics of achalasia. Gastrointest Endosc Clin N Am. 2001;11(2):235–48. v
7. Samo S, Carlson DA, Gregory DL, Gawel SH, Pandolfino JE, Kahrilas PJ. Incidence and prevalence of achalasia in Central Chicago, 2004–2014, since the widespread use of high-resolution manometry. Clin Gastroenterol Hepatol. 2016;15(3):366–73.
8. Sonnenberg A. Time trends of US hospitalization for esophageal disease. J Clin Gastroenterol. 2014;48(8):e71–5.
9. Sonnenberg A. Hospitalization for achalasia in the United States 1997–2006. Dig Dis Sci. 2009;54(8):1680–5.
10. Enestvedt BK, Williams JL, Sonnenberg A. Epidemiology and practice patterns of achalasia in a large multi-centre database. Aliment Pharmacol Ther. 2011;33(11):1209–14.
11. Stuckey BG, Mastaglia FL, Reed WD, Pullan PT. Glucocorticoid insufficiency, achalasia, alacrima with autonomic motor neuropathy. Ann Intern Med. 1987;106(1):61–3.
12. Evsyutina YV, Trukhmanov AS, Ivashkin VT. Family case of achalasia cardia: case report and review of literature. World J Gastroenterol. 2014;20(4):1114–8.
13. Gordillo-Gonzalez G, Guatibonza YP, Zarante I, Roa P, Jacome LA, Hani A. Achalasia familiar: report of a family with an autosomal dominant pattern of inherence. Dis Esophagus. 2011;24(1):E1–4.
14. Johnston BT, Colcher A, Li Q, Gideon RM, Castell JA, Castell DO. Repetitive proximal esophageal contractions: a new manometric finding and a possible further link between Parkinson's disease and achalasia. Dysphagia. 2001;16(3):186–9.
15. Moore SW. Down syndrome and the enteric nervous system. Pediatr Surg Int. 2008;24(8):873–83.
16. Zarate N, Mearin F, Hidalgo A, Malagelada JR. Prospective evaluation of esophageal motor dysfunction in down's syndrome. Am J Gastroenterol. 2001;96(6):1718–24.
17. Qualman SJ, Haupt HM, Yang P, Hamilton SR. Esophageal Lewy bodies associated with ganglion cell loss in achalasia. Similarity to Parkinson's disease. Gastroenterology. 1984;87(4):848–56.
18. Moran T, Lawlor P, Brennan M, Ravi N, Reynolds JV. Oesophageal manometry: 10-year audit from a specialist centre, and early experience with high-resolution manometry. Ir J Med Sci. 2015;184(2):379–87.
19. Kahrilas PJ, Pandolfino JE. Ineffective esophageal motility does not equate to GERD. Am J Gastroenterol. 2003;98(4):715–7.
20. Conchillo JM, Nguyen NQ, Samsom M, Holloway RH, Smout AJ. Multichannel intraluminal impedance monitoring in the evaluation of patients with non-obstructive dysphagia. Am J Gastroenterol. 2005;100(12):2624–32.
21. Goldblum JR, Whyte RI, Orringer MB, Appelman HD. Achalasia. A morphologic study of 42 resected specimens. Am J Surg Pathol. 1994;18(4):327–37.

22. Gockel I, Bohl JR, Doostkam S, Eckardt VF, Junginger T. Spectrum of histopathologic findings in patients with achalasia reflects different etiologies. J Gastroenterol Hepatol. 2006;21(4):727–33.
23. Ellis FG. The natural history of achalasia of the cardia. Proc R Soc Med. 1960;53:663–6.
24. Robertson CS, Martin BA, Atkinson M. Varicella-zoster virus DNA in the oesophageal myenteric plexus in achalasia. Gut. 1993;34(3):299–302.
25. Becker J, Niebisch S, Ricchiuto A, Schaich EJ, Lehmann G, Waltgenbach T, et al. Comprehensive epidemiological and genotype-phenotype analyses in a large European sample with idiopathic achalasia. Eur J Gastroenterol Hepatol. 2016;28(6):689–95.
26. de Oliveira RB, Rezende Filho J, Dantas RO, Iazigi N. The spectrum of esophageal motor disorders in Chagas' disease. Am J Gastroenterol. 1995;90(7):1119–24.
27. Mearin F, Garcia-Gonzalez MA, Strunk M, Zarate N, Malagelada JR, Lanas A. Association between achalasia and nitric oxide synthase gene polymorphisms. Am J Gastroenterol. 2006;101(9):1979–84.
28. Paladini F, Cocco E, Cascino I, Belfiore F, Badiali D, Piretta L, et al. Age-dependent association of idiopathic achalasia with vasoactive intestinal peptide receptor 1 gene. Neurogastroenterol Motil. 2009;21(6):597–602.
29. Grubel C, Borovicka J, Schwizer W, Fox M, Hebbard G. Diffuse esophageal spasm. Am J Gastroenterol. 2008;103(2):450–7.
30. Mittal RK, Kassab G, Puckett JL, Liu J. Hypertrophy of the muscularis propria of the lower esophageal sphincter and the body of the esophagus in patients with primary motility disorders of the esophagus. Am J Gastroenterol. 2003;98(8):1705–12.
31. Champion JK, Delise N, Hunt T. Myenteric plexus in spastic motility disorders. J Gastrointest Surg. 2001;5(5):514–6.
32. Konturek JW, Gillessen A, Domschke W. Diffuse esophageal spasm: a malfunction that involves nitric oxide? Scand J Gastroenterol. 1995;30(11):1041–5.
33. Lee JI, Park H, Kim JH, Lee SI, Conklin JL. The effect of sildenafil on oesophageal motor function in healthy subjects and patients with nutcracker oesophagus. Neurogastroenterol Motil. 2003;15(6):617–23.
34. Huang L, Pimentel M, Rezaie A. Do Jackhammer contractions lead to achalasia? A longitudinal study. Neurogastroenterol Motil. 2016;29(3). https://doi.org/10.1111/nmo.12953
35. Pandolfino JE, Gawron AJ. Achalasia: a systematic review. JAMA. 2015;313(18):1841–52.
36. Eckardt VF, Stauf B, Bernhard G. Chest pain in achalasia: patient characteristics and clinical course. Gastroenterology. 1999;116(6):1300–4.
37. Peghini PL, Johnston BT, Leite LP, Castell DO. Mucosal acid exposure sensitizes a subset of normal subjects to intra-oesophageal balloon distension. Eur J Gastroenterol Hepatol. 1996;8(10):979–83.
38. Sengupta JN. An overview of esophageal sensory receptors. AM J Med. 2000;108(Suppl 4a):87s–9s.
39. Sinan H, Tatum RP, Soares RV, Martin AV, Pellegrini CA, Oelschlager BK. Prevalence of respiratory symptoms in patients with achalasia. Dis Esophagus. 2011;24(4):224–8.
40. Gockel I, Eckardt VF, Schmitt T, Junginger T. Pseudoachalasia: a case series and analysis of the literature. Scand J Gastroenterol. 2005;40(4):378–85.
41. Eckardt VF, Aignherr C, Bernhard G. Predictors of outcome in patients with achalasia treated by pneumatic dilation. Gastroenterology. 1992;103(6):1732–8.
42. Gockel I, Junginger T. The value of scoring achalasia: a comparison of current systems and the impact on treatment–the surgeon's viewpoint. Am Surg. 2007;73(4):327–31.
43. Ren Y, Tang X, Chen Y, Chen F, Zou Y, Deng Z, et al. Pre-treatment Eckardt score is a simple factor for predicting one-year peroral endoscopic myotomy failure in patients with achalasia. Surg Endosc. 2017;31:3234–41.
44. Duranceau A, Liberman M, Martin J, Ferraro P. End-stage achalasia. Dis Esophagus. 2012;25(4):319–30.

45. Roman S, Huot L, Zerbib F, Bruley d, Varannes S, Gourcerol G, Coffin B, et al. High-resolution manometry improves the diagnosis of esophageal motility disorders in patients with dysphagia: a randomized multicenter study. Am J Gastroenterol. 2016;111(3):372–80.
46. Kahrilas PJ, Bredenoord AJ, Fox M, Gyawali CP, Roman S, Smout AJ, et al. The Chicago classification of esophageal motility disorders, v3.0. Neurogastroenterol Motil. 2015;27(2):160–74.
47. Ghosh SK, Pandolfino JE, Rice J, Clarke JO, Kwiatek M, Kahrilas PJ. Impaired deglutitive EGJ relaxation in clinical esophageal manometry: a quantitative analysis of 400 patients and 75 controls. Am J Physiol Gastrointest Liver Physiol. 2007;293(4):G878–85.
48. Pandolfino JE, Kwiatek MA, Nealis T, Bulsiewicz W, Post J, Kahrilas PJ. Achalasia: a new clinically relevant classification by high-resolution manometry. Gastroenterology. 2008;135(5):1526–33.
49. Salvador R, Costantini M, Zaninotto G, Morbin T, Rizzetto C, Zanatta L, et al. The preoperative manometric pattern predicts the outcome of surgical treatment for esophageal achalasia. J Gastrointest Surg. 2010;14(11):1635–45.
50. Bredenoord AJ, Fox M, Kahrilas PJ, Pandolfino JE, Schwizer W, Smout AJ. Chicago classification criteria of esophageal motility disorders defined in high resolution esophageal pressure topography. Neurogastroenterol Motil. 2012;24(Suppl 1):57–65.

Medical Management of Achalasia

34

Luise I. M. Pernar

Achalasia is a primary esophageal motility disorder. Achalasia is characterized by the failure of the lower esophageal sphincter (LES) to relax normally when a food bolus is propelled down the esophagus. Long-standing failure of LES relaxation leads to disordered esophageal peristalsis and esophageal dilation. Patients present with progressive dysphagia, first to solid and then progressing to even liquid food. Chest pain, regurgitation, and sensation of heartburn can also be present. The disease is rare, affecting between 1 and 3 in 100,000 new patients annually. The prevalence of achalasia is estimated near 1 in 10,000 patients. The incidence in men and women is similar; there is no racial group that is more frequently affected than another; and diagnosis is typically made between the third and sixth decade of life [1, 2].

The failure of the LES to relax is due to the near total or total loss of the normal myenteric plexus ganglion cells in the distal esophagus [3]. Evidence suggests that this loss is due in large part to an autoimmune process [4], but there may also be a hereditary or infectious component [2]. Additionally, patients with achalasia seem to have abnormal nitric oxide signaling or production, leading to failure of LES relaxation [1, 5].

All treatment modalities for achalasia are palliative, and none can reverse the underlying abnormalities. Medical management of achalasia specifically aims to decrease LES tone to allow esophageal emptying with gravity and thereby relieving the bothersome symptoms of achalasia. The classes of medications most frequently used are calcium channel blockers and nitrates. Aside from these major classes of medications, a variety of other smooth muscle relaxants have been used in an effort to ameliorate achalasia, including anticholinergic and beta-adrenergic medications as well as selective and nonselective phosphodiesterase inhibitors.

L. I. M. Pernar
Department of Surgery, Division of Minimally Invasive and Weight Loss Surgery, Boston Medical Center, Boston, MA, USA
e-mail: Luise.Pernar@bmc.org

J. Grams et al. (eds.), *The SAGES Manual of Foregut Surgery*,
https://doi.org/10.1007/978-3-319-96122-4_34

Calcium Channel Blockers

Calcium channel blockers act on calcium channels that are normally responsible for facilitating intracellular influx of calcium that is necessary for normal contraction to occur. Adverse effects include headaches, palpitations, headaches, and peripheral edema. Some gastrointestinal side effects, including nausea and vomiting, have also been described [6].

Nifedipine is the most well-studied calcium channel blocker employed in the treatment of achalasia. In numerous studies, including randomized controlled trials, nifedipine, at doses between 10 and 20 mg orally with meals, has been shown to decrease LES pressure by between 13% and 68% and improve symptoms by 53–80% [7, 8]. Effects occur between 10 and 30 min after administration and may last for up to 2 h [7].

With a relatively favorable side-effect profile when compared to nitrates, calcium channel blockers currently represent the mainstay of medical palliation of achalasia.

Nitrates

Nitrates are converted to nitric oxide after ingestion. They work by altering cyclic guanosine monophosphate (cGMP). Increased cGMP in turn decreases intracellular calcium, which contributes to smooth muscle relaxation. Adverse effects include headaches and hypotension [6].

Isosorbide dinitrate has not been evaluated in randomized trials, but studies show that its use can decrease LES pressure by 49–66% and improve symptoms by 58–87%. The typical dose is 5 mg orally with meals. Improved esophageal emptying has also been demonstrated [7, 8]. The onset of action is within 15 min and lasts between 60 and 90 min [7]. Even though nitrates are more efficacious than calcium channel blockers, their side effects are less well tolerated. Furthermore, tolerance may develop, limiting the usefulness of nitrates in management of achalasia.

Phosphodiesterase Inhibitors

Phosphodiesterase inhibitors (PDE) prevent the degradation of intracellular cyclic adenosine monophosphate (cAMP) and cGMP. As stated, this decreases intracellular calcium stores, promoting relaxation. Specific phosphodiesterase inhibitors that target the isoform 5-phosphodiesterase (PDE-5) specifically prevent changes specifically in cGMP. Concurrent use of nitrates and phosphodiesterase inhibitors potentiates the relaxing effects of these medications. Adverse effects include hypotension. If used with nitrates, hypotension can be profound and potentially life-threatening [6].

One study of the nonselective PDE aminophylline showed a decrease in LES pressure within 10 min of administration. The authors did not report a mean decrease in pressure but did report that if pressure decreased by more than 25%, which occurred in 4 of 15 patients, the mean decrease in pressure was around 45%. Esophageal emptying was unchanged [9].

More recently attention has been turned to more selective PDEs, specifically the PDE-5 sildenafil. Administration of 50 mg sildenafil decreased LES tone, residual pressure, and also esophageal contractions. LES tone decreased by roughly 50%. The effect was reached within 10–15 min and lasted for less than 1 h. Symptoms were not monitored [10].

At this time not enough is known about PDEs' effect on achalasia to recommend their use over that of calcium channel blockers.

Anticholinergics

Anticholinergic drugs selectively block the nicotinic or muscarinic acetylcholine receptors. Antimuscarinic anticholinergics, such as atropine, inhibit acetylcholine signaling, which results in smooth muscle relaxation, among other effects. These medications can act as cardio-stimulants and can cause tachycardia. Dry mouth, blurry vision, and flushing are other common side effects [11].

In nonrandomized trials, anticholinergics have been shown to have variable effects on the LES pressure. There is not enough data available to support their routine use over the previously mentioned alternatives [7, 8].

Beta-Adrenergics

Beta-adrenergic medications act directly on the beta adrenergic receptors to cause sympathomimetic effects. The beta-adrenergic medications of use in achalasia are specifically beta-2 agonists. Activation of these receptors results in relaxation of smooth muscle through cAMP signaling. Hypokalemia and tremors are among the described side effects [12].

The beta-adrenergic drug terbutaline was evaluated alongside aminophylline and showed slightly more efficacy in decreasing LES pressure, achieving a greater than 25% decrease in 8 of 15 patients with a mean decrease in that group of 43%. Likewise, esophageal emptying was improved. The effects were seen within 10–20 min of administration and lasted for around 1 h [9].

In the absence of more data, as with anticholinergics, routine use over calcium channel blockers should not be recommended.

Summary

Several drug classes have been shown to be efficacious in the palliation of achalasia, reducing LES pressure and improving symptoms. The best-studied and understood class are the calcium channel blockers. While nitrates are perhaps slightly more efficacious, the more favorable side-effect profile of calcium channel blockers makes them first-line medical therapy. Overall, however, it remains true that medical therapy for achalasia have limited utility in the treatment algorithm for achalasia. They should be considered for patients with minimally symptomatic disease or those who cannot or will not tolerate an intervention. Additionally, medications can be used as a bridge to more definitive intervention [7, 13, 14].

References

1. Ates F, Vaezi MF. The pathogenesis and management of achalasia: current status and future directions. Gut Liver. 2015;9(4):449–63.
2. Krill JT, Naik RD, Vaezi MF. Clinical management of achalasia: current state of the art. Clin Exp Gastroenterol. 2016;9:71–82.
3. Goldblum JR, Whyte RI, Orringer MB, Appelman HD. Achalasia. A morphologic study of 42 resected specimens. Am J Surg Pathol. 1994;18(4):327–37.
4. Clark SB, Rice TW, Tubbs RR, Richter JE, Goldblum JR. The nature of the myenteric infiltrate in achalasia: an immunohistochemical analysis. Am J Surg Pathol. 2000;24(8):1153–8.
5. Mearin F, Mourelle M, Guarner F, Salas A, Riveros-Moreno V, Moncada S, et al. Patients with achalasia lack nitric oxide synthase in the gastro-oesophageal junction. Eur J Clin Investig. 1993;23(11):724–8.
6. O'Shaughnessy KM. Arterial hypertension, angina pectoris, myocardial infarction and heart failure. In: Clinical pharmacology [Internet]. 11th ed. Elsevier; 2012 [cited 20 Oct 2016]. Available from: https://www-clinicalkey-com.ezp-prod1.hul.harvard.edu/#!/content/book/3-s2.0-B978070204084900063X.
7. Vaezi MF, Richter JE. Current therapies for achalasia: comparison and efficacy. J Clin Gastroenterol. 1998;27(1):21–35.
8. Bassotti G, Annese V. Review article: pharmacological options in achalasia. Aliment Pharmacol Ther. 1999;13(11):1391–6.
9. Wong RK, Maydonovitch C, Garcia JE, Johnson LF, Castell DO. The effect of terbutaline sulfate, nitroglycerin, and aminophylline on lower esophageal sphincter pressure and radionuclide esophageal emptying in patients with achalasia. J Clin Gastroenterol. 1987;9(4):386–9.
10. Bortolotti M, Mari C, Lopilato C, Porrazzo G, Miglioli M. Effects of sildenafil on esophageal motility of patients with idiopathic achalasia. Gastroenterology. 2000;118(2):253–7.
11. O'Shaughnessy KM. Cholinergic and antimuscarinic (anticholinergic) mechanisms and drugs. In: Clinical pharmacology [Internet]. 11th ed. Elsevier; 2012 [cited 20 Oct 2016]. Available from: https://www-clinicalkey-com.ezp-prod1.hul.harvard.edu/#!/content/book/3-s2.0-B9780702040849000616.
12. O'Shaughnessy KM. Adrenergic mechanisms and drugs. In: Clinical pharmacology [Internet]. 11th ed. Elsevier; 2012 [cited 20 Oct 2016]. Available from: https://www-clinicalkey-com.ezp-prod1.hul.harvard.edu/#!/content/book/3-s2.0-B9780702040849000628?scrollTo=%23hl0000196.
13. Lake JM, Wong RKH. Review article: the management of achalasia – a comparison of different treatment modalities. Aliment Pharmacol Ther. 2006;24(6):909–18.
14. Dughera L, Chiaverina M, Cacciotella L, Cisarò F. Management of achalasia. Clin Exp Gastroenterol. 2011;4:33–41.

35 Endoscopic Management of Achalasia: Botulinum Toxin and Pneumatic Dilation

Michael F. Vaezi and Brian M. Lappas

Introduction

Achalasia is the most common primary motility disorder of the esophagus. It is characterized by impaired relaxation of the lower esophageal sphincter (LES) and absent peristalsis of the esophageal body during deglutition. The incidence of achalasia is 1 in 100,000 individuals annually with a prevalence of 10 in 10,000 [1, 2]. It affects both men and women equally and has no racial predilection [3]. Diagnosis should be confirmed with high-resolution manometry only after obstruction and pseudoachalasia are excluded with esophagogastroduodenoscopy (EGD) [4]. Endoscopically there is often a dilated esophagus with puckering of gastroesophageal junction (Fig. 35.1).

Patients with achalasia most often present with dysphagia or difficulty in swallowing. Other symptoms include chest pain, regurgitation, odynophagia, aspiration, weight loss, and malnutrition [1, 2]. If left untreated, achalasia may progress to "end-stage" disease marked by a severely dilated esophagus, progressive stasis, increased risk of esophageal squamous cell carcinoma, and the need for esophagectomy [5]. The increased tonicity of the LES is caused by the loss of inhibitory interneurons in the myenteric plexus involved in facilitating LES relaxation during deglutition [6]. The etiology of neuronal disruption may be secondary to viral infection or autoimmune reaction in patients with an underlying genetic susceptibility [6–9]. Despite ongoing investigations of pathophysiology and etiology, there is no cure for achalasia.

M. F. Vaezi (✉)
Division of Gastroenterology, Hepatology and Nutrition, Vanderbilt University Medical Center, Nashville, TN, USA
e-mail: Michael.vaezi@vanderbilt.edu

B. M. Lappas
Department of Internal Medicine, Vanderbilt University Medical Center, Nashville, TN, USA

J. Grams et al. (eds.), *The SAGES Manual of Foregut Surgery*,
https://doi.org/10.1007/978-3-319-96122-4_35

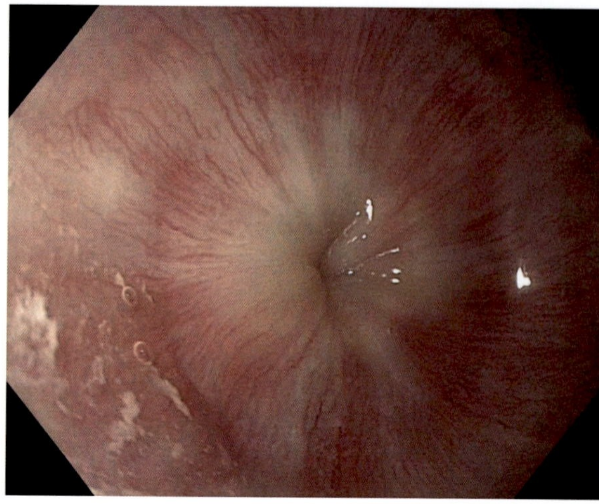

Fig. 35.1 Endoscopic view of puckered gastroesophageal junction in achalasia

Thus, treatments should aim to relieve symptoms and preventing disease progression by decreasing LES hypertonicity, reducing functional obstructions, and facilitating esophageal emptying. This may be achieved through pharmacological, endoscopic, or surgical methods. The choice of treatment depends on the patient's comorbidities, symptom severity, patient preference, and available expertise. In general, the two most effective and long-term treatments are pneumatic balloon dilation (PD) or surgical myotomy [3]. However, some patients are high-risk surgical candidates or would prefer less invasive therapies to treat achalasia symptoms.

The two most common nonoperative treatments will be discussed in this chapter: botulinum toxin (BT) injections and PD. Both treatment options provide safe and efficacious symptom relief to patients who are high-risk surgical candidates or wish to avoid surgery. The aim of this section is to provide guidance on patient selection, endoscopic instruction, and potential complications of BT injections and PD in the treatment of achalasia (Table 35.1).

Botulinum Toxin Injection

Background

Botulinum toxin (BT) is a potent paralytic of voluntary and involuntary muscles. Derived from the *Clostridium botulinum* bacteria, it cleaves the SNAP25 protein, thereby inhibiting the presynaptic vesicle release of the neurotransmitter acetylcholine. Intramuscular injections at the LES will cause relaxation of the smooth muscle allowing for easier passage of a food bolus into the gastric body. BT may induce additional pro-inflammatory mediators including nitric oxide and tumor necrosis factor alpha, which may have additional relaxation effects at the site of injection [10].

Historically, BT injection has been used to treat various maladies including muscle spasms, migraines, hyperhidrosis, and pain syndromes. Additionally, it has been used off-label in various gastrointestinal disorders including gastroparesis, anal fissures,

Table 35.1 Pros and cons of botulinum toxin injection and pneumatic dilation

Treatment	Optimal patients	Remission duration	Pros	Cons
Botox injections	Nonsurgical candidates	6–12 months	Operator friendly	Repeated treatments needed
	Elderly		Mild and rare complications	
	Type II or vigorous achalasia			
Pneumatic dilation	Must be surgical candidate	2–5 years	Efficacious and durable	Requires expertise
	Younger		Cost-effective	Surgery backup required
	Type II or vigorous achalasia			Repeated treatments needed
				Perforation risk 2–5%

sphincter of Oddi dysfunction, esophageal spasms, and achalasia [11]. BT was first studied in 1993 by Pasricha and his colleagues as a potential treatment option for achalasia with subsequent validation of symptomatic efficacy and safety [12, 13].

There are eight known serotypes of BT (A, B, C1, C2, D, E, F, and G) with two of them, type A and B, approved for medical therapy because of their lasting effects of weeks to months. There are three subtype A formulations: Botox (Allergan, Irvine, CA), Dysport (Medicis, Scottsdale, AZ), and Xeomin (Merz, Raleigh, NC). Type A formulations are prepared as a powder and require reconstitution with normal saline prior to injection (Fig. 35.2). Dosing recommendations in this chapter will refer to Botox as it is the most commonly used and well-studied formulation.

One type B formulation, Myobloc (Solstice, Louisville, KY), is approved for medical therapy. It is prepared as a vial containing 5000 units/mL in a sterile solution that also requires dilution in normal saline prior to injection. Although BT types A and B have similar reports of efficacy, animal studies generally show BT type A as having a longer duration of action [14]. The various BT subtypes and formulations have different potency requiring distinct dilutions; thus providers should be mindful of manufacturer instructions prior use.

Patient Selection and Outcomes

BT injection is a safe and efficacious treatment option for patients who may not be candidates for PD or surgery. Multiple studies have identified age > 40 years and manometric type II or III achalasia as favorable outcome variables [15–17]. Interestingly, pretreatment LES pressure, amplitude of contractions, and duration of symptoms do not predict BT treatment response. Posttreatment, a decreased LES pressure is a predictor of favorable symptom response [15]. However, many report symptomatic improvement without physiologic changes.

Most patients have symptom relief within the first month of BT injection, reported as high as 80–90% [15–18]. However, over 50% of patients will have a

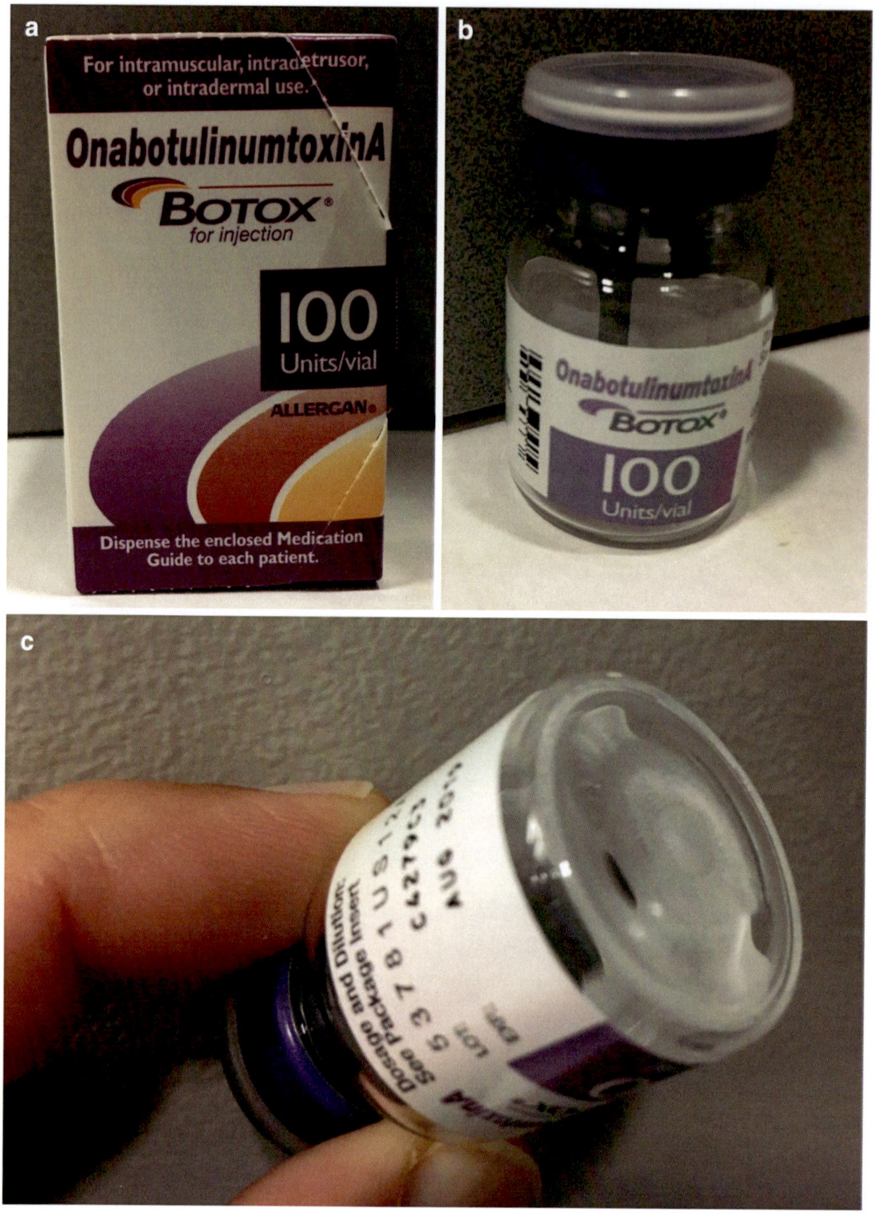

Fig. 35.2 (**a**) Botulinum toxin A (Botox) 100 units manufactured for injection in achalasia. (**b**) The vial containing botulinum toxin A (Botox) 100 units. (**c**) Thick film of botulinum toxin A at the bottom of the vial which should always be refrigerated

return of symptoms within 1 year. Thus, repeated injections are often needed at 6- to 24-month intervals as determined by symptoms [15–18]. Significant data evaluating long-term success of repeated BT injections is lacking. However, remission rate may range from 30% to 68% at 24 months [15, 18]. Elderly patients have a longer period of symptom relief, up to 1–2 years after a single injection when compared to younger patients [19]. Patients respond well to 80–100 units of Botox per session, with 20–25 units injected into four separate areas of the LES. Increasing Botox dose does not result in increased efficacy [18].

Importantly, repeated BT injections may cause localized fibrosis and increase the risk of perforation in patients undergoing subsequent PD or surgical myotomy. A study by Sweet et al. showed that preoperative treatment with BT was the only factor associated with poor outcomes postmyotomy [20]. Although, this area is controversial. Given less than optimal long-term efficacy and potential for complications of future PD or myotomy, BT injection should not be offered as initial treatment for any patient with achalasia who is a candidate for more definitive therapy. BT should be reserved for achalasia patients unlikely to undergo future PD or surgical myotomy or for those where the diagnosis is in question, and a response to BT might help determine if to proceed with more definitive therapy.

Endoscopic Steps

- Position the sedated patient in the lateral decubitus position as in preparation for an upper EGD.
- Confirm the BT type, manufacturer, and dilution instructions.
- Prepare the Botox solution by mixing 80–100 units of BT powder into 5–10 ml normal saline and draw into a 5 mm sclerotherapy needle.
- Advance the endoscope into the esophagus using direct visualization to rule out obstruction or pseudoachalasia. Gastric aspiration or lavage should be performed if retained food is found in the esophagus.
- Introduce the sclerotherapy needle through the accessory channel of the endoscope.
- Visualize the Z-line and squamocolumnar junction. Within 1 cm of the z-line, deploy the needle at 45 degrees to the surface of the esophagus.
- Inject 20–25 units of Botox (~1–2 ml) intramuscularly into each of the four quadrants of the LES. Use 80–100 units total.
- Confirm significant resistance during injection to verify intramuscular placement. Little resistance may imply injection into a superficial layer or through the esophageal wall.

Follow-Up and Complications

BT injections are outpatient procedures, and patients may be discharged 2–6 h post-intervention. Patient should be monitored for resolution of sedation and tolerate liquids without severe pain or coughing. Complications with BT injections are mild with transient side effects including chest discomfort (16–25%) or reflux (<5%) [3].

Serious complications are exceedingly rare and include mucosal ulceration, pleural effusion, mediastinitis, and allergic reactions to the egg-based protein [21]. BT injection does not increase esophageal perforation risk and is well tolerated even in patients with significant comorbidities [22–24].

Key Points

- BT injection is safe and efficacious short-term treatment for patients who are not candidates for pneumatic dilation or surgical myotomy.
- Twenty to twenty-five units of Botox total are injected into each of the four quadrants of the LES per session, 100 units total.
- Most patients (80–90%) experience short-term relief, but more than 50% of patients will have return of symptoms within 12 months. Most patients will need repeated BT injections for continued symptom control.
- Complications are mild and include chest discomfort (20%) or reflux (<5%). Patients may be discharged the same day after being observed for 2–6 h.

Pneumatic Dilation

Background

Pneumatic dilation is the most effective nonsurgical treatment option for patients with achalasia [3]. The goal of PD is to limit symptom severity and delay disease progression through mechanical disruption of the LES smooth muscle fibers. A polyethylene balloon is endoscopically deployed and filled with air creating enough radial pressure to fracture the muscularis propria. This decreases the hypertonicity of the LES, thus promoting esophageal emptying through gravity and improved peristalsis of food into the gastric body.

Forceful esophageal dilation was first reported by Sir Thomas Willis in 1674 when he used a sponge-tipped whalebone to dilate a tight LES [25]. Rigid dilators were used for centuries to treat esophageal strictures, obstruction, spasms, and symptoms of dysphagia. The technique was modernized when rigid dilators were modified with expandable balloons filled with water or air [25, 26]. Balloon dilators are less traumatic than rigid dilators as they only exert radial forces to the LES as opposed to axial forces throughout the esophagus. PD became the preferred dilation treatment in the 1980s as they can generate the 7–15 pounds per square inch (psi) needed for successful disruption of the LES smooth muscle fibers [25, 26].

Modern pneumatic dilators have sizes ranging from 3.0 to 4.0 cm. The most widely used balloon dilator is the Rigiflex (Boston Scientific, Marlborough MA) (Fig. 35.3a, b), a nonradiopaque polyethylene balloon that comes in three different diameters (3.0, 3.5, and 4.0 cm). Although deployment under fluoroscopy is recommended, direct visualization during endoscopy has gained popularity and appears to be equally effective (Fig. 35.3c) [27, 28].

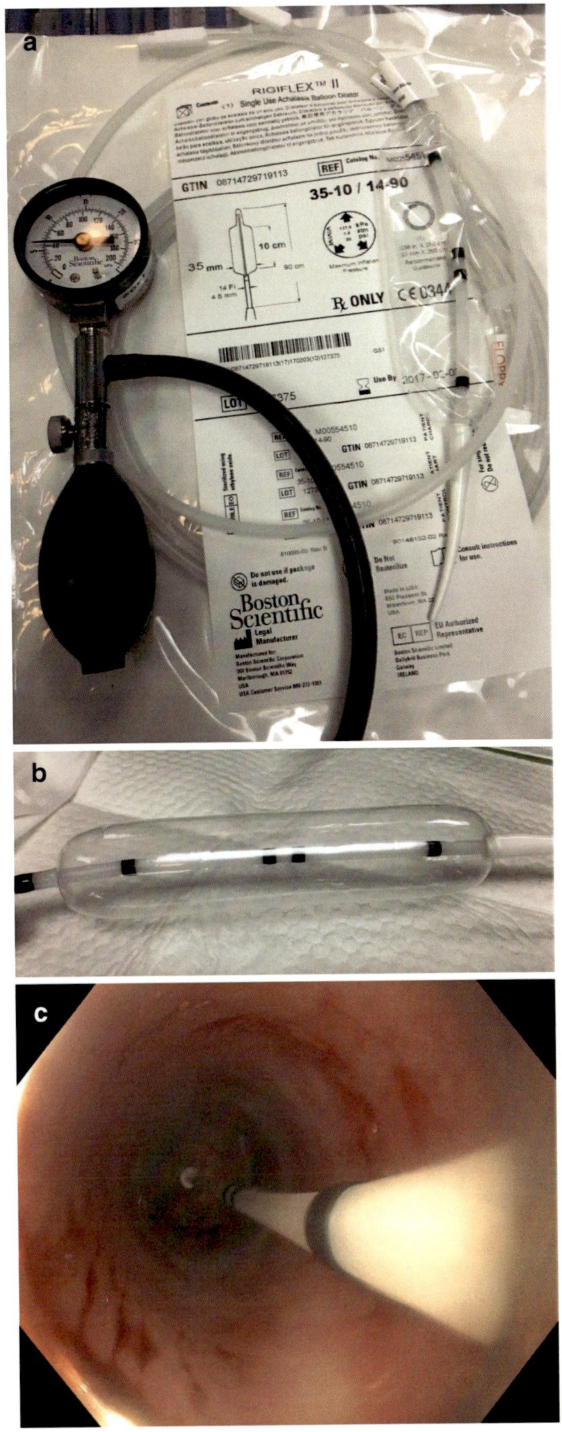

Fig. 35.3 (**a**) Pneumatic dilation assembly using the Rigiflex balloon and pressure gauge. (**b**) An example of inflated 3.5 cm Rigiflex balloon. (**c**) Pneumatic dilation employing the direct endoscopic method whereby the correct positioning of the balloon is confirmed endoscopically based on approximation of the two markers next to the gastroesophageal junction visualized through the balloon

Patient Selection and Outcomes

Pneumatic dilation is the preferred nonoperative treatment for patients as it provides good symptom relief and durability over a 5- to 10-year period. Patients may benefit from a single dilation session using a 3.0 cm balloon with one cross-sectional study with 62% showing symptomatic response at 6 months and 28% after 2 years [29]. However, we recommend a serial graded approach by repeating dilations every 4–6 weeks with increasing balloon diameters at 3.0 to 3.5 to 4.0 cm if symptoms persist. The same cross-sectional study showed a 90% response rate at 6 months and 44% at 6 years [29]. One large review analyzed 1144 patients who underwent serial dilations over a 19-month period with increasing balloon diameters: 3.0 cm followed by 3.5 cm and 4.0 cm. They found increasing remission rates of 74%, 86%, and 90%, respectively [30]. Other studies have also shown impressive long-term remission rates of 50–89% of patients over a 4-year mean follow-up interval [30–32]. Zerbib et al. showed that repeated PD provided remission in 96.8% of patients at 5 years and 93.4% of patients at 10 years [33].

Predictors of favorable clinical response include older age (>45 years old), female gender, a narrow esophagus, and type II pattern on HRM. Younger males may benefit from initial dilation of 3.5 cm if little resistance found in 3.0 cm dilation [3, 29]. Posttreatment predictors of success include decreased pressure of LES <10 mmHg, rapid recovery of symptoms, and visual confirmation of LES dilation [34, 35]. Perhaps the most powerful predictor of graded PD therapy success is patient symptomatic response in concordance with a post-procedural timed barium esophagram. Vaezi et al. found that 77% of patients who had improved symptoms and a barium column height of <5 cm remained symptom-free after 6 years. However, almost all patients with improved symptoms but a barium column height >5 cm had a return of symptoms after just 12 months [36].

Repeated dilations can be safely performed every 4–6 weeks as determined by manometry, radiographic studies, and recurrence of symptoms. The Eckardt score is a useful quantitative method used to gauge symptom severity over time [37, 38]. Using the graded approach, many patients can remain in remission for 5–10 years. If patients continue to have symptoms, surgical options should be explored, particularly in younger patients who may respond more favorably [3].

Endoscopic Steps

- Position the sedated patient in the lateral decubitus position as in preparation for an upper EGD.
- Inflate the Rigiflex balloon to check leaks or malfunction.

- Advance the endoscope into the esophagus using direct visualization to rule out obstruction or pseudoachalasia. Gastric aspiration or lavage should be performed if retained food is found in the esophagus. Take note of the distance between the incisors and LES.
- Introduce a guidewire through the accessory channel of the endoscope and into the stomach. Carefully remove the endoscope leaving the guidewire in place.
- Advance the deflated balloon over the guidewire until the center of the balloon is positioned across the LES opening. This should be the same distance from the incisors previously noted during endoscopy.
- After confirming placement (by fluoroscopy or endoscopy), attach the balloon to a pressure gauge and inflate to apply 10–15 psi over 15–60 s.
- Deflate the balloon and remove the balloon and guidewire.
- Visualize the distal esophagus for impact of dilation and examine for possible perforation.
- If perforation suspected, be prepared to place a fully covered esophageal stent and admit patient to hospital, start IV fluids and broad-spectrum antibiotics, and consult thoracic surgery as in some cases surgery may be needed.
- Otherwise discharge patient home with symptom follow-up in 1 month.

Follow-Up and Complications

Pneumatic dilation is an outpatient procedure, and patients may be discharged the same day. Potential complications include chest discomfort, aspiration pneumonia, transient fever, or intramural hematomas [39]. Up to 35% of patients may experience gastroesophageal reflux disease post-therapy and should be treated with a proton pump inhibitor [40]. Patients should be observed for 2–6 h and monitored for severe pain, coughing, or inability to tolerate liquids which may indicate an esophageal perforation, the most serious potential complication with an incidence rate of 2–5% [3].

It is important to recognize esophageal perforations and treat them early. Most perforations are small and may be managed with observation, antibiotics, or stents. However, about 1% of perforations may cause gross contamination of the mediastinum requiring surgical repair [41]. Therefore, all patients considering PD should be aware of this risk and be eligible surgical candidates. There are no predictors of perforation, but the risk may increase with repeated dilations, age over 60 [41], initial balloon diameter of 3.5 cm (as opposed to 3.0 cm) [42], and improper positioning across the LES [43]. It is recommended that patients undergo post-procedural radiographic testing with a water-based contrast (gastrografin) followed by a timed barium esophagram for both diagnostic and prognostic purposes [3].

Key Points

- Pneumatic dilation is the most preferred non-operative treatment for achalasia.
- We recommend a graded dilation strategy. Start with a 3.0 cm diameter balloon and increase to 3.5 cm or 4.0 cm as indicated by symptoms, manometry, and radiographical studies. (Males less than 45 years of age may need to be started with 3.5 cm size balloon first.)
- Repeated dilations have remission rates between 50% and 89% over 4 years. Many patients may have remission for up to 10 years, although the efficacy of repeated dilation may diminish over time.
- Esophageal perforation incidence approaches 2% with the graded strategy. All patients should be surgical candidates.
- Patients may be discharged 2–6 h post-intervention if no signs of complications.

Treatment Comparisons

Multiple randomized controlled trials (RCTs), with or without blinding, have been published directly comparing the efficacy of BT injections and PD (Table 35.2). A comprehensive Cochrane review by Leyden et al. in 2014 included seven studies in a meta-analysis with the primary endpoints of symptom relief at 4 weeks, 6 months, and 12 months [23]. There was no significant difference between remission rates within 4 weeks of intervention. However, at 12 months, PD patients had significantly higher remission rates when compared to those treated with BT injections. Overall, PD has improved clinical efficacy and is the preferred nonoperative treatment in the long term [3, 23, 44]. BT injections and PD are comparable in total cost over a 5-year period, $7011 and $7069, respectively. However, a 2002 cost-effectiveness study found that PD is more cost-effective with an incremental cost-effectiveness ratio of $1348 per quality adjusted life year [45].

Table 35.2 Randomized controlled trials directly comparing the efficacy of endoscopic pneumatic dilation and Botox injections

		1-month remission		6-month remission		12-month remission	
Author	Year	PD % (*n*)	BT % (*n*)	PD % (*n*)	BT % (*n*)	PD % (*n*)	BT % (*n*)
Vaezi et al.	1999	70% (20)	80% (20)	–	–	–	–
Ghoshal et al.	2001	–	–	80% (10)	29% (7)	70% (10)	29% (7)
Mikaeli et al.	2001	–	–	74% (19)	25% (20)	53% (19)	15% (20)
Bansal et al.	2003	94% (18)	75% (16)	–	–	89% (18)	38% (16)
Zhu et al.	2009	–	–	86% (28)	76% (29)	71% (28)	55% (29)

PD pneumatic dilation, *BT* botox injection, % percentage, *n* number of participants

Long-term outcomes between PD and surgical Heller myotomy have only recently been evaluated. Moonen et al. conducted a randomized controlled trial of 201 achalasia patients initially treated with PD or surgical myotomy and tracked symptom relief over a 5-year period. There was no statistical difference between treatments (82% vs 85%, respectively, $p = 0.92$). Of note, 5% of patients undergoing PD had esophageal perforations requiring conservative management, while 12% of surgical myotomy patients had mucosal tears requiring intraoperative repair [46].

Conclusions

Achalasia is the most common primary esophageal motility disorder with high rates of morbidity. There is no cure for achalasia, so treatment should focus on relieving symptoms and deterring disease progression. Ultimately, the choice of treatment depends on the patient's comorbidities, symptom severity, patient preference, and available expertise. Both BT injections and PD provide safe and efficacious nonoperative symptom relief for such patients. Elderly patients or those with high surgical risks should be considered for BT injections. However, if the patient is a surgical candidate, serial PD treatments and surgical myotomy are the two most definitive well-established treatment options. PD should be performed at an experienced medical center with surgical backup. Patients who do not initially respond to graded PD therapy should be referred for surgical myotomy.

Conflict of Interest Dr. Vaezi has a research grant from Sandhill Scientific, Inc. (Denver, Co, USA). Dr. Lappas has no COI.

References

1. Vaezi MF, Richter JE. Diagnosis and management of achalasia. Am J Gastroenterol. 1999;94(12):3406–1.
2. Francis DL, Katzka DA. Achalasia: update on the disease and its treatment. Gastroenterology. 2010;139(2):369–74.
3. Vaezi MF, Pandolfino JE, Vela MF. ACG clinical guideline: diagnosis and management of achalasia. Am J Gastroenterol. 2013;108(8):1238–49.
4. Kahrilas PJ, Bredenoord AJ, Fox M, Gyawali CP, Roman S, Smout AJ, Pandolfino JE. The Chicago classification of esophageal motility disorders, v3. 0. Neurogastroenterol Motil. 2015;27(2):160–74.
5. Leeuwenburgh I, Scholten P, Alderliesten J, Tilanus HW, Looman CW, Steijerberg EW, Kuipers EJ. Long-term esophageal cancer risk in patients with primary achalasia: a prospective study. Am J Gastroenterol. 2010;105(10):2144–9.
6. Clark SB, Rice TW, Tubbs RR, Richter JE, Goldblum JR. The nature of the myenteric infiltrate in achalasia: an immunohistochemical analysis. Am J Surg Pathol. 2000;24(8):1153–8.
7. Goldblum JR, Rice TW, Richter JE. Histopathologic features in esophagomyotomy specimens from patients with achalasia. Gastroenterology. 1996;111(3):648–54.
8. Villanacci V, Annese V, Cuttitta A, Fisogni S, Scaramuzzi G, De Santo E, Corazzi N, Bassotti G. An immunohistochemical study of the myenteric plexus in idiopathic achalasia. J Clin Gastroenterol. 2010;44(6):407–10.

9. Boeckxstaens GE. Achalasia: virus-induced euthanasia of neurons & quest. Am J Gastroenterol. 2008;103(7):1610–2.
10. Kim YJ, Kim JH, Lee KJ, Choi MM, Kim YH, Rhie GE, Yoo CK, Cha K, Shin NR. Botulinum neurotoxin type a induces TLR2-mediated inflammatory responses in macrophages. PLoS One. 2015;10(4):e0120840.
11. Mashimo H. Botulinum toxin for achalasia. Cham: Springer; 2016. p. 31–8.
12. Pasricha P, Ravich W, Kalloo A. Botulinum toxin for achalasia. Lancet. 1993;341(8839):244–5.
13. Pasricha PJ, Ravich WJ, Hendrix TR, Sostre S, Jones B, Kalloo AN. Treatment of achalasia with intrasphincteric injection of botulinum toxin: a pilot trial. Ann Intern Med. 1994;121(8):590–1.
14. Dressler D, Benecke R. Pharmacology of therapeutic botulinum toxin preparations. Disabil Rehabil. 2007;29(23):1761–8.
15. Pasricha PJ, Rai RU, Ravich WJ, Hendrix TR, Kalloo AN. Botulinum toxin for achalasia: long-term outcome and predictors of response. Gastroenterology. 1996;110(5):1410–5.
16. Zaninotto G, Annese V, Costantini M, Del Genio A, Costantino M, Epifani M, Gatto G, D'onofrio V, Benini L, Contini S, Molena D. Randomized controlled trial of botulinum toxin versus laparoscopic Heller myotomy for esophageal achalasia. Ann Surg. 2004;239(3):364–70.
17. Vaezi MF, Richter JE, Wilcox CM, Schroeder PL, Birgisson S, Slaughter RL, Koehler RE, Baker ME. Botulinum toxin versus pneumatic dilatation in the treatment of achalasia: a randomised trial. Gut. 1999;44(2):231–9.
18. Annese V, Bassotti G, Coccia G, Dinelli M, D'Onofrio V, Gatto G, Leandro G, Repici A, Testoni PA, Andriulli A. GISMAD achalasia study group. A multicentre randomised study of intrasphincteric botulinum toxin in patients with oesophageal achalasia. Gut. 2000;46(5):597–600.
19. Achkar E. Achalasia. Gastroenterologist. 1995;3(4):273–88.
20. Sweet MP, Nipomnick I, Gasper WJ, Bagatelos K, Ostroff JW, Fisichella PM, Way LW, Patti MG. The outcome of laparoscopic Heller myotomy for achalasia is not influenced by the degree of esophageal dilatation. J Gastrointest Surg. 2008;12(1):159–65.
21. Mac Iver R, Liptay M, Johnson Y. A case of mediastinitis following botulinum toxin type a treatment for achalasia. Nat Clin Pract Gastroenterol Hepatol. 2007;4(10):579–82.
22. Wang L, Li YM, Li L, Yu CH. A systematic review and meta-analysis of the Chinese literature for the treatment of achalasia. World J Gastroenterol. 2008;14(38):5900–6.
23. Leyden JE, Moss AC, MacMathuna P. Endoscopic pneumatic dilation versus botulinum toxin injection in the management of primary achalasia. Cochrane Database Syst Rev. 2006;(4):CD005046.
24. Tolone S, Limongelli P, del Genio G, Brusciano L, Russo A, Cipriano L, Terribile M, Docimo G, Ruggiero R, Docimo L. Recent trends in endoscopic management of achalasia. World J Gastrointest Endosc. 2014;6(9):407.
25. Cox J, Buckton GK, Bennett JR. Balloon dilatation in achalasia: a new dilator. Gut. 1986;27(8):986.
26. Kadakia SC, Wong RK. Graded pneumatic dilation using Rigiflex achalasia dilators in patients with primary esophageal achalasia. Am J Gastroenterol. 1993;88(1):34–8.
27. Lambroza A, Schuman R. Pneumatic dilation for achalasia without fluoroscopic guidance: safety and efficacy. Gastrointest Endosc. 1995;41(4):354.
28. Thomas V, Harish K, Sunilkumar K. Pneumatic dilation of achalasia cardia under direct endoscopy: the debate continues. Gastrointest Endosc. 2006;63(4):734.
29. Vela MF, Richter JE, Khandwala F, Blackstone EH, Wachsberger D, Baker ME, Rice TW. The long-term efficacy of pneumatic dilatation and Heller myotomy for the treatment of achalasia. Clin Gastroenterol Hepatol. 2006;4(5):580–7.
30. Vaezi MF, Richter JE. Current therapies for achalasia: comparison and efficacy. J Clin Gastroenterol. 1998;27(1):21–35.
31. Torbey CF, Achkar E, Rice TW, Baker M, Richter JE. Long-term outcome of achalasia treatment: the need for closer follow-up. J Clin Gastroenterol. 1999;28(2):125–30.
32. Karamanolis G, Sgouros S, Karatzias G, Papadopoulou E, Vasiliadis K, Stefanidis G, Mantides A. Long-term outcome of pneumatic dilation in the treatment of achalasia. Am J Gastroenterol. 2005;100(2):270–4.

33. Zerbib F, Thétiot V, Richy F, Benajah DA, Message L, Lamouliatte H. Repeated pneumatic dilations as long-term maintenance therapy for esophageal achalasia. Am J Gastroenterol. 2006;101(4):692–7.
34. Eckardt VF, Gockel I, Bernhard G. Pneumatic dilation for achalasia: late results of a prospective follow up investigation. Gut. 2004;53(5):629–33.
35. Alderliesten J, Conchillo JM, Leeuwenburgh I, Steyerberg EW, Kuipers EJ. Predictors for outcome of failure of balloon dilatation in patients with achalasia. Gut. 2011;60:10–6.
36. Vaezi MF, Baker ME, Achkar E, Richter JE. Timed barium oesophagram: better predictor of long term success after pneumatic dilation in achalasia than symptom assessment. Gut. 2002;50(6):765–70.
37. Gockel I, Junginger T. The value of scoring achalasia: a comparison of current systems and the impact on treatment—the surgeon's viewpoint. Am Surg. 2007;73(4):327–31.
38. Stavropoulos SN, Friedel D, Modayil R, Iqbal S, Grendell JH. Endoscopic approaches to treatment of achalasia. Ther Adv Gastroenterol. 2012;107(12):1817–25.
39. Moonen A, Boeckxstaens G. Current diagnosis and management of achalasia. J Clin Gastroenterol. 2014;48(6):484–90.
40. Krill JT, Naik RD, Vaezi MF. Clinical management of achalasia: current state of the art. Clin Exp Gastroenterol. 2016;9:71.
41. Katzka DA, Castell DO. Review article: an analysis of the efficacy, perforation rates and methods used in pneumatic dilation for achalasia. Aliment Pharmacol Ther. 2011;34(8):832–9.
42. Boeckxstaens GE, Annese V, Varannes SB, Chaussade S, Costantini M, Cuttitta A, Elizalde JI, Fumagalli U, Gaudric M, Rohof WO, Smout AJ. Pneumatic dilation versus laparoscopic Heller's myotomy for idiopathic achalasia. N Engl J Med. 2011;364(19):1807–16.
43. Metman EH, Lagasse JP, d'Alteroche L, Picon L, Scotto B, Barbieux JP. Risk factors for immediate complications after progressive pneumatic dilation for achalasia. Am J Gastroenterol. 1999;94(5):1179–85.
44. Jung HE, Lee JS, Lee TH, Kim JN, Hong SJ, Kim JO, Kim HG, Jeon SR, Cho JY. Long-term outcomes of balloon dilation versus botulinum toxin injection in patients with primary achalasia. Korean J Intern Med. 2014;29(6):738–45.
45. O'Connor JB, Singer ME, Imperiale TF, Vaezi MF, Richter JE. The cost-effectiveness of treatment strategies for achalasia. Dig Dis Sci. 2002;47(7):1516–25.
46. Moonen A, Annese V, Belmans A, Bredenoord AJ, des Varannes SB, Costantini M, Dousset B, Elizalde JI, Fumagalli U, Gaudric M, Merla A. Long-term results of the European achalasia trial: a multicentre randomised controlled trial comparing pneumatic dilation versus laparoscopic Heller myotomy. Gut. 2016;65(5):732–9.

36 Surgical Management of Achalasia: Laparoscopic Heller Myotomy

Arinbjorn Jonsson and S. Scott Davis Jr.

Indications

Achalasia is a debilitating disease characterized by absent esophageal peristalsis and failed relaxation of the lower esophageal sphincter. All patients with suspected achalasia should have a complete work-up including an upper GI series, endoscopy, and manometry. These studies are vital to rule out other causes of dysphagia such as malignancy, Schatzki rings, neurological causes, etc. While there are several treatment options for the newly diagnosed achalasia patient, it is important to note that the mean age of diagnosis is quite young, and most patients are younger than 50. Previous chapters have reviewed these topics in detail.

The laparoscopic Heller myotomy with partial fundoplication provides durable long-term relief of dysphagia and >90% patient satisfaction after 10 years [1]. It remains the gold standard of therapy [2] and should be a consideration in all patients fit for surgery. Given the low morbidity rates and excellent long-term outcomes, alternative procedures will need to be carefully and prospectively compared to laparoscopic Heller myotomy when evaluated for effectiveness.

Technique

Preoperatively Once the diagnosis is confirmed, the patient undergoes careful medical evaluation. This includes all standard preoperative considerations appropriate for low to moderate risk surgical procedures. Often times, patients with achalasia

A. Jonsson
Emory Endosurgery Unit, Emory University Hospital, Atlanta, GA, USA

S. Scott Davis Jr. (✉)
Emory Endosurgery Unit, Division of General and GI Surgery, Emory University Hospital, Atlanta, GA, USA
e-mail: sdavisj@emory.edu

J. Grams et al. (eds.), *The SAGES Manual of Foregut Surgery*,
https://doi.org/10.1007/978-3-319-96122-4_36

have been experiencing retrosternal chest pains and will need concurrent cardiac disease ruled out. The nutritional status of the patient should also be carefully considered. In many cases, there may have been clinically significant weight loss prior to surgical consultation. Occasional patients will need consideration for enteric supplemental nutrition preoperatively which can be accomplished via percutaneous gastrostomy tube, or rarely, hyperalimentation.

Perioperatively All patients will have impaired esophageal clearance which could pose an aspiration risk at the time of intubation. The surgical and anesthesia teams should be prepared for this possibility. Patients are placed on a clear liquid diet 48 h prior to surgery, and rapid sequence intubation is used.

Patients are placed in the supine position with the arms abducted to 80°. Pneumatic compression sleeves are placed. The patient is double strapped to the operating table with a footboard. Appropriate antibiotics are given prior to skin incision.

Access is gained into the abdomen using a 10 mm optical trocar inserted off Palmer's point (left subcostal midaxillary line). In this location the fascia is fixed at the costal margin decreasing the chance of visceral injury with port insertion. The patient is placed in steep reverse Trendelenburg, and three additional trocars are placed. We place a 5 mm left lateral assistant port, 12 mm midline/paramedian camera port 15 cm below the xiphoid process, a 5 mm right subcostal working port, and a subxiphoid incision for the Nathanson liver retractor (Fig. 36.1). The surgeon stands on the patient's right utilizing the two subcostal ports as

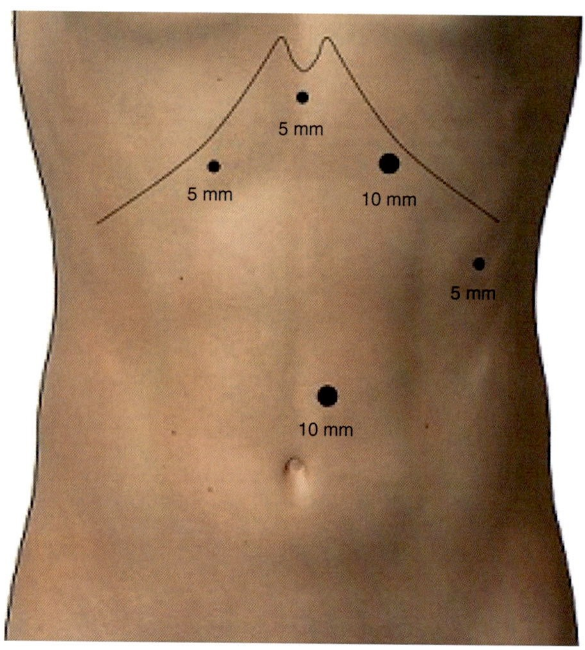

Fig. 36.1 Port placement for laparoscopic Heller myotomy

working ports, and the assistant stands on the patient's left. Alternatively, the patient may be placed in the split-leg position with the operating surgeon standing between the legs.

Step 1: Division of Short Gastric Vessels and Dissection of Left Crus

We begin the procedure by dividing the short gastric vessels using a bipolar energy device. The dissection should begin 1/3 of the way down the greater curvature to allow full mobility of the fundus while preserving as much blood supply as possible. This dissection is carried out until the left crus of the diaphragm is identified and all posterior attachments are freed. The phrenoesophageal ligament is divided, and the peritoneum medial to the left crus is entered. The hiatus is freed bluntly and as far medially as possible. This will facilitate creation of the retroesophageal window from the opposite side.

Step 2: Dissection of Right Crus, Creation of Retroesophageal Window, and Placement of Penrose Drain

The gastrohepatic ligament is opened in the bare area overlying the caudate lobe of the liver and continued to the right crus. Often times an accessory left hepatic artery is encountered within the gastrohepatic ligament. Preservation should be attempted; however, this can make the rest of the procedure cumbersome, and it can be ligated without significant consequence. Once the right crus is identified, the peritoneum is incised and the retroesophageal space is exposed. A Penrose drain is placed through the retroesophageal space and used to facilitate further dissection (Fig. 36.2).

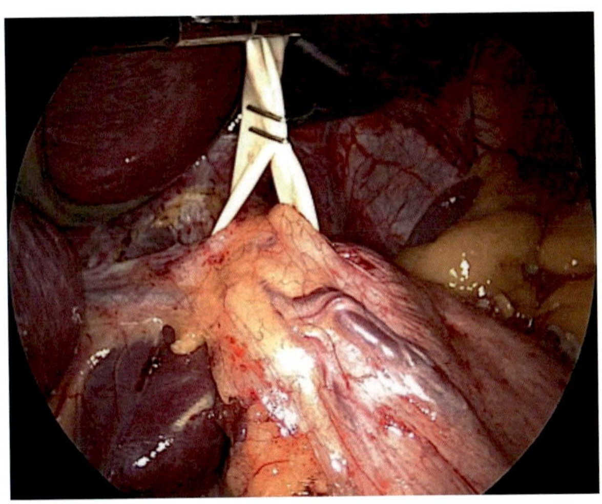

Fig. 36.2 The Penrose drain is placed around the esophagus to facilitate circumferential dissection

Step 3: Esophageal Dissection and Division of Fat Pad

With the Penrose in place, a 360°dissection of the esophagus can be completed. Care should be taken to avoid injury to the anterior vagus nerve which lies intimately within the longitudinal esophageal muscle fibers and the posterior vagus which is more separated. The mediastinal dissection should be continued until at least 3 cm of abdominal esophagus is obtained. The esophageal fat pad is then carefully dissected to expose the GE junction for preparation of the myotomy, taking care to preserve the anterior vagus nerve deep to the fat pad (Fig. 36.3).

Step 4: Creation of Myotomy

The path of the myotomy is scored using hook electrocautery. Often the anterior vagus nerve crosses directly over the trajectory of the myotomy making it necessary to dissect out the nerve to allow for retraction while performing the myotomy. It is important to perform a full myotomy encompassing 4–5 cm of distal esophagus and extending to 2–3 cm on the cardia of the stomach. A point 1–2 cm proximal to the GE junction is chosen, and the muscular layers are carefully dissected. First longitudinal and then circular fibers are divided exposing the mucosa. We have found hook cautery combined with bowel graspers to be ideal for this dissection. The bowel graspers provide traction and countertraction across the line of the myotomy giving tension to the tissues. This tension allows the hook to be used to elevate fibers easily so that the deep mucosa is not injured by cautery. Once the appropriate submucosal plane is exposed, the myotomy is continued proximally taking care to avoid injury to the underlying mucosa. We grasp the muscular fibers between short tip graspers and gently avulse the circular muscular fibers (Fig. 36.4). A gauze pad is introduced to blot the field and keep good visualization.

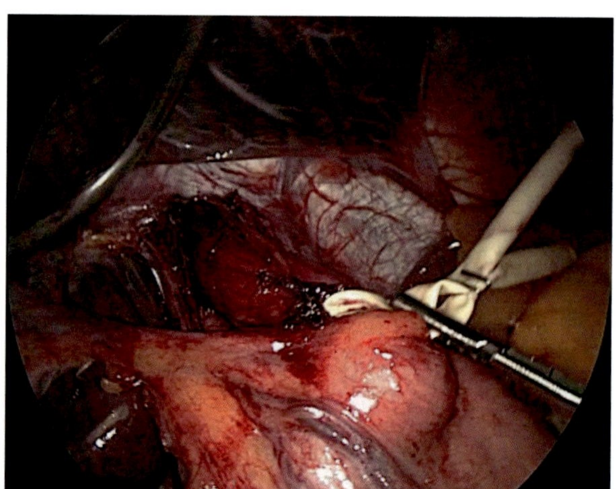

Fig. 36.3 The completed mediastinal dissection with preservation of the anterior vagus nerve and accessory left hepatic artery

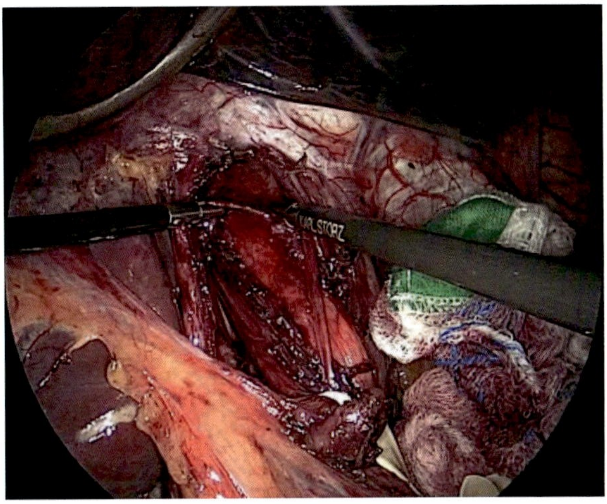

Fig. 36.4 The myotomy is performed by tearing the circular muscle fibers exposing the glistening white mucosa

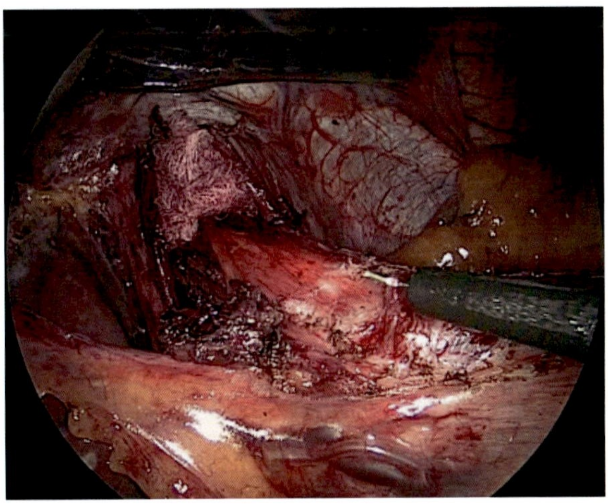

Fig. 36.5 The distal myotomy is completed using the hook electrocautery

Interestingly, we have observed less bleeding from submucosal vessels using the avulsion technique than we did when the fibers were elevated and divided with cautery. One possible explanation is that the tearing of the circular fibers causes the vessels to spasm; however, this can be a nuisance when bleeding does occur. The myotomy is continued proximally for at least 5 cm but may be continued further until the surgeon can appreciate that the thickness of the muscle is returning to a more normal caliber. Once the esophageal myotomy is complete proximally, the gastric myotomy is begun. The left hand grabs the lesser curve and provides posterior traction, while the assistant holds the greater curve and pulls it anterior. This places the stomach in a "wall" position and provides the most direct exposure for the gastric myotomy. The most distal point is dissected down to the mucosa, keeping in mind that there is an extra inner oblique layer of muscle fibers on the stomach. The hook is used to dissect and divide the muscle fibers to continue the myotomy proximally until it joins the esophageal myotomy (Fig. 36.5).

Step 5: Leak Test

The gastroscope is introduced and the myotomy is inspected for adequate length. The esophagus and stomach are insufflated to inspect for air leaks. Any leaks need to be fixed; small holes can be repaired with absorbable suture on small needles. Insufflation also facilitates exposure of any remaining circular fibers that will need to be divided. The lower esophageal sphincter should open easily with minimal insufflation, and there should be no areas of narrowing after completion of the myotomy.

Step 6: Posterior Crural Repair and Toupet Fundoplication

Once the myotomy is complete, the posterior diaphragmatic crura are closed primarily using 0 silk sutures.

We routinely perform a posterior 270° (Toupet) fundoplication to reconstruct an anti-reflux valve. The fundus is passed behind the esophagus and should lay without tension if properly mobilized (Fig. 36.6). The fundoplication is performed in standard fashion with 2-0 silk sutures. The suture should include full-thickness bites of the cut edges of the short gastric vessels on the fundus and the myotomy. Six sutures in total are used, three on either side at 1 cm intervals. Care should again be taken to avoid spearing the vagus nerve as it may course over the right side of the fundoplication.

Step 7: Completion Endoscopy

The gastroscope is again passed into the stomach, and the myotomy is inspected for leaks. A retroflex view of the wrap is performed to inspect the newly constructed valve. The omentum is draped over the myotomy to act as a barrier to the exposed mucosa.

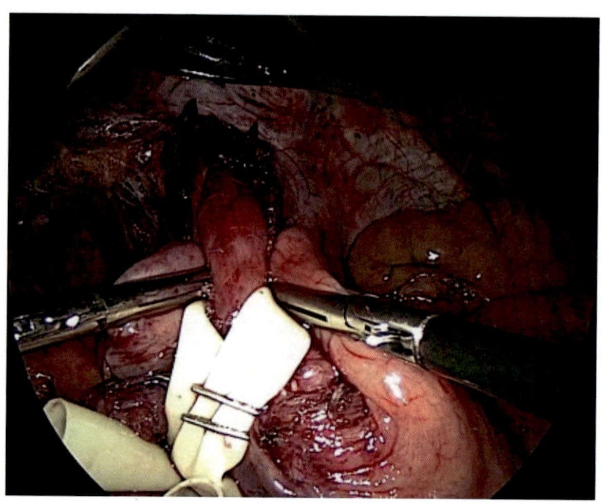

Fig. 36.6 The fundus is prepared for the posterior 270° wrap

Postop Care

Patients are kept NPO for one night after surgery. IV analgesia is necessary but PCAs are usually not. A routine UGI is performed in the morning of postoperative day 1, and clear liquids are started if there is adequate passage of contrast and no leak. Patients are advanced to full liquids and discharged home on postoperative day 2. They are advanced to a soft diet after 2 weeks.

Complications

Perforation Perforation is the most feared complication occurring in 8–15% of cases [3, 4]. It is vitally important to recognize and repair immediately. A small mucosal perforation can be repaired using a 5-0 absorbable suture. Perforations high in the mediastinum may necessitate left thoracotomy. Larger perforations are more complex problems and may require esophagectomy. After repair of a mucosal perforation, the repair can be buttressed by the fundus by switching to an anterior wrap (Dor fundoplication).

Persistent or Recurrent Dysphagia The most important factor to prevent dysphagia is careful patient selection. Preoperative manometry is mandatory, and other motility disorders or etiologies of dysphagia need to be ruled out. The most common technical failure is due to an incomplete myotomy on the gastric cardia. It is important that the myotomy continue for 2 cm on this side. Other possible etiologies include rescarring of the muscle or an overly tight fundoplication or crural closure. Patients with recurrent dysphagia undergo repeat manometry and UGI series to aid in further management. If manometry demonstrates incomplete LES relaxation, a redo myotomy should be considered. If UGI demonstrates a distinct kink or stricture from a technical failure, the patient requires revision. Most cases, however, do not require additional surgery and will respond well to pneumatic dilation. In a series of 113 undergoing LHM with partial fundoplication, 8.9% developed recurrent symptoms within the first year after surgery. These patients underwent pneumatic dilation with 78% demonstrating resolution or significant improvement. Two patients demonstrated no relief with dilation and required redo myotomies [5].

Reflux A well performed surgical myotomy along with the division of the phrenoesophageal ligament causes a permanent disruption of the LES and will lead to high reflux rates. Postoperative pH testing on these patients has demonstrated reflux rates >50%. The partial fundoplication reduces this number to <10% [6, 7]. These patients are usually well managed with proton pump inhibitors and almost never require revisions.

Outcomes

Dor Versus Toupet Fundoplication

A posterior (Toupet) wrap has the dual advantage of providing an anti-reflux valve and "stenting" open the myotomy. This theoretical advantage may prevent rescarring of the myotomy and recurrent dysphagia. Indeed, in a systematic review, patients who had a Heller myotomy with Toupet fundoplication demonstrated a decreased rate of dysphagia requiring reintervention compared with the Dor (10.1% vs. 5.9%), while reflux rates were identical [8]. For this reason we routinely perform a Toupet fundoplication. The Dor fundoplication remains a good option in cases of mucosal perforation or when a Toupet is anatomically challenging. Some surgeons prefer to perform a Dor fundoplication in all cases because it does not require posterior esophageal mobilization and therefore causes less disruption of hiatal anatomy, and this is something that is certainly acceptable.

It is important to note that Heller myotomy is not a cure for achalasia. The myotomy does not address the primary problem of underlying esophageal dysmotility. It is a palliative procedure that allows for improved swallowing. A small percentage of patients will develop progression of symptoms over time and may eventually require esophagectomy. Despite this, long-term follow-up studies have demonstrated excellent outcomes. >90% of patients are asymptomatic at full 2 years after surgery [9], and at 5 years, 91% have described their results as "good to excellent" [5].

Conclusion

Achalasia is a debilitating esophageal motility disorder characterized by aperistalsis and incomplete LES relaxation. It can lead to weight loss, regurgitation, and progressive dysphagia. While several treatment modalities exist, the laparoscopic Heller myotomy offers the best long-term success and remains the preferred treatment. Certainty of diagnosis, as well as adherence to key technical principles, assures excellent outcomes and satisfied patients.

References

1. Jeansonne LO, White BC, Pilger KE, et al. Ten-year follow-up of laparoscopic Heller myotomy for achalasia shows durability. Surg Endosc. 2007;21:1498–502.
2. Stafinidis D, Richardson W, Farrell TM, et al. SAGES guidelines for the treatment of esophageal achalasia. Surg Endosc. 2012;26:296–311.
3. Rawlings A, Soper NJ, Oelschlager B, et al. Laparoscopic Dor versus Toupet fundoplication following Heller myotomy for achalasia: results of a multicenter, prospective, randomized-controlled trial. Surg Endosc. 2012;26:18–26.
4. Huffman LC, Pandalai PK, Boulton BJ, et al. Robotic heller myotomy; a safe operation with higher postoperative quality-of-life indices. Surgery. 2007;142(4):613–8.
5. Ortiz A, Martinez de Haro LF, Parrilla P, et al. Very long-term objective evaluation of Heller myotomy plus posterior partial fundoplication in patients with achalasia of the cardia. Ann Surg. 2008;247:258–64.

6. Richards WO, Torquati A, Holzman MD, et al. Heller myotomy versus Heller myotomy with Dor fundoplication for achalasia: a prospective randomized double-blind clinical trial. Ann Surg. 2004;240:405–15.
7. Tsuboi K, Omura N, Yano F, et al. Data analyses and perspectives on laparoscopic surgery for esophageal achalasia. World J Gastroenterol. 2015;21(38):10830–9.
8. Kurian AK, Bhayani N, Sharata A, et al. Partial anterior vs. partial posterior fundoplication following transabdominal esophagocardiomyotomy for achalasia of the esophagus. JAMA Surg. 2013;148(1):85–90.
9. Gossage JA, Devitt PG, Watson DI, et al. Surveillance endoscopy at five or more years after cardiomyotomy for achalasia. Ann Surg. 2014;259(3):464–8.

Surgical Management of Achalasia: Thoracoscopic Myotomy

37

Robert E. Merritt

Introduction

Achalasia is an esophageal motility disorder that results in clinically significant dysphagia. The esophageal manometry findings are characterized by aperistalsis in the body of the esophagus and incomplete relaxation in the lower esophageal sphincter during swallowing. The etiology of achalasia is unknown, and the current therapeutic interventions target the underlying pathophysiology of the disease. Endoscopic therapies, such as pneumatic balloon dilation and botulinum toxin injection, typically only produce temporary improvement of dysphagia symptoms. The cornerstone of surgical therapy for achalasia is esophagomyotomy. The surgical myotomy for achalasia was first described by Heller in 1913 and included an anterior and posterior myotomy by an abdominal approach. Ellis described the first transthoracic esophagomyotomy through a left thoracotomy [1]. The video-assisted thoracoscopic approach for esophagomyotomy was described by Pellegrini in 1992 [2]. This chapter will describe the thoracoscopic approach for performing esophagomyotomy for the surgical management of achalasia.

Indications

Achalasia is an esophageal motility disorder that is characterized by failure of the lower esophageal sphincter (LES) to relax and the absence of esophageal peristalsis. The indications for thoracoscopic myotomy are the same as for laparoscopic myotomy. Currently, laparoscopic myotomy is the more commonly performed technique for surgical myotomy; however, the thoracoscopic myotomy would be an excellent

R. E. Merritt
The Division of Thoracic Surgery, Department of Surgery, The Ohio State University Wexner Medical Center, Columbus, OH, USA
e-mail: Robert.Merritt@osumc.edu

J. Grams et al. (eds.), *The SAGES Manual of Foregut Surgery*,
https://doi.org/10.1007/978-3-319-96122-4_37

alternative for patients who have undergone multiple abdominal operations and have extensive abdominal adhesions. Patients with achalasia often present with severe dysphagia, weight loss, regurgitation, aspiration, and chest pain. An esophageal manometry study is the gold standard for the diagnosis of achalasia and should be performed prior to any surgical myotomy. The manometry study typically demonstrates an elevated LES relaxation pressure and no evidence of peristalsis in the body of the esophagus.

In addition to manometry, a contrast esophagram and endoscopy should be performed in patients with suspected achalasia. The contrast esophagram will typically show a dilated esophagus and the classic bird's beak tapering of the distal esophagus at the esophagogastric junction in patients with achalasia. An upper endoscopy should be performed to rule out an esophageal cancer in the distal esophagus, which could mimic the symptoms of achalasia.

Technique

The objective for thoracoscopic myotomy is the effective lowering of the lower esophageal sphincter (LES) relaxing pressure, which results in the correction of the esophageal obstruction which occurs in achalasia. The complete division of the outer longitudinal fibers and the inner circular muscle fibers in the distal third of the esophagus is the cornerstone of the operation. The myotomy should be carried down onto the cardia of the stomach for a total length of 3 cm to ensure complete division of the muscle fibers at the esophagogastric junction.

Thoracoscopic myotomy requires single lung ventilation; therefore, a double lumen endotracheal tube is required. The author prefers a right thoracoscopic approach which provides complete access to the intrathoracic esophagus. The left thoracoscopic approach only provides access to the distal third of the esophagus because the aortic arch limits access to mid-esophagus at the level of the carina and azygous vein. For the right thoracoscopic myotomy, the patient is placed in the left lateral decubitus position. A total of four thoracoscopic ports are placed for the procedure (Fig. 37.1). The 12 mm thoracoscopic ports are placed in the 8th intercostal space posterior axillary line, the 7th intercostal space 3 finger breadths below the tip of the scapula, the 5th intercostal space anterior axillary line, and the 9th intercostal space posteriorly. Carbon dioxide insufflation is utilized to assist with exposure by depressing the right hemidiaphragm. The right lung is completely deflated and retracted anteriorly to expose the posterior mediastinum.

The inferior pulmonary ligament is incised with the L-hook Bovie electrocautery until the left inferior pulmonary vein is exposed. The mediastinal pleura overlying the esophagus at the level of the inferior pulmonary vein is incised with the Bovie electrocautery. The esophagus is then encircled with a Penrose drain. The distal esophagus is then circumferentially mobilized taking care not to injure the anterior and posterior vagus nerves. Once the distal esophagus is mobilized, the longitudinal muscle layer is scored longitudinally with the L-hook Bovie electrocautery. The

Fig. 37.1 The port placement for the thoracoscopic myotomy

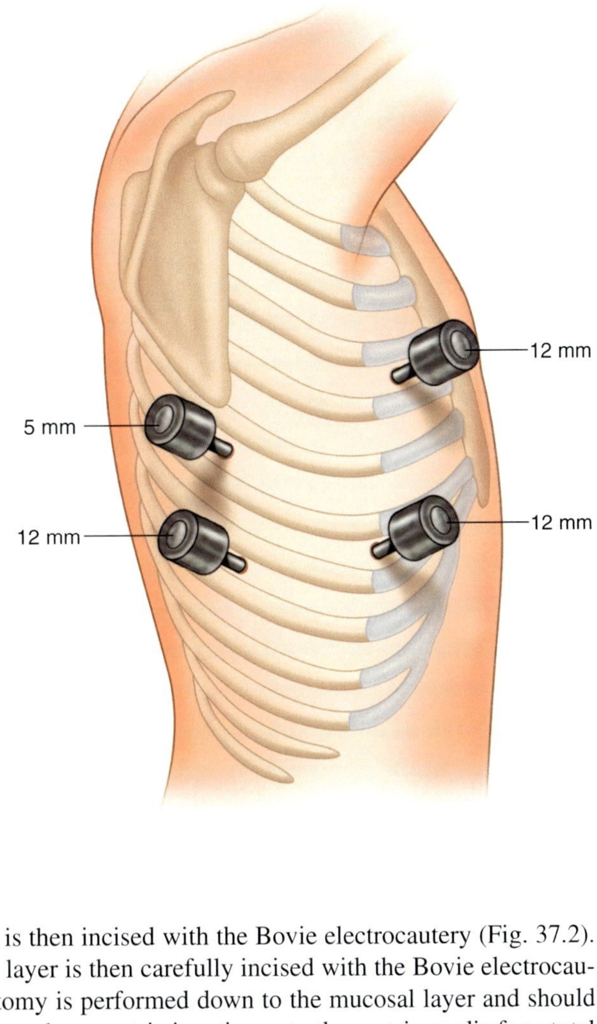

longitudinal muscle layer is then incised with the Bovie electrocautery (Fig. 37.2). The inner circular muscle layer is then carefully incised with the Bovie electrocautery. The completed myotomy is performed down to the mucosal layer and should extend distally across the esophagogastric junction onto the gastric cardia for a total length of 3 cm (Fig. 37.3). The proximal extent of the myotomy should extend approximately 7 cm in length. Laparoscopic graspers are used to tease apart the divided edges of the muscle to ensure that there is complete separation. In order to ensure that the mucosal layer was not injured during myotomy, the distal esophagus is submerged in saline solution, and air insufflation with a flexible gastroscope is performed. If a mucosal injury is detected intraoperatively, a primary suture repair should be performed. It would be advisable to consider converting to an open thoracotomy to complete the repair of the esophagus and cover the repair site with a pleural flap.

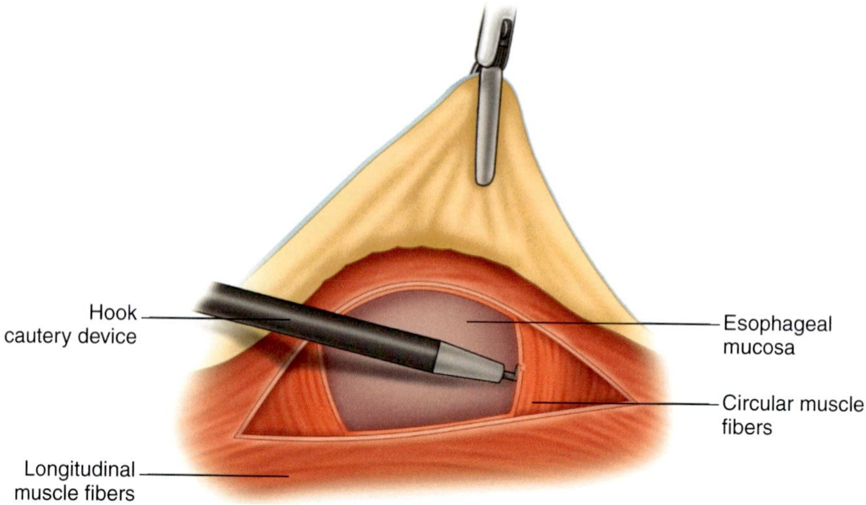

Fig. 37.2 Thoracoscopic esophagomyotomy: the division of the outer longitudinal and inner circular muscle layers of the esophagus with a hook cautery device

Fig. 37.3 The completed thoracoscopic myotomy

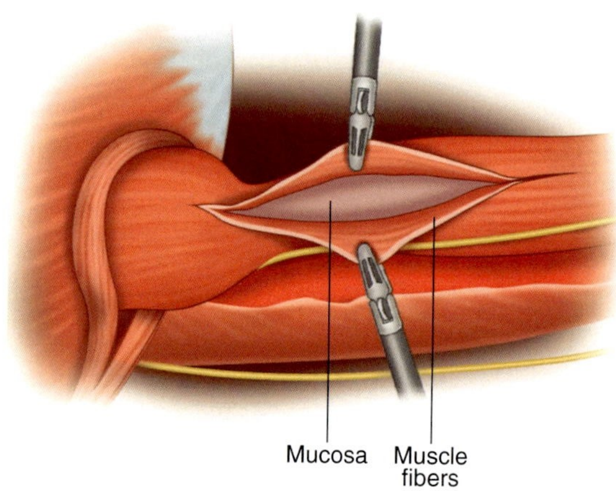

A routine partial fundoplication is not a part of the thoracoscopic myotomy; therefore, there should be minimal disruption of the hiatal esophageal attachments and the phreno-esophageal membrane. After the conclusion of the thoracoscopic myotomy, a small chest tube is inserted, and the right lung is re-expanded prior to closure. The patients are routinely extubated in the operating room at the conclusion of the operation.

Postoperative Management

After a routine thoracoscopic myotomy, patients are admitted to a regular postsurgical floor. A nasogastric tube is not routinely placed after myotomy, and patients are typically started on clear liquids as tolerated immediately after the procedure. The chest tube is removed on postoperative day number one. The author prefers to obtain a contrast esophagram on postoperative day number one to assess for emptying of the esophagus at the esophagogastric junction and an occult esophageal injury at the myotomy site. Following the contrast esophagram, patients are advanced to a full liquid diet on postoperative day number one and discharged home. Patients advance themselves to a soft mechanical diet as tolerated at home. Routine postoperative esophageal manometry is not obtained unless patients develop recurrent dysphagia and other symptoms of achalasia.

Postoperative Complications

The operative mortality rate for thoracoscopic myotomy is 0% in published reports [3]. The postoperative leak rate ranges from 0% to 5.8%. In the rare cases of postoperative leak at the myotomy site, patients can be managed with a primary repair. Postoperative atelectasis and other pulmonary complications associated with thoracotomy were not seen with the thoracoscopic approach. Other potential postoperative complications include thoracic duct injury and chyle leak, pneumonia, atelectasis, and pulmonary embolus.

Postoperative Outcomes

The results of thoracoscopic myotomy have been very good in reported series. Agrawal et al. demonstrated a significant decrease in lower esophageal sphincter pressure and in the clinical symptom score after thoracoscopic myotomy [4]. Cade compared a cohort of patients who underwent thoracoscopic or laparoscopic myotomy for achalasia [5]. In this report, there was no difference in operative time, conversion rate, or hospital length of stay. At two years, the dysphagia scores and the incidence of symptomatic reflux were the same between laparoscopic and thoracoscopic myotomy. Patti et al. reported a study comparing 30 patients undergoing thoracoscopic myotomy to 30 patients undergoing laparoscopic myotomy [6]. The patients in the laparoscopic group underwent a Dor fundoplication and reported less symptomatic reflux symptoms. However, the clinical dysphagia scores were very similar between thoracoscopic myotomy group and the laparoscopic myotomy group.

Conclusion

Achalasia is an esophageal motility disorder characterized by incomplete relaxation of the lower esophageal sphincter and impaired peristalsis of the esophagus. Thoracoscopic myotomy is an option for surgical management of achalasia. The long-term relief from dysphagia achieved with thoracoscopic myotomy is similar to the rate seen with laparoscopic myotomy.

References

1. Ellis FH Jr, Kiser JC, Schlegel JF, et al. Esophagomyotomy for esophageal achalasia: experimental, clinical, and manometric aspects. Ann Surg. 1967;166:640–56.
2. Pellegrini C, Wetter LA, Patti M, Leichter R, et al. Thoracoscopic esophagomyotomy. Initial experience with a new approach for the treatment of achalasia. Ann Surg. 1992;216:291–6.
3. Kesler KA, Tarvin SE, Brooks JA, et al. Thoracoscopy-assisted Heller myotomy for the treatment of achalasia: results of a minimally invasive technique. Ann Thorac Surg. 2004;77:385–92.
4. Agrawal D, Meekison L, Walker WS. Long-term clinical results of thoracoscopic Heller's myotomy in the treatment of achalasia. Eur J Cardiothoracic Surg. 2008;34:423–6.
5. Cade R. Heller's myotomy: thoracoscopic or laparoscopic. Dis Esophagus. 2000;13:279–81.
6. Patti MG, Arcerito M, De Pinto M, et al. Comparison of thoracoscopic and laparoscopic Heller myotomy for achalasia. J Gastrointest Surg. 1998;2:561–6.

Surgical Management of Achalasia: Peroral Endoscopic Myotomy

38

Joel Sternbach and Eric Hungness

Abbreviations

DES	Diffuse esophageal spasm
DI	Distensibility index
EGD	Esophagogastroduodenoscopy
EGJ	Esophagogastric junction
EMR	Endoscopic mucosal resection
EPT	Esophageal pressure topography
ES	Eckardt score
ESD	Endoscopic submucosal dissection
FLIP	Functional lumen imaging probe
GERD	Gastroesophageal reflux disease
HRIM	High-resolution impedance manometry
HRM	High-resolution manometry
IDQ	Impaction-dysphagia questionnaire, GERDQ
LES	Lower esophageal sphincter
NOTES	Natural orifice transluminal endoscopic surgery
POEM	Peroral endoscopic myotomy
TBE	Timed barium esophagram
VSI	Visceral sensitivity index

A novel procedure, combining the decreased invasiveness of endoscopic access with the reliability of a surgical myotomy, peroral endoscopic myotomy (POEM), represents a potential paradigm shift in the management of idiopathic achalasia and

J. Sternbach · E. Hungness (✉)
Department of Surgery, Northwestern Memorial Hospital, Chicago, IL, USA
e-mail: Eric.Hungness@nm.org

J. Grams et al. (eds.), *The SAGES Manual of Foregut Surgery*,
https://doi.org/10.1007/978-3-319-96122-4_38

other esophageal motor disorders. Comprehensive preoperative evaluation by a multidisciplinary team of gastroenterologists and surgeons is essential to confirming candidacy for POEM and appropriately counseling patients on expected outcomes and postoperative outcomes, including the lack of long-term outcome data. The key steps of the procedure are detailed, including initial EGD, safe access to the submucosal space, creation of a submucosal tunnel extending at least 3 cm onto the gastric cardia, selective myotomy of the inner circular muscle fibers, and closure of the mucosotomy. Frequently encountered complications include bleeding, inadvertent mucosotomy, full-thickness perforation, and development of capnothorax and/or capnoperitoneum.

Indications

Achalasia

Achalasia is a rare disease characterized by failure of relaxation of the lower esophageal sphincter (LES) in response to a swallow and loss of coordinated peristalsis in the distal esophageal body. The annual incidence is estimated at only 1 per 100,000 individuals, yet achalasia is the most common primary esophageal motor disorder [1]. Initially described in 1674 by Sir Thomas Willis, our current understanding of the etiology of achalasia has developed, thanks to histopathologic analysis over the last two decades. Immunohistochemical studies have suggested an autoimmune etiology, with selective loss or impairment of ganglions in the myenteric plexus resulting in unopposed cholinergic stimulation of the distal esophagus and LES [2]. Presenting symptoms include dysphagia to solids and liquids (>90%), regurgitation of undigested food and saliva (76–91%), weight loss (35–91%), and chest pain (25–64%). Patients may also report respiratory complications of aspiration such as nocturnal cough and pneumonia as well as heartburn and esophagitis secondary to stasis [3]. There is no known cure for achalasia; current treatment options are aimed at palliation of symptoms through elimination of outflow obstruction at the EGJ.

Emerging Indications

Building on the good results in treating type I and type II achalasia, POEM operators have applied the minimally invasive technique to other esophageal motor disorders including type III achalasia, diffuse esophageal spasm (DES), nutcracker esophagus, and hypertensive LES [4, 5]. In general, EGJ outflow obstruction caused by high LES pressure responds favorably to division of the obstructing muscle fibers, whereas symptoms such as chest pain, attributed to esophageal body contraction (DES and type III achalasia), have lower rates of symptom remission following myotomy [6]. POEM has also been utilized as a salvage operation following failed laparoscopic Heller myotomy (LHM), with dissection and myotomy occurring in the 4–6 o'clock position.

History/Background

In the 100 years since Dr. Heller first described the "transabdominal, extramucosal cardioplasty performed onto the anterior and posterior walls of the cardia," the procedure has been transformed by laparoscopy, modified in length, and augmented by anti-reflux procedures [7]. In the last 10 years, however, the complementary fields of natural orifice transluminal endoscopic surgery (NOTES) and endoscopic submucosal dissection (ESD) have expanded from simple proof-of-concept studies to a broad variety of fully incision-less operations in use today. Early animal models demonstrated the feasibility of both safe access to the submucosal space using the mucosal flap technique and endoscopic myotomy [8, 9]. Based on these techniques, Dr. Haru Inoue performed the first human POEM procedure in Japan in 2008 and presented his results at the 2009 Digestive Diseases Week in Chicago with subsequent publication in *Endoscopy* in 2010 [10]. Following his landmark publication in *Endoscopy* in 2010, the procedure as described by Inoue grew exponentially with an estimated number of POEM cases exceeding 2000 worldwide by the end of 2012, when the global experience in POEM was summarized in the international POEM survey (IPOEMS), conducted leading up to and during the NOSCAR conference in July 2012 [6].

Patient Selection

Symptom Assessment Questionnaires

Validated, disease-specific questionnaires can help establish the diagnosis of achalasia, assess disease severity, and establish baseline values to compare against to evaluate treatment success. The most widely used and reported instrument for achalasia is the four-item Eckardt score that evaluates the frequency of occurrence of chest pain, regurgitation, dysphagia, and amount of weight loss on a 0–3 scale [11]. Higher scores represent increasingly severe disease, while post-intervention scores less than or equal to three are associated with treatment success [12]. While simple to obtain, the ES does not measure disease impact on overall quality of life. More extensive and sensitive surveys include the Mayo Dysphagia Questionnaire-30, Achalasia Disease-Specific Quality of Life measure, Visceral Sensitivity Index, and EORTC QLQ-OES18 [13].

Physiologic Tests

Timed Barium Esophagram (TBE)

Timed barium esophagram (TBE) (Fig. 38.1), with chest radiographs obtained 1, 2, and 5 min after ingestion of 200–250 mL of dilute barium contrast, is useful for both evaluation of esophageal body and EGJ anatomy (classic appearance of the "bird-beak" esophagus) and quantification of baseline height of the barium column,

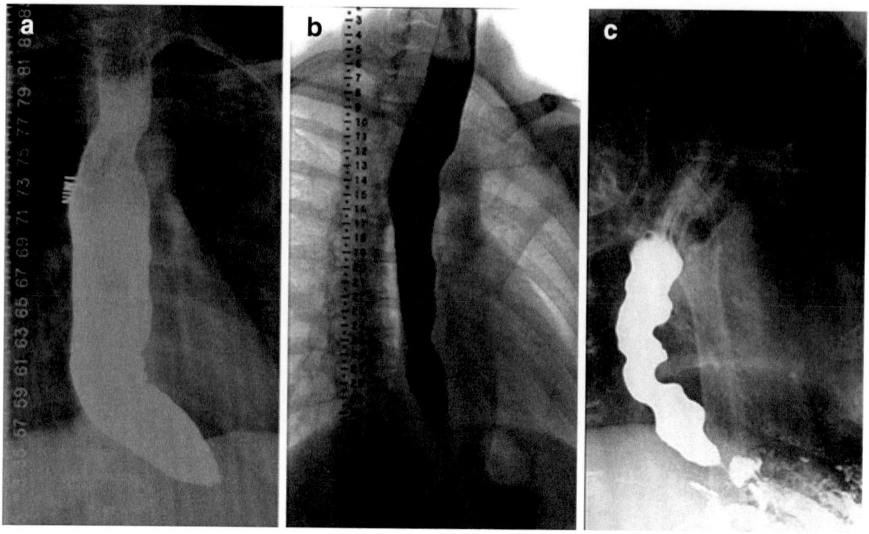

Fig. 38.1 Timed barium esophagram images for (**a**) type 1, (**b**) type 2, and (**c**) type 3 achalasia

degree of esophageal emptying, if any, and esophageal width. TBE also allows detection of sigmoid esophagus (representing the so-called end-stage achalasia), hiatus hernia, and epiphrenic diverticula.

Esophagogastroduodenoscopy (EGD)

EGD is required as part of the preoperative work-up of all patients prior to treatment for achalasia to rule out pseudo-achalasia (symptoms of EGJOO secondary to an infiltrating malignancy). If the index of suspicion remains high for pseudo-achalasia (older patients with prominent weight loss and a short duration of symptoms), despite a negative EGD, adjunctive studies such as endoscopic ultrasound or computed tomography scan should be performed [14]. EGD also allows for assessment of retained solids or liquids, stasis or reflux esophagitis, and active candidiasis.

High-Resolution Manometry (HRM)

Manometry is considered the "gold standard" for the diagnosis of idiopathic achalasia with significant improvement in resolution and evaluation of esophageal motility over the last 10 years with the introduction of solid-state, high-resolution manometry catheters utilizing 36 or more pressure sensors at 1 cm intervals. The increased resolution offered by HRM catheters has been accompanied by the development of esophageal pressure topography (EPT) to display pressure data in an accessible format. Based on manometric profiles, Pandolfino et al. proposed the

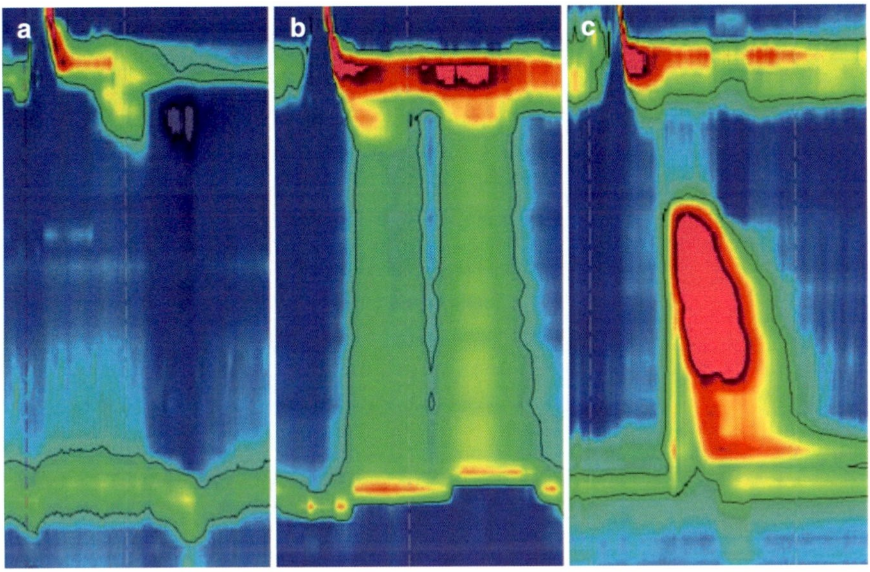

Fig. 38.2 Representative high-resolution manometry images for (**a**) type 1, (**b**) type 2 and (**c**) type 3 patterns of achalasia according to the Chicago classification

Chicago classification (Fig. 38.2), dividing patients into three subtypes of achalasia, with well-described prognostic implications [15]. Type I, or "classic" achalasia, is defined by absent peristalsis and impaired EGJ relaxation in response to swallowing, quantified as a 4-s integrated relaxation pressure (IRP) >10 mmHg. Type II achalasia is diagnosed by the presence of panesophageal pressurization (>30 mmHg) and is associated with the best outcomes following myotomy. Type III achalasia, associated with premature, spastic contractions of the distal esophagus (two or more swallows with a distal latency of <4.5 s) and impaired EGJ relaxation, has the worst prognosis [15].

EndoFLIP

The functional lumen imaging probe (Crospon, Galway, Ireland) is a novel diagnostic catheter that utilizes impedance planimetry sensors positioned at 0.5–1 cm intervals within a distensible balloon to generate a geometric representation of the lumen of the esophagus and LES (Fig. 38.3). When combined with a pressure sensor in the distal portion of the balloon, the FLIP allows quantification of the EGJ response to volumetric distention, calculated as the distensibility index (DI) = cross-sectional area/intra-balloon pressure. Recent publications have suggested a role for intraoperative EndoFLIP measurements to allow real-time evaluation of myotomy adequacy during LHM and POEM [16].

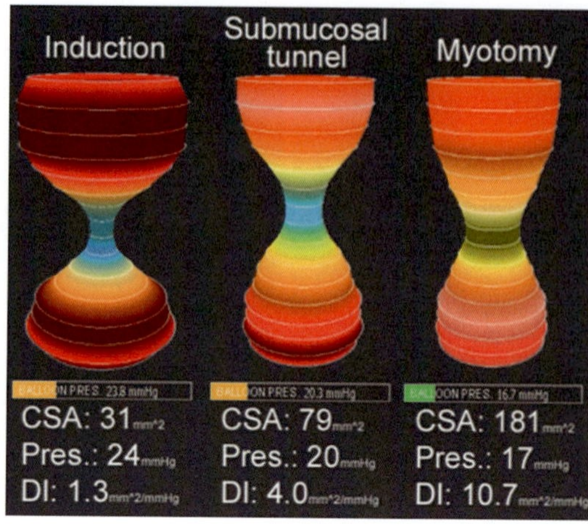

Fig. 38.3 Representative EndoFLIP images at induction, after completion of submucosal tunnel, and after completion of myotomy

Contraindications

Patient Factors

Patients should undergo evaluation in a preoperative clinic in coordination with anesthesiology and additional work-up as indicated. The less invasive nature of the POEM procedure minimizes the list of comorbidities that preclude the procedure. Absolute contraindications to POEM include the inability to tolerate general anesthesia, secondary to prohibitive cardiopulmonary disease, uncorrectable coagulopathy/thrombocytopenia, and the presence of advanced cirrhosis, with or without evidence of esophageal varices. Additionally, the POEM procedure relies on the ability to access the submucosal space, so extensive fibrosis secondary to external-beam radiation to the mediastinum, extensive mucosal ablations, and prior EMR generally prohibit the operation. Published reports have included patients ranging in age from 3 to 97 years old [6]. Prior treatments that can cause inflammation and/or fibrosis of the submucosal space such as botulinum toxin injection, pneumatic dilation, prior LHM, or prior POEM can all contribute to the difficulty of the dissection and in some cases increase the rate of inadvertent mucosotomies or duration of the procedure. While none of the prior treatment modalities, other than esophagectomy, represent absolute contraindications to POEM, the added complexity should preclude such cases from being attempted during an operator's initial learning curve (first 20–30 cases) [17].

Technical/Training

Safe conduct of the POEM procedure relies on the availability of all necessary equipment, adequately trained and well-coordinated support staff, and sufficient preclinical training. Prior experience with EMR/ESD techniques and/or NOTES procedures has been reported as helpful, as have simulations using live animal, ex vivo models, and cadavers. Most operators reported having expert proctoring during the initial human cases (median, 2; range, 1–7) [6].

Preoperative Care

Prior to surgery, a multidisciplinary team including gastroenterologists and minimally invasive surgeons should evaluate the patient.

Patient Instructions

Preoperatively, the patient is prescribed oral fluconazole for an empiric 7-day course and instructed to maintain a clear liquid diet starting 48 h and to remain NPO for 12 h, prior to surgery. Some centers report conducting routine EGD 1–3 days preoperatively to screen for candidiasis. Management of perioperative medications should be performed in consultation with the preoperative clinic, the cardiologist, and the patient's primary care provider; in general, we continue beta-blockers perioperatively, as well as aspirin when indicated for a history of stent placement, coronary artery disease, or coronary artery bypass graft. Prophylactic aspirin and clopidogrel are typically held for 7 and 5 days preoperatively, respectively, and decisions regarding management of therapeutic anticoagulation are made on an individual basis.

Anesthetic Considerations

Preoperative and intraoperative coordination with the anesthetic team are crucial to safe conduct of the POEM procedure. Issues of particular importance include positioning and securing the endotracheal tube as far laterally to the right as possible and can consider utilizing a preformed, right-angled Oral RAE™ tracheal tube (Moore Medical). Anesthesia should be aware of the potential for unplanned extubation given the frequent passage of the endoscope through the oropharynx. It is also helpful to discuss blood pressure management and specifically maintaining the systolic blood pressure below 100–110 mmHg, if safe, as this is anecdotally associated with fewer bleeding complications.

Room Setup and Equipment

For a list of equipment recommended for POEM, see Table 38.1. Sequential compression devices are utilized for thromboprophylaxis, and a second-generation cephalosporin or comparable preoperative antibiotic (Ancef/Flagyl at our institution) is given. After successful induction of general anesthesia and

Table 38.1 Equipment checklist

Equipment checklist
Forward-viewing, high-definition gastroscope with single-channel 2.8 mm working port
Clear cap with ¼″ tape to secure at the end of the gastroscope
Carbon dioxide (CO_2) insufflation system
Endoscopic cautery system
Bite block
60–90 mL syringes with saline for irrigation of esophagus +/− simethicone
Indigo carmine injection solution with epinephrine
Indigo carmine injection solution without epinephrine
Endoscopic injection needle
Triangular-tip endoscopic submucosal dissection knife
Toothbrush for cleaning knife
Additional pieces of ¼″ red tape to mark insertion depth for endoscopic instruments
QuickClip2 (Olympus) hemostatic clips for closure of mucosal defects
Instinct Hemoclips (cook) for closure of wider mucosal defects
OverStitch (Apollo endosurgery) endoscopic suturing system
Over-the-scope clip (OTSC) (Ovesco, Tübingen, Germany)
Coagrasper hemostatic forceps (Olympus)
Dilute bacitracin irrigation

secured positioning of an endotracheal tube, the patient is positioned supine, flush with the head of the OR table, the right arm is supported on an arm board, and the left arm is appropriately padded and tucked next to the torso. The bed should be lowered and step stools positioned at the head of the bed as needed to minimize strain and fatigue on the part of the operator. An endoscopy tower, equipped with a forward-viewing, 2.8 mm single-channel, high-definition flexible gastroscope (GIF-H180; Olympus America, Inc., Center Valley, PA), with carbon dioxide (CO_2) insufflation, is positioned near the midpoint of the OR table, and the cautery foot pedal is placed within reach of the operator. A minimum of one assistant is required to coordinate the operation of the injector and triangular-tip ESD knife and should be positioned to the left of the operator. A second assistant, to the right of the operator, can stabilize the endoscope at the mouth allowing simultaneous manipulation of the deflection wheels and the injector or cautery knife. The second assistant can also assist with passage of intraoperative measurement devices such as the EndoFLIP catheter. A time-out should be performed prior to the procedure to confirm patient identity, procedure, and availability of endoscopic equipment (clips, coagulation forceps, etc.) and ensure that the endoscopy tower is utilizing CO_2 insufflation and that correct electrocautery levels are set.

Operative Technique (Fig. 38.4)

Diagnostic Endoscopy

Once the anesthesiologist is satisfied with the positioning and security of the endotracheal tube, the abdomen is prepped and draped to provide access in the event that Veress needle decompression of a capnoperitoneum is required. A bite block is placed to facilitate passage of the endoscope (Fig. 38.4a). Thorough clearance of impacted food is required for complete assessment of the esophageal mucosa (Fig. 38.4b) and to minimize soilage of the submucosal tunnel. Placement of a 16 or 18 French orogastric tube can facilitate clearance, as can availability of 60–90 mL flushes or a power-flush system for the working port. Initial EGD is performed to assess for the presence of active candidiasis (Fig. 38.4d), an indication to abort the procedure and reschedule the myotomy pending resolution of the infection. It is not uncommon to encounter copious frothy sputum in the esophagus (Fig. 38.4c), a condition that resolves quickly with irrigation using dilute simethicone. Following

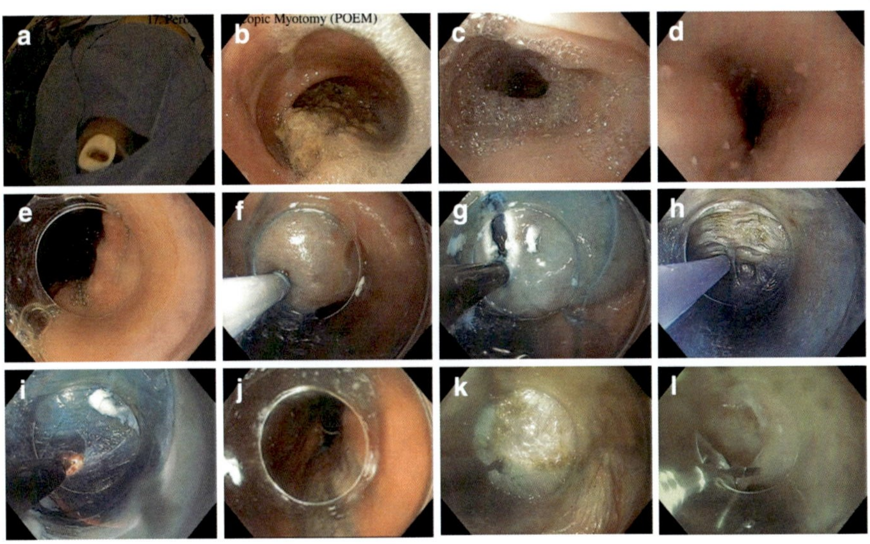

Fig. 38.4 (a–l) Illustrated steps for POEM. (**a**) Bite block is placed to facilitate passage of the endoscope. (**b**) Clearance of impacted food. (**c**) EGD to assess for active candidiasis. (**d**) Copious frothy sputum in the esophagus. (**e**) Squamocolumnar junction. (**f**) Submucosal wheal/bleb creation. (**g**) Creation of longitudinal myotomy. (**h**) Injection to hydrodissect the submucosal tunnel. (**i**) Cautery to divide the tissue of the submucosa. (**j**) Endoluminal verification of extent of tunnel onto gastric cardia. (**k**) Selective myotomy of the inner, circular muscle layer. (**l**) Mucosotomy closure with endoscopic clips

a visual inspection of the esophagus and stomach, note should be made of the location of the esophagogastric junction as determined by the distance from the incisors to the squamocolumnar junction (Fig. 38.4e) using the external markings on the endoscope for reference. In the absence of a hiatal hernia, the SCJ is typically located between 38 and 42 cm from the incisors.

Mucosal Lift and Mucosotomy

In the case of a standard-length myotomy (extending 6–7 cm proximal to the EGJ), the mucosotomy should be made 12–14 cm above the EGJ. The majority of operators participating in the IPOEMS reported creating an anterior submucosal tunnel in the 1–2 o'clock position [6]. A sclerotherapy needle is inserted just below the mucosa, and a 3–4 cm wheal is raised using 10 mL of solution containing indigo carmine (0.2 mg/mL), epinephrine (5 mcg/mL), and 0.9% saline (Fig. 38.4f). A longitudinal mucosotomy is created (using a few drops of liquid to create a meniscus to assess positioning relative to the most anterior aspect, designated 12 o'clock). Mucosotomy length should be just large enough to accommodate the clear cap on the endoscope (Fig. 38.4g), as excessive length will add time and cost to the procedure during clip closure of the mucosotomy.

Creation of Submucosal Tunnel

After the initial mucosal lift, subsequent injections during the creation of the submucosal tunnel should be diluted dye without epinephrine to limit total exposure to the adrenergic agent. Distal progression of the submucosal tunnel is facilitated by alternating hydrodissection to enlarge the submucosal space (Fig. 38.4h) and cautery to divide the thin fibers connecting the mucosa to the inner, circular muscle layer (Fig. 38.4i). Careful advancement of the endoscope and slight posterior deflection of the cap can be used to put the submucosal fibers on stretch and guide dissection. Frequent reference to fluid meniscus can help prevent spiraling as the tunnel is carried distally on the esophagus. Extra care should be taken near the EGJ as this area is prone to inadvertent mucosotomy given the increased muscular tone and anecdotally described "stickiness," attributed to prior episodes of inflammation or previous treatment modalities. Beyond the EGJ, switching back to an injection solution containing both dye and dilute epinephrine can aid in demarcating the distal extent of the submucosal tunnel. To confirm adequate extension onto the gastric cardia, the endoscope can be withdrawn from the submucosal tunnel and passed into the stomach lumen to obtain a retroflex view of the EGJ (Fig. 38.4j).

Anterior Myotomy of the Circular Muscle Layer

Using the endoscopic markings, the selective myotomy of the circular muscle layer should be initiated 6 cm proximal to EGJ for a standard length myotomy. Variations in myotomy length have been suggested when treating conditions that predominantly affect the esophageal body, such as type III achalasia or jackhammer; in these cases the myotomy can be started just proximal to the spastic segment, ensuring at least 2–3 cm of mucosal flap coverage in the submucosal tunnel [18]. Once the plane between the inner circular muscle layer and thin, outer, longitudinal muscle layer is accessed, the triangular-tip ESD knife can be used to hook the circular muscle fibers and extend the myotomy distally (Fig. 38.4k). Full-thickness myotomy or splaying of the thin, outer longitudinal muscle fibers is common, especially around the EGJ. The myotomy should be extended 2–3 cm distal to the EGJ onto the gastric cardia. At the conclusion of the myotomy, after assuring hemostasis in the tunnel, irrigation is performed with dilute bacitracin solution.

A variety of intraoperative techniques have been described to evaluate for adequacy of myotomy in relieving esophageal outflow obstruction at the level of the EGJ. These range from purely subjective, based on laparoscopic inspection or ease of passage of the endoscope during EGD post-myotomy, to quantitative but time-consuming, in the case of intraoperative manometry. At least three centers in the USA currently employ the EndoFLIP device described earlier, in the diagnostic testing section, for intraoperative assessment of myotomy adequacy as measured by an increase in EGJ distensibility index [16].

Closure of Mucosotomy

Mucosotomy width will help guide initial clip selection, with the Instinct™ Endoscopic Hemoclip (Cook Medical) being helpful in cases of wider mucosal defects and the QuickClip2 (Olympus) offering a smaller overall size following deployment (Fig. 38.4l). An alternative method of closure has been described that utilizes proprietary endoscopic suturing devices to allow a running closure of longer mucosotomy defects.

Avoiding Complications

Aspiration

Preoperative dietary restriction to clear liquids in preparation for the procedure as well as utilization of a "rapid-sequence" intubation technique by anesthesia (limited preoxygenation/bag-masking) can help minimize the risk of aspiration during induction. If needed, awake fiber-optic intubation in the upright position can be utilized in high-risk patients.

Capnothorax

Given the frequency of full-thickness myotomy or splaying of the outer, longitudinal muscle fibers, development of unilateral or bilateral capnothorax is common [6].

There is no data supporting routine postoperative chest X-rays, assuming CO_2 is utilized for insufflation in place of air. Capnothorax progressing to tension physiology or hemodynamic compromise is exceedingly rare, but the instruments should be available as well as staff capable of performing an emergent needle or tube thoracostomy, if needed. Self-limited subcutaneous emphysema is also common with expected resolution within 24 h postoperatively.

Capnoperitoneum

Roughly 50% of POEM cases are accompanied by the development of some degree of capnoperitoneum secondary to CO_2 tracking from the mediastinum or full-thickness gastric myotomy [6]. Capnoperitoneum can be differentiated from an insufflated stomach by the presence of isolated epigastric fullness in the latter; the diffuse abdominal distension of the former, when accompanied by hemodynamic instability or impaired ventilation, is an indication for decompression with a Veress needle (typically in the left upper quadrant, just inferior to the costal margin) or laparoscopic port. Desufflating the stomach with the endoscope prior to Veress needle passage ensures that capnoperitoneum is present.

Bleeding

Based on the global POEM experience to date, bleeding is most commonly encountered during dissection across and distal to the EGJ. As previously discussed, even mild hypertension will compound the bleeding risk inherent to the increased vascularity in the submucosal space of the EGJ and gastric cardia. Mild bleeding can typically be controlled with application of monopolar electrocautery. Brisker bleeding, or unavoidable division of larger bridging vessels, should be approached with coagulation forceps. Submucosal tunnel bleeding that obscures endoscopic visualization can occasionally be temporized by removal of the endoscope from the tunnel and application of direct pressure with the scope or cap from the esophageal lumen for 10–20 min. Alternative techniques include hemostatic clip application and judicious injection of dilute epinephrine. Case reports have suggested the option of utilizing tamponade devices such as Sengstaken-Blakemore, Minnesota, or Linton tubes (all Bard Medical) to staunch brisk bleeding. Given the disastrous consequences of this in the setting of a partial or full-thickness myotomy, these high-pressure balloons are contraindicated as part of the endoscopic armamentarium when approaching bleeding during the POEM procedure.

Full-Thickness Perforation

Entry into the mediastinum at the level of the mucosotomy, either during initial access of the submucosal space or subsequently, should prompt close attention to mucosal closure technique, including consideration of alternative methods of closure such as endoscopic suturing or utilization of an over-the-scope clip device [19]. Blunt dissection of the submucosal space has been described in both animal models and human case series as a means to expedite tunnel creation and decrease procedure duration. This technique is associated with increased rates of inadvertent mucosotomy, particularly in the area just proximal to the EGJ, where relative tethering of the mucosa can occur and predispose the proximal tissue to perforation when approached blindly. Significant mucosal defects that occur prior to myotomy creation should prompt consideration of aborting the procedure and/or attempting submucosal tunnel and myotomy in an alternate position on the esophagus (i.e., posterolateral). Small mucosal defects and those that occur during or after myotomy should be closed from the luminal side with endoscopic clips or suture. Note that mucosal injuries, especially in the region of the EGJ, can lead to the development of strictures and recurrent dysphagia.

Postoperative Care

At the conclusion of the case, patients are extubated in the operating room and transferred to the postanesthesia care unit (PACU). During the initial recovery phase in the PACU, patients are given standing intravenous antiemetics and analgesia as needed and kept nil per os (NPO) pending further evaluation. If the patient is sufficiently recovered from the effects of anesthesia and not experiencing chest pain, fever, or tachycardia, sips of clear liquids are initiated the evening of surgery. In the absence of concerning symptoms or signs that suggest ongoing leak, patients are given a tray of clear liquids in the morning and advanced to a full liquid diet for lunch. Discharge typically occurs in the afternoon of the first postoperative day (POD#1) after response to lunch is evaluated. Among the IPOEMS centers, the weighted mean length of stay was 3.1 days (range, 1–7), with the six US centers generally reporting earlier discharges postoperatively [6]. Patients are discharged on daily proton pump inhibitors that are continued until physiologic testing is performed at 6 months to assess for presence or degree of gastroesophageal reflux. Many centers advocate routine imaging (Gastrografin or thin barium esophagram) on POD#1 with some centers performing second-look EGD prior to diet initiation or hospital discharge [6]. During our initial experience, the postoperative care pathway included obtaining a POD#1 esophagram, but the lack of impact on patient management and low leak rate have led to abandonment of asymptomatic screening of all patients postoperatively. There are descriptions of postoperative computed tomography scans of the chest being routinely obtained; however, following the same logic that led to abandonment of routine esophagram use, there is no clear evidence to support the cost or radiation exposure associated with routine screening CT scans.

Follow-Up

Patients should be seen 2–6 weeks postoperatively to evaluate treatment response and detect potential early failures. In the absence of recurrent symptoms, full physiologic testing with TBE, HRIM, EndoFLIP, and pH impedance is postponed until the 6–9-month follow-up appointment. TBE in particular has been shown to have significant prognostic value following pneumatic dilation in detecting patients with symptomatic relief that are at increased risk for early treatment failure [20]. Patients are seen again at 1 year and then annually for life, with completion of validated questionnaires and intermittent physiologic testing to track long-term outcomes. Long-term follow-up protocols can also incorporate routine or symptom-triggered screening for esophageal malignancy.

Review of Existing Literature

Efficacy

To date, no prospective, randomized trials comparing POEM to LHM or pneumatic dilatation have been published. The IPOEMS reported overall treatment success of 98% at a mean follow-up of 9.3 months, with 40% of patients having failed prior to treatment [6]. The multicenter, prospective trial by von Renteln et al. has more recently shown a decline in success rate over time, from 97.1% at 3 months to 82.4% at 1 year [21] and 78.5% at 2 years [22]; however, the majority of failures occurred within the first ten cases at each center suggesting a learning curve. There have been several single-institution and one multicenter publication that report longer-term results [23–25]. Hungness et al. reported a 92% clinical success at 2.4-year follow-up with POEM and a 33% rate of objective reflux in patients without hiatal hernia and a BMI < 35 [23].

Rates of GERD

Richards et al. demonstrated in 2004 that in the absence of a concurrent fundoplication, complete division of the lower esophageal sphincter and gastric sling fibers during Heller's cardiomyotomy results in debilitating reflux [26]. Neither partial nor complete fundoplication is performed following POEM, and concern has been raised regarding the potential for higher long-term rates of GERD. IPOEMS study estimated the prevalence of GERD following POEM in the range of 20–46%, based on visualization of erosive esophagitis on EGD or abnormal pH studies during short-term follow-up (<1 year) [6]. Several studies with longer follow-up have confirmed this [23–25]. Comparable rates have been reported in patients undergoing LHM with anterior (Dor) fundoplication in multicenter, prospective, randomized trials [27, 28]. Similar to the argument put forth by proponents of anterior (Dor) fundoplication, the lack of posterior mediastinal dissection and preservation of the phreno-esophageal ligament during POEM may mitigate the absence of a surgical anti-reflux barrier. Preservation of the angle of His may also contribute to the anatomic anti-reflux barrier when the 1–2 o'clock position is used for myotomy during POEM, as the natural course of the esophagus (clockwise rotation and right-to-left sweep) favors dissection onto the lesser curve and division of the clasp fibers with maintenance of the sling fibers.

References

1. Mayberry JF. Epidemiology and demographics of achalasia. Gastrointest Endosc Clin N Am. 2001;11:235–48.
2. Kahrilas PJ, Boeckxstaens G. The spectrum of achalasia: lessons from studies of pathophysiology and high-resolution manometry. Gastroenterology. 2013;145(5):954–65. PMID: 23973923 PMCID: PMC3835179.
3. Moonen A, Boeckxstaens G. Current diagnosis and management of achalasia. J Clin Gastroenterol. 2014;48(6):484–90.
4. Kandulski A, Fuchs KH, Weigt J, Malfertheiner P. Jackhammer esophagus: high-resolution manometry and therapeutic approach using peroral endoscopic myotomy (POEM). Dis Esophagus. 2014;27:PMID: 24460870.
5. Minami H, Inoue H, Haji A, Isomoto H, Urabe S, Hashiguchi K, et al. Per-oral endoscopic myotomy: emerging indications and evolving techniques. Dig Endosc. 2014;27(2):175–81. [Epub ahead of print].
6. Stavropoulos SN, Modayil R, Friedel D, et al. The International Per Oral Endoscopic Myotomy Survey (IPOEMS): a snapshot of the global POEM experience. Surg Endosc. 2013;27:3322–38.
7. Fisichella PM, Patti MG. From Heller to POEM (1914–2014): A 100-year history of surgery for achalasia. J Gastrointest Surg. 2014;18(10):1870–5. [Epub ahead of print].
8. Pasricha PJ, Hawari R, Ahmed I, et al. Submucosal endoscopic esophageal myotomy: a novel experimental approach for the treatment of achalasia. Endoscopy. 2007;39:761–4.
9. Rajan E, Gostout CJ, Feitoza AB, et al. Widespread EMR: a new technique for removal of large areas of mucosa. Gastrointest Endosc. 2004;60:623–7.
10. Inoue H, Minami H, Kobayashi Y, et al. Peroral endoscopic myotomy (POEM) for esophageal achalasia. Endoscopy. 2010;42:265–71.
11. Eckardt VF. Clinical presentations and complications of achalasia. Gastrointest Endosc Clin N Am. 2001;11(2):281–92, vi. Pubmed PMID: 11319062.
12. Hungness ES, Teitelbaum EN, Santos BF, et al. Comparison of perioperative outcomes between Peroral Esophageal Myotomy (POEM) and laparoscopic Heller Myotomy. J Gastrointest Surg. 2012;17(2):228–35.
13. Harnish JL, Darling GE, Diamant NE, et al. Patient-centered measures for achalasia. Surg Endosc. 2008;22(5):1290–3.
14. Schlottmann F, Neto RML, Herbella FAM, Patti MG. Esophageal achalasia: pathophysiology, clinical presentation, and diagnostic evaluation. Am Surg. 2018;84(4):467–72.
15. Rohof WO, Salvador R, Annese V, et al. Outcomes of treatment for achalasia depend on manometric subtype. Gastroenterology. 2012;144(4):718–25. PubMed PMID: 23277105.
16. Rohof WO, Hursch DP, Kessing BF, et al. Efficacy of treatment for patients with achalasia depends on the distensibility of the esophagogastric junction. Gastroenterology. 2012;143(2):328–35.
17. Kurian AA, Dunst CM, Sharata A, Bhayani NH, Reavis KM, Swanström LL. Peroral endoscopic esophageal myotomy: defining the learning curve. Gastrointest Endosc. 2013;77(5): 719–25.
18. Kandulski A, et al. Jackhammer esophagus: high-resolution manometry and therapeutic approach using peroral endoscopic myotomy (POEM). Dis Esophagus. 2014;29(6):695–6.
19. Modayil R, Friedel D, Stavropoulos SN. Endoscopic suture repair of a large mucosal perforation during peroral endoscopic myotomy for treatment of achalasia. Gastrointest Endosc. 2014;80(6):1169–70. [Epub ahead of print] PubMed PMID: 24830579.
20. Vaezi MF, Baker ME, Achkar E, et al. Timed barium oesophagram: better predictor of long term success after pneumatic dilation in achalasia than symptom assessment. Gut. 2002;50: 765–70.
21. von Renteln D, Fuchs KH, Fockens P, et al. Peroral endoscopic myotomy for the treatment of achalasia: an international prospective multicenter study. Gastroenterology. 2013;145: 309–11.

22. Werner YB, Costamanga G, Swanstrom LL, et al. Clinical response to peroral endoscopic myotomy in patients with idiopathic achalasia as a minimum follow-up of 2 years. Gut. 2016;65:899–906.
23. Hungness EH, Sternbach JM, Teitelbaum EN, et al. Per-oral endoscopic myotomy (POEM) after the learning curve: durable long-term results with a low complication rate. Ann Surg. 2016;264:508–17.
24. Ngamruengphong S, Inoue H, Chiu PW, et al. Long-term outcomes of per-oral endoscopic myotomy in patients with achalasia with a minimum follow-up of 2 years: an international multicenter study. Gastrointest Endosc. 2016;85(5):927–933.e2.
25. Inoue H, Sato H, Ikeda H, et al. Per-oral endoscopic myotomy: a series of 500 patients. J Am Coll Surg. 2015;221:256–64.
26. Richards WO, Torquati A, Holzman MD, Khaitan L, Byrne D, Lutfi R, et al. Heller myotomy versus Heller myotomy with Dor fundoplication for achalasia: a prospective randomized double-blind clinical trial. Ann Surg. 2004;240(3):405–12.
27. Rebecchi F, Giaccone C, Farinella E, Campaci R, Morino M. Randomized controlled trial of laparoscopic Heller myotomy plus Dor fundoplication versus Nissen fundoplication for achalasia: long-term results. Ann Surg. 2008;248(6):1023–30.
28. Rawlings A, Soper NJ, Oelschlager B, et al. Laparoscopic Dor versus Toupet fundoplication following Heller myotomy for achalasia: results of a multicenter, prospective, randomized-controlled trial. Surg Endosc. 2012;26:18–26.

Surgical Management of Achalasia: Recurrent Dysphagia

39

Hope T. Jackson and Brant K. Oelschlager

Introduction

Advances in minimally invasive surgery have led to a significant shift in the surgical management of esophageal achalasia, and today, laparoscopic Heller myotomy and partial fundoplication are considered the procedures of choice [1–12]. The laparoscopic approach is the preferred approach because it provides excellent exposure of the gastroesophageal junction (GEJ) and allows for performance of a partial fundoplication [2, 13]. In addition, as a result of studies showing that a longer gastric myotomy results in improved relief of dysphagia, the length of the myotomy performed on the gastric wall has increased [4, 14]. This is facilitated by the laparoscopic approach.

This approach can achieve significant improvement in esophageal clearance in upward of 90–95% of patients [1, 4, 6, 12]. However, patients can experience persistence of their symptoms or recurrence over time with recurrent (late) dysphagia being more common than persistent (early) dysphagia. This chapter will focus on the diagnostic and therapeutic approach to patients with persistent or recurrent dysphagia following a Heller myotomy.

H. T. Jackson
University of Maryland School of Medicine, Baltimore, MD, USA

B. K. Oelschlager (✉)
Department of Surgery, University of Washington, Seattle, WA, USA
e-mail: brant@uw.edu

J. Grams et al. (eds.), *The SAGES Manual of Foregut Surgery*,
https://doi.org/10.1007/978-3-319-96122-4_39

Persistent Dysphagia

Persistent dysphagia can be defined as typically presenting immediately following a Heller myotomy or after a temporary relief of symptoms (i.e., less than 6 months). We believe there are several factors, primarily attributable to surgical technique, that are responsible for this occurrence (Table 39.1).

Inadequate Gastric Myotomy

The most common cause of persistent dysphagia is an incomplete myotomy, primarily on the gastric side of the GEJ. In the early 1990s, as minimally invasive surgery began to be applied to the treatment of achalasia, the Heller myotomy was performed through a left thoracoscopic approach that was first published by Pellegrini and colleagues [13]. A 7 cm esophageal myotomy was performed and extended for only 5 mm onto the gastric wall, without an antireflux procedure based on the conventional technique described by Ellis et al. [15]. Early experience resulted in a high incidence of dysphagia that was attributed to inadequate extension of the myotomy onto the gastric wall [13]. Because exposure of the GEJ and gastric wall was difficult through the thoracoscopic approach, the decision was made to switch to the laparoscopic approach and extend the myotomy 1–1.5 cm below the GEJ [2]. Our group had initial success with this approach with resolution of dysphagia in patients with a prior thoracoscopic myotomy and lower rates of dysphagia for primary operations, but we still had occasional patients who required reoperation. We observed that our outcomes appeared to be directly related to the length of the gastric myotomy and decided to extend the myotomy even further to 3 cm below the GEJ. We published our outcomes in a 2003 comparative study that looked at the results of a conventional myotomy (1.5 cm on the gastric wall) versus those with an extended myotomy (3 cm on the gastric wall) [14]. Those patients with an extended myotomy had significantly reduced lower esophageal sphincter pressure and incidence of dysphagia postoperatively. These results persisted in a long-term follow-up study by our group and as a result have become our standard practice [4]. Intraoperatively, surgeons can use laparoscopic instruments and/or endoscopy to help ensure that an adequate gastric myotomy length has been achieved. Laparoscopic graspers can be used to estimate the length of the gastric myotomy since an open grasper measures approximately 3 cm (Fig. 39.1). Endoscopy can also assist with

Table 39.1 Most common causes of persistent dysphagia

1. Incomplete myotomy (a) Inadequate gastric myotomy (most common) (b) Inadequate muscle fiber division
2. Lack of separation of myotomy muscle edges
3. Misconfiguration of the fundoplication
4. Tight closure of the hiatus

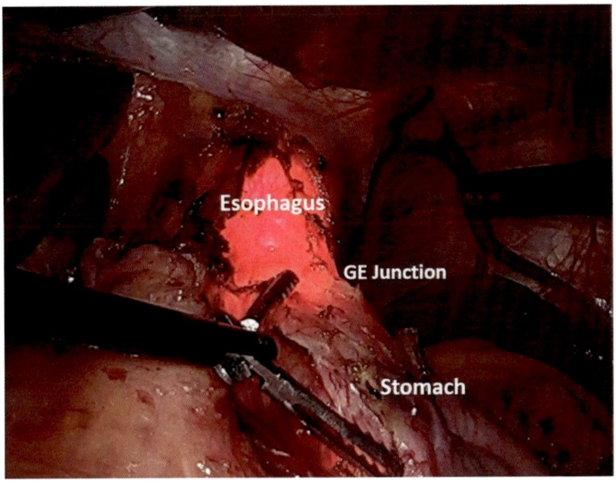

Fig. 39.1 Intraoperative picture of a Heller myotomy. An open laparoscopic grasper roughly measures 3 cm and can be used as a guide for the target length of the gastric myotomy

assessment of the entire myotomy, allows for easy identification of the squamocolumnar junction, and can confirm adequate distal extension of the myotomy onto the gastric wall.

Inadequate Division of Muscle Fibers

Incomplete division of esophageal muscle fibers can also, in theory, cause persistent dysphagia. Several studies have shown that this may occur because of scar tissue that develops at the level of the GEJ secondary to prior endoscopic treatment [16–18]. Pneumatic dilatation and intrasphincteric injection of botulinum toxin are endoscopic treatments that historically were selected as first- and second-line therapies to avoid the morbidity of open surgery. While the success of minimally invasive approaches to surgical myotomy has been well documented [2, 3, 7, 12, 13, 15, 19], pneumatic dilatation and botulinum toxin injection still continue to be offered and performed by gastroenterologists [16]. Though some studies suggest these preoperative procedures do not influence the outcome of surgical myotomy [20, 21], several studies and our own experience support the belief that these procedures, designed to cause disruption of the LES, can lead to scarring which can make the subsequent myotomy more difficult, incomplete, and prone to mucosal perforation with less predictable success rates [16, 17].

Lack of Separation of Myotomy Edges

Persistent dysphagia can also result when the myotomy edges re-approximate postoperatively and form a new scar that can result in esophageal narrowing. To decrease this occurrence, we recommend that the edges of the muscle layers are separated so that approximately 30–40% of the mucosa is uncovered [22]

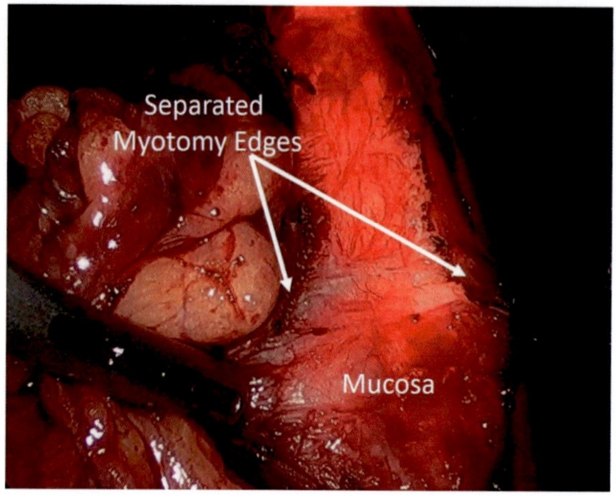

Fig. 39.2 Wide separation of the myotomy edges can prevent the postoperative re-approximation that can lead to recurrent dysphagia

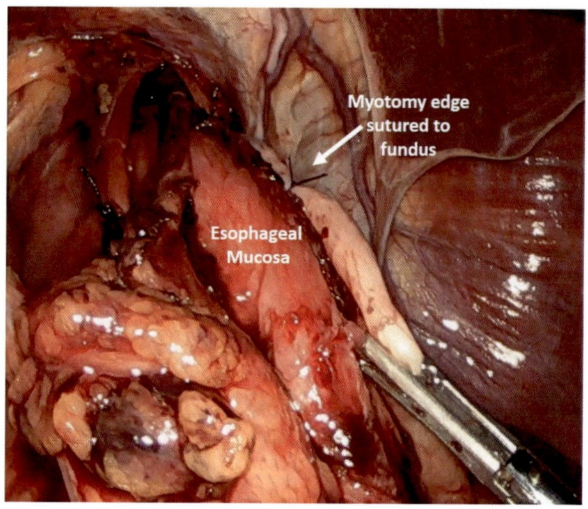

Fig. 39.3 Toupet fundoplication performed with Heller myotomy. The fundus of the stomach is sutured to the myotomy. This splays open the myotomy edges limiting re-approximation

(see Fig. 39.2). Our practice is to perform a Toupet fundoplication at the time of myotomy. The fundus of the stomach is sutured to the myotomy which splays open the myotomy edges and limits re-approximation and scarring (Fig. 39.3).

Fundoplication Misconfiguration

Our practice advocates performing a partial fundoplication following a Heller myotomy to prevent reflux. A 360-degree (Nissen) fundoplication may create a mechanical obstruction due to the lack of esophageal peristalsis that is characterized by achalasia [22]. While the type of partial fundoplication performed (anterior or

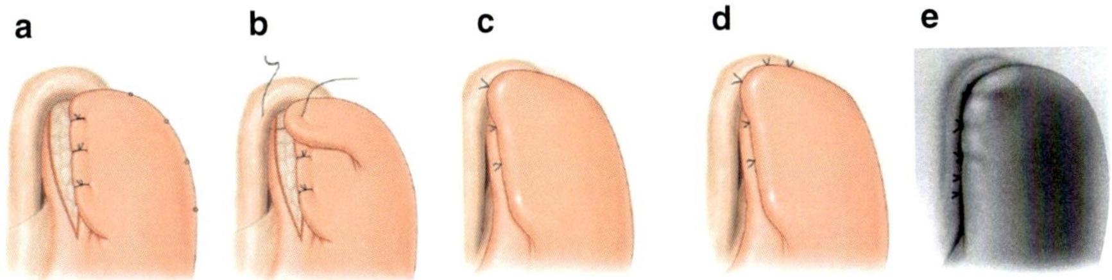

Fig. 39.4 A Dor fundoplication is created by two rows of sutures. (**a**) The first row is created by suturing the left myotomy edge to the fundus. (**b**) The fundus is then folded over the exposed mucosa, and the second row is created with three additional sutures. The first suture incorporates the fundus of the stomach, the esophagus, and the right crus. (**c**) The second and third sutures incorporate just the esophageal wall and the fundus. (**d**) Apical sutures seen in the 12 o'clock position are often placed to reduce tension. (**e**) This picture illustrates *improper* formation of the Dor fundoplication as the second row of sutures incorporates the right crus. This may lead to angulation at the GEJ and contribute to early re-approximation of the myotomy edges

posterior) may vary from center to center, poor construction of either fundoplication may lead to persistent or recurrent dysphagia, just as they can in patients who have a primary fundoplication for GERD. A Dor fundoplication is a 180-degree anterior fundoplication that is constructed with two rows of sutures. Once the first row is created on the left side (Fig. 39.4), the fundus is folded over the exposed mucosa, and three additional sutures are placed. The first suture incorporates the fundus of the stomach, the esophagus, and the right crus. The second and third sutures incorporate just the esophageal wall and the fundus, as incorporating the right crus as well may lead to angulation at the GEJ. Too many stitches at this level may cause constriction at the level of the GEJ and contribute to early re-approximation of the myotomy edges (Fig. 39.4) [7, 22, 23]. We choose a Dor fundoplication to provide coverage of a primary mucosal repair when there is an esophageal perforation. A Toupet fundoplication, our preferred partial fundoplication, is a 270-degree posterior fundoplication that may also lead to postoperative dysphagia when the fundoplication is constructed incorrectly. For example, this can occur if the posterior aspect of the fundoplication is placed under too much tension, creating an anterior angulation of the esophagus that may result in dysphagia [22].

Tight Closure of the Hiatus

Closure of the hiatal opening may impair esophageal emptying by causing constriction or creating a similar anterior angulation of the esophagus that can occur with a poorly constructed Toupet fundoplication. In general, we do not close the hiatus of the average patient with achalasia like we would with an antireflux procedure. If the patient has an associated large hiatal hernia (rare) or if the esophagus is particularly dilated or sigmoid in configuration, we recommend partial closure to avoid dysphagia.

Recurrent Dysphagia

Recurrent dysphagia is more common than persistent dysphagia and typically occurs greater than 6 months after the initial Heller myotomy. It is reported to occur in approximately 3–13 percent of patients [4, 12, 23–26]. When a patient presents for consultation, it is important to determine if the patient was asymptomatic for a period of time and was able to tolerate food. This helps to establish that the initial surgical procedure was successful and may help clarify the etiology of the recurrence. Similar to our discussion on persistent (early) dysphagia, incomplete myotomy on the gastric wall and along the esophagus is also the most common reason for recurrent (late) dysphagia. While causes of recurrence can be multifactorial, we will highlight the most common causes of recurrence that follow incomplete myotomy (Table 39.2).

Myotomy Scarring

Scarring/fibrosis at the distal edge of a properly formed myotomy can be a common cause of recurrent dysphagia following a symptom-free interval [7, 12, 22, 23, 27]. A meta-analysis performed by Campos and colleagues described an incidence of 27% [28]. We believe that the creation of a longer myotomy with a wider separation of myotomy edges should decrease the frequency of this occurrence [4, 14].

Gastroesophageal Reflux Disease

The disruption of the LES, as a result of the myotomy, places patients at risk for the development of postoperative reflux (POR). POR has an incidence of 50–60% when a myotomy is performed without a fundoplication and 2–26% when a partial fundoplication is added [4, 8, 22, 28–31]. Complications of GERD such as esophagitis, Barrett's esophagus, and peptic stricture could lead to dysphagia. Patients who develop pathologic reflux following Heller myotomy may often be asymptomatic, so it is important to perform ambulatory pH monitoring postoperatively [32]. Our practice is to perform this test at our 6-month postoperative visit. If abnormal reflux is documented, typically this is treated with acid-reducing medications if there is no abnormality with the fundoplication. In our experience, this is rare but the most common reason for severe, recurrent dysphagia.

Table 39.2 Most common causes of recurrent dysphagia

1. Incomplete myotomy (a) Inadequate gastric myotomy (most common) (b) Inadequate muscle fiber division
2. Myotomy scarring
3. Gastroesophageal reflux disease
4. Fundoplication abnormality
5. Esophageal cancer

Fundoplication Abnormality

Fundoplication herniation or movement is a less common cause of postoperative dysphagia but has a reported incidence of 10–13% [28]. Misconfiguration of the fundoplication at the time of the initial operation could make this occurrence more likely. If the fundoplication is the cause of dysphagia and the patient requires reoperation, our preference is to take down the fundoplication without reconstructing it. If it is apparent at the time of reoperation that the fundoplication was misconfigured initially (i.e., a fatal flaw such as too much fundus included in the wrap and misplaced sutures), it may be reasonable to redo both the myotomy and the fundoplication.

Esophageal Cancer

Patients with untreated achalasia are at an increased risk of developing squamous cell carcinoma. Long-term studies looking at the development of esophageal cancer following myotomy are scarce. Zaninotto and colleagues performed a retrospective review of 226 patients who received a Heller myotomy for achalasia [31]. Two percent (four) of these patients developed squamous cell carcinoma at 2, 8, 13, and 18 years following myotomy. Pathologic reflux following myotomy can result in Barrett's esophagus and adenocarcinoma which can also cause recurrent dysphagia [33]. Currently there are no precise guidelines about endoscopic follow-up in achalasia patients.

Diagnostic Evaluation

A meticulous and systematic approach to patients with dysphagia is necessary to aid the physician in choosing the most effective treatment modality. Though the etiologies of persistent and recurrent dysphagia somewhat differ, the diagnostic workup is the same (Table 39.3).

As is true for all patients, obtaining a thorough history is a crucial step in the diagnostic workup. Along with the patient's current symptoms, a review of symptoms *before* the initial operation should be elucidated as it helps establish that the initial operation was performed for the correct indication.

Table 39.3 Diagnostic workup for patients presenting with persistent/recurrent dysphagia

1. Upper gastrointestinal series
2. Upper endoscopy
3. Esophageal manometry
4. Ambulatory 24-h pH monitoring
5. Computed tomography[a]
6. Endoscopic ultrasound[a]

[a] Indicates studies that can help rule out pseudoachalasia when other studies are inconclusive

Prior manometry, endoscopy, and upper gastrointestinal (UGI) series images should be obtained along with the operative report. The operative report can provide important clues that may explain the patient's current symptoms, such as a description of scar tissue due to prior treatment, the extent of the myotomy, difficulty identifying anatomic planes, or an enlarged left lobe of the liver that precluded adequate superior extension of the myotomy [22]. In terms of imaging studies, we believe that an UGI is the most important initial study, followed by endoscopy, esophageal manometry, and then pH monitoring.

Upper GI Series

An UGI is most useful for determining if there is a persistent obstruction at the GEJ. Additionally, it can clarify the etiology of the obstruction such as a misconfigured fundoplication, incomplete gastric myotomy, scarring due to GEJ narrowing, hiatal hernia, or an overly tight hiatal closure [22, 23] (Fig. 39.5).

Independent of etiology, the grade of esophageal dilatation determined by the UGI can also help predict the success of revisional surgery. Our center looked at patients requiring a redo myotomy for recurrent dysphagia, and we found that patients with an UGI demonstrating a straight esophagus (normal or dilated, Grades 1–3) all had improved dysphagia following revisional surgery [34]. Dysphagia improvement was less consistent if the esophagus was in a sigmoid configuration (Grade 4).

Endoscopy

An upper endoscopy is the next useful diagnostic study that we recommend performing even if the etiology of dysphagia is apparent on the UGI. Endoscopy serves to identify reflux esophagitis, candida esophagitis secondary to delayed emptying, and strictures and to rule out cancer [22]. It can also reveal a malformed fundoplication and may be useful in characterizing fibrosis [23]. Additionally, at the time of endoscopy, one should consider performing a 20 mm (60 French) balloon or Savary dilatation. When performed properly it is of little risk but may provide substantial relief without proceeding to more aggressive procedures (e.g., pneumatic dilatation ≥30 mm).

Esophageal Manometry

Esophageal manometry can confirm the diagnosis of achalasia, especially if the previous two studies are inconclusive and can help identify those patients who may or may not benefit from reoperation. Chapman and colleagues showed that dysphagia is much less common in patients with a hypotensive LES pressure (less than 10 mmHg) following myotomy [35]. If postoperative manometry reveals

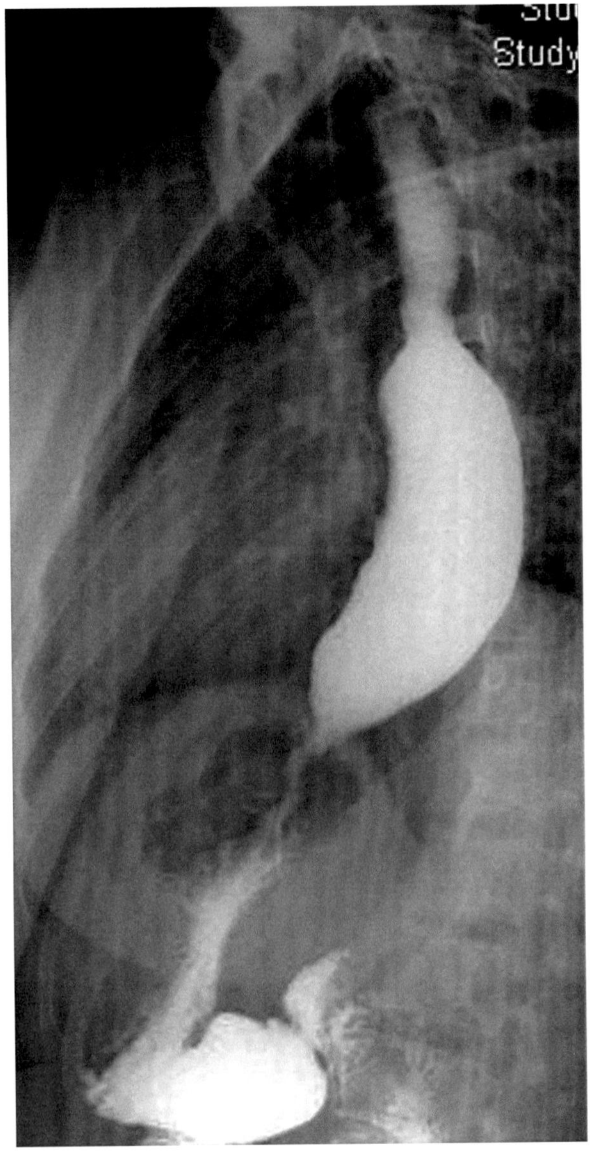

Fig. 39.5 Upper GI study in a patient presenting with recurrent dysphagia following a previous Heller myotomy with Dor fundoplication for achalasia. The patient's operative report noted a 2 cm gastric myotomy. The X-ray at presentation suggests persistent obstruction at the GE junction. This could be due to the Dor fundoplication or an inadequate gastric myotomy

persistently elevated LES pressures, this may indicate an incomplete or fibrotic myotomy that may benefit from a redo myotomy (Fig. 39.6).

Ambulatory 24-Hour pH Monitoring

GERD can lead to dysphagia and occurs frequently after myotomy, even when a fundoplication is included. The best way to confirm GERD is 24-h pH monitoring,

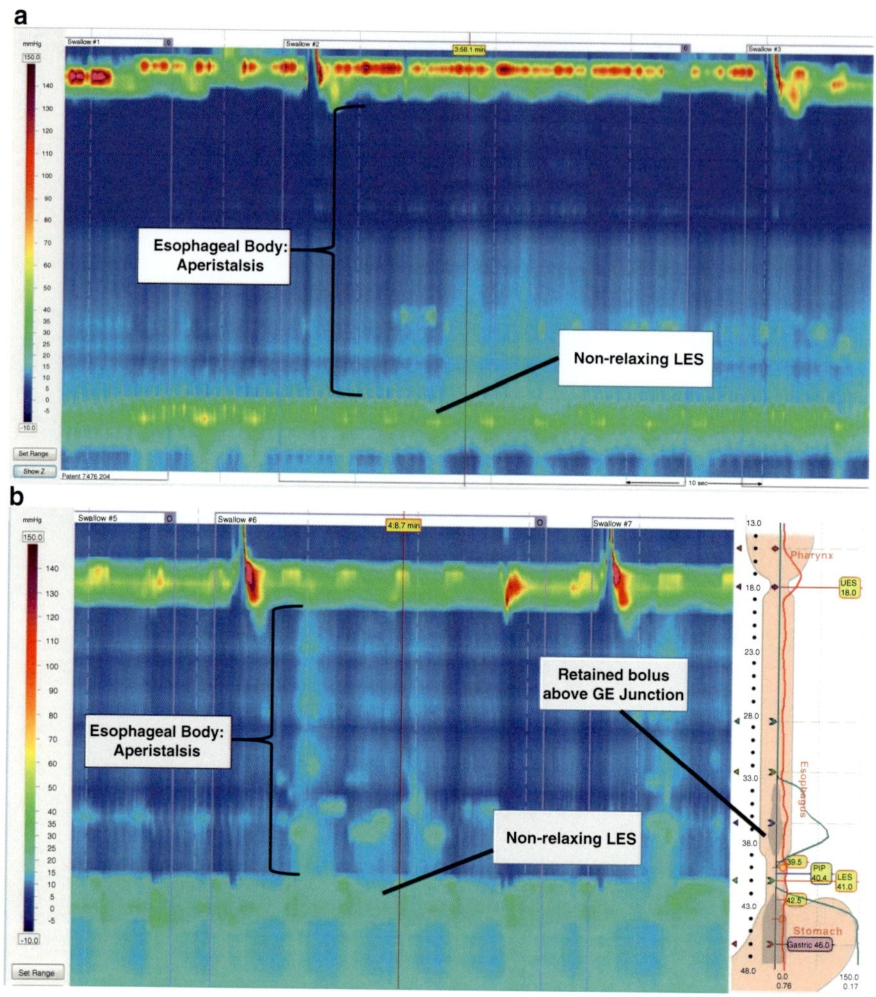

Fig. 39.6 (**a**) Classic high-resolution manometry (HRM) in a patient with type 1 achalasia. (**b**) HRM in a patient presenting with recurrent dysphagia following a Heller myotomy with Dor fundoplication. The patient still has evidence of abnormal relaxation of the LES with a LES pressure of 17 mmHg (normal post myotomy <10 mmHg) and retained bolus above the GE junction

and it should be performed in this patient population. It is important to critically review the pH tracings as there can be false positive results from stasis and fermentation. Simple review of the final composite reflux score will not reveal this, but the tracings are key in differentiating true reflux from false reflux. False reflux is secondary to the stasis of food that can occur if there is abnormal relaxation of the LES. The stasis causes "acidification" of the food as it decomposes. This is depicted on a pH tracing as a slow decrease in pH rather than the abrupt change that is seen with true reflux [23] (Fig. 39.7). There will also be long periods of the pH remaining

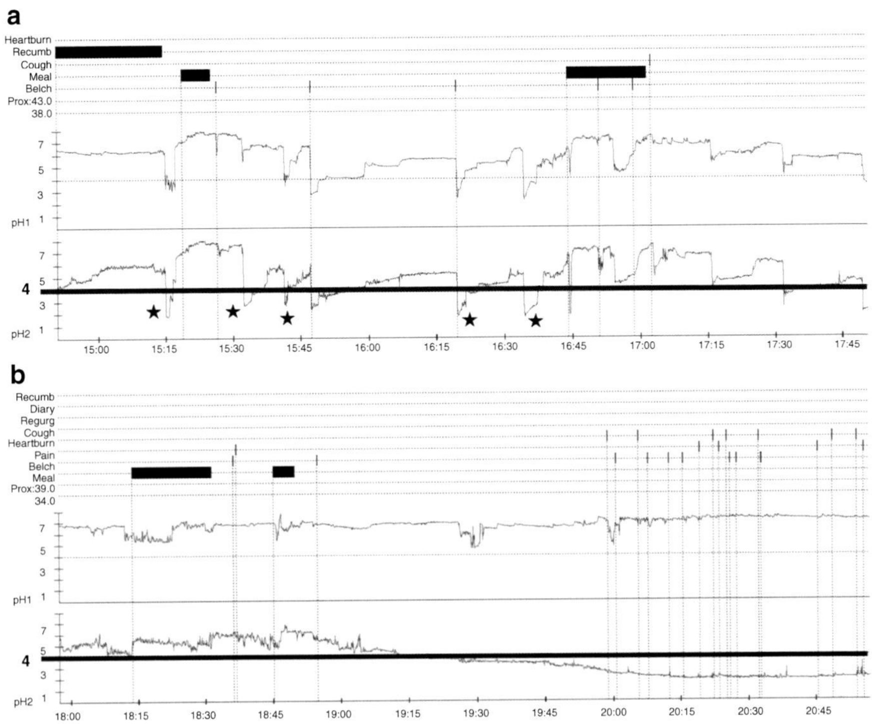

Fig. 39.7 (**a**) 24-h ambulatory pH tracing demonstrating "true" reflux with characteristic abrupt drops below a pH of 4 (stars). (**b**) A false-positive pH tracing demonstrating a slow decrease in the pH that is characteristic of food stasis and fermentation

below 4 and a very abnormal score. The key point here is that false reflux is a manifestation of poor esophageal emptying, not actual reflux. Additionally, patients with achalasia will always have an element of poor emptying as the intrinsic function of the esophagus (peristalsis) is abnormal and unable to be restored post myotomy. Those patients with true reflux may benefit from the addition of acid-reducing medications or revision/addition of a fundoplication [23]. As stated earlier in our section on GERD, reflux can often be silent, so this test should be performed routinely even on asymptomatic patients. Our center typically performs this at the time of our 6-month follow-up and if recurrent symptoms occur.

Other Studies

The workup of these patients can essentially be completed with the above studies, but rarely patients may present with postoperative dysphagia even when manometry is consistent with achalasia and when an adequate myotomy has been performed. Should this happen, computed tomography and/or endoscopic ultrasound may be useful adjuncts in identifying the unfortunate scenario of a previously missed pseudoachalasia secondary to a submucosal tumor or a tumor outside of the esophagus [36, 37].

Treatment

Endoscopic therapy, revisional surgery, esophagectomy, and newer endoscopic approaches to myotomy are all considerations for the treatment of persistent and recurrent dysphagia.

Pneumatic Balloon Dilatation

Balloon dilatation is a relatively noninvasive procedure that uses increasing intra-balloon pressure to disrupt the fibers of the LES. The balloon dilatations used in these cases are larger (30–40 mm) than the 20 mm balloon dilatations mentioned earlier in the endoscopy section so as to adequately disrupt the LES fibers. The procedure carries a low risk of perforation because the previous myotomy site is covered by the stomach if a Dor fundoplication is performed and the left lateral segment of the liver if a Toupet is performed. Dilatation to treat recurrent dysphagia following Heller myotomy has reported early success rates ranging from 30% to 80% [12, 38]. Zaninotto and colleagues performed a retrospective review of 113 patients, 9 of these patients (8%) had recurrent dysphagia following laparoscopic Heller myotomy and Dor fundoplication [25]. Seven of the nine patients were effectively treated with balloon dilatation (median, two dilatations; range, 1–4), and two patients required reoperation. Sweet et al. described similar results in patients with both persistent and recurrent dysphagia [6]. These considerations make balloon dilatation a good treatment option for patients presenting with dysphagia following myotomy.

Revisional Surgery

Revisional surgery should be considered if there is evidence of esophageal obstruction that can be improved with myotomy extension or takedown of the fundoplication, and symptoms fail to respond to pneumatic dilatation. If the patient has already undergone an extended myotomy, the need for reoperation should be rare unless there is an abnormality with the fundoplication [23]. In addition, reoperation carries a risk of irreparable damage to the esophageal mucosa that may require an esophagectomy, a high-risk procedure, even at high-volume centers.

In those patients whose diagnostic workup suggests that the original myotomy was not extended well enough onto the stomach (or the esophagus), a redo myotomy is reasonable to consider. It is also reasonable to consider a redo myotomy for those in whom we believe the main problem is fibrosis/scarring that is

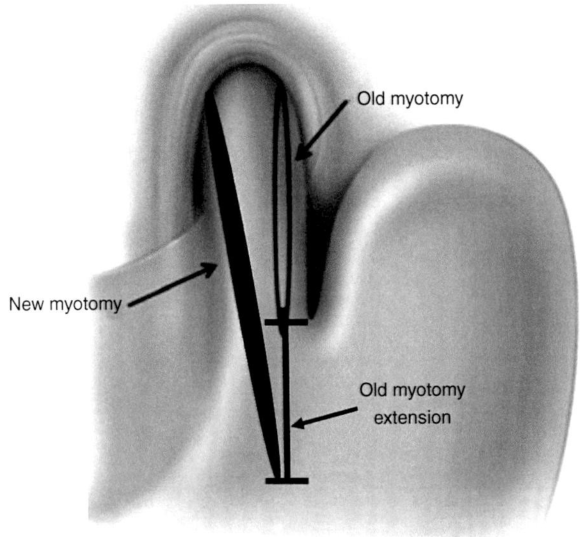

Fig. 39.8 Revisional surgery for recurrent achalasia. The surgeon can extend the prior scarred myotomy (right) or perform a new myotomy (solid oval) to the side of the old myotomy

nonresponsive to pneumatic dilatation. Intraoperatively, we either extend the prior scarred myotomy or perform the second myotomy to the side of the previous myotomy (Fig. 39.8). This allows the surgeon to take advantage of the uncut muscularis layer of the esophagus and the stomach [22, 23]. The myotomy should be extended for 3–4 cm below the GEJ and superiorly on the esophagus as far as the prior effective myotomy. Once the myotomy is completed, the surgeon should determine whether or not to perform a fundoplication. If the mucosa is inadvertently injured, performing a Dor fundoplication to buttress the repair may decrease the chance of immediate complications and prevent further reflux. In the absence of perforation, our tendency is to, in most cases, avoid performing a fundoplication in the setting of a redo operation, particularly in the presence of a dilated esophagus [22]. Our rationale is based on three concepts: (1) dysphagia, not GERD, is the primary indication for reoperation; (2) should the fundoplication fail or exacerbate dysphagia, a third operation would be increasingly difficult; and (3) abnormal reflux can be more easily treated with medications than dysphagia. This approach has been supported by several studies in the literature [34, 38–40]. However, if the esophagus is normal and there is a clear abnormality corrected (i.e., inadequate myotomy, misconfigured fundoplication), one can then consider a fundoplication if reasonably confident that it will not result in recurrent obstruction.

Peroral Endoscopic Myotomy (POEM)

Peroral endoscopic myotomy is a newer endoscopic technique for performing a LES myotomy that was developed in 2008 (Fig. 39.9). Early studies have been associated with excellent relief of dysphagia, and a recent long-term study by

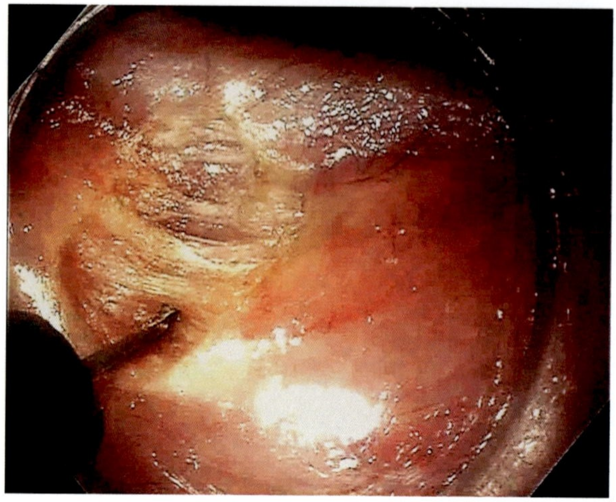

Fig. 39.9 Intraoperative photo of a POEM. This technique allows for endoscopic division of the esophageal muscle fibers, avoiding the need for laparoscopy

Hungness et al. reported symptomatic relief in 92% of patients with a low rate of complications (follow-up range 12–52 months) [41–43]. Forty percent of these patients had objective evidence of reflux. While a laparoscopic myotomy is performed on the anterior wall of the esophagus, the POEM procedure can be performed on the posterior wall of the esophagus. This makes POEM a reasonable consideration in patients presenting with persistent or recurrent dysphagia after a failed myotomy or redo operation and may allow patients to avoid an esophagectomy. One limitation of the POEM in cases of recurrent dysphagia is that it does not address the fundoplication as an etiology for the patient's dysphagia. If a fundoplication was performed at the time of initial surgery, this approach does not allow for the fundoplication to be taken down. Because of this, POEM is an ideal option in those patients without a prior fundoplication. If a POEM is performed in the setting of a prior fundoplication, and dysphagia persists, one should consider taking it down in a subsequent setting. Use of the POEM procedure is not widespread and is only available at a limited number of centers with highly trained surgical endoscopists and gastroenterologists. While the initial studies are promising, further long-term studies are needed, particularly related to recurrent dysphagia before widespread use recommendations can be made.

Esophagectomy

Esophagectomy is associated with a mortality rate between 1% and 4%, even in expert hands [44, 45]. Devaney and colleagues reported a 10% rate of anastomotic leak, 5% rate of hoarseness, and 2% rate of bleeding among 93 patients who had an esophagectomy for achalasia [45]. As a result, it should only be undertaken when all other less invasive options are exhausted. At that point, esophagectomy should be considered in patients with end-stage achalasia, characterized by a sigmoid-shaped esophagus, and those who have already failed a myotomy or redo myotomy [34].

Given the risks of an esophagectomy, the lower morbidity of a laparoscopic redo myotomy, and some success with a redo myotomy in end-stage patients [34], we tend to offer esophagectomy only to those patients who do not improve after a redo myotomy. In terms of surgical approach, the esophagus is frequently dilated with large collateral veins on the surface that make the transhiatal approach risky. Our approach in these patients is to dissect the esophagus under direct vision either thoracoscopically or via thoracotomy [22, 23].

Conclusion

Laparoscopic Heller myotomy with partial fundoplication is the procedure of choice for patients with achalasia. Persistent or recurrent dysphagia can develop over time secondary to surgical technique, fibrosis, fundoplication configuration, reflux, or esophageal cancer. A systematic and thorough approach is necessary for the diagnostic evaluation of these patients to help determine the most appropriate treatment modality. Endoscopic therapy and revisional surgery are the cornerstones of treatment, and newer endoscopic therapies may provide a more minimally invasive approach to the management of this disease. Esophagectomy, however, should be considered as a surgical option in cases that are refractory to these less invasive treatment therapies to open the LES.

References

1. Patti MG, et al. Impact of minimally invasive surgery on the treatment of esophageal achalasia: a decade of change. J Am Coll Surg. 2003;196(5):698–703; discussion 703–5.
2. Patti MG, et al. Minimally invasive surgery for achalasia: an 8-year experience with 168 patients. Ann Surg. 1999;230(4):587–93; discussion 593–4.
3. Frantzides CT, et al. Minimally invasive surgery for achalasia: a 10-year experience. J Gastrointest Surg. 2004;8(1):18–23.
4. Wright AS, et al. Long-term outcomes confirm the superior efficacy of extended Heller myotomy with Toupet fundoplication for achalasia. Surg Endosc. 2007;21(5):713–8.
5. Roll GR, et al. Excellent outcomes of laparoscopic esophagomyotomy for achalasia in patients older than 60 years of age. Surg Endosc. 2010;24(10):2562–6.
6. Sweet MP, et al. The outcome of laparoscopic Heller myotomy for achalasia is not influenced by the degree of esophageal dilatation. J Gastrointest Surg. 2008;12(1):159–65.
7. Patti MG, et al. Laparoscopic Heller myotomy and Dor fundoplication for achalasia: analysis of successes and failures. Arch Surg. 2001;136(8):870–7.
8. Richards WO, et al. Heller myotomy versus Heller myotomy with Dor fundoplication for achalasia: a prospective randomized double-blind clinical trial. Ann Surg. 2004;240(3):405–12; discussion 412–5.
9. Patti MG, Fisichella PM. Laparoscopic Heller myotomy and Dor fundoplication for esophageal achalasia. How I do it. J Gastrointest Surg. 2008;12(4):764–6.
10. Patti MG, Herbella FA. Fundoplication after laparoscopic Heller myotomy for esophageal achalasia: what type? J Gastrointest Surg. 2010;14(9):1453–8.
11. Tatum RP, Pellegrini CA. How I do it: laparoscopic Heller myotomy with Toupet fundoplication for achalasia. J Gastrointest Surg. 2009;13(6):1120–4.
12. Zaninotto G, et al. Four hundred laparoscopic myotomies for esophageal achalasia: a single centre experience. Ann Surg. 2008;248(6):986–93.

13. Pellegrini C, et al. Thoracoscopic esophagomyotomy. Initial experience with a new approach for the treatment of achalasia. Ann Surg. 1992;216(3):291–6; discussion 296–9.
14. Oelschlager BK, Chang L, Pellegrini CA. Improved outcome after extended gastric myotomy for achalasia. Arch Surg. 2003;138(5):490–5; discussion 495–7.
15. Ellis FH Jr, Gibb SP, Crozier RE. Esophagomyotomy for achalasia of the esophagus. Ann Surg. 1980;192(2):157–61.
16. Smith CD, et al. Endoscopic therapy for achalasia before Heller myotomy results in worse outcomes than heller myotomy alone. Ann Surg. 2006;243(5):579–84; discussion 584–6.
17. Snyder CW, et al. Multiple preoperative endoscopic interventions are associated with worse outcomes after laparoscopic Heller myotomy for achalasia. J Gastrointest Surg. 2009;13(12):2095–103.
18. Patti MG, et al. Effects of previous treatment on results of laparoscopic Heller myotomy for achalasia. Dig Dis Sci. 1999;44(11):2270–6.
19. Bonatti H, et al. Long-term results of laparoscopic Heller myotomy with partial fundoplication for the treatment of achalasia. Am J Surg. 2005;190(6):874–8.
20. Rakita S, et al. Esophagotomy during laparoscopic Heller myotomy cannot be predicted by preoperative therapies and does not influence long-term outcome. J Gastrointest Surg. 2005;9(2):159–64.
21. Deb S, et al. Laparoscopic esophageal myotomy for achalasia: factors affecting functional results. Ann Thorac Surg. 2005;80(4):1191–4; discussion 1194–5.
22. Warner EA, Patti MG, Allaix ME, Pellegrini CA. Revisional surgery for achalasia. In: Fisichella PM, Soper NJ, editors. Surgical management of benign esophageal disorders. London: Springer; 2014. p. 227–40.
23. Petersen RP, Pellegrini CA. Revisional surgery after Heller myotomy for esophageal achalasia. Surg Laparosc Endosc Percutan Tech. 2010;20(5):321–5.
24. Schuchert MJ, et al. Minimally-invasive esophagomyotomy in 200 consecutive patients: factors influencing postoperative outcomes. Ann Thorac Surg. 2008;85(5):1729–34.
25. Zaninotto G, et al. Etiology, diagnosis, and treatment of failures after laparoscopic Heller myotomy for achalasia. Ann Surg. 2002;235(2):186–92.
26. Cowgill SM, et al. Laparoscopic Heller myotomy for achalasia: results after 10 years. Surg Endosc. 2009;23(12):2644–9.
27. Gockel I, Junginger T, Eckardt VF. Persistent and recurrent achalasia after Heller myotomy: analysis of different patterns and long-term results of reoperation. Arch Surg. 2007;142(11):1093–7.
28. Campos GM, et al. Endoscopic and surgical treatments for achalasia: a systematic review and meta-analysis. Ann Surg. 2009;249(1):45–57.
29. Donahue PE, et al. Floppy Dor fundoplication after esophagocardiomyotomy for achalasia. Surgery. 2002;132(4):716–22; discussion 722–3.
30. Luketich JD, et al. Outcomes after minimally invasive esophagomyotomy. Ann Thorac Surg. 2001;72(6):1909–12; discussion 1912–3.
31. Zaninotto G, et al. Long-term outcome and risk of oesophageal cancer after surgery for achalasia. Br J Surg. 2008;95(12):1488–94.
32. Patti MG, Diener U, Molena D. Esophageal achalasia: preoperative assessment and postoperative follow-up. J Gastrointest Surg. 2001;5(1):11–2.
33. Lopes AB, Fagundes RB. Esophageal squamous cell carcinoma – precursor lesions and early diagnosis. World J Gastrointest Endosc. 2012;4(1):9–16.
34. Loviscek MF, et al. Recurrent dysphagia after Heller myotomy: is esophagectomy always the answer? J Am Coll Surg. 2013;216(4):736–43. discussion 743-4
35. Chapman JR, et al. Achalasia treatment: improved outcome of laparoscopic myotomy with operative manometry. Arch Surg. 2004;139(5):508–13; discussion 513.
36. Moonka R, Pellegrini CA. Malignant pseudoachalasia. Surg Endosc. 1999;13(3):273–5.
37. Moonka R, et al. Clinical presentation and evaluation of malignant pseudoachalasia. J Gastrointest Surg. 1999;3(5):456–61.

38. Grotenhuis BA, et al. Reoperation for dysphagia after cardiomyotomy for achalasia. Am J Surg. 2007;194(5):678–82.
39. Iqbal A, et al. Laparoscopic re-operation for failed Heller myotomy. Dis Esophagus. 2006;19(3):193–9.
40. Wang L, Li YM. Recurrent achalasia treated with Heller myotomy: a review of the literature. World J Gastroenterol. 2008;14(46):7122–6.
41. Swanstrom LL, et al. Long-term outcomes of an endoscopic myotomy for achalasia: the POEM procedure. Ann Surg. 2012;256(4):659–67.
42. Hungness ES, et al. Comparison of perioperative outcomes between peroral esophageal myotomy (POEM) and laparoscopic Heller myotomy. J Gastrointest Surg. 2013;17(2):228–35.
43. Hungness ES, et al. Per-oral Endoscopic Myotomy (POEM) after the learning curve: durable long-term results with a low complication rate. Ann Surg. 2016;264(3):508–17.
44. Pinotti HW, et al. Resection for achalasia of the esophagus. Hepato-Gastroenterology. 1991;38(6):470–3.
45. Devaney EJ, et al. Esophagectomy for achalasia: patient selection and clinical experience. Ann Thorac Surg. 2001;72(3):854–8.

Expert Commentary: Laparoscopic Versus Endoscopic Myotomy for Achalasia

40

Ezra N. Teitelbaum and Lee L. Swanstrom

Background and Current Standard of Care

Achalasia is the most common primary esophageal motility disorder, resulting from an immune-mediated loss of neurons of the myenteric plexus of the esophagus [1]. This neuronal death causes a failure of esophagogastric junction (EGJ) relaxation and esophageal body peristalsis with swallowing, leading to symptoms of dysphagia, regurgitation, chest pain, and weight loss. Unfortunately, there is no therapy that can restore normal EGJ and esophageal body function in patients with achalasia. Current treatment modalities seek to palliate symptoms by decreasing the resting tone of the EGJ, which allows for passive transit of food boluses into the stomach. Medications are generally ineffective in producing more than a transient and minimal improvement in symptoms, and therefore procedural interventions that mechanically disrupt the muscle fibers of the lower esophageal sphincter (LES) form the mainstay of modern treatment.

Two such procedures, endoscopic pneumatic dilation (PD) and laparoscopic Heller myotomy (LHM), have been considered standard of care for the last 20 years. The recent European Achalasia Trial randomized patients to PD or LHM and found no significant difference in symptomatic outcomes at 2 and 5 years post-procedure [2, 3]. These results have led many to view the two procedures as equivalent in efficacy, despite the fact that all patients in the PD arm received at least two dilations as part of the study protocol. A recent meta-analysis of all three randomized trials comparing PD and LHM showed that LHM results in superior symptom palliation [4], as did a meta-analysis of non-randomized trials comparing the procedures [5]. Furthermore, long-term outcomes from single institution series suggest that LHM results in more durable efficacy, with less need for reintervention for symptom

E. N. Teitelbaum
Northwestern University, Chicago, IL, USA

L. L. Swanstrom (✉)
The Oregon Clinic, Portland, OR, USA

J. Grams et al. (eds.), *The SAGES Manual of Foregut Surgery*,
https://doi.org/10.1007/978-3-319-96122-4_40

recurrence [6]. For this reason, most surgeons consider LHM to be a better initial treatment option for most patients with newly diagnosed achalasia. PD still has a role for patients who may be medically unfit or do not wish to undergo a surgical procedure and general anesthetic. PD is also useful in patients who have had a prior LHM and present with recurrent or persistent symptoms.

As described previously in this textbook, per-oral endoscopic myotomy (POEM) is a novel operation for the treatment of achalasia. POEM uses techniques of submucosal dissection to create a controlled myotomy across the LES completely endoscopically, as shown in Fig. 40.1. POEM theoretically combines the advantages of both PD (no incisions, faster recovery) and LHM (superior efficacy and durability, single intervention). While direct comparison and long-term outcome data are limited, published POEM results have thus far been promising, and the procedure is quickly being adopted by centers around the world. This commentary will review the reported outcomes after POEM, with a focus on comparisons with the current surgical standard-of-care LHM.

Perioperative Safety and Outcomes

POEM offers several theoretical advantages over LHM. The most straightforward of these is that it is a completely endoscopic procedure, without the need for skin incisions or transabdominal trocar placement. While this should result in less

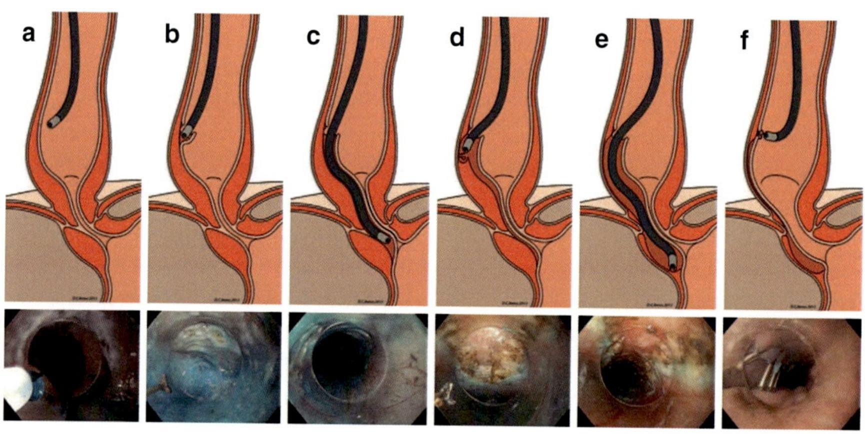

Fig. 40.1 POEM operative steps with representative endoscopic images. (**a**) A sclerotherapy needle is used to create a submucosal bleb 4–6 cm above the planned proximal extent of the myotomy. A longitudinal mucosotomy is then created, and the scope tip, with a clear dissecting cap, is advanced into the submucosal space. Using a combination of hydro, blunt, and cautery dissection, the submucosal tunnel is extended (**b**) to at least 3 cm distal to the squamocolumnar junction (SCJ) (**c**). Adequacy of the tunnel length is confirmed by retroflexion of the endoscope in the stomach and observing the extent of blue dye onto the stomach wall. A selective myotomy of the inner, circular muscle layer is then performed (**d**), extending 3 cm distal to the SCJ. After myotomy completion (**e**), the mucosotomy is closed with endoscopic clips (**f**). (Figure from Hungness et al. [7])

postoperative pain and faster return to activities, these advantages should not even be considered unless the procedure has an equivalent perioperative safety profile to the existing standards of care. Fortunately, a number of large single-center series, as well as recent meta-analyses, have demonstrated that POEM is as safe as LHM.

Professor Haruhiro Inoue was the first to perform POEM clinically in 2008 and recently published results from his first 500 cases [8]. These resulted in a complication rate of 3.2%, including pneumothorax, pleural effusion, bleeding, and mucosal perforation. However, all complications were managed either during the index POEM procedure or with conservative measures postoperatively, and no patients required reoperation. The Northwestern group reported a major complication rate of 2.7% with minor complications occurring in 15.2% of patients, of which urinary retention was the most common [7]. Our group reported an overall complication rate of 6% in the first 100 cases [9]. A recent meta-analysis of series that directly compared outcomes between POEM and LHM (all in a non-randomized fashion) showed no difference in perioperative complication rates or hospital length of stay [10]. A separate meta-analysis consisting of single-arm POEM and LHM series included 1958 and 5834 patients, respectively, and concluded that as "morbidity and mortality were extremely low for both procedures, we were not able to perform any statistical analysis regarding those outcomes" [11]. Certainly, mortality is extremely uncommon after POEM, with a systematic review showing 1 death in 1112 patients (0.09%) due to generalized cachexia from achalasia rather than a POEM-specific complication [12]. Taken together these results suggest that POEM and LHM have equivalent morbidity profiles and that when performed by experienced practitioners, POEM should no longer be considered an "experimental" operation when it comes to perioperative safety.

In most series from centers in the United States, over 90% of patients have only a 1-day hospital length of stay [7, 9], and there is some evidence that the procedure results in less pain and a quicker functional recovery than LHM. Ward and colleagues analyzed 41 patients who underwent POEM and 24 who had a LHM at the same institution and found the POEM patients to have less pain at discharge and a faster return to activities of daily living and work [13]. Given the minimal convalescence following the procedure, some centers are transitioning to performing POEM as an "outpatient" operation with same-day discharge.

Symptomatic and Physiologic Outcomes

As all current therapies for achalasia are palliative rather than curative, the main indicator of their success is symptom improvement or resolution. The most commonly used symptom measure has been the Eckardt score, which grades the frequency of dysphagia, regurgitation, and chest pain, as well as the amount of weight loss, as shown in Table 40.1. Both PD and LHM have been shown to be extremely effective in improving symptoms in the vast majority of patients. In the recent European Achalasia Trial which randomized patients between LHM and a series of at least two PDs, 90% and 86% of patients, respectively, achieved "symptomatic

Table 40.1 The Eckardt symptom score for achalasia. The final score (range 0–12) is a sum of the four component scores, with higher scores indicating more severe symptoms

	Score			
Symptom	0	1	2	3
Dysphagia	None	Occasional	Daily	With every meal
Regurgitation	None	Occasional	Daily	With every meal
Chest pain	None	Occasional	Daily	Several times a day
Weight loss (kg)	0	<5	5–10	>10

Table 40.2 Published outcomes of greater than 2 years after POEM for treatment of achalasia

Study	Number of patients	Follow-up interval (months)	Treatment success rate	Postoperative GER
Werner et al. [16]	80	29	79%	NR
Hungess et al. [7]	112	24	92%	40%
Nabi et al. [15]	172 (with 2-year follow-up)	24	91%	28%
Teitelbaum et al. [17]	23	65	83%	38%

GER gastroesophageal reflux, *NR* not reported

success" (i.e., an Eckardt score ≤ 3) at 2 years post-intervention [2]. Other LHM series have shown similar results, with approximately 85–95% of patients experiencing significant relief of dysphagia [4]. Despite the initial success of these procedures, some patients go on to develop a recurrence of symptoms years later. In the European Achalasia Trial, for example, success rates for LHM and PD decreased to 84% and 82% after 5 years [3].

From the published data to date, POEM appears to be as efficacious as LHM for palliating symptoms of achalasia. Initial case series with 6–12-month follow-up showed excellent initial efficacy, with significant symptom resolution in 90–95% of patients [14, 15]. As with LHM, there appears to be some late-term symptom recurrence after POEM. Series with longer outcomes in the 2–3-year range have reported success rates of 79–92% [7, 8, 16], shown in Table 40.2. Our own recently published results at a follow-up interval of 5 years are the longest in the literature thus far. We found sustained symptomatic success in 83% of achalasia patients treated with POEM, and none required reintervention for persistent or recurrent symptoms [17]. As with LHM, dysphagia and regurgitation are improved in almost all patients after POEM, whereas chest pain is more variable in its response to treatment.

In addition to palliating symptoms, POEM results in a dramatic improvement in esophageal physiology. Uniformly across published series, follow-up high-resolution manometry has demonstrated significant decreases in EGJ resting and relaxation pressures, and timed esophagram has shown vastly improved esophageal emptying [7, 14]. A novel measurement tool, the functional lumen imaging probe (FLIP), measures EGJ distensibility, which has been shown to be a better correlate of post-intervention symptomatic success than manometric pressure measurements in patients with achalasia [18]. Intraoperative FLIP measurements have shown that POEM actually results in a greater improvement in EGJ distensibility than LHM, a finding that may predict superior postoperative symptomatic results [19].

There was early concern that POEM would result in unacceptable rates of postoperative gastroesophageal reflux (GER), because it does not include an anti-reflux procedure as is typically performed during LHM (in the form of a partial fundoplication). Thus far, it appears that POEM may in fact cause a higher rate of GER than LHM but that the difference is likely small. When measured by follow-up 24-hour pH monitoring studies, POEM series have shown abnormal rates of esophageal acid exposure ranging from 28% to 38% [15, 17, 20]. The literature regarding the incidence of GER after LHM is extremely variable, with randomized trials reporting abnormal 24-hour pH testing in 9–42% of patients [2, 21, 22]. It is likely that preservation of the phrenoesophageal ligament and angle of His during POEM is partially protective against GER postoperatively, resulting in a smaller increase in reflux than might be expected. It is our current practice to place all patients on a proton pump inhibitor or H_2 antagonist post-POEM and then test them off therapy at 1 year. Those with normal esophageal acid exposure at that point can stop their medication, whereas those with abnormal testing remain on lifelong anti-secretory therapy.

Patient-Specific Considerations

There are some important patient-specific physiologic and anatomic factors that may favor the use of either POEM or LHM. The first is patients with spastic or hypercontractile motility disorders such as type III achalasia, distal esophageal spasm, or jackhammer esophagus. In such patients, an abnormally contracting esophageal body is likely responsible for at least some of their symptoms, most notably chest pain. This is opposed to patients with type I and II achalasia, in which impaired esophageal emptying due to a non-relaxing EGJ is the primary pathophysiologic mechanism. During LHM, the proximal extent of the myotomy is limited to 6–10 cm cephalad to the EGJ. Therefore the entire contractile segment of the esophagus cannot be addressed in patients with spastic disorders, as compared with POEM where there is no limit to the proximal extent of the myotomy. Although the data are limited, it appears that POEM may result in superior outcomes in this patient subgroup. A multi-institution analysis comparing results in patients with only type III achalasia showed a higher rate of clinical response after POEM than LHM (98% vs. 81%) [23]. Not surprisingly, the average myotomy length was twice as long (16 cm vs. 8 cm) in the POEM cases.

Another important patient subgroup to consider is those with a hiatal hernia. In such patients, the normal anatomic anti-reflux flap valve created by the phrenoesophageal ligament and angle of His has already been lost. Therefore it stands to reason that if the LES is additionally ablated by a myotomy, the patient will develop severe reflux. Although limited to just a handful of patients within larger series, it appears that patients with preoperative hiatal hernias or those who develop them postoperatively will suffer from severe GER [7]. In our series, one such patient went on to require reoperation with a laparoscopic hiatal hernia repair and Toupet fundoplication in order to definitely control his reflux [17]. Thus, if a patient is found to have a hiatal hernia preoperatively, they would likely be better served by undergoing a LHM with concurrent reduction and repair of the hernia, as opposed to POEM.

Conclusions

While POEM is a relatively new intervention for the treatment of achalasia, there have been close to 2000 reported cases in the literature, and we are beginning to gain a firm understanding of the perioperative as well as short- to medium-term outcomes after the procedure. POEM is a safe operation as LHM and likely results in less pain and faster return to activities. In terms of relief of symptoms, the two operations appear to be equivalent, with the understanding that POEM outcomes have only been reported out to 5 years. There is likely a slightly higher rate of iatrogenic GER after POEM, but almost all patients with postoperatively reflux can be managed with medical therapy. Overall, both operations are excellent treatments for achalasia. POEM should no longer be considered an experimental procedure, and physicians should facilitate in-depth discussions regarding the relative advantages and disadvantages of each modality (including PD) so that patients can choose the intervention that best suits their preferences. In the coming years, POEM, LHM, and PD will all be considered reasonable, standard-of-care treatment options. However, it is possible that POEM will rather quickly become the procedure of choice, due to its unique combination of therapeutic efficacy, durability, and minimal invasiveness.

References

1. Boeckxstaens GE, Zaninotto G, Richter JE. Achalasia. Lancet. 2014;383:83–93.
2. Boeckxstaens GE, Annese V, des Varannes SB, et al. Pneumatic dilation versus laparoscopic Heller's myotomy for idiopathic achalasia. N Engl J Med. 2011;364:1807–16.
3. Moonen A, Annese V, Belmans A, et al. Long-term results of the European achalasia trial: a multicentre randomised controlled trial comparing pneumatic dilation versus laparoscopic Heller myotomy. Gut. 2016;65:732–9.
4. Yaghoobi M, Mayrand S, Martel M, Roshan-Afshar I, Bijarchi R, Barkun A. Laparoscopic Heller's myotomy versus pneumatic dilation in the treatment of idiopathic achalasia: a meta-analysis of randomized, controlled trials. Gastrointest Endosc. 2013;78:468–75.
5. Schoenberg MB, Marx S, Kersten JF, et al. Laparoscopic Heller myotomy versus endoscopic balloon dilatation for the treatment of achalasia: a network meta-analysis. Ann Surg. 2013;258:943–52.
6. Sawas T, Ravi K, Geno DM, et al. The course of achalasia one to four decades after initial treatment. Aliment Pharmacol Ther. 2017;45:553–60.
7. Hungness ES, Sternbach JM, Teitelbaum EN, Kahrilas PJ, Pandolfino JE, Soper NJ. Per-oral Endoscopic Myotomy (POEM) after the learning curve: durable long-term results with a low complication rate. Ann Surg. 2016;264:508–17.
8. Inoue H, Sato H, Ikeda H, et al. Per-oral endoscopic myotomy: a series of 500 patients. J Am Coll Surg. 2015;221:256–64.
9. Sharata AM, Dunst CM, Pescarus R, et al. Peroral endoscopic myotomy (POEM) for esophageal primary motility disorders: analysis of 100 consecutive patients. J Gastrointest Surg. 2015;19:161–70. discussion 70
10. Awaiz A, Yunus RM, Khan S, Memon B, Memon MA. Systematic review and meta-analysis of perioperative outcomes of Peroral Endoscopic Myotomy (POEM) and Laparoscopic Heller Myotomy (LHM) for achalasia. Surg Laparosc Endosc Percutan Tech. 2017;27:123–31.

11. Schlottmann F, Luckett DJ, Fine J, Shaheen NJ, Patti MG. Laparoscopic Heller Myotomy versus Peroral endoscopic Myotomy (POEM) for achalasia: a systematic review and meta-analysis. Ann Surg. 2017;267(3):451–60.
12. Patel K, Abbassi-Ghadi N, Markar S, Kumar S, Jethwa P, Zaninotto G. Peroral endoscopic myotomy for the treatment of esophageal achalasia: systematic review and pooled analysis. Dis Esophagus. 2016;29:807–19.
13. Ward MA, Gitelis M, Patel L, Vigneswaran Y, Carbray J, Ujiki MB. Outcomes in patients with over 1-year follow-up after peroral endoscopic myotomy (POEM). Surg Endosc. 2017;31:1550–7.
14. Bhayani NH, Kurian AA, Dunst CM, Sharata AM, Rieder E, Swanstrom LL. A comparative study on comprehensive, objective outcomes of laparoscopic Heller myotomy with per-oral endoscopic myotomy (POEM) for achalasia. Ann Surg. 2014;259:1098–103.
15. Nabi Z, Ramchandani M, Chavan R, et al. Per-oral endoscopic myotomy for achalasia cardia: outcomes in over 400 consecutive patients. Endosc Int Open. 2017;5:E331–E9.
16. Werner YB, Costamagna G, Swanstrom LL, et al. Clinical response to peroral endoscopic myotomy in patients with idiopathic achalasia at a minimum follow-up of 2 years. Gut. 2016;65:899–906.
17. Teitelbaum EN, Dunst CM, Reavis KM, et al. Clinical outcomes five years after POEM for treatment of primary esophageal motility disorders. Surg Endosc. 2017;32(1):421–7.
18. Rohof WO, Hirsch DP, Kessing BF, Boeckxstaens GE. Efficacy of treatment for patients with achalasia depends on the distensibility of the esophagogastric junction. Gastroenterology. 2012;143:328–35.
19. Teitelbaum EN, Soper NJ, Pandolfino JE, et al. Esophagogastric junction distensibility measurements during Heller myotomy and POEM for achalasia predict postoperative symptomatic outcomes. Surg Endosc. 2015;29:522–8.
20. Teitelbaum EN, Soper NJ, Santos BF, et al. Symptomatic and physiologic outcomes one year after peroral esophageal myotomy (POEM) for treatment of achalasia. Surg Endosc. 2014;28:3359–65.
21. Rawlings A, Soper NJ, Oelschlager B, et al. Laparoscopic dor versus Toupet fundoplication following Heller myotomy for achalasia: results of a multicenter, prospective, randomized-controlled trial. Surg Endosc. 2012;26:18–26.
22. Richards WO, Torquati A, Holzman MD, et al. Heller myotomy versus Heller myotomy with Dor fundoplication for achalasia: a prospective randomized double-blind clinical trial. Ann Surg. 2004;240:405–12. discussion 12-5
23. Kumbhari V, Tieu AH, Onimaru M, et al. Peroral endoscopic myotomy (POEM) vs laparoscopic Heller myotomy (LHM) for the treatment of Type III achalasia in 75 patients: a multicenter comparative study. Endosc Int Open. 2015;3:E195–201.

Diagnosis and Medical Management of Other Esophageal Motility Disorders

41

Mohammed Zakari, William Hirsch, and Anthony Lembo

Diffuse Esophageal Spasm (DES)

Definition and Epidemiology

DES is characterized by uncoordinated contractions of the smooth muscle portion of the esophagus that manifest clinically with chest pain and dysphagia. DES is uncommon, occurring in only 24 (2.2%) of 1070 consecutive patients evaluated by high-resolution manometry (HRM) [1], and may occur more commonly in women and the elderly [2].

Pathophysiology and Pathogenesis

DES is believed to result from an imbalance between excitatory and inhibitory innervation of the esophagus leading to premature and simultaneous contractions. Gastroesophageal reflux disease (GERD) coexists with DES in up to 70% of patients [2, 3], though its role in the pathogenesis of DES is controversial. Thickening of the muscularis propria and lower esophageal sphincter (LES) has been reported in patients with DES [4, 5]; the significance of these findings remains unclear. Finally, DES has also been associated with opioid intake [6].

M. Zakari · W. Hirsch · A. Lembo (✉)
Division of Gastroenterology, Department of Medicine, Beth Israel Deaconess Medical Center, Boston, MA, USA
e-mail: alembo@bidmc.harvard.edu

J. Grams et al. (eds.), *The SAGES Manual of Foregut Surgery*,
https://doi.org/10.1007/978-3-319-96122-4_41

Clinical Presentation

Patients with DES typically present with dysphagia and chest pain. Among 108 consecutive patients with DES, dysphagia for solids and liquids was present in 51%, while retrosternal chest pain was present in 29% [2]. Heartburn and regurgitation are also frequently reported. Dysphagia in patients with DES appears to be secondary to bolus entrapment in the spastic segment [7]. Chest pain in patients with DES is presumed to be due to the spastic contractions [8], visceral hypersensitivity [9, 10], or potentially GERD.

Differential Diagnosis

See Table 41.1.

Diagnosis

Esophageal manometry is generally required to definitively establish the diagnosis of DES. However, additional testing may be required depending on the symptoms at the time of presentation (Table 41.1). For example, if dysphagia is present, an

Table 41.1 Differential diagnosis of esophageal symptoms. Adapted from UpToDate

Dysphagia predominant presentation	Noncardiac chest pain predominant presentation
Intrinsic mechanical lesions Benign tumors Caustic esophagitis/stricture Diverticula Malignancy Peptic stricture Eosinophilic esophagitis Infectious esophagitis Pill esophagitis Postsurgery (laryngeal, esophageal, gastric) Radiation esophagitis/stricture Rings and webs Lymphocytic esophagitis	*Gastroesophageal reflux* *Non-reflux esophagitis*, e.g., medications, infections, or radiation injury *Eosinophilic esophagitis* *Esophageal motility disorder* *Functional chest pain*
Extrinsic mechanical lesions Aberrant subclavian artery Cervical osteophytes Enlarged aorta Enlarged left atrium Mediastinal mass (lymphadenopathy, lung cancer, etc.) Postsurgery (laryngeal, spinal)	
Primary motility disorders	
Secondary motility disorders	
Chagas disease	
Functional dysphagia	

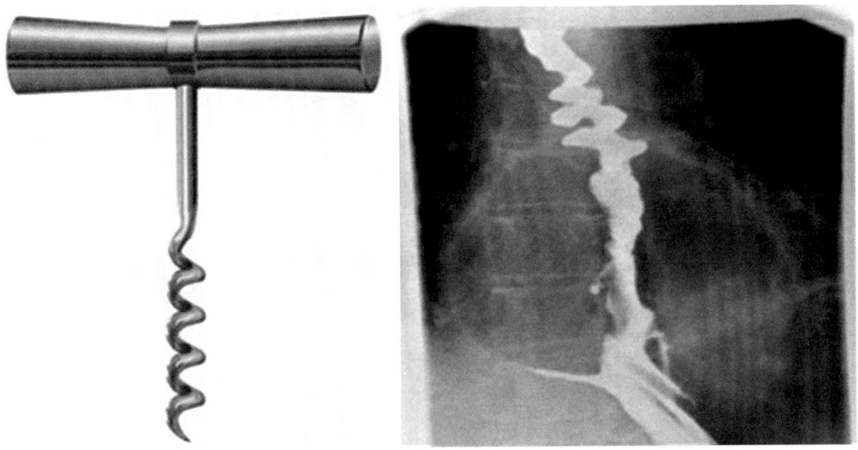

Fig. 41.1 Barium swallow shows the corkscrew esophagus (caused by multiple simultaneous contractions), which is suggestive of DES although not diagnostic

upper endoscopy should be performed to exclude structural pathologies such as stenosis, ring, neoplasia, or peptic esophagitis. An upper endoscopy is also necessary to obtain esophageal biopsies to exclude eosinophilic esophagitis. An endoscopic ultrasound is generally not required but may show thickening of the esophageal muscularis propria. It should be noted that this finding is not specific for DES [5, 11]. A barium swallow is frequently helpful in assessing bolus transit through the esophagus. The classic "corkscrew" is suggestive of DES though it is not diagnostic (Fig. 41.1) [2, 12].

Figure 41.2 demonstrates a normal swallow on high-resolution esophageal manometry. DES is defined manometrically by the presence of at least 20% wet swallows being associated with reduced distal latency (DL < 4.5 s) in the setting of normal lower esophageal sphincter (LES) relaxation (Fig. 41.3). The current Chicago V3 Classification for DES utilizes DL measurement rather than contractile velocity as the DL is more reliable in diagnosing DES [1].

Treatment

Pharmacological Treatments

Pharmacological treatment options include acid suppression therapy, smooth muscle relaxants, and neuromodulators. It should be acknowledged for all treatment options that there is a general absence of large, high-quality randomized controlled trials (Table 41.2).

Smooth Muscle Relaxants

Smooth muscle relaxants such as calcium channel blockers, nitrates, anticholinergics, sildenafil, and peppermint oil decrease smooth muscle contraction amplitude,

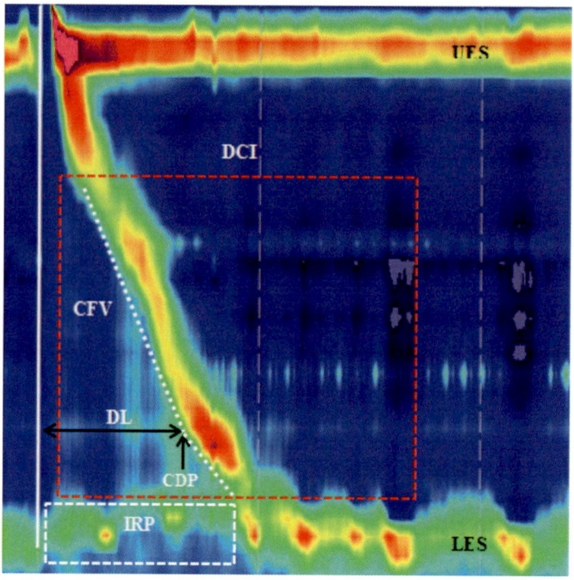

Fig. 41.2 Contractile deceleration point (CDP) represents the inflexion point in the contractile front propagation velocity in the distal esophagus. Distal latency (DL) measured from UES relaxation to the CDP (normal > 4.5 s). Integrated relaxation pressure (IRP) measures the effectiveness of the esophagogastric junction (EGJ) relaxation during swallow by measuring the average minimum pressure for 4 of the 10 s following a swallow (normal <15 mmHg). Distal contractile integral (DCI) measures the vigor of the esophageal contraction by combining the length of the esophagus with the contractile amplitude and duration (normal DCI >450 mmHg/cm/s but <8000 mmHg/cm/s). Contractile frontal velocity (CFV). Upper esophageal sphincter (UES). Lower esophageal sphincter (LES)

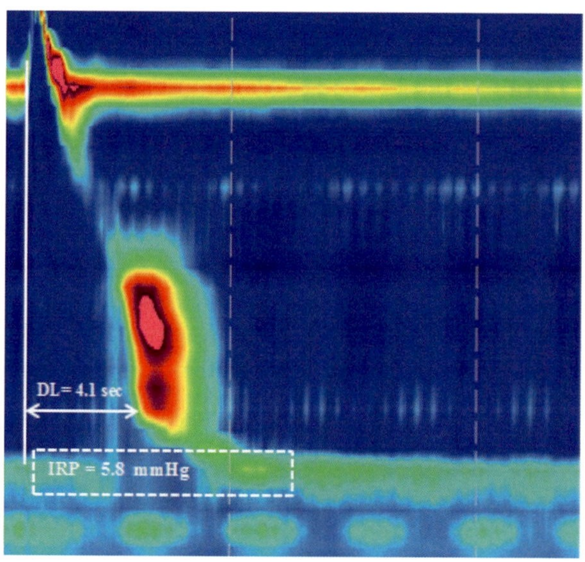

Fig. 41.3 Distal esophageal spasm (DES) is defined as a normal esophagogastric junction (EGJ) relaxation (i.e., normal IRP <15 mmHg) and at least 20% of premature contractions [distal latency (DL) < 4.5 s]

Table 41.2 Clinical trials of pharmacological treatment of diffuse esophageal spasm

Treatment	Dose	Type of study	No of patients	Outcome measure	Results
Nifedipine [13]	10 mg TID	Placebo-controlled; randomized; cross-over	20 mixed spastic esophageal motility disorders	Likert scale 0–10 (chest pain/ dysphagia)	Improvement in symptom score, LES pressure and amplitude of esophageal contractions
Nifedipine [14]	10–20 mg TID	Open-label	6	Manometry, symptom change Likert scale	5/6 (83%) at least 50% symptom relief; 60% reduction in spontaneous contractions
Nifedipine [15]	10–30 mg TID	Placebo-controlled	8	Pain or dysphagia as mild, moderate, or severe	No significant difference between frequency and severity of pain or dysphagia
Diltiazem [16]	60 mg TID	Placebo-controlled; double-blind; cross-over	8	Daily diaries using visual analogue scales for dysphagia and chest pain	Most patients had improvement in chest pain and/or dysphagia (although no significant difference between diltiazem and placebo)
Nitrates [17]	Variable doses	Consecutive	12	Symptom change	Unpredictable response in patients with GERD (7 pt), good response in the absence of GERD (5 pt)
Nitroglycerine [18]	100–200 μg/kg/hr	Consecutive	5	Symptom change and manometry	Improvement of symptom score and significant reduction in duration of contractions
Peppermint oil [19]	5 drops	Consecutive	8	Manometry	All patients had a complete elimination of spasm. Two patients reported resolution of chest pain

(continued)

Table 41.2 (continued)

Treatment	Dose	Type of study	No of patients	Outcome measure	Results
Sildenafil [20]	25–50 mg BID	Open-label	2	Manometry and symptom change	Improvement in symptoms (chest pain and dysphagia) and manometry
Trazodone [21]	100–150 mg	Placebo-controlled; double-blind	29 various motility disorders	Global improvement scores	Greater global improvement with trazodone. Resolution of chest pain
Trazodone [22]	15 mg QD followed by trazodone 50 mg QD	Placebo-controlled	9	Symptom change	5/9 psychiatric disorder; 1/9 improved on Isordil 15 mg. 8/9 improved with trazodone. Resolution of chest pain
Imipramine [23]	50 mg QHS, clonidine 0.1 mg BID	Placebo-controlled; double-blind	12	Symptom diaries, rating of chest pain	Imipramine group had 52% reduction in chest pain vs. placebo

thereby promoting esophageal relaxation. Among the calcium channel blockers, only nifedipine and diltiazem have been studied, though in small clinical trials (Table 41.2). The three trials with nifedipine have shown inconsistent clinical effects [13–15]. The only trial with diltiazem showed no difference over placebo [16]. The one trial with nitroglycerine and long-acting nitrites showed improvement in chest pain in patients with DES but not those with GERD-associated DES [17]. In an open-label case report in two patients with DES, sildenafil (25–50 mg twice daily), a phosphodiesterase type V inhibitor that potentiates endogenous nitrous oxide, improved dysphagia and chest pain as well as reduced spasm on manometry [20]. Finally, five drops of peppermint oil in 10 mL of water eliminated spasm in all eight patients, with resolution of chest pain in two of the eight patients [19].

Neuromodulator Therapy

Clouse et al. conducted a 6-week randomized, double-blind placebo-controlled trial with trazodone (100–150 mg/day) on 29 patients with DES and chest pain. The trazodone group demonstrated greater global improvement than the placebo group independent of manometric improvement [21]. In an open-label study involving nine patients with DES, the majority of which had major psychiatric disorders, only one patient responded to nitrates, while eight responded to trazodone (50 mg/day) [22].

Acid-Suppressive Medications

Currently no studies have been published specifically looking at the effect of PPIs in DES though several studies have shown PPIs to improve noncardiac chest pain [24–27], and therefore a trial of PPIs in patients with DES is generally advisable.

Endoscopic Treatment

Botulinum Toxin (BTX) Injection

By blocking the release of acetylcholine from the neurons at the neuromuscular junction in the myenteric plexus, thereby restoring the balance between excitatory and inhibitory neurotransmitters, BTX induces smooth muscle relaxation. In a prospective, double-blind, RCT in 22 patients (15 DES patients: 8 received sham, 7 received BTX), botulinum toxin resulted in significant relief in dysphagia in all 8 patients compared to patients who received saline injections [28]. Likewise, in a case report of patient with refractory DES complicated by chest pain and dysphagia, BTX injections (total of 100 U: 10 injections, starting at lower esophageal sphincter (40 U) and moving proximally along the esophagus (60 U) at 1–1.5 cm intervals) resulted in significant improvement in patient's dysphagia and chest pain [29]. It should be noted that BTX effects are generally of limited duration (i.e., approximately 6 months) and the effects of repeat BTX injections are unclear [30]. BTX injection is generally considered to be safe though complications have been reported [31].

Pneumatic Balloon Dilation

In one retrospective study from 1992 in patients with refractory DES, balloon pneumatic dilatation (rigiflex 30 mm or 35 mm) improved symptoms in 14 of 20 patients, including one patient who had an esophageal perforation [32]. Because of the associated risks and the fact that pneumatic balloon dilatation only treats the LES, this approach is generally not advised unless LES relaxation is compromised.

Surgical Treatment

Per Oral Endoscopic Myotomy (POEM)

Few case reports have demonstrated efficacy of POEM in the management of DES [33–35]. Nevertheless, long-term follow-up and randomized trials are needed to advocate this approach.

Prognosis and Complications

While evidence suggests that most patients with DES show symptomatic improvement over time [36], on occasion, significant troublesome sequels may develop in patients with DES. For example, progression from DES to achalasia has been documented in several studies [37, 38]. Potential risk factors for development to achalasia include the presence of dysphagia and simultaneous waves associated with low

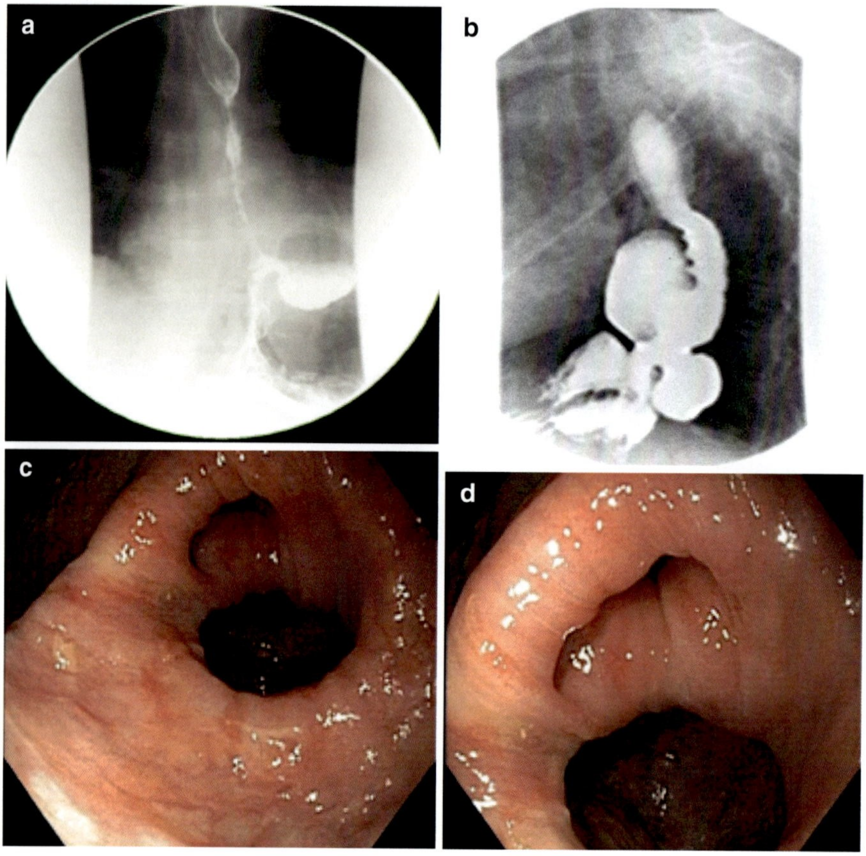

Fig. 41.4 Barium and endoscopic appearance of esophageal epiphrenic diverticulum

amplitude [38]. Likewise, esophageal epiphrenic diverticulum may develop as a consequence of DES (Fig. 41.4) [39].

Hypercontractile Esophagus (HE)

Definition

Hypercontractile esophagus (HE) is defined on high-resolution esophageal manometry by the presence of at least two swallows with very high amplitude of contractions (distal contractile integral (DCI) >8000 mmHg/sec/cm) in association with normal latency [40]. It is worth mentioning that this particular DCI value (i.e., >8000) was not seen in healthy subjects [41]. HE is often accompanied by esophageal symptoms such as dysphagia or chest pain, especially if at least two swallows have been recognized to be hypercontractile in an esophageal manometry study

[42]. In the Chicago V3 Classification of esophageal motility disorders, HE replaced "nutcracker esophagus" (NE) in its diagnostic algorithm [40] and is sometimes referred to as 'Jackhammer Esophagus'.

Epidemiology

HE is a rare esophageal motility disorder with prevalence estimate of approximately 4% [43]. Prevalence of HE seems be to slightly more common in females [43].

Pathophysiology and Pathogenesis

HE appears to arise from primary muscle hypercontractility secondary to an excess cholinergic activity [43, 44]. Increased esophageal muscle thickness has been observed [4] as well as discoordination between the contractions of the circular and longitudinal muscle layers of the esophagus [45–47]. HE is also associated with gastroesophageal junction (GEJ) obstruction [43, 48, 49]. HE may also develop as a consequence of an underlying gastroesophageal reflux [50, 51]. Eosinophilic esophagitis (EE) has rarely been associated with HE [52]. Finally, some patients with hypertensive contractions exhibit increased somatization, depression, or anxiety suggesting that psychological disorders may contribute to symptoms and potentially pathogenesis [53].

Clinical Presentation

Dysphagia and chest pain are the most common symptoms associated with HE. In a recent study, dysphagia and chest pain were reported in 67.6% and 47.1% of the patients, respectively [54].

Diagnosis

An upper endoscopy should be considered in patients presenting with dysphagia. If performed, esophageal biopsies are recommended to rule out EoE. Occasionally, robust peristaltic contractions can be seen causing, in extreme cases, difficulty in further advancement of the scope because of the resistance attributed to the hypercontractile segments [55]. EUS has a limited role though if concomitant GEJ outflow obstruction is present, it may be helpful in excluding mechanical causes for LES dysfunction [11]. Ambulatory pH testing may be helpful in understanding whether GERD is present, especially those who present with chest pain or reflux symptoms not responding to PPI therapy. Barium swallow may be helpful in patients with dysphagia to exclude subtle esophageal strictures or rings. EMS is the gold

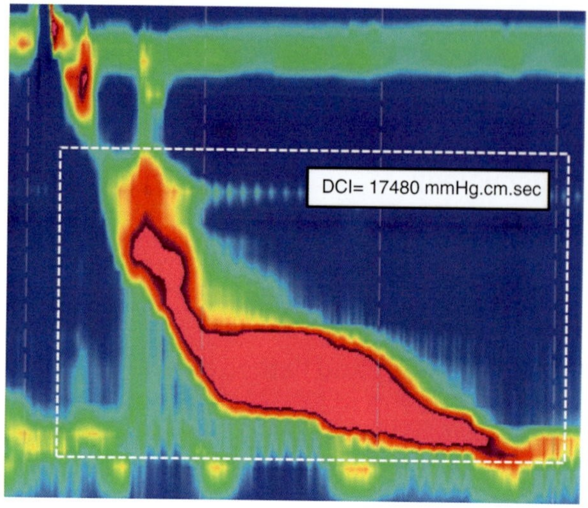

Fig. 41.5 Hypercontractile esophagus is defined as at least 20% of wet swallows associated with propagated contraction in the smooth muscle with a DCI > 8000 mmHg/cm/s with a normal distal latency (DL) and integrated relaxation pressure (IRP)

standard for diagnosing HE (Fig. 41.5) [56]. HE is defined by the presence of at least two swallows with very high amplitude of contractions in association with normal distal latency [40].

Treatment

The most effective treatment of HE has not been defined, and options include medical, endoscopic, or surgical therapy [57].

Pharmacological Treatment

Similar to other esophageal dysmotility disorders, pharmacological treatment options include nitrates, calcium channel blockers, phosphodiesterase-5 inhibitors, and proton pump inhibitors [57]. However, to date, no studies have been published with these treatments specifically in patients with HE. These medications may show potential benefits and should be attempted initially. However, they might be associated with some adverse events, and hence selection of certain treatment should be individualized and based on the patient's specific clinical presentation.

Endoscopic Treatment

Endoscopic treatment may be an alternative therapeutic option if patients do not respond to medical therapy. A recent retrospective study suggests that BTX injection (80–100 IU) in the esophageal body helps to improve symptoms in patients with HE, and this effect may last for more than 6 months [58].

Surgical Treatment

Few case reports have shown that POEM may be an effective management for HE [55, 59]. It allows for more extensive myotomy to involve the esophageal body where hypercontractility occurs [60]. Further conclusive evidence is still required to support its efficacy in HE and advocate this surgical option. Because of potential morbidity associated with POEM, this therapy should be reserved for the patients who are refractory to medical or endoscopic treatment.

Prognosis and Complications

The natural history and long-term outcomes for patients with HE are largely unknown. Several reports have documented progression of HE and nutcracker esophagus to achalasia [61]. Predictors of progression need to be determined though poorly relaxing LES (high IRP) may be implemented [62].

Absent Contractility (AC)

Definition

Absent contractility (AC) is defined in Chicago V3 Classification by complete absence of esophageal contractions in all swallows (100% failed peristalsis) with appropriate relaxation of the LES (i.e., median IRP < 15 mmHg) [40]. Since type 1 achalasia is also associated with 100% failed peristalsis, special attention to the LES is needed particularly when IRP values are borderline or when there is evidence of esophageal pressurization [40]. AC is commonly associated with systemic sclerosis (SSc) (hence the previous name "scleroderma-like motility pattern") though AC can be associated with other conditions, such as severe gastroesophageal reflux disease (GERD), diabetes mellitus, hypothyroidism, neurological conditions (e.g., Parkinson's disease, stroke), and other collagen vascular disorders (e.g., rheumatoid arthritis, systemic lupus erythematosus) (Table 41.3). Often a specific cause cannot be determined.

Patients with AC are particularly predisposed to severe gastroesophageal reflux and consequently its complications (Table 41.4). In addition, AC is characterized by poor esophageal bolus transit and therefore can be associated with significant dysphagia. Since SSc is the most frequently described and studied associated disease,

Table 41.3 Systemic disorders associated with absent contractility

Systemic lupus erythematosus
Rheumatoid arthritis
Amyloidosis
Severe gastroesophageal reflux disease (GERD)
Diabetes mellitus
Hypothyroidism
Neurological conditions (e.g., Parkinson's disease, stroke)
Post-fundoplication dysphagia
Chronic alcoholism
Severe esophageal candidiasis

Table 41.4 Predisposing factors to GERD in SSc patients

Predisposing factors
Impaired esophageal peristalsis (low or absent)
Reduced LES pressure
Delayed gastric emptying
Associated hiatal hernia (from shortening of the esophagus)
Autonomic nerve dysfunction
Associated sicca syndrome (due to reduced saliva production)
Decreased mucosal resistance

our discussion here is going to be focused on the esophageal involvement of SSc (or what commonly termed "scleroderma esophagus").

Epidemiology and Pathophysiology

The prevalence of AC appears to be more common in females than males [63]. In SSc, the smooth muscle of the distal two thirds of the esophageal body, including the lower esophageal sphincter (LES), is involved [64–68]. Patients with diffuse SSc are more likely to have AC than in those with limited SSc as well as patients with positive anti-Scl-70 antibody and negative anticentromere antibodies (ACA) [69, 70]. The cause of dysmotility in SSc is believed to result from a combination of vascular, neural, and myogenic dysfunction, leading ultimately to fibrosis and compromised smooth muscle function [71–75].

Clinical Presentation

Esophageal symptoms from AC include dysphagia (80%), heartburn, and regurgitation (78%) [76, 77]. In addition, patients with SSc are also at significant risk for complications associated with GERD (e.g., strictures and Barrett's esophagus), pill esophagitis, and candida esophagitis.

Diagnosis

Several studies can be utilized to evaluate patients with AC including barium esophagram, upper endoscopy, esophageal manometry, and 24-h pH study. However, the diagnosis is mainly established on esophageal manometry (Fig. 41.6).

Treatment

Early therapy is essential to reduce risk of developing serious complications from GERD. Anti-reflux measures such as avoidance of alcohol, smoking, NSAIDs, and dietary triggers (e.g., fatty food, chocolate, heavy meals before bed, etc.) as well as

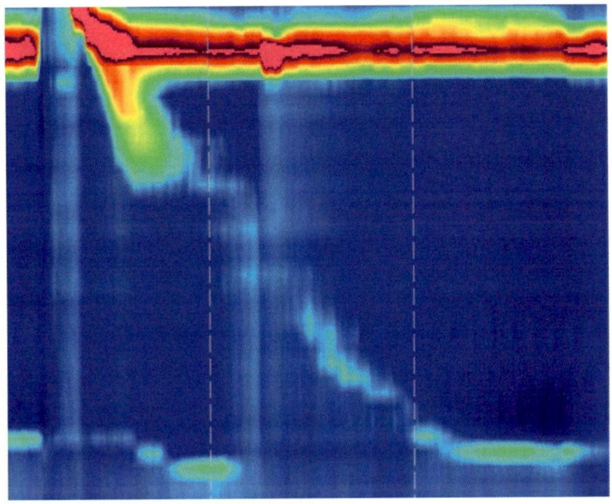

Fig. 41.6 Absent contractility (AC) is manometrically defined by failed peristalsis in 100% of swallows in association with normal EGJ relaxation (i.e., normal IRP)

sitting up during and after meals and elevating the heads of bed should be implemented. Despite these lifestyle changes, the majority of patients will require acid-reducing medications (i.e., PPIs). Most patients are adequately managed with once or twice daily dose of PPIs, though some SSc patients may require higher doses [78]. Weaning patients' PPI use to the lowest effective dose necessary to alleviate symptoms and heal esophagitis is reasonable.

Refractory patients with AC should only be considered for anti-reflux surgery when all other options fail. In general, partial fundoplication is preferred due to concerns of postoperative dysphagia.

Esophagogastric Junction Outflow Obstruction (EGJOO)

Definition

Esophagogastric junction outflow obstruction (EGJOO) is characterized by impaired EGJ relaxation (as defined by a median integrated relaxation pressure (IRP) of ten swallows that exceed the limit of normal (i.e., >15 mmHg) in association with preserved peristalsis of the esophageal body (Fig. 41.1)) [79–82]. It remains unclear whether EGJOO represents incomplete expression of an achalasia syndrome or a nonspecific finding of high-resolution manometry (HRM) measurements [83, 84].

Epidemiology

Among 790 consecutive HRM studies, 60 patients (7.6%) fulfilled the criteria for EGJOO [85]. In another study, the number of EGJOO cases increased from 1.7% in 2011 to 4.8% in 2014 [86]. EGJOO may be more common in women [6, 9].

Pathophysiology and Pathogenesis

EGJOO likely represents a heterogeneous group of conditions (Table 41.5). Undetected structural etiologies such as neoplasm, stricture, or hiatal hernia should be excluded [7, 21, 22, 24, 83, 87]. In a recently published study, among 39 patients who met the criteria for EGJOO, anatomic abnormalities were found in 21 patients (66%) [88]. Likewise, in another study among 49 patients with EGJOO, 22 patients (45%) were found to have an anatomic obstruction [86]. The size of hiatal hernias appears to correlate proportionally with the risk of outflow obstruction [86]; however, it should be noted that the crural diaphragm rather than the LES can be the cause of resistance to bolus transit resulting in outflow obstruction [79, 89].

GERD is commonly observed in patients with functional EGJOO [84] though it remains unclear whether GERD is a consequence or a cause of EGJOO [87]. The effects of opioids on esophageal motility have been evaluated in several studies [6, 90, 91]. In a new study, an increased EGJ outflow obstruction and other spastic esophageal motor abnormalities were more frequent in patients studied on opiates, suggesting that these medications may result in diminished inhibitory input [92]. Therefore, caution should be taken in interpreting esophageal manometry in patients currently taking opioids. An isolated elevated IRP value could be an artifact of the procedure. For example, the use of the 95% confidence interval to determine the normal upper value of the IRP causes 5% of normal subjects to have a high IRP [93]. In addition, diaphragmatic crural contractions due to the discomfort associated with the test can cause an elevated IRP values [94]. Other rare reported causes of EGJOO are shown in Table 41.5.

Table 41.5 Causes of EGJOO

Mechanical causes
EGJ and esophageal mucosal/submucosal neoplasm
Peptic strictures
Eosinophilic esophagitis strictures
Fibrotic stenosis (e.g., after radiotherapy/inflammation)
Sliding hiatal hernia
Paraesophageal hernia
Fundoplication wraps
Esophageal wall infiltrative process
Esophagitis dissecans superficialis
Obstructing esophageal varices
Gastric volvulus or malrotation
Functional causes
Early or incompletely expressed achalasia
GERD
Chronic opioid therapy
Technical limitations (artifacts)

Clinical Presentation

The majority of EGJOO patients have mild or intermittent symptoms of dysphagia, retrosternal pain, or regurgitation/heartburn [95]. It should be noted that a substantial number of EGJOO patients have no symptoms that can be explained by outflow obstruction [83].

Diagnosis

Evaluation of the esophagus with either upper endoscopy, barium X-ray, or both should be performed to exclude structural etiologies [96, 97]. The role of endoscopic ultrasonography (EUS) remains unclear but has been reported to identify significant lesions otherwise not seen by endoscopy or barium swallow [11, 85]. Computed tomography (CT) can also be helpful to exclude infiltrative or inflammatory disorders involving the EGJ and should be considered in patients with persistent symptoms despite negative evaluation [98, 99].

EGJOO is diagnosed on esophageal manometry by an elevated median IRP (>15 mmHg) in combination with preserved or weak peristalsis such that the criteria for achalasia are not met (Fig. 41.7) [80]. No manometric characteristics have been definitely reported to help distinguish structural from functional LES obstruction [86]. Mean IRP values appear to be higher in patients with achalasia compared to EGJOO from structural causes and lowest in the functional EGJOO group [84].

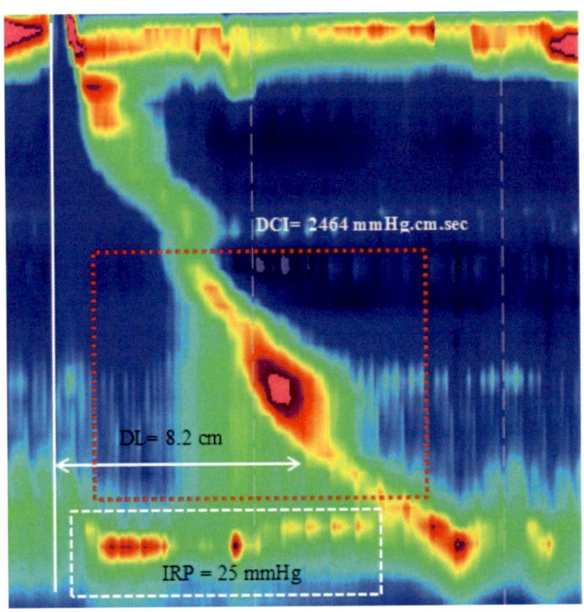

Fig. 41.7 EGJ outflow obstruction (EGJOO) is characterized by impaired EGJ relaxation as evident by an IRP >15 mmHg in association with normal peristaltic contraction

Functional lumen imaging probe (FLIP) is a new technology that offers a comprehensive evaluation of esophageal function by measuring the cross-sectional area and intraluminal pressure of the esophagus while under distension. The distensibility of the EGJ is assessed by a metric termed the EGJ distensibility index (DI), which was demonstrated to be abnormally low in treatment-naïve achalasia [100–102]. A recently published trial showed that EGJOO patients with normal EGJ-DI in the absence of radiological evidence of EGJ obstruction may follow a benign course, and subsequently expectant management is warranted [103].

Treatment

When present, anatomic abnormalities explaining the EGJOO should be corrected. Otherwise, EGJOO patients can be treated with Botox injections, pneumatic dilation (PD), or laparoscopic Heller myotomy [79, 84]. The decision of treatment should be guided by symptom nature, frequency, and severity. Importantly, a subset of EGJOO patients present with symptoms that disappear spontaneously, and waiting for some time seems reasonable before pursuing any kind of treatment [83].

A retrospective uncontrolled study assessed the effect of BTX injections into the LES in 36 patients with EGJOO and reported success with durable response for more than 6 months in 58.3% of patients, equivalent to that observed in achalasia patients treated similarly [104]. More recently, 60% rate of clinical response has been reported at 6 months in 6 patients with EGJ outflow obstruction [58]. Another study evaluating botulinum toxin injections in patients with EGJ outflow obstruction revealed symptomatic relief in 73% at 1 month [104].

Some authors perform myotomy in selected patients with functional EGJOO when early achalasia is suspected [84]. POEM was associated with better results compared to BTX injection and dilation in subjects with EGJOO [85].

Prognosis and Complications

Since EGJOO may progress to achalasia [62, 83, 105], patients should be followed closely. Future studies are needed to assess risk factors for determining which patients with EGJOO progress to achalasia.

References

1. Pandolfino JE, et al. Distal esophageal spasm in high-resolution esophageal pressure topography: defining clinical phenotypes. Gastroenterology. 2011;141(2):469–75.
2. Almansa C, et al. Esophageal spasm: demographic, clinical, radiographic, and manometric features in 108 patients. Dis Esophagus. 2012;25(3):214–21.
3. Herbella FA, et al. Primary versus secondary esophageal motility disorders: diagnosis and implications for treatment. J Laparoendosc Adv Surg Tech A. 2009;19(2):195–8.

4. Dogan I, et al. Prevalence of increased esophageal muscle thickness in patients with esophageal symptoms. Am J Gastroenterol. 2007;102(1):137–45.
5. Pehlivanov N, et al. Relationship between esophageal muscle thickness and intraluminal pressure in patients with esophageal spasm. Am J Physiol Gastrointest Liver Physiol. 2002;282(6):G1016–23.
6. Kraichely RE, Arora AS, Murray JA. Opiate-induced oesophageal dysmotility. Aliment Pharmacol Ther. 2010;31(5):601–6.
7. Behar J, Biancani P. Pathogenesis of simultaneous esophageal contractions in patients with motility disorders. Gastroenterology. 1993;105(1):111–8.
8. Tutuian R, et al. Symptom and function heterogenicity among patients with distal esophageal spasm: studies using combined impedance-manometry. Am J Gastroenterol. 2006;101(3):464–9.
9. Richter JE, Barish CF, Castell DO. Abnormal sensory perception in patients with esophageal chest pain. Gastroenterology. 1986;91(4):845–52.
10. Richter JE, Bradley LA, Castell DO. Esophageal chest pain: current controversies in pathogenesis, diagnosis, and therapy. Ann Intern Med. 1989;110(1):66–78.
11. Krishnan K, et al. Endoscopic ultrasound as an adjunctive evaluation in patients with esophageal motor disorders subtyped by high-resolution manometry. Neurogastroenterol Motil. 2014;26(8):1172–8.
12. Prabhakar A, et al. Relationship between diffuse esophageal spasm and lower esophageal sphincter dysfunction on barium studies and manometry in 14 patients. AJR Am J Roentgenol. 2004;183(2):409–13.
13. Nasrallah SM, et al. Primary esophageal motor disorders: clinical response to nifedipine. South Med J. 1985;78(3):312–5.
14. Thomas E, et al. Nifedipine therapy for diffuse esophageal spasm. South Med J. 1986;79(7):847–9.
15. Davies HA, et al. Trial of nifedipine for prevention of oesophageal spasm. Digestion. 1987;36(2):81–3.
16. Drenth JP, Bos LP, Engels LG. Efficacy of diltiazem in the treatment of diffuse oesophageal spasm. Aliment Pharmacol Ther. 1990;4(4):411–6.
17. Swamy N. Esophageal spasm: clinical and manometric response to nitroglycerine and long acting nitrites. Gastroenterology. 1977;72(1):23–7.
18. Konturek JW, Gillessen A, Domschke W. Diffuse esophageal spasm: a malfunction that involves nitric oxide? Scand J Gastroenterol. 1995;30(11):1041–5.
19. Pimentel M, et al. Peppermint oil improves the manometric findings in diffuse esophageal spasm. J Clin Gastroenterol. 2001;33(1):27–31.
20. Fox M, et al. Sildenafil relieves symptoms and normalizes motility in patients with oesophageal spasm: a report of two cases. Neurogastroenterol Motil. 2007;19(10):798–803.
21. Clouse RE, et al. Low-dose trazodone for symptomatic patients with esophageal contraction abnormalities. A double-blind, placebo-controlled trial. Gastroenterology. 1987;92(4):1027–36.
22. Handa M, et al. Antidepressant treatment of patients with diffuse esophageal spasm: a psychosomatic approach. J Clin Gastroenterol. 1999;28(3):228–32.
23. Cannon RO 3rd, et al. Imipramine in patients with chest pain despite normal coronary angiograms. N Engl J Med. 1994;330(20):1411–7.
24. Pandak WM, et al. Short course of omeprazole: a better first diagnostic approach to noncardiac chest pain than endoscopy, manometry, or 24-hour esophageal pH monitoring. J Clin Gastroenterol. 2002;35(4):307–14.
25. Fass R, et al. The clinical and economic value of a short course of omeprazole in patients with noncardiac chest pain. Gastroenterology. 1998;115(1):42–9.
26. Achem SR, et al. Effects of omeprazole versus placebo in treatment of noncardiac chest pain and gastroesophageal reflux. Dig Dis Sci. 1997;42(10):2138–45.
27. Bautista J, et al. The effect of an empirical trial of high-dose lansoprazole on symptom response of patients with non-cardiac chest pain–a randomized, double-blind, placebo-controlled, crossover trial. Aliment Pharmacol Ther. 2004;19(10):1123–30.

28. Vanuytsel T, et al. Botulinum toxin reduces dysphagia in patients with nonachalasia primary esophageal motility disorders. Clin Gastroenterol Hepatol. 2013;11(9):1115–1121.e2.
29. Patel DA, Vaezi MF. A spiraling case of persistent dysphagia. Diffuse Esophageal Spasm. Gastroenterology. 2015;149(2):298–9.
30. Miller LS, et al. Treatment of chest pain in patients with noncardiac, nonreflux, nonachalasia spastic esophageal motor disorders using botulinum toxin injection into the gastroesophageal junction. Am J Gastroenterol. 2002;97(7):1640–6.
31. van Hoeij FB, et al. Complications of botulinum toxin injections for treatment of esophageal motility disordersdagger. Dis Esophagus. 2017;30(3):1–5. https://doi.org/10.1111/dote.12491.
32. Irving JD, et al. Management of diffuse esophageal spasm with balloon dilatation. Gastrointest Radiol. 1992;17(3):189–92.
33. Minami H, et al. Peroral endoscopic myotomy (POEM) for diffuse esophageal spasm. Endoscopy. 2014;46(Suppl 1 UCTN):E79–81.
34. Louis H, et al. Distal esophageal spasm treated by peroral endoscopic myotomy. Am J Gastroenterol. 2012;107(12):1926–7.
35. Shiwaku H, et al. Successful treatment of diffuse esophageal spasm by peroral endoscopic myotomy. Gastrointest Endosc. 2013;77(1):149–50.
36. Spencer HL, Smith L, Riley SA. A questionnaire study to assess long-term outcome in patients with abnormal esophageal manometry. Dysphagia. 2006;21(3):149–55.
37. Khatami SS, et al. Does diffuse esophageal spasm progress to achalasia? A prospective cohort study. Dig Dis Sci. 2005;50(9):1605–10.
38. Fontes LH, et al. Progression of diffuse esophageal spasm to achalasia: incidence and predictive factors. Dis Esophagus. 2013;26(5):470–4.
39. Tedesco P, et al. Cause and treatment of epiphrenic diverticula. Am J Surg. 2005;190(6):891–4.
40. Roman S, Kahrilas PJ. Distal esophageal spasm. Curr Opin Gastroenterol. 2015;31(4):328–33.
41. Pandolfino JE, et al. Classifying esophageal motility by pressure topography characteristics: a study of 400 patients and 75 controls. Am J Gastroenterol. 2008;103(1):27–37.
42. Kushnir VM, Prakash Gyawali C. High resolution manometry patterns distinguish acid sensitivity in non-cardiac chest pain. Neurogastroenterol Motil. 2011;23(12):1066–72.
43. Roman S, et al. Phenotypes and clinical context of hypercontractility in high-resolution esophageal pressure topography (EPT). Am J Gastroenterol. 2012;107(1):37–45.
44. Brito EM, et al. Effect of different swallow time intervals on the nutcracker esophagus. Am J Gastroenterol. 2003;98(1):40–5.
45. Jung HY, et al. Asynchrony between the circular and the longitudinal muscle contraction in patients with nutcracker esophagus. Gastroenterology. 2005;128(5):1179–86.
46. Sugarbaker DJ, Rattan S, Goyal RK. Mechanical and electrical activity of esophageal smooth muscle during peristalsis. Am J Phys. 1984;246(2 Pt 1):G145–50.
47. Sugarbaker DJ, Rattan S, Goyal RK. Swallowing induces sequential activation of esophageal longitudinal smooth muscle. Am J Phys. 1984;247(5 Pt 1):G515–9.
48. Burton PR, et al. The effect of laparoscopic adjustable gastric bands on esophageal motility and the gastroesophageal junction: analysis using high-resolution video manometry. Obes Surg. 2009;19(7):905–14.
49. Mittal RK, et al. Modulation of feline esophageal contractions by bolus volume and outflow obstruction. Am J Phys. 1990;258(2 Pt 1):G208–15.
50. Mallet AL, et al. Prevalence and characteristics of acid gastro-oesophageal reflux disease in Jackhammer oesophagus. Dig Liver Dis. 2016;48(10):1136–41.
51. Achem SR, et al. Chest pain associated with nutcracker esophagus: a preliminary study of the role of gastroesophageal reflux. Am J Gastroenterol. 1993;88(2):187–92.
52. Melchior C, et al. Recovery of a "Jackhammer esophagus" after the treatment of an eosinophilic esophagitis. Am J Gastroenterol. 2012;107(6):952–4; author reply 954–5.
53. Song CW, et al. Inconsistent association of esophageal symptoms, psychometric abnormalities and dysmotility. Am J Gastroenterol. 2001;96(8):2312–6.

54. Herregods TV, et al. Jackhammer esophagus: observations on a European cohort. Neurogastroenterol Motil. 2016;
55. Ko WJ, et al. Jackhammer esophagus treated by a peroral endoscopic myotomy. Korean J Gastroenterol. 2014;64(6):370–4.
56. Pandolfino JE, Kahrilas PJ, A. American Gastroenterological. AGA technical review on the clinical use of esophageal manometry. Gastroenterology. 2005;128(1):209–24.
57. Roman S, Kahrilas PJ. Management of spastic disorders of the esophagus. Gastroenterol Clin N Am. 2013;42(1):27–43.
58. Marjoux S, et al. Botulinum toxin injection for hypercontractile or spastic esophageal motility disorders: may high-resolution manometry help to select cases? Dis Esophagus. 2015;28(8):735–41.
59. Kandulski A, et al. Jackhammer esophagus: high-resolution manometry and therapeutic approach using peroral endoscopic myotomy (POEM). Dis Esophagus. 2016;29(6):695–6.
60. Khashab MA, et al. Jet injection of dyed saline facilitates efficient peroral endoscopic myotomy. Endoscopy. 2014;46(4):298–301.
61. Abdallah J, Fass R. Progression of Jackhammer esophagus to type II achalasia. J Neurogastroenterol Motil. 2016;22(1):153–6.
62. Huang L, Pimentel M, Rezaie A. Do Jackhammer contractions lead to achalasia? A longitudinal study. Neurogastroenterol Motil. 2016;29(3) https://doi.org/10.1111/nmo.12953.
63. Calderaro DC, de Carvalho MA, Moretzsohn LD. Esophageal manometry in 28 systemic sclerosis Brazilian patients: findings and correlations. Dis Esophagus. 2009;22(8):700–4.
64. Ebert EC. Esophageal disease in scleroderma. J Clin Gastroenterol. 2006;40(9):769–75.
65. Ntoumazios SK, et al. Esophageal involvement in scleroderma: gastroesophageal reflux, the common problem. Semin Arthritis Rheum. 2006;36(3):173–81.
66. Szamosi S, Szekanecz Z, Szucs G. Gastrointestinal manifestations in Hungarian scleroderma patients. Rheumatol Int. 2006;26(12):1120–4.
67. Marie I, et al. Oesophageal mucosal involvement in patients with systemic sclerosis receiving proton pump inhibitor therapy. Aliment Pharmacol Ther. 2006;24(11–12):1593–601.
68. Treacy WL, et al. Scleroderma of the esophagus. A correlation of histologic and physiologic findings. Ann Intern Med. 1963;59:351–6.
69. Vischio J, et al. Progression of esophageal dysmotility in systemic sclerosis. J Rheumatol. 2012;39(5):986–91.
70. Airo P, et al. Oesophageal manometry in early and definite systemic sclerosis. Clin Rheumatol. 2005;24(4):370–6.
71. Sjogren RW. Gastrointestinal motility disorders in scleroderma. Arthritis Rheum. 1994;37(9):1265–82.
72. Kaye SA, et al. Ischaemia of the small intestine in patients with systemic sclerosis: Raynaud's phenomenon or chronic vasculopathy? QJM. 1994;87(8):495–500.
73. Pitrez EH, et al. Oesophageal dysmotility in systemic sclerosis: comparison of HRCT and scintigraphy. Br J Radiol. 2006;79(945):719–24.
74. Manetti M, et al. Severe fibrosis and increased expression of fibrogenic cytokines in the gastric wall of systemic sclerosis patients. Arthritis Rheum. 2007;56(10):3442–7.
75. Kahari VM. Activation of dermal connective tissue in scleroderma. Ann Med. 1993;25(6):511–8.
76. Santos-Navarro RR, et al. Clinical, endoscopic and manometric findings in the gastroesophageal tract of patients with systemic sclerosis. Rev Med Inst Mex Seguro Soc. 2008;46(5):503–10.
77. Abu-Shakra M, Guillemin F, Lee P. Gastrointestinal manifestations of systemic sclerosis. Semin Arthritis Rheum. 1994;24(1):29–39.
78. Hendel L, et al. Omeprazole in the long-term treatment of severe gastro-oesophageal reflux disease in patients with systemic sclerosis. Aliment Pharmacol Ther. 1992;6(5):565–77.
79. Scherer JR, et al. Functional esophagogastric junction obstruction with intact peristalsis: a heterogeneous syndrome sometimes akin to achalasia. J Gastrointest Surg. 2009;13(12):2219–25.

80. Bredenoord AJ, et al. Chicago classification criteria of esophageal motility disorders defined in high resolution esophageal pressure topography. Neurogastroenterol Motil. 2012;24(Suppl 1):57–65.
81. Ciriza-de-Los-Rios C, Canga-Rodriguez-Valcarcel F. High-resolution manometry and impedance-pH/manometry: novel techniques for the advancement of knowledge on esophageal function and their clinical role. Rev Esp Enferm Dig. 2009;101(12):861–9.
82. Kahrilas PJ, et al. The Chicago classification of esophageal motility disorders, v3.0. Neurogastroenterol Motil. 2015;27(2):160–74.
83. van Hoeij FB, Smout AJ, Bredenoord AJ. Characterization of idiopathic esophagogastric junction outflow obstruction. Neurogastroenterol Motil. 2015;27(9):1310–6.
84. Poochong Timratana MJL, Nieman DR, Han MS, Christian G, Peyre CEJ, Watson TJ, Peters JH. The clinical spectrum of esophagogastric junction outflow obstruction identified via high resolution manometry. Gastroenterolgoy. 2013;144(5, Suppl 1):S-1099.
85. Okeke FC, Raja S, Lynch KL, Dhalla S, Nandwani M, Stein EM, Chander Roland B, et al. What is the clinical significance of EGJ outflow obstruction? Evaluation of 60 patients at a tertiary referral center. Gastroenterology. 2014;146:S-101.
86. Clayton SB, Patel R, Richter JE. Functional and anatomic Esophagogastic junction outflow obstruction: manometry, timed barium Esophagram findings, and treatment outcomes. Clin Gastroenterol Hepatol. 2016;14(6):907–11.
87. Perez-Fernandez MT, et al. Characterization and follow-up of esophagogastric junction outflow obstruction detected by high resolution manometry. Neurogastroenterol Motil. 2016;28(1):116–26.
88. DeLay K, Austin GL, Menard-Katcher P. Anatomic abnormalities are common potential explanations of manometric esophagogastric junction outflow obstruction. Neurogastroenterol Motil. 2016;28(8):1166–71.
89. Kaul BK, et al. The cause of dysphagia in uncomplicated sliding hiatal hernia and its relief by hiatal herniorrhaphy. A roentgenographic, manometric, and clinical study. Ann Surg. 1990;211(4):406–10.
90. Penagini R, Bianchi PA. Effect of morphine on gastroesophageal reflux and transient lower esophageal sphincter relaxation. Gastroenterology. 1997;113(2):409–14.
91. Penagini R, Picone A, Bianchi PA. Effect of morphine and naloxone on motor response of the human esophagus to swallowing and distension. Am J Phys. 1996;271(4 Pt 1):G675–80.
92. Ratuapli SK, et al. Opioid-Induced Esophageal Dysfunction (OIED) in patients on chronic opioids. Am J Gastroenterol. 2015;110(7):979–84.
93. Weijenborg PW, et al. Normal values for solid-state esophageal high-resolution manometry in a European population; an overview of all current metrics. Neurogastroenterol Motil. 2014;26(5):654–9.
94. Mittal RK, et al. The effects of psychological stress on the esophagogastric junction pressure and swallow-induced relaxation. Gastroenterology. 1994;106(6):1477–84.
95. Galey KM, et al. Atypical variants of classic achalasia are common and currently under-recognized: a study of prevalence and clinical features. J Am Coll Surg. 2011;213(1):155–61. discussion 162-3
96. Singh S, et al. Nonobstructive dysphagia in gastroesophageal reflux disease: a study with combined ambulatory pH and motility monitoring. Am J Gastroenterol. 1992;87(5):562–7.
97. Spieker MR. Evaluating dysphagia. Am Fam Physician. 2000;61(12):3639–48.
98. Roman S, Kahrilas PJ. Challenges in the swallowing mechanism: nonobstructive dysphagia in the era of high-resolution manometry and impedance. Gastroenterol Clin N Am. 2011;40(4):823–35. ix-x
99. Ghosh SK, et al. Impaired deglutitive EGJ relaxation in clinical esophageal manometry: a quantitative analysis of 400 patients and 75 controls. Am J Physiol Gastrointest Liver Physiol. 2007;293(4):G878–85.
100. Rohof WO, et al. Efficacy of treatment for patients with achalasia depends on the distensibility of the esophagogastric junction. Gastroenterology. 2012;143(2):328–35.

101. Pandolfino JE, et al. Distensibility of the esophagogastric junction assessed with the functional lumen imaging probe (FLIP) in achalasia patients. Neurogastroenterol Motil. 2013;25(6):496–501.
102. Smeets FG, et al. Esophagogastric junction distensibility in the management of achalasia patients: relation to treatment outcome. Neurogastroenterol Motil. 2015;27(10):1495–503.
103. Carlson DA, et al. Evaluation of esophageal motility utilizing the functional lumen imaging probe. Am J Gastroenterol. 2016;111:1726.
104. Porter RF, Gyawali CP. Botulinum toxin injection in dysphagia syndromes with preserved esophageal peristalsis and incomplete lower esophageal sphincter relaxation. Neurogastroenterol Motil. 2011;23(2):139–44, e27–8.
105. Shin IS, Min YW, Rhee PL. Esophagogastric junction outflow obstruction transformed to type II achalasia. J Neurogastroenterol Motil. 2016;22(2):344–5.

Other Esophageal Motility Disorders: Role for Laparoscopic or Endoscopic Myotomy

42

Francisco Schlottmann and Marco G. Patti

Clinical Presentation

Diffuse Esophageal Spasm (DES)

DES is defined by normal peristalsis intermittently interrupted by simultaneous contractions (simultaneous contraction >20% and <100%). It was first described by Osgood [1] in 1889, who reported a series of six patients with dysphagia and severe chest pain. DES is quite rare, with a prevalence of less than 10% in patients with dysphagia and/or chest pain and 3–5% in unselected patients undergoing esophageal manometry [2]. It presents with dysphagia (80%) and regurgitation (63%), followed by heartburn (51%) and chest pain (47%) [3]. Symptoms may occur during meals or physical exertion. Unlike achalasia, dysphagia is not progressive and weight loss is rare. Chest pain may mimic myocardial infarction, and it is usually described as a crushing or squeezing pain that can radiate to the jaw, arms, or back.

Nutcracker Esophagus (NE)

NE was first described by Benjamin and Castell in 1979 [4], and it is defined by peristaltic waves of very high amplitude and duration. Patients mostly complain of severe chest pain, while dysphagia, regurgitation, and heartburn are less common.

F. Schlottmann
Surgery and Center for Esophageal Diseases and Swallowing, University of North Carolina, Chapel Hill, NC, USA

M. G. Patti (✉)
Department of Surgery and Center for Esophageal Diseases and Swallowing, University of North Carolina, Chapel Hill, NC, USA
e-mail: marco_patti@med.unc.edu

J. Grams et al. (eds.), *The SAGES Manual of Foregut Surgery*,
https://doi.org/10.1007/978-3-319-96122-4_42

In fact, NE is the most frequent esophageal dysmotility disorder present in patients with non-cardiac chest pain [5].

Hypertensive Lower Esophageal Sphincter (HTN-LES)

HTN-LES was first described by Code et al. [6], and it is characterized by a hypertensive lower esophageal sphincter with normal peristalsis. Clinically, it is associated with dysphagia (71%) and chest pain (49%) [7].

Diagnosis

Barium Esophagogram

DES It may show indentations produced by dysfunctional muscle contractions that trap barium between contracted segments. This characteristic "corkscrew" appearance, however, is not specific for DES, and manometry remains the gold standard for the diagnosis of DES [8].

NE As all patients with NE have normal propagation of peristalsis, the barium swallow is often nondiagnostic.

HTN-LES It may show non-specific findings such as narrowing of the gastroesophageal junction with delayed esophageal emptying suggesting outflow obstruction.

Upper Gastrointestinal Tract Endoscopy

All patients with dysphagia should undergo an upper endoscopy in order to rule out malignancy. Clinical features related to malignancy-induced dysphagia are age over 60 years, presence of symptoms for less than 1 year, and weight loss over 20 pounds [9]. Findings suggestive of a primary motility disorder are found in 25% of the patients with DES, 0% of the patients with NE, and 50% of the patients with HTN-LES [3].

Conventional Manometry (Richter Classification) [8]

DES Simultaneous contractions ≥20% (but less than 100%) of wet swallows, intermittent peristalsis, and contraction amplitudes >30 mmHg.

NE Normal propagation of peristaltic waves, with a mean distal amplitude >180 mmHg, and duration >6 s.

HTN-LES Resting lower esophageal sphincter pressure >45 mmHg and normal peristalsis.

High-Resolution Manometry (HRM) (Chicago Classification) [10]

DES "distal esophageal spasm" ≥20% of wet swallows with distal latency (DL) <4.5 s and mean integrated relaxation pressure (IRP) <17 mmHg.

NE "hypertensive peristalsis" Mean distal contractile integral (DCI) >5000 mmHg/s/cm (but <8000 mmHg/s/cm which defines hypercontractile esophagus) and normal DL.

HTN-LES "EGJ outflow obstruction" Mean IRP ≥ 15 mmHg with normal or weak peristalsis (Table 42.1).

Multichannel Intraluminal Impedance

This test shows that patients with HTN-LES have outflow obstruction at the gastroesophageal junction but normal esophageal bolus clearance. Patients with NE have also normal esophageal bolus transit, while patients with DES present abnormal bolus transit [11].

Table 42.1 Manometric features of primary esophageal motility disorders

	Conventional manometry	HRM
DES	Simultaneous contractions >20% (<100%) Amplitudes >30 mmHg Intermittent peristalsis	DL < 4.5 s in ≥20% of wet swallows IRP < 17 mmHg
NE	Amplitudes >180 mmHg Duration >6 s Normal peristalsis	DCI > 5000 mmHg/s/cm in ≥20% of wet swallows Normal DL
HTN-LES	Resting LES pressure > 45 mmHg Normal peristalsis	IRP ≥ 15 mmHg Normal/weak peristalsis

HRM High-resolution manometry, *DES* Diffuse esophageal spasm, *NE* Nutcracker esophagus, *HTN-LES* Hypertensive lower esophageal sphincter, *DL* Distal latency, *IRP* Integrated relaxation pressure, *DCI* Distal contractile integral

Ambulatory pH Monitoring

When a manometric profile suggesting DES or NE is present, it is important to perform an ambulatory pH monitoring in order to exclude pathologic reflux. It is indeed known that these motility patterns can be due to abnormal reflux. If GERD is present, either medical or surgical treatment should be directed toward the control of the reflux [12].

Treatment

Since the cause of these disorders is unknown, treatment is directed toward symptom relief and improvement of esophageal emptying. Medical treatment, endoscopic treatment, and surgical intervention are the available modalities.

Medical Treatment

Treatments aimed to relax esophageal smooth muscle such as nitrates, calcium channel blockers, and antimuscarinic agents may be helpful. However, these drugs have modest effect on the resting LES pressure and do not improve LES relaxation in response to swallowing. Previous reports have shown inferior outcomes of medical treatment compared to surgery [13, 14]. Hence, pharmacologic treatment is of marginal clinical value and should be considered only in patients with mild symptoms.

Endoscopic Pneumatic Dilation and Injection of Botulinum Toxin

Symptom relief may be achieved only in patients who present with dysphagia as their main complaint and in whom manometry shows a hypertensive and non-relaxing LES [15]. Injection of botulinum toxin in the distal esophagus acts by decreasing the release of acetylcholine by nerve endings of the myenteric plexus. In some patients it may improve dysphagia and chest pain [16].

Surgical Myotomy

Minimally invasive surgery has replaced open approaches to perform an esophagomyotomy. The operation can be done through a thoracoscopic or laparoscopic approach. While the initial experience was through a left thoracoscopic approach [17], the technique eventually switched into a laparoscopic myotomy with a partial fundoplication. Drawbacks of the thoracoscopic approach included the need for a double-lumen endotracheal tube, one-lung ventilation, right lateral decubitus, limited exposure of the gastroesophageal junction, postoperative discomfort, and a high rate of postoperative reflux. These problems were mostly eliminated with the laparoscopic approach (single-lumen endotracheal tube, supine position, better exposure of the gastroesophageal junction, and ability to perform a fundoplication).

Laparoscopic Heller Myotomy and Dor Fundoplication Technique

The technique is similar to that of a similar operation performed in patients with esophageal achalasia [18]. In patient with NE or DES, the myotomy is usually extended more proximally on the esophageal body. The patient is in a supine position with legs placed in stirrups with knees flexed 20–30°. Five trocars are usually used for the operation.

We start by dividing the gastrohepatic ligament and identifying the right crus of the diaphragm and posterior vagus nerve.

Subsequently the peritoneum and phrenoesophageal membrane are divided, and the left crus of the diaphragm and anterior vagus nerve are identified.

The dissection should be continued into the mediastinum, lateral and anterior to the esophagus in order to expose 7–8 cm of the esophagus. No posterior dissection is needed if a Dor fundoplication is performed after the myotomy. The short gastric vessels are routinely divided.

The myotomy is performed using a hook cautery in the 11 o'clock position. In patients with the HTN-LES, the length of the myotomy is similar to that performed for patients with achalasia. For patients with NE or DES, the myotomy is extended more proximally, for about 8–9 cm proximal to the gastroesophageal junction, and then distally onto the gastric wall for 2–2.5 cm. The muscle edges are gently separated to expose the mucosa for 30–40% of the circumference.

A Dor fundoplication is then performed as previously described [19].

Outcome of Surgical Myotomy in Motility Disorders Different from Achalasia

Patti and colleagues [3] reported that in patients with DES, dysphagia and chest pain were relieved in 86% and 80%, respectively, after laparoscopic myotomy. In these patients the myotomy was usually extended more proximally than in patients with achalasia. Regurgitation was also significantly improved. Concordantly, Leconte et al. [20] reported significant improvement for dysphagia, pain, regurgitation, and heartburn in patients with DES after an extended myotomy and anterior fundoplication.

In patients with NE and chest pain, the results of surgery were disappointing with only 50% of patients experiencing symptomatic relief [3]. Dysphagia was instead improved in 80% of patients. Champion et al. [21] reported recurrence of symptoms (dysphagia or chest pain) in 75% of patients with NE submitted to myotomy and fundoplication. Overall, it seems that myotomy would be helpful only in patients with NE whose main symptom is dysphagia or when associated pathology such as an epiphrenic diverticulum is present.

Reports on myotomy for the treatment of HTN-LES have shown good results but are limited to a small number of patients [3, 22]. Tamhankar et al. [22] presented a long-term follow-up on four patients with complete relief of symptoms (dysphagia and chest pain) and complete satisfaction after the myotomy.

These data suggest that patient selection is of paramount importance. Most patients with DES and HTN-LES who complain of dysphagia improve after a myotomy. On the other hand, patients with NE whose main complaint is chest pain often do not have relief of the pain and can even develop dysphagia as a consequence of the myotomy [3].

Per-oral Endoscopic Myotomy (POEM)

In 2010 Inoue et al. reported the result of a new technique – per-oral endoscopic myotomy (POEM) in 17 consecutive patients with achalasia [23]. Since then, this endoscopic technique has been used in thousands of patients with achalasia in every continent, and most studies, albeit with a short follow-up, have documented very good results in more than 90% of patients [24–27]. Even though this technique was initially described for the treatment of achalasia, its indications have expanded to non-achalasia motility disorders such as DES, NE, and the HTN-LES [28–31].

POEM Technique

The patient is placed supine under general anesthesia. An overtube is placed, and the site for the anterior mucosotomy is selected by correlating with HRM parameters, usually 3–4 cm proximal to the upper border of the endoscopically visualized forceful esophageal contraction, in the 1 o'clock to 2 o'clock position on the ventral aspect of the esophagus. After injection of indigo carmine into the submucosal layer, a 1.5–2 cm longitudinal mucosotomy in the mid-esophagus is performed. A submucosal tunnel is then created with blunt dissection and carbon dioxide insufflation. The tunnel is extended past the esophagogastric junction for 2–3 cm onto the gastric cardia. A proximal to distal myotomy is performed with care to preserve the longitudinal muscle layers of the esophagus and stomach. Smooth endoscope passage through the esophagogastric junction, retroflexed evaluation of the valve, and a blanched gastric mucosa (distal dissection) indicate an adequate myotomy. The mucosal entry is then closed using endoscopic clips.

Outcomes of POEM in Motility Disorders Different from Achalasia

The largest series of non-achalasia motility disorders treated by POEM was described by Sharata and colleagues [32]. The authors studied the outcome of POEM in 25 non-achalasia patients with DES (5), NE (12), and HTN-LES (8) and compared it to the outcome of POEM in 75 patients with achalasia. The study showed that dysphagia relief was better in achalasia patients (98%) than in non-achalasia patients (70%). Similarly, complete resolution of chest pain was seen in 100% of patients with achalasia but in only 75% of patients with other motility disorders. Post-POEM ambulatory pH monitoring showed abnormal reflux in 38% of patients.

Recently, Khashab et al. reported their experience with POEM for the treatment of spastic esophageal disorders refractory to medical therapy [33]. In this multicenter study (11 centers), 73 patients underwent POEM: 9 patients had DES, 10 had NE, while the remaining had type III achalasia. The mean length of stay was 3.4 days. A good clinical response was obtained in 100% of patients with DES, 96% of patients with type III achalasia, but in only 70% of patients with NE. Ambulatory pH monitoring showed pathologic reflux in 68.4% of patients. Hoppo et al. studied the utility of POEM across the spectrum of esophageal motility disorders [34]. The procedure was performed in 25 patients with achalasia and 8 patients with non-achalasia disorders. Median length of hospital stay was 3 days. At a follow-up of 7 months, dysphagia resolved in 92% of patients with achalasia and 75% of non-achalasia. Chest pain resolved in 100% of patients with achalasia and in 80% of non-achalasia.

Conclusions

Non-achalasia motility disorders are quite rare, so only a few centers have experience with their diagnosis and treatment. Few points that deserve special attention are:

- The symptoms and the manometric picture of NE and DES can be caused by GERD. Therefore, in order to have a diagnosis of "primary esophageal motility disorder," GERD must be excluded by pH monitoring. A cardiac evaluation should be routinely performed when chest pain is present.
- POEM is a relatively new procedure. As a consequence, there are no studies with long-term follow-up and no prospective and randomized trials comparing it to pneumatic dilatation or surgical myotomy.
- Many studies have shown that after POEM abnormal reflux is present in more than 50% of patients when measured objectively by pH monitoring [24, 33]. Furthermore, the multicenter study of Werner et al. of 80 patients with achalasia has shown that at a follow-up of 29 months, 3 patients had already developed Barrett's esophagus and 1 a peptic stricture [35]. The risk is that by performing POEM we might end up trading one disease process (achalasia, DES, NE, HTN-LES) with another (GERD). Contrary to what is commonly quoted by the authors of POEM studies, the incidence of GERD after myotomy and partial fundoplication is around 10% [36, 37].
- POEM has been advocated in these patients as it allows a longer myotomy onto the esophageal body. However, a long myotomy can be performed through a left thoracoscopic approach and a myotomy from the diaphragm to the thoracic inlet through a right thoracoscopic approach [3].

- Overall, we feel that the key to success is based on a complete evaluation and a careful patient selection. The best results, regardless of the technique, are in fact obtained in patients with outflow obstruction and impaired esophageal emptying, a picture similar to achalasia. In patients with NE, particularly if chest pain is the main symptom and esophageal transit is normal, the results are poor.

References

1. Osgood HA. A peculiar for of esophagismus. Boston Med Surg. 1889;120:401.
2. Katz PO, Dalton CB, Richter JE, et al. Esophageal testing of patients with non-cardiac chest pain or dysphagia. Ann Intern Med. 1987;106:593–7.
3. Patti MG, Gorodner MV, Galvani C, et al. Spectrum of esophageal motility disorders: implications for diagnosis and treatment. Arch Surg. 2005;140:442.
4. Benjamin SB, Gerhardt DC, Castell DO. High amplitude, peristaltic esophageal contractions associated with chest pain and/or dysphagia. Gastroenterology. 1979;77(3):478–83.
5. Pilhall M, Borjesson M, Rolny P, et al. Diagnosis of nutcracker esophagus, segmental or diffuse hypertensive patters and clinical characteristics. Dig Dis Sci. 2002;47:1381–8.
6. Code CF, Schlegel JF, Kelly ML Jr, et al. Hypertensive gastroesophageal sphincter. Proc Mayo Clinic. 1960;35:391–9.
7. Gockel I, Lord RV, Bremmer CG, et al. The hypertensive lower esophageal sphincter: a motility disorder with manometric features of outflow obstruction. J Gastrointest Surg. 2003;7:990–6.
8. Richter JE. Oesophageal motility disorders. Lancet. 2001;358:823–8.
9. Moonka R, Patti MG, Feo CV, et al. Clinical presentation and evaluation of malignant pseudoachalasia. J Gastrointest Surg. 1999;3(5):456–61.
10. Pandolfino JE, Kwiatek MA, Nealis T, et al. Achalasia: a new clinically relevant classification by high-resolution manometry. Gastroenterology. 2008;135:1526–33.
11. Tutuian R, Castell DO. Combined multichannel intraluminal impedance and manometry clarifies esophageal function abnormalities: study in 350 patients. Am J Gastroenterol. 2004;99(6):1011–9.
12. Herbella FA, Raz DJ, Nipomnick I, et al. Primary versus secondary esophageal motility disorders: diagnosis and implications for treatment. J Laparaoendosc Adv Surg Tech A. 2009;19(2):195–8.
13. Patti MG, Pellegrini CA, Arcerito M, et al. Comparison of medical and minimally invasive surgical therapy for primary esophageal motility disorders. Arch Surg. 1995;130(6):609–15.
14. Storr M, Allescher HD. Esophageal pharmacology and treatment of primary motility disorders. Dis Esophagus. 1999;12(4):241–57.
15. Irving JD, Owen WJ, Linsell J, et al. Management of diffuse esophageal spasm with balloon dilatation. Gastrointest Radiol. 1992;17(3):189–92.
16. Miller LS, Pullela SV, Parkman HP, et al. Treatment of chest pain in patients with noncardiac, nonreflux, nonachalasia spastic esophageal motor disorders using botulinum toxin injection into the gastroesophageal junction. Am J Gastroenterol. 2002;97(7):1640–6.
17. Pellegrini C, Wetter A, Patti MG, et al. Thoracoscopic esophagomyotomy-initial experience with a new approach for the treatment of achalasia. Ann Surg. 1992;216:291–9.
18. Patti MG, Fisichella PM. Laparoscopic Heller myotomy and Dor fundoplication for esophageal achalasia. How I do it. J Gastrointest Surg. 2008;12(4):764–6.
19. Patti MG, Herbella FA. Fundoplication after laparoscopic Heller myotomy for esophageal achalasia: what type? J Gastrointest Surg. 2010;14(9):1453–8.

20. Leconte M, Douard R, Gaudric M, et al. Functional results after extended myotomy for diffuse oesophageal spasm. Br J Surg. 2007;94(9):113–8.
21. Champion JK, Delisle N, Hunt T. Laparoscopic esophagomyotomy with posterior partial fundoplication for primary esophageal motility disorders. Surg Endosc. 2000;14(8):746–9.
22. Tamhankar AP, Almogy G, Arain MA, et al. Surgical management of hypertensive lower esophageal sphincter with dysphagia or chest pain. J Gastrointest Surg. 2003;7(8):990–6.
23. Inoue H, Minami H, Kobayashi Y, et al. Peroral endoscopic myotomy (POEM) for esophageal achalasia. Endoscopy. 2010;42(4):265–71.
24. Familiari P, Gigante G, Marchese M, et al. Peroral endoscopic myotomy for esophageal achalasia: outcomes of the first 100 patients with short-term follow-up. Ann Surg. 2016;263(1):82–7.
25. Hungness ES, Sternbach JM, Teitelbaum EN, et al. Per-oral Endoscopic Myotomy (POEM) after the learning curve: durable long-term results with a low complication rate. Ann Surg. 2016;264(3):508–17.
26. Bhayani NH, Kurian AA, Dunst CM, et al. A comparative study on comprehensive, objective outcomes of laparoscopic Heller myotomy with per-oral endoscopic myotomy (POEM) for achalasia. Ann Surg. 2014;259(6):1098–103.
27. Inoue H, Sato H, Ikeda H, et al. Per-oral endoscopic myotomy: a series of 500 patients. J Am Coll Surg. 2015;221(2):256–64.
28. Kandulski A, Fuchs KH, Weigt J, et al. Jackhammer esophagus: high-resolution manometry and therapeutic approach using peroral endoscopic myotomy (POEM). Dis Esophagus. 2016;29(6):695–6.
29. Bechara R, Ikeda H, Inoue H. Peroral endoscopic myotomy for Jackhammer esophagus: to cut or not to cut the lower esophageal sphincter. Endosc Int Open. 2016;4(5):585–8.
30. Kristensen HØ, Bjerregaard NC, Rask P, et al. Peroral endoscopic myotomy (POEM) for nutcracker esophagus. Three cases with 12 months follow-up. Scand J Gastroenterol. 2014;49(11):1285–9.
31. Shiwaku H, Inoue H, Beppu R, et al. Successful treatment of diffuse esophageal spasm by peroral endoscopic myotomy. Gastrointest Endosc. 2013;77(1):149–50.
32. Sharata AM, Dunst CM, Pescarus R, et al. Peroral endoscopic myotomy (POEM) for esophageal primary motility disorders: analysis of 100 consecutive patients. J Gastrointest Surg. 2015;19:161–70.
33. Khashab MA, Messallam AA, Onimaru M, et al. International multicenter experience with peroral endoscopic myotomy for the treatment of spastic esophageal disorders refractory to medical therapy (with video). Gastrointest Endosc. 2015;81(5):1170–7.
34. Hoppo T, Thakkar SJ, Schumacher LY, et al. A utility of peroral endoscopic myotomy (POEM) across the spectrum of esophageal motility disorders. Surg Endosc. 2016;30(1):233–44.
35. Werner YB, Costamagna G, Swanström LL, et al. Clinical response to peroral endoscopic myotomy in patients with idiopathic achalasia at a minimum follow-up of 2 years. Gut. 2016;65(6):899–906.
36. Campos GM, Vittinghoff E, Rabl C, et al. Endoscopic and surgical treatments for achalasia: a systematic review and meta-analysis. Ann Surg. 2009;249(1):47–57.
37. Salvador R, Pesenti E, Gobbi L, et al. Postoperative gastroesophageal reflux after laparoscopic Heller-Dor for achalasia: true incidence with an objective evaluation. J Gastrointest Surg. 2016;21(1):17–22. Epub ahead of print.

Evaluation of Esophageal Diverticula 43

Saad Shebrain

Pathophysiology and Etiology

Most esophageal diverticula are caused by a primary motility disorder of the esophageal body and/or motor dysfunction [1, 2]. Anatomical and structural abnormality of the upper esophageal sphincter (UES) such as a noncompliant cricopharyngeus muscle as well as a structural or functional abnormality of the lower esophageal sphincter (LES) have been documented to be contributing factors in the pathogenesis of esophageal diverticula [3]. Mediastinal inflammation has been associated with mid-esophageal diverticula.

Classification

Esophageal diverticula are commonly described in the literature using a combination of classifications (anatomic, histologic, and etiologic). According to their anatomic location, there are three types: pharyngoesophageal (Zenker's diverticulum) in the upper esophagus, parabronchial (mid-esophagus, thoracic or mediastinal), and epiphrenic (lower esophagus). Histologically, there are two types of esophageal diverticula: true (also called traction) diverticulum that contains all three layers of the esophageal wall, namely, mucosa, submucosa, and muscularis, and false (also known as pseudodiverticula or pulsion) diverticulum that consists only two layers, mucosa and submucosa, which have herniated through the muscular wall (e.g., Zenker's diverticulum). Esophageal intramural pseudodiverticulosis (EIPD) is a type of pseudodiverticula that represent dilated excretory ducts of the submucosal glands of the esophagus [3, 4, 5]. Additionally, diverticula of the esophageal body

S. Shebrain
Department of Surgery, Western Michigan University Homer Stryker MD School of Medicine, Kalamazoo, MI, USA
e-mail: Saad.shebrain@med.wmich.edu

J. Grams et al. (eds.), *The SAGES Manual of Foregut Surgery*,
https://doi.org/10.1007/978-3-319-96122-4_43

can be classified as congenital, rare, or acquired (most common). Congenital diverticula mainly occur in the mid-esophagus [1, 6].

Acquired diverticula or pulsion diverticula occur as a result of elevated intraluminal pressures in the presence of an area of weaknesses in the wall of the gastrointestinal tract. Almost all esophageal diverticula are acquired pulsion-type diverticula and commonly occur in the upper and lower parts of the esophagus. They are associated with elevated intraluminal pressure secondary to underlying motility disorder.

Zenker's Diverticulum (ZD)

Since it was first described in 1769 by Ludlow and subsequently by Zenker in 1877, posterior pharyngoesophageal diverticulum is the most common type of esophageal diverticula, occurring in 70% of cases [7, 8, 9]. ZD usually presents in older patients in the seventh to ninth decade of life. Although commonly used, the term "pharyngoesophageal" diverticula is not accurate because these diverticula arise from the hypopharynx rather than from the esophagus. ZD is an acquired pulsion diverticulum characterized by herniation of esophageal mucosa and submucosa through a defective area in the posterior wall of the hypopharynx between the oblique fibers of inferior constrictor muscle of the pharynx and the transverse fibers of cricopharyngeus muscle (Killian triangle at C5–C6 level) [10]. Elevated pressure in the oropharynx during swallowing against a closed upper esophageal sphincter (UES) leads to herniation of mucosa and submucosa through this weak zone, therefore forming ZD. The combination of noncompliant cricopharyngeus muscles as well as the aging-associated loss of tissue elasticity and muscle tone in the hypopharyngeal area plays a role in this process. Anatomically, ZD is usually located behind the upper left thyroid lobe and is in close relationship to the thyroid gland, and this should be considered when evaluating a patient with cervical dysphagia and thyroid nodules and/or when assessing a patient with recurrent laryngeal lymph nodes who have had surgery for thyroid cancer (ZD) [11].

Other rare causes of pharyngoesophageal diverticula have been reported after anterior cervical spine surgery [12, 13]. Post-thyroidectomy weakness at the Killian triangle due to upper thyroid lobe removal can facilitate herniation of the diverticulum [11].

Parabronchial (Mid-Esophagus, Mediastinal, Thoracic)

These are the least common types of esophageal diverticula and consist of 10% of cases [9]. In the mid-esophagus, these diverticula develop due to an outward traction on the esophageal wall from an inflammatory process and adenopathy in the mediastinum (fibrosing mediastinitis), e.g., in cases of pulmonary tuberculosis and histoplasmosis, sarcoidosis, and other granulomatous diseases. Mid-esophageal diverticula typically present on the right side of the chest. Although rare, pulsion (false) diverticula of the mid-esophagus as epiphrenic diverticula are caused by motility disorders of the esophageal body such as achalasia, diffuse esophageal spasm (DES), hypertensive lower esophageal sphincter, or nonspecific esophageal motility (NEM) disorder. Mid-esophageal false diverticula differ from traction diverticula, and their symptoms are related not only to their size but also to the underlying esophageal motility dysfunctions [14, 15].

Epiphrenic Diverticulum (ED)

Epiphrenic diverticula are the second most common type of esophageal diverticula and consist of 20% of cases [9]. Epiphrenic diverticula, described by Mondiere in 1833, are false pulsion diverticula, located in the distal esophagus near the gastroesophageal junction and above the diaphragm [16]. As with mid-esophageal diverticula, epiphrenic diverticula are more common on the right side and tend to be wide-neck. There is a strong association between these diverticula and esophageal motility disorders [17, 18]. The pathophysiology of ED is similar to that of ZD and is related to elevated esophageal intraluminal pressure from outflow obstruction and hypercontractility of the muscular layer in the lower esophagus leading to the formation of diverticula [19]. Most symptoms associated with ED such as dysphagia, chest pain, and heartburn are most likely due to the motility disorder rather than the diverticulum itself [20, 21].

Epiphrenic diverticula can occur in the patients with chronic gastroesophageal reflux associated with esophagitis and strictures but are rarely symptomatic [22]. Other rare causes of diverticula of the mid and distal esophagus include iatrogenic injury to the esophagus and connective tissue disorders, such as Ehlers-Danlos syndrome due to defective collagen [23].

Esophageal Intramural Pseudodiverticulosis (EIPD)

EIPD is a very rare and likely acquired condition characterized by the presence of many small outpouchings in the esophageal wall postulated to be due to dilatation of the submucosal glands that communicate with the esophageal lumen. Inflammatory processes lead to obstruction of intramural ducts with subsequent dilation of these glands. Although most patients with this condition have underlying esophageal strictures or motility disorder, EIPD has been reported following the corrosive injury to the esophagus with strictures [24, 25, 26].

Epidemiology

Age: Most esophageal diverticula present clinically in middle-aged and older people. ZDs usually present in people in their seventh and ninth decades of life.

Gender: ZD is more prevalent in men than women (4:1 ratio).

Race: Esophageal diverticula are common in Caucasians. ZD rarely occurs in Asian people [27].

Clinical Presentation

Esophageal diverticula are most commonly asymptomatic. However, large diverticula are associated with esophageal symptoms, usually dysphagia, regurgitation, or chest pain. Extraesophageal symptoms such as aspiration-related pulmonary complications, e.g., pneumonia, pose a significant risk to the patients. Patients may present with a neck mass. ZDs are the most common ones to cause symptoms.

Esophageal Symptoms

The most common symptom associated with all types of esophageal diverticula and EIPD is dysphagia. Cervical dysphagia is more common with ZD, and it is related to both solids and liquids. This typically is a result from the underlying motility disturbance rather than from the diverticulum. Dysphagia could be secondary to compression on the esophagus in cases of large diverticula especially when filled with food or a bezoar.

Regurgitation, noisy deglutition, and aspiration may be related to large diverticula at any part of the esophagus. In patients with motility dysfunction such as achalasia, aspiration is more likely to be related to a weak esophageal clearance mechanism due to hypertensive lower esophageal sphincter that fails to relax or the absence of esophageal body peristalsis in advanced cases.

Accumulation and retention of undigested food and secretions in a large diverticulum can result in food regurgitation, halitosis, nocturnal cough, and even aspiration pneumonia, chronic malnutrition, and weight loss [28].

Rare Extraesophageal Symptoms

Pulmonary symptoms: A chronic cough should raise the suspicion for the development of a bronchoesophageal fistula in a patient with mid-esophageal diverticula. A nocturnal cough is related to aspiration of diverticular contents that could occur from large-sized diverticula at any location.

Hemoptysis: While rare, it could be potentially life-threatening. It can occur in cases of mid-esophageal diverticula due to erosion of lymph nodes into the major mediastinal vessels and the bronchial tree as a result of mediastinal infectious or inflammatory process.

Hematemesis: Occurs rarely and may result from food stasis, bacterial overgrowth, or chronic inflammation of a large diverticulum [29].

Neck mass: In cases of large ZD, a mass in the neck can occasionally be detected, mainly on the left side. However, large diverticula can expand bilaterally behind both thyroid lobes [30].

Malignancy: There is a potential risk for malignant transformation of the diverticular mucosa with untreated chronic inflammation. Most reports of concomitant cancer within a diverticulum have shown squamous cell cancer [31].

Physical Examination

Physical examination is most likely to be unremarkable with no visible clinical signs in patients with symptomatic esophageal diverticula. However, a large ZD may present as a neck mass. Pulmonary findings of aspiration pneumonia may accompany the presence of large symptomatic diverticula.

Differential Diagnoses

A. Dysphagia
   (a) Functional abnormalities.
      (i) Achalasia.
      (ii) Esophageal motility disorders (EMD)
      (iii) Diffuse esophageal spasm (DES)
   (b) Anatomical abnormalities.
      (i) Gastroesophageal reflux disease (GERD) with stricture
      (ii) Esophageal cancer
B. Neck mass

Preoperative Evaluation

Evaluation of esophageal diverticulum should aim at identifying patients who may benefit from surgical intervention. Assessing the severity of the patient's symptoms such as dysphagia, regurgitation, aspiration, and other complications is important in the surgical decision-making process.

Laboratory Studies

Most laboratory testing is not necessary and may not be helpful in the diagnosis. Complete blood count may show iron-deficiency anemia in patients with upper esophageal webs [32].

Barium Esophagogram

Contrast esophagogram and upper endoscopy are the most common modalities to diagnose esophageal diverticula.

A barium esophagogram is the initial diagnostic procedure of choice. It provides an outline for the anatomy of diverticula and may provide some clues to an undiagnosed underlying motility disorder.

Zenker's diverticulum can be seen filled with barium resting posteriorly along the esophagus near the pharyngoesophageal junction. ZD is best identified during swallowing on the lateral view, and it is typically seen at the C5–C6 level [33].

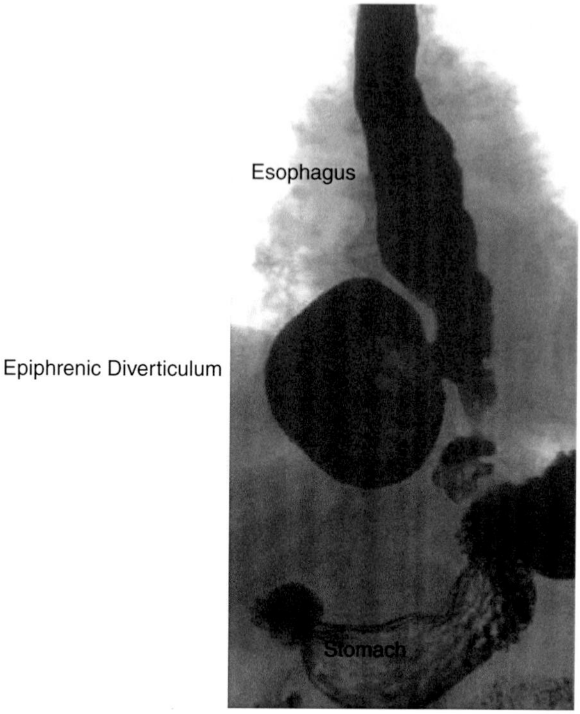

Fig. 43.1 Barium esophagogram showing epiphrenic diverticulum. (Courtesy Saad Shebrain)

In cases of epiphrenic diverticulum, the size, position, and proximity of the diverticulum to the diaphragm can be clearly delineated (Fig. 43.1). The underlying motility disorder is often identified as well. This helps dictate the approach to the diverticulum through a laparoscopic or transthoracic approach. Diverticula located more than about 10 cm proximal to the gastroesophageal junction can be treated using a transthoracic approach [34, 35]. Barium esophagogram enables diagnosis of esophageal intramural pseudodiverticulosis [25].

Esophagogastroduodenoscopy

Flexible endoscopy is a useful diagnostic modality in patients with symptoms of dysphagia or odynophagia, who have mid-esophageal and epiphrenic diverticula [33]. Endoscopy is unnecessary in a patient with Zenker's diverticula. In fact, it carries a potential risk of iatrogenic injury and perforation. An endoscopy helps evaluate for mucosal lesions, including masses, esophagitis, Barrett's esophagus, and cancer.

Esophageal Manometry (EM)

EM is the gold standard test to diagnose and classify the underlying motility disorder. It enables evaluation of lower esophageal sphincter pressure and relaxation, as well as of esophageal body function in symptomatic patients with a motility disorder such as achalasia or diffuse esophageal spasm. It has been reported that manometry results may not always be abnormal as some of these motility disorders may be episodic in nature [36]. Esophageal manometry is a prerequisite study when surgery is being considered, as it helps dictate the type of fundoplication to be performed (complete or partial) during preoperative planning.

High-Resolution Manometry (HRM)

HRM has been a revolution in the evaluation of esophageal motility disorders. It is a variant of conventional manometry. High-resolution pressure and impedance sensors spaced at 1-cm intervals from the pharynx to the stomach generate recordings that can be analyzed and presented either as "line plots" or as a "spatiotemporal plot." The data displayed in spatiotemporal plots create a "colored map" of the esophageal contraction, and this can visually distinguish clinically relevant abnormalities of motor function. This technology allows detection of segmental peristaltic defects, detecting motor defects in a higher number of patients with epiphrenic diverticula [37, 38, 39, 40].

Ultrasonography

Because of the anatomic proximity of the upper esophagus to the thyroid gland, ZD may mimic thyroid nodules on thyroid ultrasonography and can be distinguished from a thyroid nodule on ultrasound by the sign of air in the diverticulum [41, 42, 43]. In a case series in which an ultrasound was utilized, ZD appeared as a pouch-shaped structure at the posterior pharyngoesophageal junction that retained ultrasound contrast agent for longer than 3 min [44].

Computed Tomography (CT)

Large diverticulum of the esophagus and hypopharynx can be incidentally seen on computed tomography as a structure filled with gas, fluid, oral contrast material, or a mixture of these contents. A CT scan of the chest in patients with mid-esophageal diverticulum with a chronic cough or aspiration helps to make a diagnosis of a concomitant esophagobronchial fistula and to identify any mediastinal pathology.

Management

Medical Treatment

No treatment is required for patients with esophageal diverticula who are asymptomatic or minimally symptomatic. In many patients with mid-esophageal and epiphrenic diverticula, treatment of dysphagia should be directed to the motility disorder when feasible. Nonsurgical therapeutic options in cases of achalasia include pneumatic dilation and botulinum toxin injection into the lower esophageal sphincter (LES) [45]. However, surgical intervention with laparoscopic Heller esophagomyotomy remains the gold standard treatment [39]. Treatment of esophageal intramural pseudodiverticulosis is directed toward underlying strictures or dysmotility.

Surgical Treatment[1]

Symptomatic or large esophageal diverticula require intervention. The treatment ranges from minimally invasive procedures to major open surgical techniques. Treatment of Zenker's diverticulum is surgical and consists of either diverticulectomy or diverticular suspension with a myotomy of the cricopharyngeus muscle via a cervical approach [46]. Transoral rigid endoscopic stapled diverticulostomy may become the treatment of choice in patient with ZD, particularly in elderly and high-risk patients [47, 48, 49]. Flexible endoscopic treatment for Zenker's diverticulum is a feasible, safe, and effective treatment for symptomatic ZD, with a little adverse event and recurrence rates [50, 51]. Treatment of diverticula of the mid and low esophagus must consider any motor disorders or associated lesions at the time of intervention. Diverticulectomy with esophageal myotomy and an anti-reflux surgery are usually performed in cases of epiphrenic diverticula [52, 53]. Endoscopic approaches have been reported for mid-esophageal and epiphrenic diverticula and may become the standard in years to come [54].

References

1. Herbella FA, Patti MG. Modern pathophysiology and treatment of esophageal diverticula. Langenbeck's Arch Surg. 2012;397(1):29–35.
2. Jeyarajah R, Harford W. Diverticula of the hypopharynx, esophagus, stomach, jejunum, and ileum. In: Feldman M, Friedman LS, Sleisenger MH, editors. Gastrointestinal and liver disease: pathophysiology, diagnosis, management. Philadelphia: Saunders; 2002. p. 359–68.
3. Boyce HW Jr, Boyce G. Esophagus: anatomy and structural anomalies. In: Yamada T, editor. Textbook of gastroenterology. 4th ed. Philadelphia: Lippincott Williams & Wilkins; 2003. p. 1148–65.
4. Attila T, Marcon NE. Esophageal intramural pseudodiverticulosis with food impaction. Can J Gastroenterol. 2006;20(1):37–8. PMC 2538963 free to read.
5. Mahajan SK, Warshauer DM, Bozymski EM. Esophageal intramural pseudo-diverticulosis: endoscopic and radiologic correlation. Gastrointest Endosc. 1993;39(4):565–7.
6. Cassivi SD, Deschamps C, Nichols FC 3rd, et al. Diverticula of the esophagus. Surg Clin North Am. 2005;85(3):495–503, ix.
7. Ludlow A. A case of obstructed deglutition from a preternatural bag formed in the pharynx. Med Obs Inquiries. 1769;3:85–101.

[1] *Details are discussed elsewhere in this manual.*

8. Zenker FA, von Ziemssen H. Dilatations of the esophagus. In: Cyclopaedia of the practice of medicine. London: Low, Marston, Searle & Rivington; 1878. p. 46–68.
9. Carrère N, Pradère B. Esophageal diverticula. J Chir (Paris). 2004;141(2):85–92.
10. Cook IJ, Gabb M, Panagopoulos V, et al. Pharyngeal (Zenker's) diverticulum is a disorder of upper esophageal sphincter opening. Gastroenterology. 1992;103(4):1229–35.
11. Kim HK, Lee JI, Jang HW, Bae SY, Lee JH, Kim YS, et al. Characteristics of Killian-Jamieson diverticula mimicking a thyroid nodule. Head Neck. 2012;34(4):599–603.
12. Summers LE, Gump WC, Tayag EC, Richardson DE. Zenker diverticulum: a rare complication after anterior cervical fusion. J Spinal Disord Tech. 2007;20(2):172–5.
13. Tian H, Yuan W, Johnson JS, Chen H, Chen D. Pharyngoesophageal diverticulum: a delayed complication of anterior cervical spine surgery. Eur Spine J. 2011;20(Suppl 2):S211–6. https://doi.org/10.1007/s00586-010-1579-3. Epub 2010 Oct 8.
14. D'Ugo D, Cardillo G, Granone P, Coppola R, Margaritora S, Picciocchi A. Esophageal diverticula. Physiopathological basis for surgical management. Eur J Cardiothorac Surg. 1992;6(6):330.
15. Fékéte F, Vonns C. Surgical management of esophageal thoracic diverticula. Hepato-Gastroenterology. 1992;39(2):97.
16. Mondiere JT. Notes sur quelques maladies de l'oesophage. Arch Gen Med. 1833;3:28–65.
17. Melman L, Quinlan J, Robertson B, Brunt LM, Halpin VJ, Eagon JC, Frisella MM, Matthews BR. Esophageal manometric characteristics and outcomes for laparoscopic esophageal diverticulectomy, myotomy, and partial fundoplication for epiphrenic diverticula. Surg Endosc. 2009;23:1337. https://doi.org/10.1007/s00464-008-0165-9.
18. D'Journo XB, Ferraro P, Martin J, Chen LQ, Duranceau A. Lower esophageal sphincter dysfunction is part of the functional abnormality in epiphrenic diverticulum. Br J Surg. 2009;96(8):892–900.
19. Vicentine FP, Herbella FA, Silva LC, Patti MG. High-resolution manometry findings in patients with esophageal epiphrenic diverticula. Am Surg. 2011;77(12):1661–4.
20. Tedesco P, Fisichella PM, Way LW, et al. Cause and treatment of epi-phrenic diverticula. Am J Surg. 2005;190(6):891–4.
21. Herman TE, McAlister WH. Esophageal diverticula in childhood associated with strictures from unsuspected foreign bodies of the esophagus. Pediatr Radiol. 1991;21(6):410–2.
22. Toyohara T, Kaneko T, Araki H, et al. Giant epiphrenic diverticulum in a boy with Ehlers-Danlos syndrome. Pediatr Radiol. 1989;19(6–7):437.
23. Kochhar R, Mehta SK, Nagi B, et al. Corrosive acid-induced esophageal intramural pseudodiverticulosis. A study of 14 patients. J Clin Gastroenterol. 1991;13(4):371–5.
24. Long JD, Orlando RC. Esophageal submucosal glands: structure and function. Am J Gastroenterol. 1999;94(10):2818–24.
25. Herter B, Dittler HJ, Wuttge-Hannig A, et al. Intramural pseudo- diverticulosis of the esophagus: a case series. Endoscopy. 1997;29(2):109–13.
26. Ritz JP, Germer CT, Zimmer T, Isbert C, Buhr HJ. Esophageal hypermotility associated with intramural pseudo- diverticulosis. Primary esophageal disease or epiphenomena? Surg Endosc. 2000;14(7):681. https://doi.org/10.1007/s004640000139.
27. Siddiq MA, Sood S, Strachan D. Pharyngeal pouch (Zenker's diverticulum). Postgrad Med J. 2001;77(910):506.
28. Carlini M, Dell'Avanzato R, Miercadante E, Bazuroa ME, Curatola D, Castaldi F, Giovannini C. Surgical treatment of a severe, massive, symptomatic Zenker's diverticulum in a very elderly patient. Chir Ital. 2007;59(3):397–403.
29. Marcy P-Y, Benisvy D, Poissonnet G, Sadoul J-L, Thariat J. Zenker's diverticulum: the diagnostic power of ultrasound. Thyroid. 2010;20(11):1317–8. https://doi.org/10.1089/thy.2010.0140.
30. Sam AD Jr, Chaer RA, Cintron J, et al. Upper gastrointestinal bleeding caused by a "hypophrenic" diverticulum of the distal esophagus. Am Surg. 2005;71(4):333–5.
31. Bowdler DA, Stell PM. Carcinoma arising in posterior pharyngeal pulsion diverticulum (Zenker's diverticulum). Br J Surg. 1987;74(7):561–3.

32. Tobin RW. Esophageal rings, webs, and diverticula. J Clin Gastroenterol. 1998;27(4): 285–95.
33. Nuño-Guzmán CM, García-Carrasco D, Haro M, Arróniz-Jáuregui J, Corona JL, Salcido M. Zenker's diverticulum: diagnostic approach and surgical management. Case Rep Gastroenterol. 2014;8(3):346–52. https://doi.org/10.1159/000369130.
34. Fernando HC, Luketich JD, Samphire J, et al. Minimally invasive operation for esophageal diverticula. Ann Thorac Surg. 2005;80(6):2076–80.
35. Motoyama S, Maruyama K, Okuyama M, et al. Laparoscopic long esophagomyotomy with Dor's fundoplication using a transhiatal approach for an epiphrenic esophageal diverticulum. Surg Today. 2006;36(8):758–60.
36. Zaninotto G, Parise P, Salvador R, Costantini M, Zanatta L, Rella A, Ancona E. Laparoscopic repair of epiphrenic diverticulum. Sem Thorac Cardio-vasc Surg. 2012;24:218–22; Fulp SR, Castell DO. Manometric aspects of Zenker's diverticulum. Hepato-Gastroenterology. 1992;39(2):123.
37. Ghosh SK, Pandolfino JE, Zhang Q, Jarosz A, Shah N, Kahrilas PJ. Quantifying esophageal peristalsis with high-resolution manometry: a study of 75 asymptomatic volunteers. Am J Physiol Gastrointest Liver Physiol. 2006;290:G988–97.
38. Fox M, Hebbard G, Janiak P, Brasseur JG, Ghosh S, Thumshirn M, Fried M, Schwizer W. High-resolution manometry predicts the success of oesophageal bolus transport and identifies clinically important abnormalities not detected by conventional manometry. Neurogastroenterol Motil. 2004;16:533–42.
39. Clouse RE, Staiano A, Alrakawi A, Haroian L. Application of topographical methods to clinical esophageal manometry. Am J Gastroenterol. 2000;95:2720–30.
40. Aimi M, Mikami H, Izumi D, Okimoto E, Tada Y, Mishiro T, Ishimura N, Ishihara S, Kinoshita Y. Evaluation of intramural esophageal pseudo-diverticulosis using high-resolution manometry. Clin J Gastroenterol. 2016;9(5):281–4. https://doi.org/10.1007/s12328-016-0672-5. Epub 2016 Jul 13.
41. Cui XW, Ignee A, Baum U, Dietrich CF. Feasibility and usefulness of using swallow contrast-enhanced ultrasound to diagnose Zenker's diverticulum: preliminary results. Ultrasound Med Biol. 2015;41(4):975–81.
42. Pang JC, Chong S, Na HI, Kim YS, Park SJ, Kwon GY. Killian-Jamieson diverticulum mimicking a suspicious thyroid nodule: sonographic diagnosis. J Clin Ultrasound. 2009;37(9): 528–30.
43. Leboulleux S, Girard E, Rose M, Travagli JP, Sabbah N, Caillou B, Hartl DM, Lassau N, Baudin E, Schlumberger M. Ultrasound criteria of malignancy for cervical lymph nodes in patients followed up for differentiated thyroid cancer. J Clin Endocrinol Metab. 2007;92:3590–4.
44. Lixin J, Bing H, Zhang W, Binghui Z. Sonographic diagnosis features of Zenker diverticulum. Eur J Radiol. 2011;80(2):e13–9.
45. American Society for Gastrointestinal Endoscopy. Technology assessment status evaluation: botulinum toxin therapy in gastrointestinal endoscopy. November 1996. ASGE. American Society for Gastrointestinal Endoscopy. Gastrointest Endosc. 1998;47(6):569–72.
46. Bizzotto A, Iacopini F, Landi R, Costamagna G. Zenker's diverticulum: exploring treatment options. Acta Otorhinolaryngol Ital. 2013;33(4):219–29.
47. Al-Kadi AS, Maghrabi AA, Thomson D, Gillman LM, Dhalla S. Endoscopic treatment of Zenker diverticulum: results of a 7-year experience. J Am Coll Surg. 2010;211:239–43.
48. Huberty V, El Bacha S, Blero D, Le Moine O, Hassid S, Devière J. Flexible endoscopic treatment for Zenker's diverticulum: a systematic review and me-ta-analysis. Endoscopic treatment for Zenker's diverticulum: long-term results (with video). Gastrointest Endosc. 2013;77(5):701–7.
49. Wasserzug O, Zikk D, Raziel A, Cavel O, Fleece D, Szold A. Endoscopically stapled diverticulostomy for Zenker's diverticulum: results of a multidisciplinary team approach. Surg Endosc. 2009;24(3):637–41.
50. Bremner CG, DeMeester TR. Endoscopic treatment of Zenker's diverticulum. Gastrointest Endosc. 1999;49(1):126–8.

51. Visosky AM, Parke RB, Donovan DT. Endoscopic management of Zenker's diverticulum: factors predictive of success or failure. Ann Otol Rhinol Laryngol. 2008;117(7):531–7.
52. Fraiji E Jr, Bloomston M, Carey L, et al. Laparoscopic management of symptomatic achalasia associated with epiphrenic diverticulum. Surg Endosc. 2003;17(10):1600–3.
53. Del Genio A, Rossetti G, Maffetton V, et al. Laparoscopic approach in the treatment of epiphrenic diverticula: long-term results. Surg Endosc. 2004;18(5):741–5.
54. Bak YT, Kim HJ, Jo NY, et al. Endoscopic "clip and cut" diverticulectomy for a giant mid esophageal diverticulum. Gastrointest Endosc. 2003;57(6):777–9.

Cricopharyngeal Diverticulum: Open Repair

44

Kirk Withrow and Daniel Morrison

Definition

- Diverticula of the hypopharynx have been recognized for over 200 years. Zenker's diverticulum (ZD) is by far the most common with an annual incidence of 2/100,000 individuals [1]. Specifically, ZD is an outpouching of hypopharyngeal mucosa that protrudes through a weak area at the junction of the inferior constrictor muscle and the cricopharyngeus (CP) muscle, known as Killian's dehiscence (Fig. 44.1). The CP muscle is 2–5 cm long and serves as the upper esophageal sphincter. It generally exists in the contracted state except during swallowing.
- As ZD is only a mucosal sac that has herniated between the muscular layers, it is technically considered a "false" diverticulum. This is an acquired disorder that most commonly presents between the sixth and eighth decade of life and affects more men than women. In rare cases, there is a family history of ZD and evidence of genetic predisposition toward its development. Although the exact etiology of ZD remains debatable, most agree that it represents a pulsion diverticulum occurring due to a rise in intraluminal pressure relative to the resistance of the esophageal wall. While manometry data provide conflicting information about the role of CP muscle activity in ZD, functional outcomes and clinical observation support CP activity as an etiologic factor in ZD formation. This is evidenced by the fact that patients who did not undergo CP myotomy as part of their surgical management have poorer swallowing outcomes. Historically, ZD was first recognized by Abraham Ludlow in 1796 and was named after a German pathologist, Friedrich Albert Zenker, who reported a series of ZD patients in 1877 [2]. Wheeler reported the first successful open repair of a ZD in

K. Withrow · D. Morrison (✉)
Department of Otolaryngology-Head and Neck Surgery, University of Alabama-Birmingham, Birmingham, AL, USA
e-mail: kwithrow@uab.edu

J. Grams et al. (eds.), *The SAGES Manual of Foregut Surgery*,
https://doi.org/10.1007/978-3-319-96122-4_44

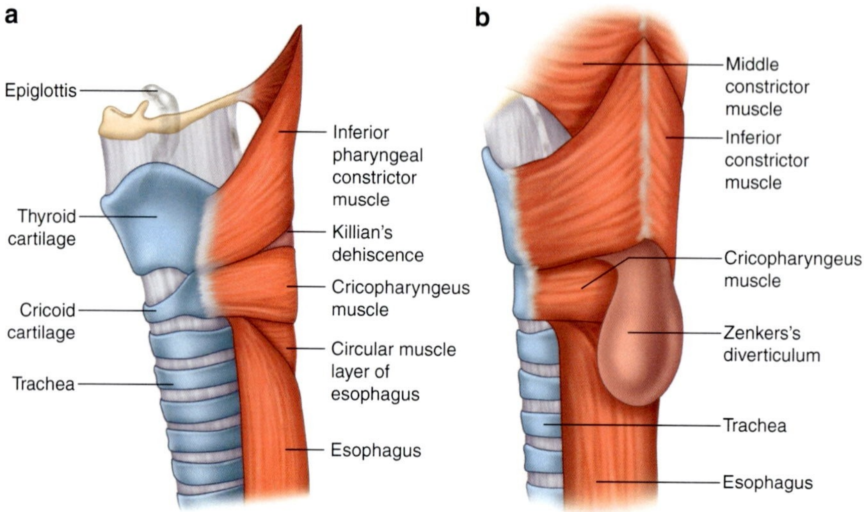

Fig. 44.1 (**a**) Anatomy of the junction of the hypopharynx and esophagus. Killian's dehiscence is located between the inferior pharyngeal constrictor and the CP muscle. (**b**) Zenker's diverticulum. The increase in intraluminal pressure during deglutition in the face of relative cricopharyngeal hypertonia leads to the formation of a mucosal outpouching just superior to CP muscle

1882 [3, 4]. In 1917, Mosher first introduced the concept of endoscopic treatment of ZD that has now seen tremendous advances with respect to both instrumentation and technique [5]. The most common method used for treatment of ZD, the endoscopic staple-assisted approach, was first reported by Collard in 1993 [6, 7]. Since then, several retrospective studies have found both open and endoscopic techniques to be highly effective with comparable complication rates and lengths of hospital stay [8, 9].

Differential Diagnosis

- Killian-Jamieson diverticulum
- Laimer's diverticulum
- Achalasia
- Esophageal cancer
- Esophageal dysmotility
- Esophageal spasm
- Esophageal stricture
- Gastroesophageal reflux disease (GERD)
- Thyroid goiter
- Myasthenia gravis
- Bulbar palsy

Patient History and Physical Findings

- Cervical dysphagia is the most common presenting symptom of ZD. Other symptoms may be quite subtle and include chronic cough, unexplained weight loss, and halitosis. As the patient swallows, the bolus preferentially enters the relatively wider mouth of the diverticular pouch rather than passing through the inappropriately closed upper esophageal sphincter into the esophagus. This in turn may lead to a sense of neck fullness and may be associated with a gurgling sound in the lower neck referred to as cervical borborygmus. Regurgitation of completely undigested food ingested minutes to hours previously is considered nearly pathognomonic for ZD. The pouch may fill and empty spontaneously during deglutition leading to coughing, choking, and possibly aspiration. Such aspiration can have insidious consequences such as chronic respiratory insufficiency or more acute manifestations, such as pneumonia and death. One must also consider the detrimental psychosocial effects of ZD including fear of choking and regurgitation during meals.
- Most ZD patients present with a normal physical exam. When an abnormality is present, it is generally a neck mass in the tracheoesophageal groove that may gurgle or decompress with palpation (Boyce's sign). Audible gurgling may be detected over the same region with swallowing. Inspection of the hypopharynx may reveal pooling of secretions. Direct visualization of the pouch generally requires esophagoscopy, and it is the authors' opinion that rigid esophagoscopy is superior to flexible endoscopy in this endeavor because of the proximal location of ZD and the increased ability to distend the cervical esophagus by displacing the larynx anteriorly.

Imaging and Other Diagnostic Studies

- Barium swallow is the primary study used in the diagnosis of ZD. A characteristic sac is noted just posterior to the esophagus (Fig. 44.2). It arises just superior to a poorly relaxing CP muscle. This phenomenon is often referred to as a CP "bar" and can lead to significant narrowing of the esophagus just distal to the ZD's take off. With this study, the surgeon can accurately size the sac and determine its location. Some authors recommend obtaining manometry testing on all ZD patients; however, that is not the practice of the author as barium swallow is usually sufficient to fully characterize the problem. Computed tomography (CT) and magnetic resonance imaging (MRI) are not generally needed, though ZD may be detected on these studies as a cyst-like mass with an air-fluid level located posterolateral to the esophagus.
- Killian-Jamieson and Laimer diverticula are differentiated from ZD based on the fact that they arise inferior to the CP muscle. The former protrudes through the anterolateral wall of the cervical esophagus via a muscular gap known as Killian-Jamieson space, which is below the CP muscle and lateral to the longitudinal muscle of the esophagus. The latter protrudes through Laimer's triangle, which is located in the posterior midline just inferior to the CP muscle and superior to the confluence of the longitudinal muscle of the esophagus.

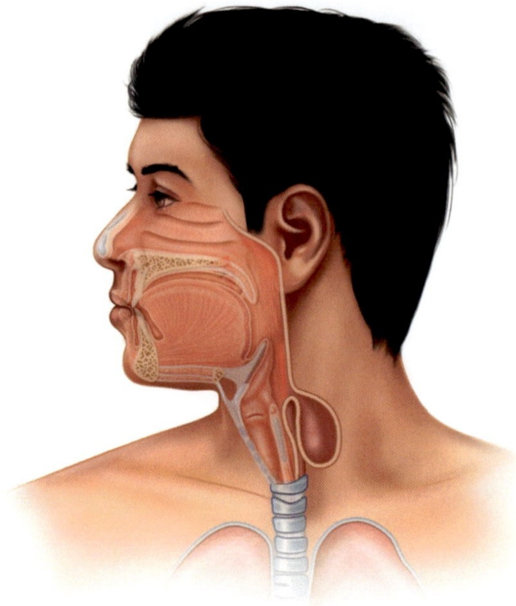

Fig. 44.2 Diagram of Zenker's diverticulum

Surgical Management

Preoperative Decision-Making

- The first decision that should be made is whether repair of a ZD is necessary. If a patient is minimally symptomatic (able to maintain nutrition with a modified diet and no history of aspiration pneumonia) and of advanced age, then continued observation may be the best course of action. Medical therapy with botulinum toxin aimed at treating CP muscle achalasia is another option, although the benefit of this in ZD is more limited than that seen in CP dysfunction without diverticulum. On the other hand, if surgery is to be offered to the patient, it is the author's opinion that the surgeon should be able to discuss the pros and cons of both open and endoscopic approaches and be capable of performing each. A detailed discussion of endoscopic treatment of ZD is found elsewhere in this text.
- Open surgery for ZD is associated with a cervical scar, longer surgical time, and a risk of superior and recurrent laryngeal nerve weakness between 0.5% and 4% [9–11]. The rate of pharyngocutaneous fistula after excision of the sac is reported to be 3–4% [12]. Compared with endoscopic repair, many authors report those treated with open repair are more likely to have complete resolution of symptoms [9, 13, 14]; other studies have not found any difference [8]. Perhaps the most notable advantage of open repair is the significantly lower rate of recurrence.

Studies have shown recurrence rates between 12% and 32% after endoscopic repair compared to rates between 0% and 4% for those treated with open repair that includes a CP myotomy [15–17]. The increased recurrence rates after an endoscopic repair are understandable as the act of dividing the common wall between the diverticular sac and the esophagus—and the CP muscle contained therein—may not result in a complete CP myotomy.

- In the author's experience, as many as 10% of patients cannot be treated via the endoscopic approach due to exposure issues related to dentition, diminished cervical spine mobility, or the presence of prominent mandibular tori. Bloom et al. reported a series of 30 patients, of which 30% could not be adequately exposed for endoscopic surgery [18]. For this reason, it is the author's practice to consent patients for both endoscopic and open approach to allow ZD to be treated in the event that endoscopic exposure is not possible.
- While no absolute size criteria exist, many surgeons argue that those with a very small or very large diverticulum (>3 cm) should be offered an open repair. Often CP myotomy without resection of diverticulum is sufficient if sac is small [19]. The concern with a very large diverticulum is that the redundant, hypotonic sac may lead to persistent dysphagia postoperatively if treated endoscopically. Visosky et al. reported a series 61 ZD patients who underwent endoscopic treatment and noted the main risk factors for recurrence were size larger than 3 cm and the associated amount of redundant mucosa noted after repair [20]. This indicates that scarring may play a role in recurrence of ZD.
- Albeit less frequently encountered, young, otherwise healthy patients with ZD should be offered an open repair due to the higher potential for recurrence with endoscopic repair, which often occurs many years later.

Surgical Technique

There are two surgical objectives when treating ZD: cricopharyngeal myotomy and management of the diverticular sac. With respect to management of the sac, focus will be placed on resection, which is the author's preference. Other options include diverticulopexy and inversion.

- *Endoscopy and dilator placement*
  - If possible, endoscopic evaluation of the diverticulum prior to open repair is strongly recommended (Fig. 44.3a). Caution must be exercised to avoid damaging the patient's dentition during this portion of the procedure. It is advisable to use a rigid tooth guard, which can be easily created using a Rolyan Aquaplast sheet (Patterson Medical, Warrenville, IL). Direct visualization of the diverticulum is possible with a variety of laryngoscopes; however, a Weerda diverticuloscope (Karl Storz, Tuttlingen, Germany) is frequently used. If exposure is not possible with that laryngoscope, the author is usually able to visualize the diverticulum using a size 4 Miller blade, a small cervical esophagoscope, or a C-MAC videolaryngoscope (Karl Storz, Tuttlingen, Germany).

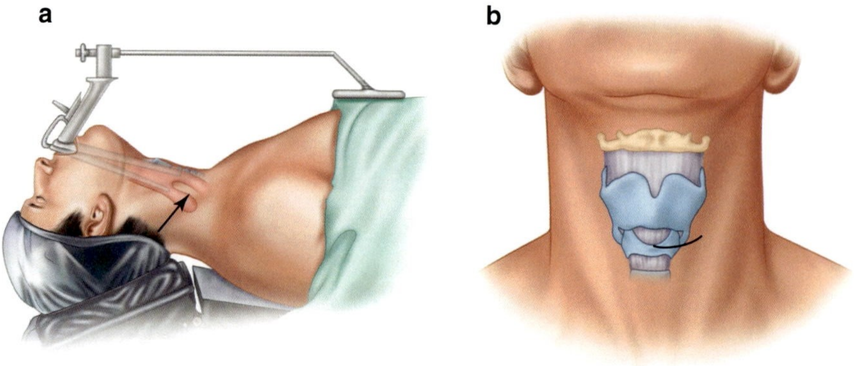

Fig. 44.3 (**a**) A Weerda diverticuloscope is used to visualize the diverticulum and esophagus. This allows packing of diverticulum with strip gauze to facilitate intraoperative identification. (**b**) Patient's head is turned slightly to the right, and an incision is marked in a skin crease on the left neck at the level of the cricoid cartilage

Visualization of the diverticulum serves several purposes including confirmation of the type and location of the diverticulum, evacuation of any food debris, and packing the diverticulum with ¼-inch strip gauze. The latter facilitates identification via transcervical approach. The end of the strip gauze should be left hanging out of the mouth to allow easy removal by an assistant during the procedure. A 36–40 Fr Maloney esophageal dilator (Teleflex Medical, Morrisville, NC) is placed in the esophagus to facilitate CP myotomy and to minimize the risk of iatrogenic esophageal stenosis during repair.

- *Positioning*
  - The patient is placed supine with the head slightly extended and turned toward the non-operative side.

- *Approach*
  - A 3–4-cm transverse incision is generally made in a natural skin crease on the left neck at the approximate level of the cricoid cartilage (Fig. 44.3b). The left side is used because the esophagus tracks toward the left in the neck and because the course of the recurrent laryngeal nerve is more vertically oriented, versus the right nerve which has a more oblique and less predictable course.
  - Subplatysmal flaps are elevated a short distance. The cervical investing fascia is then incised along the anterior border of the sternocleidomastoid muscle, which allows the muscle to be retracted posteriorly to expose the carotid sheath. Identification of the omohyoid muscle which crosses over the carotid sheath obliquely can facilitate the safe identification of the internal jugular vein, which is the most lateral structure in the sheath.
  - Inferior retraction of the omohyoid muscle generally provides adequate access to the CP muscle and ZD, but the muscle can be divided with little

clinical consequence if needed. Blunt dissection medial to the carotid sheath and lateral to the central compartment of the neck will lead to the retropharyngeal space. Caution must be exercised at this step to ensure that the superior and recurrent laryngeal nerves are not injured. While some surgeons advocate identification of these nerves, it is the author's opinion that such dissection poses unnecessary risk. Instead, approaching the retropharyngeal space at a point roughly halfway up the height of the thyroid cartilage while remaining close to the carotid artery grants the surgeon access to the CP and ZD while minimizing the risk of encountering the laryngeal nerves. The retropharyngeal space is then opened bluntly.

- *Mobilizing the diverticulum*
  - As mentioned previously, identification and mobilization of the ZD and CP are greatly facilitated by packing the diverticulum with strip gauze and placement of an esophageal dilator prior to incision. Placing a finger in the retropharyngeal space and palpating anteriorly allow the identification of the esophageal dilator. A muscular ridge can usually be felt traversing the dilator when the finger is moved in the superior and inferior directions. This ridge is at the level of the cricoid cartilage and indicates the location of the CP muscle. Provided that it was packed with ample strip gauze, the diverticulum can often be identified by palpation of a fairly firm mass arising just superior to the CP muscle.
  - Perhaps the most important step in the procedure is the complete mobilization of the diverticulum (Fig. 44.4a). With the diverticulum elevated, the CP muscle can be easily visualized. It is critical that the soft tissue attachments be separated from all sides of the diverticulum to allow it to be delivered into the surgical field. The author finds the use of Kittner dissectors to be particularly helpful in safely separating the diverticulum from the surrounding fascial attachments.
  - An assistant should remove the strip gauze at this point. Care should be taken to ensure the dilator remains in place.

- *Cricopharyngeal Myotomy*
  - A CP myotomy is performed prior to removing the diverticulum (Fig. 44.4b). The CP can be visualized and palpated as a thickened muscular band with horizontally oriented muscle fibers just inferior to the mobilized diverticulum. The CP is carefully elevated off of the underlying esophageal mucosa using a hemostat or similar dissecting clamp. Sharp incision of the entire muscle is performed, resulting in a myotomy that is at least 5 cm in length. Care must be taken to ensure that no portion of the CP muscle is left near the neck of the diverticulum. It is notable that the underlying esophageal mucosa is often thin and transparent enough to allow the surgeon to clearly see the words printed on the dilator. If the cut edges of the muscle remain in close approximation, the author will typically resect a portion of the muscle, effectively performing a myectomy, to minimize the chance of the muscle scarring back together.

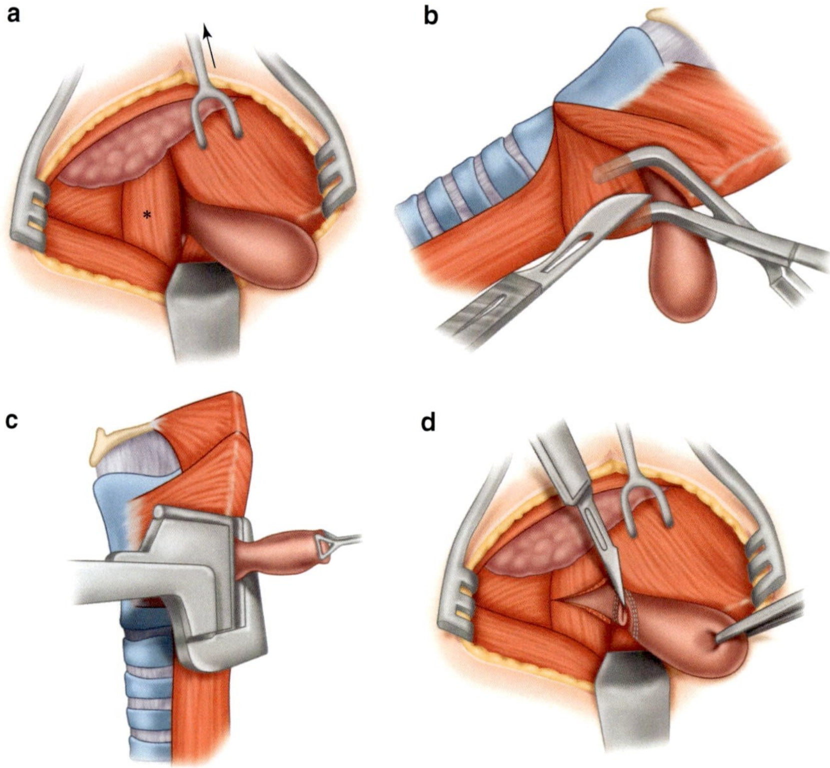

Fig. 44.4 (**a**) Zenker's diverticulum completely mobilized all the way to its neck. *Note the CP muscle inferior to the diverticulum. (**b**) CP myotomy is performed sharply after the muscle is elevated off of the underlying esophageal mucosa. The esophageal dilator is often seen through the remaining mucosal layer. (**c**) When possible, an enteral stapler is used to seal and remove the diverticulum simultaneously. Gauze packing should be removed prior to resection of the diverticulum while the dilator is left in place. (**d**) If use of a stapler is not possible, the diverticulum can be sharply excised

- *Resection of the diverticulum and mucosal repair*
  - Once the diverticulum is mobilized and the CP myotomy completed, the sac can be resected, suspended, or inverted. As mentioned previously, the author's preference is resection, and this technique will be given the most attention in this chapter.
  - If suspension is planned, the bottom of the sac is sutured superiorly to the central compartment fascia such that the mouth of the diverticulum becomes dependent. Proponents of this approach point to a decreased risk of pharyngoesophageal leak as the mucosa is not disrupted.
  - The dilator in the esophageal lumen helps minimize the risk of mucosal overresection and subsequent stenosis. It is the author's preference to use an enteral stapler in order to resect the diverticulum and close the defect simulta-

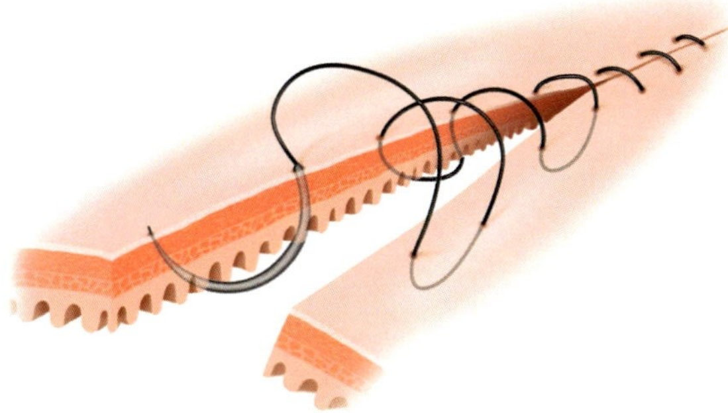

Fig. 44.5 Connell stitch used to insure inversion of mucosal edges during closure

neously (Fig. 44.4c). If this is not possible, the diverticulum is excised sharply (Fig. 44.4d). The pharyngeal defect is then closed with 3-0 Vicryl suture (Ethicon, Somerville, NJ) on a small tapered needle such as RB-1 using a running Connell stitch (Fig. 44.5). Care must be taken to ensure that all mucosal edges are inverted. If there is enough tissue to allow it to be done without causing stenosis, the first suture line will be reinforced using interrupted Lembert sutures. The dilator should remain in place until the diverticulum has been removed and the defect repaired.

- The Maloney dilator is removed and a Dobhoff tube (DHT) is placed transnasally. Palpation of the surgical site ensures that the DHT passes without difficulty.
- The wound is closed in two layers over a suction drain.

Postoperative Care

- Previous studies cite significantly longer hospitalizations and longer recovery times as well as increased complications from an open approach compared to an endoscopic approach, but this has not been the author's experience [21].
- The author's postoperative management is the same for patients treated via an open approach and an endoscopic approach. Both have a DHT placed at the conclusion of the procedure, and both are admitted overnight. A double-contrast esophagram is obtained the morning of the first postoperative day. If no leak is identified, the DHT is removed and a clear liquid diet is started. The patient is given instructions to slowly advance their diet to regular over the course of 2 weeks and is discharged without antibiotics. If, however, a leak is seen or suspected on the esophagram, the patient is kept NPO and tube feeds are initiated via DHT. The patient is still usually discharged on postoperative day 1 even with a leak but on antibiotics via DHT. A repeat esophagram is generally scheduled a week later to ensure that the leak has resolved.

Outcomes and Complications

- Verdonck and Morton performed a systematic review of the literature on the treatment of Zenker's diverticulum in 2015. They identified 71 studies that included 1990 patients treated with an open approach and 1089 treated with an endoscopic approach. Failure was seen in 4.2% of open cases compared to 18.4% of endoscopic cases. Complication rates were reported as 4.3% for open cases compared to 7.9% for endoscopic cases. These consisted of RLN weakness (3.4%) and fistula (3.7%) in the open surgical group. Emphysema (3.0%) and mediastinitis (1.2%) were the most common complications in the endoscopic group. ZD recurrence after endoscopic repair is significantly higher when compared to open approach (18.9% vs 1.9%) [12].

References

1. Scher RLP. Liana, Zenker Diverticulum. In: Cummings otolaryngology. Philadelphia: Elsevier; 2010. p. 1025–34.
2. Ludlow A. A case of obstructed deglutition from a preternatural dilatation of a bagformed in pharynx. Med Observations Inquiries. 1767;3:85.
3. Ferguson MK. Evolution of therapy for pharyngoesophageal (Zenker's) diverticulum. Ann Thorac Surg. 1991;51(5):848–52.
4. Simic A, et al. Surgical experience of the national institution in the treatment of Zenker's diverticula. Acta Chir Iugosl. 2009;56(1):25–33.
5. Hillel AT, Flint PW. Evolution of endoscopic surgical therapy for Zenker's diverticulum. Laryngoscope. 2009;119(1):39–44.
6. Collard JM, Otte JB, Kestens PJ. Endoscopic stapling technique of esophagodiverticulostomy for Zenker's diverticulum. Ann Thorac Surg. 1993;56(3):573–6.
7. Martin-Hirsch DP, Newbegin CJ. Autosuture GIA gun: a new application in the treatment of hypopharyngeal diverticula. J Laryngol Otol. 1993;107(8):723–5.
8. Narne S, et al. Endoscopic diverticulotomy for the treatment of Zenker's diverticulum: results in 102 patients with staple-assisted endoscopy. Ann Otol Rhinol Laryngol. 1999;108(8):810–5.
9. Chang CW, et al. Carbon dioxide laser endoscopic diverticulotomy versus open diverticulectomy for Zenker's diverticulum. Laryngoscope. 2004;114(3):519–27.
10. Shahawy S, et al. A comparative study of outcomes for endoscopic diverticulotomy versus external diverticulectomy. Otolaryngol Head Neck Surg. 2014;151(4):646–51.
11. Feeley MA, et al. Zenker's diverticulum: analysis of surgical complications from diverticulectomy and cricopharyngeal myotomy. Laryngoscope. 1999;109(6):858–61.
12. Verdonck J, Morton RP. Systematic review on treatment of Zenker's diverticulum. Eur Arch Otorhinolaryngol. 2015;272(11):3095–107.
13. Gutschow CA, et al. Management of pharyngoesophageal (Zenker's) diverticulum: which technique? Ann Thorac Surg. 2002;74(5):1677–82; discussion 1682–3.
14. Seth R, et al. Patient reported outcomes in endoscopic and open transcervical treatment for Zenker's diverticulum. Laryngoscope. 2014;124(1):119–25.
15. Scher RL. Endoscopic staple diverticulostomy for recurrent Zenker's diverticulum. Laryngoscope. 2003;113(1):63–7.
16. Counter PR, Hilton ML, Baldwin DL. Long-term follow-up of endoscopic stapled diverticulotomy. Ann R Coll Surg Engl. 2002;84(2):89–92.

17. Raut VV, Primrose WJ. Long-term results of endoscopic stapling diverticulotomy for pharyngeal pouches. Otolaryngol Head Neck Surg. 2002;127(3):225–9.
18. Bloom JD, et al. Factors predicting endoscopic exposure of Zenker's diverticulum. Ann Otol Rhinol Laryngol. 2010;119(11):736–41.
19. van Overbeek JJ. Meditation on the pathogenesis of hypopharyngeal (Zenker's) diverticulum and a report of endoscopic treatment in 545 patients. Ann Otol Rhinol Laryngol. 1994;103(3):178–85.
20. Visosky AM, Parke RB, Donovan DT. Endoscopic management of Zenker's diverticulum: factors predictive of success or failure. Ann Otol Rhinol Laryngol. 2008;117(7):531–7.
21. Lang RA, et al. Transoral diverticulostomy with a modified Endo-Gia stapler: results after 4 years of experience. Surg Endosc. 2007;21(4):532–6.

Zenker's Diverticulum: Transoral Repair 45

Matthew J. Skinner and Christopher C. Thompson

Pathology

Zenker's diverticulum (ZD), first described by Ludlow in 1797, is a posterior outpouching of both esophageal mucosa and submucosa penetrating immediately above the upper esophageal sphincter through Killian's triangle between the transverse cricopharyngeus muscle fibers and the oblique muscle fibers of the lower inferior constrictor (Fig. 45.1) [20]. It is hypothesized that increased upper esophageal sphincter tone in association with the anatomic weakness of Killian's triangle leads to the formation of ZD; however, direct manometric findings are inconsistent [12]. The variation in findings could be secondary to the ZD outpouching negating manometric pressure changes that lead to its formation. Other studies promote the idea that ZD may be tied to generalized esophageal dysmotility [24].

Epidemiology and Clinical Manifestations

The overall incidence of ZD is low, but higher in North America, Northern Europe, and Australia versus patients from Japan, Indonesia, or Southern Europe. The overall incidence in the United Kingdom is reported at 2 per 100,000 per year [28, 29]. The majority of patients tend to be males over the age of 60, and it occurs most commonly in the eighth decade of life [21]. Patients typically present with initial dysphagia, pulmonary aspiration, regurgitation of food, a neck mass, halitosis, and weight loss. More rarely, squamous cell carcinoma has been described within the diverticula with an incidence of 0.4 in one large case series including 1249 patients [14]. Ulceration secondary to pill retention has also been described [27].

M. J. Skinner · C. C. Thompson (✉)
Department of Surgery, Brigham and Women's Hospital, Harvard Medical School, Boston, MA, USA
e-mail: ccthompson@bwh.harvard.edu

J. Grams et al. (eds.), *The SAGES Manual of Foregut Surgery*,
https://doi.org/10.1007/978-3-319-96122-4_45

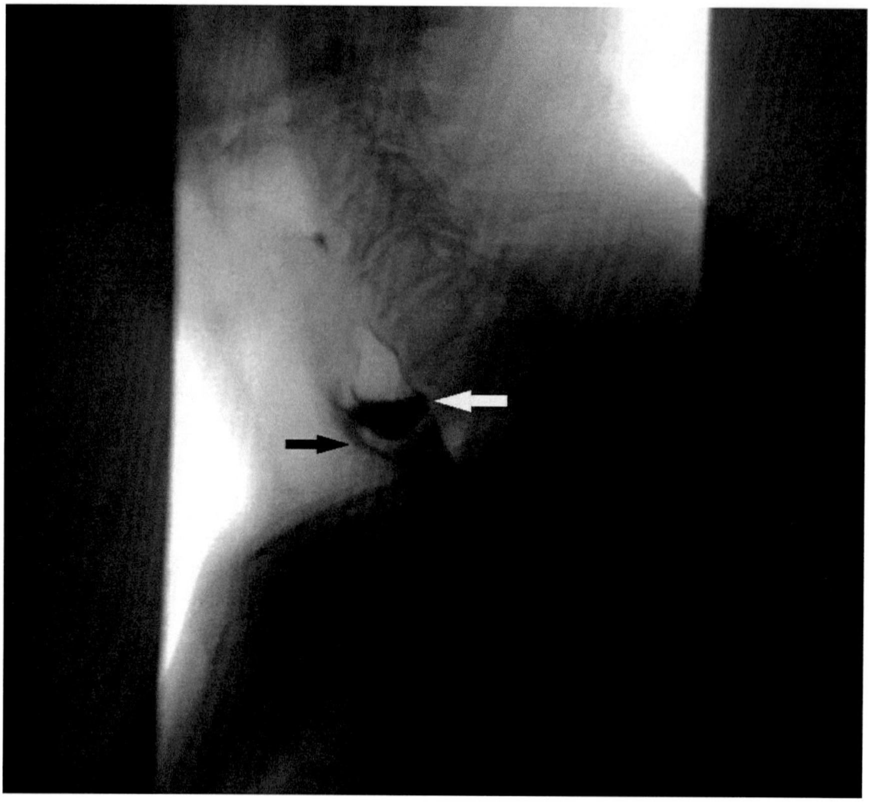

Fig. 45.1 Black arrow: esophagus. White arrow: Zenker's diverticulum

Diagnosis

ZD is typically diagnosed via barium swallow examination utilizing continuous fluoroscopy to visualize swallowing. Alternatively, cervical transcutaneous ultrasound can also be used to recognize a ZD and delineate it from other cervical pathology [19]. In the setting of smaller diverticula, evaluation by speech pathology may help exclude alternative pathology that may be causative of the patient's symptoms. Although dysmotility is felt to be etiologic of ZD, by the time the patient becomes symptomatic, alterations in anatomy make esophageal manometry findings inconsistent and thus irrelevant to diagnosis.

Treatment

The general treatment strategy of ZD involves either complete excision of ZD pouch, cricopharyngeal myotomy, or dissection of the mucosa and cricopharyngeal muscle dividing the pouch and the esophagus. The techniques employed in the treatment of ZD include open surgery via external neck incision, rigid endoscopy, and most recently flexible endoscopy.

Surgical Techniques

Open transcervical diverticulectomy was first described in 1885 and remains the "gold standard" for ZD repair. This technique is now performed with some combination of diverticulectomy, diverticulopexy, and cricopharyngeal myotomy. Myotomy is now well established as beneficial in all open procedures [9]. Open excision is often promoted as the treatment of choice in younger patients given the small but present risk of squamous cell carcinoma [14]. A systematic review including 2826 patients treated with open surgery between 2004 and 2013 demonstrated symptom resolution in 90–95% of patients [30]. The morbidity associated with open surgery was 10.5% and the mortality was 0.6% [30].

Rigid endoscopic management of ZD has been available since the 1960s. Use of a rigid endoscope requires that the patient be sedated with general anesthesia. The bridge of the ZD has been divided with electrocautery, CO_2 laser, KTP/532 laser, stapler, needle knife, and Harmonic Ace [31]. Rigid surgical success has widely varied with success rates ranging from 78.5% to 96% [11, 26]. In a meta-analysis comparing open surgery to a rigid endoscopic stapling approach between the years of 1990 and 2002, the morbidity and mortality rates were 2.6% vs 11.8% and 0.3% vs 1.6%, respectively [6]. In another literature review, the morbidity for all rigid endoscopic techniques was noted to be 8.7% and the mortality was noted at 0.2% [30]. The improvement in safety profile has led to increased utility of endoscopic techniques over the past 2 decades.

Complications associated with the use of a rigid endoscope include hyperextension injuries, dental injuries, perforation, and recurrent laryngeal nerve paralysis. Adequate field visualization using a rigid endoscope may fail with conversion to open technique reported in as high as 30% of patients [4]. Obesity, a short neck, and decreased hyomental distance are all associated with technique failure.

Flexible Endoscopic Techniques

Despite the advent of the flexible endoscope in 1957, the first cases of ZD treatment were not published until 1995 when Ishioka and Mulder published concurrent articles [17, 22]. There are a variety of techniques available; however, each is predicated on similar principles. Typically an endoscopic cap or flexible specialized ZD overtube (ZD overtube, Cook Medical, USA) is used to maintain the center of the bridge in view. Similar to rigid endoscopic techniques, the principles of coagulation and subsequent cutting of the ZD bridge apply to the endoscopic technique. Attention must be paid to coagulation given the cricopharyngeus is a muscular structure that is highly vascular. Rapid bleeding can lead to loss of visual field and failure of the procedure. Complete dissection of the bridge all the way to the base is paramount. Bridge takedown allows contents to flow directly from the ZD back into the esophagus preventing retention and subsequent complications such as aspiration.

The procedure has been performed under conscious sedation, but at our institution we utilize general anesthesia with patient intubation. The use of general anesthesia limits coughing or gagging, providing a more stable surgical field. Additionally, in the atypical case of bleeding, the trachea should be protected given the short distance from the ZD to the airway. It is our practice to perform all procedures with carbon dioxide rather than air to limit extraluminal air, optimize resorption, and improve patient comfort. All patients receive intravenous antibiotics 1 h prior to the procedure.

Intraoperatively it is imperative to preserve orientation and visualization. Frequently, ZD are large and differentiating the pouch from the esophagus can become a challenge. We will endoscopically leave a guidewire in the stomach and esophagus and after withdrawal of the endoscope, use this guidewire to place a nasogastric tube safely in the esophageal lumen. This helps preserve orientation during the procedure. To maintain the bridge of the diverticulum in the center of the visual field, a soft diverticuloscope, angled transparent cap, and straight transparent cap are most often used. Only the straight transparent cap is FDA-approved; thus, this is what is used at our institution. The soft diverticuloscope is a double-lipped transparent plastic overtube that has been approved by the Conformité Européenne (CE) but is not FDA-approved. It is placed with one lip in the diverticulum and the other in the esophageal lumen under endoscopic guidance, allowing the ZD bridge to be maintained in the center of the visual field. In a meta-analysis, diverticuloscope use was not noted to improve clinical outcomes, but one trial specifically addressing this issue demonstrated improved success rates and decreased complication rates when comparing diverticuloscope to an angled cap [8, 16]. It should be noted that the study demonstrating superiority of the diverticuloscope had a much lower overall success rate than any previous or subsequent case series [16]. The size of the diverticuloscope may limit its use in diverticula less than 2 cm.

There are a wide variety of tools that have been implemented in dissection of the ZD bridge (Fig. 45.2). Despite a decrease in procedural complications and an increase in both technical and clinical success rates over time, there are no instruments which have demonstrated superior efficacy or safety per meta-analysis [16]. At our institution, we favor using a fully rotatable insulated monopolar grasping scissor, the SB knife (Olympus, USA), in conjunction with the VIO 300 D (ERBE, Germany) using Endocut I settings. Using this device, we begin in the middle of the proximal aspect of the bridge and dissect down the midline to the base of the ZD. We use the knife to first grasp the tissue and then retract the tissue into the transparent cap if possible. Both the insulation of the knife and the cap itself are used to minimize unintended thermal damage to the tissue. After the tissue is grasped and appropriately positioned, then current can be applied for cautery and cutting. In animal models cutting with bipolar scissors results in "tissue bonding" at the edges of the divided septum that may protect against clinically significant

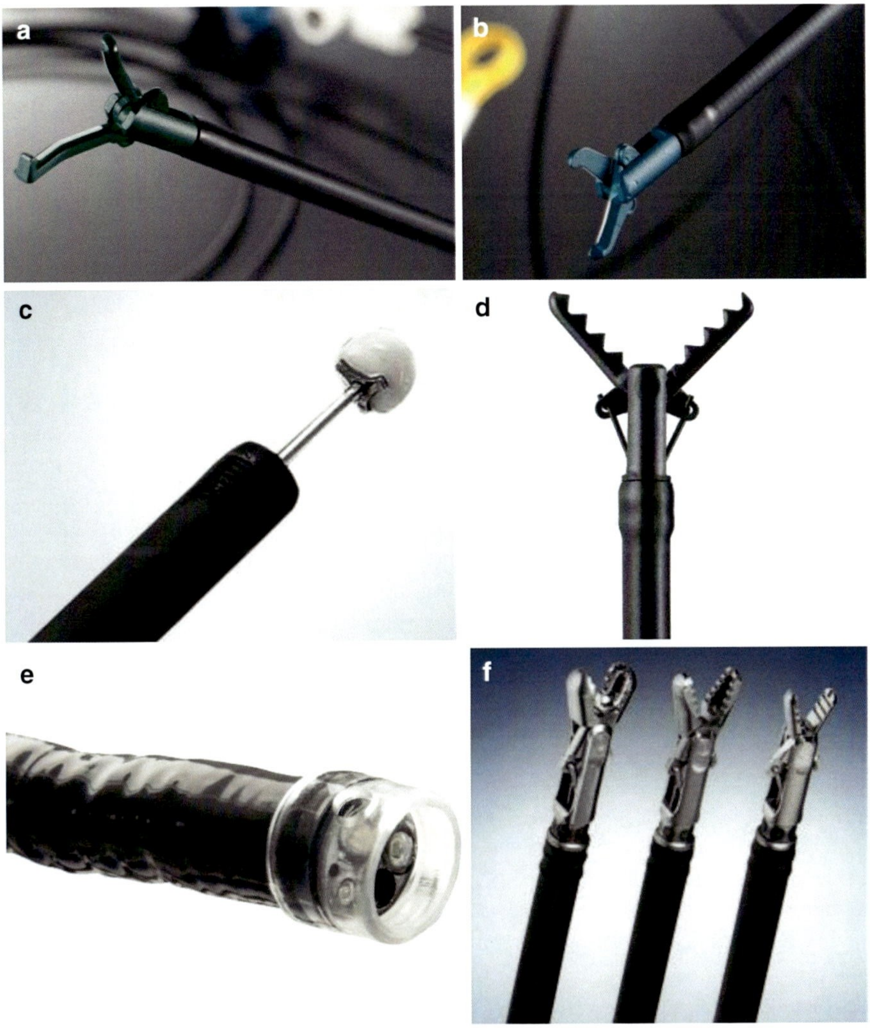

Fig. 45.2 (**a**) SB knife (Olympus, USA). (**b**) SB knife Jr. (Olympus, USA. (**c**) IT2 knife (Olympus, USA). (**d**) Clutch Cutter (Fujifilm, JP). (**e**) Transparent cap (US Endoscopy, USA). (**f**) Coagrasper (Olympus, USA)

perforation [25]. Previously we commonly used the IT2 knife (Olympus, USA), an electrocautery knife with an insulated tip. The insulated tip prevents perforation of the base and opposing esophageal wall. The Clutch Cutter (Fujifilm, Japan) is a diathermic slitter with serrated and fully rotatable jaws. Like the SB knife, it too has an insulated outer edge. Again, with any of these devices, it is important to ensure complete dissection of the mucosa and muscle layers to the base of the pouch. In small case series, there is a trend to symptom relief with size of posttreatment pouch size [7].

Needle knives, hook knives, and hot biopsy forceps have been used; however, the risk of perforation using these devices is theoretically higher [25]. Some have advocated for endoscopic tunneling to be performed into the Zenker pouch using a tunneling technique similar to that seen in a POEM [18]. After tunneling into the pocket is achieved, dissection of the cricopharyngeal muscle is performed and often extended below the base of the pouch [18]. After completion of muscle dissection, the entry point of the tunnel is then closed with clips [18]. Some institutions have advised leaving a small 2–3 mm bridge at the base to prevent perforation when using a needle knife exclusively, but this is not typically our practice. APC (ERBE VIO 300D, forced 50 W at 0.8 L/min) starting distally and moving proximally toward the bridge has also been employed in a limited case series [23].

Intraprocedural bleeding is not uncommon during the dissection of the ZD bridge. In our practice, we have found that it is important to have early hemostatic control to maintain optimal visualization and minimize procedure complications. The Coagrasper (Olympus, USA), a flexible bipolar hemostasis forceps, can be used to isolate and cauterize bleeding vessels. If these forceps are not available, clips may also be used, although this limits visualization following deployment.

Clips can be used to close microperforations. Because these typically occur at the base of the ZD, concerns over visualization are typically less applicable. Some high-volume centers place clips at the base of every dissected ZD as prophylaxis against perforation; however, this is not our practice unless perforation is evident at the end of the procedure [15]. In limited cases we have noted patient discomfort following placement of clips.

At the conclusion of the procedure, all patients are checked via physical exam for signs of perforation such as cervical crepitus. Other high-volume centers propose exclusion of perforation with barium swallow, but we reserve this for patients with symptoms [15].

If the patient does develop fever, chills, chest pain, or neck pain, a CT of the chest and neck is obtained to exclude perforation. If this is negative and symptoms persist, we then obtain a barium swallow to further evaluate for perforation.

Following the flexible endoscopic procedure, all patients are made NPO for the remainder of the day. This is followed by 1 day of clear liquids, 2 weeks of a full liquid diet, and finally 2 weeks of a pureed and semisolid diet. At our institution our dietary guidelines are detailed to ensure that the patients receive adequate nutrition in the postoperative phase to facilitate recovery. After 4 weeks, the patient can resume a regular diet.

Since we require a liquid diet following the procedure, 2 weeks prior to the procedure, all medications are converted to a crushable or liquid format to ensure tolerance of this formulation.

Patients are provided a 1-week course of an antibiotic to minimize the risk of postoperative infection. Lidocaine or benzocaine drops are prescribed to decrease the incidence of sore throat. It should be noted that some case series do not provide intraprocedural or postoperative antibiotics.

Outcomes

A meta-analysis of 813 patients between the years of 1995 and 2015 demonstrated a pooled efficacy of 91% [86%, 95%], adverse event rate of 11.3% [8%, 16%], and recurrence rate of 11% [8%, 15%] [16]. While there is typically homogeneity in outcomes in high-volume centers, success rates have been reported as low as 56% demonstrating operator influence on outcomes [8]. Among the pooled patients in the above meta-analysis, all bleeding was managed endoscopically, and perforations were typically managed conservatively by making the patient nothing by mouth, starting antibiotics, and endoscopically placing a nasogastric tube [16]. Two patients (0.2%) developed an abscess requiring surgical incision and drainage with a protracted hospital stay [5, 10]. There was no mortality associated with the procedure [16].

A case series of 31 patients using our preferred instrument, the SB knife, demonstrated technical success in all patients with no intraprocedural complications [3]. One hundred percent of patients had symptom improvement with 87.1% achieving full resolution of symptoms [3]. Patients with only partial response opted to not have further treatments [3]. The only complication (3.2%) was self-limited bleeding that did not require transfusion [3]. The median procedure time was 14 minutes [3]. Another study evaluating the same instrument in 52 patients demonstrated clinical resolution in 90.4% of patients after a single procedure [13]. These findings mirror our own institutional findings.

Flexible endoscopic diverticulotomy appears to provide durable outcomes. One study with 150 patients noted a decrease in dysphagia score from 1.88 ± 0.6 to 0.29 ± 0.71 at 1 month [15]. At a median follow-up of 43 months (range 13–121 months), the dysphagia score remained low at 0.34 ± 0.72 ($p < 0.01$) [15]. Only 1.5% of patients who underwent the procedure had an aspiration event, and 0.7% had developed pneumonia at any point following the procedure [15]. This indicates that this is a highly durable technique when performed at experienced centers.

In a systematic review comparing endoscopic therapy to surgical therapy, it has been determined that the endoscopic approach results in shorter procedure time, decreased hospitalization, lower post-procedural complications, and decreased time to diet introduction [1]. Surgery does have a lower incidence of symptom recurrence [1].

Finally, it should be noted that endoscopic ZD repair can also be used successfully following symptom recurrence after surgery [2]. One study evaluated 25 patients who had previously undergone surgery (17 endoscopic stapling, 8 cervical approach) [2]. Endoscopic dissection of the ZD resulted in symptom resolution in 84% of patients and symptom improvement in 100% [2]. Twenty percent of this cohort had recurrence which was resolved with further endoscopic ZD ablation [2].

Conclusions

ZD is a rare complication seen most commonly in elderly patients, often with multiple comorbidities. The data currently available are retrospective observational studies and case-control studies. At this stage, expert opinion is largely determinant of management. From meta-analysis of retrospective studies, it appears that flexible endoscopic therapy is the safest procedure followed by rigid endoscopic therapy and finally open surgery. Open surgery with pouch excision remains an option in younger patients in which there is a 0.4% risk of the development of squamous cell carcinoma within the pouch. Rigid endoscopic therapy is now widely available; however, anatomic considerations may limit the technique. The most commonly used tool, the endoscopic stapler, is limited in the treatment of smaller diverticula as the device has a 1 cm leading end, prohibiting dissection of the pouch fully to the base.

In our experience, flexible endoscopic therapy is highly versatile and not limited by anatomy that may prohibit rigid endoscopic access. It can be used to successfully treat small pouches. In meta-analysis, it has the lowest associated mortality. It can also be performed multiple times to ensure symptom resolution in both the setting of partial response and recurrence.

Given the wide range of therapy, treatment of ZD should be individualized based on the patient's age, comorbidities, symptom burden, and the characteristics of the ZD. An experienced surgeon/endoscopist should guide the technique selection in concert with the patient. Given the rarity of the disease, the procedure should be performed by a high-volume practitioner to maximize symptom control and minimize complications and recurrence.

References

1. Albers DV, Kondo A, Bernardo WM, Sakai P, Moura RN, Silva GL, Ide E, Tomishige T, de Moura EG. Endoscopic versus surgical approach in the treatment of Zenker's diverticulum: systematic review and meta-analysis. Endosc Int Open. 2016;4:E678–86.
2. Antonello A, Ishaq S, Zanatta L, Cesarotto M, Costantini M, Battaglia G. The role of flexible endotherapy for the treatment of recurrent Zenker's diverticula after surgery and endoscopic stapling. Surg Endosc. 2016;30:2351–7.
3. Battaglia G, Antonello A, Realdon S, Cesarotto M, Zanatta L, Ishaq S. Flexible endoscopic treatment for Zenker's diverticulum with the SB Knife. Preliminary results from a single-center experience. Dig Endosc. 2015;27:728–33.
4. Bloom JD, Bleier BS, Mirza N, Chalian AA, Thaler ER. Factors predicting endoscopic exposure of Zenker's diverticulum. Ann Otol Rhinol Laryngol. 2010;119:736–41.
5. Case DJ, Baron TH. Flexible endoscopic management of Zenker Diverticulum: the Mayo Clinic experience. Mayo Clin Proc. 2010;85:719–22.
6. Chang CY, Payyapilli RJ, Scher RL. Endoscopic staple diverticulostomy for Zenker's diverticulum: review of literature and experience in 159 consecutive cases. Laryngoscope. 2003;113:957–65.
7. Costamagna G, Iacopini F, Bizzotto A, Familiari P, Tringali A, Perri V, Bella A. Prognostic variables for the clinical success of flexible endoscopic septotomy of Zenker's diverticulum. Gastrointest Endosc. 2016;83:765–73.
8. Costamagna G, Iacopini F, Tringali A, Marchese M, Spada C, Familiari P, Mutignani M, Bella A. Flexible endoscopic Zenker's diverticulotomy: cap-assisted technique vs. diverticuloscope-assisted technique. Endoscopy. 2007;39:146–52.
9. Demeester T, Bremner CG. Selective cricopharyngeal myotomy for Zenker's diverticulum. J Am Coll Surg. 2003;196:451–2.
10. Evrard S, Moine OL, Hassid S, Devière J. Zenker's diverticulum: a new endoscopic treatment with a soft diverticuloscope. Gastrointest Endosc. 2003;58:116–20.

11. Fama AF, Moore EJ, Kasperbauer JL. Harmonic scalpel in the treatment of Zenker's diverticulum. Laryngoscope. 2009;119:1265–9.
12. Fulp SR, Castell DO. Manometric aspects of Zenker's diverticulum. Hepato-Gastroenterology. 1992;39:123–6.
13. Goelder SK, Brueckner J, Messmann H. Endoscopic treatment of Zenker's diverticulum with the stag beetle knife (sb knife) - feasibility and follow-up. Scand J Gastroenterol. 2016;51:1155–8.
14. Huang BS, Unni KK, Payne WS. Long-term survival following diverticulectomy for cancer in pharyngoesophageal (Zenker's) diverticulum. Ann Thorac Surg. 1984;38:207–10.
15. Huberty V, El Bacha S, Blero D, Le Moine O, Hassid S, Deviere J. Endoscopic treatment for Zenker's diverticulum: long-term results (with video). Gastrointest Endosc. 2013;77:701–7.
16. Ishaq S, Hassan C, Antonello A, Tanner K, Bellisario C, Battaglia G, Anderloni A, Correale L, Sharma P, Baron TH, Repici A. Flexible endoscopic treatment for Zenker's diverticulum: a systematic review and meta-analysis. Gastrointest Endosc. 2016;83:1076–1089.e5.
17. Ishioka S, Sakai P, Maluf Filho F, Melo JM. Endoscopic incision of Zenker's diverticula. Endoscopy. 1995;27:433–7.
18. Li QL, Chen WF, Zhang XC, Cai MY, Zhang YQ, Hu JW, He MJ, Yao LQ, Zhou PH, Xu MD. Submucosal tunneling endoscopic septum division: a novel technique for treating Zenker's Diverticulum. Gastroenterology. 2016;151:1071–4.
19. Lixin J, Bing H, Zhigang W, Binghui Z. Sonographic diagnosis features of Zenker diverticulum. Eur J Radiol. 2011;80:e13–9.
20. Ludlow A. A case of obstructed deglutition from a preternatural dilation of a bag formed in pharynx. Med Observations Inquiries. 1797;3:85.
21. Mulder CJ, Costamagna G, Sakai P. Zenker's diverticulum: treatment using a flexible endoscope. Endoscopy. 2001;33:991–7.
22. Mulder CJ, den Hartog G, Robijn RJ, Thies JE. Flexible endoscopic treatment of Zenker's diverticulum: a new approach. Endoscopy. 1995;27:438–42.
23. Rabenstein T, May A, Michel J, Manner H, Pech O, Gossner L, Ell C. Argon plasma coagulation for flexible endoscopic Zenker's diverticulotomy. Endoscopy. 2007;39:141–5.
24. Resouly A, Braat J, Jackson A, Evans H. Pharyngeal pouch: link with reflux and oesophageal dysmotility. Clin Otolaryngol Allied Sci. 1994;19:241–2.
25. Rieder E, Martinec D, Dunst C, Swanström L. Flexible endoscopic Zenkers diverticulotomy with a novel bipolar forceps: a pilot study and comparison with needleknife dissection. Surg Endosc. 2011;25:3273–8.
26. Rizzetto C, Zaninotto G, Costantini M, Bottin R, Finotti E, Zanatta L, Guirroli E, Ceolin M, Nicoletti L, Ruol A, Ancona E. Zenker's diverticula: feasibility of a tailored approach based on diverticulum size. J Gastrointest Surg. 2008;12:2057–64; discussion 2064–5.
27. Sharma R, Decross AJ. Zenker's diverticulitis secondary to alendronate ingestion: a rare cause of recurrent dysphagia. Gastrointest Endosc. 2011;73:368–70.
28. Siddiq MA, Sood S, Strachan D. Pharyngeal pouch (Zenker's diverticulum). Postgrad Med J. 2001;77:506–11.
29. Verhaegen VJ, Feuth T, van den Hoogen FJ, Marres HA, Takes RP. Endoscopic carbon dioxide laser diverticulostomy versus endoscopic staple-assisted diverticulostomy to treat Zenker's diverticulum. Head Neck. 2011;33:154–9.
30. Yuan Y, Zhao YF, Hu Y, Chen LQ. Surgical treatment of Zenker's Diverticulum. Dig Surg. 2013;30:207–18.
31. Zaninotto G, Rizzetto C. Optimal therapy for cricopharyngeal diverticula. In: Ferguson MK, editor. Difficult decisions in thoracic surgery: an evidence-based approach. London: Springer London; 2011.

46 Epiphrenic and Mid-Esophageal Diverticula

Lowell S. Su and Jon O. Wee

Introduction

The esophagus is an organ composed of four layers: mucosa, submucosa, muscularis propria, and adventitia. In the adult, the esophagus measures 35 cm in length and is divided into three segments: cervical, middle, and distal. The *cervical* portion extends from the cricoid cartilage to the thoracic inlet (10–18 cm from the incisors). The *middle* segment extends from the thoracic inlet to the halfway between the tracheal bifurcation and the gastroesophageal junction (19–34 cm from the incisors). The *distal* esophagus is the remaining portion that concludes in the abdomen at the gastroesophageal junction (35–42 cm from the incisors). These anatomical segments become important when classifying esophageal diverticula, as the location dictates the pathophysiology and operative treatment.

A diverticulum is defined as an abnormal sac or outpouching formed at the weak point in the esophagus. A *true* esophageal diverticulum involves all the layers of esophagus; conversely, a *false* esophageal diverticulum does not. The vast majority of esophageal diverticular disease are acquired. Esophageal diverticula can be generally classified by pathophysiology, namely, traction or pulsion type. Pulsion diverticula are the most common form and are secondary to esophageal dysmotility. They are false diverticula because they lack a muscular wall and are usually found in the cervical and distal esophagus. Traction diverticula are rare and almost exclusively occur in the mid-esophagus [1]. These are true diverticula, and as the name suggests they are caused by external forces that pull the esophagus into a conical outpouching.

Esophageal diverticula are also classified by their location. Pharyngoesophageal diverticula, commonly referred to as Zenker's [2] diverticula, are the most common diverticula and are located in the cervical esophagus. They occur at the junction between the cricopharyngeus and inferior constrictor muscles, known as *Killian's*

L. S. Su (✉) · J. O. Wee
Department of Thoracic Surgery, Brigham and Women's Hospital, Boston, MA, USA
e-mail: lssu@partners.org; jwee@bwh.harvard.edu

J. Grams et al. (eds.), *The SAGES Manual of Foregut Surgery*,
https://doi.org/10.1007/978-3-319-96122-4_46

triangle. This area between the muscle fibers is an inherent weak point that leads to diverticular formation with increased hypopharyngeal pressure. Epiphrenic diverticula are the second most common diverticula and occur at the distal esophagus. They occur most often in the right posterior wall and occur in a 1:3 ratio to pharyngoesophageal diverticula [3]. Mid-esophageal diverticula are the least common of the esophageal diverticula. Although mid-esophageal diverticula were initially thought to be caused exclusively by external traction in patients with mediastinal fibrosis, lymphadenopathy, or inflammatory conditions such as tuberculosis or histoplasmosis, there is recent increasing evidence that the majority of cases now are caused by esophageal motility disorders [4]. Most cases of congenitally acquired esophageal diverticula occur in the mid-esophagus and are a result of abortive tracheoesophageal fistula or foregut duplications [5].

This chapter focuses on the indications, preoperative preparation, minimally invasive operative technique, and postoperative outcomes for epiphrenic and mid-esophageal diverticula. Pharyngoesophageal diverticula is discussed separately in a different chapter.

Epiphrenic Diverticula

Epiphrenic diverticula (ED) are the second most common esophageal diverticula and in conjunction with mid-esophageal diverticula comprise 10–15% of esophageal diverticula. They were first described by Mondiere in 1833 [6], and overall are rare entities, occurring in 0.015% of the general population based on radiological data [7]. These diverticula occur within the distal 10 cm of the esophagus, and the majority occur on the right posterior wall. They are pulsion diverticula and represent herniation of the mucosa and submucosa through the muscular layers of the esophageal wall as a result of increased intraluminal pressure. On radiograph, these diverticula have a wide neck, rounded contour, and retain contrast during a swallow study. A radiographic study at the University of Pennsylvania found ED in their patient population to have a mean width of 4.4 cm and mean height of 3.7 cm, with a direct correlation of width and preferential filling during a barium swallow study [8]. The size also had significant correlation with development of symptoms.

Pathophysiology

With the advancement in esophageal imaging and motility studies, it is clear that these diverticula are a direct result of functional distal obstruction and dysmotility that increase luminal pressure. 66–75% of patients that develop ED have some form of functional obstruction in the form of achalasia, and the majority have esophageal dysmotility, often as a lack of coordination between the distal esophagus and lower esophageal sphincter (LES) [9]. Manometric studies in patients with ED frequently show the classic features of diffuse esophageal spasm or nonspecific motor disorders. It is inferred that increased motor activity and abnormal lower esophageal sphincter relaxation produce zones of increased intraluminal pressure through which these outpouchings occur [10, 11]. Multiple ED are found in up to a fourth of these patients [12]. When present, they are either aligned longitudinally or circumferentially along the LES. It is currently unknown whether increasing numbers of diverticula directly correlate with development of symptoms.

Signs, Symptoms, and Diagnosis

Most patients who develop epiphrenic diverticula are asymptomatic. When patients do become symptomatic, the two most common reported symptoms are dysphagia and regurgitation. Dysphagia can occur both in the setting of a hypertensive LES and a normotensive LES [13]. As the diverticulum enlarges and fills with undigested food, regurgitation occurs and worsens. Often these symptoms are easily mistaken for gastroesophageal reflux disease, but a careful history will elicit a taste of bland and not bitter food in the mouth as the regurgitated food never mixes with gastric acid. It is important to realize that the size of the diverticulum, while contributory to regurgitation, is not the most important determinant. It is now recognized that symptoms correlate better with the esophageal dysmotility characteristics than with the size of the diverticulum [14], and it is this distinguishing feature which must be taken into account when deciding upon a robust and long-lasting operative treatment. Pulmonary complications from aspiration occur in 24% to 45% of patients [15]. Ulceration, bleeding, and even perforation have been described. Though ED is correctly classified as a benign disease process, there have been reports of benign (leiomyoma) and malignant (squamous cell carcinoma) neoplasms with ED. [16–19]

The diagnosis of ED is first established by a barium swallow. Most ED are under 5 cm in width, though giant diverticulum can grow in excess of 10 cm. Best imaging results are accomplished with prone RAO oblique and upright swallow views. With a contrast swallow, it is imperative to determine the relationship between the diverticulum and the gastroesophageal junction. It is also possible to identify evidence of esophageal motility disorders and the presence of a hiatal hernia. Further diagnostic testing should proceed after initial imaging because, as stated previously, the diverticulum is the result of a functional obstruction and esophageal dysmotility. Failure to reach a diagnosis of the latter will result in sub-optimal treatment. Esophagoscopy is used to evaluate the esophagus for strictures, masses, erosions, and dysplasia (i.e., Barrett's). Special attention should be focused on the LES, noting the distance from the incisors as well as the muscle tone and possible presence of a hiatal or paraesophageal hernia. The diverticulum size and relation to the gastroesophageal junction can also be assessed directly. The stomach and proximal duodenum are also evaluated. Any abnormal finding should be documented and if necessary biopsied. Manometry and pH studies can be performed but are not required as the anatomic defect can make placement of the probes difficult and may not alter the operative plan. Often it is necessary to place it under endoscopic guidance as the catheter may otherwise coil in the diverticulum. The manometric findings may help determine the length of esophagomyotomy required to relieve the functional obstruction. The LES resting pressure, esophageal body contractile amplitudes, and contractile propagation should be measured. Twenty-four-hour pH study adds little and can be deferred as the decision for a fundoplication often is related to the operative approach.

Indications for Operative Treatment

Once a diagnosis of ED is made, there is debate concerning the indications for operative management. Patients who present with moderate-to-severe symptoms that affect lifestyle should undergo operative treatment. The controversy remains on how to manage those patients with mild symptoms or without symptoms at all. The natural history of asymptomatic ED remains widely unknown, though some reports state that less than 10% of these patients will progress to classic symptoms [20]. Proponents of treating mildly symptomatic or asymptomatic patients by medical means argue that the majority of these patients do not progress to lifestyle-limiting symptoms and the risks of surgery outweigh the benefits. Benacci et al. from the Mayo Clinic [21] reporting a series of 112 patients described the natural history of the condition in a group of 47 asymptomatic individuals who did not undergo surgical therapy. Twenty of these patients were monitored for a median of 4 years and all remained symptom-free. Fifteen additional patients had mild symptoms without surgical intervention, and in none of them did incapacitating symptoms develop during a median follow-up of 11 years. Although only half the patients with asymptomatic or mildly symptomatic disease had long-term follow-up available for review, progressive symptoms or complications did not develop in any of them. Opponents of the conservative approach state that developing symptoms can have devastating consequences. Altorki and colleagues strongly supported surgical intervention in all patients after noting aspiration in 9 of 20 patients, 3 of whom experienced life-threatening complications. Some, such as Debas et al., have argued that the size of the diverticulum guides treatment, using the arbitrary cutoff of >5 cm as an indication for operative treatment. However, as stated by Belsey himself, the size of the pouch correlates poorly with symptom severity, and it is the underlying motility disorder that should be sought after and fixed. An increasing number of asymptomatic patients are being treated surgically if found to have an underlying obstructive or motility disorder, and the results suggest that this is a safe approach with acceptable long-term outcomes.

Operative Technique

The tenets of operative treatment for ED revolve around three points:

1. Direct treatment of the diverticulum, either with diverticulectomy or diverticulopexy.
2. Esophagomyotomy.
3. Anti-reflux procedure, either full or partial esophageal wrapping.

Minimally invasive operative techniques have gained popularity and are rapidly becoming the procedure of choice for most surgeons. Recently, there have been many reports of safe and effective thoracoscopic and laparoscopic results in the literature when performed in high-volume centers by experienced surgeons. Though discussed in this chapter, the main surgical approach used until recently has been a left thoracotomy. This provides excellent access to the distal esophagus, esophagogastric junction, and the diverticulum itself. Reported morbidity from an open approach ranges from 6% to 38%, and mortality ranges from 0% to 11% [22].

Thoracoscopic Approach

The standard thoracoscopic approach is through a right video-assisted thoracoscopic surgery (VATS). The right side is chosen as the majority of ED develop from the right side of the esophagus and are adherent to the right pleura or diaphragm, or both. If there are preoperative manometric abnormalities, it is suggested that pneumatic LES dilatation be performed to help overcome the difficulty of performing a myotomy from the right chest [23]. Single-lung ventilation is preferred. The patient is placed in the left lateral decubitus position, and four thoracoscopic ports are used: one for the camera, one for retraction, and two for working instruments (Fig. 46.1). Dissection is begun by taking down the inferior pulmonary ligament and freeing the right lower lobe to the level of the inferior

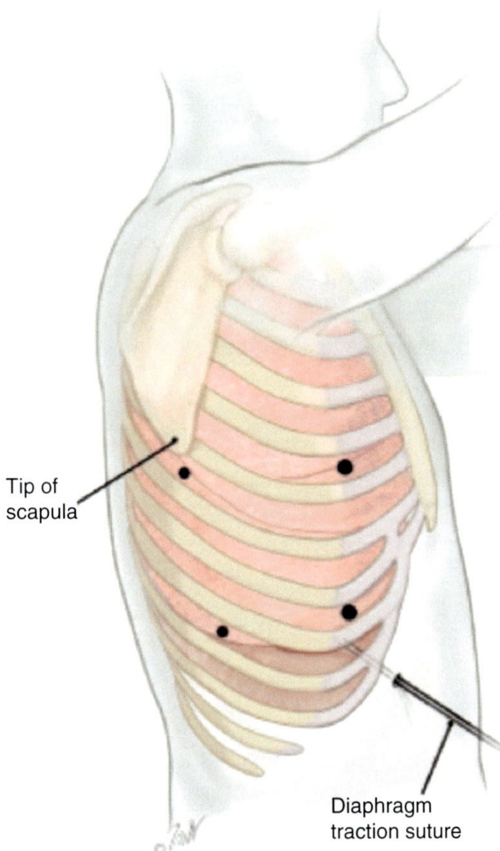

Fig. 46.1 Port placements for right video-assisted thoracoscopic surgery (VATS). (Source: Sugarbaker et al. [46]. Copyright © The McGraw-Hill Companies, Inc. All rights reserved)

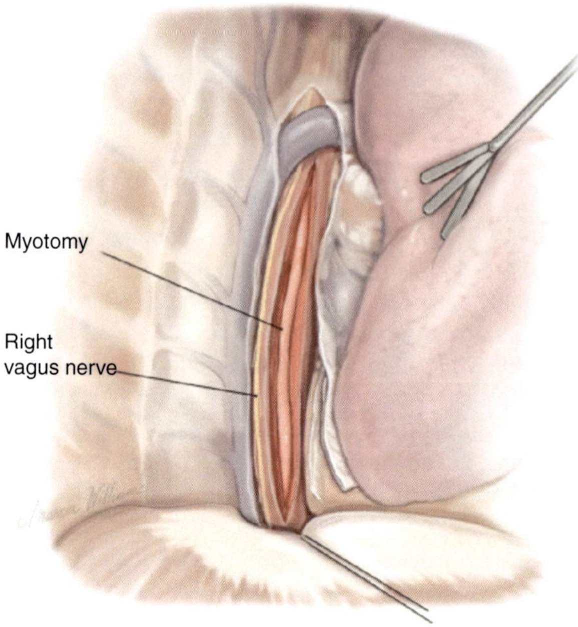

Fig. 46.2 A long myotomy is performed through a right VATS approach after resection of the epiphrenic diverticulum. (Source: Sugarbaker et al. [46]. Copyright © The McGraw-Hill Companies, Inc. All rights reserved)

pulmonary vein. Often a single retraction suture in the central tendon of the diaphragm can facilitate exposure of the distal esophagus. A fan retractor is used to retract the lung anteriorly, and division of the azygous vein is sometimes advantageous. The pleura overlying the esophagus is incised, and the right lateral aspect of the esophagus is dissected for a length of approximately 10 cm. Moderate insufflation and transillumination through an esophagoscope facilitate both dissection and resection of the diverticulum. The pouch is grasped with a clamp and gentle traction applied to facilitate identification of the diverticular neck. A myotomy must be performed either on the contralateral or ipsilateral side (Fig. 46.2). The myotomy typically extends proximal to the neck of the diverticulum and distally to an extent that is based on the preoperative and intraoperative findings. If required, the myotomy is extended across the lower esophageal sphincter (LES) and onto the stomach. A bougie or the endoscope can be used to stent the esophagus. The diverticulum is then resected using a reticulating stapler (EndoGIA), making sure that the stapler is oriented parallel to the longitudinal axis of the esophagus (Fig. 46.3). The overlying muscle and pleural layer is approximated over the mucosa staple line.

Laparoscopic Approach

The laparoscopic approach has also been advocated in an effort to simplify alignment of the stapler and facilitate performance of myotomy and fundoplication [24]. Another reported benefit of this technique includes better visualization of the distal esophagus, which is of particular importance in patients undergoing a myotomy, fundoplication, or both of these [25, 26]. The major disadvantages of the

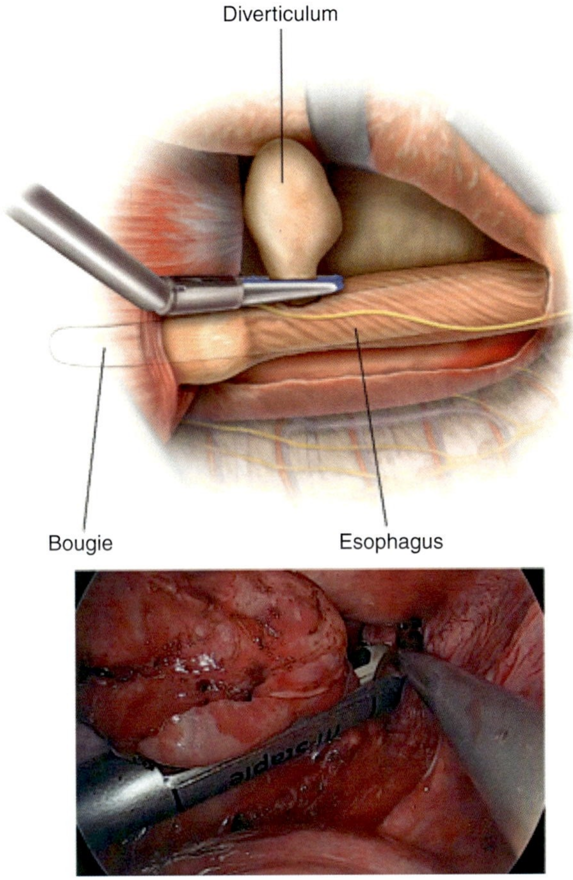

Fig. 46.3 Epiphrenic diverticulectomy. Note that the angle of the endoscopic stapler must be parallel to the neck of the diverticulum to ensure complete resection of the diverticulum and its neck

laparoscopic approach are seen in cases of diverticula that are large or inflamed with significant adhesions, both of which make adequate transhiatal dissection difficult [27, 28]. The patient is placed on the operating table supine and in reverse Trendelenburg inclination. Lithotomy positioning can be helpful. Pneumoperitoneum is established, and five operating ports are placed in the upper part of the abdomen (Fig. 46.4). The phrenoesophageal membrane is incised, and the dissection is carried up into the mediastinum to mobilize the esophagus. Mediastinal dissection is performed bluntly close to the esophageal wall until the diverticular pouch is reached. Moderate insufflation and transillumination through an endoluminal esophagoscope facilitate dissection of the diverticulum and identification of its neck. The pouch must be thoroughly cleaned of all adhesions. A Heller myotomy is performed. It is extended distally for approximately 2 cm on the gastric side and extended above the diverticulum. The endoscope is kept in the esophageal lumen to stent the esophagus. A reticulating linear endostapler is introduced through the trocar and applied parallel to the esophageal axis. Further stapler application may be necessary to remove the diverticulum. The integrity of the suture line must be

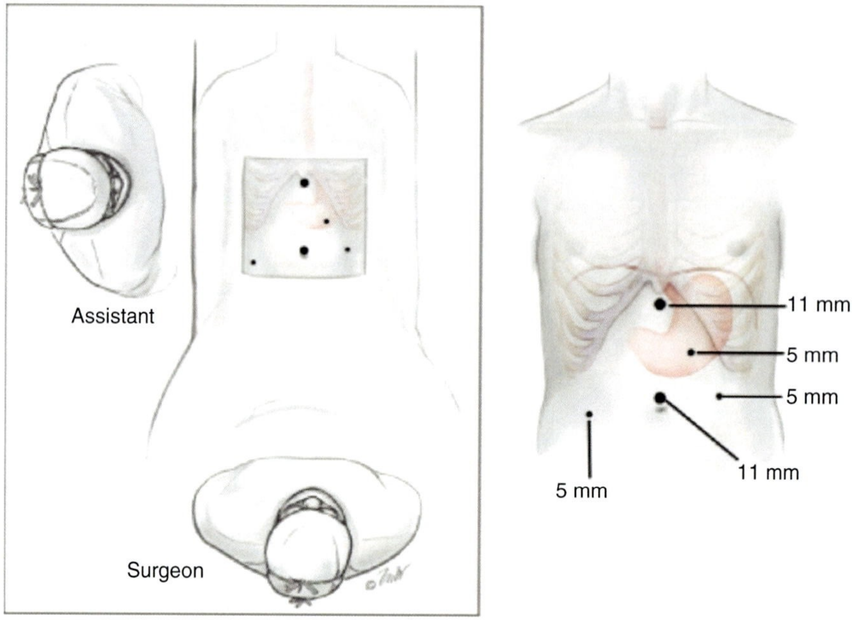

Fig. 46.4 Laparoscopic approach for epiphrenic diverticulum resection, myotomy, and fundoplication. This figure illustrates the surgeon standing in lithotomy position. (Source: Sugarbaker et al. [46]. Copyright © The McGraw-Hill Companies, Inc. All rights reserved)

checked endoscopically. A partial fundoplication is constructed by suturing the anterior fundic wall to the edges of the myotomy. The cranial sutures also attach the fundus to the anterior crus. A posterior hiatoplasty may be performed with interrupted sutures if the hiatal opening is enlarged.

Postoperative Management

A fluoroscopic swallow test is performed using Gastrografin or thin barium prior to oral feeding. This is not only to test for a leak through the staple line but to document no swallow dysfunction or aspiration. If the swallow test is reassuring for no leak, the patient is initiated on a liquid diet. An epidural is often used when a thoracoscopic approach is used to prevent postoperative splinting, and chest tubes are placed intraoperatively and usually removed 48–72 h after surgery. The median hospital stay is 5–7 days [22, 32]. Following a laparoscopic approach, patients can be advanced on a typical Nissen course.

Complications

The University of Pittsburgh reported a series of minimally invasive epiphrenic diverticula resection spanning 15 years. Patients were followed for a median of 20 months, and the median postoperative dysphagia scores were significantly reduced compared to preoperative scores ($p < 0.001$) [29]. Their overall complication rate was 30%. Major morbidity includes leak from the suture line or myotomy line, mediastinitis, fistula, recurrent laryngeal nerve injury, phrenic nerve injury, recurrence from incomplete myotomy, and development of reflux.

Controversies

There are several areas of controversy in the management of epiphrenic diverticula. The first area revolves around the choice of surgical approach. Macke et al. report that the trend of operative approach at the University of Pittsburgh has favored thoracoscopic treatment between 2003 and 2012, while the laparoscopic approach dominated between 1997 and 2002 [29]. While there are no prospective, randomized trials that compare open, laparoscopic, and thoracoscopic approaches in terms of morbidity and mortality, there are many reports in the literature of comparable results when each approach is studied individually. Hirano et al. looked at 133 patients within 25 articles published between 1995 and 2008 discussing results from laparoscopic or thoracoscopic surgery for epiphrenic diverticula. The laparoscopic approach was used in 84%, the thoracoscopic approach used in 14%, and a combined laparoscopic and thoracoscopic approach used in 2%. Overall mortality was 2%, and overall morbidity was 21%. The breakdown of complications was as follows: leak (15%), dysphagia (3%), pneumonitis (2%), symptomatic reflux (2%), and diverticulum recurrence (1%) [7]. Kilic et al. similarly looked at the operative results of 85 patients published in 10 papers who underwent minimally invasive surgery. Perioperative mortality was 1.2%, and the morbidity ranged from 0% to 45% with leaks comprising 14% [30]. While these numbers were higher than many of the more contemporary reports, many of these small series were early in the surgeons' experience with minimally invasive surgical approaches. These results were also comparable to the outcomes from open procedures reported from a large series in which mortality was 6.1% and morbidity ranged up to 38%. The authors prefer the laparoscopic approach as it gives good access to the diverticulum, allows for better extension of the myotomy distally, allows for a fundoplication, and has better pain control.

The second area which is now largely less debated is the question of performing a diverticulectomy versus a diverticulopexy. There are many reports from previous decades of varying degrees of successful diverticulopexy or imbrication for small diverticula. However, most contemporary surgeons would argue that complete resection is necessary to only prevent recurrence but also to prevent rare transformation into squamous cell carcinoma [31]. The critical step in performing a diverticulectomy is identification, exposure, and resection of the diverticular neck as failure to do so can lead to long-term recurrence. Many surgeons advocate buttressing the resection staple line. Mack and Luketich from the University of Pittsburgh found that omitting the buttressing step led to higher leak rates in an early series [32].

Another topic that has been debated in the literature is routine use of myotomy and the length of the myotomy. Belsy first stated the importance of addressing the underlying etiology leading to epiphrenic diverticular formation, namely, resolving dysmotility and over-pressurization of the esophagus. This has led to many surgeons advocating the routine use of myotomy, even if a motor disorder is not identified preoperatively [33, 34]. The counter argument is that a certain percentage of patients do not have manometric findings of dysmotility and that performing a myotomy routinely is unnecessary. However, accurate placement of the manometer can be difficult in the setting of a diverticulum, and in many cases the esophageal dysmotility can be intermittent and not captured with manometry. The Mayo Clinic reported a series where 60% of patients who were operated on for diverticular treatment had been diagnosed with esophageal dysfunction preoperatively. Varghese et al. at the University of Michigan reported preoperative identification of 82% of patients, and Nehra et al. reported 100% preoperative identification at the University of Southern California. Omitting a myotomy has led to leak and recurrence rates ranging from 10% to 20% [15, 21, 32, 35]. A closely related topic is the length of the myotomy. Streitz and colleagues advocated performing a myotomy only in the area of the motor abnormality while sparing the lower sphincter unless hypertensive [36]. Opponents to this idea state that the risk of complication is too great to omit a myotomy that extends through the lower sphincter and onto the stomach, as there are a percentage of patients with a hypertensive lower esophageal sphincter who are not diagnosed preoperatively. Currently there are no studies to conclusively state a superior myotomy length. The authors support performing a myotomy on all patients who undergo a diverticulectomy as the risk of leak and recurrence due to persistent high intraesophageal pressure remains high.

Finally, the issue of whether a fundoplication should be performed is not settled. Thomas and associates noted no difference in leak rates after myotomy with or without fundoplication (7% versus 8%), but they did report a higher rate of postoperative heartburn when a fundoplication was not performed (16% versus 9%) [37]. In a more recent series by Rossetti and coworkers, a leak rate of 24% was reported after diverticulectomy, myotomy, and complete fundoplication [38]. Most series report a fundoplication when a myotomy is performed either laparoscopically or when the myotomy is carried through the gastroesophageal junction onto the stomach. Moreover, when achalasia is present, most would favor a partial over a full fundoplication. When a thoracoscopic approach is taken, reports of not performing a fundoplication, performing a modified Belsey Mark IV, as well as adding a selective laparoscopic fundoplication have been advocated.

Mid-Esophageal Diverticula

Mid-esophageal diverticula are the least common diverticula of the esophagus. They occur between the thoracic inlet up to the distal 10 cm of the esophagus, with the majority of these outpouchings occurring within 4 cm of the carinal level (Fig. 46.5). The true etiology of mid-esophageal diverticula is unknown, but often they are considered the only true diverticula of the esophagus. There were descriptions of these types of diverticula in 1840 by Rokitansky, in 1878 by Zenker, and in 1932 by Kragh [39, 40].

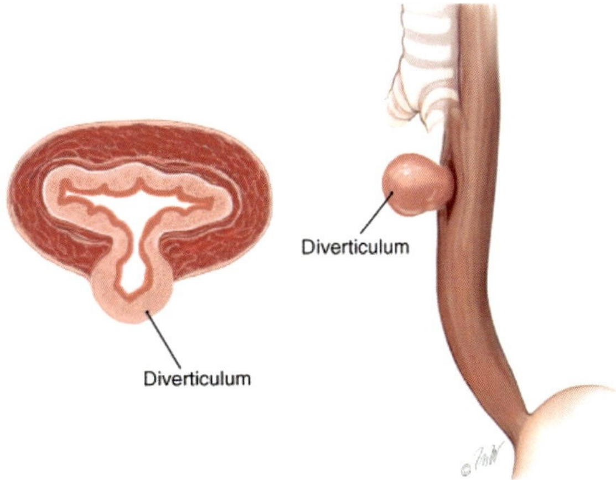

Fig. 46.5 Mid-esophageal diverticulum. Though thought to be exclusively a traction diverticulum, mid-esophageal diverticula can be pulsion type that does not involve all layers of the esophageal wall. (Source: Sugarbaker et al. [46]. Copyright © The McGraw-Hill Companies, Inc. All rights reserved)

Pathophysiology

Traditionally mid-esophageal diverticula have been associated with mediastinal lymph nodes that were pathologically altered secondary to tuberculosis, anthracosis, histoplasmosis, or other granulomatous diseases. These inflamed nodes become adherent to the esophagus, and over time the resultant scarring begins to contract and pulls the affected portion of the esophagus outward as a diverticulum. Those diverticula that arise from this outward traction are appropriately named *traction* diverticula and are true diverticula. Initially these mid-esophageal diverticula were believed to be strictly acquired, but in the early twentieth century, Ribbert began arguing a possible congenital etiology [41]. He postulated that in some patients mid-esophageal diverticula are a direct result of a closed tracheoesophageal fistula or foregut duplication cyst, and there have been reports in the literature to support this theory. Currently in the Western world there has been a steady decline in granulomatous disease of the mediastinum, and one recent review concluded that the most common etiology of these diverticula is an esophageal motor disorder [42]. Evander and associates from the University of Chicago studied a group of ten patients with mid-esophageal or epiphrenic diverticulum, and they found that whether they were traction or pulsion types, all of them had underlying esophageal motility disorders [43]. Consequently, any esophageal diverticulum should be regarded as a pulsion diverticulum until proven otherwise. There are reports of detection of squamous cell carcinoma arising from a mid-esophageal diverticulum, but this is rare [44].

Signs, Symptoms, and Diagnosis

The overwhelming majority of patients are asymptomatic, and most are discovered incidentally on imaging. This is believed to be secondary to the wide-based neck and dependent drainage distally in the esophagus. Symptoms associated with these diverticula include dysphagia, retrosternal pain, regurgitation, hemoptysis, and recurrent pneumonias and mediastinitis secondary to fistulization. Bleeding can result from erosion of the diverticulum into bronchial or esophageal arterial branches. Fistula formation between the esophagus and trachea can result in a "swallow-cough" phenomenon and recurrent aspiration pneumonias.

Any suspicion should begin with an extensive history focusing on presence of congenital tracheoesophageal fistulas or duplication cysts, previous granulomatous infections of the mediastinum, and previous lung malignancy. The workup should initially consist of chest imaging in the form of a plain X-ray and/or computed tomography (CT). The CT should help identify any mediastinal abnormalities or previous signs of disease. Esophagoscopy should be performed to visualize the diverticulum and look for other esophageal pathology. Esophageal manometry is used to diagnose any dysmotility disorders, and if the patient is having reflux symptoms, a pH study is often helpful to rule out GERD.

Indications for Operative Treatment

Unlike epiphrenic and to some extent upper esophageal diverticula, all mid-esophageal diverticula should be treated surgically. This is mainly to prevent the potentially catastrophic complications of bleeding and recurrent infection. There is no data in the literature that details the natural history of these diverticula or the percentage of patients that develop symptoms over time as this is an exceedingly rare pathologic process.

Operative Technique

The objectives for operative treatment for mid-esophageal diverticula are:

1. Resection of the diverticulum.
2. Resection of any fistula.
3. Treating an underlying esophageal motility disorder.

Thoracoscopic Approach

The optimal strategy is to approach the diverticulum from the right chest as this avoids the heart and aorta obstructing the surgeon's working field. The patient is placed in left lateral decubitus position, and four ports are used to access the chest in similar placement for a minimally invasive esophagectomy. One port is for the camera, one for a retractor, and two for working ports. Single-lung ventilation is implemented, and the inferior pulmonary ligament is taken down. The mediastinal pleura is dissected to expose the esophagus. There will be likely adhesive disease secondary to chronic inflammation and scarring, and meticulous attention must be used to preserve the anterior and posterior vagi, the phrenic nerve, and the thoracic duct. The azygous vein can be ligated if needed for exposure. Periesophageal dissection is employed for mobilization, and this can be carried to the thoracic inlet if needed in order to rotate the esophagus and display the diverticulum. Care should be taken to preserve as much of the direct arterial and venous branches to the esophagus. The diverticular neck is then exposed and a search for a fistula should ensue. If there is a fistula, the tract should be ligated and resected. A myotomy is then carried out just proximal to the diverticulum that extends 4–5 cm distal to the diverticulum. A reticulating stapler (EndoGIA) is aligned parallel to the esophagus and fired for resection. It is important to then buttress the staple line with either pleura or an intercostal muscle flap to prevent fistulization. If there is concomitant GERD or lax lower esophageal sphincter, a partial fundoplication may be added.

Endoscopic Approach

Per-oral endoscopic myotomy (POEM) has been recently used to treat mid-esophageal diverticula with short-term success [45]. Patients fast the day before the procedure, and general anesthesia is used. The esophagoscope is introduced and passed into the esophagus. The diverticulum is identified and measured from the incisors. The scope is then passed into the stomach looking for a hiatal hernia or tight lower esophageal sphincter. The scope is then passed back into the diverticulum and all debris is suctioned out. A 2-cm transverse mucosal incision is made approximately 5 cm above the diverticulum with an endoscopic knife, and a submucosal tunnel is created using repeated jet injection of normal saline mixed with methylene blue dye. Then the endoscopic knife is used to perform the myotomy proximal and distal to the diverticulum. The mucosal defect is then closed with metal clips. The scope is then passed down the natural esophageal lumen to confirm easy passage and to look for any esophageal perforation.

Postoperative Management

For patients who undergo thoracoscopic surgery, a fluoroscopic swallow test is performed to assess for esophageal leak or dysfunction. Patients who have no signs of leak or swallowing dysfunction are started on a liquid diet. The chest tubes are usually removed if there is no evidence of a leak. Patients undergoing POEM procedure are kept overnight in the hospital and undergo a contrast swallow study the next day. If there are no signs of leak or perforation, the patient is also started on a liquid diet.

Complications

The main complications that can arise are recurrent diverticulum, fistula formation, esophageal stenosis, recurrent laryngeal and phrenic nerve injury, and esophageal perforation. No long-term results have been reported for minimally invasive mid-esophageal diverticulectomy and myotomy or endoscopic myotomy.

References

1. Dukes RJ, Strimian CV, Dines DE, et al. Esophageal involvement with mediastinal granuloma. JAMA. 1976;236(20):2313–5.
2. Zenker FA, von Ziemssen H. Dilatations of the oesophagus. In: Buck AH, Ziemssen H, Peabody GL, editors. Cyclopaedia of the practice of medicine, vol. 3. London: Low, Marston, Searle & Rivington; 1878. p. 46.

3. Hammon JW, Rice RP, Postlethwait RW, et al. Esophageal intramural diverticulosis: a clinical study and pathological survey. Ann Thorac Surg. 1974;17(3):260–7.
4. Rice TW, Baker ME. Midthoracic esophageal diverticula. Semin Thorac Cardiovasc Surg. 1999;11(4):352–7.
5. Belsey R. Functional disease of the esophagus. J Thorac Cardiovasc Surg. 1966;52:164–88.
6. Mondiere JT. Notes sur quelques maladies de l'oesophage. Arch Gen Med Paris. 1833;3:28–65.
7. Hirano Y, Takeuchi H, Oyama T, et al. Minimally invasive surgery for esophageal epiphrenic diverticulum: the results of 133 patients in 25 published series and our experience. Surg Today. 2013;43(1):1–7.
8. Allen TH, Clagett OT. Changing concepts in the surgical treatment of pulsion diverticula in the lower esophagus. J Thorac Cardiovasc Surg. 1965;50(4):455–62.
9. Fasano NC, Levine MS, Rubesin SE, et al. Epiphrenic diverticulum: clinical and radiographic findings in 27 patients. Dysphagia. 2003;18:9–15.
10. Dodds WJ, Stef JJ, Hogan WJ, et al. Distribution of esophageal peristaltic pressure in normal subjects and patients with esophageal diverticulum. Gastroenterology. 1975;69(3):584–90.
11. Debas HT, Payne WS, Cameron AJ, et al. Pathophysiology of lower esophageal diverticulum and its implications for treatment. Surg Gynecol Obstet. 1980;151(5):593–600.
12. Mercantini P, Virgilio E, Petrucciani N, et al. Giant midthoracic pulsion diverticulum of the esophagus. Am Surg. 2010;76(7):782–4.
13. Nehra D, Lord RV, DeMeester TR, et al. Physiologic basis for the treatment of epiphrenic diverticulum. Ann Surg. 2002;235(3):346–54.
14. Orringer MB. Eiphrenic diverticula: fact and fable. Ann Thorac Surg. 1993;55(5):1067–8.
15. Altorki NK, Sunagawa M, Skinner DB. Thoracic esophageal diverticula: why is the operation necessary? J Thorac Cardiovasc Surg. 1993;105(2):260–4.
16. Jung JJ, Hsieh CC, Lin SC. Squamous cell carcinoma in a large epiphrenic esophageal diverticulum. Dig Dis Sci. 2009;54(6):1365–8. https://doi.org/10.1007/s10620-009-0727-2. Epub 2009 Jan 30.
17. Suzuki I, Oho K, Ariizumi K. A case report of giant esophageal leiomyoma associated with an epiphrenic esophageal diverticulum. Nihon Kyobu Geka Gakkai Zasshi. 1994;42(6):931–5.
18. Hodge GB. Esophageal leiomyoma associated with an epiphrenic diverticulum and hiatus hernia. Am Surg. 1970;36(9):538–43.
19. Eluvanthingal Muttikkal TJ, Shami VM, Jones DR. FDG positron emission tomography and computed tomography demonstration of carcinoma arising in an epiphrenic diverticulum. J Radiol Case Rep. 2014;30(11):42–6. https://doi.org/10.3941/jrcr.v8i11.2060. eCollection 2014.
20. Gust L, De Lesquen H, Ouattara M, et al. Open surgical management of oesophageal diverticulum. Multimed Man Cardiothorac Surg. 2015;2015:pii: mmv011. https://doi.org/10.1093/mmcts/mmv011. Print 2015.
21. Benacci JC, Deschamps C, Trastek VF, et al. Epiphrenic diverticulum: results of surgical treatment. Ann Thorac Surg. 1993;55(5):1109–13.
22. Varghese TK, Marshall B, Chang AC, et al. Surgical treatment of epiphrenic diverticula: a 30-year experience. Ann Thorac Surg. 2007;84:1801–9.
23. Bonavina L, Segalin A, Rosati R. Surgical therapy of esophageal leiomyoma. J Am Coll Surg. 1995;181(3):257–62.
24. Rosati R, Fumagalli U, Bona S, et al. Diverticulectomy, myotomy, and fundoplication through laparoscopy: a new option to treat epiphrenic esophageal diverticula? Ann Surg. 1998;227(2):174–8.
25. van der Peet DL, Klinkenberg-Knol EC, Berends FJ, et al. Epiphrenic diverticula: minimal invasive approach and repair in five patients. Dis Esophagus. 2001;14:60–2.
26. Del Genio A, Rossetti G, Maffetton V, et al. Laparoscopic approach in the treatment of epiphrenic diverticula: long-term results. Surg Endosc. 2004;18:741–5.
27. Rosati R, Fumagalli U, Bona S, et al. Laparoscopic treatment of epiphrenic diverticula. J Laparoendosc Adv Surg Tech A. 2001;11:371–5.

28. Neoral C, Aujeský R, Bohanes T, et al. Laparoscopic transhiatal resection of epiphrenic diverticulum. Dis Esophagus. 2002;15:323–5.
29. Macke RA, Luketich JD, Pennathur MD, et al. Thoracic esophageal diverticula: a 15-year experience of minimally invasive surgical management. Ann Thorac Surg. 2015;100:1795–803.
30. Kilic A, Schuchert MJ, Awais O, et al. Surgical management of epiphrenic diverticula in the minimally invasive era. JSLS. 2009;13(2):160–4.
31. Jordan PH, Kinner BM. New look at epiphrenic diverticula. World J Surg. 1999;23:147–52.
32. Fernando HC, Luketich JD, Samphire J, et al. Minimally invasive operation for esophageal diverticula. Ann Thorac Surg. 2005;80:2076–81.
33. D'Journo XB, Ferraro P, Martin J, et al. Lower esophageal sphincter dysfunction is part of the functional abnormality in epiphrenic diverticulum. Br J Surg. 2009;96:892–900.
34. Reznik SI, Rice TW, Murthy SC, et al. Assessment of a pathophysiology-directed treatment for symptomatic epiphrenic diverticulum. Dis Esophagus. 2007;20:320–7.
35. Vinson PP. Diverticula of the thoracic portion of the esophagus: report of 42 cases. Arch Otolaryngol. 1934;19:508–10.
36. Streitz JM, Glick ME, Ellis H. Selective use of myotomy for treatment of epiphrenic diverticula. Manometric and clinical analysis. Arch Surg. 1992;127:585–8.
37. Thomas ML, Anthony AA, Fosh BG, et al. Oesophageal diverticula. Br J Surg. 2001;88:629–42.
38. Rossetti G, Fei L, del Genio G, et al. Epiphrenic diverticula mini-invasive surgery: a challenge for expert surgeons – personal experience and review of the literature. Scand J Surg. 2013;102:129–35.
39. Zenker FA, von Ziemssen H. Cyclopedia of the practice of medicine. London: Sampson, Low, Marston, Searle and Rivinigton; 1878. p. 46–89.
40. Kragh J. Tuberculosis diverticula of the oesophagus (so-called traction diverticula). Acta Otolaryngol. 1922;4:49–62.
41. Ribbert H. Die traktionsdivertikel des oseophagus. Virchows Arch (Pathol Anat). 1904;178:351–67.
42. Borrie J, Wilson RLK. Oesophageal diverticula: principles of management and appraisal of classification. Thorax. 1980;35:759.
43. Evander A, Little AG, Ferguson MK, et al. Diverticula of the mid- and lower esophagus: pathogenesis and surgical management. World J Surg. 1986;10:820–8.
44. Nakamura T, Ota M, Marumiya K, et al. Partial esophagectomy for a superficial carcinoma arising from a mid-esophageal diverticulum. Gen Thorac Cardiovasc Surg. 2010;58:163–7.
45. Mou Y, Zeng H, Wang Q, et al. Giant mid-esophageal diverticula successfully treated by peroral endoscopic myotomy. Surg Endosc. 2016;30:335–8.
46. Sugarbaker DJ, Bueno R, Krasna MJ, Mentzer SJ, Zellos L. Adult Chest Surgery: http://www.accesssurgery.com.

A Laparoscopic Approach to Epiphrenic Diverticula

47

Jonathan Imran, Tarik Madni, and Thai Pham

Background

Epiphrenic diverticula are an uncommon form of esophageal diverticula that occur in the distal 10 cm of the esophagus [1–3]. The majority of patients have a single diverticulum, although 15–25% of patients may have multiple diverticula [4–6]. An epiphrenic diverticulum is characterized as a pulsion-type diverticulum caused by both localized weakness in the esophageal musculature and high intraluminal pressures [7]. During the mid-twentieth century, Belsey and Effler suggested that esophageal diverticula were the result of an underlying esophageal motility disorder and that treatment should focus on the motility disorder in addition to surgical resection [8, 9]. These astute observations formed the foundation for the surgical treatment of epiphrenic diverticula in the present day. Roux described the first surgical excision of an epiphrenic diverticulum through an open transabdominal approach, and in 1916 Stierling attempted transthoracic resection. Unfortunately this patient died from a leak and resultant mediastinitis [10].

As alluded to above, the pathophysiology of epiphrenic diverticula formation is likely due to a disordered contraction between the distal esophagus and the lower esophageal sphincter, which over time could lead to the development of an esophageal out-pouching containing submucosa and mucosa [11]. Recent studies have sought to identify a consistent association between esophageal motility disorders and epiphrenic diverticula. Motility disorders were found in 75–100% of patients studied with epiphrenic diverticula [2, 5, 12, 13].

J. Imran (✉) · T. Madni
University of Texas Southwestern Medical Center, Department of Surgery, Division of Burn, Trauma, and Critical Care, Dallas, TX, USA
e-mail: Jonathan.Imran@UTSouthwestern.edu

T. Pham
Section Chief of General Surgery, North Dallas VA Medical Center, Surgical Services, Dallas, TX, USA

J. Grams et al. (eds.), *The SAGES Manual of Foregut Surgery*,
https://doi.org/10.1007/978-3-319-96122-4_47

Epiphrenic diverticula are usually asymptomatic but when symptomatic can cause dysphagia, regurgitation, and chest pain [3]. There have also been reports of patients presenting with severe halitosis who are ultimately diagnosed with an epiphrenic diverticulum [14]. It is important to point out that the symptoms in patients presenting with epiphrenic diverticula are more likely due to the underlying motility disorder than the diverticulum itself [15]. In addition to the potential for severe symptoms, there is a small risk of malignancy from an epiphrenic diverticulum, estimated to be around 0.6% [16]. This is likely due to chronic inflammation that is caused by stasis and fermentation of food within the diverticulum [17].

Diagnosis and Preoperative Evaluation

A barium esophagram should be completed for diagnosis as well as to aid in surgical planning. The esophagram allows for localization and measurement of the size and dimensions of the diverticulum and its distance from the gastroesophageal junction. Upper endoscopy should also be performed to rule out malignancy. Esophageal manometry is indicated to rule out an underlying esophageal motility disorder, and 24-hour pH monitoring should be done if a patient has symptoms of gastroesophageal reflux. Once the diagnosis is confirmed, the patient should be referred for surgical consultation.

Indications for Surgery

Severe or intractable symptoms such as chest pain, dysphagia, or regurgitation are an indication for surgery. Patients are typically offered a diverticulectomy with esophagomyotomy and an anti-reflux procedure if there is an esophageal motility disorder present. Prior to surgery, a thorough history and physical examination should be performed. Appropriate preoperative imaging and manometry studies should be done as detailed above. There is, however, no consensus regarding the indications for surgery in patients with mild symptoms or patients who are asymptomatic. In a large review of 112 untreated patients with an epiphrenic diverticulum, 63% of patients were followed without symptom progression [18].

When dealing with patients who are asymptomatic or have atypical symptoms of an epiphrenic diverticulum, it is imperative to assess whether the patients have respiratory symptoms suggestive of aspiration prior to classifying them as asymptomatic. Symptoms can include night cough, asthma-like symptoms, laryngitis, or recent pneumonia. If these exist in conjunction with regurgitation, the patient likely had an aspiration event, and surgical management is warranted [3].

Controversy exists regarding some of the characteristics of the diverticulum that mandate resection. Some researchers have suggested that a diverticulum size greater than 5 cm or the presence of a dependent pouch is an indication for surgery

[19]. In a study by Fasano et al., all patients with a diverticular width greater than 5 cm were symptomatic versus only 41% of patients with diverticula less than 5 cm in width [4]. Patients with large diverticula who are symptomatic should be offered surgery if they are fit for an operation.

Technique

Minimally invasive surgical techniques that are used in the treatment of epiphrenic diverticula include the use of endoscopy, thoracoscopy, or laparoscopy. For the scope of this chapter we will only be focusing on the laparoscopic approach to epiphrenic diverticula. The standard laparoscopic approach to an epiphrenic diverticulum should be transhiatal diverticulectomy.

A laparoscopic Heller myotomy and partial fundoplication should be performed to address an underlying esophageal motility disorder if present and to prevent postoperative gastroesophageal reflux. The type of fundoplication is less important, as a Dor or Toupet fundoplication both work well to prevent postoperative reflux and dysphagia [20]. However without a fundoplication procedure, the incidence of postoperative gastroesophageal reflux after myotomy is quite high. A study of 43 patients undergoing laparoscopic Heller myotomy and esophageal diverticulectomy showed that 47% of patients had postoperative reflux without Dor fundoplication versus 9.1% of patients with fundoplication [21]. The length of the myotomy can vary, but typically should extend at least 5 cm above and 2–3 cm below the gastroesophageal junction.

The advantages of the laparoscopic approach are due to the minimally invasive nature of the procedure, as patients are able avoid a thoracotomy and the associated pain and increased hospital length of stay. The laparoscopic approach also provides an easier method to transect the diverticula along the longitudinal axis of the esophagus using an endostapler and allows for easier cardiomyotomy and fundoplication.

Description of Laparoscopic Approach (Fig. 47.1)

The patient is placed supine in the split-leg position on the operating room table with the surgeon between the legs. Alternatively, the patient can be positioned supine without the legs split. In either position, the arms can be left out or tucked. We prefer the arms tucked to allow easier placement of the bed-mounted liver retractor system. For both positions, foot boards should be utilized to decrease the risk of patients sliding, as the patient will need to be in steep reverse Trendelenburg for most of the case. The first assistant typically stands to the patient's left to assist and help drive the laparoscopic camera. Laparoscopic monitors are usually placed at eye level just over the patient's shoulders (Fig. 47.1).

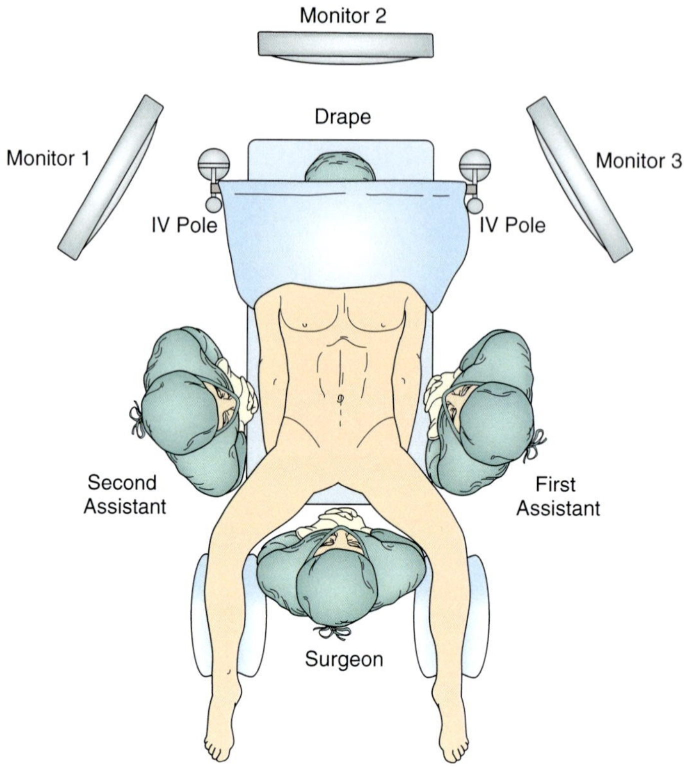

Fig. 47.1 Patient positioning [1, 20, 22]

Abdominal entry for the pneumoperitoneum can be performed according to individual preference. We typically use Veress needle technique at the level of the umbilicus or in the left upper quadrant at Palmer's point. A 10 mm camera port is usually placed at about 15 cm from the xiphoid just 1–2 cm to the patient's left of midline (Fig. 47.2). The surgeon's right-hand port is a 10 mm port that is placed about 12 cm from the xiphoid about 2–4 cm below the left costal margin. The assistant's port is a 5 mm port placed about 7–10 cm lateral from the surgeon's port in the patient's left upper quadrant. The surgeon's left hand port is a 5 mm port placed in the right upper quadrant just 7–10 cm from the xiphoid process. If the patient has a pendulous falciform ligament, this port can be placed through it to prevent obstruction by the falciform ligament during instrument exchanges. The placement of the port for the liver retractor is dependent on the type of liver retractor used. We typically use the Nathanson liver retractor, which is placed just below the xiphoid process. This is held in place with a laparoscopic iron intern that is mounted to the operating table. For other liver retraction systems, such as the fan or flexible tip liver retractors, the port would be placed in the mid or lower right quadrant of the abdomen.

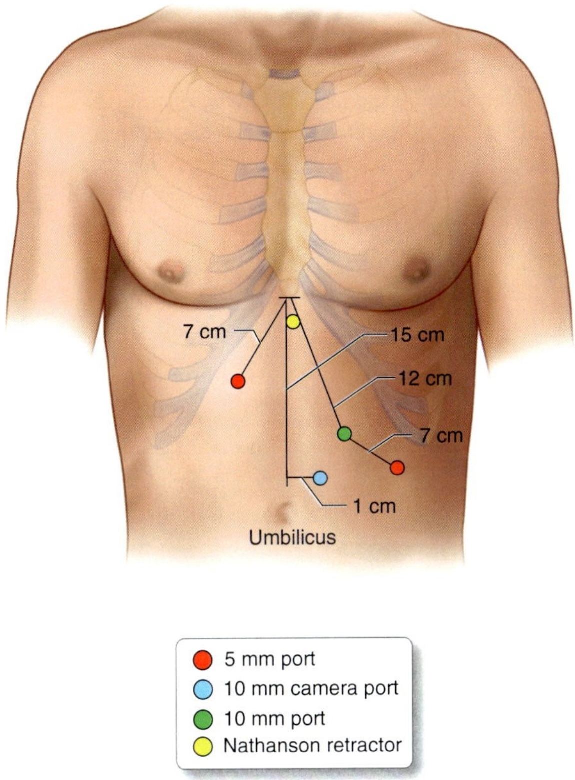

Fig. 47.2 Port placement [1, 20, 22]

Operative Details and Dissection

With the left lateral segment of the liver retracted and the patient in reverse Trendelenburg, the pars flaccida is incised and divided. Our preference is to use a vessel sealer device such as the laparoscopic Maryland (Medtronic, Minneapolis, Minn.), but other vessel sealing systems can be used instead. The pars flaccida is divided toward the right crus; if replaced or accessory left hepatic vessels are encountered, they are usually preserved, as it is difficult in this setting to determine if they are accessory or replaced. Additionally, preservation usually does not interfere with esophageal dissection or fundoplication. The hepatic branch of the vagus nerve can also be preserved, as it theoretically improves gallbladder function, but most clinical studies have not demonstrated symptomatic effect [23]. At the level of the right crus, the peritoneal attachments to the esophagus are circumferentially dissected free. During the anterior crural dissection, care should be taken to avoid injury to the anterior vagus nerve.

The short gastric vessels are divided starting at the inferior pole of the spleen. Again, a vessel sealer device can be employed and can efficiently perform this task.

The vessels are usually divided 1–2 cm from the greater curvature of the stomach. The vessels are divided up to the level of the crura and the posterior attachments of the stomach to the posterior crura are also divided. As the vessels are divided near the superior pole of the spleen, the exposure can be improved by having the assistant retract the posterior stomach medially while the surgeon retracts the greater curvature medially as well. Once this is complete, a retroesophageal window can be created and a Penrose drain can be used to encircle the esophagus and used by the assistant to retract the esophagus during mediastinal dissection.

Mediastinal attachments of the esophagus are then thinned and divided circumferentially. The diverticulum should come into view during this dissection. Mediastinal attachments to the diverticulum are then freed. Once the diverticulum is freed of its mediastinal adhesions, the diverticulum is dissected down to its neck, at the level of the esophageal longitudinal muscle.

Once dissection of the entire diverticular neck is complete, the diverticulum can be resected using an Endo GIA stapler (Medtronic, Minneapolis, Minn.). It has been reported that this mucosal staple line may be associated with higher leaks rates if left uncovered and used as the starting point of the subsequent myotomy [12]. Due to these reports, we prefer to reinforce this staple line by suturing the esophageal muscle to cover it. An esophageal myotomy is performed, starting at the level of the diverticulum and extending 2 cm onto the stomach. This myotomy is done on the side of the esophagus opposite to the diverticulectomy. An endoscope is then used to assess the adequacy of the myotomy and check for any mucosal perforations. To control gastroesophageal reflux, a partial fundoplication, typically a Dor fundoplication, is then fashioned.

On rare occasions, it may not be technically feasible to completely dissect the diverticulum free in order to resect it. As mentioned earlier, the symptoms from the diverticulum can't be distinguished from the underlying motility disorder. Recently published data have brought into question whether resection of the diverticulum is necessary. Allaix et al. compared the dysphagia symptom scores of seven patients whose epiphrenic diverticula were technically not resectable to the scores of six patients who underwent an epiphrenic diverticulectomy. Both groups had a Heller myotomy and partial fundoplication. The scores indicated a similar resolution of symptoms [24]. However, this was a small study and no other group has reported similar findings. Based on the current literature, the consensus is to perform a diverticulectomy when possible.

Postoperative Management

Patients are kept nil per os (NPO) immediately after surgery with intravenous fluids. Pain control is achieved with intravenous pain medications until they are able to tolerate oral medications. Patients are encouraged to ambulate within 24 h after surgery and appropriate DVT chemoprophylaxis is started at 12 h after surgery. Sequential compression devices are placed intraoperatively and are continued in the postoperative period. An esophagram is obtained on postoperative day 3. Patients can be started on a liquid diet if their esophagram is normal, and they are advanced as tolerated to a full liquid diet. We have found it helpful for the patients to have a consult with a nutritionist during their hospital stay to review postoperative diet restrictions. They are discharged home when they can tolerate a full liquid diet and have adequate pain control on oral pain medication. The diet is advanced to soft foods after 1 week and back to regular food by 3 weeks after surgery. We prefer to use liquid pain medication, as it can be easier for a patient to take in the early postoperative period. The patient is seen within 2 weeks of surgery for a postoperative follow-up. A repeat esophagram is not ordered unless the patient has complaints of dysphagia, nausea, emesis, or other worrisome symptoms.

Postoperative Complications

The most feared complication after laparoscopic transhiatal diverticulectomy is leakage from the staple line after transection of the diverticulum. Resultant complications include pneumonia, empyema, abscess formation, and potentially even sepsis if the leak is uncontrolled. Other complications include nausea, emesis, dysphagia, recurrence of preoperative symptoms, and port site hernia. For laparoscopic transhiatal diverticulectomy, myotomy, and partial fundoplication, the published leak rates from the largest published studies range from 9% to 23%. However, in the study with the highest leak rate, a Nissen fundoplication was performed in all patients, which may cause a partial distal obstruction that likely contributed to a higher than expected leak rate. The overall morbidity rate ranges from 0% to 50%, and the mortality rate after laparoscopic epiphrenic diverticulum repair is estimated to be 0% to 10%, which is similar to the reported rate of 0–11% through an open thoracotomy [18, 22, 25].

Postoperative Outcomes

Postoperative symptom relief can be graded using a Likert scale or a patient questionnaire. With the use of a Likert scale, patient symptom relief is stratified as excellent (complete resolution of symptoms), good (symptoms approximately once per month), fair (symptoms less than once per week), or poor (symptoms not better or worse than in the preoperative period). In a review of six recent studies, postoperative outcomes were graded as good in 85–100% of patients [11].

References

1. Zaninotto G, Parise P, Salvador R, et al. Laparoscopic repair of epiphrenic diverticulum. Semin Thorac Cardiovasc Surg. 2012;24(3):218–22.
2. Melman L, Quinlan J, Robertson B, et al. Esophageal manometric characteristics and outcomes for laparoscopic esophageal diverticulectomy, myotomy, and partial fundoplication for epiphrenic diverticula. Surg Endosc Other Interv Tech. 2009;23(6):1337–41.

3. Soares R, Herbella FA, Prachand VN, Ferguson MK, Patti MG. Epiphrenic diverticulum of the esophagus. From pathophysiology to treatment. J Gastrointest Surg. 2010;14(12):2009–15.
4. Fasano NC, Levine MS, Rubesin SE, Redfern RO, Laufer I. Epiphrenic diverticulum: clinical and radiographic findings in 27 patients. Dysphagia. 2003;18(1):9–15.
5. Nehra D, Lord RV, DeMeester TR, et al. Physiologic basis for the treatment of epiphrenic diverticulum. Ann Surg. 2002;235(3):346–54.
6. Costantini M, Zaninotto G, Rizzetto C, Narne S, Ancona E. Oesophageal diverticula. Best Pract Res Clin Gastroenterol. 2004;18(1):3–17.
7. Rosati R, Fumagalli U, Bona S, Bonavina L, Peracchia A. Diverticulectomy, myotomy, and fundoplication through laparoscopy: a new option to treat epiphrenic esophageal diverticula? Ann Surg. 1998;227(2):174–8.
8. Belsey R. Functional disease of the esophagus. J Thorac Cardiovasc Surg. 1966;52(2):164–88.
9. Effler DB, Barr D, Groves LK. Epiphrenic diverticulum of the esophagus: surgical treatment. Archives Surg (Chicago, Ill: 1960). 1959;79:459–67.
10. Kausel HW, Lindskog GE. Epiphrenic diverticulum of the esophagus; a review of its surgical treatment and report of a case. Dis Chest. 1952;21(3):334–45.
11. Fisichella PM, Jalilvand A, Dobrowolsky A. Achalasia and epiphrenic diverticulum. World J Surg. 2015;39(7):1614–9.
12. Fernando HC, Luketich JD, Samphire J, et al. Minimally invasive operation for esophageal diverticula. Ann Thorac Surg. 2005;80(6):2076–80.
13. Tedesco P, Fisichella PM, Way LW, Patti MG. Cause and treatment of epiphrenic diverticula. Am J Surg. 2005;190(6):891–4.
14. Montes de Oca Megias E, Noa Pedroso G, Martinez Alfonso MA, Perez Triana F, Seijas Cabrera O, Garcia Jorda E. Severe halitosis as presentation of epiphrenic diverticulum. *Revista espanola de enfermedades digestivas: organo oficial de la Sociedad Espanola de Patologia Digestiva.* 2016;108:756–8.
15. Varghese TK Jr, Marshall B, Chang AC, Pickens A, Lau CL, Orringer MB. Surgical treatment of epiphrenic diverticula: a 30-year experience. Ann Thorac Surg. 2007;84(6):1801–9; discussion 1801–9.
16. Herbella FA, Dubecz A, Patti MG. Esophageal diverticula and cancer. Dis Esophagus. 2012;25(2):153–8.
17. Bradley PJ, Kochaar A, Quraishi MS. Pharyngeal pouch carcinoma: real or imaginary risks? Ann Otol Rhinol Laryngol. 1999;108(11 Pt 1):1027–32.
18. Benacci JC, Deschamps C, Trastek VF, Allen MS, Daly RC, Pairolero PC. Epiphrenic diverticulum: results of surgical treatment. Ann Thorac Surg. 1993;55(5):1109–13; discussion 1114.
19. Debas HT, Payne WS, Cameron AJ, Carlson HC. Physiopathology of lower esophageal diverticulum and its implications for treatment. Surg Gynecol Obstet. 1980;151(5):593–600.
20. Rawlings A, Soper NJ, Oelschlager B, et al. Laparoscopic Dor versus Toupet fundoplication following Heller myotomy for achalasia: results of a multicenter, prospective, randomized-controlled trial. Surg Endosc. 2012;26(1):18–26.
21. Richards WO, Torquati A, Holzman MD, et al. Heller myotomy versus Heller myotomy with Dor fundoplication for achalasia: a prospective randomized double-blind clinical trial. Ann Surg. 2004;240(3):405–12; discussion 412–405
22. Del Genio A, Rossetti G, Maffettone V, et al. Laparoscopic approach in the treatment of epiphrenic diverticula: long-term results. Surg Endosc Other Interv Tech. 2004;18(5):741–5.
23. Ozdogan M, Kuvvetli A, Das K, et al. Effect of preserving the hepatic vagal nerve during laparoscopic Nissen fundoplication on postoperative biliary functions. World J Surg. 2013;37(5):1060–4.
24. Allaix ME, Borraez Segura BA, Herbella FA, Fisichella PM, Patti MG. Is resection of an esophageal epiphrenic diverticulum always necessary in the setting of achalasia? World J Surg. 2015;39(1):203–7.
25. Kilic A, Schuchert MJ, Awais O, Luketich JD, Landreneau RJ. Surgical management of epiphrenic diverticula in the minimally invasive era. JSLS (Journal of the Society of Laparoendoscopic Surgeons / Society of Laparoendoscopic Surgeons). 2009;13(2):160–4.

Evaluation of Benign Submucosal Tumors

48

Sanjay Salgado and Marvin Ryou

Introduction

Gastrointestinal submucosal tumors (SMTs) consist of a broad range of lesions which arise from the wall of the gastrointestinal tract. While commonly referred to as "submucosal" tumors, they are perhaps more accurately described as "subepithelial," as they may arise from layers of the foregut wall other than the histologic submucosa. They are generally found after the fifth decade of life, with an estimated prevalence of 0.3% [16] and equal incidence in men and women. SMTs can be generally categorized as neoplastic or nonneoplastic tumors, with the latter subdivided into epithelial and non-epithelial tumors. This chapter will focus on the evaluation of benign SMTs, potentially malignant SMTs, and nonneoplastic mimickers, paying specific attention to the tumors most likely to affect the esophagus and stomach. A more detailed discussion on the management and interventional therapies will be discussed in subsequent chapters.

As SMTs retain intact overlying mucosa, the majority are not associated with symptoms and are found incidentally during endoscopic or radiographic examinations. When symptomatic, these tumors most commonly present with non-specific abdominal discomfort, gastrointestinal bleeding, or rarely, signs of obstruction. Endoscopic evaluation of these lesions generally results in the finding of a mass or bulge covered in normal-appearing epithelium. While the size, shape, texture, and color of the lesions may aid in narrowing down the differential, endoscopy alone is usually insufficient to reach a diagnosis and is generally unable to distinguish between a foregut wall process and extrinsic compression.

Although studies have suggested that MRI has similar diagnostic yield and mitigated radiation exposure [53], contrast-enhanced CT is the preferred imaging

S. Salgado (✉) · M. Ryou
Division of Gastroenterology, Hepatology, and Endoscopy, Brigham and Women's Hospital, Boston, MA, USA
e-mail: smsalgado@bwh.harvard.edu

J. Grams et al. (eds.), *The SAGES Manual of Foregut Surgery*,
https://doi.org/10.1007/978-3-319-96122-4_48

modality to evaluate foregut masses. MRI, however, may be more diagnostically appropriate for SMTs at specific sites, including near the liver. Radiographic imaging is primarily useful in examining extrinsic tumors or determining metastatic spread, but is unable to distinguish between the layers of the gastrointestinal wall. Therefore, they have limited diagnostic value in evaluation of SMTs. Positron emission tomography (PET) measuring flurodeoxyglucose is useful for the detection of certain SMTs, with high sensitivities, but has not been adequately shown to be superior to CT imaging for diagnosis [13]. Endoscopic ultrasound (EUS) evaluation may provide further information about the layer of the wall where the lesions originate (see Table 48.1 and Fig. 48.1), as well as determine size, border irregularities, and echogenic homogeneity [61].

However, in many cases, EUS alone may not be able to differentiate between benign and malignant neoplastic lesions, necessitating the eventual need for histopathological examination. This is especially true in hypoechoic masses in the third or fourth echo layer [22], for which the differential diagnosis consists of both benign and malignant masses. There are a number of possible approaches for endoscopic biopsy. Standard forceps biopsy is primarily designed to sample mucosal tissue and is generally unable to reach sufficient depth for submucosal evaluation. However,

Table 48.1 Histologic equivalents to layers of the gastrointestinal wall identified by endoscopic ultrasound

EUS layer	Histologic equivalent	Associated SMT
1	Superficial mucosa	
2	Deep mucosa (muscularis mucosa)	Carcinoid, granular cell, fibroid polyps
3	Submucosa and interface between the submucosa and muscularis propria	Lipoma, lymphangioma, granular cell, duplication cyst, pancreatic rest, varix, fibroid polyps, Brunner gland hamartoma
4	Muscularis propria	GIST, leiomyoma, schwannoma, glomus, pancreatic rest, fibroid polyps
5	Serosa and subserosal fat	

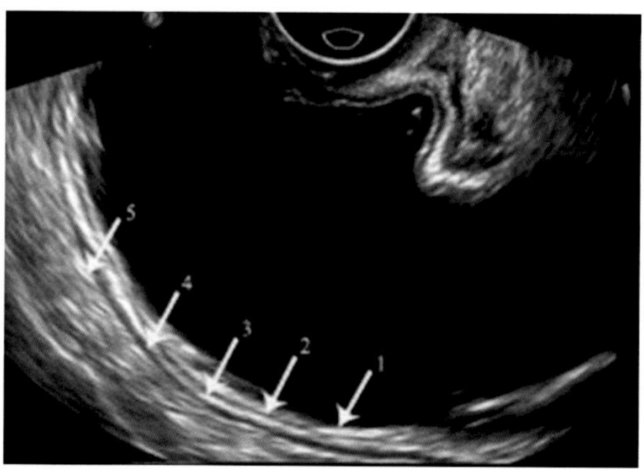

Fig. 48.1 Layers of the gastrointestinal wall identified by endoscopic ultrasound (linear array echoendoscope)

"stacked" or "tunneled" biopsies, in which multiple biopsy specimens are taken from the same site, may provide sufficient depth of tissue. However, while safe, the diagnostic yield of this test appears limited. Endoscopic mucosal resection improves this yield but comes with the risks of bleeding and perforation [21]. Newer sampling techniques, such as EUS-guided single-incision needle-knife (SINK) biopsies [6], which involved a submucosal incision followed by stacked biopsies, appear to improve the yield while limiting these adverse effects, although more study is warranted.

EUS-guided fine needle aspiration (FNA) consists of using a high-gauge needle (typically 22-gauge or 25-gauge) to aspirate cells from target lesions for cytology. While cytology is useful for distinguishing between benign and malignant lesions, it is generally difficult to differentiate between benign masses unless augmented with immunohistochemical analysis. Newer EUS-guided core biopsy needles seem to provide improved diagnostic yield by acquiring samples with intact tissue architecture for better histological analysis.

Benign Submucosal Tumors

Submucosal masses can be divided into epithelial and non-epithelial lesions. Epithelial tumors primarily include a host of malignant neoplasms, including gastric carcinomas, melanomas, and metastatic carcinomas. Non-epithelial tumors consist of primarily of mesenchymal tumors. These tumors are the most common non-epithelial benign neoplasm involving the gastrointestinal tract and constitute 1% of primary gastrointestinal cancers. Mesenchymal tumors include a wide array of benign neoplasms, including leiomyomas, lipomas, schwannomas, and lymphangiomas.

Leiomyomas

Leiomyomas are firm, well-circumscribed lesions that arise either superficially from the muscularis mucosae or from the deeper muscularis propria. Superficial leiomyomas are often found incidentally in the sigmoid colon and rectum. Deep leiomyomas are the most common mesenchymal tumor of the esophagus, and while they may occasionally be found in the stomach (see Fig. 48.2) near the gastroesophageal junction, they are rare elsewhere in the GI tract. Although superficial leiomyomas are incidentally discovered more often, it has been suggested that the overall incidence of deep leiomyomas may be higher than previously believed [1].

Clinically, the most common symptoms of leiomyomas are gastrointestinal bleeding and gastric discomfort, although a majority of these tumors are asymptomatic [4]. CT imaging demonstrates a smoothly contoured, homogeneous mass with slight enhancement and low attenuation. Endoscopic evaluation reveals a protruding mass with normal mucosa. Endoscopic ultrasound is perhaps the most accurate method for the noninvasive diagnosis of leiomyomas, demonstrating a mass that

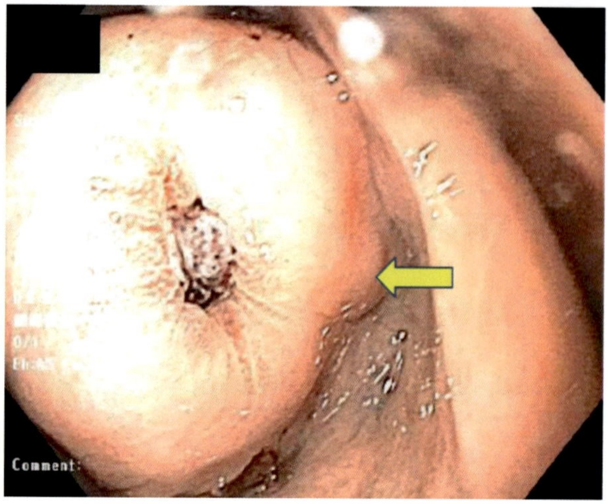

Fig. 48.2 Large ulcerated gastric subepithelial mass

arises from the fourth hypoechoic layer or rarely the second hypoechoic area. Malignant leiomyosarcomas should be considered if the lesion contains cystic spaces, has associated enlarged lymph nodes, or disrupts tissue planes.

Histologically, leiomyomas are paucicellular with fascicles of spindle cells without nuclear atypia or frequent mitoses. Leiomyomas are also more likely to grow intraluminally [5], in contrast to other SMTs, such as gastrointestinal stromal tumors (GISTs). The cellular nuclei of leiomyomas are centrally located but may be displaced by vacuole, and unlike liposarcomas and carcinomas, these vacuoles do not contain fat mucosubstances. Immunohistochemically, leiomyomas show strong positive immunoreactivity for desmin and smooth muscle actin and negative reactivity for c-kit and CD-34.

Surgical removal is considered for tumors larger than 2 cm or for any discernable symptoms. The appropriate management for smaller, asymptomatic tumors is more controversial. Histologically, leiomyomas and leiomyosarcomas are similar in appearance, leading some to recommend endoscopic resection of all such lesions. Alternatively, conservative management with serial EUS evaluations may be pursued.

Lipoma

Lipomas are well-circumscribed, homogeneous nodules consisting of mature adipose tissue. They are predominantly located in the stomach and right colon [35]. These tumors are easily identified due to their characteristic appearance of a smooth, yellow lesion with a positive "pillow sign," in which an indentation is elicited with forceps during colonoscopy. They also demonstrate the "tenting sign," where the mucosa can be easily pulled away from the underlying submucosal tumor. EUS of these tumors show a hyperechoic, homogeneous lesion arising from the third echoic layer. While the finding of a uniformly hyperechoic submucosal mass is essentially diagnostic for a lipoma, biopsies may be taken to confirm the diagnosis. A single biopsy will generally reach only the surface mucosa, while tunneled biopsies will likely result in the extrusion of underlying adipose tissue, dubbed the "naked fat sign" [36].

The majority of lipomas are asymptomatic, and in general, they can be followed without endoscopic surveillance. Excision is warranted only when there is difficulty distinguishing between lipoma and malignant neoplasms. However, lesions over 2 cm may cause abdominal pain, bowel changes, and rectal bleeding. Rarely, lipomas may ulcerate, leading to hemorrhage, obstruction, or intussusception, necessitating surgical intervention and removal. Concern for these complications may lead to elective removal of larger lipomas. While endoscopic, rather than surgical, removal may be considered in these patients, endoscopic intervention is best reserved for patients with pedunculated or superficial lesions. This is due to difficulty cauterizing adipose tissue and resultant risk of perforation. Notably, ligation with detachable nylon snares (Endoloop, Ethicon LLC) alone, or prior to endoscopic resection, may decrease this perforation risk – however, utilization of this technique will forgo the ability to procure a specimen for pathology [46, 51].

Schwannomas

Schwannomas are well-circumscribed, spherical and occasionally multinodular neuroendocrine tumors originating from the muscularis propria. They are relatively rare, account for less than 3% of mesenchymal gastrointestinal tumors, and are predominantly found in the stomach [20]. While benign, these tumors can grow to up to 10 cm in diameter. CT imaging demonstrates a homogeneous lesion with delayed enhancement, resulting in frequent misdiagnoses as GISTs [15]. Endoscopy reveals a submucosal mass with or without central ulceration. EUS demonstrates an ovoid, heterogeneously hypoechoic lesion arising from the fourth echogenic layer [64]. Microscopically, schwannomas consist of spindle cells with nuclear palisading and a nodular lymphatic cuff. While grossly schwannomas resemble GISTs, they can be distinguished by their positive immunoreactivity for S-100 and negative reactivity for desmin, actin, and c-kit.

Gastrointestinal Lymphangiomas

Lymphangiomas are benign vascular tumors that rarely affect the gastrointestinal tract, occurring in 1 per 50,000 people. They may be present anywhere in the gastrointestinal tract, although they are most frequently found in the stomach and small bowel. Like many benign submucosal tumors, they are often found incidentally. Occasionally, they can become symptomatic and usually present with vague abdominal discomfort, although some may become large enough to cause obstruction or intussusception. Endoscopy generally reveals a round, yellow-to-white nodular mass with or without a stalk. On EUS, lymphangiomas demonstrate an anechoic and septated structure, arising from the third echoic layer [23]. Histologically, these tumors demonstrate dilated lymphatics lined with endothelial cells with lymphocytic infiltrate and eosinophilic lymph [25]. As a rare tumor, there is no consensus on management, although if symptomatic, surgical or endoscopic resection is often pursued.

Potentially Malignant Submucosal Tumors

There are a number of SMTs that are potentially malignant neoplasms. They include GISTs, carcinoid tumors, granular cell tumors, and glomus tumors.

Gastrointestinal Stromal Tumors

Historically, GISTs were known as gastrointestinal smooth muscle tumors and further subclassified as leiomyoma if benign, leiomyosarcoma if malignant, and leiomyoblastoma if epithelioid. However, with the use of electron microscopy and immunohistochemical staining, these tumors were found to lack smooth muscle structure, distinguishing them from leiomyomas. Furthermore, while some had evidence of autonomic neural differentiation, these tumors also lacked microscopic features of Schwann cells. These discoveries, coupled with the discovery of the near-universal gain-of-function c-*kit* (CD177) mutation, have led to the modern conception of a GIST [37].

GISTs have an annual incidence of 14 million [47], with 4000–6000 new cases diagnosed every year in the USA alone. While the incidence of malignant GISTs is reportedly much lower (0.68 per 100,000 [56]), it is worth noting that much of this epidemiologic data is difficult to interpret in a modern context, as the definition of a "malignant GIST" was determined before GISTs had been molecularly characterized. While previously it was thought that smaller GISTs did not have malignant potential, there has been a recent shift in the understanding of the natural history of malignant GISTs, with current consensus that all GISTs, regardless of size, may have malignant transformation.

GISTs are the most common type of mesenchymal tumor of nearly every segment of the gastrointestinal tract, with the exception of the esophagus, colon, and rectum. Over 50% occur in the stomach, with another 30% detected in the jejunum or ileum. These tumors generally affect adults in the sixth or seventh decade of life with a slight male predominance. They are rare in children [37] although they are associated with certain pediatric syndromes, including Carney-Stratakis syndrome [49]. In adults, they are more common in patients with NF1 mutations or heritable mutations in the c-kit gene. Clinically, the most common symptoms are gastrointestinal bleeding and gastric discomfort. However, nearly one third are incidentally detected with radiographic imaging or endoscopy.

CT imaging findings vary depending on the size and aggressiveness of the tumor. Small benign tumors generally appear as well-defined, homogeneous masses with varying degrees of enhancement. Large size, heterogenous enhancement, regional lymphadenopathy, the presence of necrosis, or mucosal ulceration raises concern for malignancy. Endoscopic evaluation typically demonstrates a submucosal mass with normal overlaying mucosa, protruding into the lumen of the gastrointestinal tract (see Figs. 48.3 and 48.4). EUS depicts a hypoechoic, homogeneous lesion with well-defined margins. Irregular extraluminal borders, heterogeneity, cystic spaces, and echogenic foci should raise concern for malignancy. As a solid and often fibrotic mass, aspiration of sufficient cells for a histopathological diagnosis can prove difficult, resulting in a nondiagnostic sample in over 15% of cases [19]. The accuracy of EUS-FNA in diagnosis ranges from 76% to 90% [7, 31], although accuracy may increase with unroofing the overlaying mucosae prior to biopsy [28] or using EUS-guided Trucut biopsy [7].

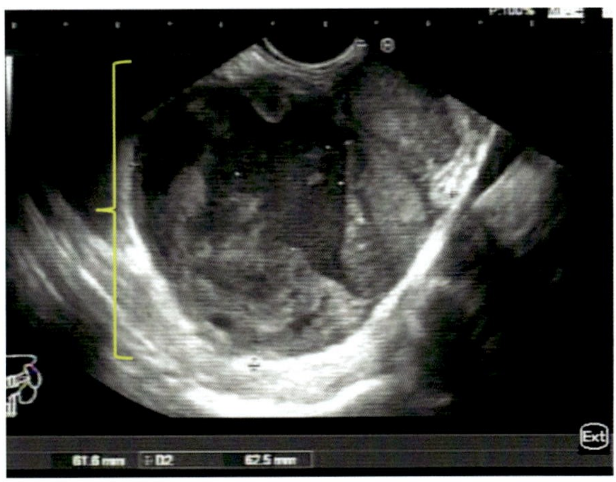

Fig. 48.3 EUS image of 6 cm exophytic gastric subepithelial mass

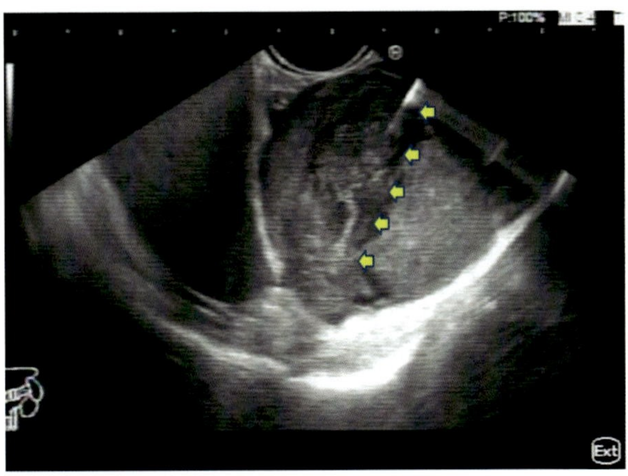

Fig. 48.4 EUS-guided fine-needle biopsy (arrows) of exophytic gastric mass. Pathology confirmed gastrointestinal stromal tumor (GIST)

Histologically, a majority of GISTs consist of spindle cells, although a minority may be epithelioid or mixed. C-kit-negative GISTs are more often epithelioid in nature[16]. In general, microscopy of GISTs tends to show hypercellularity with uniform nuclei and juxtanuclear cytoplasmic vacuoles, with cells arranged in whorls. Gastric GISTs also contain a sclerosing matrix, perinuclear vacuolization and nuclear palisading, and mitotically active morphology. Small intestinal GISTs are characterized by extracellular collagen globules, verocay bodies of neuropil-like material [37], and brightly eosinophilic stromal skeinoid fibers, which are composed of nodular tangles of collagen fibers [41]. Definitive diagnosis, however, is dependent on immunohistologic analysis.

Over 95% of GISTs are immunohistochemically positive for c-kit, and virtually all GISTs will be positive for either c-kit or anoctamin-1 (also referred to as DOG1 or ORAOV2) [40]. Furthermore, 60–70% of GISTs are positive for CD34, 30–40% are positive for smooth muscle actin, and a small minority may be positive for S-100 [52]. A vast majority of GISTs contain a gain-of-function mutation either c-kit, which codes for a tyrosine kinase receptor, or the platelet-derived growth factor receptor (PDGFRA) gene. In both cases, the resulting receptor is constitutively active, which alters cell proliferation leading to tumor growth. There appears to be no difference in downstream activation of signaling intermediates and cytogenetic changes in c-kit-driven tumors versus PDGFRA-driven tumors [17]. However, it is worth nothing that the mutation in c-kit or PDGFRA alone is likely not sufficient to cause tumor growth, and other genetic changes likely need to take place as well [10]. There are a number of different exons in the c-kit gene that maybe be affected, including exon 9, 11, 13, and 17. Understanding which exon is affected has therapeutic implications, as tumors with exon 11 mutations have been shown to respond better to imatinib therapy than other types of GISTs. It is unclear at this time whether immunohistochemical analysis informs prognosis. However, there is some data to suggest that certain mutations may be associated with aggressive phenotypes [30]. A minority of GISTs does not have a detectable c-kit or PDGFRA mutations. These wild-type GISTs include the GISTs of NF1 and Carney-Stratakis mutations and may be related to the succinate dehydrogenase gene mutations [24].

While esophageal GISTs are rare (<1%), the majority of these GISTs are malignant [39] and are generally more difficult to manage due to the inadequate confinement of the tumor by the serosal layer and the challenge of segmental resections. Because of this, esophagectomy is often necessary for larger or malignant lesions. GISTs appearing in the stomach appear to have the best prognosis [38]. Small intestinal GISTs, compared to esophageal or gastric GISTs, are more likely to present with ulceration and bleeding. As these tumors enlarge extraluminally, small bowel obstruction due to intestinal GISTs is rare and signifies particularly large tumors. While current guidelines suggest surgical removal of GISTs over 2 cm in size with potential adjuvant imatinib therapy, there is a notable lack of consensus on smaller lesions. Endoscopic removal is possible, but controversial, given risks of positive margins and perforation.

Carcinoid

Carcinoid tumors are smooth, round, nodules originating most frequently from the enterochromaffin-like cells. A neuroendocrine tumor, carcinoid can produce a variety of biologically active substances and may arise from as many as 14 different cell types. With metastatic spread, patients may develop carcinoid syndrome, which is characterized by flushing, abdominal pain, diarrhea, bronchoconstriction, and heart disease [43]. In general, carcinoid tumors are slow growing, and prognosis is better than gastrointestinal carcinomas, with high survival rates even 20 years after diagnosis [43]. However, carcinoid tumor incidence is growing [54], and the tumor is usually diagnosed late, as symptoms usually begin only after metastatic spread.

Gastrointestinal carcinoid is the most frequent type of carcinoid tumor, accounting for 70% of these tumors [45]. Interestingly, the location of carcinoid tumors in the gastrointestinal tract appears to vary based on geography, with more proximal tumors (stomach, duodenum, and rectum) presenting in Japan and more distal tumors (ileum, appendix, rectum) in the USA [14].

Among carcinoid tumors, gastric carcinoids are unique in that they have been divided into three distinct types, based on tumor characteristics, histology, association with hypergastrinemia, and biological behavior. Type 1 is the most common, comprising 70–80% of gastric carcinoid tumors [60]. They present as multiple, small, nodular lesions with or without a central ulceration. These tumors are thought to be developed by enterochromaffin-like cells exposed to high gastrin levels seen in anhydric states, such as atrophic gastritis. Type 1 gastric carcinoid tumors generally have a benign course with slow growth and rare metastasis. Notably, these tumors do not cause carcinoid syndrome. Type 2 gastric carcinoid tumors are associated with gastrinomas and account for 5% of gastric carcinoid tumors. Similar to type 1 carcinoids, these tumors present as multiple, small lesions and are associated with high gastrin levels. Unlike type 1 gastric carcinoids, these tumors are seen in high gastrin, high-acid states and occur almost exclusively in patients with MEN type 1 [60]. Type 3 gastric carcinoids account for 20% of gastric carcinoids and are not associated with MEN type 1, gastrinomas, or atrophic gastritis. They present as larger (over 1 cm) solitary lesions, and unlike the other gastric carcinoids, these are thought to develop without hyperplasia or dysplasia of the enterochromaffin-like cells [44]. While type 1 and type 2 tumors generally produce serotonin, these tumors produce 5-hydroxy-tryptophan and are associated with aggressive growth and frequent metastases. They also have a worse prognosis, with a 5-year survival under 35% [44].

On endoscopic evaluation, carcinoids are sessile or polypoid lesions with rare ulcerations. EUS of carcinoid tumors typically shows homogeneous hypoechogenicity or isoechogenicity, with the mass arising from the second echoic layer (see Fig. 48.5), with possible invasion into the third echoic layer. Histologically, these tumors consist of polygonal cells with central, round nuclei and a granular, eosinophilic cytoplasm. The cells are typically arranged in ribbon or trabecular patterns forming rosettes [34]. Management varies depending on subtype. Endoscopic resection is the treatment of choice for type 2 gastric carcinoids under 1 cm in size, with

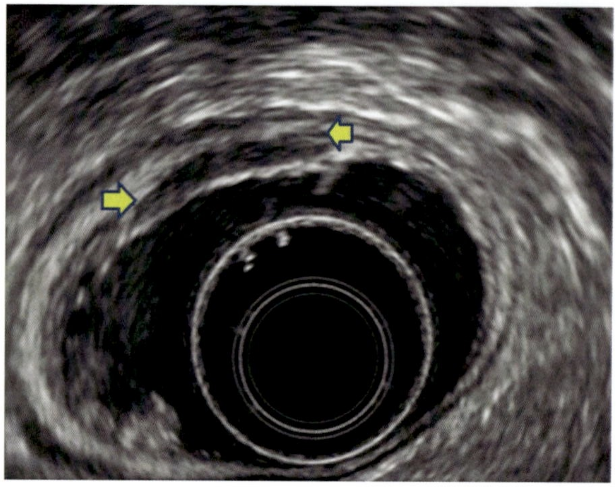

Fig. 48.5 Radial EUS view of duodenal carcinoid arising from the muscularis mucosa (second layer), denoted by arrows

surgical resection preferred in patients with larger lesions. Endoscopic resection is also preferred in type 1 gastric carcinoids with <1 cm lesions with subsequent, periodic endoscopic surveillance to exclude the formation of new lesions. Larger or multiple (>5) lesions warrant partial gastrectomy or, for patients ineligible for surgery, anti-gastrin therapies. Type 3 gastric carcinoids, if caught before metastases, may be treated with partial or total gastrectomy with lymph node resections.

Granular Cell Tumors

Granular cell tumors are firm, nodular neuroendocrine tumors which originate from the deep mucosa or submucosa. They account for 0.5% of soft tissue tumors [2] and can occur at virtually any location but are most common in the skin and/or gastrointestinal tract. In the gastrointestinal tract, they are most commonly found in the esophagus. On endoscopic evaluation, these tumors are generally firm, smooth, solitary, yellowish masses with hemispherical protrusion with a thin mucous membrane, which is sometimes referred to as a "molar tooth" or "sweet corn" appearance [2]. They are typically found in patients between the ages of 10 and 50 years old and are more common in women. On EUS, these tumors are hypoechoic, homogeneous masses with smooth margins and originate from the second or third echoic layer.

Histologically, they are characterized by plump oval or polygonal cells with a small nucleus and a PAS-positive, granular cytoplasm. Their cytology is characterized by positive immunoreactivity for S100 protein and neuron-specific enolase, and without desmin, actin, CD34, or c-kit markers, consistent with their Schwann cell origin. Close to 98% of granular cell tumors are benign, but malignancy should be suspected in tumors greater than 3 cm in size. A histopathologic classification system to identify malignant granular cell tumors has been developed, evaluating the masses for the necrosis, spindle cells, vacuolar nucleus with an enlarged nuclear body, nuclear division (2 mitoses/10HPF), an increase in the nucleoplasmic ratio, and polymorphisms to further delineate benign, atypical, or malignant lesions [9]. Management consists of local endoscopic excision or periodic surveillance with EUS.

Glomus Tumors

Glomus tumors are the most common vascular tumor of the stomach. They appear as well-defined gastric SMTs with red-blue nodules [57] and originate from the temperature-regulating glomus bodies. The majority of patients are asymptomatic, although larger lesions are associated with ulceration, GERD-like symptoms, and bleeding [50]. Mostly benign, these tumors are generally found in the gastric antrum and distal colon and consist of small, uniform, rounded glomus cells that are located in the walls of dilated vascular spaces. On CT imaging, these tumors show early enhancement and may show some degree of calcification [50]. Endoscopic biopsies many not provide much diagnostic yield, often necessitating surgical or endoscopic resection. EUS demonstrates a heterogeneous hyperechoic [3] or hypoechoic [42] solid mass arising from the fourth echoic layer. Histologically, the tumor cells have small, uniform nuclei, show positive immunoreactivity for smooth muscle actin, and are outlined by PAS-positive basement membranes. The tumor is often surrounded by hyperplastic smooth muscle cells. Immunohistochemically, these tumors are positive for smooth muscle actin, vimentin, and desmin and negative for CD34 and c-kit [58]. While generally regarded as benign, these tumors may carry malignant potential [11].

Nonneoplastic Lesions

There are a number of nonneoplastic lesions that may appear to be a submucosal tumor on endoscopic and gross evaluation including duplication cysts, pancreatic rests, varices, and inflammatory fibroid polyps.

Duplication Cysts

Duplication cysts are rare, congenital, malformations theorized to arise from abnormal budding in embryonic development. They can be subcategorized as foregut, small bowel, or large bowel cysts and commonly occur in the esophagus, ileum, and colon. They are typically discovered incidentally on imaging but may present with abdominal pain or bleeding. Notably, they may be intrinsic or extrinsic to the gastrointestinal wall and thus may be undetectable on endoscopy. Others, however, may appear as a bulge or diverticulum.

EUS is the diagnostic modality of choice, as it can distinguish between solid and cystic pathology. EUS of these lesions demonstrates hypo- or anechoic,

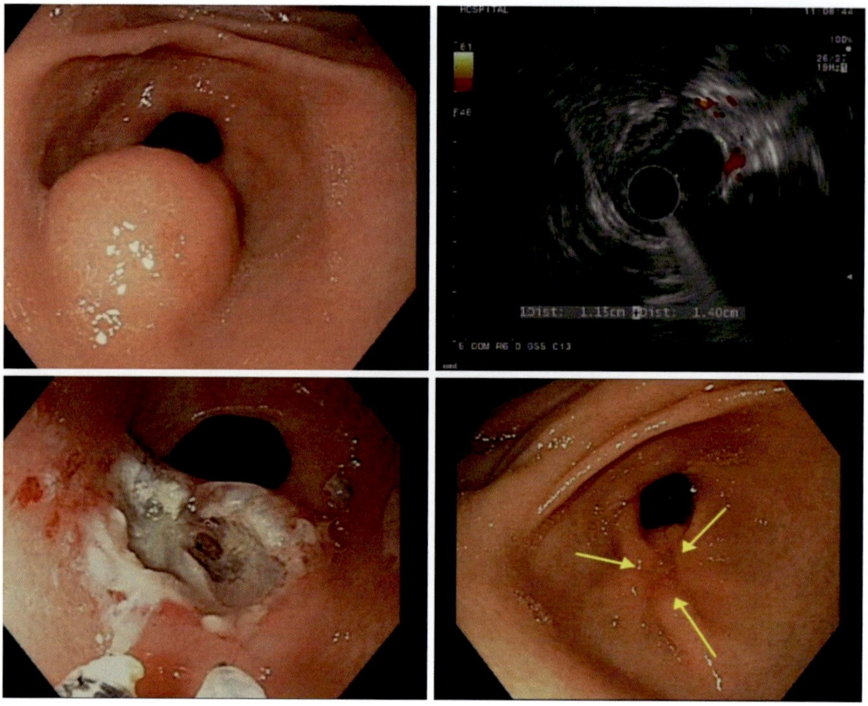

Fig. 48.6 Gastric prepyloric submucosal lesion causing outlet obstruction. Radial EUS images demonstrate a 14 mm × 12 mm duplication cyst arising from the third layer (submucosa) which was subsequently endoscopically unroofed. Three-month follow-up images demonstrate resolution which coincided with symptom resolution

homogeneous lesions with regular margins (see Fig. 48.6). Lesions intrinsic to the gastrointestinal wall typically arise from the third echogenic layer. The cyst walls typically have three to five distinct layers and may have peristaltic ring contractions, which, if seen on juxta-enteric cysts, are specific for duplication cysts [29]. FNA may be pursed with caution as there is a notable risk of infection [62]. Histologically, these cysts are lined with stratified, ciliated, or columnar epithelium. Cyst contents may include mucus, septations, and cellular debris. Detached ciliary tufts may also be present and are diagnostic of a duplication cyst [8]. Surgical resection is the preferred treatment in symptomatic patients, but endoscopic management with FNA or cystostomy has been reported [29].

Pancreatic Rests

Pancreatic rests, also known as aberrant pancreas or heterotopic pancreas, consist of ectopic pancreatic tissue. They are typically found in the distal stomach, duodenum, or jejunum and are usually discovered incidentally. On imaging, these masses have an ovoid shape, an ill-defined border, and an endoluminal growth pattern [26]. Endoscopy classically reveals a submucosal nodule with a central umbilication, due to the presence of a draining duct. EUS shows a hypoechoic heterogenous mass arising from the third or fourth echoic layer with anechoic structures corresponding to ducts. Microscopically, pancreatic rests generally display all the characteristic of normal pancreatic tissue, containing pancreatic acini, ducts, and islets. Diagnosis is made histologically, and asymptomatic lesions can be followed with endoscopic surveillance. If resection is warranted (rarely), endoscopic snaring, band ligation, or polypectomy may be utilized. Surgical resection should be considered if the muscularis propria is involved.

Varices

Gastric varices may have the appearance of submucosal lesions on endoscopy. Seen predominately in patients with end-stage liver disease or patients with vessel occlusions, endoscopic examination of these patients may show other signs of portal hypertension, such as portal gastropathy. Varices themselves have a soft consistency with a blue hue. Endoscopic ultrasound will demonstrate a round or tubular hypoechoic or anechoic structure arising from the third layer with dopplerable flow.

Inflammatory Fibroid Polyps

Gastric inflammatory fibroid polyps, occasionally referred to as eosinophilic granulomas, are benign lesions of the stomach, which appear as firm, solitary, sessile, or pedunculated and often ulcerated masses on endoscopy. EUS demonstrates hypoechoic, homogeneous masses with indistinct borders and may rise from the second, third, or fourth echogenic layer. Histologically, they consist of unencapsulated fibrous tissue with eosinophilic infiltrate with multiple penetrating blood vessels. A predominance of these vessels may lead to a slightly hyperechoic appearance on EUS. These masses arise from the deep mucosal or submucosal layer with involvement of the muscularis propria [32]. Immunohistochemical staining suggests a dendritic cell origin [48]. Furthermore, studies have found that these polyps carry gain-of-function mutations in PDGFR, similar to c-kit-negative GISTs, suggestive of a neoplastic process [55]. Extremely rare, most of the reported cases in the literature describe endoscopic or surgical resection for management.

Brunner Gland Hamartoma

Brunner glands are acinotubular glands in the submucosa of the duodenum, located mainly in the duodenal bulb. They secrete an alkaline fluid which coats the duodenum, protecting it from the acid chyme of the stomach. The pathogenesis of a Brunner gland hamartoma is unknown, with some suggesting that hyperchlorhydria may stimulate these structures to undergo hyperplasia [63], whereas others have noted a link to *Helicobacter pylori* infection [27]. Symptoms include bleeding, obstruction, and rarely, if blocking the ampulla, pancreatitis and biliary obstruction [33]. Endoscopy reveals a broad-based, sessile, or pedunculated submucosal mass [18]. Biopsies are often negative or reveal gland hyperplasia. EUS demonstrates a solid to cystic mass arising from the third echoic layer [18]. Although Brunner gland hamartomas are not considered premalignant, there have been reports of cellular atypia within the lesion [12] and subsequent development of adenocarcinoma [59]. Therefore, management with endoscopic or surgical resection is appropriate.

Conclusion

Benign foregut SMTs are potentially premalignant lesions of the gastrointestinal tract and can be subdivided into benign neoplasms, potentially malignant SMTs, and nonneoplastic lesions. The evaluation of these lesions generally begins with a CT scan, although perhaps the most sensitive imaging modality is EUS evaluation, which can provide details on size, border irregularities, echogenic homogeneity, and the layer of origin. However, definite diagnosis, and therefore appropriate management, often still requires immunohistochemical analysis of tissue, which would require surgical or endoscopic biopsy.

References

1. Abraham SC, Krasinskas AM, Hofstetter WL, et al. "Seedling" mesenchymal tumors (gastrointestinal stromal tumors and leiomyomas) are common incidental tumors of the esophagogastric junction. Am J Surg Pathol. 2007;31:1629–35. https://doi.org/10.1097/PAS.0b013e31806ab2c3.
2. Aoyama K, Kamio T, Hirano A, et al. Granular cell tumors: a report of six cases. World J Surg Oncol. 2012;10:204. https://doi.org/10.1186/1477-7819-10-204.
3. Chen K-B, Chen L. Glomus tumor in the stomach: a case report and review of the literature. Oncol Lett. 2014;7:1790–2. https://doi.org/10.3892/ol.2014.1986.
4. Chou FF, Eng HL, Sheen-Chen SM. Smooth muscle tumors of the gastrointestinal tract: analysis of prognostic factors. Surgery. 1996;119:171–7.
5. Davis GB, Blanchard DK, Hatch GF, et al. Tumors of the stomach. World J Surg. 2000;24:412–20.
6. de la Serna-Higuera C, Pérez-Miranda M, Díez-Redondo P, et al. EUS-guided single-incision needle-knife biopsy: description and results of a new method for tissue sampling of subepithelial GI tumors (with video). Gastrointest Endosc. 2011;74:672–6. https://doi.org/10.1016/j.gie.2011.05.042.
7. DeWitt J, Emerson RE, Sherman S, et al. Endoscopic ultrasound-guided Trucut biopsy of gastrointestinal mesenchymal tumor. Surg Endosc. 2011;25:2192–202. https://doi.org/10.1007/s00464-010-1522-z.
8. Eloubeidi MA, Cohn M, Cerfolio RJ, et al. Endoscopic ultrasound-guided fine-needle aspiration in the diagnosis of foregut duplication cysts: the value of demonstrating detached ciliary tufts in cyst fluid. Cancer. 2004;102:253–8. https://doi.org/10.1002/cncr.20369.
9. Fanburg-Smith JC, Meis-Kindblom JM, Fante R, Kindblom LG. Malignant granular cell tumor of soft tissue: diagnostic criteria and clinicopathologic correlation. Am J Surg Pathol. 1998;22:779–94.

10. Fletcher JA, Rubin BP. KIT mutations in GIST. Curr Opin Genet Dev. 2007;17:3–7. https://doi.org/10.1016/j.gde.2006.12.010.
11. Folpe AL, Fanburg-Smith JC, Miettinen M, Weiss SW. Atypical and malignant glomus tumors: analysis of 52 cases, with a proposal for the reclassification of glomus tumors. Am J Surg Pathol. 2001;25:1–12.
12. Fujimaki E, Nakamura S, Sugai T, Takeda Y. Brunner's gland adenoma with a focus of p53-positive atypical glands. J Gastroenterol. 2000;35:155–8.
13. Gayed I, Vu T, Iyer R, et al. The role of 18F-FDG PET in staging and early prediction of response to therapy of recurrent gastrointestinal stromal tumors. J Nucl Med Off Publ Soc Nucl Med. 2004;45:17–21.
14. Godwin JD. Carcinoid tumors. An analysis of 2,837 cases. Cancer. 1975;36:560–9.
15. Goh BKP, Chow PKH, Kesavan S, et al. Intraabdominal schwannomas: a single institution experience. J Gastrointest Surg Off J Soc Surg Aliment Tract. 2008;12:756–60. https://doi.org/10.1007/s11605-007-0441-3.
16. Hedenbro JL, Ekelund M, Wetterberg P. Endoscopic diagnosis of submucosal gastric lesions. The results after routine endoscopy. Surg Endosc. 1991;5:20–3.
17. Heinrich MC, Corless CL, Duensing A, et al. PDGFRA activating mutations in gastrointestinal stromal tumors. Science. 2003;299:708–10. https://doi.org/10.1126/science.1079666.
18. Hizawa K, Iwai K, Esaki M, et al. Endosonographic features of Brunner's gland hamartomas which were subsequently resected endoscopically. Endoscopy. 2002;34:956–8. https://doi.org/10.1055/s-2002-35849.
19. Hoda KM, Rodriguez SA, Faigel DO. EUS-guided sampling of suspected GI stromal tumors. Gastrointest Endosc. 2009;69:1218–23. https://doi.org/10.1016/j.gie.2008.09.045.
20. Hou YY, Tan YS, Xu JF, et al. Schwannoma of the gastrointestinal tract: a clinicopathological, immunohistochemical and ultrastructural study of 33 cases. Histopathology. 2006;48:536–45. https://doi.org/10.1111/j.1365-2559.2006.02370.x.
21. Hwang JH, Rulyak SD, Kimmey MB, American Gastroenterological Association Institute. American Gastroenterological Association Institute technical review on the management of gastric subepithelial masses. Gastroenterology. 2006;130:2217–28. https://doi.org/10.1053/j.gastro.2006.04.033.
22. Hwang JH, Saunders MD, Rulyak SJ, et al. A prospective study comparing endoscopy and EUS in the evaluation of GI subepithelial masses. Gastrointest Endosc. 2005;62:202–8.
23. Ishikawa N, Fuchigami T, Kikuchi Y, et al. EUS for gastric lymphangioma. Gastrointest Endosc. 2000;52:798–800. https://doi.org/10.1067/mge.2000.108292.
24. Janeway KA, Kim SY, Lodish M, et al. Defects in succinate dehydrogenase in gastrointestinal stromal tumors lacking KIT and PDGFRA mutations. Proc Natl Acad Sci U S A. 2011;108:314–8. https://doi.org/10.1073/pnas.1009199108.
25. Kim HS, Lee SY, Lee YD, et al. Gastric lymphangioma. J Korean Med Sci. 2001;16:229. https://doi.org/10.3346/jkms.2001.16.2.229.
26. Kim JY, Lee JM, Kim KW, et al. Ectopic pancreas: CT findings with emphasis on differentiation from small gastrointestinal stromal tumor and leiomyoma. Radiology. 2009;252:92–100. https://doi.org/10.1148/radiol.2521081441.
27. Kovacević I, Ljubicić N, Cupić H, et al. Helicobacter pylori infection in patients with Brunner's gland adenoma. Acta Medica Croat Cas Hravatske Akad Med Znan. 2001;55:157–60.
28. Lee CK, Chung I-K, Lee S-H, et al. Endoscopic partial resection with the unroofing technique for reliable tissue diagnosis of upper GI subepithelial tumors originating from the muscularis propria on EUS (with video). Gastrointest Endosc. 2010;71:188–94. https://doi.org/10.1016/j.gie.2009.07.029.
29. Liu R, Adler DG. Duplication cysts: diagnosis, management, and the role of endoscopic ultrasound. Endosc Ultrasound. 2014;3:152–60. https://doi.org/10.4103/2303-9027.138783.
30. Martín J, Poveda A, Llombart-Bosch A, et al. Deletions affecting codons 557-558 of the c-KIT gene indicate a poor prognosis in patients with completely resected gastrointestinal stromal tumors: a study by the Spanish Group for Sarcoma Research (GEIS). J Clin Oncol Off J Am Soc Clin Oncol. 2005;23:6190–8. https://doi.org/10.1200/JCO.2005.19.554.

31. Matsui M, Goto H, Niwa Y, et al. Preliminary results of fine needle aspiration biopsy histology in upper gastrointestinal submucosal tumors. Endoscopy. 1998;30:750–5. https://doi.org/10.1055/s-2007-1001416.
32. Matsushita M, Hajiro K, Okazaki K, Takakuwa H. Gastric inflammatory fibroid polyps: endoscopic ultrasonographic analysis in comparison with the histology. Gastrointest Endosc. 1997;46:53–7.
33. Mayoral W, Salcedo JA, Montgomery E, Al-Kawas FH. Biliary obstruction and pancreatitis caused by Brunner's gland hyperplasia of the ampulla of Vater: a case report and review of the literature. Endoscopy. 2000;32:998–1001. https://doi.org/10.1055/s-2000-9623.
34. McDermott FD, Heeney A, Courtney D, et al. Rectal carcinoids: a systematic review. Surg Endosc. 2014;28:2020–6. https://doi.org/10.1007/s00464-014-3430-0.
35. Menon L, Buscaglia JM. Endoscopic approach to subepithelial lesions. Ther Adv Gastroenterol. 2014;7:123–30. https://doi.org/10.1177/1756283X13513538.
36. Messer J, Waye JD. The diagnosis of colonic lipomas–the naked fat sign. Gastrointest Endosc. 1982;28:186–8.
37. Miettinen M, Lasota J. Gastrointestinal stromal tumors. Gastroenterol Clin N Am. 2013;42:399–415. https://doi.org/10.1016/j.gtc.2013.01.001.
38. Miettinen M, Lasota J. Gastrointestinal stromal tumors: pathology and prognosis at different sites. Semin Diagn Pathol. 2006;23:70–83.
39. Miettinen M, Sarlomo-Rikala M, Sobin LH, Lasota J. Esophageal stromal tumors: a clinicopathologic, immunohistochemical, and molecular genetic study of 17 cases and comparison with esophageal leiomyomas and leiomyosarcomas. Am J Surg Pathol. 2000;24:211–22.
40. Miettinen M, Wang Z-F, Lasota J. DOG1 antibody in the differential diagnosis of gastrointestinal stromal tumors: a study of 1840 cases. Am J Surg Pathol. 2009;33:1401–8. https://doi.org/10.1097/PAS.0b013e3181a90e1a.
41. Min KW. Small intestinal stromal tumors with skeinoid fibers. Clinicopathological, immunohistochemical, and ultrastructural investigations. Am J Surg Pathol. 1992;16:145–55.
42. Minoda Y, Akahoshi K, Oya M, et al. Gastric glomus tumor diagnosed by endoscopic ultrasound-guided fine-needle aspiration biopsy: report of a case. Fukuoka Igaku Zasshi Hukuoka Acta Medica. 2014;105:105–9.
43. Mocellin S, Nitti D. Gastrointestinal carcinoid: epidemiological and survival evidence from a large population-based study (n = 25 531). Ann Oncol mdt. 2013; 377. https://doi.org/10.1093/annonc/mdt377.
44. Modlin IM, Kidd M, Latich I, et al. Current status of gastrointestinal carcinoids. Gastroenterology. 2005;128:1717–51.
45. Modlin IM, Lye KD, Kidd M. A 5-decade analysis of 13,715 carcinoid tumors. Cancer. 2003;97:934–59. https://doi.org/10.1002/cncr.11105.
46. Murray MA, Kwan V, Williams SJ, Bourke MJ. Detachable nylon loop assisted removal of large clinically significant colonic lipomas. Gastrointest Endosc. 2005;61:756–9.
47. Nilsson B, Bümming P, Meis-Kindblom JM, et al. Gastrointestinal stromal tumors: the incidence, prevalence, clinical course, and prognostication in the preimatinib mesylate era–a population-based study in western Sweden. Cancer. 2005;103:821–9. https://doi.org/10.1002/cncr.20862.
48. Pantanowitz L, Antonioli DA, Pinkus GS, et al. Inflammatory fibroid polyps of the gastrointestinal tract: evidence for a dendritic cell origin. Am J Surg Pathol. 2004;28:107–14.
49. Pappo AS, Janeway KA. Pediatric gastrointestinal stromal tumors. Hematol Oncol Clin North Am. 2009;23:15–34, vii. https://doi.org/10.1016/j.hoc.2008.11.005.
50. Park SH, Han JK, Kim TK, et al. Unusual gastric tumors: radiologic-pathologic correlation. Radiographics. 1999;19:1435–46. https://doi.org/10.1148/radiographics.19.6.g99no051435.
51. Raju GS, Gomez G. Endoloop ligation of a large colonic lipoma: a novel technique. Gastrointest Endosc. 2005;62:988–90. https://doi.org/10.1016/j.gie.2005.08.018.
52. Rubin BP, Fletcher JA, Fletcher CDM. Molecular insights into the histogenesis and pathogenesis of gastrointestinal stromal tumors. Int J Surg Pathol. 2000;8:5–10.

53. Scarpa M, Bertin M, Ruffolo C, et al. A systematic review on the clinical diagnosis of gastrointestinal stromal tumors. J Surg Oncol. 2008;98:384–92. https://doi.org/10.1002/jso.21120.
54. Scherübl H. Rectal carcinoids are on the rise: early detection by screening endoscopy. Endoscopy. 2009;41:162–5. https://doi.org/10.1055/s-0028-1119456.
55. Schildhaus H-U, Cavlar T, Binot E, et al. Inflammatory fibroid polyps harbour mutations in the platelet-derived growth factor receptor alpha (PDGFRA) gene. J Pathol. 2008;216:176–82. https://doi.org/10.1002/path.2393.
56. Tran T, Davila JA, El-Serag HB. The epidemiology of malignant gastrointestinal stromal tumors: an analysis of 1,458 cases from 1992 to 2000. Am J Gastroenterol. 2005;100:162–8. https://doi.org/10.1111/j.1572-0241.2005.40709.x.
57. Troller R, Soll C, Breitenstein S. Glomus tumour of the stomach. BMJ Case Rep. 2016, 2016:bcr2015214135. https://doi.org/10.1136/bcr-2015-214135.
58. Vassiliou I, Tympa A, Theodosopoulos T, et al. Gastric glomus tumor: a case report. World J Surg Oncol. 2010;8:19. https://doi.org/10.1186/1477-7819-8-19.
59. Walden DT, Marcon NE. Endoscopic injection and polypectomy for bleeding Brunner's gland hamartoma: case report and expanded literature review. Gastrointest Endosc. 1998;47:403–7.
60. Wardlaw R, Smith JW. Gastric carcinoid tumors. Ochsner J. 2008;8:191–6.
61. Wiech T, Walch A, Werner M. Histopathological classification of nonneoplastic and neoplastic gastrointestinal submucosal lesions. Endoscopy. 2005;37:630–4. https://doi.org/10.1055/s-2005-870127.
62. Wildi SM, Hoda RS, Fickling W, et al. Diagnosis of benign cysts of the mediastinum: the role and risks of EUS and FNA. Gastrointest Endosc. 2003;58:362–8.
63. Zangara J, Kushner H, Drachenberg C, et al. Iron deficiency anemia due to a Brunner's gland hamartoma. J Clin Gastroenterol. 1998;27:353–6.
64. Zhong D-D, Wang C-H, Xu J-H, et al. Endoscopic ultrasound features of gastric schwannomas with radiological correlation: a case series report. World J Gastroenterol (WJG). 2012;18:7397–401. https://doi.org/10.3748/wjg.v18.i48.7397.

Thoracoscopic Management of Benign Submucosal Tumors

49

Daniel C. Thomas and Anthony W. Kim

Introduction

Benign submucosal tumors of the esophagus represent rare conditions with an incidence of less than 1% of all esophageal neoplasms [1]. Esophageal leiomyomas are the most common benign tumors of the esophagus, representing 70–80% of all benign tumors, with lesions such as hemangiomas, granular cell tumors, and lipomas occurring less frequently [2–4]. Traditionally, the standard surgical approach to resection of benign esophageal tumors has been enucleation via an open thoracotomy, often approached from the right side due to the ability to access the entire intrathoracic esophagus [2]. The use of minimally invasive approaches including the video-assisted thoracoscopic surgery (VATS) and the robotic-assisted thoracoscopic surgery (RobATS) has increased in the past decade and has become a feasible alternative to thoracotomy. Advantages to these minimally invasive approaches are operative outcomes equivalent to the open approach, reduced morbidity, decreased postoperative pain, and shorter lengths of hospital stays [5, 6].

Indications

Benign tumors of the esophagus are generally asymptomatic and are often discovered incidentally on chest imaging. Less than half of patients present with symptoms [3, 7, 8]. When present, the most common symptoms are epigastric discomfort,

D. C. Thomas
Yale School of Medicine, Yale University, New Haven, CT, USA

A. W. Kim (✉)
Department of Surgery, University of Southern California Keck School of Medicine, Los Angeles, CA, USA
e-mail: Anthony.kim@med.usc.edu

J. Grams et al. (eds.), *The SAGES Manual of Foregut Surgery*,
https://doi.org/10.1007/978-3-319-96122-4_49

atypical chest pain, and dysphagia and less frequently regurgitation and gastrointestinal bleed [3, 9].

The management of small, asymptomatic submucosal tumors remains controversial. Some surgeons have recommended resection of all tumors regardless of size, while others have advocated for observation of small tumors. An appropriate size threshold has been debated, but has varied among studies [4, 10]. Surgical resection is indicated for symptomatic tumors and to obtain a pathologic diagnosis as well as to exclude malignancy in cases of inadequate or inconclusive biopsies. Tumors that cause overlying mucosal ulceration or continue to increase in size during a period of observation should also be considered for tumor resection [11]. Previously, concern for malignant transformation of a benign esophageal tumor was cited as an indication for enucleation; however, demonstrable malignant transformation actually appears to be a rare event [3, 12]. Table 49.1 demonstrates the heterogeneous group of tumors that comprise the differential diagnosis of a submucosal lesion with benign features on endoscopy and imaging studies, and indicates the most common location of incidence in the esophagus [1, 20]. Benign leiomyoma is the most common pathologic entity, accounting for 70–80% of cases [7, 8]. The most common submucosal tumors after leiomyoma include hemangioma and granular cell tumors, each accounting for less than 5% of benign esophageal tumors, followed by a variety of rare tumor histologies [9, 10, 21].

The initial method of diagnosis for benign submucosal tumors of the esophagus depends upon the presence or absence of symptoms. Symptomatic patients are most commonly referred for evaluation of dysphagia or atypical chest pain, while asymptomatic tumors are discovered incidentally on chest radiograph or computed tomography (CT) performed for other indications. CT imaging is most helpful in ruling out any malignant potential by virtue of the absence of invasion of nearby structures and appearance of a smooth tumor; however, CT imaging is less able to distinguish the involved layers of the esophagus [22]. Contrast esophagogram is a highly sensitive and noninvasive initial evaluation to identify the level and laterality of a tumor. Benign submucosal tumors often appear as smoothly rounded filling defects on the esophagus with clear demarcation of the tumor and uninvolved esophageal border [9]. Esophagoscopy with endoscopic ultrasound (EUS) should follow esophagogram to further characterize the location, appearance, and depth of the tumor in an attempt to rule out malignant pathology. Endoscopic features of benign

Table 49.1 Differential diagnosis of a submucosal lesion with benign features in order of decreasing incidence and also describing its most common location when discovered [13–19]

Tumor pathology	Most common location
Leiomyoma	Distal 1/3
Hemangioma	Evenly distributed
Granular cell tumors	Mid-distal 2/3
Lipoma	Upper 1/3
Fibroma	Underreported
Neurofibroma	Upper-middle 2/3
Rhabdomyoma	Underreported
Lymphangioma	Lower 1/3
Hamartoma	Distal 1/3

submucosal tumors include a bulging tumor with overlying mucosa intact without ulceration, a freely mobile tumor, and tumor projecting into the lumen without stenosis or complete obstruction [11]. The most common pathology encountered, leiomyoma, appears as smooth, well-circumscribed, hypoechoic tumors of the third (submucosa) and fourth (muscularis propria) EUS layers of the esophagus [23].

Preoperative endoscopic biopsy has been demonstrated to increase the risk of intraoperative mucosal injury, and for this reason, a preoperative biopsy is not recommended when endoscopy and imaging data suggest a benign tumor [6]. Similarly, patients who are clinically diagnosed with a benign submucosal tumor can forgo preoperative positron emission tomography (PET), reserving PET scan for tumors found to be unexpectedly malignant after resection.

Technique

Surgical treatment of benign submucosal esophageal tumors most frequently involves tumor enucleation. However, segmental resections may be necessary occasionally.

Enucleation

Tumors of the intrathoracic esophagus are approached transthoracically using either the open or the minimally invasive approaches. The thoracoscopic approach was first reported by Everitt and colleagues in 1992 [24]. Tumors at or near the gastroesophageal junction can be approached transhiatally as an alternative especially if the lesion is distal and near the gastroesophageal junction. The use of RobATS can be employed for surgical enucleation of benign submucosal tumors in a fashion similar to the VATS technique described below.

For a transthoracic approach, the patient is intubated with a double-lumen endotracheal tube to allow for single lung ventilation. VATS enucleation is most often performed from the right side for tumors of the proximal two-thirds of the esophagus, while a right- or left-sided approach can be used for tumors of the distal one-third of the esophagus [2]. Owing to the access to the entire intrathoracic esophagus, the distal esophagus can also be approached from the right side, if necessary. A right- or the left-sided approach still can access lesions on the contralateral surface of the esophagus but will require additional dissection and mobilization of the esophagus to allow for complete visualization.

The VATS approach utilizes three- or four-trocar access to the pleural cavity, depending on the comfort level of the surgeon. In the left decubitus position with the right chest upward, three to four incisions to accommodate the camera port and working ports can be made using a strategy that optimizes triangulation toward the target anatomy and in keeping with the strategy that the surgeon is accustomed. Typically, these incisions may include a camera port incision between the anterior and midaxillary line in the seventh to ninth intercostal space depending on the level of the benign tumor in the esophagus. Additional incisions are made anywhere in the third to fifth intercostal space in the anterior axillary line and seventh to ninth intercostal space posterior to the posterior axillary line and the tip of the scapula. Additional incisions may be made inferior to the anterior and posterior incisions to facilitate the retraction or dissection as needed. Each of the incisions should be placed after the camera incision so that direct visualization is employed to optimize trocar placement in relation to the lesion in question. If the lesion is in the distal esophagus, a heavy monofilament suture may be placed through the central portion of the diaphragm, away from the phrenic nerves, brought out through one of the incisions, and clamped extracorporeally to move the diaphragm out of the way (Fig. 49.1).

After entering the pleural cavity, the lung is gently retracted anteriorly to expose the mediastinal pleura overlying the esophagus (Fig. 49.2). The entire extent of the tumor is assessed by palpation. Obviously, "palpation" with the minimally invasive approach entails the use of an endoscopic instrument such as a kuettner or other tool to obtain tactile feedback on the lesion itself and the extent of it in all external dimensions. If needed, intraoperative esophagoscopy can be used to determine or confirm the exact tumor location using endoscopic transillumination. The mediastinal pleura overlying the esophagus then is opened either sharply or with electrocautery (Fig. 49.3). The pleura is opened further in the cephalad and caudad direction to the extent that gaining access to the esophagus for mobilization will be feasible. If the distal esophagus is involved, the inferior pulmonary ligament may need to be divided to the level of the inferior pulmonary vein. If the proximal and middle esophagus is involved, the azygos vein may need to be divided to allow access to the tumor. Proximal and distal to the tumor, the esophagus may be circumferentially dissected so that a Penrose drain may be placed around the esophagus to facilitate retraction and exposure (Fig. 49.4).

Once the tumor is localized and the segmental esophagus is exposed, a longitudinal esophageal myotomy is made overlying the tumor (Fig. 49.5). This incision can be initiated with careful electrocautery and then continued longitudinally and

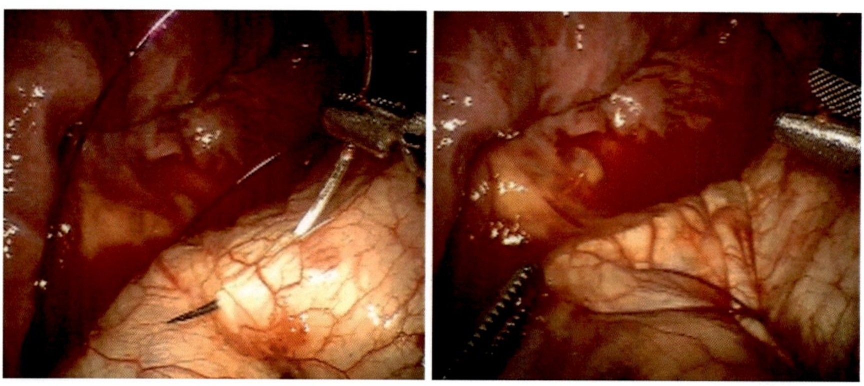

Fig. 49.1 Suture placed through the central portion of the diaphragm, brought out through an incision, and clamped extracorporeally to retract diaphragm

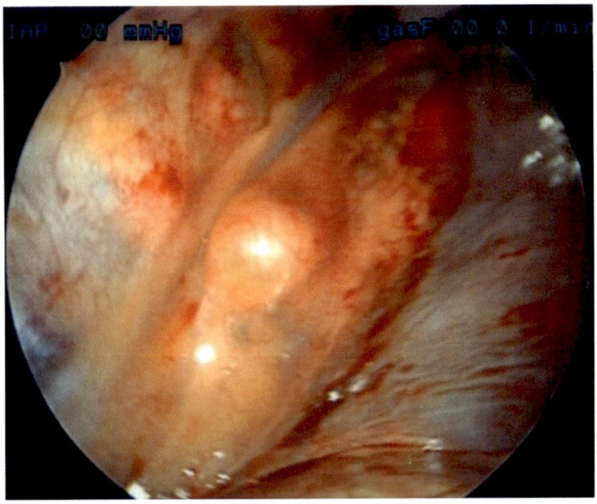

Fig. 49.2 Exposure of the benign tumor with overlying mediastinal pleura. (Courtesy of Daniel J. Boffa, M.D.)

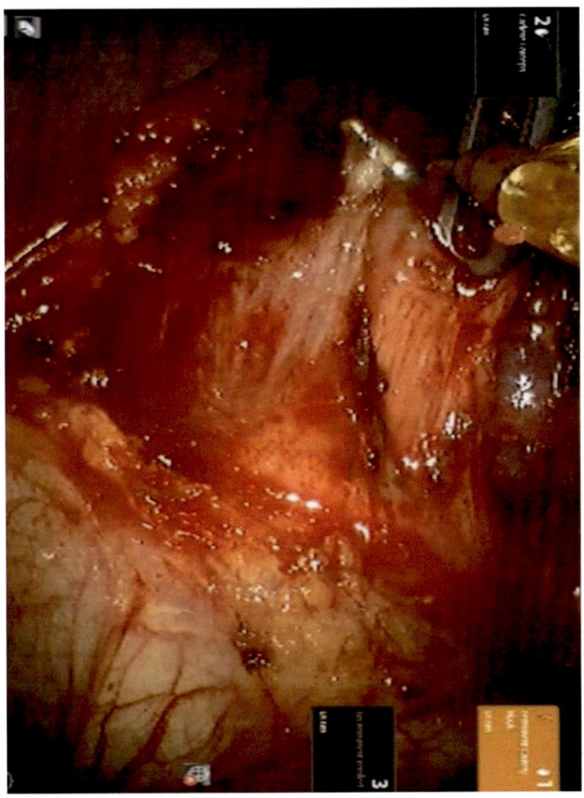

Fig. 49.3 Exposure of the involved esophagus by opening the overlying mediastinal pleura

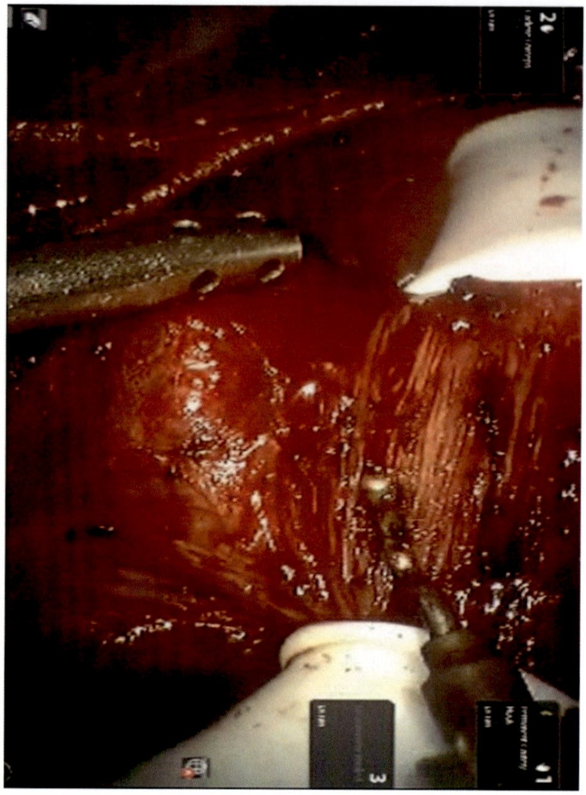

Fig. 49.4 Circumferential dissection of the esophagus with a Penrose drain providing additional retraction and tumor exposure

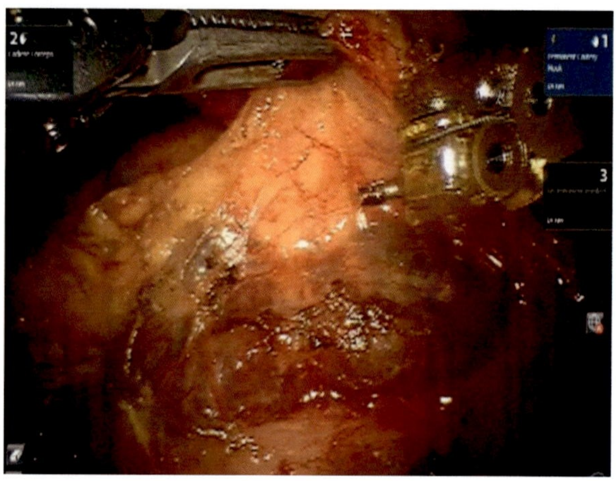

Fig. 49.5 Longitudinal esophageal myotomy made overlying the tumor

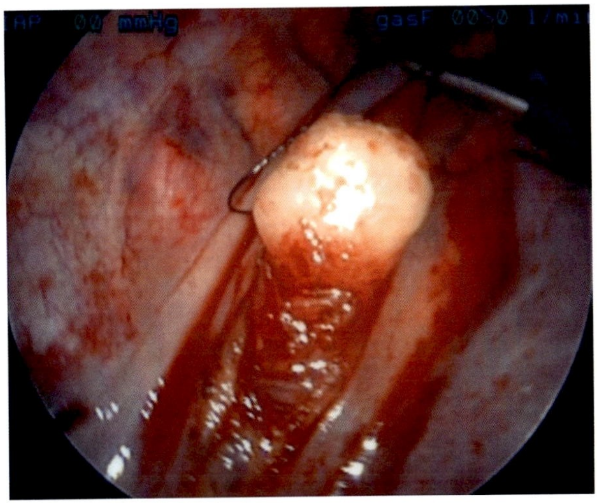

Fig. 49.6 Enucleation of the submucosal tumor by careful dissection of the tumor off the esophageal mucosal layer. (Courtesy of Daniel J. Boffa, M.D.)

toward the mucosa using blunt dissection. Staying near the "dome" of the lesion can help to avoid inadvertent injury to the mucosa. A kuettner dissector can be used for the blunt dissection and may be the preferred instrument as it can avoid thermal injury to the mucosa. Minimal sharp and electrocautery dissection can be used to facilitate exposing the lesion. Blunt dissection should be carried out around the lesion until its base or stalk at the level of the mucosa is reached. Particular care is exercised to preserve the vagus nerve trunk and its branches coursing along the esophagus. Blunt dissection is continued to separate the lesion from the mucosa until the tumor is entirely mobilized (Fig. 49.6).

After enucleation and removal of the tumor, the intraluminal mucosa is inspected for signs of thermal injury or perforation. This examination should be performed externally by close inspection and if there is greater concern of injury, then internally, by esophagoscopy. If injury or leak is suspected, the intrathoracic esophagus can be submerged in saline and a leak test performed using endoscopic insufflation [25]. Mucosal perforation is primarily repaired in two layers using an absorbable suture [10]. The longitudinal esophageal myotomy is reapproximated using an absorbable suture [11]. A chest tube is left in place and the incisions closed in the standard fashion. An additional closed suction drain may be placed in the pleural cavity also. When leaving either a chest tube or other drain, placing them near, but not directly over the surgical site, may reduce the theoretical risk of fistula formation. For the enucleation of larger tumors where a significant muscular defect remains, a tension-free reapproximation of the muscular layer may not be feasible and the enucleation site can be covered by a pedicled pleural or muscular flap [21, 26].

Segmental Resection

Segmental resection of the esophagus should be considered for benign tumors that are large (7–8 cm), circumferential tumors, or tumors causing extensive damage to the mucosa, thereby increasing the risk for postoperative leak [9, 11]. Segmental resection should also be considered intraoperatively during an enucleation procedure in cases where dissection leads to mucosal damage and an increased risk of postoperative leak [9]. For very large tumors requiring an esophagectomy or resections of circumferential tumors involving the esophagus remote from the gastroesophageal junction, the VATS approach can be utilized in a manner equivalent to that performed for other conditions such as a malignant tumor. The thoracoscopic approach provides improved visualization of the thoracic esophagus as it traverses the main airway and major vascular structures of the chest. The VATS approach also has great utility when performing an intrathoracic reconstruction such as during an Ivor Lewis minimally invasive esophagectomy or a Roux-en-Y reconstruction within the chest [27]. Since esophageal resections and reconstructions are more frequently performed for malignant disease and the technique essentially is identical to that used for benign tumors when necessary, the details of these techniques can be found where descriptions of esophageal resections for esophageal carcinoma exist.

Postoperative Management

The use of nasogastric decompression following enucleation of a benign submucosal tumor is not routinely used in straightforward cases [9]. Similarly, the routine use of postoperative contrast esophagogram studies is not recommended following enucleation especially for a straightforward operation. In cases where mucosal damage is of concern, or cases that required repair of a mucosal injury, nasogastric decompression can be used for internal drainage until postoperative contrast esophagography, commonly with barium or Gastrografin contrast, confirms that there is no ongoing esophageal leak [28]. When an esophageal disruption is not a concern, a clear liquid diet may be started. A clear liquid diet may begin on the first postoperative day for a straightforward operation without concerns of mucosal injury. Also, the tube thoracostomy may be removed early in the postoperative period depending on the absence of any perioperative issues such as mucosal injury or significant pleural space issue such as high volume pleural drain output, persistent air leak from an inadvertent visceral pleural injury, or a thoracic duct injury.

Following a more involved operation such as a segmental resection, postoperative care is more involved than following enucleation, given the invasive nature of the operation. The nasogastric tube is left in place until postoperative contrast esophagogram is performed, commonly 5–7 days after resection. If no anastomotic leak is demonstrated on contrast esophagogram, the nasogastric tube can be removed and an oral diet initiated. If a liquid diet is tolerated and there is no clinical evidence of an anastomotic leak, such as fever or leukocytosis coupled with increased chest tube output, the remaining chest drains can be removed. As with enucleation, the chest drains should remain in place in patients with high volume pleural output or persistent air leak.

Postoperative Complications

Thoracoscopic enucleation of an esophageal submucosal tumor has been demonstrated to be a safe procedure with low morbidity rates as demonstrated in several small case series [4, 6, 25, 29–35]. To date, no postoperative deaths have been reported in the literature [9, 10]. Although rare, the most distressing complication following enucleation of an esophageal tumor is a postoperative esophageal mucosal disruption secondary to intraoperative mucosal damage or impaired vascularization [36]. When identified very early in the postoperative process (typically within 24 h), a primary repair may be considered. However, when identified beyond the immediate postoperative period, conservative management with continued external drainage and internal drainage may be required [37]. Esophageal stenting may be used as either an alternative or adjunctive therapy [38]. Stent placement may not be an option for very proximal or distal disruptions owing to discomfort and reflux, respectively [39]. Also, large defects and, in particular, ones that involve a relatively substantial amount of uncovered mucosa may not be ideally suited for stent placement given the possibility of stent erosion from excessive radial force of the stent abutting an attenuated esophageal wall. There are several other issues related to the use of stents which is a topic unto itself, but stent migration and the need for reintervention should remain a concern for the surgeon [40]. Stent removal is dependent upon the healing of the disruption and the clinical condition of the patient. As a disruption heals, supplemental enteral or parenteral nutrition may be employed if the time frame is beyond 1 week [40].

Additional postoperative complications can include acid reflux esophagitis, pseudodiverticulum formation, and fistula, with frequency ranging from 0% to 33% in a number of small case series examining thoracoscopic enucleation [4, 6, 25, 29–35]. Reflux esophagitis or pseudodiverticulum formation secondary to impaired esophageal motility or laxity of the muscular layer is most commonly caused by inadequate reapproximation of the muscular layer after open thoracotomy or thoracoscopic enucleation [11]. Formation of a pseudodiverticulum has been reported after thoracoscopic enucleation, and in these cases, the myotomy was not reapproximated [6, 31]. Postoperative pseudodiverticulum formation may be asymptomatic; however, it may also present as postoperative dysphagia in larger psuedodiverticula and is typically evaluated by contrast esophagogram [6, 41]. Asymptomatic patients may be followed with endoscopy, while symptomatic pseudodiverticula should be treated with reoperation and reapproximation of the muscular layer [6].

Given the more invasive approach and extensive dissection required to perform a segmental resection compared with enucleation, these patients are at an increased risk for postoperative complications. Segmental esophageal resection can have significant postoperative morbidity, including reflux esophagitis, diarrhea, and weight loss [11, 42, 43]. These postoperative complications are thought to be secondary to disruption of the vagus nerves surrounding the esophagus, causing the loss of parasympathetic innervation to the foregut [42].

Postoperative Outcomes

Short-Term

The results of several small case series demonstrate that thoracoscopic enucleation of benign submucosal esophageal tumors is a technically feasible and safe approach [3, 5, 6, 31, 34, 36, 44]. The VATS approach is associated with reduced surgical trauma when compared with thoracotomy, with no difference in functional outcome [11]. Shorter hospital length of stay has been demonstrated in several studies comparing VATS to open thoracotomy for enucleation of benign submucosal tumors, as well as earlier removal of the tube thoracostomy [6, 10, 11, 25]. Mirroring the lung cancer surgery experience using the minimally invasive approach, VATS enucleation also is associated with reduced postoperative pain and improved cosmetic outcomes for patients [45, 46].

Long-Term

As a result of the low incidence of benign submucosal tumors, evidence for long-term outcomes of patients who undergo VATS resection is limited to several small case series in the literature. In modern series of VATS enucleation of benign tumors, follow-up has ranged from 3 months to over 10 years with no documented incidence of tumor recurrence [4, 10, 11, 30, 35]. Although the majority of patients undergo resection for asymptomatic benign submucosal tumors, the existing literature has demonstrated that those who are symptomatic at presentation experience a durable resolution of symptoms following VATS enucleation, with 89–95% of patients symptom-free at 5 years [10, 11, 30]. Symptomatic gastroesophageal reflux disease (GERD) requiring fundoplication has been demonstrated up to 3 years after surgical enucleation, in patients who had no preexisting GERD, as well as those with preoperative GERD symptoms [10, 25]. These findings highlight the need for long-term follow-up in patients following enucleation and also suggest that surgeons may consider an anti-reflux procedure at the time of enucleation in patients who are symptomatic [10]. Finally, the formation of a pseudodiverticulum during long-term follow-up has not been documented in the modern series of thoracoscopic enucleations [4, 25, 29, 30, 32–35]. Thus, the optimal strategy to address this issue remains undefined and dependent on a combination of several factors.

Conclusion

Benign submucosal tumors are rare tumors of the esophagus, with leiomyoma accounting for the majority of cases. Although the management of small asymptomatic benign submucosal tumors is debated, tumors that are symptomatic, large, or require a pathologic diagnosis to rule out malignancy should be removed by tumor enucleation. The thoracoscopic approach has been increasingly used for benign esophageal submucosal tumors and is similar to the open thoracotomy approach in many aspects without compromising exposure, mobilization, or tumor enucleation. Thoracoscopic enucleation has been demonstrated to be a technically feasible and safe alternative to the traditional thoracotomy, with shorter hospital stays, less postoperative pain, and no difference in functional outcomes.

References

1. Hatch GF 3rd, Wertheimer-Hatch L, Hatch KF, Davis GB, Blanchard DK, Foster RS Jr, et al. Tumors of the esophagus. World J Surg. 2000;24:401–11.
2. KM FMA. Benign tumors, cysts, and duplications of the esophagus. In: Shields TW, JR LC, Feins CE, et al., editors. General thoracic surgery. Philadelphia: Lippincott Williams & Wilkins; 2009. p. 7e.
3. Mutrie CJ, Donahue DM, Wain JC, Wright CD, Gaissert HA, Grillo HC, et al. Esophageal leiomyoma: a 40-year experience. Ann Thorac Surg. 2005;79:1122–5.
4. von Rahden BH, Stein HJ, Feussner H, Siewert JR. Enucleation of submucosal tumors of the esophagus: minimally invasive versus open approach. Surg Endosc. 2004;18:924–30.
5. Roviaro GC, Maciocco M, Varoli F, Rebuffat C, Vergani C, Scarduelli A. Videothoracoscopic treatment of oesophageal leiomyoma. Thorax. 1998;53:190–2.
6. Bonavina L, Segalin A, Rosati R, Pavanello M, Peracchia A. Surgical therapy of esophageal leiomyoma. J Am Coll Surg. 1995;181:257–62.
7. Seremetis MG, Lyons WS, VC dG, Peabody JW Jr. Leiomyomata of the esophagus. An analysis of 838 cases. Cancer. 1976;38:2166–77.
8. Choong CK, Meyers BF. Benign esophageal tumors: introduction, incidence, classification, and clinical features. Semin Thorac Cardiovasc Surg. 2003;15:3–8.
9. Paruch JZM, Ferguson MK. Resection of benign tumors of the esophagus. In: Sugarbaker DJ, Bueno R, Colson YL, Jaklitsch MT, Krasna MJ, Mentzer SJ, et al., editors. Adult chest surgery. New York: McGraw-Hill Education; 2009. p. 2e.
10. Samphire J, Nafteux P, Luketich J. Minimally invasive techniques for resection of benign esophageal tumors. Semin Thorac Cardiovasc Surg. 2003;15:35–43.
11. Lee LS, Singhal S, Brinster CJ, Marshall B, Kochman ML, Kaiser LR, et al. Current management of esophageal leiomyoma. J Am Coll Surg. 2004;198:136–46.
12. Arnorsson T, Aberg C, Aberg T. Benign tumours of the oesophagus and oesophageal cysts. Scand J Thorac Cardiovasc Surg. 1984;18:145–50.
13. Hanel K, Talley NA, Hunt DR. Hemangioma of the esophagus: an unusual cause of upper gastrointestinal bleeding. Dig Dis Sci. 1981;26:257–63.
14. Palazzo L, Landi B, Cellier C, Roseau G, Chaussade S, Couturier D, et al. Endosonographic features of esophageal granular cell tumors. Endoscopy. 1997;29:850–3.
15. Coutinho DSS, Soga J, Yoshikawa T, Miyashita K, Tanaka O, Sasaki K, et al. Granular cell tumors of the esophagus: a report of two cases and review of the literature. Am J Gastroenterol. 1985;80:758–62.
16. Akiyama S, Kataoka M, Horisawa M, Inoue S, Sakai M, Ito K, et al. Lipoma of the esophagus—Report of a case and review of the literature. Jpn J Surg. 1990;20:458–62.
17. Nishikawa K, Omura N, Yuda M, Tanaka Y, Matsumoto A, Tanishima Y, et al. Video-assisted thoracoscopic surgery for localized neurofibroma of the esophagus: case report and review of the literature. Int Surg. 2013;98:461–5.
18. Yoon YH, Kim KH, Baek WK, Kim JT, Son KH, Han JY, et al. Lymphangioma of the esophagus: surgical treatment. Ann Thorac Surg. 2004;78:e51–e3.
19. Everett C, Volberg F, Ulshen M, Murray G. Intramural esophageal hamartoma: A report of two cases and review of the literature. Gastrointest Radiol. 1980;5:317–9.

20. Kim AW, Korst RJ, Port JL, Altorki NK, Lee PC. Giant cavernous hemangioma of the distal esophagus treated with esophagectomy. J Thorac Cardiovasc Surg. 2007;133:1665–7.
21. Rijcken E, Kersting CM, Senninger N, Bruewer M. Esophageal resection for giant leiomyoma: report of two cases and a review of the literature. Langenbeck's Arch Surg. 2008;394:623.
22. Yang PS, Lee KS, Lee SJ, Kim TS, Choo I-W, Shim YM, et al. Esophageal leiomyoma: radiologic findings in 12 patients. Korean J Radiol. 2001;2:132–7.
23. Rice TW. Benign esophageal tumors: esophagoscopy and endoscopic esophageal ultrasound. Semin Thorac Cardiovasc Surg. 2003;15:20–6.
24. Everitt NJ, Glinatsis M, McMahon MJ. Thoracoscopic enucleation of leiomyoma of the oesophagus. Br J Surg. 1992;79:643.
25. Kent M, d'Amato T, Nordman C, Schuchert M, Landreneau R, Alvelo-Rivera M, et al. Minimally invasive resection of benign esophageal tumors. J Thorac Cardiovasc Surg. 2007;134:176–81.
26. Aurea P, Grazia M, Petrella F, Bazzocchi R. Giant leiomyoma of the esophagus. Eur J Cardiothorac Surg. 2002;22:1008–10.
27. Jobe BA, Hunter JG, Watson DI. Esophagus and diaphragmatic hernia. In: Brunicardi FC, Andersen DK, Billiar TR, Dunn DL, Hunter JG, Matthews JB, et al., editors. Schwartz's principles of surgery. 10e ed. New York: McGraw-Hill Education; 2014.
28. Vogel SB, Rout WR, Martin TD, Abbitt PL. Esophageal perforation in adults: aggressive, conservative treatment lowers morbidity and mortality. Ann Surg. 2005;241:1016–21. discussion 21–3
29. Nguyen NT, Reavis KM, El-Badawi K, Hinojosa MW, Smith BR. Minimally invasive surgical enucleation or esophagogastrectomy for benign tumor of the esophagus. Surg Innov. 2008;15:120–5.
30. Jiang G, Zhao H, Yang F, Li J, Li Y, Liu Y, et al. Thoracoscopic enucleation of esophageal leiomyoma: a retrospective study on 40 cases. Dis Esophagus. 2009;22:279–83.
31. Bardini R, Asolati M. Thoracoscopic resection of benign tumours of the esophagus. Int Surg. 1997;82:5–6.
32. Palanivelu C, Rangarajan M, Madankumar MV, John SJ, Senthilkumar R. Minimally invasive therapy for benign tumors of the distal third of the esophagus – a single institute's experience. J Laparoendosc Adv Surg Tech A. 2008;18:20–6.
33. Fisichella PM, Soper NJ, Pellegrini CA, Patti MG. Surgical management of benign esophageal disorders. London: Springer; 2014.
34. Luh S-P, Hou S-M, Fang C-C, Chen C-Y. Video-thoracoscopic enucleation of esophageal leiomyoma. World J Surg Oncol. 2012;10:52.
35. Obuchi T, Sasaki A, Nitta H, Koeda K, Ikeda K, Wakabayashi G. Minimally invasive surgical enucleation for esophageal leiomyoma: report of seven cases. Dis Esophagus. 2010;23:E1–4.
36. Vallbohmer D, Holscher AH, Brabender J, Bollschweiler E, Gutschow C. Thoracoscopic enucleation of esophageal leiomyomas: a feasible and safe procedure. Endoscopy. 2007;39:1097–9.
37. Brinster CJ, Singhal S, Lee L, Marshall MB, Kaiser LR, Kucharczuk JC. Evolving options in the management of esophageal perforation. Ann Thorac Surg. 2004;77:1475–83.
38. Blackmon SH, Santora R, Schwarz P, Barroso A, Dunkin BJ. Utility of removable esophageal covered self-expanding metal stents for leak and fistula management. Ann Thorac Surg. 2010;89:931–7.
39. Wu JT, Mattox KL, Wall MJ Jr. Esophageal perforations: new perspectives and treatment paradigms. J Trauma. 2007;63:1173–84.
40. Dasari BV, Neely D, Kennedy A, Spence G, Rice P, Mackle E, et al. The role of esophageal stents in the management of esophageal anastomotic leaks and benign esophageal perforations. Ann Surg. 2014;259:852–60.
41. Zaninotto G, Portale G, Costantini M, Rizzetto C, Salvador R, Rampado S, et al. Minimally invasive enucleation of esophageal leiomyoma. Surg Endosc. 2006;20:1904–8.
42. Banki F, Mason RJ, DeMeester SR, Hagen JA, Balaji NS, Crookes PF, et al. Vagal-sparing esophagectomy: a more physiologic alternative. Ann Surg. 2002;236:324–36.

43. Watson TJ, DeMeester TR, Kauer WK, Peters JH, Hagen JA. Esophageal replacement for end-stage benign esophageal disease. J Thorac Cardiovasc Surg. 1998;115:1241–7. discussion 7-9
44. Nguyen NT, Alcocer JJ, Luketich JD. Thoracoscopic enucleation of an esophageal leiomyoma. J Clin Gastroenterol. 2000;31:89.
45. Boffa DJ, Dhamija A, Kosinski AS, Kim AW, Detterbeck FC, Mitchell JD, et al. Fewer complications result from a video-assisted approach to anatomic resection of clinical stage I lung cancer. J Thorac Cardiovasc Surg. 2014;148:637–43.
46. Shigemura N, Yim AP. Variation in the approach to VATS Lobectomy: effect on the evaluation of surgical morbidity following VATS lobectomy for the treatment of stage I non–small cell lung cancer. Thorac Surg Clin. 2007;17:233–9.

50 Benign Esophageal and Gastric Tumors: Laparoscopic Management of Benign Submucosal Tumors

Riley K. Kitamura and Brian Jacob

Introduction

Submucosal tumors (SMT) are protuberant lesions covered by intact mucosa in the gastrointestinal tract [1–5]. Often asymptomatic and discovered incidentally, they are commonly diagnosed after the fifth decade of life, occur equally in men and women, and are most commonly found in the stomach, followed by the esophagus, duodenum, and colon.

Benign esophageal tumors are rare with prevalence rates of 0.17–0.5%. Sixty-five percent of these are leiomyomas, followed by esophageal cysts, fibrovascular polyps, and granular cell tumors [2].

Nearly half of all gastric SMT are gastrointestinal stromal tumors (GISTs), which may be benign or malignant (Fig. 50.1). Gastric leiomyomas are the next most common SMT, though they are infrequent overall with prevalence rates near 13%, followed by gastric lipomas and fibromas/fibromyomas [6, 7]. Overall, benign gastric SMT are rare and represent less than 5% of all gastric tumors [8].

Symptomatic tumors should be excised. Surveillance of asymptomatic patients is acceptable; however, there is a hypothetical risk of malignant transformation, rapid growth, or development of severe obstruction and/or bleeding. Therefore, if the nature of the tumor remains doubtful, resection is advised [9].

R. K. Kitamura · B. Jacob (✉)
Department of Surgery, Icahn School of Medicine at Mount Sinai, New York, NY, USA
e-mail: Brian.Jacob@mountsinai.org

J. Grams et al. (eds.), *The SAGES Manual of Foregut Surgery*,
https://doi.org/10.1007/978-3-319-96122-4_50

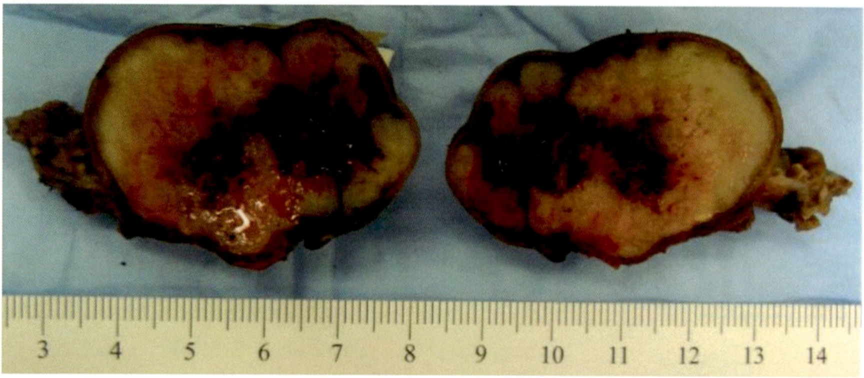

Fig. 50.1 Encapsulated gastric SMT (GIST) in cross section with central hemorrhage

Principles of Resection

The operative goal is tumor resection without altering gastrointestinal function. Therefore, surgeons should equip themselves with a thorough knowledge of the relevant anatomy, common pitfalls, and alternative operative approaches to avoid unnecessary complications.

Surgical approach depends on SMT location, which is variable (Fig. 50.2). Thus, preoperative imaging with endoscopy, endoscopic ultrasound, and abdominopelvic computed tomography (CT) is critical to assess adjacent structure involvement, length of resection, and the need for multiple-modality approaches (concomitant endoscopic and laparoscopic procedures) and to anticipate variant anatomy (replaced or accessory hepatic arteries, proximate splenic artery) [10].

Needle biopsy is not contraindicated; however, it infrequently reveals the final pathology and can complicate future submucosal dissection as well as predispose for fistula formation later [2].

In regard to surgical approach, laparoscopic is equally effective compared to open resection; however, laparoscopic (minimally invasive surgery) is associated with less pain, inflammation, blood loss, earlier diet tolerance, and shorter hospital stay [7, 11–14]. Common indications for open conversion are uncontrolled hemorrhage and tumor rupture. Additionally, conversion should be strongly considered when there is evidence of tumor invasion or other signs of undiagnosed malignancy [9, 12]. Conversion rates are 0–22%, though this is expected to lower as laparoscopic techniques are more commonly used [8].

During the operation, optimal exposure within each step is paramount and facilitates working in the correct plane, as well as prevents inadvertent thermal injury to healthy tissue.

SMTs can be small, endophytic, and hard to localize with tactile or visual sensation. Therefore, laparoscopic sonography and intraoperative endoscopy are

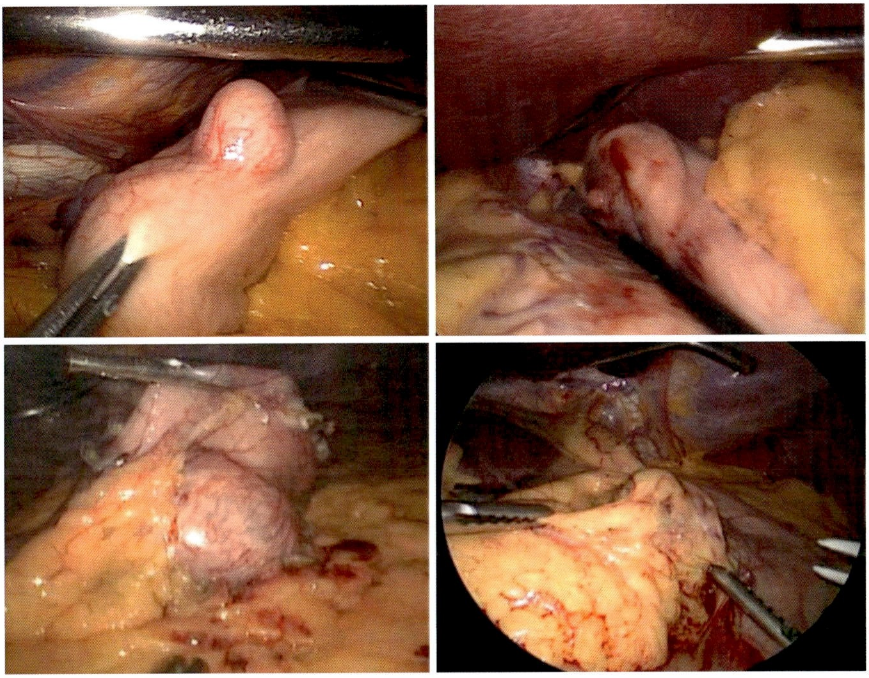

Fig. 50.2 Exophytic gastric SMT of the greater curvature (top left), fundus (top right), posterior antrum (bottom left), lesser curvature (bottom right)

Fig. 50.3 Endoscopic localization of endophytic, small, or otherwise difficult to localize SMT by laparoscopy alone

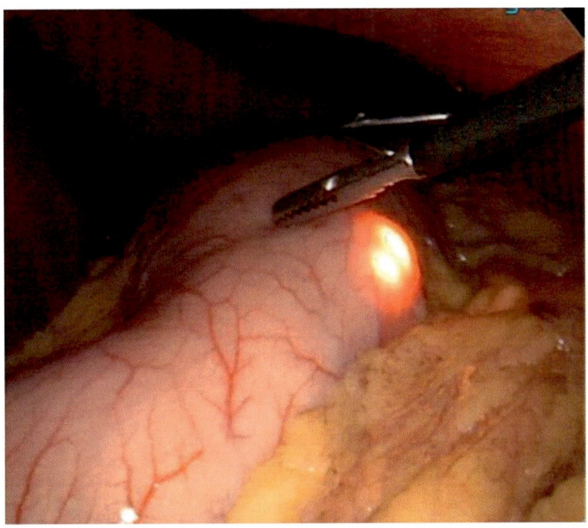

constructive adjuncts for localization and preventing postoperative stenosis or leak (Fig. 50.3) [16, 17]. Additionally, we advise resection over a 36–40 French bougie if there is any question of luminal compromise.

Finally, while there are no reports of tumor dissemination after benign SMT resection [7], there is a hypothetical risk of occult malignancy. Therefore, oncologic principles of tumor resection (i.e., avoid repeated insufflation, spillage of intragastric content, direct tumor manipulation, tumor capsule rupture or disruption of lymphatic vessels, and use a specimen retrieval bag) should be maintained.

Equipment List

Laparoscopic tower and instruments
Endoscopic tower and instruments
36–40 French bougie
5 mm trocar × 3, 12–15 mm trocar × 1
Nathanson or other liver retractor
Harmonic scalpel (Ethicon Endo-Surgery, J & J Medical Ltd, Cincinnati, USA)
Laparoscopic linear stapler
Laparoscopic specimen bag

Surgical Technique

After induction of general anesthesia, our practice is to position the patient in the supine or split-leg position. Foley catheterization is reserved for complicated cases.

Pneumoperitoneum is produced through a left upper quadrant incision using the closed 5 mm bladeless optical trocar. The abdomen is inspected for variant anatomy and adhesions, and subsequently additional working ports are placed under direct vision. A periumbilical port is upsized to a 12–15 mm port to facilitate stapling later. A liver retractor through the subxiphoid port assists with full visualization of the esophageal hiatus and proximal stomach (Fig. 50.4).

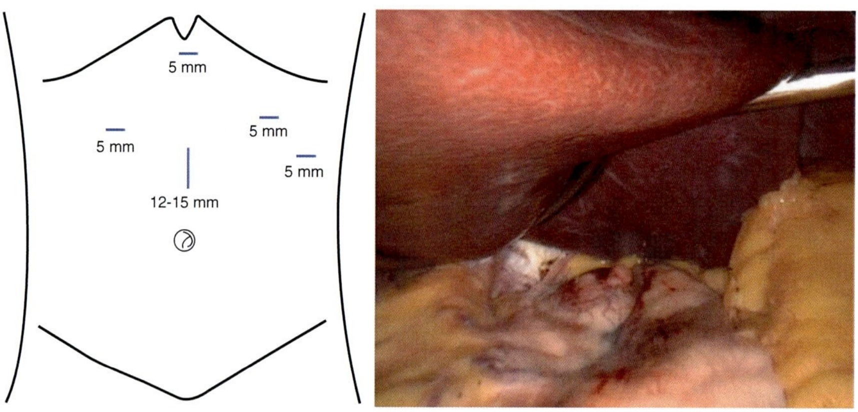

Fig. 50.4 Example of port placement (left), and exposure after placement of Nathanson retractor (right)

Following port placement, the stomach is mobilized by entering the lesser sac 1 centimeter away from the gastroepiploic vessels. The greater curvature is mobilized proximally until the left crus of the diaphragm or distally toward the pylorus depending on the location of the lesion.

Esophagogastric Junction Tumor

Resection of esophagogastric and prepyloric lesions is particularly challenging and high risk for postoperative luminal stenosis. In such cases, conversion to a more radical approach (partial or total gastrectomy) should be considered particularly if the nature (benign versus malignant) of the tumor is unclear [8].

If the tumor is small and not directly involving the esophagogastric junction, transgastric resection or enucleation are acceptable options [8]. The transgastric approach is performed through an anterior gastrotomy and subsequent eversion of the tumor through the gastric opening. A laparoscopic linear stapler is directed perpendicularly to the longitudinal axis of the stomach, and the mass is resected en bloc. The anterior gastrotomy is either sewn or stapled closed (Figs. 50.5, 50.6 and 50.7) [18].

The drawback of transgastric resection is the high potential for intra-abdominal gastric fluid contamination and posterior extraluminal organ injury. Both can be avoided with careful inspection of surrounding structures prior to firing the stapler. This approach also provides poor visualization of the cardioesophageal junction and is therefore not ideal for very proximal lesions [19].

Proximal gastrectomy is discouraged due to a high rate of complications including stricture, reflux esophagitis, and leak [15].

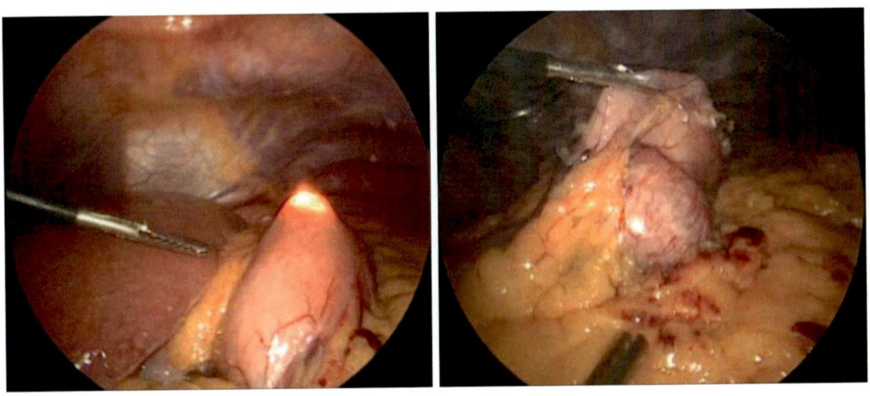

Fig. 50.5 Endoscopic (left), followed by laparoscopic (right), localization of a posterior gastric SMT

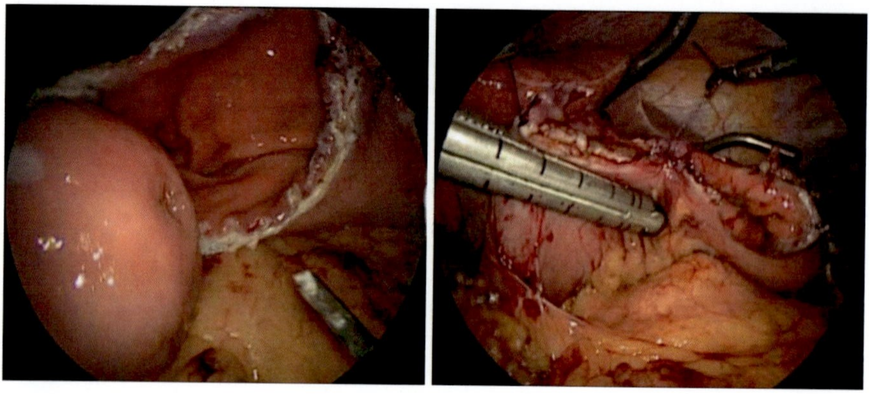

Fig. 50.6 Transgastric SMT resection (left), followed by closure of the gastrotomy via laparoscopic stapling

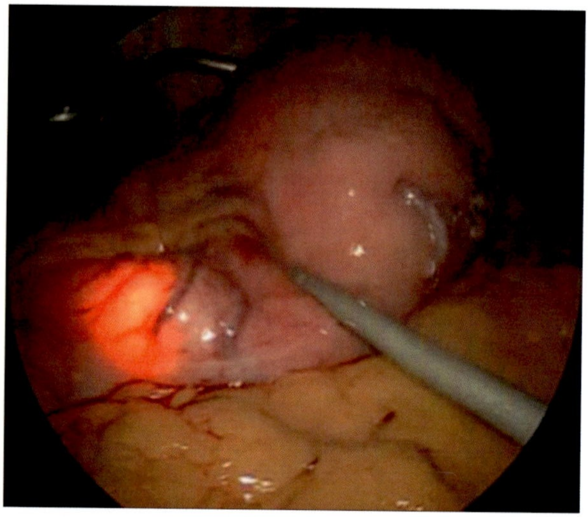

Fig. 50.7 Endoscopic intraluminal evaluation and leak test

Gastric Fundus or Antrum

Lesions of the gastric fundus or antrum are relatively straightforward and may be approached through a simple wedge resection with the linear stapler once adequate mobilization of the stomach is achieved. Risk for stenosis or staple line tension is lower, though care must be taken to avoid excessive traction, and the linear stapler should be directed perpendicular to the longitudinal axis of the stomach—minimizing the risk of postoperative stenosis/obstruction (Fig. 50.8) [7].

Posterior Wall

Tumors of the posterior wall are challenging and approached through several methods. The transgastric approach is described above.

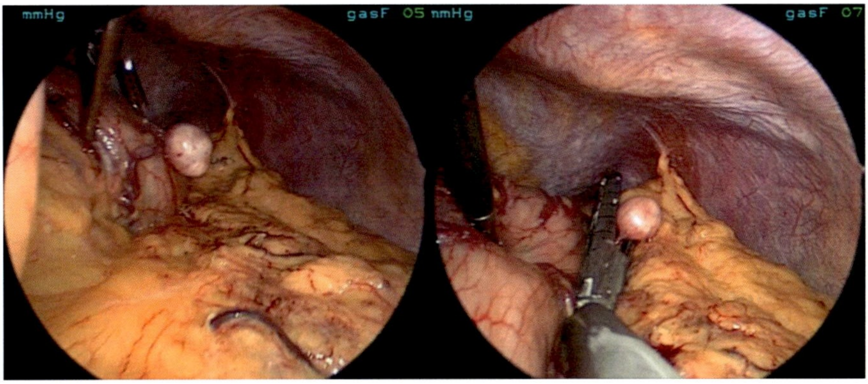

Fig. 50.8 Stapled resection of an exophytic SMT on the greater curvature of the stomach

With large exophytic posterior lesions, laparoscopic extraluminal resection is the optimal approach. The gastric body and greater curvature is completely mobilized and axially rotated. The lesion is then similarly retracted away from the lumen followed by full-thickness wedge resection. Again, care must be given to ensure the interspace between the fundus and spleen is dissected free of attachments and that the cardioesophageal junction is not narrowed [20].

Intragastric approaches are not well-studied in the USA; however, they may be ideal in lesions near the cardioesophageal junction. Tagaya et al. describe an intragastric approach where the stomach is brought to the abdominal wall, and balloon-tipped trocars are placed through the anterior abdominal and gastric wall into the gastric lumen. The tumor is subsequently enucleated or resected under vision [21]. Similar to this, Na et al. have reported single-incision laparoscopic surgery (SILS) where the stomach is brought anteriorly and entered through a multichannel umbilical port. The resection is completed laparoscopically and appears to be feasible for small tumors [22]. The authors report less spillage of gastric contents and continuous visualization of the esophagogastric junction. The drawbacks of this technique are limited range of resection and higher incidence of splenic injury if the short gastric vessels are not divided. Lateral tension can otherwise exacerbate splenic capsular injury or gastric laceration.

Antrum and Prepyloric Lesions

The prepyloric/antral area of the stomach can be a technically demanding area with high risk of stenosis due to low distensibility of the stomach as well as risk of vagal nerve injury. This may manifest as postoperative functional gastric outlet obstruction and delayed gastric emptying. Thus, local resection followed by intra- or extracorporeal suturing is recommended to minimize the amount of healthy tissue taken (Fig. 50.9). If the lumen becomes stenosed, the procedure may be converted to distal gastrectomy with Billroth I or II reconstruction.

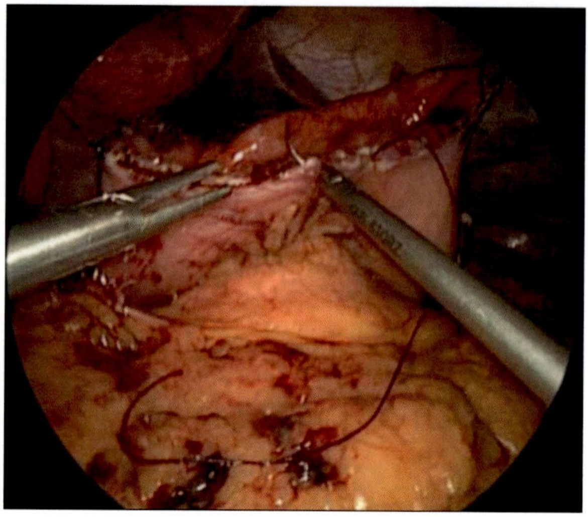

Fig. 50.9 Intracorporeal suture closure of gastrotomy

Advanced Techniques

Reduced Port

Several options for port reduction have been described for benign SMT resection but are not well-studied for long-term outcomes. Single-incision laparoscopic surgery (SILS) for favorably located lesions such as the anterior wall or greater curvature has been successful [23]. Double-bended instruments to assist with instrument conflict have also been used successfully for a posteriorly located lesion [24]. Intragastric SILS (described previously) have been reported in small series with some success [22], and a two-port option using a 25 mm multi-port trocar and 2 mm working port have also been attempted, although many of these techniques are still being developed [25].

Hybrid Approaches

Combined endoscopic and laparoscopic approaches is ideal for endophytic, small, and difficult to localize lesions. Endoscopic assistance may result in less radical resection margins, lower rate of postoperative bleeding, perforation, and stenosis [26]. Small intramural tumors can be localized with endoscopic ultrasound with a diagnostic precision of 92% [8]. With the aid of an experienced endoscopist, SMT can be suctioned or grasped providing countertraction as well to assist with subserosal dissection.

Staged endoscopic-laparoscopic dissection techniques are also under development to minimize the amount of heathy tissue sacrificed. For example, laparoscopic-endoscopic cooperative surgery (LECS) is a sequential procedure in which endoscopic submucosal dissection (ESD) is performed, followed by laparoscopic seromuscular layer dissection. Laparoscopic linear staplers are then applied for resection of tumor and closure of the gastric wall simultaneously via an eversion method, ultimately minimizing the amount of healthy resected tissue and potential for postoperative stenosis [26].

Laparoscopy-assisted endoscopic full-thickness resection (LAEFR) is a staged full-layer endoscopic dissection, followed by laparoscopic suture repair of the gastric defect [1]. Nonexposed endoscopic wall-inversion surgery (NEWS) is performed by laparoscopic seromuscular dissection followed by oversewing of the dissection line. The dissected area is endoscopically invaginated and resected using the ESD technique. This minimizes healthy tissue removal, abdominal contamination, and the potential of peritoneal spread [27, 28]. Critiques of endoscopic dissection are that it is challenging to achieve R0 resection margins and difficult to remove the specimen as one piece or avoid disruption of the tumor capsule. Additionally, it may be more difficult to control bleeding, ESD carries risk of perforation, and it requires an experienced endoscopist [3]. Further studies of endoscopic technique are needed but have thus far shown promising results.

Robotic-Assisted Surgery

Robotic-assisted surgery offers surgeons the ability to perform gastric SMT resection, intracorporeal suturing, and complex gastrointestinal reconstructions with greater comfort and control while achieving similar standards to laparoscopy. Long-term outcomes of robotic versus laparoscopic resection are not yet available.

Postoperative Management

For gastric wedge resections, our practice is to begin a clear liquid diet the following day, and the patient is advised to take frequent but small sips to maintain adequate hydration. Alternatively, an esophogram prior to starting a diet may be sought if there is concern for obstruction or leak. The diet is slowly advanced as tolerated and a proton-pump inhibitor or H2 antagonist is added to decrease gastric secretions.

Patients who undergo a more radical resection involving subtotal or total gastrectomy are typically kept NPO with nasogastric tube decompression for one to two postoperative days and undergo upper GI swallow study prior to starting a diet.

Postoperative Complications

Complications specific to laparoscopic resection of benign submucosal tumors include but are not limited to anastomotic leak, bleeding, gastrointestinal lumen stenosis, missed injury to adjacent structures, surgical site infection, and port-site hernias.

Conclusion

Laparoscopic approach is an effective and safe technique for benign gastric SMT resection. Lesions of the posterior wall, as well as large tumors near the cardia or pylorus, are often more difficult to locate and/or resect without affecting GI tract function. As a result, multiple laparoscopic (transgastric, intragastric, extraluminal) approaches have been developed, and many innovative laparoscopic-endoscopic cooperative approaches have evolved.

References

1. Abe N, Takeuchi H, Yanagida O, Masaki T, Mori T, Sugiyama M, Atomi Y. Endoscopic full thickness resection with laparoscopic assistance as hybrid NOTES for gastric submucosal tumor. Surg Endosc. 2009;23:1908–13.
2. Camp P Jr, Lukanich J. Resection of benign tumors of the esophagus. In: Sugarbaker DJ, Bueno R, Colson YL, Jaklitsch MT, Krasna MJ, Mentzer S, Williams M, Adams A, editors. Adult chest surgery. 2nd ed. New York: McGraw-Hill Medical; 2014.
3. Lee CM, Kim H-H. Minimally invasive surgery for submucosal (subepithelial) tumors of the stomach. World J Gastroenterol. 2014;20(36):13035–43.
4. Nishida T, Kawai N, Yamaguchi S, Nishida Y. Submucosal tumors: comprehensive guide for the diagnosis of gastrointestinal submucosal tumors. Dig Endosc. 2013;25(5):479–89.
5. Nakachi A, Miyazato H, Oshiro T, Shimoji H, Shiraishi M, Muto Y. Granular cell tumor of the rectum: a case report and review of the literature. J Gastroenterol. 2000;35:631–4.
6. Bouillot J-L, Bresler L, Fagniez P, Samama G, Champault G, Parent Y. Laparoscopic resection of benign submucosal gastric tumors. A report of 65 cases. Gastroenterol Clin Biol. 2003;27:272–6.
7. Palanivelu C, Rangarajan M, Parthasarathi R, Senthilkumar R. Laparoscopic resection for benign tumors of the stomach. JSLS. 2007;11(1):81–6.
8. Palanivelu C. Laparoscopic gastric resection for benign tumors. In: Palanivelu C, editor. Art of laparoscopic surgery. New Delhi: Jaypee Brothers; 2007. p. 495–507.
9. Ponsaing L, Hansen M. Therapeutic procedures for submucosal tumors in the gastrointestinal tract. World J Gastroenterol. 2007;13:3316–22.
10. Palazzo L, Landi B, Cellier C, Roseau G, Chaussade S, Couturier D, Barbier J. Endosonographic features of esophageal granular cell tumors. Endosocpy. 1997;29:850–3.
11. De Volgelaere K, Hoorens A, Haentjens P, Delvaux G. Laparoscopic versus open resection of gastrointestinal stromal tumors of the stomach. Surg Endosc. 2013;27:1546–54.
12. Matthews B, Walsh R, Kercher K, Sing R, Pratt B, Answini G, Heniford B. Laparoscopic vs open resection of gastric stromal tumors. Surg Endosc. 2002;16(5):803–7.
13. Morinaga N, Sano A, Katayama K, Suzuki K, Kamisaka K, Asao T, Kuwano H. Laparoscopic transgastric tumor-everting resection of the gastric submucosal tumor located near the esophagogastric junction. Surg Laparosc Endosc Percutan Tech. 2004;14(6):344–8.
14. Yahchouchy E, Etienne J, Fagniez P, Adam R, Fingerhut A. A new "no-touch" technique for the laparoscopic treatment of gastric stromal tumors. Surg Endosc. 2002;16:962–4.
15. Ahn S, Jung do H, Son S, Lee C, Park do J, Kim H. Laparoscopic double-tract proximal gastrectomy for proximal early gastric cancer. Gastric Cancer. 2014;17(3):562–70.
16. Cugar E, Hoyuela C, Rodriguez-Santiago J, Marco C. Laparoscopic ultrasound guidance for laparoscopic resection of benign gastric tumors. J Laparoendosc Adv Surg Tech A. 1999;9(1):63–7.

17. Wilhelm D, Delius S, Burian M, Schneider A, Frimberger E, Meining A, Feussner H. Simultaneous use of laparoscopy and endoscopy for minimally invasive resection of gastric subepithelial masses – analysis of 93 interventions. World J Surg. 2008;32:1021–8.
18. Choi Y, Oh S. Laparoscopy in the management of gastric submucosal tumors. Surg Endosc. 2000;16(14):741–5.
19. Watson D, Game P, Devitt P. Laparoscopic resection of benign tumors of the posterior gastric wall. Surg Endosc. 1996;10:540–1.
20. Zhong-Wei K, Cheng-Zhu Z, Ming-Gen H, Dan-Lei C. Laparoscopic resection of submucosal-tumor on posterior wall of gastric fundus. World J Gastroenterol. 2004;10(19):2850–5853.
21. Tagaya N, Mikami H, Kubota K, Hosoya Y, Nagai H. Laparoscopic intragastric stapled resection of gastric submucosal tumors located near the esophagogastric junction. Surg Endosc. 2002;16:177–9.
22. Na J, Lee S, Noh S. The single incision laparoscopic intragastric wedge resection of gastric submucosal tumor. J Gastric Cancer. 2011;11:225–9.
23. Sasaki A, Koeda K, Nakajima J, Obuchi T, Baba S, Wakabayashi G. Single-incision laparoscopic gastric resection for submucosal tumors: report of three cases. Surg Today. 2011;41:133–6.
24. Henckens T, Van de Putte D, Van Renterghem K, Ceelen W, Pattyn P, Van Nieuwenhove Y. Laparoendoscopic single-site gastrectomy for gastric GIST using double-bended instruments. J Laparoendosc Adv Surg Tech A. 2010;20(5):469–71.
25. Hirano Y, Watanabe T, Uchida T, Yoshida S, Kato H, Hosokawa O. Laparoendoscopic single site partial resection of the stomach for gastrointestinal stromal tumor. Surg Laparosc Endosc Percutan Tech. 2010;20:262–4.
26. Hiki N, Yamamoto Y, Fukunaga T, Yamaguchi T, Nunobe S, Tokunaga M, Miki A, Ohyama S, Seto Y. Laparoscopic and endoscopic cooperative surgery for gastrointestinal stromal tumor dissection. Surg Endosc. 2008;22:1729–35.
27. Mitsui T, Niimi K, Yamashita H, Goto O, Aikou S, Hatao F, Wada I, Shimizu N, Fujishiro M, Koike K, Seto Y. Non-exposed endoscopic wall-inversion surgery as a novel partial gastrectomy technique. Gastric Cancer. 2014;17:594–9.
28. Goto O, Mitsui T, Fujishiro M, Wada I, Shimizu N, Seto Y, Korke K. New method of endoscopic full thickness resection: a pilot study of non-exposed endoscopic wall-inversion surgery in an ex vivo porcine model. Gastric Cancer. 2011;14:183–7.

Endoscopic Management of Benign Submucosal Tumors

51

Ran Bill Luo and Garth R. Jacobsen

Introduction

Benign submucosal tumors in the upper gastrointestinal (GI) tract are typically discovered incidentally on either routine or surveillance upper endoscopies. Unless the lesions are near the gastroesophageal junction or the pylorus, the patient may not have symptoms given the slow-growing benign nature of these lesions. As imaging resolution and endoscopic technologies improve, the ability to perform minimally invasive endoscopic resections for these lesions becomes increasingly feasible. Incision-less per-oral endoscopic resections for benign lesions allow for faster recovery, decreased pain, and lower surgical morbidity for patients. Submucosal tumors discovered in the upper GI tract can be leiomyomas, lipomas, carcinoids, cysts, and ectopic pancreas tissue.

Diagnostic Testing

Endoscopic ultrasound (EUS) is one of the most important preoperative imaging studies prior to treatment decision [1]. Assessment of the depth of lesion penetration is necessary prior to consideration for endoscopic intervention. The main contraindication for endoscopic mucosal or submucosal resection of benign tumors is the presence of suspicious lymph nodes seen on EUS or the presence of distance metastases. If these are discovered on initial work-up, then re-evaluation of the lesion is necessary as the index of suspicion for malignancy is much higher and repeat stacked

R. B. Luo (✉)
Division of Minimally Invasive Surgery, Department of General Surgery, UC San Diego Health Systems, La Jolla, CA, USA
e-mail: r4luo@ucsd.edu

G. R. Jacobsen
Department of Surgery, University of California San Diego, Rancho Santa Fe, CA, USA

J. Grams et al. (eds.), *The SAGES Manual of Foregut Surgery*,
https://doi.org/10.1007/978-3-319-96122-4_51

biopsies should be obtained at the time of the EUS. Depending on the pathology discovered, radiologic work-up can also be obtained either with computer tomography (CT) or magnetic resonance imaging (MRI) of the abdomen and pelvis.

Preoperative Preparations

The patients should receive preoperative health evaluation and laboratory testing to be able to undergo general anesthesia. General anesthesia may be preferred as the procedures can be much longer than most standard endoscopic interventions and would allow for the conversion to operative surgical management in case the lesion is unable to be removed with the endoscopic approach.

Operative Technique

As with surgical resection, the goal with endoscopic therapy is to completely remove the lesion and provide tissue for pathology for assessing the true depth of penetration. Currently, the two most common techniques for endoscopic excision of benign lesions are endoscopic mucosal resection (EMR), which is used for masses smaller than 2 cm, and endoscopic submucosal dissection (ESD), which is utilized for resection of masses larger than 2 cm [1, 5]. Two alternative techniques of unroofing and enucleation are less commonly employed but appear effective.

Operative Equipment

Therapeutic upper endoscope with a 3.7 mm inner channel.

Dual-channel therapeutic upper endoscope with 2.8 mm and 3.7 mm inner channels – useful for specific techniques of resection (i.e., grasper and a snare technique of EMR)

Power irrigation

Injection needle

SPOT™(*GI Supply, Camp Hill, PA*) for tattooing the lesion in case a laparoscopic approach is necessary in the future

Small and large endoscopic snares with electrosurgery capabilities

Endoscopic graspers

Endoscopic caps – either oblique viewing or straight caps

Band ligation device

Endoscopic needle knife – hook knife, triangle-tip (TT) electrosurgery knife, or dual knife

(*Olympus Optical Co., Tokyo, Japan*)

Epinephrine (1:20,000) solution

Through-the-scope hemoclips or endoscopic clips or over-the-scope clips in case of full-thickness perforation or bleeding

Endoscopic Mucosal Resection (EMR)

EMR has been traditionally utilized in mucosal lesions and submucosal masses are likely not amenable to EMR. If the mass clearly arises from the submucosal layer, then ESD should be performed. However, if the lesion begins in the mucosa and there is uncertainty on EUS regarding involvement into the submucosa, then EMR can be attempted initially with ESD as a readily available rescue technique. The various techniques of EMR are depicted in Fig. 51.1. The initial step of EMR involves a saline lift in order to elevate the mass away from the muscularis propria in order to avoid possible full-thickness perforation. The injection needle should be angled and care should be taken to avoid full-thickness penetration with the needle and normal saline is injected to perform the lift. Endoscopic caps may or may not be used based on surgeon preference. An angled cap is useful in the esophagus, while a straight cap is easier to work with for gastric lesions. The cap can be taped onto the endoscope to avoid accidental dislodgement while performing the procedure. Suction is applied to the lesion in order to elevate it further, and eventually a cautery snare is introduced into the endoscope and energy is applied to the base of lesion. The mass is then either snare retrieved or suctioned into a suction trap for pathologic analysis.

If a cap is not utilized, then placing a band ligation initially can be helpful in raising tissue and aiding in cautery snaring of the lesion. If further elevation of the mass is necessary, then a grasper may be used to elevate the lesion in combination with either band ligation or cautery snare. This ensures that there is adequate tissue retracted into the scope to ensure negative oncologic margins.

Endoscopic Submucosal Dissection (ESD)

For benign submucosal lesions, ESD is much likely to be the better option compared to EMR given the tissue layer of origin for the masses. For lesions greater than 2 cm in size, ESD should be the standard treatment of choice. ESD allows for an en bloc resection of the mass, thus preserving depth as well as lateral margins appropriately for pathologic analysis.

The steps for ESD are listed below and depicted in Fig. 51.2:

1. Circumferential marking of the mucosa surrounding the mass with electrocautery – either a hook knife or a triangle-tip knife (TT knife).
2. Injection lift with normal saline, glycerol solution, or sodium hyaluronate mixture. Addition of epinephrine (1:20,000) useful for hemostasis.
3. Mucosal incision is created allowing access into the submucosal space.
4. An endoscopic cap is then mounted on the tip of the endoscope, and the space is dissected with a combination of insufflation and electrocautery.

Throughout this process the patient can be repositioned as needed and maneuvered in order to allow for gravity to aid in the dissection. It is important to maintain

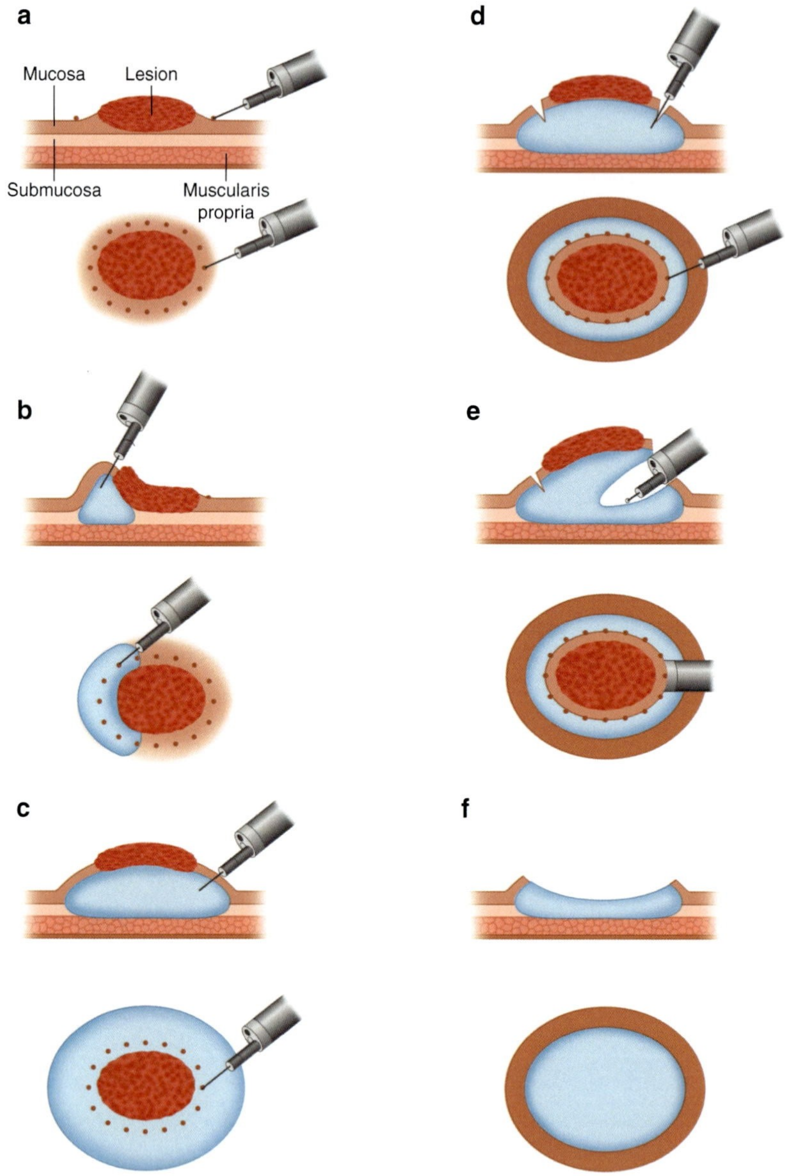

Fig. 51.1 Schematic representation of endoscopic submucosal dissection. (**a**) Mucosal markings for incision line. (**b**) Submucosal injections of a solution. (**c**) Complete elevation of the lesion by injecting a solution into the submucosal space. (**d**) Mucosal incision around the mucosal markings. (**e**) Submucosal dissection with a needle knife through the cap attached on the tip of endoscope. (**f**) En bloc resection of the tumor. M mucosa, SM submucosa, MP muscularis propria

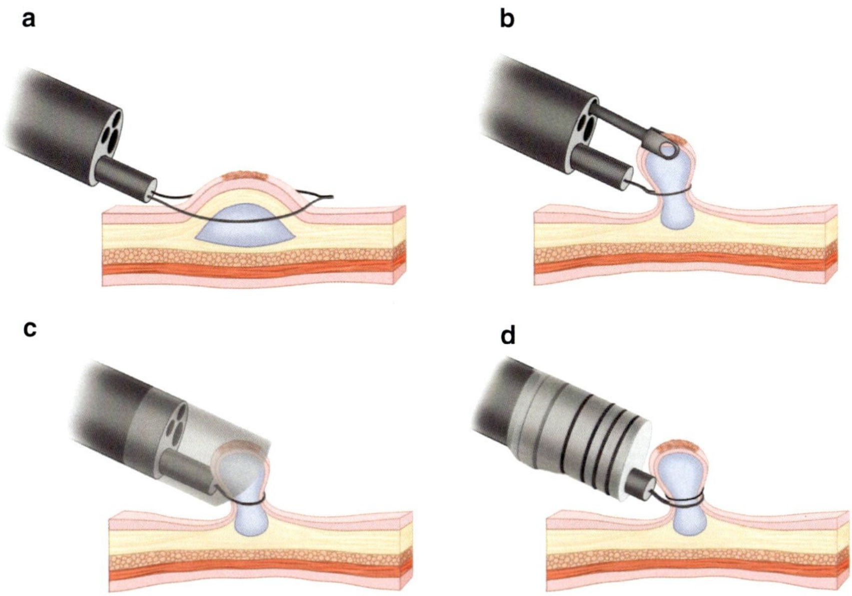

Fig. 51.2 Four types of endoscopic mucosal resection (EMR) techniques. (**a**) Snare polypectomy. (**b**) Strip biopsy technique. (**c**) The cap resection technique. (**d**) The ligate-and-cut technique

orientation so that the dissection is not carried out past the circumferential lift. This avoids taking unnecessary tissues past the borders of the lesion as well as the increased risk of perforation in the tissue layers that did not receive an injection lift. Frequent visualization of the borders outside of the created submucosal tunnel will help with reorientation. If the tumor does not appear to lift despite 5–10 cc of injection, then high consideration to aborting the endoscopic approach should be given, as the depth of invasion is likely much greater than the submucosa.

Unroofing

The unroofing technique is currently used only in cases of submucosal lipomas and cyst lymphangiomas. The confirmation of the preoperative diagnosis should be made on frozen pathology and the area tattooed in case the diagnosis changes on final pathology and ESD is required to complete the resection. Unroofing utilizes the snare technique; however, only the upper half of the mass is resected. Large masses that may otherwise be extremely difficult to resect with EMR or ESD can utilize the unroofing technique as the lower portion of the mass that is left in situ should resolve on its own if the pathology is correct. There is no long-term data for this technique or comparing unroofing with EMR/ESD, and only case reports and small case series are available in the literature [2, 3].

Enucleation

Enucleation is a combination of the unroofing technique with a variation of ESD. The surface of the tumor is unroofed with either snare cautery or a needle knife, and the tumor is then again snared or the base is cauterized and removed [4]. This technique may be useful for tumors deeper than the submucosa as it allows for full evaluation of the margins after unroofing the mucosa prior to excision. However, there is no longer-term data comparing this method to the more frequently utilized EMR and ESD.

Postoperative Management [5]

Patients that undergo EMR can typically be discharged home on the day of surgery. Depending on the ESD area of dissection and location, patients are observed for 1 day in the hospital and discharged with strict instructions to notify their surgeon with delayed symptoms of pain, fever, melena, or hematochezia. Patients should undergo endoscopic surveillance depending on the pathology at 6 months to 1 year.

Postoperative Complications [5]

The most feared complication after EMR or ESD is full-thickness perforation at the area of electrocautery. Depending on the location of injury, patients may present with a variety of symptoms that may include chest or abdominal pain, fevers, nausea, emesis, or food intolerance. Computer tomography with oral and intravenous contrast or an upper gastrointestinal swallow study should be performed to diagnose the perforation and leak. Rapid return to the operating room is important to treat the perforation, which can typically be managed with endoscopic clips or suturing. If endoscopic closure is unsuccessful, then laparoscopic repair with primary closure and/or omental patch buttressing should be performed.

Bleeding risks are low with the proper initial EMR or ESD techniques, but treatment for postoperative bleeding is endoscopic therapy with electrocautery, epinephrine 1:10,000 injection, and hemoclips. Patients should also have proper resuscitation with balanced blood product transfusions and be admitted to the ICU for invasive monitoring as needed. Surgical exploration is reserved for refractory bleeding in the hemodynamically unstable patient that fails endoscopic interventions.

References

1. Shim CS, Jung IS. Endoscopic removal of submucosal tumors: preprocedure diagnosis, technical options, and results. Endoscopy. 2005;37(7):646–54.
2. Fukuda S, Yamagata R, Mikami T, et al. Gastric lipoma successfully treated by endoscopic unroofing. Dig Endosc. 2003;15:228–31.

3. Kopáčová M, Rejchrt S, Bureš J. Unroofing technique as an option for the endoscopic treatment of giant gastrointestinal lipomas. Acta Med (Hradec Kralove). 2015;58(4):115–8.
4. Park YS, Park SW, Kim TI, et al. Endoscopic enucleation of upper GI submucosal tumors by using an insulated–tip electrosurgical knife. Gastrointest Endosc. 2004;59(3):409–15.
5. Lee KJ, Kim GH, Park DY, et al. Endoscopic resection of gastrointestinal lipomas: a single-center experience. Surg Endosc. 2014;28(1):185–92.

The Evolution of Management of Peptic Ulcer Disease

52

Jeffrey L. Ponsky and Andrew T. Strong

There is no dispute. The role that infection of the gastric lining with the bacteria *Helicobacter pylori* is a well-recognized etiological risk factor for peptic ulcer disease. Colonization with *H. pylori* approaches 80% in some endemic areas of the globe, which, when combined with patient factors, produces peptic ulcers in a thankfully small minority [1]. *H. pylori* bacterial infestation interferes with normal protective defenses of the gastric mucosa and alters the diffusion of hydrogen ions, leading to localized gastritis and resultant ulceration. Proper treatment of the peptic ulcer disease appropriately involves *H. pylori* eradication with antibacterial medications, in combination with protection of the gastric mucosa and acid suppression. For the *H. pylori*-negative patient, alteration of native mucosal protection by nonsteroidal anti-inflammatory medications, leading to peptic ulceration, is the leading etiology.

But, such knowledge is just several decades old, preceded by more than a century of medical thought predicated upon elevated acid secretion as the prime causative factor in peptic disease. For many decades, the German phrase coined by Karle Schwarz "Ohne saureen Magesaft kein eptisches Geschwür" translated to "no acid, no ulcer" was dictum in surgical wards worldwide [2]. Current understanding still clings to elements of this maxim.

Despite the fact that surgery was never considered first-line therapy for peptic ulcer disease, the position of peptic ulcer disease within the history of modern general surgery is profound. Three Nobel Prizes in Medicine have been directly related to advances in understanding of gastric physiology and pathophysiology that underlie peptic ulcer disease. Ivan Pavlov was recognized in 1904 for "his work on the physiology of digestion, through which knowledge on vital aspects of the subject

J. L. Ponsky (✉) · A. T. Strong
Department of General Surgery, Cleveland Clinic, Cleveland, OH, USA
e-mail: ponskyj@ccf.org; stronga@ccf.org

J. Grams et al. (eds.), *The SAGES Manual of Foregut Surgery*,
https://doi.org/10.1007/978-3-319-96122-4_52

has been transformed and enlarged" [3]. Elements of this work are detailed below. Sir James W. Black shared a Nobel Prize in Medicine in 1988, in part for his discovery of cimetidine, the first commercially available pharmaçologic therapy to reduce acid secretion for the treatment of peptic ulcer disease [4]. Just over a century after Pavlov received his prize, Barry J. Marshall and J. Robin Warren shared the Nobel Prize in Medicine in 2005 for "their discovery of the bacterium *Helicobacter pylori* and its role in gastritis and peptic ulcer disease" [5]. That discovery was the strongest driving factor away from surgery.

Surgical therapy for peptic ulcer disease was always intended to address the complications, namely, hemorrhage, obstruction, perforation, and intractability. The evolution of surgical techniques to accomplish these ends evinces contemporary advances in anesthesia, bacteriology, discoveries in physiology and endocrinology, and rediscovery of the fine points of anatomy over the past several decades. Current surgical therapy blends understanding garnered from each of these disciplines into surgical and increasingly medicinal therapies.

In the late nineteenth century, anesthesia was in its infancy. Inhaled ether provided the first reasonable anesthetic which could be used to perform intra-abdominal surgery [6]. There were no respirators, no blood transfusion, no antibiotics. Successful surgical management was intentionally simple and performed expeditiously. Recognizing these operating conditions, and believing that intra-gastric acid was primarily responsible for peptic ulceration, surgeons of the time sought a means to rapidly evacuate gastric acid. Thus gastroenterostomy was the first operation to be used to treat peptic ulcer disease. It could be carried out rapidly and with low morbidity (see Fig. 52.1) [7]. It was in this era that techniques described by Theodor Billroth and Lord Moynihan gained significant traction. Unfortunately, these operations had a recurrence rate approaching 50%, with the jejunal side of the anastomosis bearing most of the recurrences, called marginal ulcers.

Concluding that rapid drainage of acidic gastric contents was insufficient, surgeons next proposed that removal of the acid source, the stomach, in the form of a subtotal gastrectomy would be therapeutic (see Fig. 52.2). While effective in reducing ulcer recurrences (less than 1%), subtotal gastrectomy addled patients with significant morbidity and mortality. In addition, there were adverse effects of removing the pylorus and creating a long gastroenterostomy [8]. Some patients developed abdominal cramping, diaphoresis, and hypotension about in the first hour or two after eating This is now recognized as "early dumping syndrome" and thought to be due to inappropriate release of a gastrointestinal hormone, vasoactive intestinal peptide (VIP), from the pancreatic islet delta cells [9, 10]. Other patients developed the same symptoms from 4 to 6 h after meals. This is called "late dumping" and now believed to be secondary to an imbalance in insulin release from the pancreatic islet beta cells with an excess of insulin remaining after 4 hours causing the symptoms of insulin shock [11].

Application of surgical gastroenterostomy and subtotal gastrectomy occurred concurrent with laboratory work in physiology that provided the underpinnings of the next two major advances in management of peptic ulcer disease. Laboratory work by Pavlov in dogs outlined the phases of digestion. What Pavlov initially

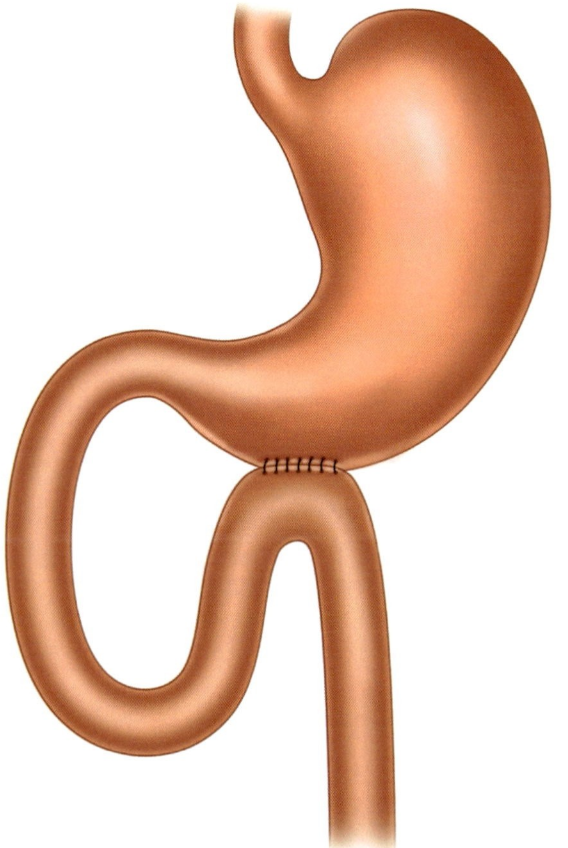

Fig. 52.1 Gastroenterostomy

termed "psychic reflex" has since become known as the cephalic phase of digestion. This first phase of digestion is primarily mediated by gustatory and olfactory properties of ingested food, but sight and anticipation have been shown to induce similar vagal stimulation of oral enzyme secretion, gastric acid production, and gastric motility [12, 13]. The second phase of digestion, the gastric phase, is principally mediated by gastrin. Pavlov and colleagues knew this only as a secretogogue, but decades of careful biochemical and physiological experimentation have shown gastrin is a 17-amino acid polypeptide secreted from the G cells of the gastric antrum. Gastrin secretion is mediated by mechanical distention of the antrum by the ingested food bolus and by chemical stimulation from the presence of intraluminal protein fragments known as peptones [14]. It should be noted that that pentapeptide comprising the N-terminus of gastrin is identical to that of cholecystokinin, explaining the coincident effects those hormones have. Gastrin then binds to G-protein-coupled receptors on parietal cells (CCK-2 receptor), causing direct release of intraluminal acid, and by binding to G-protein coupled receptors (CCK-2 receptors) on enterochromaffin-like cells to release histamine, which in turn strongly induces acid

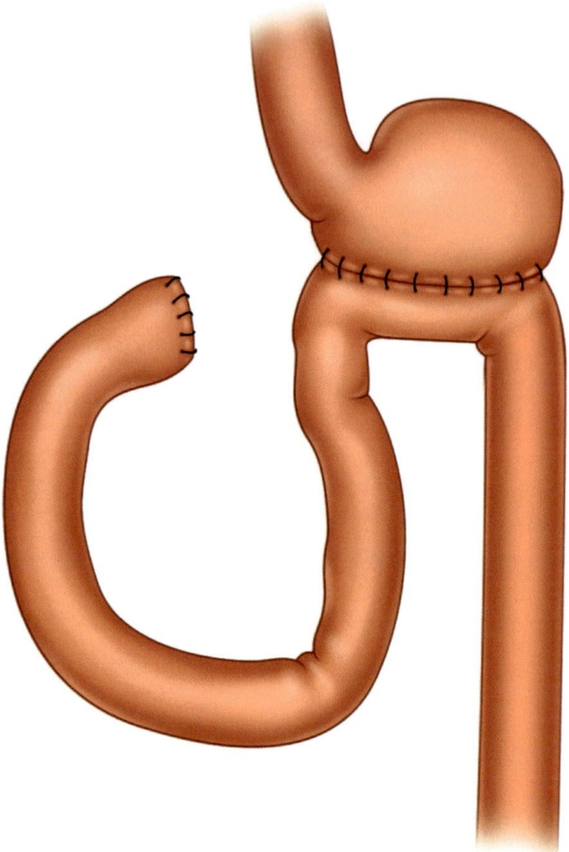

Fig. 52.2 Subtotal gastrectomy

production by parietal cells [14]. Taken together, vagal stimulation of acid production and the importance of gastrin and cholecystokinin illumine the next phase in surgical and medical therapy for ulcer disease.

While current thought identifies André Latarjet as a surgical innovator, his contemporaries failed to be convinced that vagotomy with gastroenterostomy, reported first in 1922, would be an effective operation for peptic ulcer disease [15]. The lack of experimental evidence produced by Latarjet contemporaneously met bombastic acolytes of Billroth and Moynihan advocating subtotal gastrectomies for ulcer disease and relegated Latarjet's procedure to a fringe status at the time [16]. Lester Dragstedt is identified as the individual who integrated the concepts of the cephalic phase of digestion and vagal innervation with pathophysiology of ulcer disease. He reported in 1943 on a supradiaphragmatic vagotomy in a patient with a bleeding duodenal ulcer [17]. Interestingly, that patient's consent to the experimental operation was predicated on his refusal of a subtotal gastrectomy, based on his father's perioperative mortality following the same procedure [16]. The patient had complete symptom relief within 9 days.

Despite remarkable success in some patients relieving peptic ulcer symptoms, truncal vagotomy resulted in an atonic stomach with impaired gastric emptying, a fact initially noted by Latarjet nearly two decades prior to Dragstedt's work [16]. The need for a concomitant gastric drainage procedure with vagotomy became obvious. Initially, gastroenterostomy was again employed to drain the stomach, largely based upon familiarity with this operation (see Fig. 52.3). Pyloroplasty for emptying was later introduced in combination with truncal vagotomy, as described by both Heineke-Mikulicz and Weinburg (see Fig. 52.4) [18, 19]. Truncal vagotomy with a drainage procedure was found to be very effective in the reduction of gastric acid and had a reasonable recurrence rate (about 15%) while being safe and relatively easy to perform. This operation was the most commonly performed in the midportion of the twentieth century.

Unintended adverse effects attendant to proximal vagotomy illustrated nuances in nervous system anatomy as well. Section of the vagal trunks resulted in denervation of the liver (hepatic branch) and the small bowel (celiac branch). Some patients

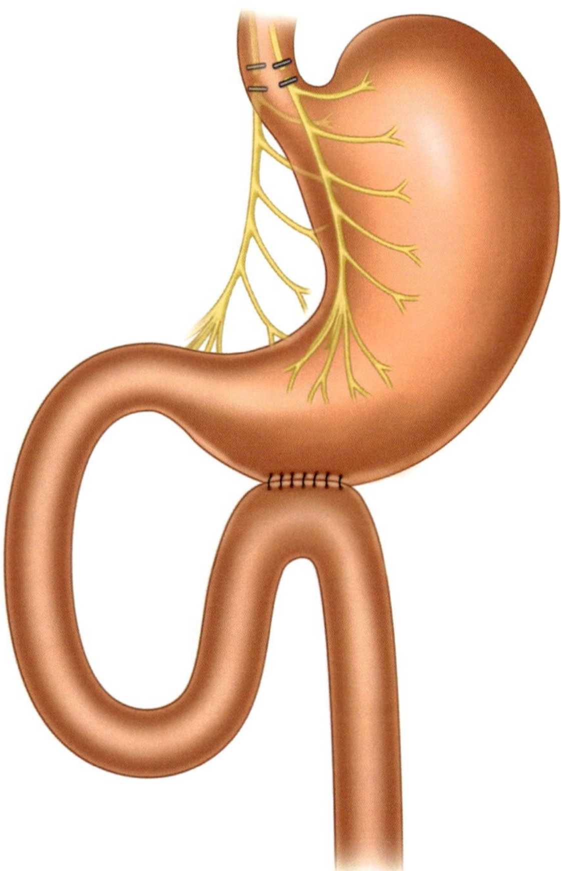

Fig. 52.3 Truncal vagotomy and gastroenterostomy

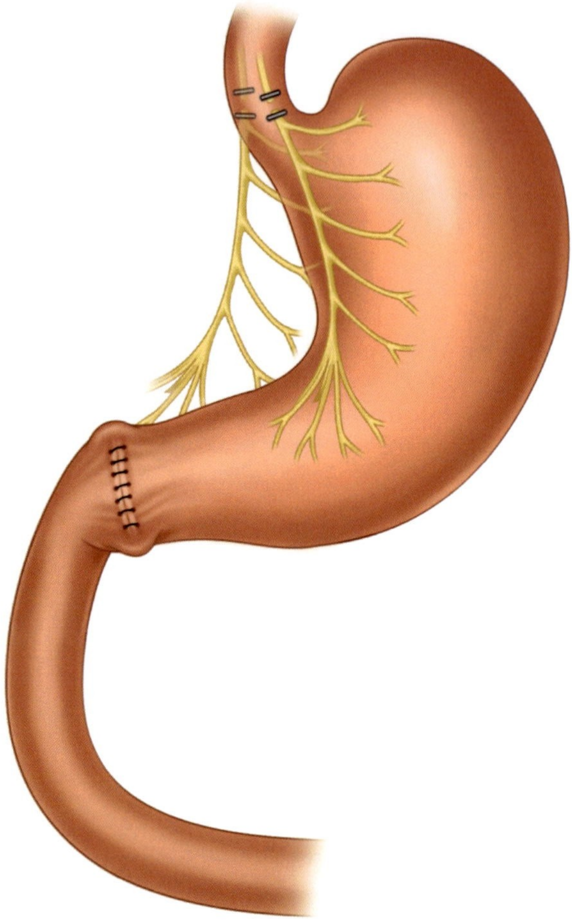

Fig. 52.4 Truncal vagotomy and pyloroplasty

developed gallstones, while others had severe disabling diarrhea. Because the pylorus was bypassed or destroyed, a good number of patients developed dumping syndrome. Finally, there were still patients in whom the disease was inadequately treated and recurrence developed.

The latter situation led to the development of procedures aimed at ablation of the gastric phase of digestion. These all involved combining the truncal vagotomy to ablate the cephalic phase and antrectomy to remove the G cells. The combination of vagotomy and antrectomy was extremely effective in preventing ulcer recurrence, with recurrence rates less than 2%. The gastric remnant could be reconnected to the duodenum (Billroth I reconstruction; see Fig. 52.5) or to a looped jejunum (Billroth II reconstruction; see Fig. 52.6). Later, Roux-en-Y reconstruction became popular, partly driven by the popularity of that operation for weight loss.

While the evolution of peptic ulcer surgery had produced effective operations with low ulcer recurrence rates, the postsurgical side effects proved troublesome in

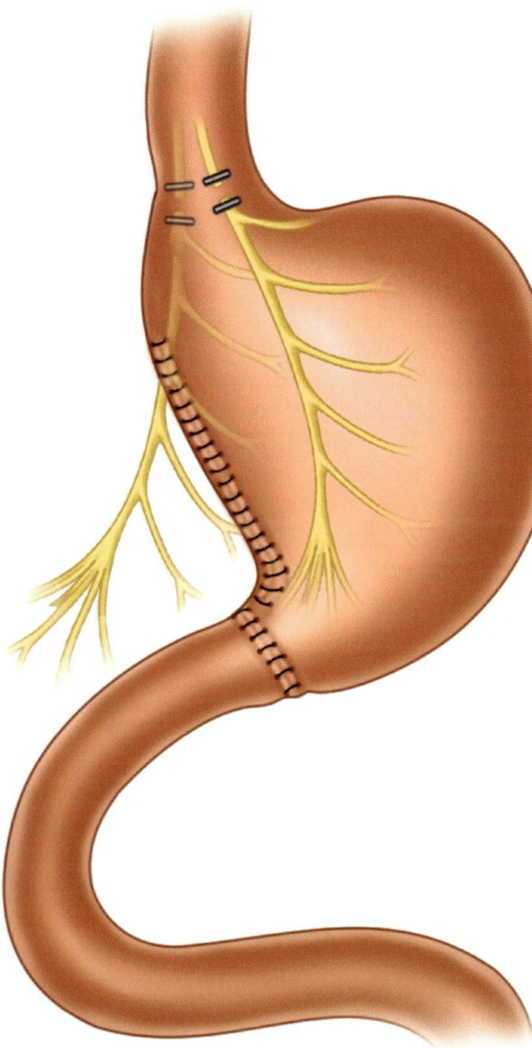

Fig. 52.5 Truncal vagotomy and antrectomy with Billroth I (gastroduodenostomy) anastomosis

many patients. Gallstones, secondary to hepatic denervation, gastroparesis, diarrhea, and dumping continued to plague many patients. Correspondingly the enthusiasm with which many surgeons applied vagotomy faded somewhat. In some ways it is remarkable that more than a decade passed with surgeons performing vagotomies with undesirable side effects, without improvement. An Irish surgeon, Terence Kennedy, wrote: "No surgeon wishing to denervate the soleus muscle for intermittent claudication would divide the whole sciatic nerve in the thigh; yet most surgeons using vagotomy for duodenal ulcer unthinkingly divide the whole of both vagus nerves immediately below the diaphragm, thus depriving all abdominal

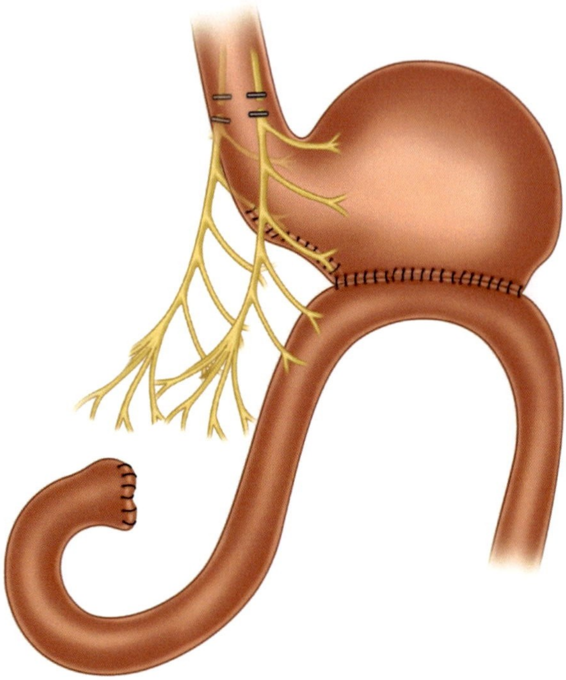

Fig. 52.6 Truncal vagotomy and antrectomy with Billroth II (gastrojejunostomy)

viscera, except the distal colon, of their para-sympathetic nerve supply" [20]. He and his colleagues in the Belfast school were some of the early promoters of new surgical approaches with lesser physiologic perturbations.

Popularized in the 1970s, new operative techniques based upon the anatomy of the vagal nerve were developed. It was noted that after delivering branches to the stomach, a branch of the vagal nerve went to the liver (hepatic branch) and one to the small bowel (celiac branch). Selective vagotomy was developed and preserved these branches without totally denervating the stomach (see Fig. 52.7). This operation still required a drainage procedure but obviated the side effects of small bowel and hepatic denervation. Dumping, however, remained a problem because the pylorus was either removed or rendered permanently patent. Finally, another look at the anatomy of the vagus nerve at the gastric wall revealed that the final gastric branch to the antrum, which looked like a crow's foot and which was previously named the nerve of Latarjet, could not possibly produce gastric acid from the parietal cells as the parietal cells were in the body and fundus of the stomach and not in the antrum. Thus, the nerve of Latarjet was discovered to be responsible for antral motility. An operation was then devised, highly selective vagotomy or parietal cell vagotomy, which divided all of the vagal nerve branches to the stomach proximal to the nerve of Latarjet and preserved the latter (see Fig. 52.8) [16]. In this case, no drainage procedure was necessary. In a landmark publication in 1975, data from 5539 patients was aggregated across Europe and the United States who had undergone highly

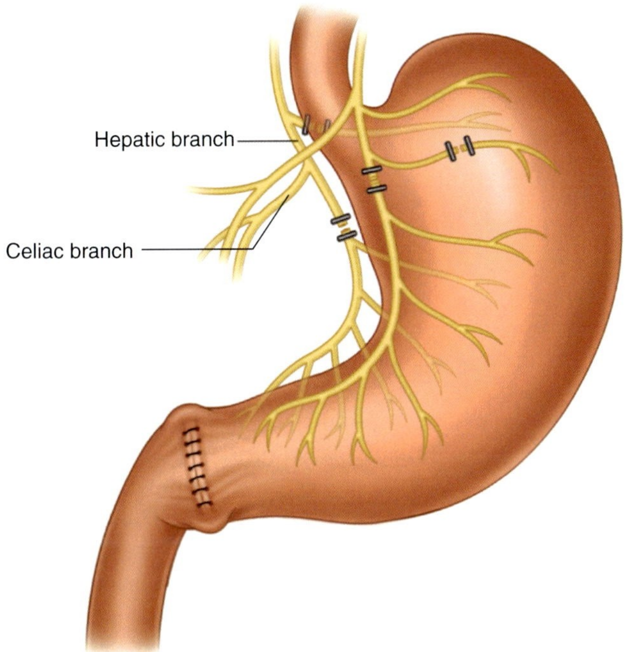

Fig. 52.7 Selective vagotomy and pyloroplasty

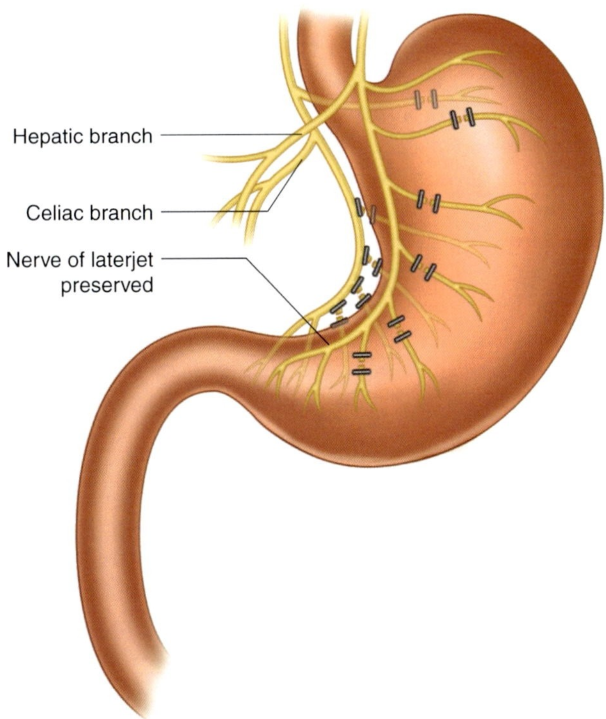

Fig. 52.8 Highly selective (parietal cell) vagotomy

selective vagotomy. They reported a ~5% recurrence with low incidence of gastric stasis, dumping syndrome, and mortality [21]. This recurrence rate was on par with truncal vagotomy, with an improved complication profile, and no need for an emptying procedure and resultant anastomosis. This operation became extremely popular and was widely used for intractable ulcer disease.

Enthusiasm for highly selective vagotomy was tempered slightly a few years later with new evidence recurrences increased over time; however, it was still the most effective operation available. With the notable exception of the application of laparoscopic techniques to vagotomy and gastric drainage procedures, development of surgical concepts for peptic ulcer disease largely ceased at this point. The commercially available cimetidine and later proton pump inhibitors gave surgeons a bevy of medical therapies to treat recurrent ulcer disease. Shortly thereafter, the discovery of *H. pylori* organisms and the uncovering of the role bacterial colonization plays in the development of many gastric ulcers was the next major development. The series of experiments in both animals and humans that identified, and eventually described, these mechanisms similarly spans the bulk of the nineteenth and twentieth centuries up to and including a bold experiment in self-inoculation by then gastroenterology fellow, now Nobel laureate, Barry Marshall [18].

Heretofore discussion of surgical management has been focused upon treatment of the non-perforated ulcer; we would be remiss to conclude this chapter without acknowledging the body of surgical thought targeting treatment of perforations. The youngest daughter of King Charles I of England, Henriette-Anne, at the age of 26 had acute onset abdominal pain lasting roughly 1 day prior to her sudden death [22]. While not attributed to a peptic ulcer until decades later, her demise from a perforated peptic ulcer was a topic in the second volume of the *British Medical Journal* [23].

Fundamentally treatment of perforated peptic ulcers has not significantly changed since Mikulicz proposed that any physician faced with a potential gastric or duodenal perforation should consider "opening the abdomen, sewing up the hole, and averting a possible inflammation by careful cleansing of the abdominal cavity" [22]. While non-operative treatment is occasionally successful with gastric decompression and antibiotic therapy, this is the exception. Roscoe Graham is credited with the first free omentoplasty to seal a perforated gastric ulcer without primary suture closure [24]. It was Cecil Cellan-Jones that reported a pedicled omentoplasty to buttress a primarily closed perforation, which is commonly referred to as the Graham patch [25]. Minor variations on this technique exist, but precious little surgical innovation has occurred in this arena. Despite more than eight decades of increased medical understanding, perforated gastric ulcer remains a premorbid condition in 16% of cases.

Today we have a variety of operations available for the treatment of peptic ulcer complications and select that procedure which best meets the needs of the patient. Certainly, highly selective vagotomy has a role when disease is persistent and medical therapy unsuccessful or poorly tolerated. For perforation, omentoplasty patch remains an effective initial approach and is often combined with *H. pylori* eradication and acid suppression with proton pump inhibitors. For patients with chronic obstruction of the pylorus and massive gastric distention, subtotal gastrectomy is still a very effective approach. In patients with severe disease or recalcitrant bleeding, vagotomy and pyloroplasty with suture of the bleeding vessel or vagotomy and antrectomy are still employed. Some surgeons, realizing the adverse effects of vagotomy, are choosing to perform pyloroplasty and combine this with medication instead of vagotomy.

The history of the evolution of peptic ulcer surgery is a saga of procedures developed based upon available thought and science of the time. Currently there is renewed attention to management of recalcitrant peptic ulcer disease. Partially this is being driven by concerns about long-term effects of anti-secretory medications. But, there is also now a generation of surgeons currently in training, or having recently finished, with a paucity of exposure to operations to manage peptic ulcer disease. As it has seemed to be the pattern with this disease process, where revisiting prior thought leads to greater clarity in terms of surgical treatment, we may be collectively sitting at the cusp of significant innovation. As further refinements in physiologic understanding and new techniques in endoscopic therapy for peptic ulcer disease come forth, they join a rich history in the development of surgical decision-making, surgical techniques, and innovation – a rich history that commands reverent consideration by any practicing general surgeon or endoscopist.

References

1. Leja M, Axon A, Brenner H. Epidemiology of Helicobacter pylori infection. Helicobacter. 2016;21(Suppl 1):3–7. https://doi.org/10.1111/hel.12332.
2. Schwarz K. Uber penetrierende magen-und jejunalgeschwüre. Beitr Klin Chir. 1910;67:96–128.
3. The Nobel Prize in Physiology or Medicine. 1904. Nobel Media AB. Available at: https://www.nobelprize.org/prizes/medicine/1904/pavlov/biographical. Accessed 28 Feb 2018. Updated 2018.
4. The Nobel Prize in Physiology or Medicine. 1988. Nobel Media AB. Available at: https://www.nobelprize.org/prizes/medicine/1988/black/facts/. Accessed 28 Feb 2018. Updated 2018.
5. The Nobel Prize in Physiology or Medicine. 2005. Nobel Media AB. Available at: https://www.nobelprize.org/prizes/medicine/2005/marshall/facts/. Accessed 28 Feb 2018. Updated 2018.
6. Campbell GG. III. Ether Anaesthesia; Clinical notes on 300 cases. Ann Surg. 1894;20:676–704.
7. Balfour DC. Results of gastroenterostomy for ulcer of the duodenum and stomach. Ann Surg. 1930;92:558–62.
8. Berg AA. The mortality and late results of subtotal gastrectomy for the radical cure of gastric and duodenal ulcer. Ann Surg. 1930;92:340–66.
9. Hertz AF. The cause and treatment of certain unfavourable after-effects of gastro-enterostomy. Proc R Soc Med. 1913;6:155–63.
10. MacGregor I, Parent J, Meyer JH. Gastric emptying of liquid meals and pancreatic and biliary secretion after subtotal gastrectomy or truncal vagotomy and pyloroplasty in man. Gastroenterology. 1977;72:195–205.
11. Tack J, Arts J, Caenepeel P, et al. Pathophysiology, diagnosis and management of postoperative dumping syndrome. Nat Rev Gastroenterol Hepatol. 2009;6:583–90. https://doi.org/10.1038/nrgastro.2009.148.
12. Pavlov I. The work of the digestive glands. 2nd ed. London: Charles Griffin & Co., Ltd.; 1910.
13. Zafra MA, Molina F, Puerto A. The neural/cephalic phase reflexes in the physiology of nutrition. Neurosci Biobehav Rev. 2006;30:1032–44. https://doi.org/10.1016/j.neubiorev.2006.03.005.
14. Schubert ML. Gastric acid secretion. Curr Opin Gastroenterol. 2016;32:452–60. https://doi.org/10.1097/MOG.0000000000000308.

15. Latarjet A. Resection des nerfs de l'estomac: technique operatoire; Resultats cliniques. Bull Académie Natl Médecine Académie Médecine. 1922;87:681–91.
16. Waisbren SJ, Modlin IM, Lester R. Dragstedt and his role in the evolution of therapeutic vagotomy in the United States. Am J Surg. 1994;167:344–59.
17. Dragstedt LR, Owens FM Jr. Supradiaphragmatic section of vagus nerves in treatment of duodenal ulcer. Proc Soc Exp Biol Med. 1943;53:152–4.
18. Gustafson J, Welling D. "No acid, no ulcer" – 100 years later: a review of the history of peptic ulcer disease. J Am Coll Surg. 2010;210:110–6. https://doi.org/10.1016/j.jamcollsurg.2009.08.014.
19. Weinberg JA, Stempien SJ, Movius HJ, Dagradi AE. Vagotomy and pyloroplasty in the treatment of duodenal ulcer. Am J Surg. 1956;92:202–7.
20. Kennedy T. Evaluation of selective vagotomy. Vagotomy Trial. 1973.
21. Johnston D. Operative mortality and postoperative morbidity of highly selective vagotomy. Br Med J. 1975;4:545–7.
22. Bertleff MJOE, Lange JF. Perforated peptic ulcer disease: a review of history and treatment. Dig Surg. 2010;27:161–9. https://doi.org/10.1159/000264653.
23. Gee S. The Bradshaw lecture on the signs of acute peritoneal diseases. Br Med J. 1892;2:1041–6.
24. Graham RR. The treatment of perforated duodenal ulcers. Surg Gynecol Obstet. 1937;64:235–8.
25. Cellan-Jones CJ. A rapid method of treatment in perforated duodenal ulcer. Br Med J. 1929;36:1076–7.

Evaluation of Peptic Ulcer Disease

53

Thomas C. Tsai and David C. Brooks

Peptic ulcers are defects in the gastric or duodenal mucosa through the muscularis mucosa. Unlike erosions or gastritis which are small or superficial lesions that involve only the mucosa, peptic ulcers can vary from as small as 5 mm to several centimeters, and the depth of injury may lead to life-threatening complications such as GI bleeding, perforation, or gastric outlet obstruction.

Traditionally, peptic ulcer disease was thought to be secondary to acid hypersecretion. However, recent evidence suggests that the pathogenesis of peptic ulcers is multifactorial and due to an imbalance of inciting factors and protective factors. The paradigm shift in the evaluation of peptic ulcer disease occurred in the 1984 with the discovery of *Helicobacter pylori* by Marshall and Warren. Since then, a robust literature has shown that eradication of *H. pylori* can reduce the rate of ulcer recurrence. Additionally, the use of nonsteroidal anti-inflammatory drugs (NSAIDs) and aspirin have also been closely linked to the formation of peptic ulcers due to the inhibition of cyclooxygenase-1 (COX-1) which results in impaired mucosal healing. Evaluation of peptic ulcer disease now largely rests on the diagnosis of these two predisposing factors of *H. pylori* infection and impaired mucosal healing from NSAID use.

T. C. Tsai
Department of Surgery, Brigham and Women's Hospital, Harvard Medical School, Boston, MA, USA

D. C. Brooks (✉)
Division of General and Gastrointestinal Surgery, Brigham and Women's Hospital, Harvard Medical School, Boston, MA, USA
e-mail: dbrooks@bwh.harvard.edu

J. Grams et al. (eds.), *The SAGES Manual of Foregut Surgery*,
https://doi.org/10.1007/978-3-319-96122-4_53

Epidemiology

Prevalence of peptic ulcer disease in the general population has been estimated to be about 5–10% with an incidence of 0.1–0.3% per year [1]. There continues to be a sharp decrease in the incidence of peptic ulcer disease in the past 20–30 years with a concomitant reduction in the prevalence of *H. pylori* infections [2, 3]. Significantly, hospitalizations for peptic ulcer disease have dramatically decreased in the USA and other countries. In an analysis of the Nationwide Inpatient Sample, the incidence of hospitalization for peptic ulcer disease decreased by 30% from 1993 to 2006 [4]. The ulcer incidence among *H. pylori*-infected individuals is approximately 1% per year, a rate six- to tenfold higher than among non-infected individuals [5, 6].

Pathogenesis

Peptic ulcer disease is related to two primary factors—presence of *H. pylori* infection and use of NSAIDs. Both factors disrupt normal mucosal repair mechanisms, leading to increased susceptibility to gastric acid. This imbalance leads to the formation of peptic ulcers, and accordingly, suppression of gastric acid secretion through proton-pump inhibitors (PPI) or histamine receptor 2 (H2) blockers can restore the balance of mucosal injury and repair. Peptic ulcers arising from gastrin-secreting tumors, such as in Zollinger-Ellison syndrome, are extremely rare and account for fewer than 1% of patients with duodenal ulcers. Stress-related mucosal disease is generally encountered in the critical care setting. Clinical factors related to peptic ulcer disease arising from physiologic stress include sepsis, acute respiratory distress syndrome, renal failure, trauma with central nervous system injury (Cushing's ulcer), or extensive burns (Curling's ulcer). Cigarette smoking may also promote the development of ulcers through mechanisms of mucosal ischemia and increasing susceptibility to acid.

Recent studies have suggested that a proportion of peptic ulcers may be idiopathic in origin. The proportion of peptic ulcers non-related to *H. pylori*, NSAID use, or other known factors may be as high as 20–44%, with a meta-analysis of published clinical trials suggesting that 27% of duodenal ulcers are idiopathic [7]. Idiopathic ulcers especially appear to be more common in older patients with comorbid conditions. Especially for peptic ulcer disease that manifests as gastrointestinal bleeding, the presence of multiple or significant comorbidities was associated with an odds ratio of 2.26 [8].

H. pylori

H. pylori is a spiral Gram-negative bacterium. *H. pylori* produces urease to create an alkaline environment to enable its survival in the gastric mucosa. The majority of infected persons remain asymptomatic, but 10–15% of infected persons develop peptic ulcer disease during their lifetime [9]. Development of peptic ulcer disease is secondary to a complex interaction between bacterial and host factors, which determines the severity of gastric inflammation and gastric secretion. For example, the cytotoxic-associated gene A (CagA) positive strains have been shown to interact with gastric tissue and promote inflammation [10]. Eradication of *H. pylori* infection is a mainstay of the initial medical management of peptic ulcer disease, and studies have shown that PPI alone are inferior to a strategy employing PPI and antibiotics for peptic ulcer disease. In cases of upper gastrointestinal bleeding from peptic ulcer disease, failure to eradicate *H. pylori* is associated with a 26% rebleeding rate at 1-year follow-up, whereas incidence of rebleeding of peptic ulcers is 1.3% following confirmed *H. pylori* eradication [11].

NSAIDs

NSAIDs can damage the gastroduodenal mucosa through the inhibition of prostaglandins derived from COX-1. Reduced mucosal prostaglandins are associated with lower mucous and bicarbonate secretion and decreased mucosal blood flow. NSAIDs increase the complications of peptic ulcer disease fourfold, and similarly aspirin can increase the complications twofold [1, 12, 13]. Many patients with *H. pylori* infection may concomitantly take NSAIDs, thereby compounding the risk of peptic ulcer disease and its complications. Compared with *H. pylori*-negative individuals not taking NSAIDs, the relative risk of peptic ulcer disease in *H. pylori*-infected NSAID takers was estimated to be 61-fold higher. Among those with *H. pylori* infection, use of NSAIDs increased the risk of peptic ulcer disease greater than threefold [14]. Eradication of *H. pylori* among patients taking NSAIDs for musculoskeletal pain has been shown to significantly decrease the occurrence of and complications arising from peptic ulcers [15, 16]. Furthermore, if NSAIDs cannot be stopped, double-blind trials have shown that COX-2 selective NSAIDs and PPI result in significantly lower rebleeding rates from peptic ulcers than with a COX-2 selective NSAID alone [17].

Classification of Peptic Ulcers

Although originally described in 1965 and predating the discovery of *H. pylori* and epidemiological studies linking peptic ulcer disease to NSAID use, Johnson's classification of gastric ulcers remains a useful paradigm for understanding the anatomic location of ulcers and the role of surgical management in complicated peptic ulcer disease [18]. While endoscopic and interventional radiology techniques have largely replaced surgical management of bleeding peptic ulcers, perforated peptic ulcers remain a surgical disease. In a recent study using the Nationwide Inpatient Sample to analyze the burden of emergency general surgery, operations for either bleeding or perforated peptic ulcer disease accounted for the fourth-highest emergency surgical burden when considering the combined impact of hospital costs, morbidity, and mortality [19].

Type I ulcers are located near the incisura of the lesser curvature. These are the most common and comprise approximately 60% of benign gastric ulcers. Type I ulcers historically have been described as arising from impaired mucosal defense. *H. pylori* infection is often found in patients with type I ulcers. Surgical management typically would involve distal gastrectomy with Billroth I or II reconstruction.

Type II ulcers are ulcers concomitantly located along the lesser curvature and the duodenum, whereas type III ulcers are prepyloric ulcers. These ulcers are typically associated with acid hypersecretion, and as such in medically refractory cases, antrectomy with vagotomy may be indicated.

Type IV ulcers are located along the lesser curvature near the gastroesophageal junction. Given the location along the lesser curve, these ulcers can be considered a subset of type I ulcers, but the location near the GE junction poses unique surgical challenges. In medically refractory cases, a variety of different surgical procedures are available, including the Csendes procedure (subtotal gastrectomy including the ulcer with Roux-en-Y reconstruction to remnant gastric fundus), Pauchet procedure (distal gastrectomy with extension along the lesser curve to include the ulcer), and Kelly-Madlener procedure (distal gastrectomy distal to the ulcer with truncal vagotomy), which may be indicated based on location of ulcer relative to the GE junction.

Type V ulcers can be located anywhere in the stomach and are due to NSAID or steroid use. These ulcers typically respond to withdrawal of the inciting medication and respond to proton-pump inhibitor therapy and endoscopic intervention in the setting of bleeding. Surgical options in the setting of refractory GI bleeding can include anterior gastrostomy and oversewing of bleeding sites or with embolization by interventional radiology.

Clinical Manifestation

Uncomplicated peptic ulcer disease classically presents as epigastric pain, but symptoms generally are non-specific. Patients with gastric ulcers typically present with postprandial abdominal pain, nausea, emesis, and weight loss. In contrast, patients with duodenal ulcers may feel hungry or have nocturnal pain. Duodenal ulcers are associated with initial relief from ingestion of milk, food, or antacids, but the pain typically recurs 2–4 h later. These symptoms can wax and wane due to spontaneous healing of ulcers. The main complications of peptic ulcer disease include bleeding, perforation, and gastric outlet obstruction. Bleeding can occur suddenly without proceeding symptoms and can manifest as either hematochezia or melena. Perforation typically presents with acute onset of sharp epigastric pain and can rapidly progress to intra-abdominal sepsis. As many as 60% of patients presenting with perforated peptic ulcer disease may not have had a prior diagnosis of peptic ulcer disease, and mortality can be as high as 10% [20]. Gastric outlet obstruction is rare but in most cases can respond to medical management with PPI and *H. pylori* eradication after temporary nasogastric decompression.

Diagnostic Workup

Endoscopy is the gold standard for the diagnosis of peptic ulcer disease, especially for those greater than 55 years of age. Endoscopy offers the benefit of both direct examination and biopsies that aid in the diagnosis of *H. pylori* or underlying malignancy. Up to 5% of gastric ulcers may be malignant. For giant ulcers greater than 3 cm in diameter, the risk of malignancy can be as high as 30%. Malignant ulcers may appear as an ulcerated mass or possess thickened, irregular edges. Multiple biopsies (one from each quadrant with jumbo forceps) of the ulcer edge as well as the base should be taken. Benign peptic ulcers generally have smooth, regular, rounded edges with a flat ulcer base that can be filled with exudative material.

Biopsy of benign-appearing gastric ulcers is controversial, with some advocating for biopsy at the index endoscopy to rule out malignancy and others electing to forego biopsy if a patient's history and risk factors suggest a low risk of gastric cancer. Antral biopsies can be sent for histologic analysis, and polymorphonuclear leukocytes are suggestive of *H. pylori* gastritis. Specialized stains can also be employed to directly detect the presence of *H. pylori*. Rapid urease testing of antral biopsies is also sensitive as well as specific. While *H. pylori* can be cultured from biopsy specimens, it is usually reserved for medically refractory cases to determine antibiotic susceptibility.

Patients with suspected peptic ulcer disease presenting with alarming symptoms such as weight loss or GI bleeding should undergo prompt endoscopic evaluation. Patients with multiple ulcers on exam, refractory ulcers, ulcers in unusual locations such as in the distal duodenum, or diarrhea should undergo testing for Zollinger-Ellison syndrome with a fasting gastrin and secretin stimulation test. As *H. pylori* is the most common cause of peptic ulcer disease, a test-and-treat approach with a noninvasive test for *H. pylori* has been advocated for patients under the age of 55 [21, 22]. With the test-and-treat approach, follow-up is crucial, and further evaluation with endoscopy may be needed if symptoms do not resolve after discontinuation of NSAIDs, cessation of smoking, or initiation of antisecretory medications such as a PPI or H2 blocker.

Laboratory testing for *H. pylori* involve several methods and can vary by institutional preference (Table 53.1). All patients with peptic ulcer disease should undergo testing for *H. pylori* infection. Options for testing include urea breath test, serologic enzyme-linked immunosorbent assay (ELISA), and stool antigen test. Urea breath test is highly sensitive even in the acute hospital setting or with active GI bleeding [11, 23]. Sensitivity however decreases after induction of PPI therapy. Stool antigen can similarly test for false negative in the setting of PPI or if there is blood in the specimen due to cross-reactivity of the test [24]. Serology can be used to detect exposure to *H. pylori*, but is less useful for monitoring eradication after treatment. As most recommended treatment regimens now consist of a 14-day course of triple or quadruple therapy, repeat urea breath or stool testing should be performed 4 weeks after initiation of treatment to allow for completion of the regimen as well as 2 weeks off PPI to improve specificity. Patients can be switched to H2 blockers

Table 53.1 Diagnostic tests for *H. pylori*

Test	Sensitivity (%)	Specificity (%)	Comments
Noninvasive tests			
Serologic ELISA	85	79	Detects exposure to *H. pylori* but cannot be used to confirm eradication of infection
Urea breath test	95–100	91–98	Recommended for both screening and confirmation of eradication of infection. Antibiotics and PPIs can increase false-negative results
Stool antigen test	91–98	94–99	Can be used for both screening and confirmation of eradication of infection
Invasive tests (endoscopy with biopsy)			
Histology	>95	95–98	Sensitivity can be improved by taking at least 2 biopsies from antrum and 1 from the body of the stomach
Rapid urease test	93–97	95–100	Reduced accuracy in patients with active GI bleeding
Culture	70–80	100	Technically demanding and sensitivity may vary by laboratory

Adapted from Greenberger et al. [28]. Table 15.2

prior to retesting to minimize false-negative results [25]. Repeat endoscopy should be performed in 12 weeks to assess resolution of the ulcer.

The use of fluoroscopic upper GI study with barium has a limited role in the evaluation of peptic ulcer disease. Endoscopic evaluation is preferred when available due to the ability to biopsy for both *H. pylori* testing as well as for malignancy. Barium radiography can evaluate for gastric outlet obstruction, but this would also be seen on endoscopy. Ulcers appear round or oval on barium radiograph with secondary changes including deformities of the affected region due to edema or scarring [26, 27].

Summary

Despite decreasing prevalence in the last few decades, peptic ulcer disease remains a common and morbid condition that can manifest as GI bleeding, perforation, or gastric outlet obstruction if undiagnosed and untreated. The two primary inciting factors include *H. pylori* infection and NSAID use. The mainstay of evaluation of peptic ulcer disease is esophagogastroduodenoscopy with laboratory testing for *H. pylori*. After completion of treatment with either treatment for *H. pylori* or withdrawal of offending agents such as NSAIDs or smoking, repeat testing and EGD should be performed to ensure adequate resolution of peptic ulcer disease.

References

1. Lanas A, Chan FK. Peptic ulcer disease. Lancet. 2017;390(10094):613–24.
2. Sandler RS, Everhart JE, Donowitz M, et al. The burden of selected digestive diseases in the United States. Gastroenterology. 2002;122:1500–11.
3. Sung JJ, Kuipers EJ, El-Serag HB. Systematic review: the global incidence and prevalence of peptic ulcer disease. Aliment Pharmacol Ther. 2009;29:938–46.
4. Wang YR, Richter JE, Dempsey DT. Trends and outcomes of hospitalizations for peptic ulcer disease in the United States, 1993 to 2006. Ann Surg. 2010;251:51–8.
5. Kuipers EJ, Thijs JC, Festen HP. The prevalence of Helicobacter pylori in peptic ulcer disease. Aliment Pharmacol Ther. 1995;9(Suppl 2):59–69.
6. Sipponen P, Varis K, Fraki O, Korri UM, Seppala K, Siurala M. Cumulative 10-year risk of symptomatic duodenal and gastric ulcer in patients with or without chronic gastritis. A clinical follow-up study of 454 outpatients. Scand J Gastroenterol. 1990;25:966–73.
7. Charpignon C, Lesgourgues B, Pariente A, et al. Peptic ulcer disease: one in five is related to neither Helicobacter pylori nor aspirin/NSAID intake. Aliment Pharmacol Ther. 2013;38:946–54.
8. Crooks CJ, West J, Card TR. Comorbidities affect risk of nonvariceal upper gastrointestinal bleeding. Gastroenterology. 2013;144:1384–93. 93 e1–2; quiz e18–9.
9. Cover TL, Blaser MJ. Helicobacter pylori in health and disease. Gastroenterology. 2009;136:1863–73.
10. Yamaoka Y. Mechanisms of disease: Helicobacter pylori virulence factors. Nat Rev Gastroenterol Hepatol. 2010;7:629–41.
11. Gisbert JP, Abraira V. Accuracy of Helicobacter pylori diagnostic tests in patients with bleeding peptic ulcer: a systematic review and meta-analysis. Am J Gastroenterol. 2006;101:848–63.
12. Lanas A, Carrera-Lasfuentes P, Arguedas Y, et al. Risk of upper and lower gastrointestinal bleeding in patients taking nonsteroidal anti-inflammatory drugs, antiplatelet agents, or anticoagulants. Clin Gastroenterol Hepatol. 2015;13:906–12. e2.
13. Lanas A, Garcia-Rodriguez LA, Arroyo MT, et al. Risk of upper gastrointestinal ulcer bleeding associated with selective cyclo-oxygenase-2 inhibitors, traditional non-aspirin non-steroidal anti-inflammatory drugs, aspirin and combinations. Gut. 2006;55:1731–8.
14. Huang JQ, Sridhar S, Hunt RH. Role of Helicobacter pylori infection and non-steroidal anti-inflammatory drugs in peptic-ulcer disease: a meta-analysis. Lancet. 2002;359:14–22.
15. Chan FK, To KF, Wu JC, et al. Eradication of Helicobacter pylori and risk of peptic ulcers in patients starting long-term treatment with non-steroidal anti-inflammatory drugs: a randomised trial. Lancet. 2002;359:9–13.
16. Labenz J, Blum AL, Bolten WW, et al. Primary prevention of diclofenac associated ulcers and dyspepsia by omeprazole or triple therapy in Helicobacter pylori positive patients: a randomised, double blind, placebo controlled, clinical trial. Gut. 2002;51:329–35.
17. Chan FK, Wong VW, Suen BY, et al. Combination of a cyclo-oxygenase-2 inhibitor and a proton-pump inhibitor for prevention of recurrent ulcer bleeding in patients at very high risk: a double-blind, randomised trial. Lancet. 2007;369:1621–6.
18. Johnson HD. Gastric ulcer: classification, blood group characteristics, secretion patterns and pathogenesis. Ann Surg. 1965;162:996–1004.
19. Scott JW, Olufajo OA, Brat GA, et al. Use of national burden to define operative emergency general surgery. JAMA Surg. 2016;151:e160480.
20. Sarosi GA Jr, Jaiswal KR, Nwariaku FE, Asolati M, Fleming JB, Anthony T. Surgical therapy of peptic ulcers in the 21st century: more common than you think. Am J Surg. 2005;190:775–9.
21. Agreus L, Talley NJ, Jones M. Value of the "Test & Treat" strategy for uninvestigated dyspepsia at low prevalence rates of Helicobacter pylori in the population. Helicobacter. 2016;21:186–91.
22. Delaney BC, Qume M, Moayyedi P, et al. Helicobacter pylori test and treat versus proton pump inhibitor in initial management of dyspepsia in primary care: multicentre randomised controlled trial (MRC-CUBE trial). BMJ. 2008;336:651–4.

23. Gisbert JP, Esteban C, Jimenez I, Moreno-Otero R. 13C-urea breath test during hospitalization for the diagnosis of Helicobacter pylori infection in peptic ulcer bleeding. Helicobacter. 2007;12:231–7.
24. Lin HJ, Lo WC, Perng CL, et al. Helicobacter pylori stool antigen test in patients with bleeding peptic ulcers. Helicobacter. 2004;9:663–8.
25. Laine L. Upper gastrointestinal bleeding due to a peptic ulcer. N Engl J Med. 2016;375:1198.
26. Dooley CP, Larson AW, Stace NH, et al. Double-contrast barium meal and upper gastrointestinal endoscopy. A comparative study. Ann Intern Med. 1984;101:538–45.
27. Glick SN. Duodenal ulcer. Radiol Clin N Am. 1994;32:1259–74.
28. Greenberger NJ, Blumber RS, Burakoff R. Current diagnosis and treatment: gastroenterology, hepatology, & endoscopy. 3rd ed. New York: McGraw-Hill Education; 2016.

Risk Factor Modification in Patients with Peptic Ulcer Disease

54

Ioana Baiu and Dan E. Azagury

Introduction

A "peptic ulcer" refers to a defect in the gastric or duodenal mucosa and submucosa caused by an imbalance between injurious factors and defense mechanisms in the GI tract. Injury to the gastric or duodenal lining can be caused by a number of factors that alter the delicate acid equilibrium. These include infections, medications, acid hypersecretion, and environmental aggressors such as smoking, alcohol, and diet. Although the incidence of uncomplicated PUD is approximately 1 case per 1000 person-year [1], it accounted for nearly 4000 deaths in 2004 in the United States alone [2]. The economic impact of PUD reaches \$6 billion per year in the United States [3]. The burden of disease is much higher globally than in the United States [4]. Unlike many other medical conditions, PUD has been very clearly linked to a limited number of causative factors. Prevention, early identification, and treatment of these injurious mechanisms can significantly decrease the morbidity and mortality in affected patients. In this chapter, we discuss the main risk factors that predispose to peptic ulcer disease and management of these conditions.

I. Baiu
Department of Surgery, Stanford Health Care, Stanford, CA, USA

D. E. Azagury (✉)
Bariatric & Minimally Invasive Surgery, Department of Surgery, Stanford University School of Medicine, Stanford, CA, USA
e-mail: dazagury@stanford.edu

J. Grams et al. (eds.), *The SAGES Manual of Foregut Surgery*,
https://doi.org/10.1007/978-3-319-96122-4_54

Pathophysiologic Risk Factors

Infection

Perhaps one of the most clearly elucidated causes of peptic ulcer disease is the infection with *Helicobacter pylori*, a Gram-negative microaerophilic bacterium that is nearly ubiquitous in the general population. The prevalence of infection depends on age, socioeconomic status, and country and is estimated to be anywhere from 20–50% in industrialized countries and 50–80% in developing countries [5]. The infection is transmitted via oral ingestion and clusters within families. *H. pylori* is thought to be responsible for 90% of PUD development and is the leading cause of chronic gastritis and gastric cancer [6]. While the acidic environment of the gastric mucosa allows protection from most bacterial infections, *H. pylori* has developed sophisticated mechanisms to avoid the host defense systems. These include specialized proteins that allow it to manipulate host signaling cascades, bind to gastric epithelial cells, and evade the immune system, while causing low-grade inflammation [7]. With time, and depending on a variety of host factors, this chronic inflammation can lead to metaplasia, dysplasia, and subsequently carcinoma. The World Health Organization classifies *H. pylori* as a class I carcinogen because of its strong association with gastric adenocarcinoma and lymphoma [8, 9].

While the pathogenesis of *H. pylori* infection is quite complex and beyond the scope of this textbook, there are several mechanisms that are clinically important to understand as they contribute to the development of gastric and duodenal ulcers. Chief among them is the production of the enzyme urease, which converts urea into bicarbonate and ammonia. This creates an alkaline buffer around the organism that protects it from the bactericidal activity of the stomach. The ammonia that is produced as a result is damaging to the mucosal lining. Furthermore, the bacterium has been shown to inhibit the secretion of somatostatin from the antral D-cells; somatostatin is an inhibitor of G-cell gastrin secretion. The result is hypergastrinemia and acid hypersecretion, leading to parietal cell hyperplasia and gastric metaplasia. Infection in the duodenum leads to a decrease in the normal bicarbonate secretion in response to acidic chyle, leading to duodenal metaplasia [7, 10].

Although a majority of the population is infected with *H. pylori*, only a small percentage will develop complications. As such, the American College of Gastroenterology recommends testing for *H. pylori* only in specific circumstances, arguing against routine screening for the population at large [11]. In general, all patients with PUD should be tested for *H. pylori*. Table 54.1 illustrates the current indications for diagnosis and treatment.

The diagnosis of *H. pylori* is relatively inexpensive and can be performed either via noninvasive methods or invasive tests, depending on the clinical scenario. The noninvasive methods include urea breath test, stool antigen assays, and serologic tests. These tests are ideal for detecting uncomplicated PUD. With a sensitivity and specificity of >90%, the urea breath test is a qualitative study that detects active infection and relies on high urease activity during active infection in the stomach. It is a good initial screen as well as an easy means of confirming eradication following

Table 54.1 Current indications for diagnosis and treatment of *H. pylori*

Established
Active peptic ulcer disease (gastric or duodenal ulcer)
Confirmed history of peptic ulcer disease (not previously treated for *H. pylori*)
Gastric MALT lymphoma (low grade)
After endoscopic resection of early gastric cancer
Uninvestigated dyspepsia (depending upon *H. pylori* prevalence)
Controversial
Nonulcer dyspepsia
Gastroesophageal reflux disease
Persons using nonsteroidal antiinflammatory drugs
Unexplained iron deficiency anemia
Populations at higher risk for gastric cancer

Source: American College of Gastroenterology guideline on the management of Helicobacter pylori infection [11]

treatment. Similarly, stool antigen testing has a sensitivity of 89–98% and specificity >90% [12]. This assay can also be used to confirm eradication, with the caveat that at least 8 weeks must pass between completion of treatment and retesting. Serologic testing for IgG against *H. pylori* is highly sensitive (90–100%) but not specific (76–96%), and the positive predictive is highly dependent on the prevalence of infection within a certain population [13]. This is not a practical test in countries such as the United States where the prevalence is relatively low, and a positive test would not be indicative of an active infection. One scenario in which serologic testing may be useful is to confirm eradication of infection by proving seroconversion from positive to negative serology [14]; however, at least 18 months must pass after completion of treatment and the sensitivity of detecting seroconversion was only 60%. Other testing modalities such as PCR, salivary assays, urinary assays, and ^{13}C-urea breath test exist, but none of them have been shown to be of particular value and are rarely used.

Invasive testing, such as endoscopy, is indicated in clinical scenarios where patients present with gastrointestinal bleeding or anemia. Active infection can be detected using a biopsy urease test, bacterial culture, or histology. The biopsy urease test relies on the bacterium's ability to secrete urease and create an alkaline buffer around itself. The sensitivity is 90–95% and specificity 95–100% [11]. Bacterial culture has not proven to be an initial test of choice because *H. pylori* is notoriously difficult to grow. However, it may be useful in patients with refractory infection, as there are reports of resistance to treatment. Lastly, histological diagnosis allows for detection of the bacteria as well as screening for secondary changes associated with infection such as dysplasia or metaplasia. Not surprisingly, any diagnostic testing that relies on biopsies is subject to sampling error; furthermore, the accuracy of these tests is decreased in patients taking proton pump inhibitors (PPIs). Lastly, it is important to recognize that repeat endoscopy is not recommended to test for eradication for simple peptic ulcers, and other noninvasive tests can be used instead if necessary. However, in patients with refractory PUD, repeat endoscopy is warranted to increase sampling opportunities, document healing, or identify the presence of neoplasms.

Hormonal Factors

Any process that leads to a pathologic increase in acid secretion can predispose to ulcer formation. The most classic hormonal imbalance that contributes to PUD is caused by gastrinomas. As the name suggests, these are functional neuroendocrine tumors that secrete gastrin, which causes excessive amounts of acid to be secreted. This leads to damage to the GI mucosa as well as malabsorption secondary to inactivation of bicarb and other digestive enzymes. The constellation of symptoms associated with these tumors are also referred to as Zollinger-Ellison (ZE) syndrome. Suspicion for these tumors should be raised when patients present with weight loss, diarrhea, steatorrhea, multiple ulcers, ulcers in the setting of negative *H. pylori* and NSAID use, or a family history of multiple endocrine neoplasia type I (MEN I) [15].

Gastrinomas are typically located in the pancreas (60%) or the duodenum (30%) and represent an important cause of duodenal ulcers. The diagnosis can be made by measuring a fasting gastrin level that is typically tenfold the upper limit of normal [16]. If the gastrin level is normal but there is persistent high suspicion for gastrinoma, a secretin test can be performed. Whereas normal gastric G cells are inhibited by secretin, gastrinoma tumor cells have an exaggerated gastrin release that can be diagnostic in these patients [17]. There are rare conditions of gastric G-cell hyperplasia or retained antrum syndrome after surgical gastrectomy. Both conditions can present with hypergastrinemia and PUD, but in neither case would there be a significant response to secretin stimulation test. It is worth mentioning that the widespread use of PPIs has led both to a delay in diagnosis and an increase in false-positive rates during secretin stimulation [18]. Patients with mild symptoms can be temporarily transitioned to a high-dose H_2 receptor antagonist for one week prior to the secretin stimulation test; in patients with severe symptoms of Zollinger-Ellison syndrome, the risk of interrupting antacid medications and having a massive GI bleed or perforation from a duodenal ulcer is too great and not recommended [19].

Patient Comorbidities

"Stress ulcers" are essentially peptic ulcers that occur in critically ill patients. Traditionally, these are seen in patients with severe burns, trauma, sepsis, or multiorgan failure on mechanical ventilation. Recent data suggest that even stressors associated with hospital admissions can lead to GI mucosal injury. The relationship between critically ill patients and gastric erosions is determined by mucosal blood flow to the GI tract. Hypotension or inadequate perfusion leads to decreases in blood flow to areas of the gut that are important for maintaining the mucosal barrier and buffer from the damaging effects of acid. Refluxed bile salts and uremic toxins can also contribute to gastrointestinal mucosal damage.

Inflammatory or infiltrative diseases such as sarcoidosis, Crohn's disease, eosinophilic gastroduodenitis, systemic mastocytosis, hypersecretory duodenal ulcer have also been associated with peptic ulcer development, although the mechanisms are not entirely clear. Similarly, organ transplantation, diabetes mellitus, cirrhosis, and renal disease have also been implicated as risk factors for gastroduodenal ulcer development. However, some of these associations may be confounded by the effects of medications used to treat these conditions. Radiation therapy has also been shown to cause both gastric and duodenal ulcerations. Lastly, there is a very small proportion of patients who present with "idiopathic ulcers," in which none of the abovementioned factors can be diagnosed.

Environmental Risk Factors

Medications

Nonsteroidal anti-inflammatory drugs (NSAIDs), including aspirin, represent 60% of the over-the-counter sales for analgesics in the United States. At least 70% of people over age 65 take NSAIDs, and half of them take at least 7 doses/week [20]. It has been shown that nearly half of patients who use these medications regularly have gastric erosions and that up to 30% of them have ulcers on endoscopy [21]. Despite this, the FDA accredits only 1–4% per year risk of a significant gastrointestinal event such as bleeding, perforation, or pyloric obstruction in patients who routinely use NSAIDs. Risk factors for developing PUD in patients who use NSAIDs include not only the dose, duration of action, and duration of therapy but also extrinsic elements such as age, concomitant treatment with other medications (e.g., steroids, anticoagulants, selective serotonin reuptake inhibitors, alendronate), comorbidities including *H. pylori* infection, and even genetic polymorphisms that predispose to ulcerogenic side effects [21].

NSAIDs lead to ulcer formation through several mechanisms, including direct damage to the mucosa, suppression of prostaglandin synthesis, reduction of gastric mucosal blood flow, inhibition of mucosal regeneration, and delay in healing [22].

Steroids alone have not been specifically shown to cause PUD. However, they do increase the risk of bleeding in patients with existing ulcers. Even a short 7-day course of glucocorticoids has been shown to increase the risk of bleeding in patients with existing ulcers [23]. This effect was even higher in patients taking NSAIDs or aspirin.

Smoking

Epidemiologically, the risk of PUD is twice as high in smokers compared to nonsmokers. The effects of nicotine on the development of gastroduodenal ulcers are manyfold and include stimulation of gastric acid secretion via activation of H_2 receptors, decrease in gastric mucus production and defense mechanisms, oxidative stress, and inhibition of gastric cell renewal to name a few [24]. In addition, smoking potentiates the ulcerogenesis associated with the use of NSAIDs, as well as *H. pylori* infection, and alcohol. It is important to mention that although alcohol is often mentioned as a risk factor for peptic ulcer development, there is no confirmatory data to support this claim.

Other Risk Factors

There are many other risk factors associated with the development of peptic ulcer disease. These include mechanical causes such as magnet and battery ingestions. Vascular compromise caused by use of cocaine and methamphetamines has also been shown to be linked to gastric and duodenal erosions.

Management

H. pylori Treatment

It is important to remember that, despite its prevalence and pathogenicity, only 3% of people infected with *H. pylori* develop PUD [25]. The goal of therapy is eradication of the infection, although up to 20% of patients will likely redevelop ulcers in the future [26]. Because the antibiotic treatments are needed to work within highly acidic gastric mucosa and many of them are inactivated in this environment, antacids such as proton pump inhibitors and H_2 blockers are used to increase effectiveness of the treatment. In addition, in order to prevent the development of resistance in the versatile genome of *H. pylori*, two antibiotic regiments are typically used. Hence, the treatment of *H. pylori* is commonly referred to as "triple therapy," meaning two antibiotics and an antacid used together to effectively maximize therapeutic potential with minimal induction of bacterial resistance. Table 54.2 illustrates current treatment recommendations for *H. pylori* [27].

First-line therapies include a PPI, such as omeprazole or lansoprazole, and two antibiotics such as amoxicillin and clarithromycin or metronidazole or a nitroimidazole and clarithromycin. Multiple randomized controlled trials have shown equivalence of any of the above regimens [28]. The recommended duration of therapy is 14 days to achieve 80% cure rate based on intention-to-treat analyses [28]. Ranitidine bismuth citrate with clarithromycin and bismuth with metronidazole and tetracycline are also valid options [13]. Persistence of infection despite initial treatment is due either to non-adherence or antibiotic resistance. The latter is problematic as cultures are not routinely performed, and, thus, susceptibility data is typically not available. As such, a second course of triple therapy can be prescribed, ideally using different antibiotics than in the initial regimen.

Table 54.2 2017 American College of Gastroenterology guidelines for treatment of *H. pylori* [27]

Clarithromycin, amoxicillin or metronidazole, PPI x 14 days*

- OR –

Bismuth, Tetracycline, nitroimidazole, PPI x 10-14 days**

- OR –

Clarithromycin, amoxicillin or nitroimidazole, PPI x 10-14 days

- OR –

Amoxicillin and PPI x 5-7 days, followed by clarithromycin, nitroimidazole, PPI x 5-7 days

- OR –

Amoxicillin and PPI x 7 days, followed by amoxicillin, clarithromycin, nitroimidazole and PPI x7 days

- OR –

Levofloxacin, amoxicillin, PPI x 10-14 days

- OR –

Amoxicillin and PPI x 5-7 days, followed by fluoroquinolone, nitroimidazole, PPI x 5-7 days

* if clarithromycin resistance <15%

** in patients allergic to penicillin

Managing Hormonal Causes of PUD

In patients who present with peptic ulcers caused by acid hypersecretion from an underlying gastrinoma, the treatment focuses on treating the underlying etiology. Acid suppression with proton pump inhibitors is paramount to preventing mortality and morbidity in patients with Zollinger-Ellison syndrome [15]. Surgical options are also available and should be considered in patients without metastases. Radiation therapy is available for those who are not surgical candidates.

Patient Comorbidities

With the advent of PPIs and H_2 blockers, stress ulcer prophylaxis has dramatically decreased the incidence of peptic ulcer disease in critically ill patients. The latest guidelines for prophylaxis in severe illness recommend the use of PPIs in the presence of a history of GI ulceration within the past year, mechanical ventilation × 48 h or more, coagulopathy (platelet count <50,000/m^3 [3], INR > 1.5 or PTT > 60), traumatic brain injury, spinal cord injury or burn injury, or two of the following: sepsis, ICU stay >7 days, GI bleeding, or use of steroids. Nevertheless, cautious use should be enforced as the latest data emphasize the risk of nosocomial pneumonia, *Clostridium difficile* infection, drug interactions, and thrombocytonemia associated with unnecessary use of antacids [29].

Medications Use

Patients with risk factors for development of peptic ulcer disease should avoid the use of NSAIDs. COX-2 inhibitors have been linked to a lower risk of PUD compared to NSAIDs, but the risk is still higher than placebo [30]. Furthermore, both classes of medications inhibit ulcer healing and therefore are contraindicated in patients with PUD. Ideally, the use of such medications should be paused during treatment of PUD to allow for adequate healing. The same is valid for antiplatelet agents such as clopidogrel and aspirin.

The interaction between NSAIDs and *H. pylori* in patients with PUD is complex and not yet fully elucidated. Numerous studies that investigated this relationship have shown correlation, but not causation of increased risk of PUD in this patient population. Nevertheless, the American College of Gastroenterology agrees that there is a potential synergy between NSAID use and *H. pylori* infection. The current recommendations are to test and treat the infection prior to initiation of long-term NSAID therapy, particularly in patients with other risk factors for PUD.

Environmental Risk Factor Management

The prevention of peptic ulcer disease caused by environmental factors focuses on avoidance of injurious insults. Smoking cessation, avoidance of mechanical injurious entities, and abstinence from any drugs that can lead to vascular compromise can be equally important in prevention of PUD.

Conclusion

While the majority of peptic ulcers are caused by infection with *H. pylori* or NSAID use, there are many other risk factors that deserve consideration. Prophylaxis or treatment against these various injurious elements can significantly decrease morbidity and mortality in affected patients.

References

1. Lin KJ, García Rodríguez LA, Hernández-Díaz S. Systematic review of peptic ulcer disease incidence rates: do studies without validation provide reliable estimates? Pharmacoepidemiol Drug Saf. 2011;20(7):718–28.
2. Sonnenberg A. The burden of digestive diseases in the United States. Chapter 15: Peptic ulcer disease. In: Everhart JE, editor. US Dep Health Hum Serv Public Health Serv Natl Inst Health Natl Inst Diabetes Dig Kidney Dis Wash DC US Gov Print Off 2008 NIH Publ. 1994;09(6443):257–408.
3. Sonnenberg A, Everhart JE. Health impact of peptic ulcer in the United States. Am J Gastroenterol. 1997;92(4):614.
4. Global Burden of Disease Study 2013 Collaborators. Global, regional, and national incidence, prevalence, and years lived with disability for 301 acute and chronic diseases and injuries in 188 countries, 1990–2013: a systematic analysis for the Global Burden of Disease Study 2013. Lancet. 2015;386(9995):743–800.
5. Brown L. Helicobacter pylori: epidemiology and routes of transmission. Epidemiol Rev. 2000;22(2):283–97.
6. Chong J, Marshall BJ, Barkin JS, McCallum RW, Reiner DK, Hoffman SR, O'Phelan C. Occupational exposure to Helicobacter pylori for the endoscopy professional: a sera epidemiological study. Am J Gastroenterol. 1994;89(11):1987–92.
7. Backert S, Neddermann M, Maubach G, Naumann M. Pathogenesis of Helicobacter pylori infection. Helicobacter. 2016;21(1):19–25.
8. Parsonnet J, Isaacson PG. Bacterial infection and MALT lymphoma. N Engl J Med. 2004;350:213–5.
9. Ferreira AC, Isomoto H, Moriyama M, Fujioka T, Machado JC, Yamaoka Y. Helicobacter and gastric malignancies. Helicobacter. 2008;13(1):28–34.
10. Lina TT, Alzahrani S, Gonzalez J, Pinchuk IV, Beswick EJ, Reyes VE. Immune evasion strategies used by Helicobacter pylori. World J Gastroenterol. 2014;20(36):12753–66.
11. Chey WD, Wong BC. American College of Gastroenterology guideline on the management of Helicobacter pylori infection. Am J Gastroenterol. 2007;102(8):1808.
12. Graham DY, Qureshi WA. Markers of infection. In: Mobley HLT, Mendz GL, Hazell SL, editors. Helicobacter pylori: physiology and genetics. Washington, D.C: ASM Press; 2001. p. 499–510.
13. Malfertheiner P, Megraud F, O'Morain C, Bazzoli F, El-Omar E, Graham D, Hunt R, Rokkas T, Vakil N, Kuipers EJ. Current concepts in the management of Helicobacter pylori infection: the Maastricht III Consensus Report. Gut. 2007;56(6):772–81.
14. Feldman M, Cryer B, Lee E, Peterson WL. Role of seroconversion in confirming cure of Helicobacter pylori infection. JAMA. 1998;280(4):363.
15. Meko JB, Norton JA. Management of patients with Zollinger-Ellison syndrome. Annu Rev Med. 1995;46:395.
16. Berna MJ, Hoffmann KM, Serrano J, Gibril F, Jensen RT. Serum gastrin in Zollinger-Ellison syndrome: I. Prospective study of fasting serum gastrin in 309 patients from the National

Institutes of Health and comparison with 2229 cases from the literature. Medicine (Baltimore). 2006;85(6):295.
17. Metz DC, Jensen RT. Gastrointestinal neuroendocrine tumors: pancreatic endocrine tumors. Gastroenterology. 2008;135(5):1469–92.
18. Corleto VD, Annibale B, Gibril F, et al. Does the widespread use of proton pump inhibitors mask, complicate and/or delay the diagnosis of Zollinger-Ellison syndrome? Aliment Pharmacol Ther. 2001;15:1555–61.
19. Poitras P, Gingras MH, Rehfeld JF. The Zollinger-Ellison syndrome: dangers and consequences of interrupting antisecretory treatment. Clin Gastroenterol Hepatol. 2012;10(2):199–202.
20. Talley NJ, Evans JM, Fleming KC, Harmsen WS, Zinsmeister AR, Melton LJ III. Nonsteroidal antiinflammatory drugs and dyspepsia in the elderly. Dig Sci. 1995;40:1345–50.
21. Laine L. Approaches to nonsteroidal anti-inflammatory drug use in the high-risk patient. Gastroenterology. 2001;120:594.
22. Wallace JL. How do NSAIDs cause ulcer disease? Baillieres Best Pr Res Clin Gastroenterol. 2000;14(1):147–59.
23. Tseng CL, Chen YT, Huang CJ, Luo JC, Peng YL, Huang DF, Hou MC, Lin HC, Lee FY. Short-term use of glucocorticoids and risk of peptic ulcer bleeding: a nationwide population-based case-crossover study. Aliment Pharmacol Ther. 2015 Sep;42(5):599–606.
24. Maity P, Biswas K, Roy S, Banerjee RK, Bandyopadhyay U. Smoking and the pathogenesis of gastroduodenal ulcer – recent mechanistic update. Mol Cell Biochem. 2003;253(1–2):329–38.
25. Feldman RA. Epidemiologic observations and open questions about disease and infection caused by Helicobacter pylori. In: Helicobacter Pylori Mol Cell Biol. Wymondham: Horizon Scientific Press; 2001. p. 29–51.
26. Laine L, Hopkins R, Girardi L. Has the impact of Helicobacter pylori therapy on ulcer recurrence in the United States been overstated? A meta-analysis of rigorously designed trials. Am J Gastroenterol. 1998 Sep;93(9):1409–15.
27. Chey WD, Leontiadis GI, Howden CW, Moss SF. ACG clinical guideline: treatment of Helicobacter pylori infection. Am J Gastroenterol. 2017;112:212–38.
28. Laheij RJ, Rossum LG, Jansen JB, Straatman H, Verbeek AL. Evaluation of treatment regimens to cure Helicobacter pylori infection – a meta-analysis. Aliment Pharmacol Ther. 1999;13:857–64.
29. MacLaren R, Reynolds PM, Allen RR. Histamine-2 receptor antagonists vs proton pump inhibitors on gastrointestinal tract hemorrhage and infectious complications in the intensive care unit. JAMA Intern Med. 2014;174(4):564–74.
30. Hooper L, Brown TJ, Elliott R, Payne K, Roberts C, Symmons D. The effectiveness of five strategies for the prevention of gastrointestinal toxicity induced by non-steroidal anti-inflammatory drugs: systematic review. BMJ. 2004;329(7472):948.

Medical Management of Peptic Ulcer Disease

55

Ashley H. Vernon

Introduction

Peptic ulcers remain a common pathology found in the USA. With the identification of *Helicobacter pylori* and nonsteroidal anti-inflammatory drugs (NSAIDs) as major contributing factors in the formation of peptic ulcers, targeted medical management has become much more effective in mitigating severe complications [1]. The widespread use of H_2 receptor antagonists (H_2RAs), proton pump inhibitors (PPIs), and *H. pylori* eradicating regimens has significantly decreased the need for surgical intervention [2–4]. Due in large part to these advancements, there has also been a significant decline in the number of hospitalizations for peptic ulcer disease (PUD) in the USA decreasing from 222,000 to 156,000 (29.9%) from 1993 to 2006 [1].

Treatment

H. pylori Ulcers

Helicobacter pylori infection is the most common etiology of peptic ulcer disease. Ulcers associated with *H. pylori* may resolve spontaneously; however, many will persist or worsen without treatment. Although *H. pylori* ulcers may heal with the use of anti-secretory therapy alone, most will recur if the *H. pylori* infection is not treated [5]. Treatment with an *H. pylori* eradication regimen is highly effective at healing ulcers and preventing recurrence [6, 7]. The most effective treatment regimens utilize at least a triple-drug therapy which typically includes the use of

A. H. Vernon
Department of Surgery, Brigham and Women's Hospital, Harvard Medical School, Boston, MA, USA
e-mail: avernon@bwh.harvard.edu

J. Grams et al. (eds.), *The SAGES Manual of Foregut Surgery*,
https://doi.org/10.1007/978-3-319-96122-4_55

antibiotics with a proton pump inhibitor (PPI). The use of concomitant antacid therapy is critical to the effectiveness of the regimen as the elevation in gastric pH encourages *H. pylori* to enter a replicative state which increases antibiotic effectiveness [8]. A major challenge to successful management of *H. pylori* infection is the increasing rate of antibiotic resistance emerging worldwide, especially to the classically used drug clarithromycin [9].

Historically in the USA, the first-line therapy involved a triple-drug regimen which is comprised of clarithromycin 500 mg BID and amoxicillin 1 g BID plus standard-dose PPI (omeprazole 20 mg or pantoprazole 40 mg) administered twice daily for 10–14 days. Multiple meta-analyses have demonstrated that 14-day triple-therapy regimens increase cure rates when compared to 7- or 10-day alternatives [10–13]. However, with the rise of clarithromycin resistance, eradication rates of less than 80% are now being documented throughout the globe. As the USA is now considered to be an area of high clarithromycin resistance (15–40%), the majority of US clinicians favor the use of a quadruple drug regimen as first-line therapy [14].

The most commonly prescribed "quadruple regimen" contains bismuth and is recommended as second-line therapy in areas without clarithromycin resistance; however, in areas with high rates of clarithromycin resistance, the "quadruple regimen" should be considered as the therapy of choice. The dosing for the "quadruple regimen" is bismuth subsalicylate 525 mg QID, metronidazole 250 mg QID, and tetracycline 500 mg QID plus standard-dose PPI twice daily for 10–14 days [14]. A non-bismuth-containing quadruple regimen described as concomitant therapy may also be considered as first- or second-line options especially in areas of high clarithromycin and metronidazole resistance. Concomitant therapy includes a 14-day course of amoxicillin 1 g BID, clarithromycin 500 mg BID, and metronidazole 500 mg BID plus standard-dose PPI twice daily. Quadruple regimens have been shown to provide *H. pylori* cure rates of greater than 90% when used as first-line therapy [15, 16].

Alternative regimens include fluoroquinolone-based therapies as well as sequential therapies. The most commonly used fluoroquinolone-based regimen involves levofloxacin 500 mg BID and amoxicillin 1 g BID plus twice-daily standard-dose PPI for 10–14 days. Given increasing rates of fluoroquinolone resistance, this regimen is not recommended for use as an option for first-line therapy [14]. As a second-line regimen, cure rates of ~80% are seen [17]. Sequential therapy is another option that can be utilized in those who fail first-line therapy. It refers to a split regimen which consists of two consecutive periods of 5–7-day treatments. This regimen typically involves a twice-daily standard-dose PPI and amoxicillin 1 gm daily for the first treatment period and then standard-dose PPI BID, clarithromycin 500 mg BID, and metronidazole 500 mg BID for the next period of 5–7 days. Sequential therapy has been shown to reach higher cure rates than 7- or 10-day triple therapies, but it has not been shown to be as efficacious as 14-day triple therapy [18, 19].

Proton pump inhibitors should be continued for 8–12 weeks in patients with any gastric ulcer triple/quadruple therapy and in patients with complicated duodenal ulcers for 4–8 weeks. No further PPI therapy is typically needed in patients with uncomplicated duodenal ulcers after the antibiotic regimen. Over one in five treated with an *H. pylori* eradication regimen will fail to clear the infection [20]. Therefore, 4 or more weeks after treatment, it is vital to confirm the eradication of *H. pylori* in all patients, typically with a urea breath test; however, fecal antigen testing is an option, especially useful for patients with an excluded stomach such as Roux-en-Y gastric bypass [14].

NSAID Ulcers

NSAIDs cause ulcers through a variety of mechanisms including a topical irritant effect on the epithelium and interference with mucosal barrier properties. The management of NSAID-associated ulcers should begin with the termination of the NSAID therapy, if at all possible. If the NSAID cannot be discontinued, the lowest possible effective dose should be prescribed and an attempt should be made to consider a change to the least ulcerogenic medication. Indomethacin, naproxen, diclofenac, and piroxicam have been shown to have higher rates of ulcer formation among the NSAIDs [21]. Alternatively, tenoxicam, ibuprofen, and meloxicam are considered some of the less ulcerogenic NSAIDs; however, ulcer formation can still occur with high-dose usage and in high-risk populations, especially the elderly [21]. Selective COX-2 inhibitors can also be used to reduce the risk of ulcer recurrence or exacerbation [22]. These NSAIDs specifically target cyclooxygenase-2. This is an advantage over nonselective NSAIDs which also inhibit cyclooxygenase-1 which is important in gastrointestinal mucosal barrier protection. The widespread use of COX-2 inhibitors, however, is limited by a possible increased risk of thromboembolic events [23].

In all instances, a PPI should be started to assist in ulcer healing because intraluminal acid impairs ulcer healing. Multiple studies have demonstrated the superiority of PPIs over H_2 receptor antagonists (H_2RA) especially in the setting of continued NSAID use [24, 25]. In the ASTRONAUT trial, 541 patients with NSAID-associated ulcers were randomized to groups treated with omeprazole 20 mg or 40 mg daily or ranitidine 150 mg BID for 8 weeks. At 8 weeks, the ulcer healing rate was significantly improved in both groups taking omeprazole 80% for the 20 mg group and 79% for the 40 mg group compared to 63% for the ranitidine group [25]. In another double-blind, randomized study from Agrawal et al., 315 patients with NSAID-associated gastric ulcers were treated with lansoprazole 15 mg or 30 mg daily or ranitidine 150 mg BID for 8 weeks. After 8 weeks, there was also a significantly increased rate of healed ulcers among the PPI group (69% in the 15 mg group and 73% in the 30 mg group) as compared to the H_2RA group (53%) [24]. In summary, patients with NSAID ulcers should remain on PPIs for at least 8 weeks after discontinuing NSAID usage. If patients cannot discontinue NSAIDs, they should remain on PPI therapy, if possible, to prevent ulcer recurrence.

Idiopathic Ulcers

Patients with non-*H. pylori*, non-NSAID ulcers should be treated with at least a 4–8-week regimen of PPIs. If no cause can be identified, these patients may require high-dose maintenance therapy to prevent ulcer complication and recurrence [26]. Sucralfate now plays a minor role in the treatment of peptic ulcers but maybe helpful in treating severe refractory non-*H. pylori*, non-NSAID ulcers in combination with PPIs. This medication is most often used as prophylaxis against stress ulceration. Sucralfate is generally ingested orally forming a cross-linking, viscous paste in acidic environments that creates a physical barrier over the gastrointestinal tract protecting the mucosa from further damage from acid, pepsin, and bile. It has also been shown to stimulate angiogenesis as well as the formation of granulation tissue [27].

All smokers with ulcers should be encouraged to quit indefinitely given its effects on gastrointestinal microcirculation and impairment of ulcer healing.

Complications

Bleeding

Bleeding peptic ulcers are associated with high morbidity as well as mortality. It is the most common complication identified in patients with PUD. Patients may present with hematemesis, melena, dizziness, syncope, and hemodynamic compromise. It is vital that these patients are adequately resuscitated with fluids and/or blood products immediately. All anticoagulants should be stopped, and any coagulopathy should be corrected. These patients should undergo upper endoscopy within 24 h of presentation with the goal of diagnosing as well as possibly treating the source of bleeding. Endoscopic options for control of ulcer bleeding include epinephrine injection, vessel coagulation, and hemostatic clipping. In patients with endoscopic findings concerning for a high risk of rebleed such as active spurting, active oozing, a nonbleeding visible vessel, and adherent clot, endoscopic therapy should be administered and a PPI infusion should be given for at least 72 h [28]. In the absence of treatment, significant bleeding will ensue in ~25% of patients with active oozing, ~35% of patients with a nonbleeding visible vessel, and ~60% of those with active spurting [29]. Endoscopic therapy is generally unnecessary for ulcers with a flat pigmented spot or clean base as they are at low risk of recurrent bleeding. The first time the ulcer rebleeds, endoscopy should be repeated. In the small number of patients with persistent or recurrent bleeding despite endoscopic therapy, interventional angiography should be considered. The use of transarterial embolization is a significantly less invasive and less morbid alternative to surgery. However, surgery will be required in the event of therapeutic failure or the absence of interventional radiology.

Perforation

Perforations due to PUD occur only in about 10% of cases in developed countries [30]. Ulcer perforation tends to occur more in those with duodenal as compared to gastric ulcers, NSAID and aspirin users, and cigarette smokers. Patients frequently present with sudden, severe upper abdominal pain and subsequent peritonitis due to leakage of air and intraluminal contents into the peritoneal cavity. This pain may initially improve; however, typically the pain will again worsen significantly after several hours. Upright chest and abdominal plain films may demonstrate free air; however, currently the diagnosis of perforation is often made by CT scan. Patients are treated with an IV PPI and broad-spectrum antibiotics. The decision will be made to take many of these patients to surgery; however, some patients may be effectively managed conservatively if stable, without peritonitis, and have evidence of a perforation which is contained. In a retrospective review by Tanaka et al., 183 patients were identified to have a perforated gastric ulcer. Of the 57 patients that underwent conservative management, 41 (72%) were successfully treated [31]. In a prospective randomized trial by Crofts et al., 83 patients were identified with perforated peptic ulcers, and 40 of these patients were randomized to a conservative treatment group with nasogastric tube suction, IV antibiotics, and ranitidine, while the remaining 43 patients underwent laparotomy. The mortality was the same in both groups with two deaths in each. Among the patients in the conservative treatment group, 28 percent required surgery as a result of failure to improve after 12 h. The remainder of the conservative group, however, were successfully managed [32].

Gastric Outlet Obstruction

In developed countries, gastric outlet obstruction (GOO) is a rare complication of peptic ulcer disease seen in less than 3% of cases. Nevertheless, it is still the most common indication for surgical intervention of PUD in the developing world. GOO often results as a consequence of severe pyloric channel or duodenal ulceration. The obstruction occurs due to a combination of fibrosis, inflammation, and spasm. Patients may present with postprandial emesis, upper abdominal pain, early satiety, and abdominal distension. Due to persistent vomiting, a hypokalemic, hypochloremic metabolic alkalosis may be present and should be corrected with intravenous normal saline. The diagnosis of GOO may be achieved through abdominal CT scan and upper endoscopy. Biopsies should be obtained if there is evidence of GOO on endoscopy to rule out malignancy and to evaluate for *H. pylori*. Patients should undergo nasogastric decompression and treatment with IV PPIs. If symptoms continue despite medical management, patients may require endoscopic balloon dilatation therapy. Historically, long-term outcomes after balloon dilatation have been poor; however, many of these studies were completed prior to the development of PPIs and the discovery of *H. pylori* as a major etiological agent in PUD [33, 34]. In a more recent observational study by Cherian et al., 23 patients with PUD-associated GOO were managed conservatively with *H. pylori* eradication if indicated and PPIs with favorable outcomes. Twenty-one patients were successfully treated with balloon dilatation with no further symptoms at a median follow-up of 43 months [35].

References

1. Wang YR, Richter JE, Dempsey DT. Trends and outcomes of hospitalizations for peptic ulcer disease in the United States, 1993 to 2006. Ann Surg. 2010;251:51–8. https://doi.org/10.1097/SLA.0b013e3181b975b8.
2. Espat NJ, Ong ES, Helton WS, Nyhus LM. 1990-2001 US general surgery chief resident gastric surgery operative experience: analysis of paradigm shift. J Gastrointest Surg. 2004;8:471–8. https://doi.org/10.1016/j.gassur.2004.02.002.
3. Gralnek IM, Barkun AN, Bardou M. Management of acute bleeding from a peptic ulcer. N Engl J Med. 2008;359:928–37. https://doi.org/10.1056/NEJMra0706113.
4. Schwesinger WH, Page CP, Sirinek KR, et al. Operations for peptic ulcer disease: paradigm lost. J Gastrointest Surg. 2001;5:438–43.
5. Bardhan KD. Intermittent treatment of duodenal ulcer for long term medical management. Postgrad Med J. 1988;64(Suppl 1):40–6.
6. Leodolter A, Kulig M, Brasch H, et al. A meta-analysis comparing eradication, healing and relapse rates in patients with Helicobacter pylori-associated gastric or duodenal ulcer. Aliment Pharmacol Ther. 2001;15:1949–58.
7. Ford AC, Delaney BC, Forman D, Moayyedi P. Eradication therapy in Helicobacter pylori positive peptic ulcer disease: systematic review and economic analysis. Am J Gastroenterol. 2004;99:1833–55. https://doi.org/10.1111/j.1572-0241.2004.40014.x.
8. Marcus EA, Inatomi N, Nagami GT, et al. The effects of varying acidity on *Helicobacter pylori* growth and the bactericidal efficacy of ampicillin. Aliment Pharmacol Ther. 2012;36:972–9. https://doi.org/10.1111/apt.12059.
9. Thung I, Aramin H, Vavinskaya V, et al. Review article: the global emergence of Helicobacter pylori antibiotic resistance. Aliment Pharmacol Ther. 2016;43:514–33. https://doi.org/10.1111/apt.13497.
10. Ford A, Moayyedi P. How can the current strategies for Helicobacter pylori eradication therapy be improved? Can J Gastroenterol Hepatol. 2003;17:36B–40B. https://doi.org/10.1155/2003/714124.
11. Calvet X, García N, López T, et al. A meta-analysis of short versus long therapy with a proton pump inhibitor, clarithromycin and either metronidazole or amoxycillin for treating Helicobacter pylori infection. Aliment Pharmacol Ther. 2000;14:603–9. https://doi.org/10.1046/j.1365-2036.2000.00744.x.
12. Flores HB, Salvana A, Ang ELR, et al. M1138 duration of proton-pump inhibitor-based triple therapy for Helicobacter pylori eradication: a meta-analysis. Gastroenterology. 2010;138:S-340. https://doi.org/10.1016/S0016-5085(10)61564-8.
13. Fischbach LA, Goodman KJ, Feldman M, Aragaki C. Sources of variation of Helicobacter pylori treatment success in adults worldwide: a meta-analysis. Int J Epidemiol. 2002;31:128–39.
14. Malfertheiner P, Megraud F, O'Morain CA, et al (2016) Management of Helicobacter pylori infection—the Maastricht V/Florence consensus report. Gut. gutjnl-2016-312288. https://doi.org/10.1136/gutjnl-2016-312288.
15. Laine L, Hunt R, El-Zimaity H, et al. Bismuth-based quadruple therapy using a single capsule of bismuth biskalcitrate, metronidazole, and tetracycline given with omeprazole versus omeprazole, amoxicillin, and clarithromycin for eradication of Helicobacter pylori in duodenal ulcer patients: a prospective, randomized, multicenter, North American trial. Am J Gastroenterol. 2003;98:562–7. https://doi.org/10.1111/j.1572-0241.2003.t01-1-07288.x.
16. Salazar CO, Cardenas VM, Reddy RK, et al. Greater than 95% success with 14-day bismuth quadruple anti- Helicobacter pylori therapy: a pilot study in US Hispanics. Helicobacter. 2012;17:382–90. https://doi.org/10.1111/j.1523-5378.2012.00962.x.
17. O'Connor A, Molina-Infante J, Gisbert JP, O'Morain C. Treatment of helicobacter pylori infection 2013. Helicobacter. 2013;18:58–65. https://doi.org/10.1111/hel.12075.
18. Liou J-M, Chen C-C, Chen M-J, et al. Sequential versus triple therapy for the first-line treatment of Helicobacter pylori: a multicentre, open-label, randomised trial. Lancet. 2013;381:205–13. https://doi.org/10.1016/S0140-6736(12)61579-7.

19. Gatta L, Vakil N, Vaira D, Scarpignato C. Global eradication rates for Helicobacter pylori infection: systematic review and meta-analysis of sequential therapy. BMJ. 2013;347:f4587. https://doi.org/10.1136/bmj.f4587.
20. Vakil N. Primary and secondary treatment for Helicobacter pylori in the United States. Rev Gastroenterol Disord. 2005;5:67–72.
21. Coxib and traditional NSAID Trialists (CNT) Collaboration, Bhala N, Emberson J, Merhi A, Abramson S, Arber N, Baron JA, et al. Vascular and upper gastrointestinal effects of non-steroidal anti-inflammatory drugs: meta-analyses of individual participant data from randomised trials. Lancet. 2013;382:769–79. https://doi.org/10.1016/S0140-6736(13)60900-9.
22. Rostom A, Muir K, Dubé C, et al. Gastrointestinal safety of cyclooxygenase-2 inhibitors: a Cochrane Collaboration systematic review. Clin Gastroenterol Hepatol. 2007;5:818–28, 828.e1–5; quiz 768. https://doi.org/10.1016/j.cgh.2007.03.011.
23. Kearney PM, Baigent C, Godwin J, et al. Do selective cyclo-oxygenase-2 inhibitors and traditional non-steroidal anti-inflammatory drugs increase the risk of atherothrombosis? Meta-analysis of randomised trials. BMJ. 2006;332:1302–8.
24. Agrawal NM, Campbell DR, Safdi MA, et al. Superiority of lansoprazole vs ranitidine in healing nonsteroidal anti-inflammatory drug–associated gastric ulcers: results of a double-blind, randomized, multicenter study. Arch Intern Med. 2000;160:1455–61. https://doi.org/10.1001/archinte.160.10.1455.
25. Yeomans ND, Tulassay Z, Juhász L, et al. A comparison of omeprazole with ranitidine for ulcers associated with nonsteroidal antiinflammatory drugs. N Engl J Med. 1998;338:719–26. https://doi.org/10.1056/NEJM199803123381104.
26. Gisbert JP, Calvet X. Review article: Helicobacter pylori-negative duodenal ulcer disease. Aliment Pharmacol Ther. 2009;30:791–815. https://doi.org/10.1111/j.1365-2036.2009.04105.x.
27. Tarnawski A, Tanoue K, Santos AM, Sarfeh IJ. Cellular and molecular mechanisms of gastric ulcer healing. Is the quality of mucosal scar affected by treatment? Scand J Gastroenterol Suppl. 1995;210:9–14.
28. Barkun AN, Bardou M, Kuipers EJ, et al. International consensus recommendations on the management of patients with nonvariceal upper gastrointestinal bleeding. Ann Intern Med. 2010;152:101–13. https://doi.org/10.7326/0003-4819-152-2-201001190-00009.
29. Laine L, Jensen DM. Management of patients with ulcer bleeding. Am J Gastroenterol. 2012;107:345–60. https://doi.org/10.1038/ajg.2011.480.
30. Behrman SW. Management of complicated peptic ulcer disease. Arch Surg Chic Ill 1960. 2005;140:201–8. https://doi.org/10.1001/archsurg.140.2.201.
31. Tanaka R, Kosugi S, Sakamoto K, et al. Treatment for perforated gastric ulcer: a multi-institutional retrospective review. J Gastrointest Surg. 2013;17:2074–81. https://doi.org/10.1007/s11605-013-2362-7.
32. Crofts TJ, Park KG, Steele RJ, et al. A randomized trial of nonoperative treatment for perforated peptic ulcer. N Engl J Med. 1989;320:970–3. https://doi.org/10.1056/NEJM198904133201504.
33. Lau JY, Chung SC, Sung JJ, et al. Through-the-scope balloon dilation for pyloric stenosis: long-term results. Gastrointest Endosc. 1996;43:98–101.
34. Kuwada SK, Alexander GL. Long-term outcome of endoscopic dilation of nonmalignant pyloric stenosis. Gastrointest Endosc. 1995;41:15–7.
35. Cherian PT, Cherian S, Singh P. Long-term follow-up of patients with gastric outlet obstruction related to peptic ulcer disease treated with endoscopic balloon dilatation and drug therapy. Gastrointest Endosc. 2007;66:491–7. https://doi.org/10.1016/j.gie.2006.11.016.

Surgical Management: Truncal, Selective, and Highly Selective Vagotomy

56

Leena Khaitan and Adil Haleem Khan

Introduction

Peptic ulcer disease is a common cause of epigastric pain. Every general surgeon must be familiar with the treatment options available to manage the disease. In the past, surgical management of ulcer disease was a common practice. However, since the advancement in medical therapy and its success in managing patients with PUD, the number of surgical procedures being performed for ulcer disease has dramatically decreased. Historically, indications for surgical management of PUD included intractable pain, obstruction, bleeding, and perforation. In recent times, medical management has made surgery almost obsolete for the first two indications with surgery being performed primarily for the latter two scenarios in an emergency setting [1, 2].

It is not possible to understand the concept of surgical vagotomy without having some basic knowledge of gastric acid secretion and the anatomy of the vagus nerves and its branches.

Gastric Acid Secretion

Secretion of gastric acid is divided into three phases. The cephalic phase starts with mere sight or smell of food. It is primarily mediated by the vagus nerve. The vagus nerve then activates chief cells to release acid. It also activates

L. Khaitan (✉)
Metabolic and Bariatric Program, Department of Surgery, University Hospitals, Cleveland, OH, USA
e-mail: Leena.Khaitan@UHhospitals.org

A. H. Khan
Department of Surgery, University Hospitals, Cleveland Medical Center, Cleveland, OH, USA

J. Grams et al. (eds.), *The SAGES Manual of Foregut Surgery*,
https://doi.org/10.1007/978-3-319-96122-4_56

enterochromaffin-like cells (ECL) and G-cells in the antrum to stimulate release of gastric acid by releasing histamine and gastrin, respectively. This phase is responsible for about 25% of acid output. Next is the gastric phase which is responsible for the majority of gastric acid output. It is also primarily mediated by the vagus nerve and also by local activation of stimulatory peptides by breakdown products in chyme. The last phase is the intestinal phase which is responsible for only 5–10% of acid secretion and is primarily mediated through chemical stimulation of peptides and amino acids entering the small bowel [3] (Fig. 56.1).

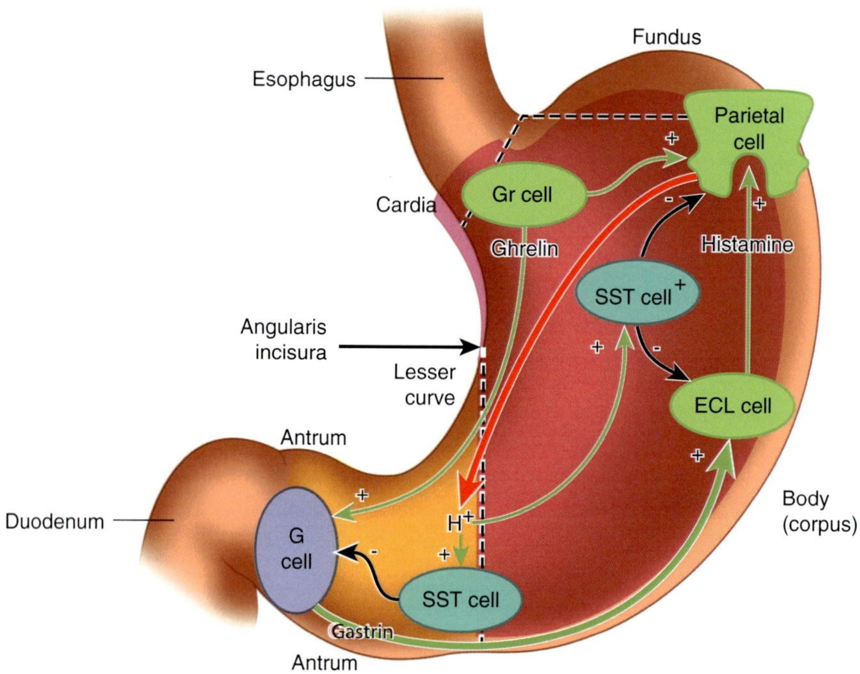

Anatomic areas	Functional areas
Cardia fundus body	Oxyntic gland area (80%)
Antrum	Pyloric gland area (20%)

Fig. 56.1 Gastric acid secretion

Anatomy of Vagus Nerves

The right and left vagus nerves are located posterior and anterior to the esophagus, respectively, due to the embryological clockwise rotation of the foregut. Both nerves descend along the esophagus and enter the abdomen through diaphragmatic hiatus. The anterior vagus nerve is closely adherent to the esophagus and can have one or more trunk or form a plexus at the level of the hiatus. The posterior vagus nerve can be up to one centimeter away from the esophagus and usually has only one trunk. The anterior vagus nerve gives off two terminal branches. These include the hepatic branch that runs in the gastrohepatic ligament and the principal gastric branch or nerve of Latarjet that runs along the lesser curve. The nerve of Latarjet gives off five to seven gastric branches that supply the stomach and have a characteristic crow's foot appearance along the lesser curve. This nerve continues off to supply the pylorus. The posterior vagus gives off a sizeable branch right after emerging through the hiatus or sometimes above the hiatus called the criminal nerve of grassi. This must be identified during vagotomy as this is believed to result in ulcer recurrence if not sacrificed during the procedure. It also gives branches to the celiac axis and then continues down as the posterior nerve of Latarjet [4, 5].

Surgical Management

As mentioned previously, the surgical management of ulcer disease has been largely limited to emergency management of complications including bleeding and perforation. Obstructions still do occasionally occur due to ulcer disease. In the past vagotomy was recommended at the time of surgical management of ulcer complications to decrease risk of recurrence. Nowadays, preference is given to emergency management, diagnosis and treatment of *H. pylori*, and acid blocking medications before planning vagotomy to avoid the complications of vagotomy.

Three types of vagotomies are described: truncal vagotomy (TV), selective vagotomy (SV), and highly selective vagotomy (HSV). The schematic diagram shows location for these three types of vagotomies (Fig. 56.2).

While these operations were classically performed as open procedures, successful cases of laparoscopic vagotomies have been described in literature [6, 7]. We describe details of the laparoscopic approach to these vagotomies.

Port Placement

Port placement is key to successful foregut surgery. We utilize five incisions. The initial port is a 10 mm trocar which is placed 15 cm below the xiphoid just to the left of midline using a direct cutdown technique. This is the camera port. The abdomen is insufflated to allow placement of the remaining ports under direct visualization. A subxiphoid incision is used for placement of a Nathanson liver retractor. A 12 mm

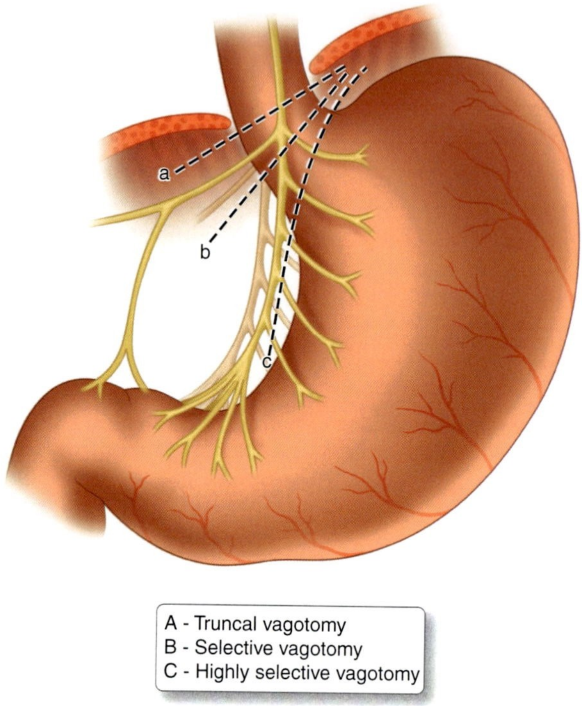

Fig. 56.2 Anatomy of vagus nerves and their branches

port is placed 10 cm from xiphoid process in subcostal area in the left midclavicular line off of the costal margin. A 5 mm port is placed in the left anterior axillary line off of the left costal margin. Finally a 5 mm port is placed 4 fingerbreadths from xiphoid process on the right side with entry at the base of the falciform below the left lobe of the liver.

Exposure

The abdomen is entered using an open Hasson technique and insufflated with CO2 to a pressure of 15 mm Hg. A liver retractor is placed to retract left lobe of the liver and expose the hiatus. Using hook electrocautery, we incise the pars flaccida and open it in a horizontal fashion above the hepatic branch of the vagus. It is opened in a transverse fashion below the hepatic branch. We preserve the hepatic branch of the vagus routinely. The peritoneum overlying the medial border of the right crus is opened and we enter the mediastinum. A retroesophageal window is created to expose the left crus. The esophagus is mobilized in a circumferential fashion by dissecting along the border of the crura. At this point the anterior vagus can be identified overlying the esophagus. The posterior vagus is noted along the posterior esophagus.

Vagotomy Techniques

After adequate dissection, traction with a Penrose is used on the esophagus to expose the anterior and posterior vagi. For truncal vagotomy, 2–3 cm of each nerve is clipped and transected above the level of GE junction (Fig. 56.2). These transected segments should be sent to pathology to confirm that the nerves have been transected. Since this procedure also interrupts the motor fibers to the pylorus and can lead to gastric outlet obstruction, it must be combined with a drainage procedure such as a pyloroplasty. Alternatively one can resect the gastric antrum to decrease acid output. With distal gastrectomy, reconstruction is accomplished with either Billroth I or Billroth II reconstruction. The details of these procedures are described in another chapter.

For selective vagotomy, the vagal nerves are transected distal to the LES (Fig. 56.2). Gastric emptying is also a concern with these procedures and a drainage procedure is usually added.

For highly selective vagotomy, the hiatal dissection is omitted, and trocar placement is the same as described. Highly selective vagotomy (HSV) divides only the gastric branches of the vagus nerves and preserves the innervation to the pylorus, thereby obviating need for any drainage procedure (Fig. 56.2). It is performed by identifying nerves of Latarjet and then dividing the nerves supplying the stomach. These branches are present in the classic crow's foot configuration and are 5–7 in number. Usually transection is started 5–6 cm proximal to the pylorus and is carried along the way up to 5 cm distal to the GE junction. Great attention must be paid to criminal nerve of grassi in any of these procedures as sparing this nerve leads to a high recurrence rate.

Postsurgical Management

The patient is admitted to the hospital for postoperative recovery. A liquid diet is started on POD # 1 and advanced as tolerated. If a drainage procedure is performed, then an upper GI study is done to rule out any leaks prior to resuming oral intake. Oral pain medications are started, and patient can be discharged home once tolerating adequate oral intake.

Outcomes and Complications

The three procedures have variable effectiveness in control of acid secretion. While studies have shown that TV and SV have almost comparable decrease in basal acid output (BAO) and maximal acid output (MAO), HSV is less effective in this regard [8]. This difference is further accentuated over long-term follow-up, and recurrence rate for patients with HSV is much higher compared to other two types of vagotomies. Oftentimes, the procedure selection is based more on the possible complications versus the success in controlling acid secretion.

The incidence of various morbidities is variable depending on the type of vagotomy procedure and also the type of drainage procedure performed. Overall, the

Table 56.1 Complications after ulcer operations [10, 12]

Percent of patients with	HSV	TV + D	TV + A
Epigastric fullness	14.3	19.1	36.2
Early dumping	0	8.5	12.8
Late dumping	0	4.3	8.5
Nausea	6.1	8.5	8.5
Vomiting (food)	6.1	0	2.1
Vomiting (bile)	0	0	4.3
Heartburn	8.2	8.5	17
Flatulence	18.4	21.3	29.8
Diarrhea	10.2	14.9	21.3

HSV highly selective vagotomy, *TV + D* truncal vagotomy and drainage with pyloroplasty, *TV + A* truncal vagotomy and antrectomy

incidence of recurrent ulcer is lowest with TV and highest with HSV. On the other hand, the incidence of postoperative morbidities is higher with TV and SV and lower with HSV. One of the largest prospective studies reporting these complications was published in 1989 with 248 patients that had follow-up to 11–15 years [10, 11]. The incidence of recurrent ulceration was 28.5%, 37.4%, and 39.3% for TV, SV, and HSV, respectively. The incidence of diarrhea was 9.8%, 11.8%, and 4.4%; incidence of dyspepsia was 18.4%, 20.5%, and 8.6%; and incidence of dumping was 5.9%, 19.6%, and 2.2% for TV, SV, and HSV, respectively [9]. Patients who underwent TV with antrectomy (to remove the G-cells) had the lowest ulcer recurrence but higher morbidity compared to TV with pyloroplasty [10, 11]. A study done 6 years prior demonstrated TV with antrectomy had no case of recurrent ulceration but was associated with the highest incidence of postoperative complications compared with other procedures (Table 56.1) [10].

We describe these post-op morbidities in further detail below.

Diarrhea The incidence of diarrhea is variable depending on type of vagotomy. The incidence is 25% after truncal vagotomy and only about 5% after highly selective vagotomy [13]. Different etiological explanations are given for cause of diarrhea including rapid transit of food through the bowel, disturbance in bile acid metabolism, and dysregulation of enteral hormones. The diarrhea is usually self-limiting in most cases and rarely requires surgical intervention.

Dumping syndrome This is one of the common and oftentimes most debilitating outcomes after gastric ulcer surgery. It consists of symptoms that occur after ingestion of food. Two forms are recognized. Early dumping occurs 20–30 min after ingestion of food. Patients complain of epigastric fullness, cramping abdominal pain, nausea, explosive diarrhea, and cardiovascular manifestations including palpitations, tachycardia, flushing, and diaphoresis. This is believed to occur due to the sudden shift of fluid as hyperosmotic chyme enters the small bowel. Later dumping syndrome occurs 2 to 3 h after food ingestion. Rapid gastric emptying leads to hyperinsulinemia in response to sudden appearance of large quantities of food in the small bowel. The resulting hyperinsulinemia leads to manifestation of hypoglycemia including tremors, sweating, light headedness, and confusion. Dietary changes and use of somatostatin analogues help ameliorate symptoms in majority of patients.

Gastric atony The vagus nerve has a major role in gastric emptying. After truncal and selective vagotomy, gastric emptying is significantly affected and needs a drainage procedure as mentioned earlier. Unfortunately, even after a drainage procedure, some patients will continue to have delayed emptying of solids. On the other hand, emptying of liquids can increase due to loss of receptive fundic relaxation. This can usually be managed with prokinetic agents after other causes of delayed gastric emptying are ruled out.

Bile reflux gastritis This is a common problem after antrectomy and reconstruction. Patients have epigastric pain and bilious vomiting. Diagnosis is confirmed on upper endoscopy which reveals inflamed mucosa and superficial ulcerations. Classically this syndrome does not respond well to medical therapy, and conversion to Roux-en-Y gastrojejunostomy is required.

Afferent loop syndrome This syndrome can result from a variety of causes, including kinking of the afferent limb, internal herniation, or stenosis of the gastrojejunal anastomosis. It can present as an acute or chronic syndrome. In case of the latter patients may present with megaloblastic anemia due to deficiency of vitamin B-12 from bacterial overgrowth. In both acute and chronic afferent loop syndrome, surgery is indicated. Options include shortening of afferent limb, conversion of Billroth II to Billroth I anastomosis, creation of enteroenterostomy past the stoma, or conversion to Roux-en-Y gastric bypass.

Efferent loop syndrome This syndrome is relatively uncommon. It usually results from herniation of efferent limb behind the anastomosis. Patients present with abdominal pain and bilious vomiting. Diagnosis is usually established with a CT scan with oral contrast. It reveals failure of contrast to enter the efferent limb. Treatment is surgical with reduction of hernia and closure of defect to prevent herniation in the future.

Conclusion

Vagotomies have mostly become procedures of the past due to excellent medical options, available now for the treatment of PUD. However, surgeons should be familiar with the anatomy and physiology of this region of the foregut. There are still some situations such as obstruction, perforation, or bleeding due to PUD that are not responsive to medical therapy where these procedures may still be considered.

References

1. Martin RF. Surgical management of ulcer disease. Surg Clin North Am. 2005;85(5):907–29.
2. Steger AC. Remaining indications for vagotomy with drainage or antrectomy in duodenal ulcer. Ann R Coll Surg Engl. 1987;69(1):24–6.
3. Soybel DI. Anatomy and physiology of the stomach. Surg Clin North Am. 2005;85(5):875–94.
4. Baccaro LM, et al. Anatomy of the anterior vagus nerve: an anatomic description and its application in surgery. Anat Physiol. 2013;3:2161-0940.
5. Jackson RG. Anatomy of the vagus nerves in the region of the lower esophagus and the stomach. Anat Rec. 1949;103(1):1–18.
6. Casas AT, Gadacz TR. Laparoscopic management of peptic ulcer disease. Surg Clin North Am. 1996;76(3):515–22.
7. Laws HL, JB MK. Endoscopic management of peptic ulcer disease. Ann Surg. 1993;217(5):548–55.
8. Thompson JC, Fender HR, Watson LC, Villar HV, et al. Ann Surg. 1976;183(5):599–608.
9. Hoffmann J, Jensen HE, Christiansen J, Olesen A, Loud FB, Hauch O. Prospective controlled vagotomy trial for duodenal ulcer. Results after 11-15 years. Ann Surg. 1989;209(1):40–5.
10. Koo J, Lam SK, Chan P, Lee NW, Lam P, Wong J, Ong GB. Proximal gastric vagotomy, truncal vagotomy with drainage and truncal vagotomy with antrectomy for chronic duodenal ulcer. A prospective, randomized controlled trial. Ann Surg. 1983;197(3):265–71.
11. Herrington JL Jr, Sawyers JL. Results of elective duodenal ulcer surgery in women: comparison of truncal vagotomy and antrectomy, gastric selective vagotomy and pyloroplasty, proximal gastric vagotomy. Ann Surg. 1978;187(5):576–82.
12. Taylor TV. Postvagotomy and cholecystectomy syndrome. Ann Surg. 1981;194(5):625–9.
13. Goligher JC, Hill GL, Kenny TE, Nutter E. Proximal gastric vagotomy without drainage for duodenal ulcer: results after 5-8 years. Br J Surg. 1978;65(3):145–51.

Surgical Management: Vagotomy and Pyloroplasty

57

Nathan G. LaFayette and Jennifer S. Schwartz

Indications

Most indications for vagotomy and pyloroplasty (VP) are of historical importance, with the widespread use of proton pump inhibitors (PPIs) and eradication of *H. pylori* making the aforementioned procedures rare. There are, however, certain clinical scenarios that still employ these procedures. Instances when a vagotomy and pyloroplasty may be indicated include ulcer disease refractory to medical therapy with extensive scarring that makes a formal antrectomy impossible. The most common reason to perform a VP is a bleeding duodenal ulcer, which was first described by Jan Mikulicz-Radecki in 1887 [1]. It is the most common presentation of complicated ulcer disease, indication for surgery, and common cause of mortality related to peptic ulcer disease. Typically, surgery is sought after failed endoscopic attempts at control of bleeding or unavailable angiographic embolism of the gastroduodenal artery. The indications for surgical management of a bleeding ulcer are massive hemorrhage leading to shock/instability, continuing transfusion >6 units in 48 h, recurrent bleeding during medical therapy or after endoscopic therapy, and recurrent hemorrhage requiring rehospitalization. Peptic ulcer disease causing gastric ulcers typically has low acid production, and therefore, VP is rarely indicated [2].

A second indication for VP is a perforated duodenal/gastric ulcer. The most common location is in the prepyloric anterior wall, in which this can be incorporated into the pyloroplasty. VP is currently only indicated in stable patients with minimal spillage who are resistant or allergic to PPIs or those with high recurrence potential, such as heavy smokers or patients on chronic nonsteroidal anti-inflammatory drugs [3].

A third indication is an obstructing pyloric channel/duodenal ulcer, which was first described by Walter Hermann von Heineke in 1886. Prior to surgical

N. G. LaFayette · J. S. Schwartz (✉)
Department of Surgery, The Ohio State University Wexner Medical Center, Columbus, OH, USA
e-mail: jennifer.schwartz@osumc.edu

J. Grams et al. (eds.), *The SAGES Manual of Foregut Surgery*,
https://doi.org/10.1007/978-3-319-96122-4_57

intervention, it is prudent to allow approximately 72 h of gastric decompression and correction of electrolyte abnormalities. VP may be considered at the index procedure or after failed medical and endoscopic therapies such as dilation [4].

Technique(S) (Fig. 57.1) [5]

The techniques for truncal, selective, and highly selective vagotomy were described in the previous chapter. A pyloroplasty is performed in conjunction with the denervation procedure to overcome the gastric stasis and potential functional gastric outlet obstruction created with vagotomy. One of the benefits of a pyloroplasty is that it decreases the possibility of marginal ulceration occasionally seen after gastrojejunostomy secondary to bile reflux. The Heineke-Mikulicz approach is most commonly used for routine cases, whereas the Finney pyloroplasty is best suited for a J-shaped stomach laying in the longitudinal axis. The latter is also preferred when ulcers are located in the second portion of the duodenum or when the duodenum and pylorus have been displaced secondary to extensive inflammation. In the most severe cases of inflammation and scarring of the pylorus, a Jaboulay gastroduodenostomy may be employed which bypasses the pylorus entirely. All described pyloroplasties may be accomplished laparoscopically, and each technique mirrors the open approach. Finally, consideration may be given to a decompressive gastrostomy and feeding jejunostomy at the time of operation depending on the clinical status of the patient.

Heineke-Mikulicz Pyloroplasty

1. Laparoscopic port placement or upper abdominal incision (transverse vs. vertical)
2. Traction sutures placed at the superior and inferior margins of the pyloric ring.
   (a) These should be placed in a position to ligate the pyloric vein if needed.
3. ~4 cm longitudinal full-thickness incision starting on prepyloric antrum halfway between the greater and lesser curvature – extended into the duodenum, transecting the pylorus (which should be the midpoint).
4. 3–0 silk interrupted seromuscular transverse closure.
   (a) Alternatively, this can be accomplished using a TA 30 stapler.
5. Test the suture line – compress distal duodenum and insufflate air via endoscopy or into NGT while suture line is submerged. Additional seromuscular sutures as needed.
6. Omental flap tacked over suture line (optional).

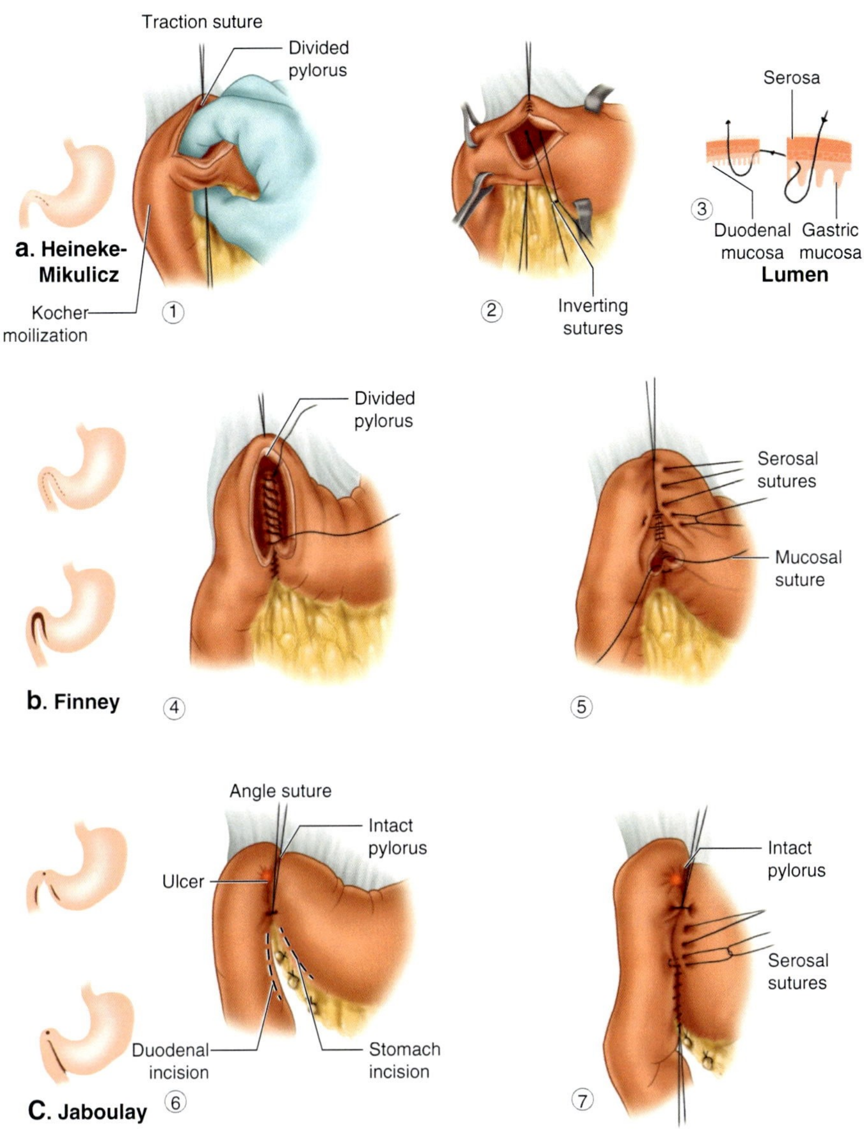

Fig. 57.1 Three alternative pyloroplasty procedures: (**a**) Heineke-Mikulicz – longitudinal opening with transverse closure. (**b**) Finney – incorporates the pylorus at the apex of the anastomosis. (**c**) Jaboulay gastroduodenostomy – completely bypasses the pylorus [5]

Finney U-Shaped Pyloroplasty (First Described 1902)

1. Laparoscopic port placement or upper abdominal incision (transverse vs. vertical).
2. Kocher maneuver.
3. 10–12 cm longitudinal gastroduodenostomy, transecting the pylorus, which should be at the midpoint of the incision.
4. Close in two layers as a side-to-side anastomosis with the pylorus at the apex.
   (a) Running silk on posterior outer layer, running absorbable suture on the inner layer, and then interrupted silk on the outer front layer.
5. Test the suture line – compress distal duodenum and insufflate air via endoscopy or into NGT while suture line is submerged.
6. Omental flap tacked over suture line (optional).

Jaboulay Gastroduodenostomy (First Described 1892)

1. Laparoscopic port placement or upper abdominal incision (transverse vs. vertical).
2. May require takedown of the hepatic flexure of the colon for exposure and wide Kocher maneuver.
3. Side-to-side 4–5 cm anastomosis between the greater curvature of the stomach and anterior proximal duodenum in the same two-layer fashion as the Finney.
   (a) May staple with a 45 mm linear cutting stapler and TA 30.
4. Test the suture line – compress distal duodenum and insufflate air via endoscopy or into NGT while suture line is submerged.
5. Omental flap tacked over suture line (optional).

Postoperative Management [6]

Continuous gastric suction is maintained until the third postoperative day or until there is clinical evidence of gastric emptying. An upper GI series may be considered if no progress has been made after that third postoperative day to evaluate for a potential leak and to objectively document gastric emptying. The usual care is that of any major foregut procedure and includes DVT prophylaxis, PPIs, and antiemetics. Once it has been determined clinically appropriate, six small feedings should be initiated in order to counter the distention that may occur with a denervated, atonic stomach. Occasionally, a self-limited diarrhea will develop. Clinically relevant and studied medications available to ameliorate this include cholestyramine, loperamide, and codeine. It has been suggested that sweet juice, as well as hot and cold liquids, should be avoided, especially at breakfast. Caffeinated beverage consumption should be minimized until the patient is symptom-free. The return to an unrestricted diet is determined by the patient's progress and resolution of symptoms. All attempts to eliminate smoking must be taken.

Postoperative Complications [7–9]

Complications of vagotomy have been described in the previous chapter; these include *injury to the phrenic vein*, *esophageal perforation*, *injury to the spleen*, *pneumothorax*, *aortic injury*, *injury to the thoracic duct*, *post-vagotomy diarrhea*, and *dysphagia*.

Complications related to the pyloroplasty are as follows:

Dumping Syndrome

Early dumping is considered if vasomotor symptoms of tachycardia, sweating, lightheadedness, and weakness accompanied by abdominal cramping and diarrhea occur within 30 min after eating. This phenomenon is caused by rapid bolus of hypertonic food bolus into the small bowel and is often relieved with recumbent positioning and diet modifications. Late dumping manifests as symptomatic hypoglycemia 2–3 h after eating and is caused by an initial postprandial hyperglycemic insulin surge. Typically this is alleviated by limiting high sugar foods in the diet.

Bile Reflux Gastritis

Most commonly this can be medically managed with metoclopramide or other prokinetic agents to increase gastric emptying or the addition of cholestyramine to bind bile acids. If medical management fails to resolve the symptoms, an additional operation – typically a Roux-en-Y gastrojejunostomy – is completed for bile reflux gastritis.

Inadequate Drainage Versus Delayed GI Function

Typically this is a self-limited problem, but if it continues, medical management with metoclopramide or other prokinetic agents to increase gastric emptying is employed. Similarly to bile reflux, if medical management fails to resolve the symptoms, an additional operation – typically a Roux-en-Y gastrojejunostomy – is completed.

Anastomotic Leak

Contained leaks in a stable patient are often treated with drainage (either by interventional radiology or in the operating room) and antibiotics. If uncontained or if the patient is unstable, early re-exploration with primary repair vs. diversion and/or Roux-en-Y gastrojejunostomy is the appropriate intervention.

Postoperative Outcomes

Acid reduction with vagotomy has been found to be upward of 70% basal and 50% stimulated; however these numbers are from a series of studies when maximal acid suppression therapy and *H. pylori* eradication were not the standard of care. The same holds true for the ulcer recurrence rate of 12% [10].

The first large series reported by Weinberg et al. in 1956 revealed a mortality rate of <0.5% with a recurrence risk of 7.3% up to 8 years after vagotomy and pyloroplasty [11]. A number of prospective, randomized trials comparing the various surgical options have a reported mortality rate of 0.5%–0.8% for the same procedure. The addition of pyloroplasty invites the potential complication of mild dumping in approximately 10% of patients, while only about 1% found this to be disabling. Separately, diarrhea was found to be mild and limited in 25% of patients, while 2% had continued disabling diarrhea [10].

References

1. Lagoo J, Pappas TN, Perez A. A relic or still relevant: the narrowing role for vagotomy in the treatment of peptic ulcer disease. Am J Surg. 2014;207(1):120–6.
2. de la Fuente SG, Khuri SF, Schifftner T, et al. Comparative analysis of vagotomy and drainage versus vagotomy and resection procedures for bleeding peptic ulcer disease: results of 907 patients from the Department of Veterans Affairs National Surgical Quality Improvement Program database. J Am Coll Surg. 2006;202:78.
3. Jordan PH Jr, Thornby J. Perforated pyloroduodenal ulcers. Long-term results with omental patch closure and parietal cell vagotomy. Ann Surg. 1995;221:479.
4. Csendes A, Maluenda F, Braghetto I, et al. Prospective randomized study comparing three surgical techniques for the treatment of gastric outlet obstruction secondary to duodenal ulcer. Am J Surg. 1993;166:45.
5. Zollinger RM, Zollinger RM. Atlas of surgical operations. New York: McGraw-Hill, Health Professions Division; 1993.
6. Evans SR, Chahine AA. Surgical pitfalls: prevention and management. Philadelphia, PA: Saunders/Elsevier; 2009.
7. Johnston D. Operative mortality and postoperative morbidity of highly selective vagotomy. Br Med J. 1975;4:545.
8. Hejazi RA, Patil H, McCallum RW. Dumping syndrome: establishing criteria for diagnosis and identifying new etiologies. Dig Dis Sci. 2010;55:117.
9. Frederiksen HJ, Johansen TS, Christiansen PM. Postvagotomy diarrhoea and dumping treated with reconstruction of the pylorus. Scand J Gastroenterol. 1980;15:245.
10. Greenfield LJ, Mulholland MW. Surgery: scientific principles and practice. Philadelphia: Lippincott Williams & Wilkins; 2001.
11. Weinberg JA, Stempien SJ, Movius HJ, Dagradi AE. Vagotomy and pyloroplasty in the treatment of duodenal ulcer. Am J Surg. 1956;92(2):202–7.

Surgical Management: Billroth I

58

Patrick James McLaren and James Patrick Dolan

Introduction

The surgical treatment of peptic ulcer disease (PUD) has declined significantly in recent decades due to the advent of *H. pylori* treatment, acid-suppressing medications, and endoscopic therapies [1]. Uncomplicated PUD can often be treated successfully with medical interventions. However, surgical management of ulcer disease still plays a role in refractory and complicated ulcer disease. The first large gastric resection with reconstruction was described by Theodor Billroth in 1885. In the following years, Dr. Billroth and colleagues conceived a number of surgical techniques for reconstruction following gastric resection. Among the most widely adopted and still used in practice today is the Billroth I gastroduodenostomy (B-I). The B-I procedure is a hemigastrectomy with gastroduodenostomy that restores the native configuration of the gastrointestinal tract. In this chapter we will discuss the indications, technique, management, complications, and expected outcomes of B-I reconstruction for PUD.

Indications

Surgical treatment of PUD is most often indicated for complications such as hemorrhage, perforation, and obstruction (Table 58.1) [1, 2]. Prepyloric and pyloric channel ulcers are the best candidates for antrectomy with B-I reconstruction [1]. Generally, antrectomy is reserved for Type II and III peptic ulcers and some distal Type I ulcers [1]. Antrectomy may be inadequate for NSAID-induced ulcers, GE

P. J. McLaren · J. P. Dolan (✉)
Department of Surgery, Division of Gastrointestinal and General Surgery, Oregon Health and Science University, Portland, OR, USA
e-mail: dolanj@ohsu.edu

J. Grams et al. (eds.), *The SAGES Manual of Foregut Surgery*,
https://doi.org/10.1007/978-3-319-96122-4_58

Table 58.1 Surgical indications for peptic ulcer disease

Surgical indications
Bleeding antral or duodenal ulcer
Perforated antral or duodenal ulcer
Large ulcer or ulcer causing gastric outlet obstruction
Ulceration refractory to medical management
Recurrent ulcer

junction ulcers, and proximal lesser curvature ulcers [1]. Furthermore, antrectomy may not address the underlying pathophysiology of these ulcers as they are not related to high acid secretion.

Elective indications for surgical resection include large ulcers, nonhealing ulcers, recurrent ulcers, and failure of medical management [1]. An ulcer causing obstructive symptoms should be expeditiously resected. Unnecessary delay to attempt medical management in the setting of obstruction may lead to worse outcomes due to poor nutrition. For acutely presenting bleeding or perforated ulcers, the decision to perform a gastric resection [1] depends on the stability of the patient. In an unstable patient, it is acceptable to delay definitive gastrectomy in favor of hemostasis, washout, simple patch closure, and resuscitation. When performing a gastric resection for PUD, a concurrent vagotomy should also be considered. The specifics of the proper vagotomy technique are discussed in previous chapters in this manual.

The B-I reconstruction offers some advantages over other popular reconstruction techniques. B-I is a simple reconstruction with a single anastomosis, without the need for an intestinal bypass or a blind loop. The gastroduodenal anastomosis of a B-I is less prone to marginal ulceration than the gastrojejunal anastomoses constructed in Billroth II (B-II) and Roux-en-Y configurations. Furthermore, some studies have demonstrated improved perioperative outcomes for B-I compared to Roux-en-Y [3, 4]. However, improved long-term outcomes like reflux esophagitis and alkaline gastritis are highest with a B-I reconstruction [5–9]. If adhesions, scarring, or patient anatomy does not allow for a tension-free gastroduodenal anastomosis, an alternative reconstruction technique should be used. No one gastric reconstruction is definitively superior, so the decision often depends on the clinical scenario and surgeon's preference.

Open Surgical Technique: Billroth I

Positioning and Exposure

The patient should be laid in the supine position, and a nasogastric an (NG) tube should be placed. Access to the peritoneum is gained through an upper midline incision extending from the xiphoid to the umbilicus. A self-retaining abdominal wall retractor is useful to maintain exposure. Slight reverse Trendelenberg positioning may aid in exposure [1, 10].

Mobilize the Stomach

In order to minimize tension on the gastroduodenal anastomosis, adequate mobilization of the stomach and duodenum is crucial. We recommend mobilization of the proximal stomach first. This is done by dividing the gastrophrenic and gastrosplenic ligaments. Care should be taken not to place too much traction on the spleen. Next, enter the lesser sac through the gastrocolic ligament approximately midway along the greater curvature. Divide any adhesions of the posterior gastric wall to pancreas sharply. Take care to minimize trauma to the pancreas, as this can lead to subsequent inflammation and postoperative complications. Carry the dissection distally along the greater curve between the gastric wall and the gastroepiploic artery in order to maintain this collateral blood supply to the future gastroduodenal anastomosis. Serially clamp and divide branches of the gastroepiploic artery as the dissection proceeds distally to the pylorus. Next, mobilize the lesser curvature. Enter the lesser omentum midway on the lesser curve. Proceed distally with the dissection ligating small branch vessels as they are encountered as close to the gastric wall as possible. Continue dissection until encountering the main branch of the right gastric artery. Divide and doubly ligate the right gastric artery using suture [1, 10].

Mobilize the Duodenum

Circumferentially mobilize the proximal 1 cm duodenum at the distal extent of your gastric dissection. Identify the common bile duct, gastroduodenal artery, and pancreas in order to avoid injury to these structures. Next perform a Kocher maneuver. Divide the lateral peritoneal attachments from the epiploic foramen proceeding inferiorly. The duodenum and head of the pancreas can then be elevated and rotated medially off the underlying vena cava, which marks the extent of the dissection. At this point both the stomach and duodenum should be freely mobile and a tension-free gastroduodenal anastomosis possible [1, 10].

Identify the Points of Gastric and Duodenal Division

We suggest a line of gastric division extending from the third vein distal to the gastroesophageal (GE) junction on the lesser curvature to the midpoint of the greater curvature where the gastroepiploic artery comes closest to the gastric wall. This technique is an approximately 40–50% gastrectomy [10]. There is significant anatomic variation between patients in distribution of the antral cells, but this technique should confidently remove the entire antrum. The distal line of division is in the first portion of the duodenum within 1 cm of the pylorus (Fig. 58.1) [1, 10].

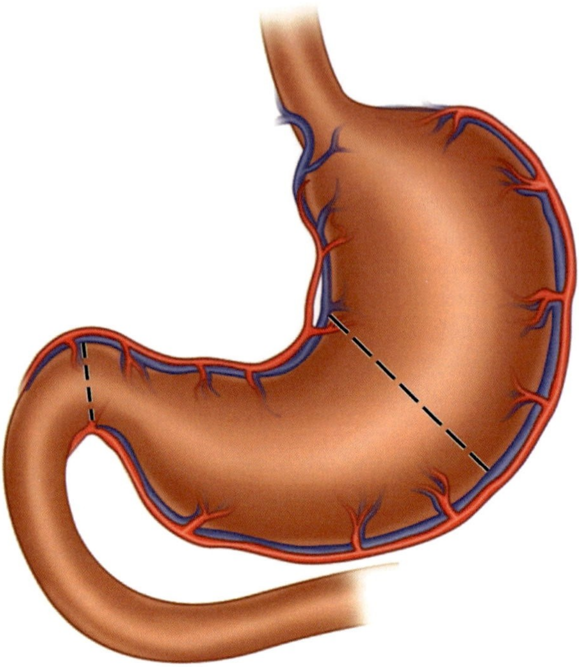

Fig. 58.1 The lines of gastric and duodenal division are depicted with dashed lines

Divide the Stomach and Duodenum

Instruct anesthesia to pull back the NG tube as the surgeon manually confirms the NG tube is proximal to the line of transection. The duodenum is then divided using a GIA stapler. Next, proceed to division of the stomach. Fire a stapling device along the predetermined line of gastric division, and remove the specimen from the field [1, 10].

Create the Gastroduodenal Anastomosis

The gastroduodenostomy is created in two layers, with an inner absorbable Vicryl and outer seromuscular silk sutures. First, with interrupted seromuscular silk sutures, approximate the posterior duodenal wall with the posterior gastric wall (Fig. 58.2). Excise the duodenal staple line and the inferior corner of the gastric staple line to create a gastrotomy with a diameter equal to the duodenum. Place a full-thickness inner layer of running absorbable suture (Fig. 58.3). Complete the anastomosis with an anterior layer of silk Lembert stitches.

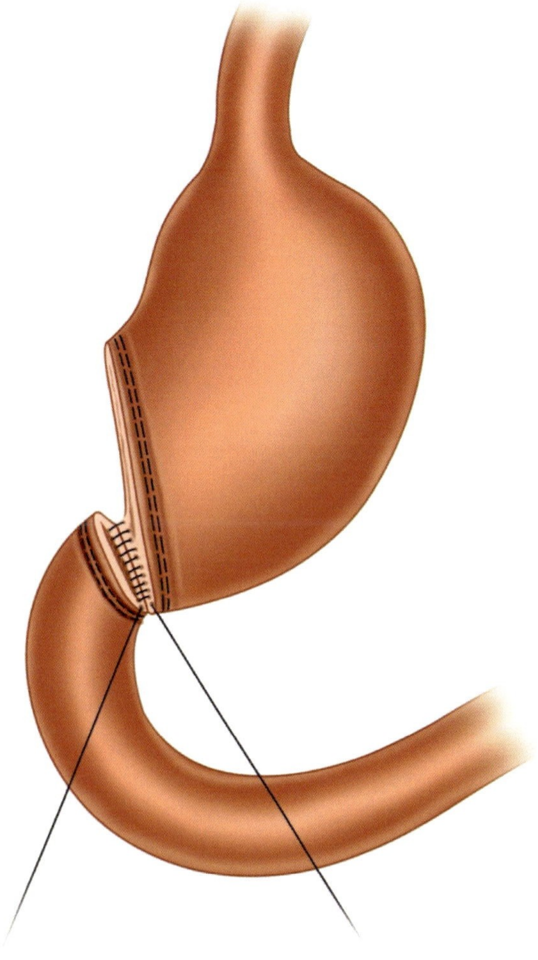

Fig. 58.2 The posterior walls of the duodenum and stomach are approximated with interrupted silk suture

The point where staple line and suture lines meet is sometimes prone to leakage and often called the "Angle of Sorrow." We recommend reinforcing this point with seromuscular bites of the duodenum and both sides of the lesser curvature with silk. Hemostasis and patency of the anastomosis should be checked endoscopically. A leak test can be performed with the anastomosis submerged and the stomach insufflated. If a leak is detected, additional sutures can be placed at this time. Once satisfied with the anastomotic integrity, the abdomen can be closed in standard fashion [1, 10].

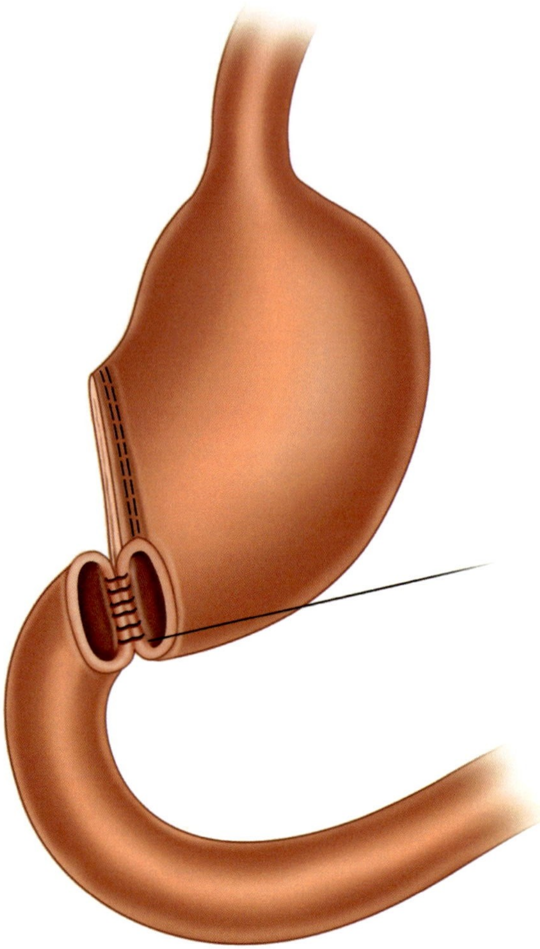

Fig. 58.3 The inner layer of the anastomosis is created with full-thickness running absorbable suture

Laparoscopic Surgical Technique: Billroth I

Patient Positioning and Port Placement

The patient is placed in the supine split-leg position with monitors at the head of the bed. The split-leg position allows the surgeon to operate from below and minimizes crowding at the operating table. Reverse Trendelenberg positioning is used to facilitate exposure. Port placement can vary and should be determined by patient body habitus. Figure 58.4 depicts our general guide for gastrectomy port placement [11].

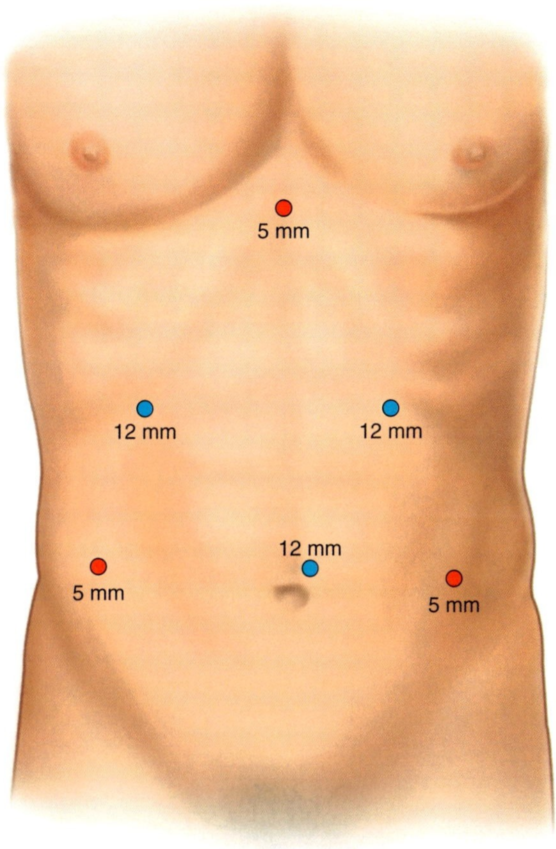

Fig. 58.4 Six ports are placed for laparoscopic gastrectomy. (Camera port 17 cm inferior to the xiphoid and just left of the umbilicus (12 mm). Left subcostal working port 12 cm from xiphoid and 2 cm below the costal margin (12 mm). Right subcostal working port 11 cm from xiphoid and 2 cm below the costal margin (12 mm). Subxiphoid port for a Nathanson liver retractor (5 mm). Right lateral working port (5 mm). Left lateral working port (5 mm))

Mobilize the Stomach and Duodenum

The initial mobilization of the stomach and duodenum do not differ greatly from the open procedure. Begin first by mobilizing the proximal stomach, then performing a Kocher maneuver. Using a laparoscopic vessel-sealing energy device, enter the lesser sac through the gastrocolic ligament, then retract the stomach cephalad and anteriorly, and divide pancreatic adhesions until the entire posterior wall is free. The greater curve can be dissected to level of the pylorus at this time [11].

Divide the Stomach

Lines of transection are the same as described previously. On the greater curve, the gastroepiploic vessels are divided using an energy device or stapler at the point of transection. A window in the gastro-hepatic ligament is made at the point of transection on the lesser curve. The stomach is then divided using a laparoscopic GIA stapler. This may require multiple staple loads to complete. Once the stomach is transected, the dissection is carried distally along the lesser curve toward the pylorus using a vessel-sealing energy device. The distal stomach can be reflected to the patient's right to aid exposure of the pylorus and duodenum. Dissection along the lesser curve is complete when the right gastric artery is identified and divided. The duodenum is then divided just distal to the pylorus using an endo-GIA stapler. The location of the gastroduodenal artery and common bile duct should be identified prior to division of the duodenum in order to avoid injury to these structures. A laparoscopic specimen bag can then be used to remove the specimen through a 12 mm trocar site. The fascial defect may require enlargement to allow removal of the specimen [11].

Laparoscopic Gastroduodenal Anastomosis

For laparoscopic B-I reconstruction, we prefer a stapled anastomosis. Using atraumatic laparoscopic graspers, bring the duodenal stump adjacent to the posterior gastric wall, and align the duodenal staple line with the inferior edge of the gastric staple line. Using electrocautery, create enterotomies in the stomach and duodenum. The enterotomies should be just large enough to accommodate the anvil and jaws of an endo-GIA stapler. Fire the stapler to create the anastomosis between the duodenum and stomach. The single common enterotomy is then closed using two layers running absorbable suture. Perform an endoscopic leak test as described above. De-sufflate the abdomen and close facial defects at all trocar sites larger than 10 mm [11].

Postoperative Management

The B-I patient can usually be managed on the surgical ward barring any major comorbidities. Standard DVT prophylaxis should be continued until discharge. Prophylactic postoperative antibiotics are not indicated, and Foley catheter can be removed on postoperative day #1. Early ambulation within postoperative day #1 and aggressive incentive spirometry is encouraged to minimize pulmonary complications. Postoperative intravenous fluid and electrolyte replacement should be provided until an oral diet is tolerated. A nasogastric tube is not necessary in all patients, but may be used in select cases for nausea or postoperative ileus. NG tube removal can be attempted on postoperative day #1. Clear liquid diet can usually be tolerated on postoperative day #1 and should be advanced slowly to six small meals per day [12]. Once tolerating PO intake, meals should be high in protein and fat but relatively low in carbohydrates to minimize dumping syndrome that can follow gastrectomy. We recommend the patient consult with a nutritionist prior to discharge to familiarize themselves with their dietary restrictions.

Postoperative Complications and Expected Outcomes

If maintained on acid-suppressing medications, antrectomy and vagotomy for PUD is permanently curative for ulcer disease in 97–98% of cases [1, 12]. However, between 5 and 15% of patients may experience some postoperative complication [1, 8, 11].

Early Complications

Early complications following gastrectomy include bleeding, ileus, and anastomotic leak [1, 2, 12]. Bleeding after antrectomy is usually intraluminal at the gastroduodenal anastomosis. Bright red blood in the nasogastric suction canister in conjunction with hematocrit drop or hemodynamic changes warrant an upper endoscopy. Bleeding from the anastomosis can usually be controlled with endoscopic coagulation or epinephrine injections. Rarely re-exploration in the operating room may be needed to control hemorrhage. Anastomotic leak is rare and occurs in less than 2% of patients [8]. A leak generally presents as tachycardia and abdominal pain followed by other signs of systemic inflammatory response. An ileus lasting more than 5 days postoperatively warrants workup for other causes. Contrast studies and plain film X-rays are the initial studies of choice to evaluate for obstruction and leak as potential sources of prolonged ileus.

Late Complications

Late complications include delayed gastric emptying, gastric dumping syndrome, alkaline reflux, and recurrent ulceration [1]. Delayed gastric emptying occurs in about 2% of patients but can usually be managed with prokinetic agents like metoclopramide [1]. Up to 15% of vagotomy and antrectomy patients experience some postprandial discomfort or dizziness, but clinically significant gastric dumping occurs in only 1–2% of patients [1]. High-fat, high-protein, and low-carbohydrate diets are usually successful in treating most cases of dumping syndrome. Somatostatin analogs may also be beneficial in refractory cases [2]. Alkaline reflux of duodenal contents into the stomach can cause gastritis in 5–15% of patients [1]. Symptoms include postprandial pain, nausea, and epigastric discomfort. Endoscopy demonstrates inflamed

Table 58.2 Postoperative complications following B-I resection for PUD

Early
Bleeding
Ileus
Anastomotic leak
Late
Delayed gastric emptying
Gastric dumping syndrome
Alkaline reflux
Recurrent ulceration

mucosa and bile in the stomach. Management is generally dietary modification, bile acid chelators, and antacids [2]. If severe pain persists, a revision with Roux-en-Y gastrojejunostomy should be considered. Finally, recurrent ulcers can occur in approximately 2–3% of patients who undergo a vagotomy and antrectomy [1]. Marginal ulceration on the intestinal side of anastomosis is more common with gastrojejunal anastomoses compared to the B-I configuration. The most common symptom of recurrent ulceration is abdominal pain that is worse with eating and relieved with antacid medications. Diagnosis is made via endoscopy; treatment is acid suppression and surgical revision if severe (Table 58.2).

References

1. Nussbaum M. Master techniques in surgery: gastric surgery: Wolters Kluwer Health; 2012.
2. Soriano IS, Dempsey DT. Chap. 21. Benign gastric disorders. In: Zinner MJ, Ashley SW, editors. Maingot's abdominal operations. New York: The McGraw-Hill Companies; 2013. p. 12e.
3. Imamura H, Takiguchi S, Yamamoto K, et al. Morbidity and mortality results from a prospective randomized controlled trial comparing Billroth I and Roux-en-Y reconstructive procedures after distal gastrectomy for gastric cancer. World J Surg. 2012;36(3):632–7.
4. Kumagai K, Hiki N, Nunobe S, et al. Different features of complications with Billroth-I and Roux-en-Y reconstruction after laparoscopy-assisted distal gastrectomy. J Gastrointest Surg. 2011;15(12):2145–52.
5. Inokuchi M, Kojima K, Yamada H, et al. Long-term outcomes of Roux-en-Y and Billroth-I reconstruction after laparoscopic distal gastrectomy. Gastric Cancer. 2013;16(1):67–73.
6. Kojima K, Yamada H, Inokuchi M, Kawano T, Sugihara K. A comparison of Roux-en-Y and Billroth-I reconstruction after laparoscopy-assisted distal gastrectomy. Ann Surg. 2008;247(6):962–7.
7. Lee MS, Ahn SH, Lee JH, et al. What is the best reconstruction method after distal gastrectomy for gastric cancer? Surg Endosc. 2012;26(6):1539–47.
8. Xiong JJ, Altaf K, Javed MA, et al. Roux-en-Y versus Billroth I reconstruction after distal gastrectomy for gastric cancer: a meta-analysis. World J Gastroenterol. 2013;19(7):1124–34.
9. Mai C, Tang Y, Zhao H, Tang H. Comparison of long-term outcomes between Billroth-I and Roux-en-Y reconstruction after distal gastrectomy. Zhonghua Wei Chang Wai Ke Za Zhi. 2014;17(5):449–52.
10. Skandalakis LJ, Skandalakis JE, Skandalakis PN. Surgical anatomy and technique : a pocket manual. 3rd ed. New York: Springer; 2009.
11. Hawn M. Operative techniques in foregut surgery: Wolters Kluwer Health; 2015.
12. Newman EL, Mulholland MW. Chap. 6. Operative management of gastric lesions. In: Minter RM, Doherty GM, editors. Current procedures: surgery. New York: The McGraw-Hill Companies; 2010.

Surgical Management: Billroth II

59

Jaclyn Wierzbicki and Peter Nau

Introduction

Partial gastrectomy is performed for a number of reasons including carcinoma, ulcer disease, and gastric outlet obstruction. Removal of a portion of the stomach is followed by a reconstruction to restore intestinal continuity. Several options exist, including Bilroth I (BI), Bilroth II (BII), and Roux-en-Y (REY). The BII gastrojejunostomy is the focus of this chapter. While the BI maintains the normal anatomic configuration, the resulting tension created by a gastroduodenostomy can be troublesome as it increases risk of leak or may lead surgeons to perform an inadequate resection in order to preserve proximal gastric length [1]. As a result of these concerns, the BII reconstruction was developed as a tension-free anastomosis between the stomach and jejunum brought up as a loop. This option was not without its own challenges, and a third option was conceived to ameliorate these issues. The REY, which seems less fraught with the complications seen in BII reconstruction, has become favored in recent literature. Despite concerns regarding the BII and the sequelae of this procedure, it still has a role in the armamentarium of the foregut surgeon. Individual patient factors must be taken into account when selecting a method for reconstruction, and the situations in which a BII may be the better option are outlined below.

J. Wierzbicki · P. Nau (✉)
Department of Surgery, The University of Iowa Hospitals and Clinics, Iowa City, IA, USA
e-mail: Peter-nau@uiowa.edu

J. Grams et al. (eds.), *The SAGES Manual of Foregut Surgery*,
https://doi.org/10.1007/978-3-319-96122-4_59

Advantages of the Billroth II Reconstruction

When choosing between procedures for restoring the continuity of the GI tract, the surgeon must weigh the pros and cons of each technique (Table 59.1). There are several patient-centered considerations that would favor the BI reconstruction. Performing intestinal reconstructions on the multiply operated abdomen can be problematic. Incidence of adhesions increases with number of abdominal operations, and the risk of inadvertent enterotomy is 6% when adhesiolysis must be performed [2]. The Billroth II is a technically straightforward procedure to perform in the setting of extensive abdominal adhesions limiting small bowel mobility. The jejunal loop selected must be able to reach the stomach, while other adhesions can be left in place. For a REY reconstruction, adhesiolysis must be performed to accurately measure the afferent and efferent limbs and also to achieve the necessary length for a tension-free anastomosis. In the event that adhesions are particularly dense and unintentional bowel injury is a concern, a BII is a reasonable alternative to avoid much of the obligatory adhesiolysis. Additionally, the prognosis and vitality of the patient may be a factor to consider. If a patient has limited physiologic reserve and expeditious completion of the case is necessary, the speed of a BII reconstruction may be the preferred approach.

In addition to patient-oriented decision, technical concerns may favor the application of a BII reconstruction. The BII classically entails a single anastomosis. Unlike a REY which requires both a gastrojejunostomy (GJ) and a jejunojejunostomy (JJ), the GJ can be performed alone. With that said, in order to avoid alkaline reflux from the afferent limb, a Braun enteroenterostomy between the afferent and efferent limbs is recommended when performing a BII [3]. Thus the appeal of the single anastomosis may only be advantageous in situations where the benefit of limiting new bowel connections outweighs the risk of reflux. The anatomy of a BII may be preferable when endoscopic access to the biliary tree is anticipated. Following partial gastrectomy, the classic transgastric approach to the proximal duodenum can be prohibitively difficult outside of a BI reconstruction. When the extent of gastric resection prohibits use of this method, BII or REY are the remaining options. Though laparoscopic access to a remnant stomach has allowed endoscopic retrograde cholangiopancreatography (ERCP) to be performed in patients with gastric bypass, the REY reconstruction in the setting of partial gastric resection lacks even this option. ERCP in this population becomes difficult if not impossible as the endoscope must be directed down the Roux limb, through the jejunojejunostomy and retrograde through the biliopancreatic limb. With BII reconstruction, endoscopic intubation of the afferent limb provides a direct path to the

Table 59.1 Advantages and disadvantages of Billroth II reconstruction

Advantages	Disadvantages
Simpler in setting of multiply operated abdomen with adhesions	Bile reflux
Access of biliary tree	Afferent loop syndrome
Avoidance of complications associated with REY	Ulcers
	Gastric remnant carcinoma

biliopancreatic tree. Though the approach in either case is still from the distal duodenum and opposite of conventional ERCP, it is a more direct route with BII anatomy compared with REY.

When choosing between surgical options, it is also necessary to consider complications of the alternate reconstruction options. The morbidities of a BII will be discussed later in this chapter. With that said, it is important to note that the REY does have complications not seen in BII. Roux stasis is isolated to the REY anatomy. Symptoms include abdominal pain, nausea, vomiting, and postprandial bloating. It is estimated to occur in up to 30% of patients and is thought to result from disruption of electrical signaling involved in bowel motility [4]. Though evidence for this is debated, it prompts careful consideration of the reconstructive options in the setting of a patient with known bowel motility issues. When the REY is not an option, deciding between Billroth I and II is usually based on the extent of the resection. While BI maintains the normal physiologic path for food to travel, the more stomach taken for adequate resection translates to increased likelihood of tension on a BI anastomosis and thus higher chance of leak [1]. Certainly there is no option that is free of potential morbidity. Given this, it is important to consider the specific issues with each alternative prior to committing to an operation.

Technique

A Billroth II gastrojejunostomy can be approached both laparoscopically and open. Gastric surgery is increasingly being performed with minimally invasive techniques and has been proven safe even in the setting of gastric cancers.

Laparoscopy

Patients undergoing partial gastrectomy with Billroth II reconstruction laparoscopically are placed supine. The legs can be kept straight or in split-leg position depending on the surgeon's preference to stand on the patient's right or between the legs. The decision to tuck arms is also at the discretion of the surgeon. Preoperative endoscopy may be performed to localize pathology and orient port sites. A 12 mm port for a 30 ° laparoscope is utilized through a site just cephalad and to the left of the umbilicus. Working ports are selected based on the operative plan and moved further to the left and superiorly if more proximal dissection of the stomach is needed. After placement of the camera port, additional working ports are oriented to allow for unhindered access to the pathology in the left upper quadrant (Fig. 59.1). Once the ports are in place, the patient is placed in steep reverse Trendelenburg, and a liver retractor is positioned to optimize visualization of the foregut [5].

Given the variety of indications for a distal gastrectomy and the associated extent of lymph node harvest, a complete discussion on the technique of a partial gastrectomy is beyond the scope of this chapter. In short, the greater curve of the stomach is mobilized from the gastrocolic ligament distally toward the pylorus and proximally

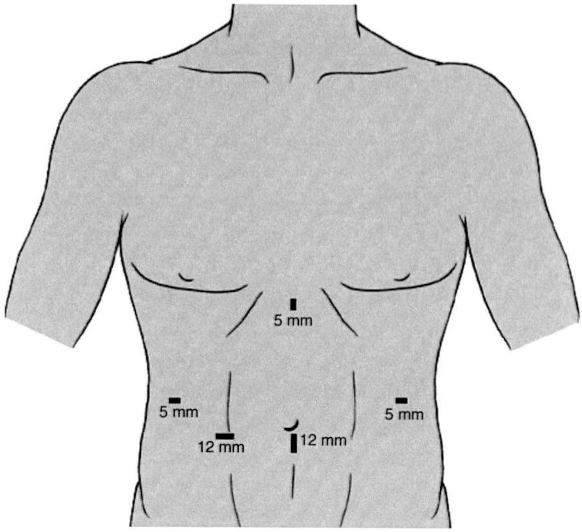

Fig. 59.1 Port placement for laparoscopic Billroth II anastomosis. 12 mm camera port near umbilicus. Lateral 12 mm port on right for stapling and suturing devices. 5 mm right-sided port for operating surgeon. 5 mm assist port on left. Optional 5 mm liver retractor port in the epigastrium

beyond the lesion to be resected. The gastrohepatic ligament is opened to enter the lesser sac, and the lesser curve is similarly dissected toward the pylorus and GE junction. Posterior attachments to the stomach are divided to free the stomach. Endoscopic staplers are used to divide the stomach distal to the pylorus. The location for division of the proximal stomach is determined by pathology and is also performed with linear staplers. Several loads may be needed and depend on the level at which the transection is performed. Once the stomach is resected, reconstruction is performed [5].

For an intracorporeal Billroth II, a jejunal loop can be brought up in a retrocolic or antecolic fashion. Antecolic is the preferred technique as it eliminates creation of an additional site for internal hernia through the transverse mesocolon and avoids risk of injury to colonic blood supply. The antecolic technique does pose a risk for additional tension as the loop must travel over the bulk of the colon. To decrease this possibility, the omentum is divided and a path for the jejunal loop is created. This division of the omentum is continued cephalad toward the transverse colon and then laterally, splitting it into two tongues to create adequate space anterior to the colon for the jejunal loop to reach the proximal stomach staple line.

Having divided the omentum, the ligament of Treitz is again identified, and a site for the gastrojejunostomy is selected approximately 35 cm distal to this landmark. The jejunal limb is brought over the colon between the divided omentum. The jejunal limb is oriented so that it is isoperistaltic. A stay suture is placed between the jejunum and gastric staple line. A posterior suture line is created from left to right with an absorbable suture. Next, a gastrotomy and an enterotomy are made on the medial aspect of the suture line. The interior row of the anastomosis is created with a linear stapler fired through these defects. The common gastroenterostomy is closed with a running absorbable suture. An imbricating anterior row is performed in a running fashion with absorbable suture. Once complete, a leak test is performed by insufflating via an orogastric tube or endoscope while submerging the anastomosis under saline.

Open

In the open technique, the stomach is approached through a midline incision with the patient supine. Dissection and mobilization of the stomach mirrors that which is performed using a laparoscopic technique. The distal margin of the partial gastrectomy is typically two centimeters past the pylorus, and the proximal extent of the resection is dictated by the pathology. With a BII gastrojejunostomy, there is much less tension than a BI, and the proximal extent of resection is decided based on pathology and is free from the conflicting goals of an adequate margin and tension-free reconstruction. Division of the stomach is performed using a linear stapler. Currently, there is no consensus as to the utility of oversewing the duodenal stump and the stomach staple lines. At the time of resection, concurrent truncal vagotomy can be considered in the case of ulcer disease secondary to acid hypersecretion.

The BII reconstruction is performed by bringing a jejunal loop to the greater curve of the remaining stomach. The jejunum is measured from the ligament of Treitz and a site 35 cm distal to this structure is selected. This loop can be brought either retrocolic or antecolic and the gastrojejunostomy is performed. There are several described techniques including anastomoses that are handsewn or fashioned with stapling devices. Prior to closure of the GJ, a nasogastric tube can be advanced past the anastomosis if needed [1].

Braun Enterostomy

Once the BII GJ anastomosis is completed, a Braun enteroenterostomy between the ascending and descending loops can be considered. The enteroenterostomy is created 30 cm distal to the gastrojejunostomy. This second anastomosis connects the afferent to the efferent limb and is utilized to prevent bile reflux and direct alkaline contents away from the stomach. This can be performed in a side-to-side fashion by either open or laparoscopic technique [1].

Postoperative Management

Immediately following a BII reconstruction, the patient is initially kept NPO. Nasogastric decompression is most beneficial in the setting of gastric outlet obstruction as a degree of transient gastroparesis is often seen in this population. With that said, a nasogastric tube may be placed at the discretion of the surgeon based upon patient risk factors. Perioperative antibiotics should be administered according to Surgical Care Improvement Program (SCIP) Guidelines. Redosing of antibiotics should be completed based on operative time. Typically no drains are required. The gastric tube can be removed in 1–2 days if placed, and PO liquids can generally be started around postoperative day 2. In the situation where a patient is unable to take oral intake, an NGT advanced beyond the anastomosis can be used as early feeding access [1].

Postoperative Complications

The mortality of a partial gastrectomy is approximately 1–2% and is independent of the reconstruction type. Mortality increases if the procedure is done emergently. Gastric resections performed for ulcer disease may be complicated by ulcer recurrence 1–4% of the time. Bleeding occurs in 2% of cases and anastomotic leak ranges from 1 to 4% [1]. Postgastrectomy morbidities may occur when a Billroth II reconstruction is performed. Many of these complications are not unique to the BII, though the frequency may vary between reconstruction options.

Nutritional Deficiency

Following removal of the stomach or a portion of it, nutritional deficiencies such as iron, calcium, vitamin B12, and folate are common (Table 59.2). Microcytic anemia from iron deficiency is the most common cause of anemia after gastric resection. It is related to bypassing the duodenum which is the primary site of iron absorption and is seen in both BII and REY reconstructions. Decreased gastric acidity is also thought to have a role. Ferritin levels are an accurate indicator of deficiencies and oral supplementation with elemental iron effectively treats the deficit. Megaloblastic anemia can also be seen after gastrectomy. Intrinsic factor (IF) produced in the stomach is decreased after gastrectomy. Decreased availability of IF to bind with

Table 59.2 Nutritional deficiencies

Nutrient	Site of absorption	Clinical presentation	Monitoring	Treatment
Iron	Duodenum	Microcytic anemia	Serum ferritin	PO elemental iron
Calcium	Duodenum, proximal jejunum	Osteoporosis, osteopenia, osteomalacia	Serum calcium, Serum 25-OHD vitamin D, Bone mineral density (DEXA)	PO calcium and PO vitamin D
B12	Terminal ileum, requires IF binding	Megaloblastic anemia, lassitude, fatigability, chills, numbness in extremities, dizziness, and neurological symptoms	Serum vitamin B12	PO or IM vitamin B12
Folate	Jejunum	Megaloblastic anemia	RBC folate, Vitamin B12 should be checked to avoid masking deficiency by folate supplementation	PO folate
Copper	Proximal duodenum	Ataxia, myelopathy, peripheral neuropathy	Serum copper	IV and PO copper supplements

B12 leads to malabsorption in the terminal ileum. Folate deficiency, another cause of megaloblastic anemia, can also be seen after gastrectomy, and supplementation of both is recommended to avoid masking a deficiency of the other. The BII and REY reconstructions both lead to increased bone disease like osteoporosis related to impaired calcium absorption when the duodenum is bypassed. Patients should be given calcium supplements as well as vitamin D [6]. Copper deficiency can occur since it is absorbed in the proximal duodenum leading to ataxia, myelopathy, and peripheral neuropathy [7]. Due to the nutritional implications of gastrectomy, close follow-up is necessary, and patients should have baseline nutritional labs checked before surgery with periodic monitoring post-op.

Dumping Syndrome

Loss of gastric regulation can cause rapid gastric emptying and can occur early or late. Early gastric emptying occurs within 30 min of a meal and manifests as crampy abdominal pain, diarrhea, lightheadedness, and tachycardia. It results from hyperosmolar solute emptying into the small intestine and is reproducible with oral glucose challenge. Late gastric emptying happens approximately 2 h after meal ingestion and is related to hypoglycemia subsequent to inappropriately high levels of insulin secreted in response to ingested glucose loads. This syndrome can occur not just in BII but with any reconstruction, though the incidence may be lower in those with a REY [4]. Patients with dumping syndrome can alleviate symptoms with dietary modifications including small frequent meals, avoiding sweets and avoidance of liquids with meals [1]. Symptoms of hypoglycemia can be managed with medications like acarbose in cases of late dumping. Somatostatin analogs can help both early and late dumping as it has a variety of effects including inhibiting insulin release. Severe cases may require conversion to a REY [7].

Afferent Loop Syndrome

Afferent loop syndrome is unique to BII anatomy. Patients with this rare syndrome present with colicky right upper quadrant pain which progressively worsens and culminates with vomiting that provides instantaneous pain relief. Imaging may demonstrate a chronically dilated afferent limb, or postprandial ultrasound can confirm the diagnosis of acute distension of the afferent limb. Treatment is conversion to Roux-en-Y if technically feasible. An alternative would be Braun enterostomy if revision of the gastrojejunostomy is prohibitively difficult [4].

Delayed Gastric Emptying

Severe delays in gastric emptying are quite rare. In those who undergo a truncal vagotomy in addition to partial gastrectomy, the incidence of gastric stasis is 3–5%.

Patients report postprandial bloating and fullness that lasts hours after oral intake. They may also regurgitate undigested food hours to days later. Patients can develop bezoars and bacterial overgrowth and demonstrate intolerance to solids while liquids empty normally or rapidly [6]. Endoscopic evaluation of patients with previous gastrectomy shows retained food in 21% after an overnight fast. The incidence is highest in those with B1 reconstruction, though the significance is unclear. Diet modification or prokinetic drugs can be tried but have variable success. Patients rarely go on to require completion gastrectomy for this condition [4].

Bile Reflux Esophagitis

Patients with this syndrome present with abdominal pain, bilious vomiting, and even weight loss. The symptoms result from the reflux of alkaline fluid into the stomach leading to gastritis. Aside from inflammation seen on endoscopy, the diagnosis can also be made with a technetium biliary scan which demonstrates bile reflux into the stomach. The syndrome is overwhelmingly associated with BII anatomy, occurring in approximately 70% of patients. Repeated studies have shown that bile reflux is significantly decreased in REY reconstruction compared with both BI and BII. Though bile reflux occurs quite frequently, not all patients have debilitating effects related to it. Medical management includes many strategies including bile absorption with cholestyramine, antacid therapy, and coating medications like sucralfate [8]. Symptoms may also be managed by changing bile acid composition with ursodeoxycholic acid [9]. The effectiveness of these treatments is debated, but for patients who suffer significantly, conversion to REY often alleviates their symptoms. Other surgical options include Braun enterostomy and jejunal interposition loop [4].

Ulcers

Anastomotic ulcers can occur in both BII and REY reconstruction. Patients may present with epigastric pain, bloating, and nausea. Bleeding can result in anemia and occult blood in the stool. Recurrent ulcers in patients with peptic ulcer disease are possible and may result from incomplete vagotomy. Nonsteroidal anti-inflammatory drugs (NSAIDs) and exposure to tobacco use can also cause ulcers. Less common reasons include Zollinger-Ellison syndrome and retained antrum. In the latter scenario, antral G cells present in the duodenal stump are bathed in alkaline fluid which results in continued gastrin production. Gastrin prompts parietal cells in the proximal stomach to continuously secrete acid. The jejunal side of the gastrojejunostomy lacks protective agents produced by gastric mucosa and is prone to marginal ulcer formation [4]. The diagnosis can be made by checking serum gastrin levels and a [99mTc] pertechnetate scan. While more invasive, endoscopy with biopsy of the duodenal stump can also establish the diagnosis. Medical treatment focuses on acid reduction with medications such as proton pump inhibitors. In the setting of persistent symptoms, revision may be required in the form of duodenal cuff resection [7]. The retained-antrum syndrome remains quite rare but is a reminder that care should be taken to ensure all gastric tissue is resected. Outside of this condition, ulcers should be managed nonoperatively with acid suppression and avoidance of inciting factors such as very acidic foods, NSAIDs, and tobacco exposure. Symptoms can be managed with coating agents like sucralfate.

Gastric Remnant Carcinoma

The risk of developing gastric remnant cancer has been investigated for many years, and several studies have endeavored to establish a difference in the risk profile for this morbidity between reconstruction types. Though it has been difficult to tease out the true risk associated with each, it does seem that, regardless of reconstruction type, patients who underwent resections performed for ulcer disease are at higher risk compared with other benign indications. A Swedish study did show an increased risk of developing cancer in the remnant when a BII is performed compared with B1. This was thought to be due to alkaline exposure which has been shown to increase risk of cancer in animal models [4].

Conclusion

A review of the recent literature investigating reconstruction options after partial gastrectomy appears to favor Roux-en-Y. Though REY has improved quality of life measures and decreased incidence of certain complications when compared with the BII, it is not always the best option for every patient requiring partial gastrectomy. The Billroth II reconstruction is still a useful adjunct for the foregut surgeon, and in the setting of dense adhesive disease, need for biliary access or other patient-specific circumstances remains a relevant reconstructive option which can be performed with either open or laparoscopic techniques. Furthermore, though REY may be favored in the future, there remains a large patient population with Billroth II anatomy. Understanding the complications seen in Billroth II reconstruction remains relevant to surgeons who may provide care for these patients.

References

1. Bumm R, Siewert JR. Distal gastrectomy with Billroth I or Billroth II reconstruction. Mastery of surgery. 6th ed; p. 986–95. Philadelphia: Wolters Kluwer, 2011.
2. ten Broek RP, Issa Y, van Santbrink EJ, et al. Burden of adhesions in abdominal and pelvic surgery: systematic review and met-analysis. BMJ. 2013;347:f5588.
3. Vogel SB, Drane WE, Woodward ER. Clinical and radionuclide evaluation of bile diversion by Braun enteroenterostomy: prevention and treatment of alkaline reflux gastritis. An alternative to Roux-en-Y diversion. Ann Surg. 1994;219(5):458–65; discussion 65–6.
4. Bolton JS, Conway WC II. Postgastrectomy syndromes. Surg Clin N Am. 2011;91:1105–22.
5. Yang H, Kong S, Hope W, Kercher K, Heniford BT. Laparoscopic resection for gastric adenocarcinoma. Mastery of endoscopic and laparoscopic surgery. 4th ed; p. 235–55. Philadelphia: Lippincott Williams and Wilkins, 2014.

6. Radigan AE. Post-gastrectomy: managing the nutrition fall-out. Practical gastroenterology, Nutrition issues in gastroenterology, series #18; p. 63–75. New York: Mahl, 2004.
7. Kate V, Kalayarasan R, Elamurugan TP, Ananthakrishnan N. Surgery for peptic ulcer disease. Textbook of surgical gastroenterology. p. 283–99. New Delhi: Jaypee Brothers Medical Publishers, 2016.
8. Madura JA. Primary bile reflux gastritis: diagnosis and surgical treatment. Am J Surg. 2001;186:269–73.
9. Stefaniwsky AB, Tint GS, Speck J, Shefer S, Salen G. Ursodeoxycholic acid treatment of bile reflux gastritis. Gastroenterology. 1985;89(5):1000–4.

Surgical Management: Roux-en-Y Reconstruction

60

Leonard K. Welsh Jr. and Kenric M. Murayama

Introduction

History

Peptic ulcer disease was once the most common indication for gastric surgery until the development and adoption of potent antisecretory medications [1]. Partial gastrectomy removes the portion of the stomach containing the ulcer, the gastrin-producing cells that stimulate acid secretion, and a variable number of acid-producing parietal cells depending upon the extent of the resection. Reconstruction of the stomach is necessary following partial gastrectomy to re-establish gastrointestinal continuity. The Billroth I, Billroth II, and Roux-en-Y reconstruction techniques are the most common.

The Roux-en-Y gastrointestinal anastomosis is a valuable and versatile technique used in the reconstruction and drainage of the stomach, esophagus, and biliary tree. The Swiss surgeon César Roux first published the operation in 1893 in a case series of 29 gastrectomies performed between 1888 and 1893 with the intent of relieving gastric outlet obstruction [2]. He would later describe his reconstruction as the "ANSA en Y" anastomosis in an 1897 article detailing his first 50 gastroenterostomies, describing his observations from all 50 patients, along with general discussion of the surgical indications, approaches, and problems particularly observed with the gastroenterostomy.

The operation remained relatively unchanged for over a century; however, due to the high rate of marginal ulcers, the Roux-en-Y was largely abandoned by surgeons during the first half of the twentieth century and subsequently left out of many surgical textbooks. It has been readopted for treatment of postgastrectomy complications

L. K. Welsh Jr. · K. M. Murayama (✉)
Department of Surgery, University of Hawaii John A. Burns School of Medicine, Honolulu, HI, USA
e-mail: kenricm@hawaii.edu; http://jabsom.hawaii.edu

J. Grams et al. (eds.), *The SAGES Manual of Foregut Surgery*,
https://doi.org/10.1007/978-3-319-96122-4_60

after advances in gastric physiology led to surgical control of gastric acidity with vagotomy and acid-reducing medications [3]. The operation, currently widely performed for many indications, has gained increasing popularity and notoriety by the general public due to its application in bariatric surgery.

This chapter will discuss some indications for a Roux-en-Y reconstruction related to peptic ulcer disease and gastric outlet obstruction, common techniques, and subsequent management.

Indications

Elective surgery is uncommon for peptic ulcer disease in light of current medical treatments. The most common indications for elective and emergency surgery include bleeding, perforation, obstruction, intractable disease, and suspected malignancy [4].

Bleeding is the most common complication of peptic ulcer disease requiring hospitalization occurring in nearly 75% of patients compared to 9% and 3% for perforation and obstruction, respectively [5]. Most patients with acute bleeding can be managed with fluid resuscitation and transfusion, acid suppression therapy, and endoscopic intervention. For those who fail these efforts, surgery may become necessary.

Ulcer perforation may be suspected in patients with a history consistent with peptic ulcer disease who develop the sudden onset of severe, diffuse abdominal pain. Once a diagnosis of perforation is established, surgical intervention is indicated.

Peptic ulcer disease was once the most common cause of gastric outlet obstruction, accounting for up to 90 percent of cases, but is now the least common [6–8]. Both acute and chronic ulcers can result in obstruction, and surgical consultation is obtained for chronic partial obstruction that is refractory to medical treatment or those found to have complete gastric outlet obstruction. Surgery is usually reserved for patients that fail to respond to conservative medical management and endoscopic therapy.

Failure of medical treatment as an indication for elective gastric surgery is increasingly unusual. Severe symptoms, failure to heal on medical therapy, and relapse while on acid reduction therapy may indicate the need for surgical intervention. Noncompliance with proton pump inhibitors, persistent *H. pylori* infection, continued smoking, and nonsteroidal anti-inflammatory use all contribute to refractory ulcerative disease [9]. Gastrinoma should be excluded before performing elective surgery [10], and malignancy should be suspected for a gastric ulcer that has failed to heal after 12 weeks of medical therapy. Resection is indicated even if biopsies are benign [11].

Historically the Roux-en-Y gained popularity as a reconstructive operation after gastrectomy yet, unfortunately, fell out of favor due to high complication rates. Gastric cancer is one of the most common cancers worldwide, and surgical resection remains the only option for definitive treatment of this malignant disease [12]. Laparoscopic gastrectomy for gastric cancer has increased in popularity due to advances in surgical techniques, and recent studies have demonstrated similar oncologic results with laparoscopic gastrectomies compared to open approaches [13–17].

Gastrectomy Reconstruction

The three main reconstruction techniques after distal or subtotal gastrectomy are gastroduodenal anastomosis (Billroth I), gastrojejunal anastomosis (Billroth II), and Roux-en-Y gastrojejunostomy. Billroth II and Roux-en-Y anastomoses are recognized as standard reconstruction procedures after distal gastrectomy. The Billroth I reconstruction is often complicated by gastroesophageal and duodenogastric reflux [18] in addition to severe gastritis, esophagitis, and recurrent gastric cancer [19, 20]. Additionally, a Billroth I is not indicated after a subtotal gastrectomy due to anastomotic tension. In many situations a Roux-en-Y reconstruction after a distal gastrectomy has become increasingly more common as the procedure is successful in preventing reflux and has proven suitable for laparoscopy [21]. It is the reconstruction method of choice in total gastrectomy [22] as the advantages of improved postoperative quality of life and decreased morbidity supersede the potential postoperative complications due to two gastrointestinal anastomoses and increased operating time [23].

Despite this data, many surgeons continue to choose a Billroth II reconstruction likely due to concerns about morbidity as a Roux-en-Y reconstruction is commonly viewed as a complicated procedure with more anastomoses and a duodenal stump [22]. Although Roux-en-Y patients experience less reflux than noted in Billroth reconstructions, patients report dumping symptoms to a greater extent.

Conversion for Bile Reflux

Postgastrectomy bilious vomiting and abdominal pain have been described since the first successful procedures were performed in the late 1800s by Theodor Billroth. Bile reflux gastritis is most commonly seen after Billroth II reconstruction as a consequence of a nonfunctional pyloric channel and exposure of the gastric mucosa to bile, pancreatic secretions, and duodenal contents. Bile reflux incidence following Billroth II anastomosis in published series ranges from 40% to 79% [24, 25]. It is known that the syndrome can also occur after subtotal gastrectomy and Billroth I anastomosis, as well as following truncal vagotomy and drainage with either a pyloroplasty or gastrojejunostomy [25].

Symptoms include burning epigastric pain, bilious emesis, oral aversion, and weight loss. Pain is unrelieved by acid suppression and is aggravated by both oral intake and the recumbent position. Bile reflux gastritis is often a diagnosis of exclusion owing to the low specificity of endoscopic and histologic findings [25].

In healthy individuals, many anatomical structures play a role in preventing gastroesophageal reflux including the lower esophageal sphincter, diaphragm, abdominal esophagus, and the corrugation of the esophagogastric mucosal junction [26]. These reflux-preventive systems are disrupted by gastric surgery leading to reflux into the esophagus. Alkaline reflux is caused by reflux of pancreatic secretions and bile. In patients undergoing distal gastrectomy for gastric cancer, gastric hydrochloric acid secretion is generally reduced because of extensive resection of the glandular gastric fundus and dissection of the vagus nerve due to lymph node dissection. Therefore, the main aggravating factor for reflux esophagitis is believed to be duodenal reflux into the stomach [27]. A Roux-en-Y anastomosis with an appropriate 40 cm length Roux limb results in almost no reflux of duodenal secretions into the stomach and is unlikely to cause reflux esophagitis [27, 28]. Medical management of bile reflux gastritis typically includes prokinetic agents, cholestyramine, and dietary modification. The aim of surgery is to divert duodenal contents away from the gastric remnant and can be accomplished by creation or conversion to Roux-en-Y gastrojejunostomy with a Roux limb of at least 40 cm [27]. This is associated with symptomatic relief in up to 85% of patients [28].

Technique

Gastrectomy with Roux-en-Y Reconstruction

Preoperative work-up will vary depending on the appropriate indication and diagnosis. Endoscopic studies may be required in addition to imaging. Preoperative systemic antibiotics should be given according to established guidelines. The blood volume should be restored, especially in patients with long-standing complaints and loss of considerable weight.

In the setting of a gastrectomy for carcinoma or other indications and a Roux-en-Y reconstruction has been selected, a proper exploration to rule out metastatic disease and adequate dissection and division of the stomach should be performed. Subsequently a segment of jejunum approximately 20 cm distal to the ligament of Treitz is selected. A window in the mesentery is created and the bowel is divided with a linear stapler. The distal limb of the intestine is again brought either antecolic or through a mesenteric defect behind the transverse colon to the gastric remnant. The mesentery usually needs to be divided perpendicular to the bowel to create enough length while preserving adequate blood supply to the bowel. A gastrojejunostomy can be constructed with absorbable sutures in a full-thickness single-layer anastomosis or in two layers with an inner layer of running 3-0 absorbable suture and imbricated with an outer layer of interrupted silk sutures. A stapled gastrojejunostomy anastomosis is also acceptable.

The pancreatobiliary anastomosis is constructed by identifying a segment of the jejunum approximately 40–45 cm distal from the gastrojejunostomy. This anastomosis is most easily performed in a side-to-side fashion, either stapled or hand sewn depending on surgeon preference.

Billroth Conversion

The skin of the lower chest as well as the abdomen is prepared in a routine manner, and for an open approach, the incision may be made through an old scar from the previous operation. The incision may need to extend cephalad for adequate exposure and exploration of the gastroesophageal junction to determine the adequacy of a previous vagotomy. Even when a previous vagotomy has been performed, it is advisable to search for overlooked vagal fibers, especially the posterior vagus nerves, unless firm adhesions between the undersurface of the left lobe of the liver and upper stomach make such a search too hazardous. The previous gastrojejunostomy is freed to permit careful inspection and palpation for evidence of ulceration or stenosis or evidence of long loop, angulations, or partial obstruction of the jejunostomy.

The extent of the previous resection must be determined to be certain that the antrum has been resected for prevention of retained-antrum syndrome. A complete vagotomy as well as antrectomy is recommended as a safeguard against recurrent ulceration [29–31].

When a Billroth I procedure is to be converted, it is essential to carefully dissect the anastomosis both anterior and posterior before applying clamps. Often mobilization and medial rotation of the duodenum were previously performed to reduce tension on the suture line, and it is important to maintain as much duodenum as possible while minimizing the amount of further mobilization in order to reduce the risk of injury to the ampulla in the first portion of the duodenum. The proximal duodenum can then be transected with either a linear cutting stapler or with a row of interrupted sutures. This suture line is then reinforced with a second layer of interrupted silk sutures.

A section of the jejunum 40–50 cm distal from the ligament of Treitz is selected and transected with either a linear cutting stapler or with a scalpel and closed with a double layer of sutures. The suture or staple line is imbricated again with interrupted silk sutures. Special care should be taken to ensure that the corners are securely approximated. A retrocolic anastomosis can be created by passing the distal limb through an opening in the mesocolon to the left of the middle colic vessels. While a retrocolic anastomosis appears more anatomic, there is support for an antecolic anastomosis with data suggesting increased incidence of obstruction and Roux stasis syndrome with a retrocolic configuration [32, 33]. However, antecolic anastomoses have been associated with increased rate of marginal ulcers [34].

After it is certain that all of the antrum has been removed, the gastrojejunostomy is made with either an end-to-side or side-to-side configuration by a two-layer hand-sewn method or with a stapler device. If a retrocolic configuration was selected, the defect in the mesocolon is closed with interrupted sutures to avoid a possible internal hernia and avoid a twist or angulations of the jejunal limb.

For non-bariatric procedures, the jejunojejunal anastomosis should be at least 40 cm from the gastrojejunal anastomosis. Either stapled or two-layer hand-sewn anastomosis can be chosen depending on surgeon preference. Mesenteries defects should be closed to reduce internal hernia risk. A nasogastric tube can then be directed through the anastomosis and advanced into the duodenum to ensure decompression of the duodenal stump.

Postoperative Complications

Postoperative complications following Roux-en-Y reconstruction can be loosely grouped into early and late complications. Early complications typically occur within the immediate perioperative period, namely, within the first 2 weeks. Late complications typically arise after the second postoperative week. Medical complications, such as deep vein thromboses, pulmonary embolism, and myocardial infarctions, can occur following any operative intervention. Early complications include anastomotic or staple line leak, postoperative hemorrhage, bowel obstruction and internal hernias, and incorrect Roux limb reconstructions. Delayed complications include anastomotic stricture, stomal and marginal ulcer formation, and Roux stasis syndrome.

Anastomotic Leaks

Anastomotic or staple line leaks are a dreaded and potentially devastating complication of any procedure [35]. Fortunately, the incidence of anastomotic leak is relatively low at 0.4%–5.2% [36–38], and it has been suggested that surgeon experience plays an important role in lowering leak rates. A large retrospective series revealed an almost 40% reduction in leaks as the surgeons became more adept using the technique [35]. Appropriate training, mentorship, and meticulous adherence to operative techniques contribute to a decreased incidence [38]. Anastomotic leaks occur most frequently at the gastrojejunal anastomosis [37, 39], and early recognition of anastomotic leaks is critical to avoid further adverse outcomes [35]. The diagnosis of an anastomotic leak is typically based on clinical presentation, with or without the help of radiographic studies [40]. Clinical signs, such as tachycardia, fever, abdominal pain, purulent drain output, oliguria, and nausea or vomiting, are harbingers of a leak [39, 40]. Early operative management is the mainstay of treatment to confirm and repair the leak, remove extraluminal enteric contents, and place closed-suction drains. The repair of the leak may be challenging, due to friability of the acutely inflamed tissues. In such cases, placement of drains may be the safest option. Placement of a distal feeding jejunostomy could also be considered, as this would allow for continued enteral nutrition, while bowel rest is maintained at the site of the leak.

Hemorrhage

Postoperative bleeding is a serious early complication following surgery. In a systematic review comparing open versus laparoscopic Roux-en-Y gastric bypass patients, it was noted that the frequency of gastrointestinal tract hemorrhage was significantly higher in the laparoscopic cohort [41]. Overall incidence of post Roux-en-Y hemorrhage is difficult to generalize due to the vast settings and indications. In general there are two types of postoperative hemorrhage—bleeding into the abdominal cavity (intra-abdominal) and intraluminal bleeding. Once again, reliance on clinical parameters and laboratory work-up become crucial. Features such as a large quantity of bloody fluid from the drains, tachycardia, drops in hemoglobin levels, bright red blood per rectum, hematemesis, and melena can be indicative of acute postoperative hemorrhage [40]. Re-exploration may be necessary in patients with significant hemorrhage or instability with the operative goal to evacuate the clot, to identify and control the site of hemorrhage, or to oversew staple lines [42].

Obstruction and Hernias

Internal hernias are a common cause of small bowel obstruction following Roux-en-Y reconstructions [43, 44]. As previously discussed, the gastrojejunostomy can be accomplished using either an antecolic or retrocolic approach; thus a number of potential mesenteric defects are created. The retrocolic approach creates an additional defect through the transverse mesocolon in addition to one at site of the jejunojejunostomy. A Petersen defect is created by the space between the Roux limb mesentery and the transverse mesocolon and acts as a site of potential internal herniation and obstruction. The antecolic approach eliminates the defect created in the transverse mesocolon, and it has been debated whether the additional defect contributes to an increased incidence of internal hernia [45]. Many argue that internal hernia complications were relatively rare during the era of open Roux-en-Y reconstructions and have become more frequent with the adoption of minimally invasive approaches [46]. Some groups suggest that the reduced bowel manipulation and peritoneal irritation with a laparoscopic approach causes fewer adhesions and thus results in reduced fixation of the Roux limb to help close mesenteric defects [46]. Inadequate closure of mesenteric defects is often blamed as a factor leading to strong support of closing all defects in an attempt to reduce herniation potential [45–48]. Internal hernias can pose a life-threatening risk to patients due to the possibility of strangulation of bowel loops trapped within the hernia. Unfortunately, internal hernias remain difficult to diagnose clinically or with radiographic imaging. Symptoms are typically sporadic and can range from non-focal colicky pain and distention to nausea, vomiting, and ultimately peritonitis and sepsis. A high index of suspicion must be maintained in patients exhibiting suspicious symptoms with a low threshold for surgical exploration.

Roux-en-O Configuration

Another rare but devastating complication of laparoscopic Roux-en-Y reconstructions involves the inadvertent anastomosis of the proximal biliopancreatic limb of the jejunum to the stomach in conjunction with a misplaced jejunojejunostomy. This so- called Roux-en-O construction gives rise to a blind loop [49]. This is a rare complication; however, it deserves mentioning as it can easily be avoided and the consequences can be profound. Patients with the Roux-en-O configuration typically present with early postoperative abdominal pain, biliary emesis, esophagitis, and severe dehydration. This vague constellation of symptoms can cause diagnostic difficulty. Sherman et al. discovered that ultimately, hepatobiliary iminodiacetic acid (HIDA) scanning was able to facilitate the diagnosis by revealing reflux of radioactive tracer from the duodenum to the esophagus [49]. Prevention remains the best management strategy. It is recommended that the pancreaticobiliary limb be no longer than 50 cm, thus reducing its redundancy and the ease with which it can be connected incorrectly to the stomach. Additionally, marking the different limbs with a suture for identification aides in differentiation. As a final safety measure, the pancreaticobiliary limb should be traced back to the ligament of Treitz so that proper orientation is assured before completing the gastrojejunostomy.

Roux Stasis Syndrome

About 30% of patients who have a Roux-en-Y gastrojejunostomy after gastrectomy suffer from early satiety, abdominal pain, nausea, vomiting, and bloating [50]. This syndrome, called Roux stasis syndrome, is caused by a motility disorder of the Roux limb. Transection of the jejunum separates the limb from the natural small intestinal pacemaker located in the duodenum. Ectopic pacemakers in the jejunum trigger retrograde contractions in its proximal portion, slowing transit through the limb and result in stasis. Current nonsurgical treatment of the syndrome includes the use of prokinetic agents such as metoclopramide or erythromycin or intestinal pacing, neither of which has demonstrated long-term benefits [51].

Similar symptoms can be experienced with gastric dysmotility or anastomotic stricture. Failure to improve with medical and endoscopic management may indicate surgical intervention. Promising results have been demonstrated with a near-total gastrectomy, especially if gastric dysmotility is suspected. Tu et al. demonstrated effective prevention by the use of an “uncut” Roux limb to preserve myoneural continuity between the duodenal pacemaker and the Roux limb [52, 53]. Studies have also noted that longer length (41 cm versus 36 cm) of the Roux limb was associated with higher rates of Roux stasis syndrome, but this must be balanced against the risk of afferent loop syndrome [50, 54].

Ulcers

Stomal ulcers are a concern because there is less alkaline bile reflux into the stomach and the jejunum is vulnerable to acid. It has been acknowledged that Roux-en-Y anatomy contradicts the physiological principle that the mucosa of the small intestine should not be exposed to acidic peptic juice in the absence of alkaline secretions. However, a distal gastrectomy usually results in reduced gastric acid secretion because dissection of the anterior vagal trunk [55] and the glandular gastric fundus is often resected. In a study of European and American patients, the primary disease in stomal ulcer was duodenal ulcer in 95% of cases compared to gastric ulcers in 3%

of cases [56]. Conversely, in Japan the primary disease was duodenal ulcer in 65.9% of cases and gastric or gastroduodenal in 34% [57]. These findings show that preoperatively duodenal ulcers are frequently the primary disease in stomal ulcers and that gastric ulceration secondary to cancer is a relatively rare cause. However, it is important to note that these studies were conducted before the Roux-en-Y reconstruction was widely adopted for reconstruction after a distal gastrectomy for gastric cancer. In summary, these findings indicate that stomal ulcers can be avoided in a Roux-en-Y reconstruction if the acid-secreting region is resected, a complete antrectomy is carried out, and a proper vagotomy is performed [54].

Cholelithiasis: ERCP Access

Cholelithiasis occurs in 10%–20% of all patients undergoing a gastric resection, typically within 3 years after surgery [54]. The involvement of the hepatic branch of the vagus nerve and the hepatic branch which connects with the celiac branch is strongly associated with the development of gallstones, as is delayed gastric evacuation due to the decreased movement of the residual stomach after a gastrectomy [58]. Other factors that affect gallbladder motility include changes in the secretion of gut hormones such as cholecystokinin (CCK) and a decreased sensitivity of CCK receptors in the gallbladder wall. The reconstructed anatomy also makes it difficult to perform either diagnostic or therapeutic endoscopic procedures. Although there is currently no consensus regarding the need for a prophylactic cholecystectomy in most gastrectomy procedures, it has been suggested for consideration in procedures requiring extensive lymph node dissection, total gastrectomy, vagal trunk dissection, or vagotomy [59].

The challenges in patients with Roux-en-Y anatomy are threefold. One challenge involves the altered anatomy in terms of reaching the major papilla. Although better endoscopes have recently become available, the distance involved is a significant challenge. The second challenge involves orientation. Endoscopists use front-viewing scopes; however, the papilla is usually in an upside-down configuration, which is the opposite of what endoscopists are used to. These scopes often do not have elevators; therefore, scope positioning must be precise in order to maneuver the instruments in the correct orientation. The third challenge involves the instruments. The currently available instruments that were actually designed for the long endoscopes required for performing ERCP in these patients are very few and extremely limiting.

Multiple techniques have been described to access the pancreaticobiliary limb. Surgery-assisted ERCP can be performed in the operating room by having the surgeon bring the excluded portion of the stomach and to access percutaneously with a laparoscopic trocar through which a standard side-viewing duodenoscope is advanced and a standard ERCP is then performed [60]. Another alternative includes using a single-balloon or double-balloon enteroscope through the mouth, through the Roux limb to the jejunojejunostomy, and then up the pancreaticobiliary limb retrograde, where the papilla is identified and accessed. This technique is more demanding. The therapeutic success rates of the laparoscopy-assisted and balloon enteroscopy-assisted approaches are 100 and 59 percent, respectively. Interestingly, in patients with a Roux plus pancreaticobiliary limb length less than 150 cm, balloon enteroscopy-assisted ERCP has a success rate of over 85 percent [61].

Conclusion

Since César Roux's first 50 cases in the late nineteenth century, the Roux-en-Y operation has become a standard in gastrointestinal surgery with well-defined applications and effectiveness. The choice of reconstruction following gastric resection for ulcer disease or distal gastrectomy for tumor depends upon the remnant anatomy available for reconstruction. It is the reconstruction of choice of many surgeons for gastric resections [22]. Although complication rates are similar, a meta-analysis of 15 randomized trials comparing reconstructions following gastrectomy demonstrated that a Roux-en-Y reconstruction is better tolerated and leads to a better quality of life with less reflux compared to Billroth reconstructions [62, 63]. Limitations exist including leaks, internal hernias, and Roux stasis syndrome. Over time the operation has proven safe, effective, and feasible for many surgeons. It is effective in reducing reflux gastritis and esophagitis, decreasing risks of recurrent gastric cancer [54, 62, 63]. The operation remains a staple in the armamentarium of general surgeons around the world and commonplace due to its application in bariatric surgery.

References

1. Kauffman GL Jr. Duodenal ulcer disease: treatment by surgery, antibiotics, or both. Adv Surg. 2000;34:121–35.
2. Roux C. Chirurgie gastronintestinale. Rev Chir. 1983;13:402–3.
3. Deitel M. Cesar roux and his contribution. Obes Surg. 2007;17(10):1277–8.
4. Chung KT, Shelat VG. Perforated peptic ulcer - an update. World J Gastrointest Surg. 2017;9(1):1–12.
5. Wang YR, Richter JE, Dempsey DT. Trends and outcomes of hospitalizations for peptic ulcer disease in the United States, 1993 to 2006. Ann Surg. 2010;251(1):51–8.
6. Goldstein H, Boyle JD. The saline load test--a bedside evaluation of gastric retention. Gastroenterology. 1965;49(4):375–80.
7. Shone DN, Nikoomanesh P, Smith-Meek MM, Bender JS. Malignancy is the most common cause of gastric outlet obstruction in the era of H2 blockers. Am J Gastroenterol. 1995;90(10):1769–70.
8. DiSario JA, Fennerty MB, Tietze CC, Hutson WR, Burt RW. Endoscopic balloon dilation for ulcer-induced gastric outlet obstruction. Am J Gastroenterol. 1994;89(6):868–71.
9. Bardhan KD, Nayyar AK, Royston C. History in our lifetime: the changing nature of refractory duodenal ulcer in the era of histamine H2 receptor antagonists. Dig Liver Dis. 2003;35(8):529–36.
10. Annibale B, De Magistris L, Corleto V, et al. Zollinger-ellison syndrome and antral G-cell hyperfunction in patients with resistant duodenal ulcer disease. Aliment Pharmacol Ther. 1994;8(1):87–93.
11. Whiting JL, Sigurdsson A, Rowlands DC, Hallissey MT, Fielding JW. The long term results of endoscopic surveillance of premalignant gastric lesions. Gut. 2002;50(3):378–81.
12. Kim JP. Current status of surgical treatment of gastric cancer. J Surg Oncol. 2002;79(2):79–80.

13. Lin JX, Huang CM, Zheng CH, et al. Surgical outcomes of 2041 consecutive laparoscopic gastrectomy procedures for gastric cancer: a large-scale case control study. PLoS One. 2015;10(2):e0114948.
14. Kitano S, Iso Y, Moriyama M, Sugimachi K. Laparoscopy-assisted Billroth I gastrectomy. Surg Laparosc Endosc. 1994;4(2):146–8.
15. Kitano S, Shiraishi N, Fujii K, et al. A randomized controlled trial comparing open vs laparoscopy-assisted distal gastrectomy for the treatment of early gastric cancer: an interim report. Surgery. 2002;131(1 Suppl):S306–11.
16. Oh SY, Kwon S, Lee KG, et al. Outcomes of minimally invasive surgery for early gastric cancer are comparable with those for open surgery: analysis of 1,013 minimally invasive surgeries at a single institution. Surg Endosc. 2014;28(3):789–95.
17. Lee JH, Han HS, Lee JH. A prospective randomized study comparing open vs laparoscopy-assisted distal gastrectomy in early gastric cancer: early results. Surg Endosc. 2005;19(2):168–73.
18. Paakkonen M, Aukee S, Syrjanen K, Mantyjarvi R. Gastritis, duodenogastric reflux and bacteriology of the gastric remnant in patients operated for peptic ulcer by Billroth I operation. Ann Clin Res. 1985;17(1):32–6.
19. Richter JE. Duodenogastric reflux-induced (alkaline) esophagitis. Curr Treat Options Gastroenterol. 2004;7(1):53–8.
20. Miwa K, Hasegawa H, Fujimura T, et al. Duodenal reflux through the pylorus induces gastric adenocarcinoma in the rat. Carcinogenesis. 1992;13(12):2313–6.
21. Kojima K, Yamada H, Inokuchi M, Kawano T, Sugihara K. A comparison of roux-en-Y and Billroth-I reconstruction after laparoscopy-assisted distal gastrectomy. Ann Surg. 2008;247(6):962–7.
22. Kumagai K, Shimizu K, Yokoyama N, et al. Questionnaire survey regarding the current status and controversial issues concerning reconstruction after gastrectomy in Japan. Surg Today. 2012;42(5):411–8.
23. Xiong JJ, Altaf K, Javed MA, et al. Roux-en-Y versus billroth I reconstruction after distal gastrectomy for gastric cancer: a meta-analysis. World J Gastroenterol. 2013;19(7):1124–34.
24. Ritchie WP. Alkaline reflux gastritis: a critical reappraisal. Gut. 1984;25(9):975–87.
25. Ritchie WP Jr. Alkaline reflux gastritis. Gastroenterol Clin N Am. 1994;23(2):281–94.
26. Szentpali K, Eros G, Kaszaki J, et al. Microcirculatory changes in the canine oesophageal mucosa during experimental reflux oesophagitis: comparison of the effects of acid and bile. Scand J Gastroenterol. 2003;38(10):1016–22.
27. Rea T, Bartolacci M, Leombruni E, Brizzi F, Picardi N. Study of the antireflux action of the roux-en-Y jejunal loop in reconstruction after gastrectomy and nutritional status in the follow-up. Ann Ital Chir. 2005;76(4):343–51.
28. Zobolas B, Sakorafas GH, Kouroukli I, et al. Alkaline reflux gastritis: early and late results of surgery. World J Surg. 2006;30(6):1043–9.
29. Lundell L. Acid secretion and gastric surgery. Dig Dis. 2011;29(5):487–90.
30. Abdel-Salam WN, Katri KM, Bessa SS, El-Kayal eA. Laparoscopic-assisted truncal vagotomy and gastro-jejunostomy: trial of simplification. J Laparoendosc Adv Surg Tech A. 2009;19(2):125–7.
31. Herrington JL Jr, Scott HW Jr, Sawyers JL. Experience with vagotomy--antrectomy and roux-en-Y gastrojejunostomy in surgical treatment of duodenal, gastric, and stomal ulcers. Ann Surg. 1984;199(5):590–7.
32. Otsuka R, Natsume T, Maruyama T, Tanaka H, Matsuzaki H. Antecolic reconstruction is a predictor of the occurrence of roux stasis syndrome after distal gastrectomy. J Gastrointest Surg. 2015;19(5):821–4.
33. Escalona A, Devaud N, Perez G, et al. Antecolic versus retrocolic alimentary limb in laparoscopic roux-en-Y gastric bypass: a comparative study. Surg Obes Relat Dis. 2007;3(4):423–7.
34. Ribeiro-Parenti L, Arapis K, Chosidow D, Marmuse JP. Comparison of marginal ulcer rates between antecolic and retrocolic laparoscopic roux-en-Y gastric bypass. Obes Surg. 2015;25(2):215–21.

35. Ballesta C, Berindoague R, Cabrera M, Palau M, Gonzales M. Management of anastomotic leaks after laparoscopic roux-en-Y gastric bypass. Obes Surg. 2008;18(6):623–30.
36. Fernandez AZ Jr, DeMaria EJ, Tichansky DS, et al. Experience with over 3,000 open and laparoscopic bariatric procedures: multivariate analysis of factors related to leak and resultant mortality. Surg Endosc. 2004;18(2):193–7.
37. Marshall JS, Srivastava A, Gupta SK, Rossi TR, DeBord JR. Roux-en-Y gastric bypass leak complications. Arch Surg. 2003;138(5):520–3; discussion 523–4.
38. Fullum TM, Aluka KJ, Turner PL. Decreasing anastomotic and staple line leaks after laparoscopic roux-en-Y gastric bypass. Surg Endosc. 2009;23(6):1403–8.
39. Gonzalez R, Sarr MG, Smith CD, et al. Diagnosis and contemporary management of anastomotic leaks after gastric bypass for obesity. J Am Coll Surg. 2007;204(1):47–55.
40. Bellorin O, Abdemur A, Sucandy I, Szomstein S, Rosenthal RJ. Understanding the significance, reasons and patterns of abnormal vital signs after gastric bypass for morbid obesity. Obes Surg. 2011;21(6):707–13.
41. Podnos YD, Jimenez JC, Wilson SE, Stevens CM, Nguyen NT. Complications after laparoscopic gastric bypass: a review of 3464 cases. Arch Surg. 2003;138(9):957–61.
42. Nguyen NT, Rivers R, Wolfe BM. Early gastrointestinal hemorrhage after laparoscopic gastric bypass. Obes Surg. 2003;13(1):62–5.
43. Iannelli A, Buratti MS, Novellas S, et al. Internal hernia as a complication of laparoscopic roux-en-Y gastric bypass. Obes Surg. 2007;17(10):1283–6.
44. Champion JK, Williams M. Small bowel obstruction and internal hernias after laparoscopic roux-en-Y gastric bypass. Obes Surg. 2003;13(4):596–600.
45. Steele KE, Prokopowicz GP, Magnuson T, Lidor A, Schweitzer M. Laparoscopic antecolic roux-en-Y gastric bypass with closure of internal defects leads to fewer internal hernias than the retrocolic approach. Surg Endosc. 2008;22(9):2056–61.
46. Higa KD, Ho T, Boone KB. Internal hernias after laparoscopic roux-en-Y gastric bypass: incidence, treatment and prevention. Obes Surg. 2003;13(3):350–4.
47. Carmody B, DeMaria EJ, Jamal M, et al. Internal hernia after laparoscopic roux-en-Y gastric bypass. Surg Obes Relat Dis. 2005;1(6):543–8.
48. Madan AK, Lo Menzo E, Dhawan N, Tichansky DS. Internal hernias and nonclosure of mesenteric defects during laparoscopic roux-en-Y gastric bypass. Obes Surg. 2009;19(5):549–52.
49. Sherman V, Dan AG, Lord JM, Chand B, Schauer PR. Complications of gastric bypass: avoiding the roux-en-O configuration. Obes Surg. 2009;19(8):1190–4.
50. Gustavsson S, Ilstrup DM, Morrison P, Kelly KA. Roux-Y stasis syndrome after gastrectomy. Am J Surg. 1988;155(3):490–4.
51. Petrakis J, Vassilakis JS, Karkavitsas N, et al. Enhancement of gastric emptying of solids by erythromycin in patients with roux-en-Y gastrojejunostomy. Arch Surg. 1998;133(7):709–14.
52. Tu BN, Kelly KA. Motility disorders after roux-en-Y gastrojejunostomy. Obes Surg. 1994;4(3):219–26.
53. Tu BN, Kelly KA. Elimination of the roux stasis syndrome using a new type of "uncut roux" limb. Am J Surg. 1995;170(4):381–6.
54. Hoya Y, Mitsumori N, Yanaga K. The advantages and disadvantages of a roux-en-Y reconstruction after a distal gastrectomy for gastric cancer. Surg Today. 2009;39(8):647–51.
55. Khadzhibaev AM, Mekhmanov AM, Bakirov DB, Tursunov BK, Kutlikov SI. Resection of the stomach with excision of the small curvature and selective vagotomy in primary and reconstructive surgery of gastroduodenal ulcers. Khirurgiia (Mosk). 2005;(1):25–8.
56. Turnage RH, Sarosi G, Cryer B, et al. Evaluation and management of patients with recurrent peptic ulcer disease after acid-reducing operations: a systematic review. J Gastrointest Surg. 2003;7(5):606–26.
57. Akimoto H, Kashiwagi H, Ito A, et al. Problems in ulcer surgery after the introduction of H2-receptor antagonists. Nihon Geka Gakkai Zasshi. 1992;93(9):1067–70.
58. Kobayashi T, Hisanaga M, Kanehiro H, et al. Analysis of risk factors for the development of gallstones after gastrectomy. Br J Surg. 2005;92(11):1399–403.

59. Akatsu T, Yoshida M, Kubota T, et al. Gallstone disease after extended (D2) lymph node dissection for gastric cancer. World J Surg. 2005;29(2):182–6.
60. Lopes TL, Clements RH, Wilcox CM. Laparoscopy-assisted ERCP: Experience of a high-volume bariatric surgery center (with video). Gastrointest Endosc. 2009;70(6):1254–9.
61. Schreiner MA, Chang L, Gluck M, et al. Laparoscopy-assisted versus balloon enteroscopy-assisted ERCP in bariatric post-roux-en-Y gastric bypass patients. Gastrointest Endosc. 2012;75(4):748–56.
62. Zong L, Chen P. Billroth I vs. billroth II vs. roux-en-Y following distal gastrectomy: a meta-analysis based on 15 studies. Hepato-Gastroenterology. 2011;58(109):1413–24.
63. Hirao M, Takiguchi S, Imamura H, et al. Comparison of billroth I and roux-en-Y reconstruction after distal gastrectomy for gastric cancer: one-year postoperative effects assessed by a multi-institutional RCT. Ann Surg Oncol. 2013;20(5):1591–7.

Postgastrectomy Syndromes

61

George Z. Li and Stanley W. Ashley

Introduction

Due to the development of effective medical therapy for peptic ulcer disease (PUD) [1, 2] and a decreasing incidence of gastric cancer [3], gastric resections are now less commonly performed in the USA. Nevertheless, over 3000 operations were performed during hospitalizations for PUD in 2006 [4], and there will still be an estimated 26,370 new cases of gastric cancer in the USA in 2016 [5]. Furthermore, the shift in demographics toward older cancer patients and those who require urgent or emergent surgery for complicated PUD means that gastrectomies are now performed on a higher-risk population than ever before [6]. Thus, it remains crucial for the general surgeon and the surgical oncologist to be familiar with gastrectomy and its associated complications.

Gastric operation results in a variety of physiological disturbances. Two key contributors to postoperative gastrointestinal dysfunction are resection or division of the pylorus, which removes the normal barrier to gastric outflow, and vagal denervation, which disrupts regulation of gastrointestinal motility and bile secretion. These derangements can manifest as one of several "postgastrectomy syndromes," and this chapter discusses the pathophysiology, diagnosis, and management of each of these syndromes. In section "Complications After Bariatric Surgery", we also briefly discuss complications after surgery for morbid obesity, which has now become the most common indication for elective gastric surgery. In fact, similar mechanisms may contribute to symptoms and even weight loss after these procedures [6, 7].

G. Z. Li
Department of Surgery, Brigham and Women's Hospital, Boston, MA, USA

S. W. Ashley (✉)
Brigham and Women's Hospital, Harvard Medical School, Boston, MA, USA
e-mail: sashley@partners.org

J. Grams et al. (eds.), *The SAGES Manual of Foregut Surgery*,
https://doi.org/10.1007/978-3-319-96122-4_61

Types of Gastric Operations

Gastric resections can be classified as partial or total. Partial gastrectomy, which consists of any resection that does not remove the entire stomach, encompasses wedge resection, sleeve gastrectomy, distal gastrectomy, and segmental pylorus-preserving gastrectomy. Total gastrectomy involves removal of the entire stomach, including the gastroesophageal junction and the pylorus. Vagotomy and drainage operations do not involve gastric resection but can also cause postgastrectomy syndromes. A vagotomy can be truncal, in which the main vagal trunks are divided at the distal esophagus, or highly selective, in which only the terminal vagal branches to the corpus and fundus are divided, sparing the "crow's foot" that innervates the antrum and pylorus. Truncal vagotomy leads to delayed gastric emptying unless a drainage operation is also performed [8]. The simplest is a Heineke-Mikulicz pyloroplasty, which involves making a longitudinal incision along the pylorus then closing it transversely, resulting in a less competent pylorus. Highly selective vagotomy does not require routine drainage.

Postgastrectomy syndromes occur when the pylorus is resected or divided and/or the vagus nerve or its branches are transected, although symptoms of early satiety, a component of several syndromes, can develop after any gastric resection. As such, postgastrectomy syndromes are typically associated with distal gastrectomy, total gastrectomy, or vagotomy and/or drainage alone. Wedge resection and sleeve gastrectomy do not usually cause postgastrectomy syndromes, though sleeve gastrectomy is effective because it reduces the gastric remnant and can cause various other complications. Segmental gastrectomy is a pylorus-sparing option for proximal early-stage gastric cancers that is commonly associated with delayed gastric emptying. However, it is primarily performed in Japan and South Korea, where the incidence of early-stage gastric cancers is much higher due to screening programs [9, 10]. Segmental gastrectomy is uncommon in the USA, where most surgeons favor total gastrectomy for proximal cancers.

Types of Reconstruction After Distal or Total Gastrectomy

After resection of the pylorus, several options exist to restore gastrointestinal continuity. As described in detail in the previous chapters, the three main techniques are the Billroth I, the Billroth II, and the Roux-en-Y.

The Billroth I can be performed after a distal gastrectomy by creating an end-to-end anastomosis between the remnant stomach and the duodenum (Fig. 61.1a). Advantages of the Billroth I include the preservation of gastroduodenal passage of food, which theoretically protects against malabsorption, and the need for only one suture/staple line. However, patients who have had a Billroth I are at risk for dumping syndrome and alkaline reflux gastritis [11], which will both be discussed in section "Postgastrectomy Syndromes". Furthermore, a Billroth I is not feasible if the relatively immobile duodenum cannot reach the stomach remnant without tension.

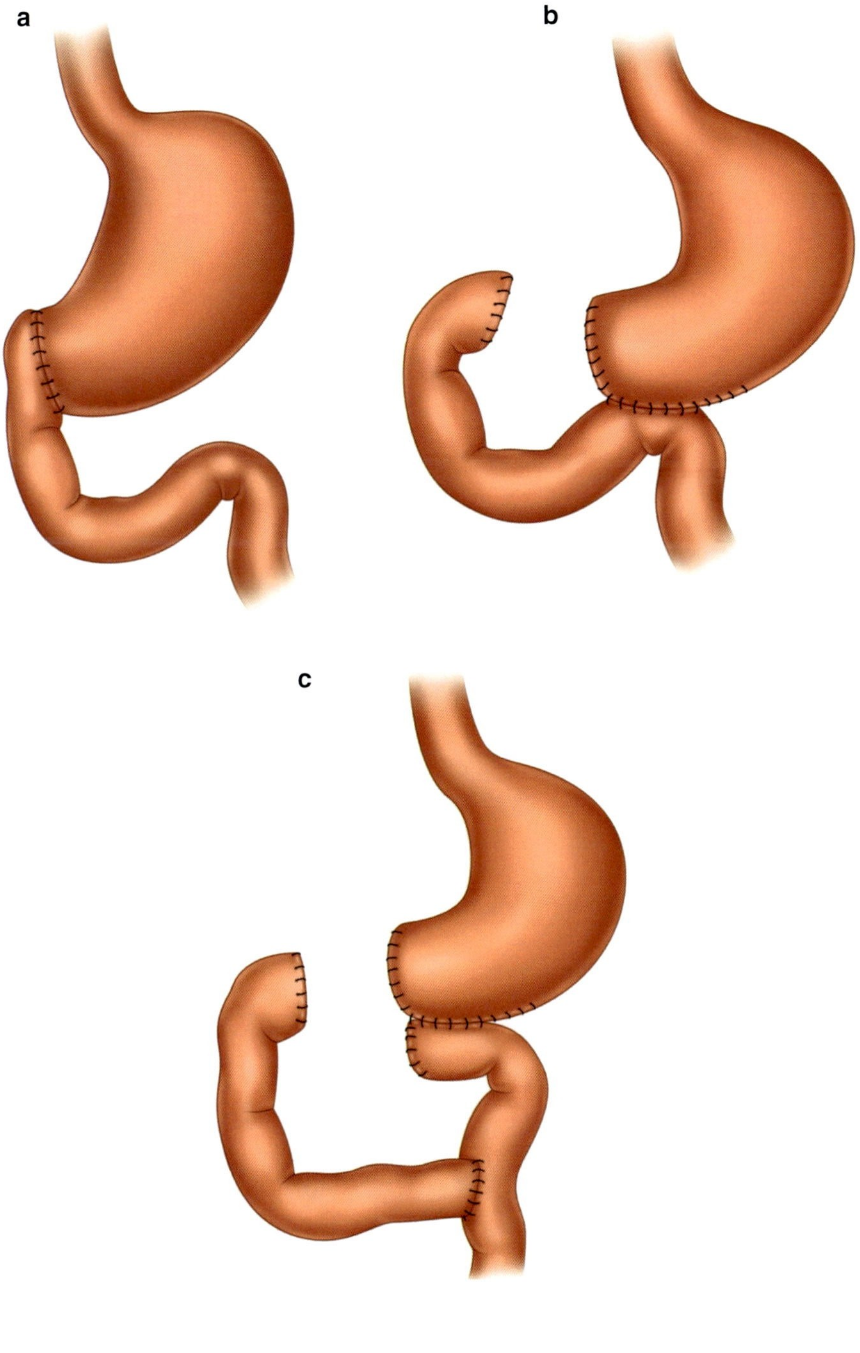

Fig. 61.1 Reconstruction options after a partial gastrectomy include (**a**) Billroth I, (**b**) Billroth II, or (**c**) Roux-en-Y

The Billroth II is performed by bringing up a loop of proximal jejunum to the stomach to create an end-to-side gastrojejunal anastomosis (Fig. 61.1b). This creates an afferent limb and efferent limb. The afferent limb is the duodenojejunal segment proximal to the gastrojejunostomy into which the pancreatic and common bile ducts drain, and the efferent limb is the jejunal limb distal to the gastrojejunostomy. The Billroth II can be performed after more extensive gastric resections that do not allow for a Billroth I due to excessive tension. However, it leads to formation of a duodenal stump, which can leak and lead to significant morbidity and mortality [12–14]. In addition, the afferent limb can become kinked or obstructed [15]. Finally, the Billroth II increases the risk of malabsorption due to loss of gastroduodenal continuity, and patients are also at risk of dumping syndrome and alkaline reflux gastritis.

The Roux-en-Y is the third reconstructive option and is most commonly used after a total or near-total gastrectomy. After division of the jejunum, two anastomoses are performed: one connecting the distal jejunum to the remnant stomach or esophagus to form the Roux limb and another connecting the proximal jejunum to the Roux limb to produce a Y-shaped configuration (Fig. 61.1c). The Roux-en-Y creates the most separation between the common bile duct and the stomach and has the lowest risk of alkaline reflux gastritis. However, it is more prone to slow-transit syndromes than the Billroth I or II due to the inherent dysmotility of the Roux limb [16].

Postgastrectomy Syndromes

The majority of evidence attributes the development of postgastrectomy syndromes to derangements caused by loss of pyloric function and/or normal vagal innervation. Postgastrectomy syndromes can be broadly categorized into rapid- and slow-transit syndromes. Rapid-transit syndromes include dumping syndrome and post-vagotomy diarrhea, and slow-transit problems include delayed gastric emptying, alkaline reflux gastritis, and Roux limb stasis.

Dumping Syndrome

One of the first descriptions of dumping syndrome was published by Dr. Arthur Hertz in 1913, who described "too rapid drainage of the stomach" after gastroenterostomy as seen on barium swallow [17]. The syndrome encompasses a constellation of gastrointestinal and vasomotor symptoms that patients experience following a meal. Dumping is further sub-categorized as early dumping or late dumping. Early dumping, which is the most common, occurs 15–30 min after a meal. Symptoms include flushing, palpitations, diaphoresis, nausea, bloating, and diarrhea. Late dumping, which occurs in 25% of cases, occurs several hours after eating and is characterized by palpitations, dizziness, and a strong desire to lie down [18]. After distal gastrectomy, approximately 10–20% of patients initially experience dumping syndrome [18, 19], though it can also occur after total gastrectomy or drainage procedures such as pyloroplasty.

The pathophysiology of dumping syndrome has not been completely defined, but is thought to be primarily due to loss of pyloric function as well as decreased gastric accommodation in response to distension [20]. As a result, there is rapid emptying of hyperosmolar gastric contents into the small bowel after a meal. The osmotic gradient pulls excess fluid into the intestinal lumen, which can cause intestinal distension and hypermotility leading to nausea, bloating, and diarrhea. In addition, the prematurely emptied gastric contents contain abnormally high levels of carbohydrates, which stimulate release of hormones such as neurotensin and vasoactive intestinal polypeptide to produce flushing, palpitations, and diaphoresis [21]. Finally, this carbohydrate load also stimulates an insulin surge that leads to postprandial hypoglycemia [22], which is thought to be the cause of late dumping.

Diagnosis of dumping syndrome is primarily clinical and is based on a history of the above symptoms in a postgastrectomy patient. If the diagnosis is uncertain, one can employ a monitored glucose challenge to see if dumping symptoms can be reproduced. After a 50-gram glucose challenge in a patient who has been fasting for at least 10 h, a rise in heart rate by at least 10 beats per minute within the first hour is considered diagnostic [23]. A gastric emptying study or an upper gastrointestinal series can also be used to demonstrate rapid emptying of gastric contents and help exclude alternative diagnoses (Table 61.1).

Table 61.1 Differential diagnosis and diagnostic evaluation of postgastrectomy syndromes

	Differential diagnosis	Diagnostic studies
Dumping syndrome	Post-vagotomy diarrhea Irritable bowel syndrome Lactose intolerance Gastroenteritis	Fasting glucose challenge Upper GI series Nuclear gastric emptying study
Post-vagotomy diarrhea	Dumping syndrome Irritable bowel syndrome Lactose intolerance Gastroenteritis	Diagnosis of exclusion, rule out other etiologies
Delayed gastric emptying	Mechanical obstruction Postoperative ileus Roux limb stasis (RY) Anastomotic stricture Ulcer	Upper GI series Upper endoscopy Nuclear gastric emptying study
Alkaline reflux gastritis	Delayed gastric emptying Afferent loop obstruction (BII) Ulcer	Upper endoscopy Gastric pH monitoring Cholescintigraphy
Roux limb stasis	Delayed gastric emptying Mechanical obstruction Postoperative ileus Anastomotic stricture Ulcer	Upper GI series Upper endoscopy Nuclear gastric emptying study

RY Roux-en-Y, *BII* Billroth II, *GI* gastrointestinal

Management of dumping syndrome, both early and late, is primarily conservative. Most patients can be successfully managed with changes in dietary habits. Frequent small meals, meals high in protein and fiber and low in carbohydrates, and separation of liquid and solid foods during meals have all been effective [18]. Patients who are refractory to dietary modifications may benefit from octreotide, a somatostatin analog that inhibits secretion of insulin and various other gut-derived hormones and also slows gastric emptying and small bowel motility. Octreotide has been demonstrated to be superior to placebo in improving dumping symptoms as well as stabilizing fasting glucose levels. Short-term relief occurs in almost 100% of treated patients, and long-term symptom control occurs in up to 80% of patients at 3 months [24–27]. Side effects include diarrhea and steatorrhea, and the drug is still only available in subcutaneous injection form. For patients with late dumping, acarbose, an α-glycoside hydrolase, may be effective as well based on evidence from small series [28]. Acarbose delays carbohydrate digestion and thus blunts the insulin surge that causes late dumping symptoms.

For the small group of patients with intractable dumping syndrome refractory to both dietary changes and medical therapy, reoperation may be indicated. In patients with a Billroth II, revision to a Roux-en-Y may help relieve dumping. The Roux limb has impaired motility, which may help slow the transit of chyme from the stomach to the remainder of the small bowel.

Post-Vagotomy Diarrhea

Twenty-five percent of patients who have undergone truncal vagotomy develop post-vagotomy diarrhea [29]. Fortunately, most cases are self-limited and resolve over time. The pathophysiology is not entirely clear, but may be due to excess secretion of unconjugated bile salts due to vagal denervation of the biliary system [30].

The diagnosis is made clinically, and it may be difficult to distinguish from the dumping syndrome discussed above. Dietary modifications, such as small frequent meals and addition of fiber, may help some patients. A trial of cholestyramine, an oral bile salt binder, may also be effective [29, 30]. For the small group of patients with intractable diarrhea refractory to medical management, creation of an antiperistaltic jejunal segment has been employed with at least anecdotal success. In this technique, a 10 cm segment of jejunum 100 cm distal to the ligament of Treitz is reversed and re-anastomosed end-to-end (Fig. 61.2a) [31].

Delayed Gastric Emptying

On the opposite side of the spectrum, some patients who have undergone partial gastrectomy suffer from delayed gastric emptying. Contributing factors are thought to include denervation of the stomach remnant, postoperative gastric atony, and another underlying exacerbating factor such as a marginal ulcer. Symptoms include fullness and early satiety, abdominal pain, nausea, and non-bilious emesis of

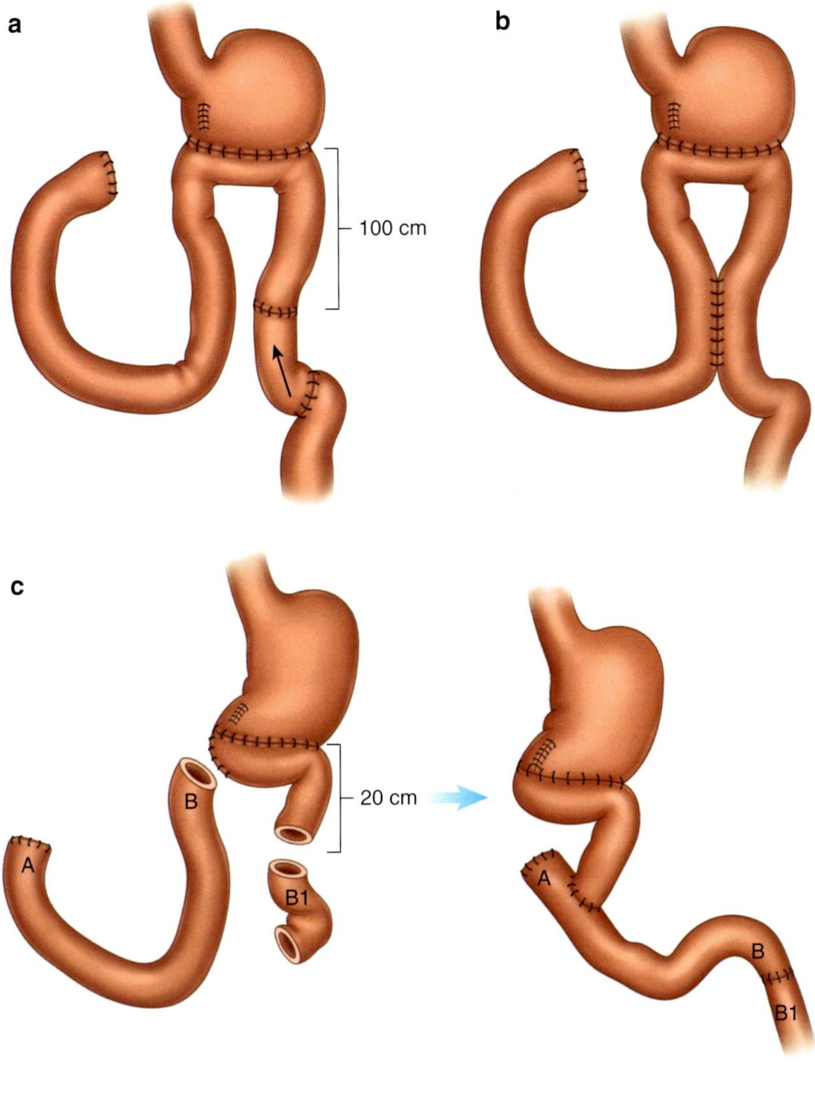

Fig. 61.2 (**a**) Antiperistaltic jejunal interposition for treatment of refractory post-vagotomy diarrhea. (**b**) Braun enteroenterostomy and (**c**) Henley jejunal interposition for treatment of alkaline reflux gastritis

undigested food. While 32% of patients may have evidence of prolonged gastric food retention on upper endoscopy 1 year after a Billroth I or II reconstruction (with higher rates after a Billroth I) [32], clinically significant delayed gastric emptying affects a much smaller proportion of patients.

In evaluating a patient with delayed gastric emptying, one must exclude a mechanical obstruction and also evaluate for additional underlying pathology. An upper gastrointestinal series should be performed to rule out obstruction, and upper endoscopy should be performed to evaluate for anastomotic stricture or marginal ulcers. A nuclear medicine gastric emptying test can also demonstrate impaired gastric emptying.

Many patients improve over time with conservative treatment, which consists of small, frequent meals to limit gastric volume. Prokinetic agents such as metoclopramide and erythromycin may be useful as well. A few select centers offer gastric pacing [33], but this is currently considered experimental therapy.

Surgery is indicated for patients who fail conservative and medical therapy. In general, the goal is to reduce the size of the remnant stomach. A partial gastrectomy can be converted to a subtotal gastrectomy or completion gastrectomy with esophagojejunostomy. If possible, a Billroth II reconstruction is preferred over a Roux-en-Y reconstruction, because the Roux limb itself is thought to contribute to slow transit.

Alkaline Reflux Gastritis

After removal of the pylorus, bile can reflux into the stomach. This is much more common after a Billroth I or II than after a Roux-en-Y, since the intestinal length between the common bile duct and the gastro- or esophago-enterostomy is the greatest after a Roux-en-Y. There is evidence that bile salts can damage gastric mucosa and cause foveolar hyperplasia and chronic atrophic gastritis [34] and that bile salts lead to gastroesophageal cancer in animal models [35]. However, the clinical significance of bile reflux in humans is more controversial, as while the majority of patients without pyloric function have bile reflux, only a small proportion develop clinical symptoms of burning epigastric discomfort or nausea.

The diagnosis of alkaline reflux involves demonstrating objective evidence of bile reflux in a postgastrectomy patient and excluding alternative diagnoses. Bile reflux can be demonstrated by upper endoscopy with or without biopsy, gastric pH monitoring demonstrating alkaline reflux, or cholescintigraphy demonstrating gastric reflux of bile. Upper endoscopy can also identify other etiologies of epigastric pain and nausea, such as anastomotic stricture or ulceration.

There are several medical treatment options available, with ursodeoxycholic acid and sucralfate having the most success in small trials. Ursodeoxycholic acid significantly improved symptoms but not histologic features, while sucralfate improved histologic features but not symptoms [13, 36]. Definitive management of clinically significant alkaline reflux gastritis is surgical, though the choice of operation depends upon the patient's anatomy. A Billroth I or II can be revised to a Roux-en-Y reconstruction to increase the distance between the common bile duct and the gastroenterostomy [37]. For patients with a Billroth II, other options include a Braun enteroenterostomy placed 30 cm from the gastroenterostomy to divert bile away from the stomach (Fig. 61.2b) [38] or a Henley jejunal interposition, which involves placing a 20 cm isoperistaltic jejunal segment between the gastric remnant and the duodenum (Fig. 61.2c) [39].

Roux Limb Stasis

After Roux-en-Y reconstruction, up to 30% of patients may develop Roux limb stasis [40]. This syndrome is thought to occur due to antiperistalsis in the Roux limb that propels intestinal contents retrograde toward the stomach as opposed to antegrade toward the common channel [41]. Roux limb stasis does not seem to be associated with vagotomy but is associated with longer Roux limb length [40]. Patients with Roux limb stasis experience symptoms similar to those of other slow-transit syndromes, such as epigastric fullness and pain, nausea, vomiting, and weight loss.

Diagnostic evaluation for suspected Roux limb stasis is similar to that of delayed gastric emptying, and it is again crucial to rule out mechanical obstruction. Both an upper gastrointestinal series and a nuclear gastric emptying study may show similar findings to patients with delayed gastric emptying but can also show a dilated and/or flaccid Roux limb. Upper endoscopy should also be performed to rule out other diagnoses.

Once the diagnosis is established, medical therapy consists of prokinetic agents such as metoclopramide or erythromycin. Patients refractory to medical therapy should undergo reoperation, which usually involves resecting the dysfunctional Roux limb and redoing the Roux-en-Y reconstruction. Alternatively, total gastrectomy may be of benefit in some patients.

Other Postgastrectomy Conditions

Afferent Loop Syndrome

Afferent loop syndrome can occur after a Billroth II if the afferent limb becomes obstructed from kinking, postoperative adhesions, volvulus, intussusception, or anastomotic stricture. Patients may present acutely with severe abdominal pain and vomiting or chronically with postprandial episodic epigastric pain followed by bilious vomiting that relieves the pain. An acute obstruction requires emergent reoperation, because the patient is at imminent risk for bowel ischemia and a duodenal stump blowout. Chronic obstruction can be treated electively with a Braun entero-enterostomy to decompress the afferent limb into the efferent limb, revision of the Billroth II anastomosis to correct a mechanical obstruction, or conversion to a Roux-en-Y [6, 42].

Gastric Remnant Carcinoma

As discussed in section "Postgastrectomy Syndromes: Alkaline Reflux Gastritis", the gastric remnant is more exposed to bile and pancreatic secretions after a Billroth I or II, which in animal models seem to be carcinogenic. There is indeed also evidence that humans who have had a partial gastrectomy for benign disease may be at increased risk for carcinoma in the gastric remnant [43, 44]. However, these studies found that the increased risk does not appear until 10–20 years after surgery. Furthermore, this risk does not seem high enough to justify mandatory endoscopic surveillance for all patients.

Malnutrition

Patients who have had gastroduodenal bypass with a Billroth II or Roux-en-Y can develop deficiencies in minerals absorbed in the duodenum and proximal jejunum such as calcium, iron, copper, and zinc. Patients who have had a total gastrectomy are also at risk for vitamin B12 deficiency due to loss of parietal cells and intrinsic factor production. Postoperatively, patients should be provided with an appropriately tailored regimen of oral supplements, which at high enough doses usually overcome malabsorption. Patients who develop clinical symptoms of malnutrition or do not tolerate oral supplementation may require parenteral supplementation via the intravenous or intramuscular routes.

Complications After Bariatric Surgery

Here we briefly discuss several complications after bariatric surgery. Laparoscopic sleeve gastrectomy and laparoscopic Roux-en-Y gastric bypass are the two most common procedures performed in the USA [45], so the sequelae of these two operations will be the focus of the discussion. Laparoscopic adjustable gastric banding, which was popular in the past, has declined precipitously in use, and biliopancreatic diversion with duodenal switch is no longer performed at most US centers [45].

Dumping Syndrome and Malnutrition

Dumping syndrome, as discussed in section "Postgastrectomy Syndromes: Dumping Syndrome", can also occur in up to 75% of patients after Roux-en-Y gastric bypass [46], since food is rerouted past both the pylorus and the vast majority of the stomach. The clinical presentation, diagnosis, and management are identical to non-bariatric patients, except that surgery for refractory dumping in this population usually involves bypass reversal. Fortunately, most patients improve with dietary modifications. Gastric bypass, which by design is a malabsorptive weight-loss procedure, also predictably puts patients at risk for malnutrition (see section "Other Postgastrectomy Conditions: Malnutrition"), as food no longer flows past the distal stomach, duodenum, or proximal jejunum. Appropriate monitoring of labs such as iron studies, complete blood count, and vitamin B12 levels is crucial, and multivitamin and mineral supplementation should be tailored accordingly.

Marginal Ulcer

Ulcers, adjacent to the gastrojejunostomy can occur after Roux-en-Y gastric bypass, or after gastrectomy with Billroth II or Roux-en-Y reconstructions, due to exposure of the jejunum to acid. Marginal ulcers are associated with use of nonsteroidal anti-inflammatory drugs (NSAIDs), smoking, and gastro-gastric fistulas in bypass patients, since the excluded gastric remnant contains the vast majority of acid-producing cells [47]. Patients often present with nausea, pain, or symptoms of bleeding such as hematochezia or iron-deficiency anemia. The diagnosis can be confirmed by upper endoscopy, and patients should also be tested for *H. Pylori* and treated appropriately if positive. Management consists of avoidance of NSAIDs, smoking cessation, and therapy with proton pump inhibitors (PPIs) plus sucralfate. Patients with persistent symptoms, refractory bleeding, or signs of perforation require surgery, which involves revision of the gastrojejunostomy plus a truncal vagotomy.

Internal Hernia

Internal hernia is a dreaded complication after any Roux-en-Y reconstruction. The Roux-en-Y creates up to three potential internal herniation sites: (1) a space between the transverse mesocolon and small bowel limb mesentery (Petersen's defect), (2) a space between the two jejunal limb mesenteries near the jejunojejunostomy, and (3) a defect in the transverse mesocolon if a retrocolic Roux limb is used. Patients present with signs of bowel obstruction, including nausea, vomiting, and abdominal pain. An abdominal CT scan should be obtained in any patient suspected of having an internal hernia. Management involves emergent reoperation to reduce the hernia and resect any necrotic small bowel. The risk of internal hernia can be reduced with careful closure of all mesenteric defects at the initial operation.

Gastric Stricture

Gastric strictures can develop after sleeve gastrectomy, most commonly at the gastroesophageal junction or incisura angularis [48]. Contributing technical factors include using a bougie that is too small or excessive oversewing of the gastric staple line. Strictures may also develop after scarring from a staple line leak.

Patients present with nausea, vomiting, epigastric pain, and heartburn. The diagnosis is made with an upper gastrointestinal series, and initial management consists of serial endoscopic dilations. Patients refractory to endoscopic therapy may require reoperation, which consists of gastric stricturoplasty, resection of the strictured segment with gastrogastrostomy, or conversion to a Roux-en-Y gastric bypass.

Gastroesophageal Reflux

A sleeve gastrectomy increases intragastric pressure [49], which can predispose patients to developing gastroesophageal reflux. After ruling out anatomic causes, such as a stricture, with upper endoscopy or an upper gastrointestinal series, patients with reflux symptoms should be trialed on PPIs. Patients who cannot be managed medically usually require conversion to a Roux-en-Y gastric bypass.

Summary

Following distal or total gastrectomy or vagotomy with or without drainage, either rapid- or slow-transit postgastrectomy syndromes can develop due to the effects of pyloric resection and/or vagal denervation. The different gastric reconstruction options each carry different risks of causing the various postgastrectomy syndromes. The gastric surgeon should be well aware of the pathophysiology and clinical

Table 61.2 Summary of management of postgastrectomy syndromes

	Dietary/medical management	Surgical management
Dumping syndrome	Small, frequent meals Low-carbohydrate diet Avoid liquid with solid meals Octreotide Acarbose (late dumping)	Conversion to RY (BI, BII)
Post-vagotomy diarrhea	Frequent small meals, fiber Small, frequent meals Cholestyramine	Antiperistaltic jejunal interposition
Delayed gastric emptying	Small meals Metoclopramide Erythromycin	Conversion of a partial to a near-total or total gastrectomy
Alkaline reflux gastritis	Ursodeoxycholic acid Sucralfate	Conversion to RY (BI, BII) Braun enteroenterostomy (BII) Henley loop interposition (BII)
Roux limb stasis	Metoclopramide Erythromycin	Redo RY

RY Roux-en-Y, *BI* Billroth I, *BII* Billroth II

presentation of each syndrome, the necessary studies to conduct, and the medical and surgical management options available for patients (Table 61.2).

References

1. NIH consensus conference. Helicobacter pylori in peptic ulcer disease. NIH consensus development panel on helicobacter pylori in peptic ulcer disease. JAMA. 1994;272(1):65–9.
2. Yeomans ND, Tulassay Z, Juhasz L, Racz I, Howard JM, van Rensburg CJ, Swannell AJ, Hawkey CJ. A comparison of omeprazole with ranitidine for ulcers associated with nonsteroidal antiinflammatory drugs. Acid suppression trial: ranitidine versus omeprazole for NSAID-associated ulcer treatment (ASTRONAUT) study group. N Engl J Med. 1998;338(11):719–26. https://doi.org/10.1056/NEJM199803123381104.
3. Anderson WF, Camargo MC, Fraumeni JF Jr, Correa P, Rosenberg PS, Rabkin CS. Age-specific trends in incidence of noncardia gastric cancer in US adults. JAMA. 2010;303(17):1723–8. https://doi.org/10.1001/jama.2010.496.
4. Wang YR, Richter JE, Dempsey DT. Trends and outcomes of hospitalizations for peptic ulcer disease in the United States, 1993 to 2006. Ann Surg. 2010;251(1):51–8. https://doi.org/10.1097/SLA.0b013e3181b975b8.
5. Siegel RL, Miller KD, Jemal A. Cancer statistics, 2016. CA Cancer J Clin. 2016;66(1):7–30. https://doi.org/10.3322/caac.21332.
6. Bolton JS, Conway WC 2nd. Postgastrectomy syndromes. Surg Clin North Am. 2011;91(5):1105–22. https://doi.org/10.1016/j.suc.2011.07.001.
7. Livingston EH. The incidence of bariatric surgery has plateaued in the U.S. Am J Surg. 2010;200(3):378–85. https://doi.org/10.1016/j.amjsurg.2009.11.007.
8. Thompson BW, Read RC. Long-term randomized prospective comparison of Finney and Heineke-Mikulicz pylorplasty in patients having vagotomy for peptic ulceration. Am J Surg. 1975;129(1):78–81.
9. Ishikawa K, Arita T, Ninomiya S, Bandoh T, Shiraishi N, Kitano S. Outcome of segmental gastrectomy versus distal gastrectomy for early gastric cancer. World J Surg. 2007;31(11):2204–7. https://doi.org/10.1007/s00268-007-9192-2.
10. Park DJ, Lee HJ, Jung HC, Kim WH, Lee KU, Yang HK. Clinical outcome of pylorus-preserving gastrectomy in gastric cancer in comparison with conventional distal gastrectomy with Billroth I anastomosis. World J Surg. 2008;32(6):1029–36. https://doi.org/10.1007/s00268-007-9441-4.
11. Fukuhara K, Osugi H, Takada N, Takemura M, Higashino M, Kinoshita H. Reconstructive procedure after distal gastrectomy for gastric cancer that best prevents duodenogastroesophageal reflux. World J Surg. 2002;26(12):1452–7. https://doi.org/10.1007/s00268-002-6363-z.
12. Barnett WO, Tucker FH Jr. Management of the Difficult Duodenal Stump. Ann Surg. 1964;159:794–801.
13. Burch JM, Cox CL, Feliciano DV, Richardson RJ, Martin RR. Management of the difficult duodenal stump. Am J Surg. 1991;162(6):522–6.
14. Degiuli M, Sasako M, Ponti A, Soldati T, Danese F, Calvo F. Morbidity and mortality after D2 gastrectomy for gastric cancer: results of the Italian Gastric Cancer Study Group prospective multicenter surgical study. J Clin Oncol. 1998;16(4):1490–3.
15. Wells CA, Macphee IW. The afferent-loop syndrome: bilious regurgitation after subtotal gastrectomy and its relief. Lancet. 1952;2(6747):1189–93.
16. van der Mijle HC, Kleibeuker JH, Limburg AJ, Bleichrodt RP, Beekhuis H, van Schilfgaarde R. Manometric and scintigraphic studies of the relation between motility disturbances in the Roux limb and the Roux-en-Y syndrome. Am J Surg. 1993;166(1):11–7.

17. Hertz AF. The cause and treatment of certain unfavourable after-effects of gastro-enterostomy. Proc R Soc Med. 1913;6(Surg Sect):155–63.
18. Ukleja A. Dumping syndrome: pathophysiology and treatment. Nutr Clin Pract. 2005;20(5):517–25.
19. Eagon JC, Miedema BW, Kelly KA. Postgastrectomy syndromes. Surg Clin North Am. 1992;72(2):445–65.
20. Azpiroz F, Malagelada JR. Gastric tone measured by an electronic barostat in health and post-surgical gastroparesis. Gastroenterology. 1987;92(4):934–43.
21. Sirinek KR, O'Dorisio TM, Howe B, McFee AS. Neurotensin, vasoactive intestinal peptide, and Roux-en-Y gastrojejunostomy. Their role in the dumping syndrome. Arch Surg. 1985;120(5):605–9.
22. Holdsworth CD, Turner D, McIntyre N. Pathophysiology of post-gastrectomy hypoglycaemia. Br Med J. 1969;4(5678):257–9.
23. van der Kleij FG, Vecht J, Lamers CB, Masclee AA. Diagnostic value of dumping provocation in patients after gastric surgery. Scand J Gastroenterol. 1996;31(12):1162–6.
24. Geer RJ, Richards WO, O'Dorisio TM, Woltering EO, Williams S, Rice D, Abumrad NN. Efficacy of octreotide acetate in treatment of severe postgastrectomy dumping syndrome. Ann Surg. 1990;212(6):678–87.
25. Hopman WP, Wolberink RG, Lamers CB, Van Tongeren JH. Treatment of the dumping syndrome with the somatostatin analogue SMS 201-995. Ann Surg. 1988;207(2):155–9.
26. Mackie CR, Jenkins SA, Hartley MN. Treatment of severe postvagotomy/postgastrectomy symptoms with the somatostatin analogue octreotide. Br J Surg. 1991;78(11):1338–43.
27. Vecht J, Lamers CB, Masclee AA. Long-term results of octreotide-therapy in severe dumping syndrome. Clin Endocrinol. 1999;51(5):619–24.
28. Hasegawa T, Yoneda M, Nakamura K, Ohnishi K, Harada H, Kyouda T, Yoshida Y, Makino I. Long-term effect of alpha-glucosidase inhibitor on late dumping syndrome. J Gastroenterol Hepatol. 1998;13(12):1201–6.
29. Duncombe VM, Bolin TD, Davis AE. Double-blind trial of cholestyramine in post-vagotomy diarrhoea. Gut. 1977;18(7):531–5.
30. Ayulo JA. Cholestyramine in postvagotomy syndrome. Preliminary report. Am J Gastroenterol. 1972;57(3):207–25.
31. Herrington JL Jr, Sawyers JL. A new operation for the dumping syndrome and post-vagotomy diarrhea. Ann Surg. 1972;175(5):790–801.
32. Jung HJ, Lee JH, Ryu KW, Lee JY, Kim CG, Choi IJ, Kim YW, Bae JM. The influence of reconstruction methods on food retention phenomenon in the remnant stomach after a subtotal gastrectomy. J Surg Oncol. 2008;98(1):11–4. https://doi.org/10.1002/jso.21076.
33. Forster J, Sarosiek I, Delcore R, Lin Z, Raju GS, McCallum RW. Gastric pacing is a new surgical treatment for gastroparesis. Am J Surg. 2001;182(6):676–81.
34. Bechi P, Amorosi A, Mazzanti R, Romagnoli P, Tonelli L. Gastric histology and fasting bile reflux after partial gastrectomy. Gastroenterology. 1987;93(2):335–43.
35. Attwood SE, Smyrk TC, DeMeester TR, Mirvish SS, Stein HJ, Hinder RA. Duodenoesophageal reflux and the development of esophageal adenocarcinoma in rats. Surgery. 1992;111(5):503–10.
36. Stefaniwsky AB, Tint GS, Speck J, Shefer S, Salen G. Ursodeoxycholic acid treatment of bile reflux gastritis. Gastroenterology. 1985;89(5):1000–4.
37. Kennedy T, Green R. Roux diversion for bile reflux following gastric surgery. Br J Surg. 1978;65(5):323–5.
38. Vogel SB, Drane WE, Woodward ER. Clinical and radionuclide evaluation of bile diversion by Braun enteroenterostomy: prevention and treatment of alkaline reflux gastritis. An alternative to Roux-en-Y diversion. Ann Surg. 1994;219(5):458–65; discussion 465–456
39. Herrington JL Jr, Sawyers JL, Whitehead WA. Surgical management of reflux gastritis. Ann Surg. 1974;180(4):526–37.
40. Gustavsson S, Ilstrup DM, Morrison P, Kelly KA. Roux-Y stasis syndrome after gastrectomy. Am J Surg. 1988;155(3):490–4.

41. Miedema BW, Kelly KA, Camilleri M, Hanson RB, Zinsmeister AR, O'Connor MK, Brown ML. Human gastric and jejunal transit and motility after Roux gastrojejunostomy. Gastroenterology. 1992;103(4):1133–43.
42. Mitty WF Jr, Grossi C, Nealon TF Jr. Chronic afferent loop syndrome. Ann Surg. 1970;172(6):996–1001.
43. Lundegardh G, Adami HO, Helmick C, Zack M, Meirik O. Stomach cancer after partial gastrectomy for benign ulcer disease. N Engl J Med. 1988;319(4):195–200. https://doi.org/10.1056/NEJM198807283190402.
44. Viste A, Bjornestad E, Opheim P, Skarstein A, Thunold J, Hartveit F, Eide GE, Eide TJ, Soreide O. Risk of carcinoma following gastric operations for benign disease. A historical cohort study of 3470 patients. Lancet. 1986;2(8505):502–5.
45. Surgery ASfMaB. Estimate of bariatric surgery numbers. 2011-2015. 2016. https://asmbs.org/resources/estimate-of-bariatric-surgery-numbers. Accessed 10 Oct 2016.
46. Mallory GN, Macgregor AM, Rand CS. The influence of dumping on weight loss after gastric restrictive surgery for morbid obesity. Obes Surg. 1996;6(6):474–8. https://doi.org/10.1381/096089296765556368.
47. Patel RA, Brolin RE, Gandhi A. Revisional operations for marginal ulcer after Roux-en-Y gastric bypass. Surg Obes Relat Dis. 2009;5(3):317–22. https://doi.org/10.1016/j.soard.2008.10.011.
48. Dapri G, Cadiere GB, Himpens J. Laparoscopic seromyotomy for long stenosis after sleeve gastrectomy with or without duodenal switch. Obes Surg. 2009;19(4):495–9. https://doi.org/10.1007/s11695-009-9803-0.
49. Yehoshua RT, Eidelman LA, Stein M, Fichman S, Mazor A, Chen J, Bernstine H, Singer P, Dickman R, Beglaibter N, Shikora SA, Rosenthal RJ, Rubin M. Laparoscopic sleeve gastrectomy--volume and pressure assessment. Obes Surg. 2008;18(9):1083–8. https://doi.org/10.1007/s11695-008-9576-x.

Evaluation and Management: Recurrent Peptic Ulcer Disease

62

Kamran Samakar and Adrian B. Dobrowolsky

Management of Refractory or Recurrent Peptic Ulcer Disease

The major causes of peptic ulcer disease (PUD) are smoking, nonsteroidal anti-inflammatory drug (NSAID) use, and *Helicobacter pylori (H. pylori)* infection. The vast majority of peptic ulcers respond to antimicrobial therapy for *H. pylori* infection, treatment with antisecretory therapy, and withdrawal of inciting factors. However, not all peptic ulcers are easily eradicated and may persist. A refractory or recurrent peptic ulcer is defined as an endoscopically proven ulcer greater than 5 mm that does not heal after 12 weeks of appropriate treatment or recurs after complete healing of the previous site [1]. In this chapter, we will focus our discussion on the management of refractory and recurrent peptic ulcers.

Endoscopic Evaluation

Routine management of benign gastric ulcers relies on eradication of *H. pylori*, withdrawal of inciting factors such as smoking and NSAID use, and treatment with antisecretory therapy. Endoscopic evaluation after initial therapy for gastric ulcers should be individualized but is generally recommended after 8–12 weeks of treatment in patients affected by gastric ulcers [2]. Importantly, however, repeat endoscopy may not be necessary in patients with benign appearing ulcers with a determined etiology or resolution of symptoms after a course of appropriate therapy [3–5]. After initial treatment, refractory or recurrent gastric ulcers should undergo

K. Samakar · A. B. Dobrowolsky (✉)
Department of Upper GI, General, and Bariatric Surgery, USC Keck Medical Center, Los Angeles, CA, USA
e-mail: Adrian.dobrowolsky@med.usc.edu

J. Grams et al. (eds.), *The SAGES Manual of Foregut Surgery*,
https://doi.org/10.1007/978-3-319-96122-4_62

multi-quadrant biopsies including both the edges and the base of the ulcer along with testing for *H. pylori*. Routine surveillance after treatment of duodenal peptic ulcers is not recommended due to the exceedingly low malignancy rate and the fact that the vast majority of duodenal ulcers respond within 4 weeks to appropriate antisecretory therapy [6, 7]. Repeat endoscopy should be considered in patients with duodenal ulcers experiencing persistent symptoms despite appropriate therapy.

Etiology and Management

The presence of refractory ulcers on repeat endoscopy after 8–12 weeks of treatment prompts further evaluation for underlying risk factors and other etiologies for PUD. Up to 10% of peptic ulcers are refractory to initial treatment, and up to 20% recur within 6 months despite eradication of *H. pylori* and concomitant antisecretory treatment [8]. Failure of *H. pylori* eradication with first-line triple therapy should be followed by bismuth-quadruple therapy or levofloxacin triple therapy. *H. pylori* eradication should be confirmed in patients with refractory peptic ulcer disease with posttreatment testing [9]. Persistent infection may result from failure of therapy, false negative testing, or poor patient compliance. Similarly, continued NSAID use is a leading cause of recurrent and refractory peptic ulcer disease [10]. Patients should be counseled on lifestyle modification including smoking and tobacco cessation, NSAID use, and medication compliance including therapy for *H. pylori* eradication. Maintenance therapy with a PPI should be continued in patients with high-risk peptic ulcer disease defined as having ulcers greater than 2 cm and age >50 years, failure to eradicate *H. pylori*, recurrent and/or refractory peptic ulcers, and patients with PUD that are *H. pylori* negative in the absence of NSAID use.

Acid hypersecretion or inadequate inhibition of acid secretion may both contribute to cases of refractory or recurrent peptic ulcer disease. Inadequate inhibition of acid secretion may be secondary to suboptimal therapy or poor patient compliance. Proton pump inhibitors have been shown to be more effective than H2 receptor antagonists in the treatment of peptic ulcer disease and should be used as first-line therapy [11]. Patients with refractory peptic ulcers should be treated with double-dose PPI therapy, and consideration should be given to an alternative PPI regimen [12]. When trying to determine the etiology of acid hypersecretion causing refractory and recurrent peptic ulcer disease, one must entertain the possibility of Zollinger-Ellison syndrome (ZES). ZES is defined by the presence of a gastrin-secreting neuroendocrine tumor that manifests clinically with symptoms of abdominal pain, PUD, diarrhea, gastroesophageal reflux, and dyspepsia. Testing for ZES involves measuring fasting serum gastrin levels in the setting of low gastric pH. Serum gastrin levels help differentiate ZES from other disorders such as atrophic gastritis with hypochlorhydria when the gastrin levels are above 1000 pg/mL or basal acid outputs are greater than 15 mEq/h [13]. Also, to aid in diagnosing a gastrinoma, one may perform a secretin stimulation test in which the gastrin levels are serially measured after administration of intravenous secretin with a positive result with an increase in gastrin levels of ≥120 pg/mL [14]. Additionally, multiple endocrine neoplasia type I (MEN I) is typically associated with pituitary, parathyroid, and pancreatic neoplasms, most commonly insulinoma, but gastrinoma is the second most common manifestation of the disease. Therefore, additional testing for the other manifestations of MEN I must be ruled out if one confirms a gastrinoma. Somatostatin receptor scintigraphy along with endoscopic ultrasound may be useful in identifying the tumor site. When identified, a gastrinoma is treated by acid suppression, surgical resection, and therapy of metastatic disease. In the absence of ZES, idiopathic gastric acid hypersecretion should be considered for patients with acid hypersecretion.

Rare and unusual cases of refractory peptic ulcer disease account for a small proportion of cases but should be considered in the absence of a clear etiology. There are a number of medications that may cause or contribute to the development of PUD including acetaminophen, bisphosphonates, glucocorticoids, clopidrogel, sirolimus, spironolactone, selective serotonin reuptake inhibitors, and chemotherapeutic agents [5, 15–18]. Chronic disease states such as liver cirrhosis, chronic kidney disease, Crohn's disease, organ transplantation, sarcoidosis, lymphoma, mesenteric ischemia, and diabetes mellitus can also contribute to refractory or recurrent PUD [19–21]. Infectious etiologies include tuberculosis, syphilis, cytomegalovirus, IgG4-related sclerosing disease, strongyloidiasis, cytomegalovirus, and herpes virus [12, 21–24].

Surgery

Due to advances in antisecretory therapy and the recognition that treatment of *H. pylori* can eliminate most ulcers, surgical intervention is rarely needed as an elective therapy for PUD. More commonly, surgery is necessary to deal with the sequelae of PUD including bleeding, perforation, and obstruction [25–27]. One main indication for elective surgical intervention for recurrent or refractory PUD is the failure of ulcer healing after adequate therapy for 12–24 weeks. Patients with intractable symptoms, relapse, and the suspicion of malignancy should prompt consideration of surgical intervention. The general principles of surgery for PUD are reduction of acid secretion, treatment of ulcer disease, and minimization of postoperative sequelae from surgery [28]. The extent of resection for ulcers that may harbor malignancy should be tailored to the patient based on location, size, and their overall physiologic status.

Typically, gastric ulcers are treated according to the type, location, and features of the ulcer. Type I gastric ulcers are not associated with hyperacidity and are often treated with distal gastrectomy to include the ulcer in the resected specimen. Type I ulcers can be resected and reconstructed using either a Billroth I or Billroth II reconstruction. Type II and III gastric ulcers are associated with acid hypersecretion and are generally treated with antrectomy and vagotomy. Some surgeons prefer vagotomy in these cases as an option for patients who are noncompliant with antisecretory therapy or have a history of complicated or recurrent disease [29]. Type IV gastric ulcers present a technical challenge owing to the fact that they are typically located close to the gastroesophageal junction. Approaches for type IV ulcers include the Pauchet procedure, Kelly-Madlener procedure, Csendes procedure, and esophagogastrojejunostomy. Laparoscopic approaches should be considered for all elective surgical interventions for refractory and recurrent PUD [30–35].

A vagotomy is indicated for patients with acute complications of PUD or those affected by recurrent and refractory disease. Typically, a vagotomy is added to a primary procedure by transecting or removing the vagus nerve or branches of the vagus nerve in order to provide an antisecretory measure. Various techniques have been established including truncal vagotomy, highly selective vagotomy, posterior truncal vagotomy and anterior serosal myotomy (Taylor procedure), and posterior truncal vagotomy and anterior highly selective vagotomy (Hill-Barker procedure) (Figs. 62.1, 62.2 and 62.3) [36–38]. Postoperative complications of vagotomy include delayed gastric emptying and possible ulcer disease recurrence due to inadequate or incomplete vagotomy. Due to the risk for delayed gastric emptying, vagotomy is most often performed in conjunction with a drainage procedure or surgical resection. The decision to perform a vagotomy for refractory or recurrent peptic ulcer disease should be determined by the indication for surgery, the patient's ability to tolerate medical antisecretory therapy, and the surgeon's familiarity and expertise with the various techniques.

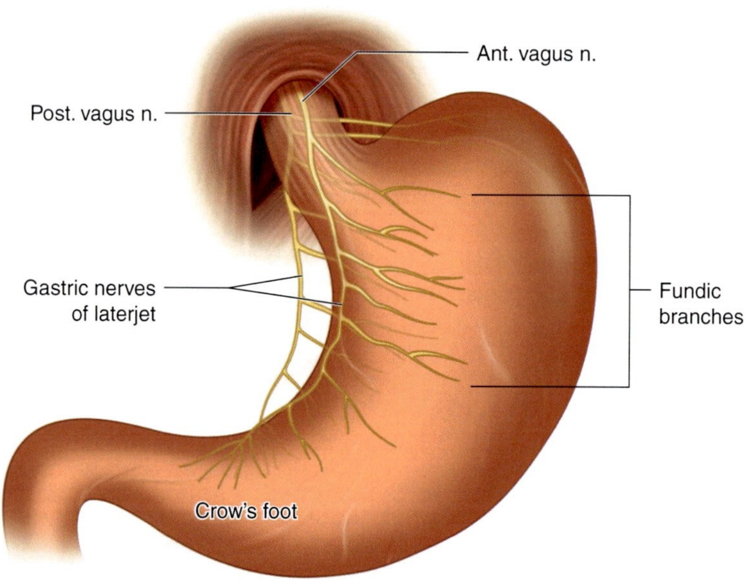

Fig. 62.1 Anatomical landmarks in highly selective vagotomy

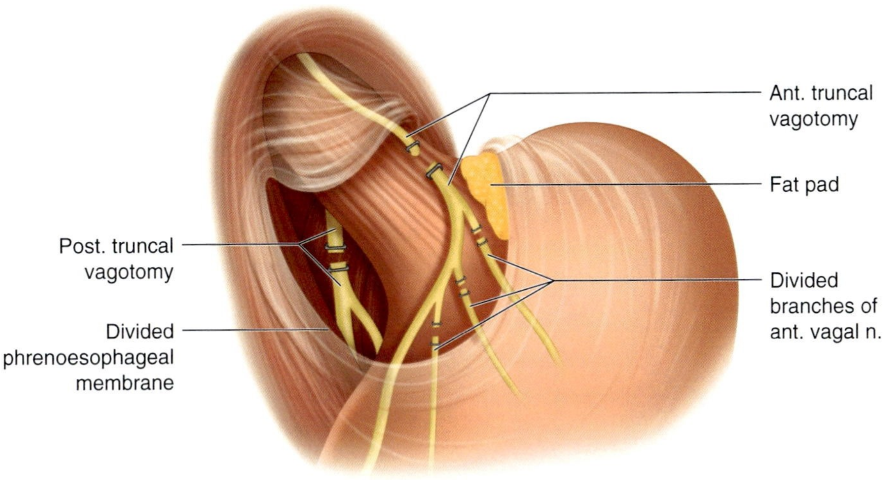

Fig. 62.2 Bilateral truncal vagotomy. Ensure adequate cephalad dissection above the branch point for the "criminal" nerve branches of Grassi off the posterior vagal trunk

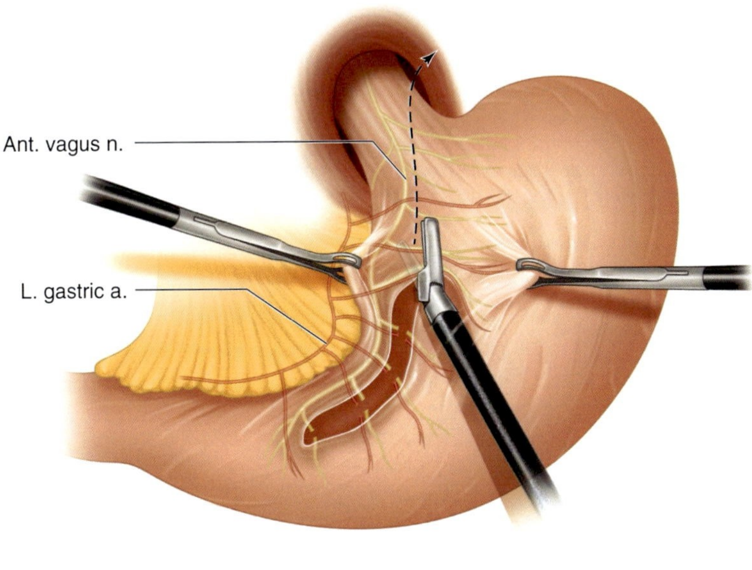

Fig. 62.3 Highly selective vagotomy

Special Considerations

For the purposes of this chapter, we have limited our discussion to the treatment of chronic refractory and recurrent PUD. The approach to acute complications of PUD such as bleeding, perforation, and gastric outlet obstruction may vary drastically from non-emergent management of chronic PUD. Likewise, we have not discussed the management of ulcerations that occur after gastric surgery. In the setting of Billroth II or Roux-en-Y reconstruction, ulcerations of the gastroenteric anastomoses require special consideration to determine the best therapeutic course.

References

1. Vakil N, Grover S. Approach to refractory or recurrent peptic ulcer disease. UpToDate. 04/23/2015.
2. ASGE Standards of Practice Committee, Banerjee S, Cash BD, et al. The role of endoscopy in the management of patients with peptic ulcer disease. Gastrointest Endosc. 2010;71(4):663–8.
3. Whiting JL, Sigurdsson A, Rowlands DC, Hallissey MT, Fielding JW. The long term results of endoscopic surveillance of premalignant gastric lesions. Gut. 2002;50(3):378–81.
4. Hosokawa O, Watanabe K, Hatorri M, Douden K, Hayashi H, Kaizaki Y. Detection of gastric cancer by repeat endoscopy within a short time after negative examination. Endoscopy. 2001;33(4):301–5.
5. Vakil N, Grover S. Peptic ulcer disease: management. UpToDate. 07/23/2015.
6. Liang XY, Gao Q, Gong NP, Tang LP, Wang PL, Tao XH. Comparison of esomeprazole enteric-coated capsules vs esomeprazole magnesium in the treatment of active duodenal ulcer: a randomized, double-blind, controlled study. World J Gastroenterol. 2008;14(12):1941–5.
7. Lanza F, Goff J, Scowcroft C, Jennings D, Greski-Rose P. Double-blind comparison of lansoprazole, ranitidine, and placebo in the treatment of acute duodenal ulcer. Lansoprazole study group. Am J Gastroenterol. 1994;89(8):1191–200.
8. Laine L, Hopkins RJ, Girardi LS. Has the impact of helicobacter pylori therapy on ulcer recurrence in the United States been overstated? A meta-analysis of rigorously designed trials. Am J Gastroenterol. 1998;93(9):1409–15.
9. Malfertheiner P, Megraud F, O'Morain CA, et al. Management of helicobacter pylori infection – the Maastricht IV/Florence consensus report. Gut. 2012;61(5):646–64.
10. Lanas A, Remacha B, Sainz R, Hirschowitz BI. Study of outcome after targeted intervention for peptic ulcer resistant to acid suppression therapy. Am J Gastroenterol. 2000;95(2):513–9.
11. Yeomans ND, Tulassay Z, Juhasz L, et al. A comparison of omeprazole with ranitidine for ulcers associated with nonsteroidal antiinflammatory drugs. Acid suppression trial: ranitidine versus omeprazole for NSAID-associated ulcer treatment (ASTRONAUT) study group. N Engl J Med. 1998;338(11):719–26.
12. Kim HU. Diagnostic and treatment approaches for refractory peptic ulcers. Clin Endosc. 2015;48(4):285–90.
13. Nieto JM, Pisegna JR. The role of proton pump inhibitors in the treatment of zollinger-ellison syndrome. Expert Opin Pharmacother. 2006;7(2):169–75.
14. Berna MJ, Hoffmann KM, Long SH, Serrano J, Gibril F, Jensen RT. Serum gastrin in zollinger-ellison syndrome: II. prospective study of gastrin provocative testing in 293 patients from the national institutes of health and comparison with 537 cases from the literature. evaluation of diagnostic criteria, proposal of new criteria, and correlations with clinical and tumoral features. Medicine (Baltimore). 2006;85(6):331–64.
15. Dall M, Schaffalitzky de Muckadell OB, Lassen AT, Hansen JM, Hallas J. An association between selective serotonin reuptake inhibitor use and serious upper gastrointestinal bleeding. Clin Gastroenterol Hepatol. 2009;7(12):1314–21.

16. Shike M, Gillin JS, Kemeny N, Daly JM, Kurtz RC. Severe gastroduodenal ulcerations complicating hepatic artery infusion chemotherapy for metastatic colon cancer. Am J Gastroenterol. 1986;81(3):176–9.
17. Smith AD, Bai D, Marroquin CE, et al. Gastrointestinal hemorrhage due to complicated gastroduodenal ulcer disease in liver transplant patients taking sirolimus. Clin Transpl. 2005;19(2):250–4.
18. Verhamme K, Mosis G, Dieleman J, Stricker B, Sturkenboom M. Spironolactone and risk of upper gastrointestinal events: population based case-control study. BMJ. 2006;333(7563):330.
19. Kim JH, Moon JS, Jee SR, et al. Guidelines of treatment for peptic ulcer disease in special conditions. Korean J Gastroenterol. 2009;54(5):318–27.
20. Fireman Z, Sternberg A, Yarchovsky Y, et al. Multiple antral ulcers in gastric sarcoid. J Clin Gastroenterol. 1997;24(2):97–9.
21. Diaz L, Hernandez-Oquet RE, Deshpande AR, Moshiree B. Upper gastrointestinal involvement in crohn disease: histopathologic and endoscopic findings. South Med J. 2015;108(11):695–700.
22. Lohr JM, Nelson JA, Oldstone MB. Is herpes simplex virus associated with peptic ulcer disease? J Virol. 1990;64(5):2168–74.
23. Hori K, Fukuda Y, Tomita T, Kosaka T, Noda S. Cytomegalovirus-associated gastritis. Gastrointest Endosc. 2004;59(6):692–3.
24. Jo J, Kim H, Heo S. A case of gastric syphilis diagnosed by PCR test: a case report. J Med Life Sci. 2014;11:43–7.
25. Sachdeva AK, Zaren HA, Sigel B. Surgical treatment of peptic ulcer disease. Med Clin North Am. 1991;75(4):999–1012.
26. Towfigh S, Chandler C, Hines OJ, McFadden DW. Outcomes from peptic ulcer surgery have not benefited from advances in medical therapy. Am Surg. 2002;68(4):385–9.
27. Jamieson GG. Current status of indications for surgery in peptic ulcer disease. World J Surg. 2000;24(3):256–8.
28. Vernon A, Ferzoco S, Ashley S, Chen W. Surgical management of peptic ulcer disease. UpToDate. 08/24/2015.
29. Lightner A, Brunicardi C. In: Cameron J, Cameron A, editors. The management of benign gastric ulcers. 12th ed. Philadelphia: Elsevier; 2017. p. 79–82.
30. Katkhouda N, Heimbucher J, Mouiel J. Laparoscopic posterior vagotomy and anterior seromyotomy. Endosc Surg Allied Technol. 1994;2(2):95–9.
31. Croce E, Azzola M, Golia M, et al. Laparoscopic posterior truncal vagotomy and anterior proximal gastric vagotomy. Endosc Surg Allied Technol. 1994;2(2):113–6.
32. Cadiere GB, Himpens J, Bruyns J. Laparoscopic proximal gastric vagotomy. Endosc Surg Allied Technol. 1994;2(2):105–8.
33. Katkhouda N. Advanced laparoscopic surgery: techniques and tips. In: second ed. New York: Springer; 2010.
34. Dallemagne B, Weerts JM, Jehaes C, Markiewicz S, Lombard R. Laparoscopic highly selective vagotomy. Br J Surg. 1994;81(4):554–6.
35. Zittel TT, Jehle EC, Becker HD. Surgical management of peptic ulcer disease today--indication, technique and outcome. Langenbeck's Arch Surg. 2000;385(2):84–96.
36. Taylor TV, Lythgoe JP, McFarland JB, Gilmore IT, Thomas PE, Ferguson GH. Anterior lesser curve seromyotomy and posterior truncal vagotomy versus truncal vagotomy and pyloroplasty in the treatment of chronic duodenal ulcer. Br J Surg. 1990;77(9):1007–9.
37. Petrakis I, Vassilakis SJ, Chalkiadakis G. Anterior lesser curve seromyotomy using a stapling device and posterior truncal vagotomy for the treatment of chronic duodenal ulcer: Longterm results. J Am Coll Surg. 1999;188(6):623–8.
38. Croce E, Olmi S, Russo R, Azzola M, Mastropasqua E, Golia M. Laparoscopic treatment of peptic ulcers. A review after 6 years experience with hill-barker's procedure. Hepato-Gastroenterology. 1999;46(26):924–9.

63 Peptic Ulcer Disease: Deciding What Procedure When

Benjamin R. Veenstra and Daniel J. Deziel

There are elegant operations to be done for peptic ulcer disease (PUD), operations that eliminate the source and stimulation of acid secretion according to the best anatomic and physiologic principles. Acid is a necessary component of PUD, as seminally articulated by Karl Schwarz in 1910: "Ohne saueren Magensaft kein peptisches Geschwur" ("Without acidic gastric juice, no peptic ulcer") [1]. However, acid is not necessarily a sufficient cause. Recognition of the multifactorial etiology of PUD, particularly the contributory roles of infection with *Helicobacter pylori* and the use of nonsteroidal anti-inflammatory drugs (NSAIDs), has enabled successful nonoperative management in a majority of cases. The frequency of hospital admissions and of operations for PUD has declined [2–4]. Current surgical trainees have limited exposure to definitive anti-ulcer procedures. Hence, these elegant curative operations have nearly become a historical teaching point. Nevertheless, urgent operations for the complications of PUD remain a steadfast scenario for surgeons.

The contemporary indications for surgery in PUD, by order of decreasing frequency, are generally perforation, bleeding, obstruction, failed medical management (intractability, recurrence), and concern for malignancy. When an operation for PUD is indicted, there are multiple options to consider with various types of resection, vagotomy, and reconstruction. The goals are to treat any immediate ulcer complication, to promote ulcer healing, to prevent ulcer recurrence, and to minimize undesirable sequelae. The choice of operation is always a balance between curative treatment of the ulcer disease and postoperative consequences. Surgical management of PUD is thus a compromise, albeit a life-saving one.

B. R. Veenstra (✉) · D. J. Deziel
Department of Surgery, Division of MIS and Bariatrics, Rush University Medical Center, Chicago, IL, USA
e-mail: Benjamin_Veenstra@Rush.Edu

J. Grams et al. (eds.), *The SAGES Manual of Foregut Surgery*,
https://doi.org/10.1007/978-3-319-96122-4_63

The rational selection of an operation for PUD depends upon these factors:

1. Understanding of the specific disease process (diagnosis/ulcer location, etiology)
2. Suitable operative conditions (inflammation, contamination, prior interventions, tissue characteristics)
3. Suitable patient (hemodynamic stability, comorbidities, potential for compliance)
4. Suitable surgeon (a surgeon's personal experience and capability)
5. Local resources (assistants, equipment, support services)

This chapter provides some comments on the selection of the operation in various ulcer scenarios and offers what we most typically do in our own practice. Operations for PUD can be satisfactorily accomplished by either laparoscopic or open methods. The approach should be determined according to the surgeon's experience, the local environment, and the pathology at hand. Emergent operations should be conducted properly and with dispatch.

Perforation

Perforation is the most frequent complication of PUD that prompts surgery in the United States [5, 6]. Perforation has the highest mortality rate of ulcer complications, especially perforated gastric ulcer [7]. The preferred operative management is largely dictated by ulcer location but must be tempered by local pathologic conditions and by the status of the patient. Approximately one-half of perforated ulcers are in the first portion of the duodenum, and the other half are pyloric, prepyloric, antral, or in the gastric body.

For duodenal perforations, the primary goal is closure and peritoneal washout. Closure is accomplished by use of a Graham patch of omentum or with the falciform ligament. We prefer to place the sutures as seromuscular bites in healthy tissue with one bite taken on each side of the perforation away from the friable edge. Graham's original article illustrates through and through sutures passed from one side of the perforation to the other, into which a free or attached piece of omentum is incorporated [8].

The operation is limited to patch closure alone for patients with shock, delayed presentation and significant peritoneal contamination and for most patients who have not previously been treated for PUD. Given the prevalence of *H. pylori* and of NSAID use, there has been a trend in some settings toward repair of the perforation alone without a definitive antiulcer operation for essentially all patients with perforated duodenal ulcer. This approach is based on the assumption that subsequent medical management will be sufficient for ulcer healing and prevention of recurrence. This is a leap of faith. Surgeons must understand some key considerations before blindly adopting this strategy.

Among patients requiring urgent operations for perforated PUD, fewer than one-half of those who are tested for *H. pylori* will prove positive, and only about one-half will have a history of NSAID use [5, 6, 9]. One-third of patients undergoing urgent PUD operations have already been receiving ulcer treatment at the time of the complication [6]. PUD may be refractory or recurrent for numerous reasons including persistent *H. pylori*, inability to eliminate use of NSAIDs or other ulcerogenic medications, inadequate pharmacologic acid suppression, and continued smoking. Unfortunately, much of this may not be known at the time of an emergent or urgent operation. When operative conditions permit, we consider whether a definitive operation may be beneficial. If the determination is yes, we usually extend the perforation and perform a pyloroplasty with truncal vagotomy. If the patient and peritoneal cavity permit and the surgeon is experienced, we perform a highly selective vagotomy following closure of the perforation.

Local ulcer characteristics also influence the choice of operation. So-called "giant"' (>2 cm) duodenal ulcers and ulcers with considerable fibrosis are associated with a higher risk for complications and recurrence. For these ulcers, we recommend truncal vagotomy and antrectomy with a Billroth II reconstruction if the patient is stable.

Perforated pyloric or pyloric channel ulcers often do not do well following closure alone. Therefore, we recommend pyloroplasty with either a truncal vagotomy or a highly selective vagotomy when conditions are suitable [10].

Perforated gastric ulcers pose a highly morbid situation. The preferred operation is gastric resection. Unfortunately, the condition of the patient may only allow a limited procedure. When formal gastrectomy is not prudent, the ulcer is excised or generously biopsied, and patch or primary closure is carried out as a compromise. When possible, we perform a subtotal gastrectomy to include resection of the ulcer and add truncal vagotomy for patients who have type II (combined duodenal and gastric ulcers) or type III (prepyloric) gastric ulcers.

Hemorrhage

Bleeding is the most frequent complication of PUD that results in hospital admission [2]. *H. pylori* and NSAID use are risk factors that contribute to bleeding, as they do to perforation. Patients that come to operation for bleeding PUD are typically on intense acute antisecretory therapy and have failed one or more endoscopic attempts to control hemorrhage, with or without additional angiographic interventions. Accordingly, a definitive acid-reducing operation is advisable once the bleeding has been stopped.

Duodenal ulcer hemorrhage is controlled through a longitudinal duodenotomy over the first portion of the duodenum. The bleeding vessels will be the superior and inferior aspects of the gastroduodenal artery and the transverse pancreatic artery. These are secured by direct suture ligation with multiple sutures. The gastroduodenal artery can also be separately ligated outside the duodenum. If not already done, the duodenotomy is extended across the pylorus, and pyloroplasty and truncal vagotomy are performed. If it has been possible to secure the vessels through a duodenotomy with an intact pylorus, highly selective vagotomy is an option for an experienced surgeon with a stable patient.

Bleeding gastric ulcer disease that requires operation is preferably treated by gastric resection and Billroth II reconstruction. Vagotomy is not necessary, although it is not objectionable. For compromised patients who fail nonoperative control but cannot tolerate a formal gastrectomy, the chance for a successful outcome is guarded. Ulcer oversewing or excision (due to risk of malignancy) with truncal vagotomy and pyloroplasty is an option if it can be performed expediently.

Gastric Outlet Obstruction

Patients who require an operation for PUD complicated by gastric outlet obstruction have chronic disease with significant fibrosis. Most frequently this is consequent to ulceration of the duodenum or pyloric channel, but gastric cancer must be excluded. The optimal operation will depend upon the findings at the time of surgery and the fitness of the patient. In our current experience, distal gastrectomy with truncal vagotomy and Billroth II reconstruction provides satisfactory relief for many patients. Vagotomy is not done when there has been prolonged obstruction with gastric atony. Likewise, Roux-en-Y reconstruction is a poor choice as it may compound delayed gastric emptying with the roux stasis syndrome.

At operation, prior to embarking on resection, an assessment must be made as to whether the duodenum can be safely mobilized and divided and securely closed. Ulcer disease with obstruction is often associated with considerable anatomic distortion. Injury to the bile ducts, pancreas, and major adjacent vessels is an inherent risk. Combined operative injury to the main pancreatic duct and bile duct has most frequently occurred during gastrectomy.

Some method for gastric drainage must be established if resection is not feasible. Fibrosis that is so pronounced as to prohibit resection will also usually render pyloroplasty untenable. However, if healthy enough tissue is accessible, a Jaboulay gastroduodenostomy might be accomplished. Otherwise, a gastrojejunostomy is created on the posterior aspect of the stomach. Concurrent placement of a gastrostomy tube for drainage and a feeding jejunostomy is advisable and may alone be the safest surgical option for the most infirm patients.

Occasionally, patients undergoing operation for gastric outlet obstruction are found to have a limited pyloroduodenal stenosis. This can be remedied with pyloroplasty in Heineke-Mikulicz fashion or with a version of gastroduodenostomy (Jaboulay, Finney).

We perform a truncal vagotomy in conjunction with either pyloroplasty or gastrojejunostomy, except when there is concern for gastric motility. Some have successfully coupled highly selective vagotomy with Jaboulay gastroduodenostomy [11] or gastrojejunostomy [12].

Intractability

Elective operations for intractable PUD are infrequent these days. For a variety of reasons however, ulcers may be refractory or recurrent with nonoperative management or after prior ulcer operations. These patients remain a challenge for which the properly selected and executed operation can be reparative. The choice of procedure is predicated on patient factors, pharmacologic factors, physiologic factors, and pathologic factors. The operation is a balance between the risk for ulcer recurrence and for postoperative digestive disturbances including diarrhea, dumping, and bile reflux.

In the current era, patients with medically intractable duodenal ulcer are unusual and usually have pronounced pathologic changes with ulcers that are deep, penetrating, or extensive. Antrectomy with truncal vagotomy remains our surgical standard for this group.

For patients with less severe pathologic disruption and intractable disease, a highly selective vagotomy is preferred. This includes division of the branches from the nerves of Latarjet to the parietal call mass along the anterior and posterior lesser curvature, dissection of the gastroesophageal junction and distal esophagus with division of the upper short gastric vessels and any posterior vagal branches to the fundus (nerves of Grassi), and division of the right gastroepiploic vessels and accompanying recurrent vagal fibers (nerve of Rosetti). As this can be tedious laparoscopically, some prefer a laparoscopic posterior truncal vagotomy and anterior seromyotomy (Taylor procedure), although that has not been our practice.

Elective management of intractable gastric ulcer must exclude cancer. We perform ulcer resection by subtotal distal gastrectomy and Billroth II reconstruction. Truncal vagotomy is also done for type II or III ulcers. Type IV ulcers high on the lesser curvature can be included in the resection by a variety of configurations or by separate excision. Care must be exercised to avoid compromise of the gastroesophageal junction and to obtain a sound anastomosis.

Summary

The number of operations necessary for PUD has declined substantially over recent decades. However, urgent operations for perforation and bleeding are still required with some regularity. Elective operations for refractory disease and gastric outlet obstruction are far less common but can be curative. A spectrum of classic ulcer operations must remain in the surgical armamentarium for properly selected patients.

References

1. Schwarz K. Uber penetrierende Magen-und jejunalgeschure. Beitr Klin Chir. 1910;67:96–128.
2. Wang YR, Richter JE, Dempsey DT. Trends and outcomes of hospitalizations for peptic ulcer disease in the United States, 1993 to 2006. Ann Surg. 2010;251:51–8.

3. Smith BR, Stabile BE. Emerging trends in peptic ulcer disease and damage control surgery in the H. pylori era. Am Surg. 2005;71:797–801.
4. Schwesinger WH, Page CP, Sirinek KR, et al. Operations for peptic ulcer disease: paradigm lost. J Gastrointest Surg. 2001;5:438–43.
5. Sarosi GA Jr, Jaiswal KR, Nwariaku FE, et al. Surgical therapy of peptic ulcers in the 21st century: more common than you think. Am J Surg. 2005;190:775–9.
6. Zelickson MS, Bronder CM, Johnson BL, et al. Helicobacter pylori is not the predominant etiology for peptic ulcers requiring operation. Am Surg. 2011;77:1054–60.
7. Hermansson M, Stael von Hostein C, Zilling T. Surgical approach and prognostic factors after peptic ulcer perforation. Eur J Surg. 1999;165:566–72.
8. Graham RR. The treatment of perforated duodenal ulcers. Surg Gynecol Obstet. 1937;64:235–8.
9. Gunshefski L, Flancbaum L, Brolin RE, Frankel A. Changing patterns in perforated peptic ulcer disease. Am Surg. 1990;56:270–4.
10. Jordan PH Jr, Thornby J. Perforated pyloroduodenal ulcers. Long term results with omental patch and parietal cell vagotomy. Ann Surg. 1995;221:479–86.
11. Dittrich K, Blauensteiner W, Schrutka-Kolbl C, et al. Highly selective vagotomy plus Jaboulay: a possible alternative in patients with benign stenosis secondary to duodenal ulceration. J Am Coll Surg. 1995;180:654–8.
12. Csendes A, Maluenda F, Braghetto I, et al. Prospective randomized study comparing three surgical techniques for the treatment of gastric outlet obstruction secondary to duodenal ulcer. Am J Surg. 1993;166:45–9.

Etiology and Diagnosis of Gastric Outlet Obstruction

64

Michael Paul Meara

Etiology

The general etiology of gastric outlet obstruction can be broken into two encompassing groups, benign and malignant. While historically benign causes of gastric outlet obstruction occupied the majority of the causes of this clinical presentation, malignancy now overshadows this group [1–3]. We will explore these two realms as well as delve into the more uncommon diagnoses, which may also contribute to this disease.

Benign

Peptic Ulcer Disease

This term refers to any disease process that leads to ulceration or injury of the gastric mucosa, most notably in the pre-pylorus, pylorus, and the duodenal bulb. Historically, peptic ulcer disease accounted for as much as 80–90% of gastric outlet obstructions [4, 5]. This disease was originally attributed to acid hypersecretion, either intrinsic or secondary to excessive gastrin secretion. Stress was also incorrectly attributed as a causative agent of ulcer disease. Recognition of the bacterium *Helicobacter pylori* and its treatment has led to a dramatic decrease in this disease and its complications [6, 7].

Multiple nonsteroidal anti-inflammatory drugs have also been linked to peptic ulcer disease. Common over-the-counter formulations including ibuprofen,

M. P. Meara
Department of Surgery, The Ohio State University Wexner Medical Center, Columbus, OH, USA
e-mail: michael.meara@osumc.edu

J. Grams et al. (eds.), *The SAGES Manual of Foregut Surgery*,
https://doi.org/10.1007/978-3-319-96122-4_64

naproxen, and aspirin have all been implicated in peptic ulcer disease. The damaging effects of NSAIDs are multifactorial. Mechanisms that have been implicated in ulcer formation include direct irritation to the gastric lining, damage to the buffering mechanism of the gastric mucosa, suppression of prostaglandin synthesis, and decrease in gastric blood flow impeding repair [8–10].

Recognition of *Helicobacter pylori*, recognition of the harmful effects of NSAIDs, and the liberal usage of proton pump inhibitors have further decreased the prevalence of peptic ulcer disease. Gastric outlet obstruction now only accounts for 2% of complications related to peptic ulcer disease [4, 9, 11, 12].

Gastric Volvulus

Mechanical obstruction secondary to gastric volvulus can be acute or chronic in nature. Volvulus is defined as any abnormal rotation of the stomach. Chronically, this can involve rotation into defects in the diaphragm, either congenital or acquired – most frequently traumatically. Nomenclature defining volvulus includes organoaxial and mesenteroaxial rotations. Organoaxial rotations are defined as rotations along the long axis of the stomach, while rotations perpendicular to the stomach are defined as mesenteroaxial rotations. These rotations are thought to be permitted by failure of formation of restrictive gastric ligaments to other surrounding structures or secondary to adhesive disease from previous operative interventions. In the setting of acute gastric volvulus, such rotations can result in gastric outlet obstruction and mucosal ischemia. Acute volvulus and gastric outlet obstruction should be treated as a surgical emergency. In such cases, the stomach requires reduction and evaluation for preservation and fixation versus resection [13, 14].

Caustic Injury

Either accidental or intentional ingestion of caustic chemicals can result in fibrosis and stricturing of the stomach resulting in gastric outlet obstruction. The most commonly injured digestive organ in these cases is the esophagus, but the stomach is often also affected. Stricture of the esophagus is relatively common, happening in one quarter of cases of caustic ingestion, while stricturing from fibrosis in the stomach can occur in up to 5% of patients. Injury after ingestion happens immediately, but subsequent fibrosis from injury occurs anywhere from 6 to 12 weeks after ingestion. The subsequent fibrosis is the ultimate causative agent of gastric outlet obstruction. Ingestion of both alkali and acidic materials can be equally severe despite the commonly held belief that alkali materials may be better tolerated secondary to the acidic buffering qualities of the stomach [15–18].

Pancreatitis

Both acute and chronic pancreatitis can be contributory to gastric outlet obstruction, though relatively rarely. Reports have noted obstruction related to pancreatitis on the order of 1–5%. Acute pancreatitis can result in obstruction secondary to the profound inflammatory response resulting in a tremendous amount of local inflammation and edema. This can be further exacerbated by acute pancreatitis that goes on to overt pancreatic necrosis. Despite this cascade, duodenal obstruction in the acute setting remains rare [19].

Repeat bouts of pancreatitis can result in chronic fibrosis, scarring, and pseudocyst formation of the pancreas. This can be associated with stricturing of the duodenum, pancreatic ducts, and bile ducts. Often this presentation results in a thorough work-up to rule out malignancy prior to further intervention [20].

Crohn's Disease

Crohn's disease is an inflammatory bowel disease that can affect any component of the digestive tract, from mouth to anus. Despite this pan-gastrointestinal involvement, Crohn's disease affecting the stomach and duodenum is relatively rare, occurring in only 5% of individuals who have Crohn's disease. In individuals who have gastroduodenal Crohn's disease, pyloric and duodenal stricture can be causative agents of gastric outlet obstruction with individuals who ultimately require operative intervention [21–23].

Other Benign Causes

1. Gastric Polyps
   Quite rarely, large gastric polyps can result in gastric outlet obstructions. These may be secondary to their sheer size or may be pedunculated and intussuscept into the pyloric channel. Reports of these phenomena are case reports and small case series [24–26].
2. Gastrostomy Tube Migration
   Similar in nature to prolapse of a gastric polyp, balloon gastrostomy tubes can be carried by the peristalsis of the stomach down into the pyloric channel and into the duodenum. This can result in an acquired obstruction secondary to the size of the balloon if the balloon does not allow for appropriate egress of liquids out of the stomach [27–29].
3. Gastric Tuberculosis
   Gastroduodenal tuberculosis is a rare manifestation of systemic tuberculosis infection, only affecting 2–3% of individuals with the disease. In this small subset of individuals with this disease, gastric outlet obstruction is relatively common, occurring in greater than 50% of patients. Obstruction can be secondary to mucosal invasion or from external compression of surrounding structures and adenopathy [30–33].
4. Gastric Bezoar
   A bezoar is any concretion of undigested material. This can form in any area of stagnation in the intestinal tract but most commonly accumulates in the stomach. As the concretion continues to grow in size, it can ultimately become an obstructing mass within the stomach resulting in gastric outlet obstruction. This manifestation is more commonly observed in children and in patients who have undergone bariatric surgery [34, 35].

Malignant

Pancreatic Adenocarcinoma

Pancreatic adenocarcinoma currently occupies the single most common causative agent of gastric outlet obstruction in modern time. This typically results from focal invasion of the duodenum or the stomach secondary to the mass. The gastric outlet obstruction is commonly complicated by biliary and/or pancreatic obstruction as well. Up to 25% of individuals with locally advanced pancreatic cancer will have clinical evidence of gastric outlet obstruction [3, 36, 37].

Gastric Adenocarcinoma

Gastric adenocarcinoma is second in number only to pancreatic adenocarcinoma as the cause of gastric outlet obstruction. Gastric cancers causing outlet obstruction typically arise from the distal portion of the stomach and are relatively advanced. Primary gastric adenocarcinomas are responsible for up to 35% of gastric outlet obstructions currently reported [38–40].

Other Malignant Diseases

Other less commonly observed causes of malignant obstruction include untreated gastric lymphoma, invasive cholangiocarcinomas (with similar mechanisms of obstruction as pancreatic adenocarcinoma), and primary duodenal malignancies. These all represent uncommon causes of gastric outlet obstruction but must be thoroughly evaluated when gastric outlet obstruction is identified.

Clinical Presentation

Patient Presentation

The primary patient presentation of gastric outlet obstruction is nausea and vomiting. The degree and nature of the vomitus is primarily predicated on the stage of presentation and disease. In early or partial obstruction, vomiting can be intermittent and may be present with solid foods but absent with liquids. Vomitus is typically described as non-bilious in nature. As the disease progresses, vomitus will progress to undigested food particles with both liquids and solids. As the disease further evolves, gastric outlet obstruction may also be associated with epigastric pain and bloating. Patients often also complain of early satiety and weight loss further in the disease state. Upon complete obstruction, the patients may present in extremis with projectile vomiting.

Physical Examination

Physical examination can vary widely dependent on the stage of presentation, but a component of malnutrition with dehydration is not uncommon with patients with gastric outlet obstruction. In patients with advanced partial obstructions or complete obstructions, the abdominal exam can demonstrate bloating in the epigastrium and right upper quadrant. There may also be an associated finding of tympany secondary to recent retained food and liquid. While the gastric distention can be disconcerting to the patient, it is infrequent that peritonitis is present on exam.

If gastric outlet obstruction is suspected, the examining provider may elicit a "succussion splash." a succussion splash is performed by placing the provider's stethoscope over the epigastrium or right upper quadrant. The patient is then rocked gently using the torso and hips. Appreciation of a splash can be representative of gastric outlet obstruction. Sensitivity of the "succussion splash" was noted to near 50% in one study examining gastric outlet obstruction [41].

Diagnosis

Laboratory Findings

Upon initial presentation, specific laboratory abnormalities may range from normal to profoundly deranged. In patients with early stages of obstruction, labs may appear normal in nature, and complaints may be entirely clinical. As the disease progresses, overt dehydration and malnutrition will manifest. Laboratory values will include high BUN and creatinine levels on metabolic panels. Serum albumin levels and nutrition labs may also be low in advanced disease. In patients with protracted vomiting secondary to severe obstruction, hypochloremic, hypokalemic metabolic alkalosis is frequently observed. Care should be taken to ensure correction of these electrolytes is slow and methodical to avoid complications secondary to overzealous correction [42–44].

Radiographic Tests

Plain Films

Despite being somewhat nonspecific in nature, plain films can provide a wealth of knowledge to direct further studies. In patients with advanced disease, an enlarged gastric bubble is not an uncommon finding on chest X-rays or abdominal films. Scattered calcification of the pancreas and retroperitoneum can be observed in cases of chronic pancreatitis. In rare cases of Bouveret's syndrome – Gastric outlet obstruction secondary to large calcific gallstone observed with associated choledoudenal fistula – A calcific stone may be appreciated on radiographic examination [20, 45].

Upper Gastrointestinal Series

The use of contrast studies when gastric outlet obstruction is suspected may be helpful to determine the underlying cause of obstruction. This may demonstrate extrinsic compression versus mucosal ingrowth. Failure of passage of contrast may be indicative of a complete obstruction. Likewise, slow transit may be indicative of non-obstructive disease such as diabetic gastroparesis.

Computed Tomography/MRI

Similar to plain films, computed tomography will demonstrate gastric distention to the degree the gastric outlet obstruction has worsened. With the additional detail that these modalities can provide, the study may shed light as to the potential causative disease process. If the inciting disease is malignant, this imaging may assist in further diagnosis and prognosis in the setting of malignant disease [46].

Endoscopy

Upper endoscopy is critical in establishing a diagnosis as to the etiology of the gastric outlet obstruction. Endoscopy also provides the unique opportunity for both diagnostic and therapeutic procedures to aid with the clinical diagnosis of the causative mechanism of gastric outlet obstruction. Prior to proceeding with upper endoscopy, attempts should be made to decompress the stomach. This is routinely performed with a large bore nasogastric tube. Care should be taken during placement of the nasogastric tube as patients with large volume contents in the stomach are prone to aspiration. After allowing for adequate time for decompression, the patient should be brought for endoscopy. Dependent on the degree of distension, endoscopy can be attempted under moderate conscious sedation or may be performed under general anesthesia.

Traditional caliber endoscopes can be employed, but consideration should be lent to large bore or dual lumen endoscopes that may allow for more adequate clearance of residual food and liquid in the setting of gastric outlet obstruction. Thorough clearance of the stomach should be attempted to allow for complete examination and increase the possibility for therapeutic intervention. After adequate clearance has been obtained, a standard examination of the upper intestinal tract should be undertaken including the esophagus, stomach, and the proximal portion of the duodenum. Despite this intention, the endoscopist may or may not be able to traverse the pylorus dependent on the degree of obstruction. Gentle attempts should be made to traverse the restriction, but may not be entirely necessary for diagnosis. The ability to pass into the duodenum may be facilitated by a small caliber endoscope, like a nasopharyngeal scope.

Endoscopic biopsies should be performed to aid in definitive diagnosis. These should include permanent pathology for malignancy as well as stains to evaluate for the presence of *Helicobacter pylori*. Despite convincing endoscopic evidence of disease, biopsies may return negative in nature. If suspicion remains high, further interrogations should be undertaken and may include endoscopic ultrasound, CT-guided biopsy, or endoscopic mucosal resection [29, 37, 46, 47]. Rarely, surgical resection may be necessary for definitive diagnosis. This may be the case in gastroduodenal tuberculosis, as traditional endoscopic biopsies may prove to be non-diagnostic [32, 33].

Conclusion

Despite advances in medical management of peptic ulcer disease, gastric outlet obstruction remains a clinically significant diagnosis. This is most commonly observed in malignancy with the two predominate causes being pancreatic and gastric adenocarcinoma. Various other benign causative mechanisms exist, but each remains relatively rare. Plain film and advanced imaging techniques such as CT and MRI may be employed to assist in the diagnosis of the underlying disease state. Endoscopy is essential to provide tissue diagnosis and provide the possibility of endoscopic interventions when possible.

References

1. S Ian Gan M, FRCP(C). Gastric Outlet Obstruction in Adults http://www.uptodate.com: UpToDate; 2016 [updated 05/27/2016; cited 2017 05/03/2017].
2. Lichtman MA. A bacterial cause of Cancer: an historical essay. Oncologist. 2017;22:542.
3. Poruk KE, Wolfgang CL. Palliative Management of Unresectable Pancreas Cancer. Surg Oncol Clin N Am. 2016;25(2):327–37.
4. Chowdhury A, Dhali GK, Banerjee PK. Etiology of gastric outlet obstruction. Am J Gastroenterol. 1996;91(8):1679.
5. Johnson CD. Gastric outlet obstruction malignant until proved otherwise. Am J Gastroenterol. 1995;90(10):1740.
6. Diaz Blasco J, Garcia Valriberas R. [Resolution of a case of gastric outlet obstruction after eradication of Helicobacter pylori]. Rev Esp Enferm Dig 1998;90(12):890–891.
7. de Boer WA, Driessen WM. Resolution of gastric outlet obstruction after eradication of Helicobacter pylori. J Clin Gastroenterol. 1995;21(4):329–30.
8. Wallace JL. How do NSAIDs cause ulcer disease? Baillieres Best Pract Res Clin Gastroenterol. 2000;14(1):147–59.
9. Shim YK, Kim N. [Nonsteroidal Anti-inflammatory Drug and Aspirin-induced Peptic Ulcer Disease]. Korean J Gastroenterol. 2016;67(6):300–312.
10. Ong TZ, Hawkey CJ, Ho KY. Nonsteroidal anti-inflammatory drug use is a significant cause of peptic ulcer disease in a tertiary hospital in Singapore: a prospective study. J Clin Gastroenterol. 2006;40(9):795–800.
11. Papatheodoridis GV, Sougioultzis S, Archimandritis AJ. Effects of Helicobacter pylori and nonsteroidal anti-inflammatory drugs on peptic ulcer disease: a systematic review. Clin Gastroenterol Hepatol. 2006;4(2):130–42.
12. Tang CL, Ye F, Liu W, Pan XL, Qian J, Zhang GX. Eradication of Helicobacter pylori infection reduces the incidence of peptic ulcer disease in patients using nonsteroidal anti-inflammatory drugs: a meta-analysis. Helicobacter. 2012;17(4):286–96.
13. Tabib SM, Assadipoya K, Mansorian R, Nasehy N, Assadi M. Acute gastric volvulus presenting with gastric outlet obstruction and upper gastrointestinal bleeding. Turk J Gastroenterol. 2013;24(3):293–5.
14. Yau KK, Siu WT, Cheung HY, Yang GP, Li MK. Acute gastric volvulus: an unusual cause of gastric outlet obstruction. Minim Invasive Ther Allied Technol. 2005;14(1):2–5.
15. Ahmed Z, Mohyuddin Z. Complete gastric outlet obstruction following acid ingestion complicated by acute pancreatitis and disseminated intravascular coagulation. Postgrad Med J. 1997;73(861):421–3.
16. Sood A, Midha V, Sood N. Gastric outlet obstruction as a late complication of ingestion of diazinon. Indian J Gastroenterol. 2003;22(3):106–7.
17. Wilson WH, Winegarner FG, Jesseph JE. Gastric outlet obstruction following alkali ingestion. Ohio State Med J. 1969;65(10):1000–3.

18. Lebeau R, Coulibaly A, Kountele Gona S, Koffi Gnangoran M, Kouakou B, Yapo P, et al. Isolated gastric outlet obstruction due to corrosive ingestion. J Visc Surg. 2011;148(1):59–63.
19. Reddy RY, Arun AC, Siddappa PK, Sinha SK, Kochhar R. Inflammatory gastric outlet obstruction after acute pancreatitis: a novel method of treatment. Gastrointest Endosc. 2015;81(3):775–6.
20. Taylor SM, Adams DB, Anderson MC. Duodenal stricture: a complication of chronic fibrocalcific pancreatitis. South Med J. 1991;84(3):338–41.
21. Spisni R, Giusti S, Iacconi C, Giusti P, Berti P, Conte M, et al. Duodenal Crohn's disease. Ann Ital Chir. 2007;78(5):439–41.
22. Shapiro M, Greenstein AJ, Byrn J, Corona J, Greenstein AJ, Salky B, et al. Surgical management and outcomes of patients with duodenal Crohn's disease. J Am Coll Surg. 2008;207(1):36–42.
23. Tonelli F, Alemanno G, Bellucci F, Focardi A, Sturiale A, Giudici F. Symptomatic duodenal Crohn's disease: is strictureplasty the right choice? J Crohns Colitis. 2013;7(10):791–6.
24. Aydin I, Ozer E, Rakici H, Sehitoglu I, Yucel AF, Pergel A, et al. Antral hyperplastic polyp: a rare cause of gastric outlet obstruction. Int J Surg Case Rep. 2014;5(6):287–9.
25. Vlacancich R, Sultan M, Al-Kawas F. Gastric outlet obstruction caused by prolapsed gastric polyp into the pyloric channel. Clin Gastroenterol Hepatol. 2014;12(5):A27–8.
26. Kosai NR, Gendeh HS, Norfaezan AR, Razman J, Sutton PA, Das S. Prolapsing gastric polyp causing intermittent gastric outlet obstruction. Int Surg. 2015;100(6):1148–52.
27. Fonseca J, Nunes G, Patita M, Barosa R, Santos CA. Catheter traction and gastric outlet obstruction: a repeated complication of using a Foley catheter for gastrostomy tube replacement. Nutr Hosp. 2017;34(2):499–501.
28. Feldstein RC, Leong J, Devito B. Gastric outlet obstruction caused by replacement gastrostomy tube. Clin Gastroenterol Hepatol. 2008;6(7):A26.
29. Than MM, Witherspoon J, Tudor G, Saklani A. Gastric outlet obstruction secondary to percutaneous endoscopic gastrostomy tube placement. Endoscopy. 2012;44(Suppl 2 UCTN):E269–70.
30. Kalpande S, Pandya JS, Tiwari A, Adhikari D. Gastric outlet obstruction: an unusual case of primary duodenal tuberculosis. BMJ Case Rep. 2017;2017.
31. Ecka RS, Wani ZA, Sharma M. Gastric tuberculosis with outlet obstruction: a case report presenting with a mass lesion. Case Rep Med. 2013;2013:169051.
32. Upadhyaya VD, Kumar B, Lal R, Sharma MS, Singh M. Rudramani. Primary duodenal tuberculosis presenting as gastric-outlet obstruction: its diagnosis. Afr J Paediatr Surg : AJPS. 2013;10(2):83–6.
33. Arabi NA, Musaad AM, Ahmed EE, Ibnouf MM, Abdelaziz MS. Primary gastric tuberculosis presenting as gastric outlet obstruction: a case report and review of the literature. J Med Case Rep. 2015;9:265.
34. Guner A, Kahraman I, Aktas A, Kece C, Reis E. Gastric outlet obstruction due to duodenal bezoar: a case report. Int J Surg Case Rep. 2012;3(11):523–5.
35. Lu L, Zhang XF. Gastric outlet obstruction--an unexpected complication during Coca-Cola therapy for a gastric bezoar: a case report and literature review. Intern Med. 2016;55(9):1085–9.
36. Sugiura T, Okamura Y, Ito T, Yamamoto Y, Ashida R, Yoshida Y, et al. Prognostic scoring system for patients who present with a gastric outlet obstruction caused by advanced pancreatic adenocarcinoma. World J Surg. 2017;41:2619.
37. Oh SY, Edwards A, Mandelson M, Ross A, Irani S, Larsen M, et al. Survival and clinical outcome after endoscopic duodenal stent placement for malignant gastric outlet obstruction: comparison of pancreatic cancer and nonpancreatic cancer. Gastrointest Endosc. 2015;82(3):460–8.e2.
38. Otabor IA, Abdessalam SF, Erdman SH, Hammond S, Besner GE. Gastric outlet obstruction due to adenocarcinoma in a patient with ataxia-telangiectasia syndrome: a case report and review of the literature. World J Surg Oncol. 2009;7:29.
39. Shyr YM, Su CH, Wu CW, Lui WY. Prospective study of gastric outlet obstruction in unresectable periampullary adenocarcinoma. World J Surg. 2000;24(1):60–4; discussion 4–5.

40. Matsumoto T, Wada M, Imai Y, Inokuma T. A rare cause of gastric outlet obstruction: gastritis cystica profunda accompanied by adenocarcinoma. Endoscopy. 2012;44(Suppl 2 UCTN):E138–9.
41. Lau JY, Chung SC, Sung JJ, Chan AC, Ng EK, Suen RC, et al. Through-the-scope balloon dilation for pyloric stenosis: long-term results. Gastrointest Endosc. 1996;43(2 Pt 1):98–101.
42. Rune SJ. The metabolic alkalosis following aspiration of gastric acid secretion. Scand J Clin Lab Invest. 1965;17(4):305–10.
43. Vaziri ND, Byrne C, Barton CH, Robertson D, Jay K, McDonald L. Prevention of metabolic alkalosis induced by gastric fluid loss using H2 receptor antagonist. Gen Pharmacol. 1985;16(2):141–4.
44. Ludtke FE, Bertus M, Voth E, Lepsien G. [Long-term results following conservative and surgical treatment of infantile hypertrophic pyloric stenosis]. Helv Chir Acta 1989;56(1–2):15–17.
45. Yau KK, Siu WT, Li MK. An unusual cause of gastric outlet obstruction. Diagnosis: Bourevet's syndrome. Gut. 2006;55(3):373. 87
46. Awan A, Johnston DE, Jamal MM. Gastric outlet obstruction with benign endoscopic biopsy should be further explored for malignancy. Gastrointest Endosc. 1998;48(5):497–500.
47. Nakai Y, Hamada T, Isayama H, Itoi T, Koike K. Endoscopic management of combined malignant biliary and gastric outlet obstruction. Dig Endosc. 2017;29(1):16–25.

Medical and Endoscopic Management of Gastric Outlet Obstruction

65

Cheyenne C. Sonntag and Eric M. Pauli

Introduction

The term gastric outlet obstruction (GOO) describes the end result of a variety of disease processes in which the gastric antrum, pylorus, or bulbar duodenum becomes an impediment to gastric emptying. Presenting symptoms of GOO vary depending on etiology of the obstruction, but common symptoms include abdominal pain, nausea, vomiting, and weight loss. Patients may also experience sensation of early satiety or bloating.

Prior to introduction and widespread use of histamine-receptor antagonists in the 1970s, benign peptic ulcer disease was the most common cause of GOO [1, 2]. Today, malignancy is the most common cause in adults, frequently due to adenocarcinoma of the stomach, duodenum, or pancreas [2, 3]. The number of adult patients with benign disease resulting in GOO, however, remains significant. Benign disease is most commonly due to peptic ulcer disease (PUD), caustic ingestion, postoperative scarring, or anastomotic stricture. It may also be related to inflammatory causes (e.g., Crohn's disease, acute and chronic pancreatitis), benign tumors, tuberculosis, Bouveret's syndrome, and more [4–11] (Table 65.1).

This chapter will discuss the evaluation, medical management, and diagnosis of GOO, as well as explore endoscopic management options for both benign and malignant disease. A more detailed discussion specific to medical management of PUD can be found in Chap. 55. Surgical pyloroplasty techniques are covered in detail in Chap. 57.

C. C. Sonntag · E. M. Pauli (✉)
Division of Minimally Invasive and Bariatric Surgery, Department of Surgery, Penn State Hershey Medical Center, Hershey, PA, USA
e-mail: epauli@hmc.psu.edu

J. Grams et al. (eds.), *The SAGES Manual of Foregut Surgery*,
https://doi.org/10.1007/978-3-319-96122-4_65

Table 65.1 Malignant and benign causes of gastric outlet obstruction

Malignant	Benign
Pancreatic adenocarcinoma	Peptic ulcer disease
Gastric adenocarcinoma	Caustic ingestion
Duodenal adenocarcinoma	Benign tumors
Linitis plastica	Inflammatory polyp
Gastric lymphoma	Acute pancreatitis
Periampullary carcinoma	Chronic pancreatitis
Local extension of gallbladder carcinoma	Pancreatic pseudocyst
Local extension of cholangiocarcinoma	Gastroduodenal Crohn's disease
Metastatic disease	Eosinophilic gastroenteritis
	Nonsteroidal anti-inflammatory-related strictures
	Postsurgical scarring/anastomotic stricture
	Postvagotomy pylorospasm
	Gastric tuberculosis
	Annular pancreas
	Adult hypertrophic pyloric stenosis
	Bezoar
	Intramural duodenal hematoma
	Gastric volvulus
	Gastrostomy tube migration

Evaluation, Diagnosis, and Medical Management

A detailed history and physical examination should be performed, with attention being paid to the chronicity of symptoms, history of PUD, prior operations, or history of caustic ingestion (both acute and remote). As malignancy is the most common cause of GOO, a detailed family history of cancer should be obtained and a high index of suspicion maintained.

It is important to assess the patient's oral intake beyond when the last meal was eaten. Use of the Gastric Outlet Obstruction Scoring System (GOOSS), developed by Adler and Baron, allows for an objective determination of the patient's ability to eat as well as a measure for comparison following any intervention [12]. The GOOSS score ranges from 0 to 4, with 0 being no oral intake, 1 liquid only, 2 soft solids, and 3 a low-residue or full diet.

Patients presenting with clinical symptoms of GOO of unknown etiology should be considered for hospital admission, especially in the setting of recurrent vomiting where fluid imbalance and electrolyte abnormalities such as hypokalemia and hypochloremic metabolic alkalosis may be present. Appropriate IV fluid resuscitation and electrolyte replacement should be administered, with periodic measurement of electrolytes to ensure normalization.

On admission, patients should be kept *nil* per os (NPO) and early nasogastric tube decompression with a large bore tube should be initiated. Gastric evacuation alleviates symptoms of abdominal pain and nausea and also begins patient preparation for imaging studies and endoscopic evaluation. Initiation of nasogastric decompression prior to administration of contrast for imaging may additionally reduce the risk of aspiration event. Early initiation of parenteral proton pump inhibitor (PPI) should be considered even in absence of known etiology for the GOO.

An abdominal CT scan with enteral contrast can clarify both the extent of the obstruction (complete vs incomplete) and provide clues to its etiology (e.g., by evaluation for mural thickening, enlarged lymph nodes, and general state of the pancreas, biliary tree, and retroperitoneum as well as possible evidence of extrinsic compression by mass or pseudocyst) (Fig. 65.1).

All patients with persistent symptoms of GOO should undergo endoscopic evaluation to establish diagnosis and obtain tissue biopsies to determine etiology (Fig. 65.2). Biopsy allows for histological diagnosis of specific diseases as well as pathologic evaluation to confirm or rule out malignancy. In the presence of an extrinsic compressive mass on CT, endoscopic ultrasound may aid in tissue acquisition (Fig. 65.3). If malignant diagnosis is made following endoscopic evaluation and biopsy, additional imaging may be required to complete staging.

Subsequent treatment of the GOO varies greatly depending on the etiology of the obstruction. Acute GOO due to edema and inflammation may improve with enteric decompression and acid suppression. Patients with ulcer disease who are found to have *Helicobacter pylori* should undergo triple therapy (PPI, amoxicillin, and clarithromycin) and confirmatory eradication testing (see Chap. 55 for complete treatment guidelines and recommendations). Patients with tuberculosis, infection, or evidence of gastroduodenal Crohn's disease should similarly receive appropriate medical treatment. *Helicobacter pylori* eradication therapy may be considered first-line treatment for gastric mucosa-associated lymphoid tissue

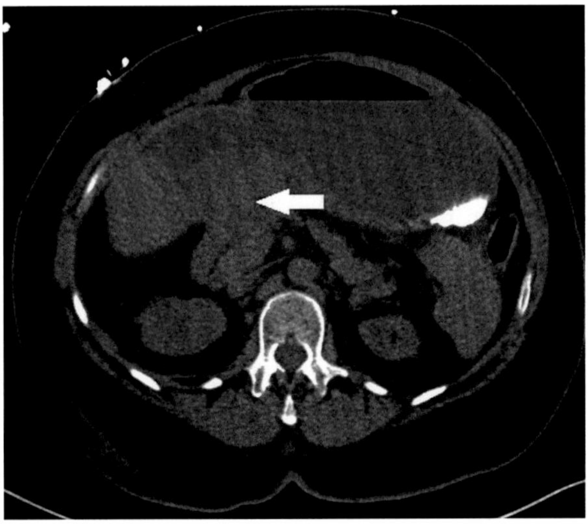

Fig. 65.1 CT scan of a patient with GOO due to an obstructing pancreatic mass (arrow) with profound dilation of the stomach and well as duodenum

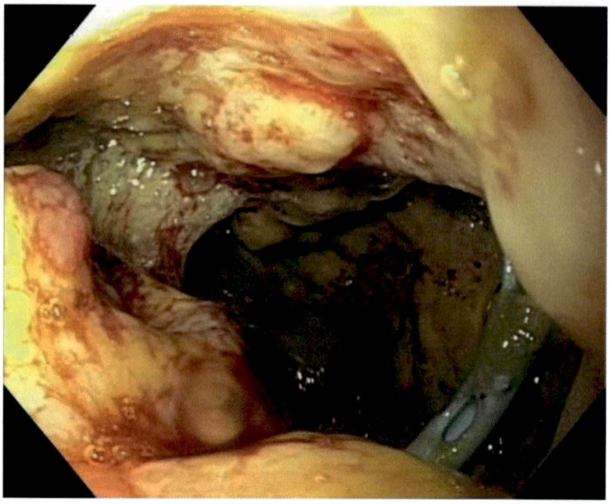

Fig. 65.2 Endoscopic evaluation of obstructing duodenal lesion, found to be metastatic colorectal malignancy on biopsy pathology

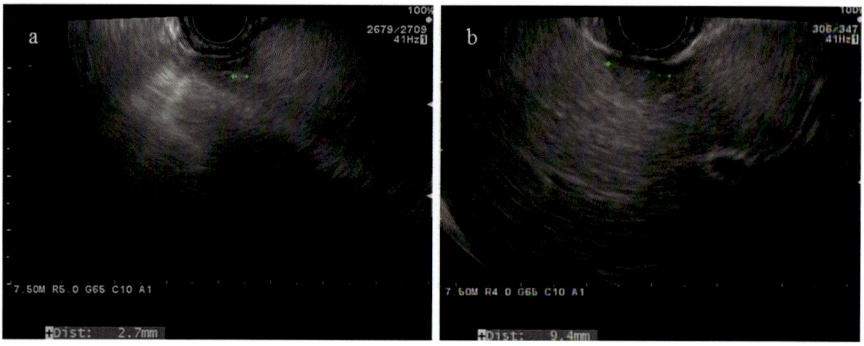

Fig. 65.3 (**a**) EUS assessment of obstructing duodenal mass. (**b**) Further EUS examination of same patient demonstrated evidence of metastatic lesions within the liver parenchyma

(MALT) lymphoma, regardless of infection status or disease stage [13]. Chemotherapy remains the mainstay of treatment for primary gastrointestinal non-Hodgkin lymphoma, with some evidence to suggest that surgery may play a role in survival benefit as well [14].

Patients with more chronic obstructive symptoms should undergo nutritional assessment and optimization, as malnutrition is an established risk factor for morbidity if surgical intervention is ultimately required. Depending on degree of obstruction, it may be feasible to obtain temporary nasojejunal feeding access with endoscopic assistance while maintaining more proximal gastric decompression, such as with a percutaneous endoscopic gastrostomy tube and jejunal feeding extension (PEG-J) [15]. In cases where distal enteric feeding access cannot be obtained, total parenteral nutrition may need to be considered until more definitive intervention to relieve the obstruction can be performed.

Therapeutic Endoscopic Interventions in Benign Disease

The conventional treatment for persistent or irreversible benign GOO has been surgery, but such interventions are not without risk [16, 17]. Surgical intervention for ulcer-related GOO is associated with significant morbidity as well as potential postoperative sequelae including anemia, dumping syndrome, and malabsorption [18, 19]. The advancement of endoscopic technologies has led to the development of less invasive treatment options in select patients with benign GOO, with high therapeutic and clinical success.

Endoscopic Balloon Dilation

Overview and Patient Selection

Prior to advent and acceptance of endoscopic balloon dilation (EBD), up to 90–98% of patients with chronic peptic ulcer-related gastric outlet obstruction and 67–68% of patients with acute gastric outlet obstruction required surgical intervention [16, 17]. Chronic gastric sequelae from caustic substance ingestion was also managed surgically [5]. Endoscopic guidewire placement with over-the-wire balloon dilation under fluoroscopy for peptic gastric outlet obstruction was first reported by Benjamin et al. in 1981 [20]. Although early studies questioned success of long-term remission of obstructive symptoms in PUD with balloon dilation, several subsequent studies have shown balloon dilation to be an effective alternate to surgery for corrosive ingestion and anastomotic stricture in addition to GOO due to ulcer disease [19, 21–25]. Endoscopic balloon dilation in patients with obstructive Crohn's disease has shown variable success, with two failures of three reported cases [26–28]. Balloon dilation in four patients with chronic pancreatitis associated GOO by Kochhar et al. was similarly unsuccessful [23].

Hydrostatic and pneumatic balloon dilators are available in over-the-wire and through-the-scope forms. Available controlled radial expansion (CRE) balloon dilators dilate in three 1.0–1.5 mm intervals to pressure-controlled diameters and exert large radial dilating force along the entire balloon length [29]. The use of a CRE balloon minimizes number of balloons necessary for the procedure as well as time spent on instrument exchange. The luminal diameter of the stricture may be assessed endoscopically using commercially available endoscopic measuring devices or may be assessed using the open jaw of endoscopic biopsy forceps. Initial dilator size should be approximately the same diameter as the strictured lumen.

Fluoroscopy is sometimes used during dilation procedures, but it is not required. When strictures are too narrow to be traversed with an endoscope, fluoroscopy may be particularly useful to delineate length of stricture, ensure normal lumen beyond the GOO, and confirm correct of passage of the guidewire into the lumen distal to the stricture (Fig. 65.4). Fluoroscopic visualization of the balloon dilation using dilute water-soluble radiopaque contrast allows for proper balloon positioning as well as confirmation of complete balloon inflation by observing waist ablation

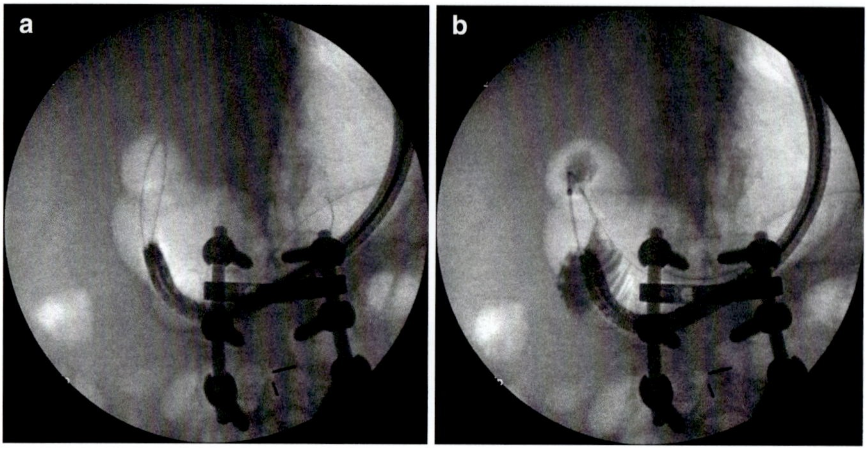

Fig. 65.4 Fluoroscopic delineation of stricture location and extend. (**a**) Guidewire passage beyond stricture under fluoroscopic guidance. (**b**) ERCP catheter passed over the guidewire permits contrast injection; here delineating normal bulb and D2 with a stricture present in D1

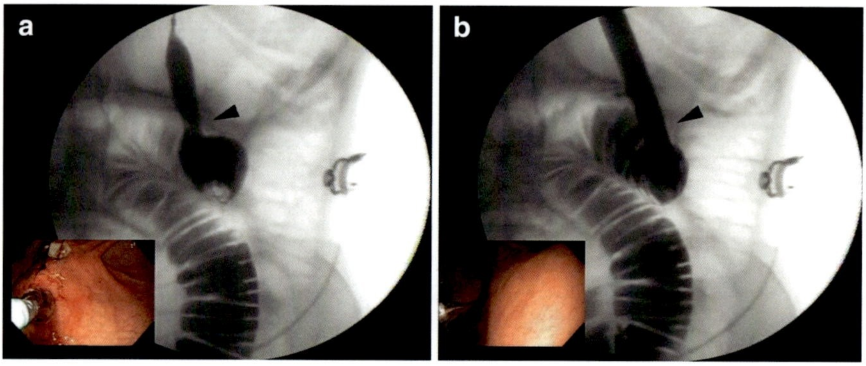

Fig. 65.5 Fluoroscopic images of through-the-scope balloon dilation demonstrating the "waist" at the stricture (**a**) and its ablation on complete balloon dilation (**b**). (Image Credit: Pauli and Marks [123])

(Fig. 65.5). Despite these advantages, there is no difference in perforation rates with EBD performed with or without fluoroscopy, and the endoscopist must balance the risks of ionizing radiation with the procedural guidance benefits noted above.

Patient Preparation

Patients should fast the night prior to procedure. Coagulopathy, if present, should be corrected (goal International Normalizing Ration of less than 1.3) and anticoagulation held for the procedure. Although bacteremia may occur with endoscopic procedures, current consensus recommendations do not support the use of prophylactic antibiotics [30–32]. This procedure may be accomplished under conscious sedation with patients in the left lateral decubitus position; however, for patient comfort and to minimize aspiration risk in obstructed patients, the procedure can be performed under general anesthesia with endotracheal intubation in the supine position.

Technique: Through-the-Scope (TTS) Balloon Dilation

Upper endoscopy is performed and the location and diameter of the stricture documented. If possible, the endoscope should be passed through the stricture for complete evaluation; the use of a pediatric or slim adult endoscope may allow traversal of smaller strictures. Available TTS balloon sizes range from 6 to 20 mm (18–54 French). After endoscopic evaluation, an appropriate-sized TTS balloon is selected and passed through the endoscope channel. If there is difficulty passing the balloon sheath beyond the stricture due to anatomy, the balloon may be passed over a 0.035″ (0.89 mm) guidewire. The endoscope should be positioned just proximal to stricture, with the stricture situated at the midpoint of the balloon (Fig. 65.6).

To minimize prograde and retrograde migration of the balloon during inflation, the sheath of the balloon should be held tightly at the control section of the endoscope, and the endoscope held firmly against the bite block. Dilute contrast material may be used to inflate the balloon rather than water, which allows the inflation and waist ablation to be viewed with fluoroscopy. The balloon is then inflated to nominal diameter as determined by atmospheres of pressure on the package insert. If a CRE balloon is used, it may be dilated to three different diameters by alteration of the pressure. Following dilation, the endoscope should be used to traverse the stricture. Inspection for bleeding and overt signs of perforation (e.g., the presence of a full-thickness defect, omental or retroperitoneal fat, or difficulty insufflating) should

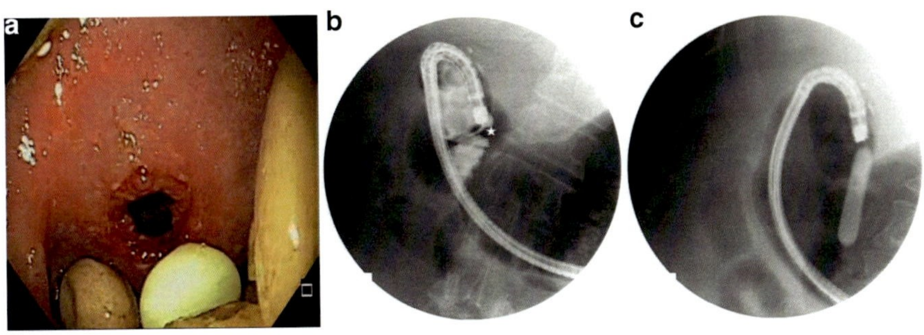

Fig. 65.6 (**a**) Endoscopic evaluation of a peptic stricture demonstrates pills within the duodenal bulb just proximal to the stenosis, (**b**) contrast injection delineates the stricture (star) (**c**) fully dilated balloon centered at stricture midpoint

be undertaken. If fluoroscopy is available, contrast injection can be employed to further evaluate for leak.

Outcomes

EBD is successful for both immediate and long-term symptomatic relief in patients with benign causes of GOO. Solt et al. demonstrated immediate symptom relief in 80% of patients with sustained relief in 70% at 3 months [26]. Several stepwise dilation sessions may be required to reach the desired dilation endpoint in patients, and reported rates of recurrent stenosis requiring reintervention vary by cause.

Balloon dilation for treatment of GOO caused by anastomotic stricture has reported long-term symptom resolution rates of 91–100% with mean follow-up of 13.5–98 months [26, 33, 34]. One large study followed 30 patients with successful dilations for caustic injury for a median of 21 months (range 3–72) with no recurrence of symptoms [35]. Several studies have shown 78.6–100% long-term remission rates (median follow-up range 14–43 months) in patients with GOO related to peptic ulcer disease treated with EBD when combined with medical treatment (treatment for *H. pylori,* PPI, smoking/NSAID cessation) [22, 36, 37].

Unfortunately, the results of EBD for GOO due to gastroduodenal Crohn's disease are less encouraging. Solt et al. and Murthy each report attempted treatment of patients with duodenal Crohn's, both with failure to respond to multiple dilations [26, 27]. However, Rana et al. report successful dilation of one patient with duodenal Crohn's, but the patient's symptoms returned whenever systemic steroids or immunosuppressive medications were held due to complications. After incorporation of intralesional steroid injections with dilation, along with maintenance injections at 3 month intervals, they were able to achieve a 14-month asymptomatic follow-up [34].

Complications

Bleeding, perforation, and self-limited pain are the most common complications of dilation therapy for GOO. Perforation rates for dilation of pyloric or gastric outlet obstructions are low and were reported to be between 2.2% and 8% [26, 34, 38, 39]. Studies suggest that perforation is related to the maximum diameter of the balloon and more often observed when diameters greater than 15 mm are used [37, 39]. Historically a goal of 15 mm dilation has been used based on the frequency of perforations reported when digital dilation using the index finger up to the proximal interphalangeal joint (estimated diameter of 20 mm) was performed during surgical interventions [40], and several recent studies continue to use 15 mm as their dilation endpoint with few incidents of perforation [22, 23, 25, 35, 41].

Endoscopic Steroid Injection

Overview and Patient Selection

Steroids interfere with collagen synthesis and reduce fibrotic healing, inflammation, and scar formation. Intralesional steroid injections have been described as an adjunct therapy with EBD for gastric corrosive strictures where cicatrization of the stomach can result in GOO symptoms by antral or pyloric stenosis [42]. Additionally, it has been documented as an adjunct to EBD in treatment for upper GI strictures due to Crohn's disease [34, 43].

Patient Preparation

As intraluminal steroid injection occurs as an adjunct procedure to endoscopic balloon dilation, patient preparation is the same as endoscopic balloon dilation described above.

Technique

Upper endoscopy and complete evaluation of the stricture are performed, including traversal of the stricture with the endoscope if possible. The use of a pediatric or slim adult endoscope for initial evaluation may be beneficial. Under direct visualization, using a TTS sclerotherapy needle, the lesion is injected in four quadrants with triamcinolone acetate in 0.25–1 mL aliquots at 10–40 mg/mL. This is to be followed by endoscopic balloon dilation of the lesion as described above.

Outcomes

Three cases reported by Kochhar et al. of intralesional triamcinolone injections and EBD in patients with distal antral and pyloric stenosis following corrosive ingestion remained asymptomatic at follow-up ranging from 12 to 39 months, with no noted complications [42]. In a study by Singh et al. that combined EBD and four-quadrant triamcinolone injections in 11 Crohn's disease strictures (including 3 upper GI strictures), the recurrence rate 5 months after stricture dilation was 10%, with no complications noted among those with upper GI strictures and the 3 UGI strictures maintaining a 100% long-term success rate (range 17–48 months) [43].

Complications

As intralesional steroid injections occur most often in tandem with EBD, the complication profile is similar: perforation, bleeding, and self-limited pain. Additionally, with injection lies a theoretical risk of intramural infection or bleeding.

Botulinum Toxin A Injection

Overview and Patient Selection

Botulinum toxin A (BTA), a potent acetylcholine inhibitor, has long been employed in the gastrointestinal tract for treatment of achalasia, esophageal spasm, and anal fissures to relax muscle tone [44–46]. Pyloric dysfunction consisting of pyloric restriction or spasm may result in functional gastric outlet obstruction and contribute to gastroparesis symptoms in some patients [47].

Initial evaluation of possible candidates for endoscopic BTA injection includes barium fluoroscopy, which may suggest a functional pyloric obstruction. Manometry studies may demonstrate prolonged localized contraction. Upper endoscopy should also be performed for visual inspection of the pylorus to rule out lesions and may yield visual confirmation of constriction or spasm of the sphincter.

Patient Preparation

Patient preparation is similar to that of endoscopic balloon dilation described above.

Technique

After endoscopic evaluation, BTA (typically diluted in 4 ml of injectable saline) is delivered in four quadrants circumferentially into the pyloric sphincter using a sclerotherapy needle under direct visualization, with care that the injections are intramuscular (Fig. 65.7). The endoscopist should observe for any sign of leak into the lumen or of mucosal lift, both of which suggest that the needle is not positioned

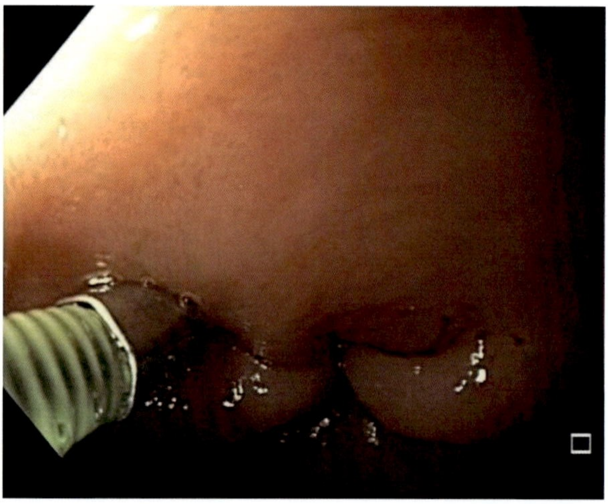

Fig. 65.7 Injection of botulinum toxin into pyloric sphincter using sclerotherapy needle

deeply enough. Once all four injections have been performed, an additional 1 ml of saline should be injected at the original injection site to flush the remaining BTA from the sclerotherapy needle.

A 2009 study by Coleski et al. suggests that higher botulinum toxin dose of 200 units may significantly improve clinical response of patients undergoing injection for gastroparesis compared to 100 unit dosing [48]; however, successful dosages reported elsewhere in the literature for treating pylorospasm have ranged from 80 to 200 units [49–51].

Outcomes

While endoscopic intrapyloric injection of botulinum toxin for gastroparesis has not been shown reliably effective in randomized control trials and is not endorsed by the American College of Gastroenterology, there may be a subset of patients with documented pylorospasm in which the therapy may offer benefit [47, 52]. Botulinum toxin injection has also been reported therapy for refractory postoperative pyloric spasm in patients post truncal vagotomy with pyloroplasty and following pylorus-preserving duodenopancreatectomy [50]. Successful endoscopic treatment with pylorus BTA injections for stomach dysmotility and pylorospasm, resulting from division of the vagus nerves during esophagectomy, has also been described [49]. It should be noted, however, that BTA injection is not an effective treatment option for hypertrophic pyloric stenosis [53].

Complications

Complications of BTA injection include tissue inflammatory response and potential scarring with repeated procedures. The effect of the toxin is short-lived, and as such patients that benefit from this intervention may require frequent injections. In one study, symptom response was observed for an average of 4.9 months in women and 3.5 months in male patients following botulinum toxin exposure [54].

Self-Expanding Metal Stents (SEMS)

Overview and Patient Selection

Self-expanding metal stents (SEMS) were first utilized in 1989 for the treatment of malignant obstruction of the biliary tract [55] and since have found wide use within the upper and lower GI tract to address obstruction. SEMS used for treatment of gastric outlet obstruction are composed of alloys such as nitinol (nickel and titanium) and elgiloy (cobalt, nickel, and chromium). Approved stents come in covered and uncovered variations, with the covering membranes composed of plastic or silicone and deployed diameters of 20–22 mm, although off-label use of stents designed for esophageal or vascular use has been described. It is important to note that all currently available stents have some degree of shortening on deployment and appropriate stent sizing and selection are necessary for good clinical outcome.

Endoscopic stenting of benign lesions causing GOO may be indicated in patients who previously failed endoscopic balloon dilation and are poor surgical candidates [56–58]. Few studies evaluating endoscopic stenting have included patients with benign etiology of gastroduodenal obstruction along with the larger malignant populations, and little data is available for this patient subset separate from malignant cases. The small numbers described are likely due to the good success rate of other previously described endoscopic therapy modalities that do not leave a foreign body at risk for migration.

Patient Preparation

For pre-procedural planning, cross-sectional imaging is useful to assess lesion localization and offers a good estimate of lesion length to be stented. Patients should fast the evening prior to the procedure, and any coagulopathy should be corrected. Prophylactic antibiotics are not currently recommenced [30–32]. As with balloon dilation, this procedure may be performed under conscious sedation with the patient in the left lateral decubitus position; however, providers may elect to perform the procedure under general endotracheal anesthesia with the patient in supine position to minimize aspiration risk or for patient comfort.

Technique

Upper endoscopy should be performed with documentation of the diameter and length of the obstruction. Ideal stent length allows for 2 cm coverage both proximal and distal to the lesion, with total stent length 4 cm longer than the lesion. If lumen diameter permits, the region of obstruction should be traversed to evaluate distal anatomy and assist with visualized wire passage; a pediatric or slim adult endoscope may be utilized for smaller lumen diameters. With the endoscope in place distal to the lesion, a stiff guidewire with a floppy tip, such as 0.038″ Savory type wire, is advanced into the jejunum 15–20 cm beyond the lesion. If a lesion is unable to be traversed endoscopically, an ERCP catheter with preloaded guidewire can be used, with the biliary wire passed under fluoroscopic guidance. The biliary catheter can then be advanced and a water-soluble contrast study obtained to confirm passage of the wire beyond the lesion. Blind passage of a guidewire is not recommended. The biliary wire may be exchanged for a stiffer 0.038″ Savory type wire, or the biliary wire itself may then be used to guide stent insertion. If a nontherapeutic scope was used in preceding steps, an over-the-wire exchange to a therapeutic endoscope with at least a 3.8 mm working channel is required to facilitate the 10 Fr TTS stent delivery systems. The enteral stent is then advanced through the endoscopic channel over the wire and deployed under endoscopic and fluoroscopic guidance (Fig. 65.8).

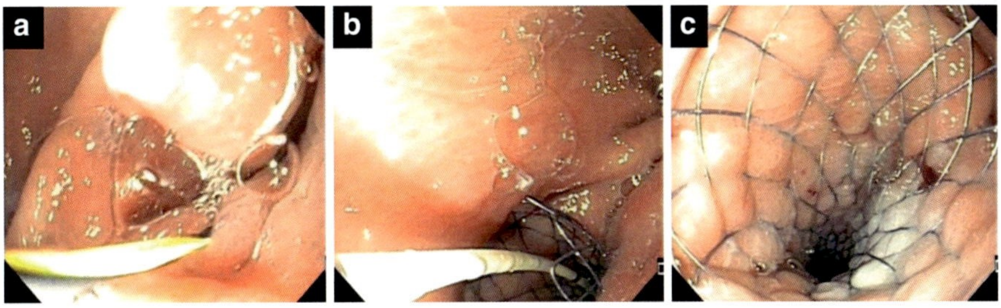

Fig. 65.8 (**a**) Endoscopic images showing passage of wire beyond obstructing lesion. (**b**) Stent deployment over the stent delivery system. (**c**) Incomplete expansion of stent immediately following deployment but with restortion of patent lumen

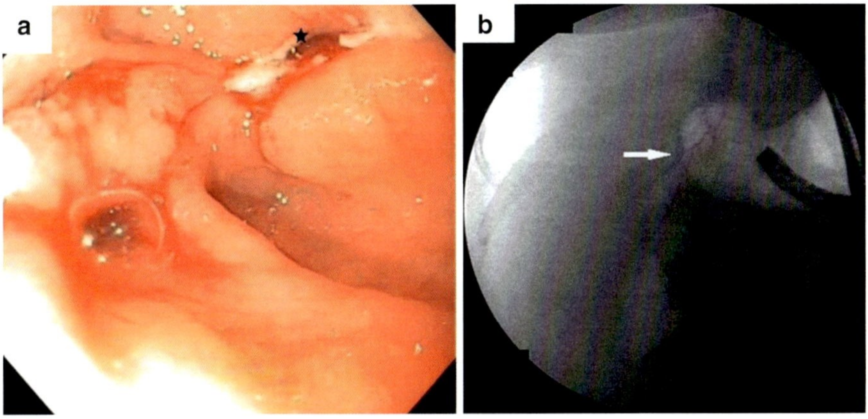

Fig. 65.9 (**a**) Endoscopic image of nearly obstructed pylorus (star) between two large peptic ulcers. (**b**) Fluoroscopic image showing incompletely expanded fully covered stent (arrow) across aforementioned peptic lesion

As with TTS balloon dilation, the endoscope should be positioned just proximal to the obstructing lesion, with the lesion situated at the midpoint of the stent. Stents exhibit varying amount of shortening with deployment and as such may require constant adjustment during deployment to ensure proper positioning, with the goal of 2 cm overlap beyond the lesion on both sides. For longer lesions, a second stent may be required. Following deployment, confirmation of luminal patency and evaluation for inadvertent perforation are assessed with injection of water-soluble contrast under fluoroscopy.

Stents will continue to expand radially for 24–48 h post-deployment, and as such immediate post-deployment balloon dilation is not recommended if the stent does not appear maximally expanded on immediate post-deployment imaging [59, 60] (Fig. 65.9).

Outcomes

The majority of outcomes data regarding SEMS in gastric outlet obstruction pertains to stenting in the setting of malignancy and is discussed in detail in "Endoscopic Stenting with SEMS in Malignant GOO" below. With regard to benign disease, two patients treated by Pinto Pabon et al. for benign disease resistant to balloon dilation and considered poor surgical candidates were reported to have clinical success [56]. Binkert et al. included two patients with benign obstruction in their stent series, with one patient with peptic pyloric stenosis experiencing retention symptoms on post-procedure day 5 and imaging showing the distal end of the stent abutting the duodenal wall [57]. Bae et al. describe treatment of a duodenojejunal anastomotic stricture with placement of a temporary PTFE-covered nitinol stent for a period of 2 months and observed continued favorable results at 6 months following stent removal [58].

Complications

As studies specific to stenting in benign gastric outlet obstruction are lacking, the majority of the data regarding complications with stenting gastric outlet obstruction come from deployment in the setting of malignant disease. Please refer to the Complications section for "Endoscopic Stenting with SEMS in Malignant GOO" below.

Palliative Endoscopic Interventions in Malignant Disease

Gastric outlet obstruction is commonly associated with advanced malignancies involving the upper GI tract, and palliative intervention to address symptoms and improve quality of life is an important aspect of patient care. Average life expectancy for patients presenting with malignant gastroduodenal obstruction is 3–6 months [61–64]. Surgical palliation for malignancy is any procedure that is performed with the intent to relieve symptoms due to malignancy or with the aim of improving quality of life [65]. Palliative procedures utilized in malignant GOO include operative open or laparoscopic gastrojejunostomy and nonoperative endoscopic therapies such as stenting and gastric decompression. In choosing which palliative intervention is most appropriate for obstruction in advanced malignancy, several factors should be considered, including extent of disease, patient medical condition and comorbidities, details of symptomatology and quality of life, patient's goals and expectations, and prognosis and life expectancy [59, 65].

Endoscopic Stenting with SEMS in Malignant GOO

Overview and Patient Selection

Stenting is indicated for patients with non-resectable obstructing disease and patients with tumor recurrence at previous surgical anastomosis presenting with

GOO. While operative gastrojejunostomy is associated with better long-term patency and with fewer repeat interventions compared to endoscopic stenting, stenting has been shown to have lower procedure-related mortality, shorter hospital stay, and quicker return to oral intake and is less invasive [61, 62, 64, 66–70]. As such, endoscopic stenting may be more appropriate in patients with short life expectancy (<6 months). Differences in overall complication and reintervention rates for uncovered and fully covered stents have not been found significant [71–73]. Uncovered stents are more commonly used than fully covered stents in palliation of malignant obstruction due to their lower migration rate [74–76]. This has been suggested as related to their incorporation into the wall of the organ in 3–6 weeks [59, 77, 78]. This lower migration rate, however, may be a trade-off with a higher reobstruction rate due to tumor ingrowth [66, 71, 73, 74, 79], though some studies have shown longer patency of uncovered to covered stents [72, 73, 80]. Covered stents may be deployed in event of leak or reobstruction from tissue ingrowth within an uncovered stent—the radial pressure of the covered stent deployed within the uncovered stent results in necrosis of the ingrown tissue and resolution of obstruction [60].

If biliary obstruction is present or likely to occur with disease progression, endoscopic placement of a biliary stent should be strongly considered prior to gastroduodenal stenting (Fig. 65.10). Endoscopic biliary access may be difficult if not impossible after gastroduodenal stent placement and result in need for percutaneous transhepatic biliary drainage [65, 69]. Concomitant or subsequent biliary obstruction with stenting in malignant GOO has been reported in up to 44% of cases [12]. Duodenal obstructions from malignancy should not be routinely dilated prior to SEMS placement as dilation caries risk of perforation [60, 69]. Dilation may be necessary, however, in patients who also require biliary stent placement to allow for passage of the larger duodenoscope required for endoscopic retrograde cholangiography.

Long segment stenosis, multilevel intestinal obstructive disease (as often seen in peritoneal carcinomatosis), and poor functional status are predictive of ineffective stenting, and such patients are less likely to see symptomatic relief [64, 75]. GI perforation is a contraindication to palliative stent placement.

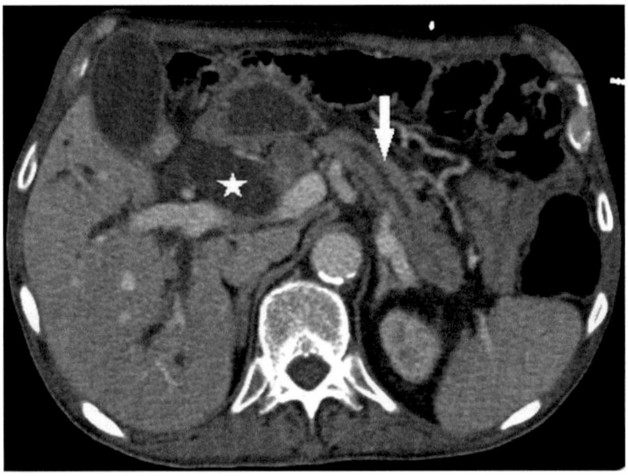

Fig. 65.10 CT scan showing duodenal obstruction by malignancy with severely dilated common bile duct (star) and dilated pancreatic duct (arrow) due to concomitant malignant biliary obstruction

Patient Preparation

Patient preparation for endoscopic stenting in malignant GOO is the same as discussed above for stenting in benign disease. Pre-procedural cross-sectional imaging remains useful for procedural planning. Care should be taken to correct coagulopathy, as this may be exacerbated by malnutrition in patients with more chronic obstruction. Current guidelines do not support preoperative antibiotic administration [30–32]. Patients should fast the evening prior to the procedure; however, large gastric residuals may still require gastric decompression prior to the procedure. Patient comfort and aspiration risk may predispose providers to perform endoscopic stenting under general endotracheal anesthesia; however, it is also possible to perform the procedure under conscious sedation with the patient positioned in the left lateral decubitus position.

Technique

Technique for endoscopic self-expanding metal stent placement for gastric outlet obstruction in setting of malignancy is equivalent to stent deployment in benign disease (outlined above). Typically uncovered stents are selected for primary intervention, with covered stents utilized for reobstruction due to tissue ingrowth in a stent-in-stent fashion.

Outcomes

Endoscopic stenting in malignant GOO has high technical and clinical success. Dormann et al., in large systematic review of over 6000 patients, found 97% underwent technically successful stenting and 89% had clinical symptom relief and oral intake improvement [81]. A meta-analysis by Minata et al. similarly found technical and clinical success rates of 95% and 90%, respectively [71]. Covered and uncovered stents have been shown to have comparable technical and clinical success rates, as well as overall patency rates [73, 74, 80].

Reported rates of resumption of oral food intake following uncovered gastroduodenal stenting for malignant obstruction are in the range 73–87.4% [12, 56, 75, 82]. Significant improvement in GOOSS in 86% of stented patients was measured by Adler et al., with 58% of patients able to resume oral intake within 24 h of the procedure [12]. Similarly a small series of 8 patients by Binkert et al. report 78% of stented patients reported quality of life improvement with return of oral intake and relief of vomiting, as well as a 100% patency rate in patients who received uncovered stents for GOO of the duodenum and stomach over follow-up of 1–52 weeks (mean 17 weeks) or until patient death [57].

Complications

Reintervention rate for both covered and uncovered stents has been reported as high as 20–25% of patients [12, 71]. Early major complication rate from stent placement has been reported at 7%, due to stent dysfunction, migration, aspiration, bleeding, or perforation [12, 83]. The late complication rate (>7 days following stent placement) is reportedly higher at 18%, predominantly due to reobstruction, stent migration, bleeding, and perforation [62, 63, 83–85]. A more distal location of malignant GOO has been shown to be predictive of stent occlusion [76, 86]. Restenosis secondary to tumor ingrowth is higher in patients with uncovered SEMS [73, 74]. Overall perforation rate after stenting in a large retrospective multicenter cohort study was reported at 2.2%, with deployment of two stents in the same procedure the single predictive factor for perforation ($p < 0.01$), suggesting that longer stenosis and the increased axial force of overlapping stents may contribute to perforation risk [75].

Higher incidence of stent migration is seen in fully covered stents compared to uncovered SEMS [59, 73–75, 79]. Additional factors related to stent migration include to lesion location, initial undersizing of the stent diameter, or reduction in lesion size with treatment of underlying process such as chemotherapy in malignancy. Partial stent migration may be addressed with repositioning or insertion of an overlapping stent if anatomy allows. Complete migration of the stent from initial placement location is addressed with stent retrieval and replacement if it is within reach of an endoscope. Distal migration of stents may require surgical retrieval (Fig. 65.11). Stent migration is a common occurrence with endoscopic

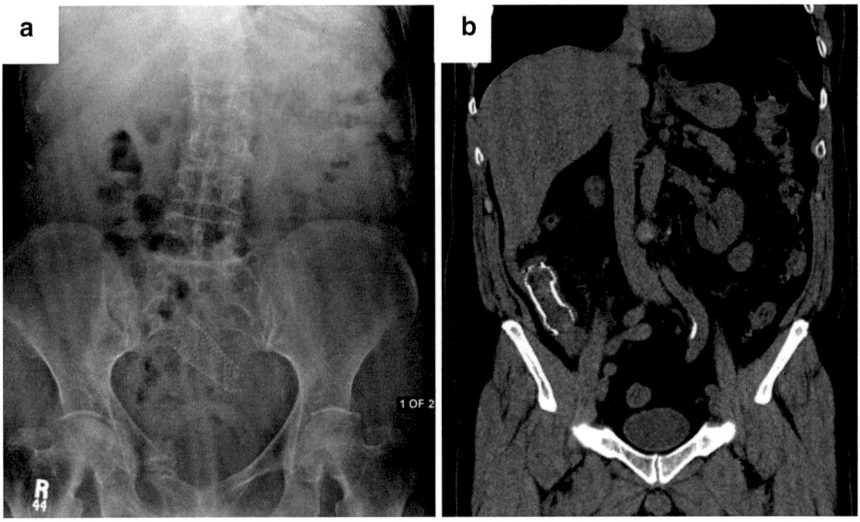

Fig. 65.11 (**a**) Abdominal X-ray image showing migration of an uncovered duodenal stent into the distal small bowel. (**b**) CT image showing fully covered duodenal stent migration in another patient. Both patients required operative intervention for stent removal

stenting, and endoscopic clipping of the proximal stent to the mucosa has been shown to reduce risk of early stent migration in patients with malignant gastric outlet obstruction [87].

Stent kinking, collapse, breakage, and occlusion due to food impaction combined are reported at 2.8% [75]. Food impaction resulting in obstruction may be addressed endoscopically. Low-residue diet, with avoidance of leafy greens, is recommended by some to prevent this complication [65, 88]. Obstruction due to ingrowth of malignancy or granulation tissue may be addressed with placement of a second stent within the lumen of the first. The radial tension of the second stent, usually a fully covered stent, results in tissue necrosis of the accumulated tissue and reopening of the lumen.

Decompressive Percutaneous Endoscopic Gastrostomy (PEG) Tube

Overview and Patient Selection

Placement of a percutaneous decompressive gastrostomy (PEG) tube is appropriate for patients with obstructing malignancy in whom surgery or stent placement is not possible [89–91]. Patients will often undergo nasogastric tube (NGT) decompression first to more quickly address symptoms of intractable nausea and emesis in GOO; however, long-term NGT use is not recommended due to risk of erosion in the nasal passages as well as patient discomfort associated with the tube. Symptomatic response to NGT decompression, however, may be a good predictor of decompressive PEG response; one retrospective study by Issaka et al. found that patients with a clinical response to NGT decompression prior to PEG placement had zero hospitalizations for obstructive symptoms following decompressive PEG [92].

Presence of malignant ascites, diffuse carcinomatosis, or tumor encasing the stomach may make placement of a PEG tube more difficult; however, they are not absolute contraindications to the procedure [89, 92].

Patient Preparation

As discussed above, patients may benefit from a trial of NGT decompression prior to PEG placement; however, at the least patients should fast the evening prior to procedure. Coagulopathy, if present, should be corrected. Prophylactic antibiotics with coverage for skin flora should be administered within 1 h of the procedure as this is associated with significant reduction in peristomal and abdominal wall infections [93]. Percutaneous endoscopic gastrostomy tube placement is performed in the supine position. For patient comfort and to reduce the risk of aspiration, general endotracheal anesthesia may be utilized, but is not required.

Technique

Upper endoscopy should be performed with documentation of the obstructing lesion and location. The endoscope is then withdrawn into the stomach and any residual food or fluid within the stomach evacuated. Full gastric insufflation is then performed to approximate the stomach with the anterior abdominal wall. Procedure room lights are dimmed, and identification of optimal PEG placement site on the abdominal wall is identified by the location of maximal transillumination, as this represents the region where the stomach is most close to the abdominal wall without intervening viscera. The site is confirmed with finger compression of the abdominal wall beginning at 2 cm below the costal margin near the midline until the endoscopist can clearly visualize this palpation of the abdominal wall. Ideal placement is between the greater and lesser gastric curves to avoid major vasculature and distal in the stomach body or proximal antrum in as dependent a position as feasible to promote gravity drainage.

Difficulty with transillumination may occur in patients with malignant ascites, tumor involvement of the abdominal wall, or in patients with multiple prior abdominal operations, and the use of fluoroscopy may aid in defining appropriate placement [94] (Fig. 65.12). If difficulty with transillumination is due to malignant

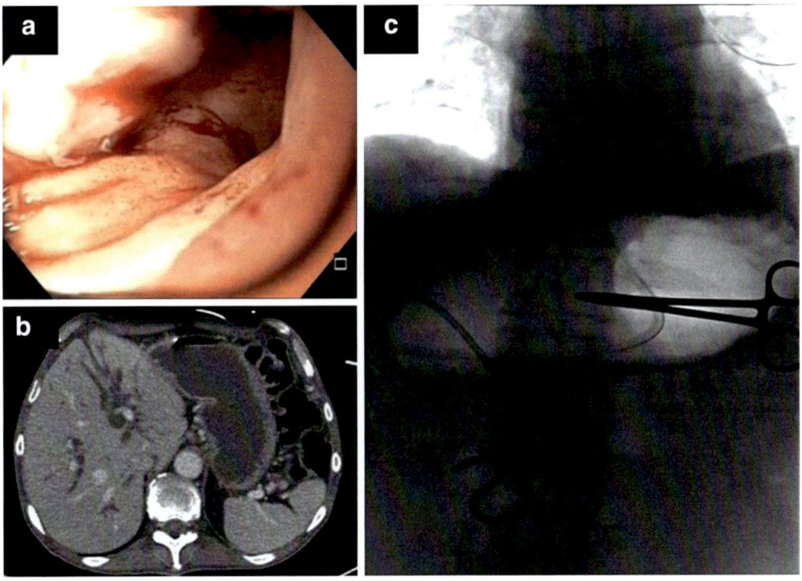

Fig. 65.12 (**a**) Endoscopic image of a metastatic ovarian lesion resulting in complete duodenal obstruction in a patient requiring decompressive PEG. (**b**) Involvement of gastric wall and the altered anatomy due to tumor burden seen on CT complicate traditional PEG placement methods. (**c**) Fluoroscopy was utilized for optimal placement. Surgical instrument placed on the abdomen was used to mark ideal decompressive PEG placement location. Percutaneous transhepatic biliary drain is seen in situ

ascites, drainage of ascites fluid with insertion of a peritoneal catheter may increase visibility. If used, the peritoneal catheter should remain in place for several days post procedure to allow for continued ascites management to allow the gastrostomy site to heal [92].

Once the insertion site is identified, the skin is prepared with an antiseptic preparation, the region infiltrated with local anesthetic, and the sight confirmed with the "safe tract" technique, for which an assistant is necessary. A small caliber needle attached to a syringe partly filled with fluid is advanced with negative pressure applied to the syringe plunger, while the endoscopist directly visualizes needle entry into the stomach. The endoscopist should visualize needle entry at the same moment that the assistant sees air withdrawn into the syringe. If air is seen in the syringe before the endoscopist sees the needle (indicating passage into small bowel or colon) or if blood is withdrawn (indicating likely liver puncture or epigastric or gastroepiploic vessel), location needs to be re-evaluated.

After "safe tract" confirmation, a small skin incision is made transversely over the "safe tract" site. When a PEG is placed for GOO, we elect to place gastrointestinal T-anchors around the PEG site (Fig. 65.13). T-anchors help oppose the gastric body to the abdominal wall, which may reduce the risk of PEG leak in this high-risk population. Leak may occur in PEGs placed for GOO due to the high volume of gastric contents, the presence of malignant ascites, or from malnutrition from chronic gastric obstruction.

The endoscopist should ensure that the stomach remains fully insufflated. A snare is inserted into the working channel and opened adjacent to the anticipated needle entry site. The introducer needle and cannula are then inserted through the abdominal wall at the incision site into the gastric lumen under direct visualization, and the snare used to secure the cannula with the introducer needle removed (Fig. 65.13). The assistant then inserts a looped guidewire through the cannula and the wire grasped with the snare. The endoscope, snare, and wire are then withdrawn in unison by the endoscopist through the patient's mouth.

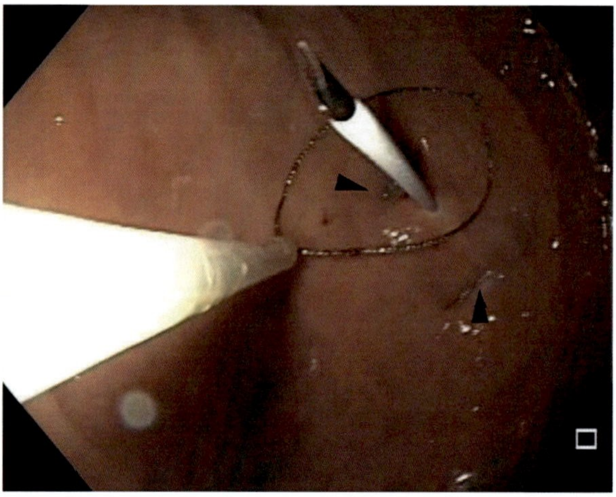

Fig. 65.13 Endoscopic image during PEG placement, showing snare positioned around the introducer needle and catheter. Gastrointestinal T-anchors (arrowheads) may be used in patients with malignant GOO to help oppose gastric body to the abdominal wall and reduce risk of leak

The "pull technique" is then employed for tube insertion. Tube sizes ranging from 15 to 24 Fr have shown good results with decompression [91, 94], and Duncan et al. have demonstrated that increased tube size does not decrease tube blockage rates [95]. The PEG tube is attached to the guidewire by the endoscopist at the mouth, and the endoscopist may elect to use the snare to grasp the PEG internal retention bumper in an in-line manner to allow the endoscope to be advanced into the stomach while the assistant pulls the wire at the abdomen to pull the PEG tube into place. The assistant should apply constant gentle pressure to the abdominal end of the guidewire to advance the tube into the stomach until the tapered portion of the PEG tube has exited the abdominal wall and the internal bumper is engaged with the stomach wall (Fig. 65.14).

The assistant next attaches the external bumper to the tube and the endoscopist confirms hemostasis and that the tube assembly is not too tight—that the internal retention bumper can spin easily. The centimeter marking at the skin should be recorded for future reference, and any remaining kit clamps and adaptors attached. The tube should be left open to gravity drainage at the conclusion of the procedure. Patients and caregivers should receive hands-on education in tube care and proper venting.

For patients in whom malignant ascites or bulky abdominal tumor burden precludes PEG placement, a percutaneous transesophageal gastrostomy (PTEG) technique can be considered [96, 97]. With the patient in a supine position, a rupture free balloon is advanced into the esophagus and confirmed fluoroscopically. Under ultrasound guidance, a needle is advanced through the left neck and into the balloon. A guidewire is placed transcervically and advanced into the distal esophagus. A 16 Fr sheath dilator is used to dilate the cervical tract, and a long decompressive tube is advanced into the stomach. The guidewire is removed and the tube is secured to the neck with suture.

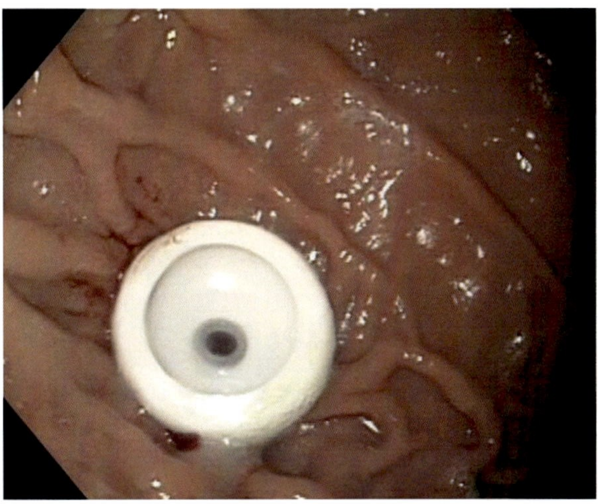

Fig. 65.14 Endoscopic visualization of PEG tube internal bumper engaged with stomach wall and hemostasis following insertion

Outcomes

Decompressive percutaneous gastrostomy tubes successfully resolve symptoms in 84–97% of patients in malignant intestinal obstruction, and technical success rates are high (up to 93%) [89, 91, 92, 98]. Additionally, many patients with more distal intestinal lesions are able to resume liquids and occasionally soft foods with decompressive gastrostomy tubes left to gravity drainage, which for many offers quality-of-life benefit from being able to engage in the social activity of eating [89].

Complications

Minor complications associated with PEG tube insertion include infection, local pain at insertion site, peristomal leakage, skin excoriation, tube migration, and tube blockage and have reported incidence of 5–13% [99]. A retrospective review by Issaka et al. found infectious complications in decompressive percutaneous gastrostomy tube placement were more common in patients with malignant ascites, with a trend toward fewer infectious events if ascites was drained prior to decompressive PEG placement [92]. Major complications, including peritonitis, tube dislodgement, fasciitis, and tumor implantation at the gastrostomy tube site, occur in 1.3–3% of patients [99].

Novel Therapeutic Endoscopic Interventions for GOO

Peroral Endoscopic Pyloromyotomy

Endoscopic division of the pyloric muscle complex (so-called peroral pyloromyotomy (POP) or gastric peroral endoscopic myotomy (G-POEM) is a novel technique that applies principles learned from esophageal peroral endoscopic myotomy (POEM) cases. Briefly, a submucosal bleb is created with a saline solution and a mucosal incision is created. The endoscope is advanced into the submucosal space and a tunnel is dissected toward the pylorus. When the pyloric ring is reached, the inner circular and oblique fibers of the muscle complex are divided with electrosurgical energy. The scope is subsequently withdrawn from the submucosal tunnel, and the mucosal entry site is closed with endoscopically placed clips.

Kawai et al. first reported feasibility of endoscopic pyloromyotomy using submucosal tunneling technique in porcine models in 2012 [100], followed by the first human report of its use by Kashab et al. in a patient with refractory diabetic gastroparesis who refused surgical intervention in 2013 [101]. Early successful use of peroral endoscopic pyloromyotomy was described in cases of post-esophagectomy gastric outlet obstruction, postsurgical or idiopathic gastroparesis, and a case of adult primary pyloric stenosis [102–104].

Two larger retrospective studies evaluating efficacy and safety of G-POEM in patients with gastroparesis refractory to previous therapeutic measures who underwent G-POEM have recently been reported by Gonzalez et al. (12 patients) and Kashab et al. (30 patients.) Both report 100% technical success rate and good clinical responses with 85% and 86% of patients showing symptom improvement or resolution during follow-up of 3 and 5.5 months, respectively [105, 106]. Additionally Kashab et al. showed normalization of gastric emptying scan in 46% and improvement in another 35% of 17 patients who underwent repeat scan following intervention [106]. Gonzalez et al. report a greater normalization of 75% of gastric emptying scans performed at 2 months following G-POEM [105]. The cohort evaluated by Gonzales et al. reports zero adverse events, and Kashab et al. report an adverse event rate of 6.7% (two patients) due to capnoperitoneum managed by intraprocedure needle drainage (one patient) and prepyloric ulcer on second-look enteroscopy that was medically treated (one patient) [105, 106]. Limitations of these studies include retrospective methodologies and patient numbers (12 and 30 patients); nonetheless, they strengthen the evidence for technical feasibility as well as clinical efficacy of G-POEM in patients with gastroparesis. Further experiences with prospective, sham-controlled trials of G-POEM/POP for gastroparesis are needed to better identify which patients will have highest probability of response, but thus far it appears a promising technique for treatment of refractory gastroparesis [107].

GJ Anastomosis with Magnets

With evidence of prolonged patency in gastrojejunostomy compared to enteral stenting for palliation for malignant gastric outlet obstruction, there is increased interest in development of endoluminal entero-enteral bypass systems that may be utilized in those deemed too high risk for laparoscopic surgery. Compression anastomoses utilizing magnets have been described in porcine models; however, results were initially limited by transoral delivery methods resulting in small anastomosis and subsequent poor long-term patency rates [108–110]. Incorporation of enteral stents results in increased patency but is associated with obstruction, migration, and bleeding as well as retained foreign object [111, 112]. Recently, Ryou et al. have developed a purely endoscopic smart magnet system that self-assembles into an open macro-configuration that when paired with another mate in an adjacent lumen results in a portal for either immediate enterostomy or fusion over several days followed by the magnets sloughing off and being naturally expelled, leaving behind a large caliber anastomosis [113, 114]. They have most recently demonstrated anastomosis durability and long-term patency of the technology in porcine models [115].

GJ Anastomosis with Lumen-Apposing Metal Stents (LAMS Gastrojejunostomy)

Endoscopic ultrasound-guided gastrojejunostomy using fully covered lumen-apposing biflanged metal stents (LAMS) has recently become an option for symptomatic management in benign and malignant gastric outlet obstruction. The goal of the procedure is to produce a fully functional anastomosis without the need for open procedure and has been described successfully in individual cases and small studies [116–121].

A recent multicenter retrospective study by Tyberg et al. of 26 patients with benign and malignant disease who underwent ultrasound-guided gastrojejunostomy with lumen-apposing stents reported technical success in 92% of patients, with clinical success in symptom resolution and ability to tolerate oral diet in 85% [118]. Of the 22 patients with clinical success, 19 had had failure of previous endoscopic intervention for their GOO. Overall adverse event rate was 11.5% and included two patients with failed distal LAMS placement, one of whom had extensive malignant disease and developed peritonitis and died the following day. The second patient with LAMS misplacement was salvaged with deployment of SEMS, however developed post-procedure bleeding requiring transfusion.

Retrospective study by Chen et al. compared outcomes of EUS-guided gastrojejunostomy to endoscopic stenting in patients with malignant gastric outlet obstruction and showed no significant difference between clinical and technical success or adverse and severe adverse events between the two modalities [122]. Their adverse event rate for EUS-guided gastrojejunostomy was 16.7%, comparable to the rate reported by Tyberg et al., and included three misdeployments of the stent into the peritoneum. Endoscopic stenting was noted to have a significantly greater reintervention rate over the follow-up period compared to EUS-guided gastrojejunostomy [122]. These studies suggest promising results for use of EUS-gastrojejunostomy in gastric outlet obstruction; however, further studies of prospective nature of long-term outcomes as well as larger prospective comparative studies are still needed.

Conclusion

The most common cause of gastric outlet obstruction has shifted from benign causes to malignancy since the introduction of H2 blockers and medical therapy for *H. pylori* infection. As such, thorough evaluation and workup for malignancy, including endoscopic evaluation and biopsy, are necessary for all patients presenting with gastric outlet obstruction. Treatment of GOO is dependent on specific etiology of the obstruction; however, all patients presenting with acute obstruction will benefit from NGT decompression and fluid and electrolyte replacement. Several endoscopic therapies are now available for symptomatic management of gastric outlet obstruction—TTS balloon dilations, injections of steroids and botulinum toxin, self-expanding metal stents, and decompressive PEG tubes—each appropriate in different etiologies. The continuing advancement of endoscopic technologies will likely lead to the development and implementation of still more novel interventions.

References

1. Ellis H. The diagnosis of benign and malignant pyloric obstruction. Clin Oncol. 1976;2(1):11–5.
2. Johnson CD, Ellis H. Gastric outlet obstruction now predicts malignancy. Br J Surg. 1990;77(9):1023–4.
3. Khullar SK, DiSario JA. Gastric outlet obstruction. Gastrointest Endosc Clin N Am. 1996;6(3):585–603.
4. Milosavljevic T, et al. Complications of peptic ulcer disease. Dig Dis. 2011;29(5):491–3.
5. Chaudhary A, et al. Elective surgery for corrosive-induced gastric injury. World J Surg. 1996;20(6):703–6. discussion 706
6. Reynolds HL Jr, Stellato TA. Crohn's disease of the foregut. Surg Clin North Am. 2001;81(1):117–35. viii
7. Scheck SM, et al. Crohn's disease presenting as gastric outlet obstruction. J Surg Case Rep. 2014;2014(12):1–3.
8. Padmanabhan H, Rothnie A, Singh P. An unusual case of gastric outlet obstruction caused by tuberculosis: challenges in diagnosis and treatment. BMJ Case Rep. 2013;2013:1–5.
9. Weil BR, Howard TJ, Zyromski NJ. Spontaneous duodenal hematoma: a rare cause of upper gastrointestinal tract obstruction. Arch Surg. 2008;143(8):794–6.
10. Dean PG, et al. Hyperplastic gastric polyp causing progressive gastric outlet obstruction. Mayo Clin Proc. 1998;73(10):964–7.
11. Qasaimeh GR, Bakkar S, Jadallah K. Bouveret's syndrome: an overlooked diagnosis. A case report and review of literature. Int Surg. 2014;99(6):819–23.
12. Adler DG, Baron TH. Endoscopic palliation of malignant gastric outlet obstruction using self-expanding metal stents: experience in 36 patients. Am J Gastroenterol. 2002;97(1):72–8.
13. Asano N, et al. Helicobacter pylori-negative gastric mucosa-associated lymphoid tissue lymphomas: a review. World J Gastroenterol. 2015;21(26):8014–20.
14. Lightner AL, et al. Primary gastrointestinal non-Hodgkin's lymphoma of the small and large intestines: a systematic review. J Gastrointest Surg. 2016;20(4):827–39.
15. Pauli EM, Marks JM, editors. Percutaneous Endoscopic Gastrostomy (PEG): techniques, effectiveness, and potential complications. New York: Nova Biomedical; 2016. p. 125–39.
16. Jaffin BW, Kaye MD. The prognosis of gastric outlet obstruction. Ann Surg. 1985;201(2):176–9.
17. Weiland D, et al. Gastric outlet obstruction in peptic ulcer disease: an indication for surgery. Am J Surg. 1982;143(1):90–3.
18. Johnston D, et al. Highly selective vagotomy without a drainage procedure in the treatment of haemorrhage, perforation, and pyloric stenosis due to peptic ulcer. Br J Surg. 1973;60(10):790–7.
19. Kozarek RA, Botoman VA, Patterson DJ. Long-term follow-up in patients who have undergone balloon dilation for gastric outlet obstruction. Gastrointest Endosc. 1990;36(6):558–61.
20. Benjamin SB, Cattau EL, Glass RL. Balloon dilation of the pylorus: therapy for gastric outlet obstruction. Gastrointest Endosc. 1982;28(4):253–4.
21. Hogan RB, Hamilton JK, Polter DE. Preliminary experience with hydrostatic balloon dilation of gastric outlet obstruction. Gastrointest Endosc. 1986;32(2):71–4.
22. Cherian PT, Cherian S, Singh P. Long-term follow-up of patients with gastric outlet obstruction related to peptic ulcer disease treated with endoscopic balloon dilatation and drug therapy. Gastrointest Endosc. 2007;66(3):491–7.
23. Kochhar R, Kochhar S. Endoscopic balloon dilation for benign gastric outlet obstruction in adults. World J Gastrointest Endosc. 2010;2(1):29–35.
24. Solt J, Hertelendi A, Szilagyi K. Balloon catheter dilatation of lower gastrointestinal tract stenoses: long-term results. Orv Hetil. 2002;143(31):1835–40.
25. Boylan JJ, Gradzka MI. Long-term results of endoscopic balloon dilatation for gastric outlet obstruction. Dig Dis Sci. 1999;44(9):1883–6.

26. Solt J, et al. Long-term results of balloon catheter dilation for benign gastric outlet stenosis. Endoscopy. 2003;35(6):490–5.
27. Murthy UK. Repeated hydrostatic balloon dilation in obstructive gastroduodenal Crohn's disease. Gastrointest Endosc. 1991;37(4):484–5.
28. Kim JH, et al. Benign duodenal strictures: treatment by means of fluoroscopically guided balloon dilation. J Vasc Interv Radiol. 2005;16(4):543–8.
29. Goldstein JA, Barkin JS. Comparison of the diameter consistency and dilating force of the controlled radial expansion balloon catheter to the conventional balloon dilators. Am J Gastroenterol. 2000;95(12):3423–7.
30. Committee, A.S.o.P., et al. Antibiotic prophylaxis for GI endoscopy. Gastrointest Endosc. 2015;81(1):81–9.
31. Geist SM, Fitzpatrick S, Geist JR. American Heart Association 2007 guidelines on prevention of infective endocarditis. J Mich Dent Assoc. 2007;89(9):50–6.
32. Nishimura RA, et al. ACC/AHA 2008 guideline update on valvular heart disease: focused update on infective endocarditis: a report of the American College of Cardiology/ American Heart Association Task Force on Practice Guidelines: endorsed by the Society of Cardiovascular Anesthesiologists, Society for Cardiovascular Angiography and Interventions, and Society of Thoracic Surgeons. Circulation. 2008;118(8):887–96.
33. Kim JH, et al. Gastric outlet obstruction caused by benign anastomotic stricture: treatment by fluoroscopically guided balloon dilation. J Vasc Interv Radiol. 2005;16(5):699–704.
34. Rana SS, et al. Endoscopic balloon dilatation without fluoroscopy for treating gastric outlet obstruction because of benign etiologies. Surg Endosc. 2011;25(5):1579–84.
35. Kochhar R, et al. Early endoscopic balloon dilation in caustic-induced gastric injury. Gastrointest Endosc. 2010;71(4):737–44.
36. Kochhar R, et al. Endoscopic balloon dilatation of benign gastric outlet obstruction. J Gastroenterol Hepatol. 2004;19(4):418–22.
37. Lam YH, et al. Endoscopic balloon dilation for benign gastric outlet obstruction with or without Helicobacter pylori infection. Gastrointest Endosc. 2004;60(2):229–33.
38. Ukleja A, et al. Outcome of endoscopic balloon dilation of strictures after laparoscopic gastric bypass. Surg Endosc. 2008;22(8):1746–50.
39. Lau JY, et al. Through-the-scope balloon dilation for pyloric stenosis: long-term results. Gastrointest Endosc. 1996;43(2 Pt 1):98–101.
40. Kirk RM. The size of the pyloroduodenal canal: its relation to the cause and treatment of peptic ulcer. Proc R Soc Med. 1970;63(9):944–6.
41. Perng CL, et al. Characteristics of patients with benign gastric outlet obstruction requiring surgery after endoscopic balloon dilation. Am J Gastroenterol. 1996;91(5):987–90.
42. Kochhar R, et al. Intralesional steroid injections for corrosive induced pyloric stenosis. Endoscopy. 1998;30(8):734–6.
43. Singh VV, Draganov P, Valentine J. Efficacy and safety of endoscopic balloon dilation of symptomatic upper and lower gastrointestinal Crohn's disease strictures. J Clin Gastroenterol. 2005;39(4):284–90.
44. Pasricha PJ, Ravich WJ, Kalloo AN. Botulinum toxin for achalasia. Lancet. 1993;341(8839):244–5.
45. Bashashati M, et al. Botulinum toxin in the treatment of diffuse esophageal spasm. Dis Esophagus. 2010;23(7):554–60.
46. Jost WH, Schimrigk K. Use of botulinum toxin in anal fissure. Dis Colon Rectum. 1993;36(10):974.
47. Clarke JO, Snape WJ Jr. Pyloric sphincter therapy: botulinum toxin, stents, and pyloromyotomy. Gastroenterol Clin N Am. 2015;44(1):127–36.
48. Coleski R, Anderson MA, Hasler WL. Factors associated with symptom response to pyloric injection of botulinum toxin in a large series of gastroparesis patients. Dig Dis Sci. 2009;54(12):2634–42.
49. Kent MS, et al. A pilot study of botulinum toxin injection for the treatment of delayed gastric emptying following esophagectomy. Surg Endosc. 2007;21(5):754–7.

50. Wiesel PH, et al. Botulinum toxin for refractory postoperative pyloric spasm. Endoscopy. 1997;29(2):132.
51. Arts J, et al. Clinical trial: a randomized-controlled crossover study of intrapyloric injection of botulinum toxin in gastroparesis. Aliment Pharmacol Ther. 2007;26(9):1251–8.
52. Camilleri M, et al. Clinical guideline: management of gastroparesis. Am J Gastroenterol. 2013;108(1):18–37. quiz 38
53. Heinen F, et al. Lack of response to botulinum toxin A in patients with hypertrophic pyloric stenosis. Eur J Pediatr. 1999;158(5):436.
54. Bromer MQ, et al. Endoscopic pyloric injection of botulinum toxin A for the treatment of refractory gastroparesis. Gastrointest Endosc. 2005;61(7):833–9.
55. Huibregtse K, et al. Endoscopic placement of expandable metal stents for biliary strictures – a preliminary report on experience with 33 patients. Endoscopy. 1989;21(6):280–2.
56. Pinto Pabon IT, et al. Gastric and duodenal stents: follow-up and complications. Cardiovasc Intervent Radiol. 2001;24(3):147–53.
57. Binkert CA, et al. Benign and malignant stenoses of the stomach and duodenum: treatment with self-expanding metallic endoprostheses. Radiology. 1996;199(2):335–8.
58. Bae JI, et al. Treatment of a benign anastomotic duodenojejunal stricture with a polytetrafluoroethylene-covered retrievable expandable nitinol stent. J Vasc Interv Radiol. 2004;15(7):769–72.
59. Baerlocher MO, et al. Interdisciplinary Canadian guidelines on the use of metal stents in the gastrointestinal tract for oncological indications. Can Assoc Radiol J. 2008;59(3):107–22.
60. Mangiavillano B, et al. Role of stenting in gastrointestinal benign and malignant diseases. World J Gastrointest Endosc. 2015;7(5):460–80.
61. Brimhall B, Adler DG. Enteral stents for malignant gastric outlet obstruction. Gastrointest Endosc Clin N Am. 2011;21(3):389–403. vii-viii
62. Jeurnink SM, et al. Surgical gastrojejunostomy or endoscopic stent placement for the palliation of malignant gastric outlet obstruction (SUSTENT study): a multicenter randomized trial. Gastrointest Endosc. 2010;71(3):490–9.
63. Miyazaki Y, et al. Treatment of gastric outlet obstruction that results from unresectable gastric cancer: current evidence. World J Gastrointest Endosc. 2016;8(3):165–72.
64. Lopera JE, et al. Gastroduodenal stent placement: current status. Radiographics. 2004;24(6):1561–73.
65. Potz BA, Miner TJ. Surgical palliation of gastric outlet obstruction in advanced malignancy. World J Gastrointest Surg. 2016;8(8):545–55.
66. Maetani I, et al. Metallic stents for gastric outlet obstruction: reintervention rate is lower with uncovered versus covered stents, despite similar outcomes. Gastrointest Endosc. 2009;69(4):806–12.
67. Ly J, et al. A systematic review of methods to palliate malignant gastric outlet obstruction. Surg Endosc. 2010;24(2):290–7.
68. Bian SB, et al. Palliative therapy for gastric outlet obstruction caused by unresectable gastric cancer: a meta-analysis comparison of gastrojejunostomy with endoscopic stenting. Chin Med J. 2016;129(9):1113–21.
69. Kochar R, Shah N. Enteral stents: from esophagus to colon. Gastrointest Endosc. 2013;78(6):913–8.
70. Tsauo J, et al. Partially-covered stent placement versus surgical gastrojejunostomy for the palliation of malignant gastroduodenal obstruction secondary to pancreatic cancer. Abdom Radiol (NY). 2016;41(11):2233–40.
71. Minata MK, et al. Stents and surgical interventions in the palliation of gastric outlet obstruction: a systematic review. Endosc Int Open. 2016;4(11):E1158–70.
72. Kim JW, et al. Comparison between uncovered and covered self-expandable metal stent placement in malignant duodenal obstruction. World J Gastroenterol. 2015;21(5):1580–7.
73. Pan YM, et al. Covered versus uncovered self-expandable metallic stents for palliation of malignant gastric outlet obstruction: a systematic review and meta-analysis. BMC Gastroenterol. 2014;14:170.

74. Kim CG, et al. Covered versus uncovered self-expandable metallic stents for palliation of malignant pyloric obstruction in gastric cancer patients: a randomized, prospective study. Gastrointest Endosc. 2010;72(1):25–32.
75. Yamao K, et al. Factors predicting through-the-scope gastroduodenal stenting outcomes in patients with gastric outlet obstruction: a large multicenter retrospective study in West Japan. Gastrointest Endosc. 2016;84(5):757–63. e6
76. Jung K, et al. Outcomes of endoscopically inserted self-expandable metal stents in malignancy according to the type of stent and the site of obstruction. Surg Endosc. 2016;30(9):4001–10.
77. Bethge N, et al. Human tissue responses to metal stents implanted in vivo for the palliation of malignant stenoses. Gastrointest Endosc. 1996;43(6):596–602.
78. Vakil N. Expandable metal stents: principles and tissue responses. Gastrointest Endosc Clin N Am. 2011;21(3):351–7. vii
79. Maetani I, Isayama H, Mizumoto Y. Palliation in patients with malignant gastric outlet obstruction with a newly designed enteral stent: a multicenter study. Gastrointest Endosc. 2007;66(2):355–60.
80. Woo SM, et al. Comparison of uncovered and covered stents for the treatment of malignant duodenal obstruction caused by pancreaticobiliary cancer. Surg Endosc. 2013;27(6):2031–9.
81. Dormann AJ, Deppe H, Wigginghaus B. Self-expanding metallic stents for continuous dilatation of benign stenoses in gastrointestinal tract – first results of long-term follow-up in interim stent application in pyloric and colonic obstructions. Z Gastroenterol. 2001;39(11):957–60.
82. Johnsson E, Thune A, Liedman B. Palliation of malignant gastroduodenal obstruction with open surgical bypass or endoscopic stenting: clinical outcome and health economic evaluation. World J Surg. 2004;28(8):812–7.
83. Gaidos JK, Draganov PV. Treatment of malignant gastric outlet obstruction with endoscopically placed self-expandable metal stents. World J Gastroenterol. 2009;15(35):4365–71.
84. Jeurnink SM, et al. Stent versus gastrojejunostomy for the palliation of gastric outlet obstruction: a systematic review. BMC Gastroenterol. 2007;7:18.
85. No JH, et al. Long-term outcome of palliative therapy for gastric outlet obstruction caused by unresectable gastric cancer in patients with good performance status: endoscopic stenting versus surgery. Gastrointest Endosc. 2013;78(1):55–62.
86. Grunwald D, et al. The location of obstruction predicts stent occlusion in malignant gastric outlet obstruction. Therap Adv Gastroenterol. 2016;9(6):815–22.
87. Kim ID, et al. Prevention of covered enteral stent migration in patients with malignant gastric outlet obstruction: a pilot study of anchoring with endoscopic clips. Scand J Gastroenterol. 2010;45(1):100–5.
88. Baron TH. Expandable metal stents for the treatment of cancerous obstruction of the gastrointestinal tract. N Engl J Med. 2001;344(22):1681–7.
89. Dolan EA. Malignant bowel obstruction: a review of current treatment strategies. Am J Hosp Palliat Care. 2011;28(8):576–82.
90. Schmidt C, et al. A prospective observational study examining quality of life in patients with malignant gastric outlet obstruction. Am J Surg. 2009;198(1):92–9.
91. Teriaky A, Gregor J, Chande N. Percutaneous endoscopic gastrostomy tube placement for end-stage palliation of malignant gastrointestinal obstructions. Saudi J Gastroenterol. 2012;18(2):95–8.
92. Issaka RB, et al. Palliative venting percutaneous endoscopic gastrostomy tube is safe and effective in patients with malignant obstruction. Surg Endosc. 2014;28(5):1668–73.
93. Lipp A, Lusardi G. Systemic antimicrobial prophylaxis for percutaneous endoscopic gastrostomy. Cochrane Database Syst Rev. 2013;11:CD005571.
94. Campagnutta E, et al. Palliative treatment of upper intestinal obstruction by gynecological malignancy: the usefulness of percutaneous endoscopic gastrostomy. Gynecol Oncol. 1996;62(1):103–5.
95. Duncan HD, et al. Prospective randomized comparison of two different sized percutaneous endoscopically placed gastrostomy tubes. Clin Nutr. 1996;15(6):317–20.

96. Udomsawaengsup S, et al. Percutaneous transesophageal gastrostomy (PTEG): a safe and effective technique for gastrointestinal decompression in malignant obstruction and massive ascites. Surg Endosc. 2008;22(10):2314–8.
97. Oishi H, et al. A nonsurgical technique to create an esophagostomy for difficult cases of percutaneous endoscopic gastrostomy. Surg Endosc. 2003;17(8):1224–7.
98. Brooksbank MA, Game PA, Ashby MA. Palliative venting gastrostomy in malignant intestinal obstruction. Palliat Med. 2002;16(6):520–6.
99. McClave SA, Ritchie CS. The role of endoscopically placed feeding or decompression tubes. Gastroenterol Clin N Am. 2006;35(1):83–100.
100. Kawai M, et al. Endoscopic pyloromyotomy: a new concept of minimally invasive surgery for pyloric stenosis. Endoscopy. 2012;44(2):169–73.
101. Khashab MA, et al. Gastric peroral endoscopic myotomy for refractory gastroparesis: first human endoscopic pyloromyotomy (with video). Gastrointest Endosc. 2013;78(5):764–8.
102. Chung H, et al. Endoscopic pyloromyotomy for postesophagectomy gastric outlet obstruction. Endoscopy. 2014;46 Suppl 1 UCTN:E345–6.
103. Pham KD, et al. Peroral endoscopic pyloromyotomy for primary pyloric stenosis. Endoscopy. 2015;47(Suppl 1):E637–8.
104. Shlomovitz E, et al. Early human experience with per-oral endoscopic pyloromyotomy (POP). Surg Endosc. 2015;29(3):543–51.
105. Gonzalez JM, et al. Gastric per-oral endoscopic myotomy with antropyloromyotomy in the treatment of refractory gastroparesis: clinical experience with follow-up and scintigraphic evaluation (with video). Gastrointest Endosc. 2017;85(1):132–9.
106. Khashab MA, et al. Gastric per-oral endoscopic myotomy for refractory gastroparesis: results from the first multicenter study on endoscopic pyloromyotomy (with video). Gastrointest Endosc. 2017;85(1):123–8.
107. Camilleri M, Szarka LA. POEMs for gastroparesis. Gastrointest Endosc. 2017;85(1):129–31.
108. Pichakron KO, et al. Magnamosis II: magnetic compression anastomosis for minimally invasive gastrojejunostomy and jejunojejunostomy. J Am Coll Surg. 2011;212(1):42–9.
109. Jamshidi R, et al. Magnamosis: magnetic compression anastomosis with comparison to suture and staple techniques. J Pediatr Surg. 2009;44(1):222–8.
110. Gonzales KD, et al. Magnamosis III: delivery of a magnetic compression anastomosis device using minimally invasive endoscopic techniques. J Pediatr Surg. 2012;47(6):1291–5.
111. Chopita N, et al. Endoscopic gastroenteric anastomosis using magnets. Endoscopy. 2005;37(4):313–7.
112. Cope C, et al. Stent placement of gastroenteric anastomoses formed by magnetic compression. J Vasc Interv Radiol. 1999;10(10):1379–86.
113. Ryou M, Agoston AT, Thompson CC. Endoscopic intestinal bypass creation by using self-assembling magnets in a porcine model. Gastrointest Endosc. 2016;83(4):821–5.
114. Ryou M, et al. Smart Self-Assembling MagnetS for ENdoscopy (SAMSEN) for transoral endoscopic creation of immediate gastrojejunostomy (with video). Gastrointest Endosc. 2011;73(2):353–9.
115. Ryou M, Aihara H, Thompson CC. Minimally invasive entero-enteral dual-path bypass using self-assembling magnets. Surg Endosc. 2016;30(10):4533–8.
116. Barthet M, et al. Natural orifice transluminal endoscopic surgery gastroenterostomy with a biflanged lumen-apposing stent: first clinical experience (with videos). Gastrointest Endosc. 2015;81(1):215–8.
117. Tyberg A, et al. EUS-guided gastrojejunostomy after failed enteral stenting. Gastrointest Endosc. 2015;81(4):1011–2.
118. Tyberg A, et al. Endoscopic ultrasound-guided gastrojejunostomy with a lumen-apposing metal stent: a multicenter, international experience. Endosc Int Open. 2016;4(3):E276–81.
119. Khashab MA, et al. EUS-guided gastroenterostomy: the first U.S. clinical experience (with video). Gastrointest Endosc. 2015;82(5):932–8.
120. Itoi T, et al. Technical review of endoscopic ultrasonography-guided gastroenterostomy in 2017. Dig Endosc. 2017;29(4):495–502.

121. Itoi T, et al. Novel EUS-guided double-balloon-occluded gastrojejunostomy bypass. Gastrointest Endosc. 2016;83(2):461–2.
122. Chen YI, et al. EUS-guided gastroenterostomy is comparable to enteral stenting with fewer re-interventions in malignant gastric outlet obstruction. Surg Endosc. 2017;31(9):3765.
123. Pauli EM, Marks JM. Endoscopic tools and techniques for strictures and stenoses. In: Principles of flexible endoscopy for surgeons. New York: Springer; 2013. https://doi.org/10.1007/978-1-4614-6330-6_10.

Surgical Management: Resection and Reconstruction Versus Drainage

66

Anupamaa J. Seshadri and Douglas S. Smink

Indications for Surgical Management

Historically, peptic ulcer disease was the leading cause of benign gastric outlet obstruction, necessitating surgical management to restore the ability for oral intake [1]. With better understanding of the underlying causes of peptic ulcer disease and improved medical therapies, gastric outlet obstruction from peptic ulcer disease has become more rare. Current data suggest that gastric outlet obstruction occurs in 2–8% of patients with peptic ulcer disease [2–4]. In spite of declining rates of surgical procedures related to peptic ulcer disease (Fig. 66.1), gastric outlet obstruction still remains a significant problem that requires surgical expertise. There are estimates that obstruction necessitates operative management in approximately 2000 peptic ulcer disease patients per year in the United States [3]. Therefore, the surgeon must be not only comfortable with the operative techniques for management of this entity but also have an in-depth knowledge of the decision-making required to determine the best operation for each individual patient. In this chapter, we discuss the strategy of resection and reconstruction in comparison to drainage procedures and outline the relative advantages and disadvantages of each procedure.

Resection and Reconstruction

Procedure Options

Definitive treatment for gastric outlet obstruction in peptic ulcer disease is resection of the obstructed area, typically consisting of an antrectomy, as well as a vagotomy

A. J. Seshadri · D. S. Smink (✉)
Department of Surgery, Brigham and Women's Hospital, Boston, MA, USA
e-mail: dsmink@bwh.harvard.edu

J. Grams et al. (eds.), *The SAGES Manual of Foregut Surgery*,
https://doi.org/10.1007/978-3-319-96122-4_66

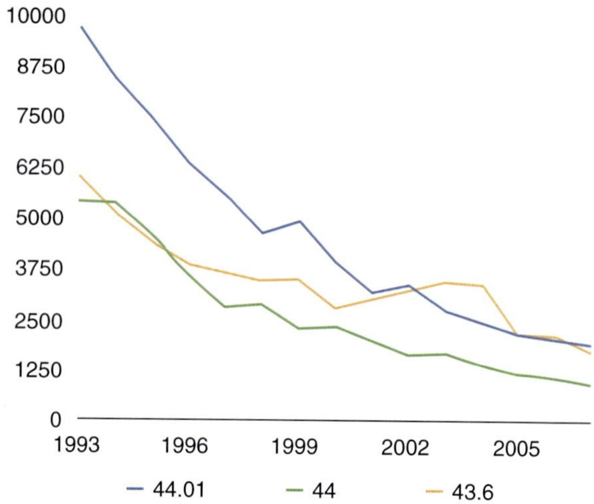

Fig. 66.1 Decreasing incidence of procedures related to peptic ulcer disease. The lines represent different ICD-9 CM procedure codes: 44.01 truncal vagotomy, 44 vagotomy not otherwise specified, 43.6 partial gastrectomy with anastomosis to duodenum. (Adapted from Basinskaya et al. [39])

to prevent recurrent peptic ulcer disease. A number of options exist for reconstruction, including a Billroth I, Billroth II, or Roux-en-Y reconstruction. The technical details of these operations have been discussed in prior chapters and will therefore not be discussed here.

Advantages

Vagotomy and antrectomy have several benefits in the management of gastric outlet obstruction for patients with peptic ulcer disease, the most important of which is that antrectomy provides definitive therapy by resecting the area of obstruction. Antrectomy also eliminates gastrin release from the antrum, thus decreasing acid secretion [5]. Vagotomy at the time of the resection further reduces subsequent acid production, leading to only a 5% risk of recurrent ulceration [5–7]. Finally, resection and reconstruction enable the pathologist to definitively identify or rule out malignancy in the area of ulceration and obstruction.

Disadvantages and Complications

A main disadvantage of vagotomy and antrectomy is the risk of anastomotic leak and the morbidity associated with this. This risk is particularly relevant in this patient population, as gastric outlet obstruction can lead to malnutrition, which hinders anastomotic healing. Further risk factors for anastomotic leak include patient smoking, steroid medications, long operative time, and gross spillage [8]. Anastomotic leak can be managed operatively or with percutaneous drainage depending on the nature of the leak and the hemodynamic stability of the patient.

Another potentially catastrophic complication is duodenal stump blowout, which can occur in 1–6% of patients who are reconstructed with a Billroth II technique [9]. As the name suggests, this is caused by breakdown of the staple line at the proximal duodenum. This can be caused by ischemia of the duodenal stump secondary to mobilization, or from afferent loop syndrome, where there is distention of the duodenum and jejunum of the afferent limb of the Billroth II reconstruction secondary to obstruction from adhesions, internal herniation, volvulus, or an edematous or tight gastrojejunostomy [10, 11]. This complication can cause devastating sepsis and is associated with a mortality rate of 5–16% [12]. To prevent duodenal stump blowout, a duodenostomy tube can be placed at the time of the operation for decompression of the duodenal stump [10, 13]. Alternatively, a nasogastric tube can be placed through the gastrojejunostomy into the afferent loop at the time of surgery to allow for early decompression [11]. Once it occurs, duodenal stump blowout may need to be managed operatively, and the underlying cause of afferent loop syndrome, if present, should be addressed at that time.

Delayed gastric emptying can also occur after vagotomy and antrectomy. Thirteen percent of all gastroparesis cases are postsurgical, and while not all of these cases are related to vagotomy and antrectomy, they are commonly associated [14]. There are multiple explanations for this postoperative gastroparesis, including vagotomy-induced gastric atony and neuromuscular dysfunction, decreased mechanical digestion of food in the stomach after antrectomy, and potential disruption of the migrating motor complex in the setting of Billroth II or Roux-en-Y reconstruction [15–17]. The management of postoperative gastroparesis is initially supportive, as it can often resolve without further intervention. This is potentially because of vagal reinnervation or adaptation by the enteric nervous system [18]. Medical therapy with erythromycin, metoclopramide, or other prokinetic agents may also be attempted [19, 20]. For those patients who do not improve with medical management and at least a year of expectant management, further procedures may be required. Completion gastrectomy is one option, but the success rate reported in the literature ranges widely from 40% to 80% [21, 22]. Conversion to Roux-en-Y gastrojejunostomy can be performed but should include resection of the atonic stomach. This has a reported success rate of only 66%, likely because of potential continued stasis secondary to a denervated Roux efferent limb [23, 24]. Finally, gastric electrical stimulation can be attempted, although this is not yet commonly performed in this patient population [22, 25].

Conversely, patients after vagotomy and antrectomy can develop dumping syndrome, with rapid emptying of the stomach after a meal. This is classified into early (within 10–30 min of a meal) and late (1–3 h after a meal) forms, with the majority of patients affected having early dumping and only approximately 25% of patients experiencing late dumping [25, 26]. The mechanisms behind dumping syndrome are multifactorial. These include a reduced stomach reservoir size, altered emptying patterns, and change in neural and hormonal feedback postoperatively that lead to rapid emptying of osmotically active chyme into the small intestine. Dumping results in bowel distention and osmotic shifts that can lead to abdominal pain, nausea, bloating, tachycardia, and dizziness [25]. Dumping syndrome has been found to be most prevalent with a Billroth II reconstruction, with a reported frequency of 7–29% [26, 27]. Similar to postoperative delayed gastric emptying, the preferred treatment for dumping syndrome is nonoperative because the majority of patients will improve over time. Nonoperative management of dumping syndrome includes change in diet to several small meals per day, as well as medical therapies including acarbose and octreotide [25]. Should the patient fail nonoperative management after 1 year, surgical intervention may be pursued, including narrowing the gastrojejunal stoma or converting the patient's reconstruction to a Billroth I or a Roux-en-Y reconstruction. However, there are no clear data about the efficacy of these conversions or as to which procedure has the best outcomes [25, 28].

Alkaline or bile reflux gastritis can occur, specifically after a Billroth I or II reconstruction. The reflux of bile salts and other intestinal contents into the stomach can cause damage to the gastric mucosa, leading to abdominal pain and bilious emesis [29, 30]. Medical management of bile reflux gastritis includes administration of cholestyramine, H2 blockers, proton pump inhibitors, sucralfate, or promotility agents, but these treatments are often unsuccessful [31]. Typically, treatment of bile reflux requires reoperation with conversion to a Roux-en-Y configuration, although performing a Braun enteroenterostomy (Fig. 66.2) can also assist in diversion of bile from the stomach in those patients that have had a Billroth II reconstruction [29, 32].

Finally, while resection and reconstruction is definitive therapy for gastric outlet obstruction, there is a risk that the patient could develop restenosis and recurrent

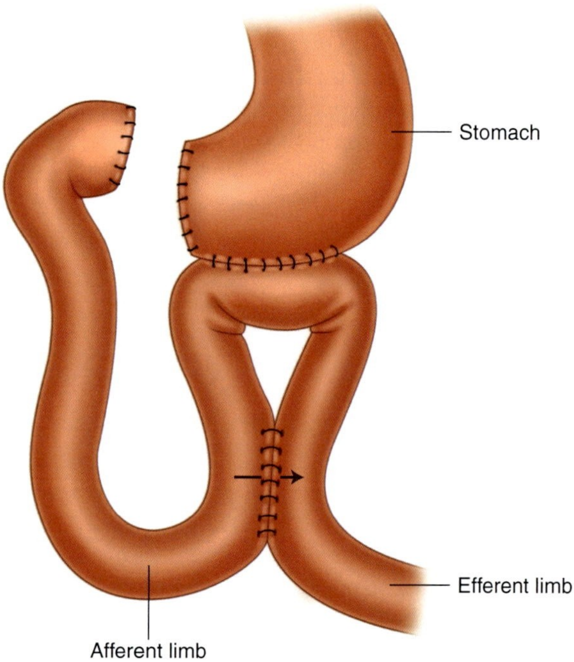

Fig. 66.2 Braun enteroenterostomy as part of a Billroth II reconstruction, for prevention of bile reflux

obstruction. There is a reported restenosis rate of 5–8% after resection and reconstruction in this patient population [33].

Drainage Procedures

Procedure Options

Drainage procedures are an option for surgical management of gastric outlet obstruction in peptic ulcer disease, in conjunction with vagotomy to treat the underlying excess acid production. These procedures include pyloroplasty and gastrojejunostomy without resection. Pyloroplasty techniques will be discussed in more detail in the following chapter; here, we will focus on the management advantages and disadvantages conveyed by drainage as opposed to technical details of the procedure.

Advantages

Both pyloroplasty and gastrojejunostomy without resection have a distinct advantage in being a shorter, less involved surgery than any of the resection and reconstruction procedures discussed in the previous section. Furthermore, these procedures require less dissection of the inflamed and scarred tissue, making inadvertent injury to vital structures less likely and therefore conveying a safety advantage [3]. These procedures also have fewer staple lines and anastomoses than those required for resection and reconstruction, and in this patient population that often suffers from malnutrition, this decreases the risk of potentially severe anastomotic leak. Either drainage procedure would be performed with vagotomy, so they retain the same advantage of decreasing ulcer recurrence that vagotomy supplies in resection and reconstruction procedures.

Disadvantages and Complications

The most prominent disadvantage of pursuing drainage as opposed to resection and reconstruction in patients with gastric outlet obstruction in the setting of peptic ulcer disease is the potential for recurrence. Ulcer recurrence with repeat obstruction has been reported to occur in up to 50% after drainage procedures, although these data are from prior to our modern understanding of *H. pylori* [4]. Indeed, one prospective randomized study comparing techniques for treatment of gastric outlet obstruction secondary to duodenal ulcer found that vagotomy and gastrojejunostomy had equivalent outcomes to vagotomy and antrectomy, although vagotomy and Jaboulay gastroduodenostomy patients did have some recurrence of ulcer disease [34].

Bile reflux is also a potential complication of drainage procedures [35]. This can be treated through the modalities described in the previous section, but as there is significantly less bile reflux gastritis in those patients who undergo Roux-en-Y reconstruction, drainage with a primary Roux-en-Y configuration may be preferred to avoid this complication [36].

Afferent loop syndrome can occur in patients who undergo gastrojejunostomy without resection for drainage. In the absence of antrectomy, there is no risk for duodenal stump leak although eventual perforation of originally intact bowel may occur because of progressive distention and bowel ischemia. The symptoms caused by afferent loop syndrome include abdominal pain, nausea, and emesis and require operative management to treat the underlying cause, whether it is volvulus, adhesions, or internal herniation [10].

Dumping syndrome can also occur in those patients who undergo drainage procedures, although some studies demonstrate a lower rate than in resection and reconstruction procedures [37, 38]. It is equally difficult to manage in this patient population, with the same strategy to be employed of a prolonged trial of nonoperative management and with no convincing data on which surgical procedure is best should an operation be required.

Decision-Making

While gastric outlet obstruction in patients with peptic ulcer disease has become less common with improvements in medical therapy, it remains a problem that the surgeon may encounter and requires focused decision-making to ensure the best outcome for the patient. Vagotomy and antrectomy remain the gold standard for management of gastric outlet obstruction in this patient population, as it is a definitive treatment with low recurrence. However, the procedure can be long, requires multiple staple lines and anastomoses, and may be difficult in the patient with chronic ulcer disease that has significant inflammation and scarring in the operative field. Therefore, drainage procedures remain a useful option in patients who cannot tolerate a longer operation due to frailty or comorbidities and in patients who have inflammation and fibrosis that distort the operative anatomy, making resection unsafe. As a result, a discussion with the patient preoperatively about the potential need to convert from a planned resection to drainage is critical, as a patient who appears to be a good candidate for resection may have unexpectedly hostile anatomy discovered intraoperatively. It is also important to optimize the nutrition of any patient who is undergoing a surgical procedure for gastric outlet obstruction preoperatively to assist in their postoperative healing.

References

1. Goldstein H, et al. The saline load test – a bedside evaluation of gastric retention. Gastroenterol. 1965;49(4):375–80.
2. Appasani S, et al. Benign gastric outlet obstruction – spectrum and management. Trop Gastroenterol. 2011;32(4):259–66.
3. Behrman SW. Management of complicated peptic ulcer disease. Arch Surg. 2005;140(2):201–8.

4. Zittel TT, et al. Surgical management of peptic ulcer disease today – indication, technique, and outcome. Langenbeck's Arch Surg. 2000;385(2):84–96.
5. Norton J, et al. Essential practice of surgery: basic science and clinical evidence. New York: Springer; 2003.
6. Gibson JB, et al. Gastric outlet obstruction resulting from peptic ulcer disease requiring surgical intervention is infrequently associated with helicobacter pylori infection. J Am Coll Surg. 2000;191(1):32–7.
7. Lagoo J, Pappas TN, Perez A. A relic or still relevant: the narrowing role for vagotomy in the treatment of peptic ulcer disease. Am J Surg. 2014;207(1):120–6.
8. Evans S. Surgical pitfalls: prevention and management. Philadelphia: Saunders; 2009.
9. Ali BI, et al. Outcomes of non-operative treatment for duodenal stump leakage after gastrectomy in patients with gastric cancer. J Gastric Cancer. 2016;16(1):28–33.
10. Kutlu OC, et al. The successful use of simple tube duodenostomy in large duodenal perforations from varied etiologies. Int J Surg Case Rep. 2013;4(3):279–82.
11. Raman RS, et al. A technique to prevent duodenal blowout after difficult gastrectomies. Indian J Gastroenterol. 2013;32(1):60–1.
12. Vasiliadis K, et al. Delayed duodenal stump blow-out following total gastrectomy for cancer. Int J Surg Case Rep. 2014;5(12):1229–33.
13. Nussbaum MS, et al. Management of giant duodenal ulcer. Am J Surg. 1985;149(3):357–61.
14. Camilleri M, et al. Clinical guideline: management of gastroparesis. Am J Gastroenterol. 2013;108(1):18–37.
15. Britton JP, et al. Gastric emptying and clinical outcome after Roux-en-Y diversion. Br J Surg. 1987;74(10):900–4.
16. Fich A, et al. Stasis syndromes following gastric surgery: clinical and motility features of 60 symptomatic patients. J Clin Gastroenterol. 1990;12(5):505–12.
17. Kalbasi H, et al. Gastric emptying following vagotomy and antrectomy and proximal gastric vagotomy. Gut. 1975;16(7):509–13.
18. Phillips RJ, et al. Long-term regeneration of abdominal vagus: efferents fail while afferents succeed. J Comp Neurol. 2003;455(2):222–37.
19. Petrakis J, et al. Enhancement of gastric emptying of solids by erythromycin in patients with Roux-en-Y gastrojejunostomy. Arch Surg. 1998;133(7):709–14.
20. Rayner CK, et al. New management approaches for gastroparesis. Nat Clin Pract Gastroenterol Hepatol. 2005;2(10):454–62.
21. Shafi MA, et al. Post-surgical and obstructive gastroparesis. Curr Gastroenterol Rep. 2007;9:280–5.
22. Jones MP, et al. A systematic review of surgical therapy for gastroparesis. Am J Gastroentrol. 2003;98(10):2122–9.
23. Karlstrom L, Kelly KA. Roux-Y gastrectomy for chronic gastric atony. Am J Surg. 1989;157(1):44–9.
24. Camilleri M, Parkman HP, Shafi MA, Abell TL, Gerson L. Clinical guideline: management of gastroparesis. Am J Gastroenterol. 2013;108(1):18–38.
25. Li FY, et al. Clinical application prospects of gastric pacing for treating postoperative gastric motility disorders. J Gastroenterol Hepatol. 2007;22(12):2055–9.
26. Ukleja A. Dumping syndrome: pathophysiology and treatment. Nutr Clin Pract. 2005;20(5):517–25.
27. Berg P, et al. Dumping syndrome: a review of the current concepts of pathophysiology, diagnosis, and treatment. Dig Dis Sci. 2016;61(1):11–8.
28. Fisher J. Mastery of surgery. Philadelphia: Lippincott Williams & Wilkins; 2007.
29. Rostas JW 3rd, et al. Gastric motility physiology and surgical intervention. Surg Clin North Am. 2011;91(5):983–99.
30. Madura J. Primary bile reflux gastritis: diagnosis and surgical treatment. Am J Surg. 2003;186(3):269–73.
31. Hoare AM, et al. A prospective randomized study of effect of proximal gastric vagotomy and vagotomy and antrectomy on bile reflux, endoscopic mucosal abnormalities and gastritis. Surg Gastroenterol. 1984;3(2):54–9.

32. Zobolas B, et al. Alkaline reflux gastritis: early and late results of surgery. World J Surg. 2006;30:1043–9.
33. Vogel SB, et al. Clinical and radionuclide evaluation of bile diversion by Braun enteroenterostomy: prevention and treatment of alkaline reflux gastritis. Ann Surg. 1994;219(5):458–65.
34. Makela J, et al. Gastric outlet obstruction caused by peptic ulcer disease – analysis of 99 patients. Hepato-Gastroenterology. 1996;43(9):547–52.
35. Csendes A, et al. Prospective randomized study comparing three surgical techniques for the treatment of gastric outlet obstruction secondary to duodenal ulcer. Am J Surg. 1993;166(1):45–9.
36. Earlam R. Bile reflux and the roux en Y anastomosis. Br J Surg. 1983;70:393–7.
37. Lunde O-C, et al. Proximal gastric vagotomy and pyloroplasty for duodenal ulcer with pyloric stenosis: a thirteen-year experience. W Jour Surg. 1985;9(1):165–70.
38. Bowers RF, et al. Dumping syndrome following pyloroplasty. Arch Surg. 1966;92(1):39–43.
39. Basinskaya B, et al. Trends in peptic ulcer disease and the identification of Helicobacter Pylori as a causative organism: population-based estimates from the US nationwide inpatient sample. J Glob Infect Dis. 2011;3(4):366–70.

Surgical Management: Pyloroplasty Options

67

Andrea M. Stroud and Jacob A. Greenberg

Indications

Surgical intervention for benign gastric outlet obstruction (GOO) may be considered as primary therapy or after failed pneumatic dilation (PD). Current data suggest that *H. pylori*-negative patients respond poorly to PD alone [1]. Thus in patients with recurrent symptoms after two dilations or those found to be *H. pylori* negative, surgery should be strongly considered. There are a variety of surgical interventions available for the treatment of GOO, including drainage procedures as well as procedures requiring resection with reconstruction. In this chapter we will focus on surgical options for pyloroplasty. Pyloroplasty facilitates gastric emptying through incision of the pyloric muscle and reconstruction of the pyloric channel [2]. This approach results in low recurrence rates for GOO as well as low incidence of post-gastrectomy pathophysiology [1]. Pyloroplasty may be performed via an open, laparoscopic, robotic, or endoscopic approach.

Operative Technique

Open Techniques

Open techniques for pyloroplasty include the Heineke-Mikulicz (HM) and Finney procedures. Also described is the Jaboulay pyloroplasty, which technically is a gastroduodenostomy as the incision does not extend through the pylorus. Additional

A. M. Stroud
University Hospital, Madison, WI, USA

J. A. Greenberg (✉)
Department of General Surgery, University Hospital, Madison, WI, USA
e-mail: greenbergj@surgery.wisc.edu

J. Grams et al. (eds.), *The SAGES Manual of Foregut Surgery*,
https://doi.org/10.1007/978-3-319-96122-4_67

modifications of the traditional HM pyloroplasty have been described and are mentioned briefly. The choice of pyloroplasty should be based on the condition and quality of the tissue. Even in the presence of fibrosis and inflammation, the HM pyloroplasty is often feasible. In the presence of an inflexible duodenum, a Finney or Jaboulay pyloroplasty should be considered. This decision should be made prior to gastroduodenal incision, given that the optimal incision differs between procedures (Fig. 67.1).

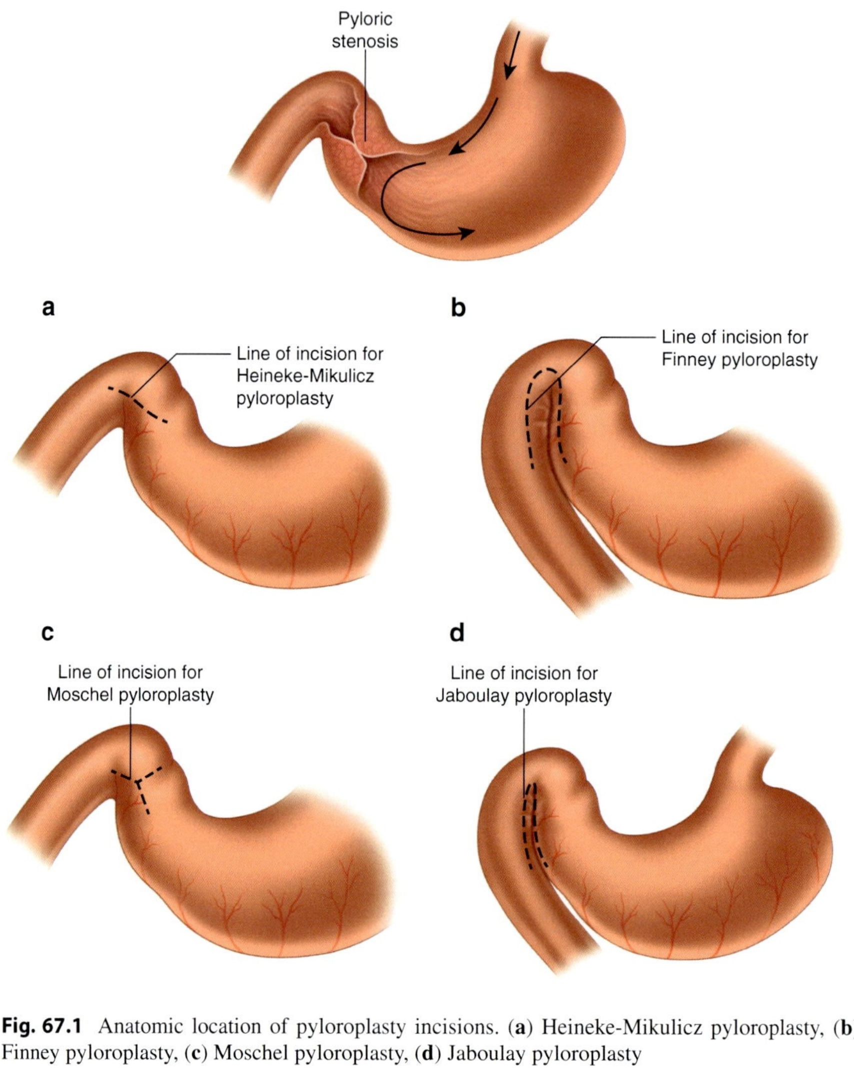

Fig. 67.1 Anatomic location of pyloroplasty incisions. (**a**) Heineke-Mikulicz pyloroplasty, (**b**) Finney pyloroplasty, (**c**) Moschel pyloroplasty, (**d**) Jaboulay pyloroplasty

General Considerations

The patient is positioned supine on the operating room table. A general anesthetic is required. A prophylactic dose of preoperative antibiotics with appropriate coverage for upper gastrointestinal flora is administered, along with 5000 units of subcutaneous unfractionated heparin. A Foley catheter can be omitted, unless the surgeon suspects that patient factors may prolong the expected operative time. A standard midline laparotomy prep and drape is performed. An upper midline laparotomy incision is utilized. In the majority of cases, a generous Kocher maneuver is required for adequate maneuverability of the tissues. The anterior surface of the pylorus should be minimally involved in the inflammatory process to allow for a healthy, tension-free closure.

Heineke-Mikulicz Pyloroplasty

After obtaining exposure and performing a Kocher maneuver, an incision is made along the anterior portion of the pylorus, which extends both proximally onto the distal antrum and distally onto the first portion of the duodenum. The incision should be approximately 5–7 cm and is made with a monopolar electrocautery to prevent bleeding. Traction sutures are then placed on the cranial and caudal aspects at the midpoint of the incision. The sutures are then distracted in a cranial-caudal direction to align the incision transversely. This transverse closure provides a patulous lumen for gastric emptying (Fig. 67.1a).

Various techniques have been described to close the pyloroplasty. To keep the outlet diameter sufficient, we recommend a single-layer closure in a continuous fashion with absorbable suture. This should be accomplished with deep seromuscular sutures. As compared to full-thickness sutures, this technique avoids everting the mucosa between sutures [3]. Alternately, a Gambee stitch can be utilized, which is both hemostatic and inverting. A single layer of interrupted full-thickness or a double-layered closure may be preferred by some surgeons; whichever method is used, care must be taken not to narrow the reconstructed gastric outlet.

The gastroduodenostomy can also be closed using a surgical stapler. Apply Allis clamps to approximate mucosa to mucosa along the length of the incision. Apply and fire a linear stapling device just inferior to the row of Allis clamps.

An omentoplasty sutured loosely over the pyloroplasty can help protect against free intraperitoneal leakage from the suture line. The omentum can also help prevent adhesion between the suture line and the undersurface of the liver. If there is any concern for a potential leak, a closed suction drain should be left in the vicinity of the closure.

Finney Pyloroplasty

This technique is well suited for a J-shaped stomach with a pylorus that is retracted and fixed. Prior to making the gastrointestinal incision, place a posterior row of sutures. This avoids excessive tension on the anterior suture line. In contrast to the anterior midline incision of the Heineke-Mikulicz pyloroplasty, the incision for the Finney pyloroplasty is made in close proximity to the greater curve of the stomach and the pancreatic side of the first portion of the duodenum (Fig. 67.1b). Thus, begin by placing a layer of Lembert sutures, which approximates the greater curve of the stomach to the proximal duodenum, close to the junction of the duodenum and pancreas (Fig. 67.2a). Create a suture line that is approximately 5–6 cm from the pylorus.

After completion of the posterior suture line, make an inverted U-shaped incision along a line 0.5 cm anterior to the suture line. This incision is made full thickness, exposing both the gastric and duodenal mucosa. The pyloroplasty is then closed beginning the suture line at the apex of the inferior portion of the divided pylorus. Continue the suture line in a full-thickness continuous locking fashion caudally until the inferior most aspect of the incision is reached (Fig. 67.2b, c). Pass the needle from inside to outside on the gastric side of the suture line, and continue the anterior closure as a continuous Connell (or Cushing) suture (Fig. 67.2d). Finally, close the anterior seromuscular layer with another row of Lembert sutures. Verify that the lumen can accommodate the surgeon's two fingers.

Jaboulay Pyloroplasty

As mentioned above this procedure is not a true pyloroplasty but rather a gastroduodenostomy as the incision does not extend through the pyloric muscle. The steps of the procedure are essentially the same as that described for the Finney, except that the incision is not extended onto the pylorus (Fig. 67.1d). Following placement of a posterior row of sutures, make one incision on the distal antrum and a second incision on the proximal duodenum. Close the resulting gastroduodenomtomy, beginning with the posterior adjacent walls with a continuous seromuscular suture, which is continued onto the anterior wall of the gastroduodenotomy. Alternatively, a linear gastrointestinal stapler can be used to form the common channel, and the common enterotomy can be approximated with sutures or TA stapler.

Moschel Pyloroplasty

This modification of the classic HM plyoroplasty uses a Y-shaped incision, with the arms of the Y extending onto the gastric antrum (Fig. 67.1c). The technique aims to maintain an adequate blood supply to the antral advancement flap. Similarly to the HM pyloroplasty, close the pyloroplasty transversely, as a single running layer, suturing the antral flap to the duodenum.

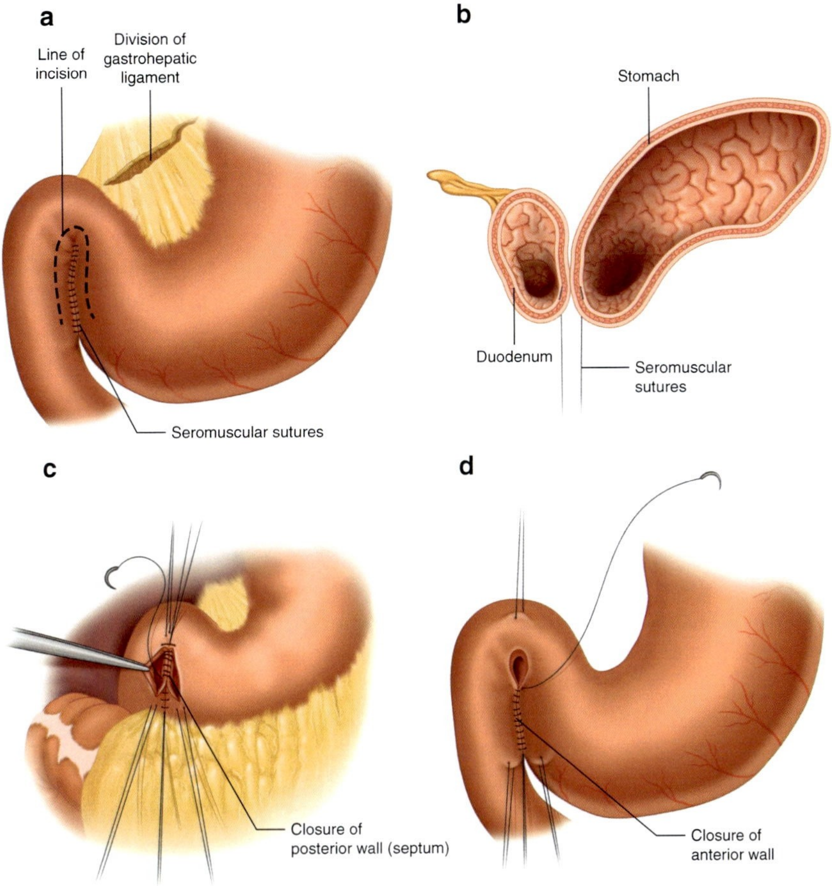

Fig. 67.2 Finney pyloroplasty. (**a**) A posterior row of sutures is placed to avoid excessive tension on the anterior suture line. The dotted line marks the planned inverted U-shaped pyloroplasty incision. (**b**) Full-thickness seromuscular sutures are used to approximate the gastric antrum to the duodenum. (**c**) The pyloroplasty is then closed beginning at the apex of the inferior portion of the divided pylorus, continuing the suture line until the inferior most aspect of the incision is reached. (**d**) The anterior closure is performed as a continuous Connell (or Cushing) suture

Circular Stapled Pyloroplasty

This modification, developed by Potter et al., utilizes a circular stapler without a pyloric incision [4]. Make a transverse gastrotomy on the anterior surface of the stomach approximately 6 cm proximal to the pylorus. The gastrotomy must be large enough to accommodate the head of the circular stapler. Insert the stapler through the gastrotomy, and advance the stapler distally through the pylorus. Proper positioning of the stapler is critical. Bring the head of the stapler into the gastric outlet, and wedge the anvil firmly against the proximal border of the pyloric sphincter. Open the stapler, advancing the anvil portion through the pyloric sphincter. As the anvil clears the distal border of the pyloric sphincter, a "popping" sensation is felt. Visualize the sphincter within the gap between the anvil and the staple cartridge. Place a transverse suture across the mid-sphincter. Next approximately two thirds of the pylorus is fed into the gap of the stapler, using the previously placed suture while applying equal pressure on both sides of the suture. Close and fire the stapler. After removal of the stapler, inspect the resulting "half-moon" piece of pyloric muscle in the circular stapler. Palpate for a patent gastric outlet. Close the gastrotomy with a linear stapler.

Laparoscopic Techniques

Modified Heineke-Mikulicz

Position the patient supine and place four or five ports in the standard arrangement for foregut surgery. Begin by mobilizing the pylorus from its cranial and caudal peritoneal attachments to facilitate maneuverability of the pylorus. When necessary, perform a Kocher maneuver to allow for complete visualization and a tension-free closure. This is particularly important in patients with prior cholecystectomy. Make a full-thickness pyloromyotomy using an ultransonic shear (Fig. 67.3). As with the open procedure, the myotomy is approximately 5 cm in length, centered on the anterior surface at the midpoint of the pylorus. Close the pyloromyotomy in a transverse fashion, beginning at the center, and work toward the cranial and caudal apexes (Fig. 67.4). Close using a running continuous single layer of 2–0 monofilament absorbable suture. After completion of the suture line, perform a leak test, using endoscopic insufflation under saline irrigation. We perform a sutured omentoplasty. Some surgeons elect to leave a closed suction drain adjacent to the suture line [5, 6].

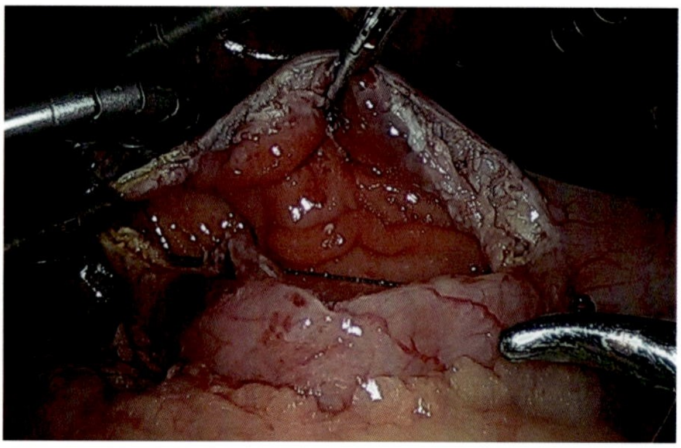

Fig. 67.3 Intraoperative photograph demonstrating laparoscopic pyloroplasty incision

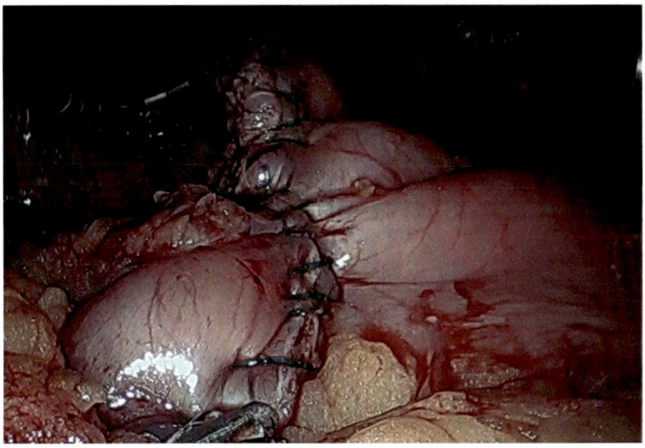

Fig. 67.4 Intraoperative photograph demonstrating laparoscopic pyloroplasty closure with full-thickness running continuous suture

Laparoscopic Transoral Flexible Endoscopic Stapled Pyloroplasty

Pass a flexible 21 mm circular powered stapler (Power Medical Interventions, Langhorn, PA) transorally into the stomach, and position the stapler across the pylorus with laparoscopic assistance. Pass a suture across the anterior midline of the pylorus, and hold this between two graspers. Open the anvil on the circular stapler, and use the suture to position the pylorus. Compress the pylorus into the stapler and close the stapler. Firing the stapler results in a partial pylorectomy involving the anterior wall of the pylorus, this increases the luminal diameter of the gastric outlet [5].

Endoscopic Pyloromyotomy

The endoscopic approach utilizes a pyloromyotomy rather than a true plyoroplasty. The technique applies the same basic principles as the endoscopic submucosal dissection and myotomy used in the setting of peroral endoscopic myotomy (POEM) for treatment of achalasia. This technique has been primarily described in the setting of gastroparesis but may provide a less invasive, incisionless alternative compared to standard plyoroplasty [7].

This technique requires a high-definition forward-viewing gastroscope, outfitted with a transparent dissection cap and carbon dioxide insufflation. Begin by carefully inspecting the stomach and duodenum. Lavage any retained gastric contents. Advance a gastric overtube over the gastroscope well into the gastric body. Locate the pylorus and select a site for mucosotomy, approximately 5 cm proximal to the pylorus and on the anterior wall of the stomach. Perform a submucosal lift with 5–10 cc of lift solution (500 cc of normal saline mixed with 0.5 cc of 1:1000 epinephrine and 3–4 drops of methylene blue dye). Using a triangle-tip (TT) knife, make a 1–2 cm longitudinal mucosal incision. Enter the submucosal space with the dissecting cap, and begin to create a submucosal tunnel with the TT knife by dividing the loose submucosal areolar tissue. To facilitate tunneling, repeat submucosal injections with the lift solution. During dissection, care is taken not to cause thermal injury to the overlying mucosa. The dissection is carried out in the sm3 level, adjacent to the muscularis layer of the gastric wall. Continue the tunnel past the pylorus and onto the proximal duodenal bulb. Confirm the length of the submucosal tunnel by observing the dissection length from the gastric lumen. Next the myotomy is performed, beginning 2 cm proximal to the pylorus. The myotomy is a full-thickness myotomy, through all muscle layers down to the serosa. The myotomy is continued until the visible pyloric muscle is completely divided. Take great care at the distal extent of the myotomy to avoid inadvertent perforation or thermal injury of the duodenal mucosa. Inspect the tunnel for hemostasis. At the completion of the dissection and myotomy, the mucosotomy is closed with endoscopic clips or an endoscopic suturing device.

Postoperative Management

Following pyloroplasty the patient is admitted and kept nil per os overnight. Gastric drainage should be performed on an individual patient basis. A nasogastric tube can be used for temporary gastric drainage. However, in patients with long duration of symptoms and a relatively dilated stomach, gastric emptying may be significantly impaired. In these cases, a gastrojejunostomy, with gastric port for decompression and jejunal port for feeding should be considered [8]. A gastrografin upper gastrointestinal series can be performed prior to oral intake to confirm that no gastrointestinal leak is present. Some surgeons leave a surgical drain at the time of pyloroplasty and measure drain amylase levels. A leak is defined as drain amylase >1000. If no leak is present, the patient is advanced to a puree diet until follow-up in 2–3 weeks.

Postoperative Complications

Complications following pyloroplasty are rare. Given the gastrointestinal incision, suture line leak is possible but rare given the ample blood supply and the general lack of tension on the suture line. Incomplete division of the pyloric sphincter or inadvertent narrowing of the suture line may result in recurrent obstruction. Dumping syndrome can occur following interruption of the pyloric sphincter mechanism. Clinically significant dumping occurs rarely after pyloroplasty. Although the pathophysiologic mechanism is incompletely understood, the syndrome is believed to be the result of rapid transit of a high osmolar load into the proximal small bowel. Symptoms include gastrointestinal discomfort, nausea, vomiting, diarrhea, diaphoresis, palpitations, and flushing, approximately 15–30 min after a meal. Rarely, patients may suffer from reflux alkaline gastritis due to reflux of duodenal fluid into the stomach [8].

References

1. Gibson JB, Behrman SW, Fabian TC, Britt LG. Gastric outlet obstruction resulting from peptic ulcer disease requiring surgical intervention is infrequently associated with Helicobacter pylori infection. J Am Coll Surg. 2000;191(1):32–7.
2. Soreide JA, Soreide K. Pyloroplasty. Oper Tech General Surg. 2003;5(2):65–72.
3. Scott-Conner CEH. Pyloroplasty (Heineke-Mikulicz and Finney) operation for bleeding duodenal ulcer. In: Chassin's operative strategy in general surgery. 3rd ed; 2012. p. 244–51.
4. Potter SD, Spiro SA, Nance FC. An alternative method to traditional Pyloroplasty using a circular stapler. J Am Coll Surg. 1995;180(6):742–4.
5. Hibbard ML, Dunst CM, Swanstrom LL. Laparoscopic and endoscopic pylorplasty for gastroparesis results in sustained symptom improvement. J Gastrointest Surg. 2015;15:1513–9.
6. Shada AL, Dunst CM, Pescarus R, Speer EA, Cassera M, Reavis KM, Swanstrom LL. Laparoscopic pyloroplasty is a safe and effective first-line surgical therapy for refractory gastroparesis. Surg Endosc. 2016;30:1326–32.
7. Shlomovitz E, Pescaru R, Cassera MA, Sharata AM, Reavis KM, Dunst CM, Swanstrom LL. Early human experience with per-oral endoscopic pyloromyotomy (POP). Surg Endosc. 2015;29:543–51.
8. Soreide MG, Soreide JA. Pyloroplasty for benign gastric outlet obstruction – indications and techniques. Scaninavian J Surg. 2006;95:11–6.

Evaluation and Classification of Gastroparesis

68

Michael B. Goldberg and Eric G. Sheu

Introduction

Gastroparesis, a chronic disorder of the stomach characterized by delayed emptying without mechanical obstruction, is an underrecognized and often undertreated disease. Gastroparesis affects an estimated 9.6 per 100,000 men and 38 per 100,000 women in the United States [1]. It is estimated that at least four million American adults suffer from the disorder [2]. Patients with gastroparesis typically present with nausea, vomiting, and early satiety and can also experience bloating, epigastric fullness, and abdominal pain. These symptoms vary in severity and duration and, in the most severe cases, can lead to malnutrition, dehydration, and weight loss.

Aside from these somatic symptoms, gastroparetics typically have diminished physical and social functioning and reduced well-being [2]. In a recent survey-based study from Lacy and colleagues including questionnaires from 250 gastroparetics, the disease led to a striking reduction in quality of life. Responses to a validated quality of life survey were analogous to those from patients with other serious chronic medical conditions and depression. Furthermore, gastroparesis was found to lower annual income in 28.5% of patients and placed 11% on disability from work [3].

In this chapter, we will discuss the evaluation, workup, and classification of gastroparesis.

M. B. Goldberg
Department of Surgery, Brigham and Women's Hospital, Boston, MA, USA

E. G. Sheu (✉)
Assistant Professor of Surgery, Harvard Medical School; Associate Surgeon, Division of General and Gastrointestinal Surgery, Brigham and Women's Hospital, Boston, MA, USA
e-mail: esheu@bwh.harvard.edu

J. Grams et al. (eds.), *The SAGES Manual of Foregut Surgery*,
https://doi.org/10.1007/978-3-319-96122-4_68

Pathophysiology

The pathophysiology of gastroparesis is still not completely understood, but it includes derangements of normal gastric motor function caused by a number of etiologic factors which are discussed in the following section. Impairments may be seen in gastric accommodation to food via a nitric oxide pathway [4], antral hypomotility [5], elevated pyloric tone [6], duodenal dysmotility [7], or a lowered gastric sensory threshold to pressure distention [8]. These abnormalities are most likely caused by problems with the autonomic nervous system, smooth muscle cells of the stomach, enteric neurons, and the interstitial cells of Cajal that are responsible for gastric pacemaker activity [9]. Histologic examination of the stomach in gastroparetic patients commonly demonstrates increased concentration of lymphocytes in the myenteric plexus which may represent an inflammatory-mediated destruction of nerves. Similar histologic findings are seen in other enteric dysmotility disorders including achalasia and chronic intestinal pseudoobstruction [10].

Etiology

There are several conditions associated with gastroparesis, listed in Table 68.1. In a recent multicenter study of 146 patients, the most common etiologies were idiopathic (36%), diabetes (29%), and postsurgical (13%) [11]. In approximately one-half of gastroparetics, there is no identifiable cause [12]. Other causes include connective tissue disorders such as scleroderma and lupus, Raynaud's disease, Parkinson's disease, endocrinopathies such as hypothyroidism and critical illness, and medications including narcotics and anticholinergics.

Diabetes is the most commonly diagnosed comorbidity in patients with gastroparesis. Up to 50% of patients with long-standing type 1 diabetes and 30% of those with type 2 diabetes have delayed gastric emptying which is thought to be from damage to the vagus nerve and its branches from hyperglycemia [2]. Other theories exist as to the role of diabetes in gastroparesis, including abnormal postprandial gastric accommodation and contraction, dysfunctional antral motor function, and oxidative stress [13]. Gastric emptying can often be accelerated by hypoglycemia and delayed by hyperglycemia in diabetics. Typically,

Table 68.1 Major etiologies of gastroparesis

Diabetes
Postsurgical
Idiopathic
Connective tissue disorders
Neurologic illness
Endocrine disorders
Critical illness
Medications
Post-viral

gastrointestinal complaints occur in patients who have had diabetes for greater than 5 years and are often seen in conjunction with diabetic neuropathy and other diabetes-related microvascular pathology [14].

Postsurgical gastroparesis is usually present after foregut surgery, most likely caused by division or traction injury to the vagus nerve [9]. Although vagotomy for peptic ulcer disease is less commonly being performed, postsurgical gastroparesis can be associated with fundoplication, bariatric surgery, subtotal gastrectomy, pancreatic surgery, and even thoracic and cardiac operations such as pneumonectomy and heart transplant [15].

Patients without any known etiology of their delayed gastric emptying are diagnosed with idiopathic gastroparesis. This form of the disease is often suggested to be the most common. While there are many postulated etiologies for the disease, idiopathic gastroparesis is a diagnosis of exclusion. Therefore, a thorough evaluation to exclude all other known, potential causes of gastroparesis must be completed before arriving at a diagnosis of idiopathic gastroparesis. Several rare causes of gastroparesis are discussed below.

Gastroparesis is sometimes preceded by an infectious prodrome such as gastroenteritis or an upper respiratory infection which may cause viral injury to the nerves of the stomach [16]. Several case reports document delayed gastric emptying in association with Norwalk virus and Rotavirus. While post-viral gastroparesis is typically self-limited, patients with cytomegalovirus, Epstein-Barr virus, and varicella may have more chronic symptoms from autonomic denervation. Autoimmune gastroparesis has been described either independently or in conjunction with a neoplasm, typically small cell lung cancer. These patients may have slow intestinal transit and pelvic floor dysfunction in addition to delayed gastric emptying.

Gastroparesis can be associated with systemic illness. This includes neurologic dysfunction (Parkinson's disease, stress, stroke, multiple sclerosis), rheumatologic/inflammatory conditions (scleroderma, lupus, Raynaud's disease, amyloidosis), and hypothyroidism. Delayed gastric emptying is a common side effect of several medications listed in Table 68.2, most commonly narcotic analgesics. Finally, much less common causes of gastroparesis include Stiffman syndrome, Charcot-Marie-Tooth syndrome, Waardenburg syndrome, paraneoplastic syndromes, and systemic mastocytosis.

Table 68.2 Medications associated with delayed gastric emptying

Alpha-2-adrenergic agonists
Amylin analogues
Calcium channel blockers
Cholinergic receptor antagonists
Cyclosporine
Dopamine agonists
Glucagon-like peptide agonists
Octreotide
Phenothiazines
Tricyclic antidepressants

Differential Diagnosis

A broad differential is important when evaluating a patient with nausea, vomiting, early satiety, and abdominal pain. It is particularly important to distinguish delayed gastric emptying from a mechanical gastric outlet obstruction. Obstruction can be caused by an intra- or extraluminal neoplasm or less commonly by median arcuate ligament or SMA syndrome. Small bowel obstruction can present with similar symptoms as well.

Psychiatric disease such as depression, anxiety, eating disorders, and psychogenic vomiting may be the sole cause of a patient's presentation or may be present in conjunction with gastroparesis. Rumination syndrome consists of daily effortless regurgitation of undigested food within minutes of eating a meal and can often be seen in adolescents and adults. Cyclic vomiting syndrome is characterized by recurrent episodes of nausea and vomiting separated by symptom-free intervals. Finally, functional dyspepsia has similar presenting symptoms to gastroparesis: however the majority of these patients have normal gastric emptying.

Clinical Presentation

The dominant presenting symptoms of gastroparesis are heterogeneous. Most commonly, nausea and vomiting are reported in rates that range from 40 to over 90% [17, 18]. Patients with idiopathic and diabetic gastroparesis frequently report the feeling of fullness or early satiety, which causes inability to finish a normal meal and can lead to weight loss. Bloating is also experienced by up to 60% of patients [11].

Abdominal pain is reported in many functional gastrointestinal disorders and is the presenting symptom in only ~ 20% of patients with gastroparesis. The pain is usually in the epigastric region, and it is described as vague, burning, and/or crampy. Pain may be exacerbated by meals and can interfere with sleep [19]. Pain in gastroparesis is believed to arise from visceral hypersensitivity or exaggerated pain response to visceral stimulation such as gastric distension [18]. Patients presenting with abdominal pain as their predominant symptom should trigger the provider to consider alternative diagnosis.

Workup/Diagnosis

As described earlier, it is prudent to rule out all causes of nausea, vomiting, bloating, and abdominal pain in the workup of a patient with suspected gastroparesis. A careful history must include personal history of comorbid illness and a detailed list of medications. A full physical exam may uncover manifestations of systemic diseases associated with gastroparesis, including scleroderma, Parkinson's disease, and diabetes. Neurologic examination may uncover signs of autonomic dysfunction, including orthostatic hypotension and the absence of the pupillary reaction to light.

To aid in the diagnosis of gastroparesis, mechanical causes of nausea and vomiting must be excluded. Mechanical gastric outlet obstruction from an intrinsic mass or inflammatory process, as well as distal or extrinsic causes of obstruction (SMA syndrome, non-GI tumors), can be ruled out with a computed tomographic (CT) scan with oral contrast. Upper endoscopy should also be performed to evaluate the mucosa to rule out neoplasm, peptic ulcer disease, and other causes of obstruction. Once mechanical obstruction is ruled out by imaging and upper endoscopy, gastric emptying should be evaluated.

Baseline laboratory values should be obtained in patients undergoing workup for gastroparesis, including a complete blood count, electrolytes, and nutritional parameters. It is always important to consider the nutritional status of any patient with nausea and vomiting, especially these patients who may require nutritional support. Laboratory testing may help identify the cause of gastroparesis in patients who are found to have delayed gastric emptying without a known cause. Fasting plasma glucose and HbA1c can assess glycemic control, and thyroid studies and antinuclear antibody titers can help identify metabolic or rheumatologic causes of delayed gastric emptying.

Gastric emptying scintigraphy (Fig. 68.1) is a noninvasive and quantitative measurement of gastric emptying and is considered the gold standard for diagnosis of gastroparesis. While this test varies by institution, it typically involves ingestion of solid food bound to a radiolabeled isotope (technetium Tc 99 m-labeled low-fat egg white with jam and toast) with imaging at 0, 1, 2, and 4 h. Delayed gastric emptying is defined as greater than 60% retention of tracer in the stomach at 2 h after the meal

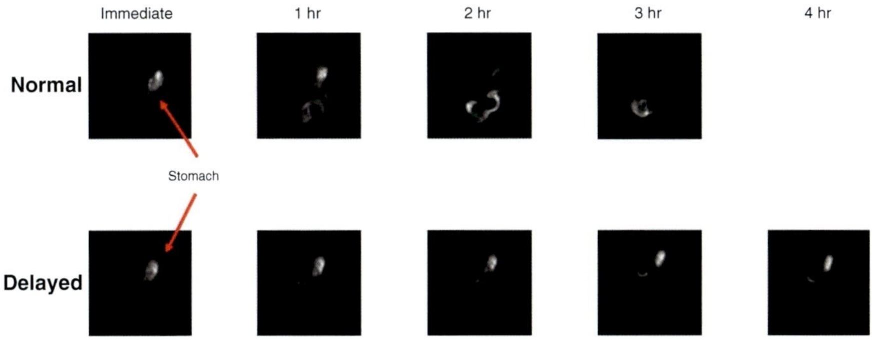

Fig. 68.1 Gastric emptying scintigraphy of patients with both normal and delayed emptying after ingestion a radiolabeled meal. In the "Normal" images, food has entered the small bowel by 1 h and the stomach is almost completely empty by 2 h. In the "Delayed" images, a significant amount of the meal remains in the stomach at 4 h

and/or greater than 10% retention at 4 h. Further, delayed gastric emptying is classified based on the extent of retention at 4 h: mild delay 10–15% retention, moderate 15–35%, and severe greater than 35%. Normal values for retained food in the stomach are 37–90% at 1 h, 30–60% at 2 h, and 0–10% at 4 h [20]. All of this data is used to calculate a $T_{1/2}$, or gastric emptying half-life time. While gastric emptying scintigraphy can be used to diagnose gastroparesis, results should not be used to grade the severity of clinical symptoms as they typically do not correlate to scintigraphy results [21].

An alternative to gastric emptying scintigraphy uses a wireless motility capsule that quantifies gastric pH and pressure [22]. This study is useful as it measures motility of the small bowel and colon as well as the stomach. As the capsule passes from the stomach to the duodenum, it detects an increase in luminal pH. Emptying of the capsule should relate to the end of emptying for a solid meal [23], and generally 5 h is considered the cutoff time between normal and delayed emptying with both a sensitivity and specificity of 83% [24]. Another alternative to gastric scintigraphy is CO_2 breath testing. Patients ingest a meal with [13]CO_2-labeled octanoate (a medium-chain triglyceride) which is subsequently absorbed by the small intestine, metabolized in the liver, and ^{13}C is excreted from the lungs during respiration. Measuring the concentration of ^{13}C in breath samples indirectly estimates gastric emptying [25]. This test is rarely used in clinical practice.

While measuring gastric emptying is necessary for the diagnosis of gastroparesis, it has some limitations. Gastric emptying rates can vary greatly in an individual and are also highly variable among patients. It is unclear whether this test truly captures what is occurring chronically in gastroparetics as it only signifies delayed emptying of solids at one point in time. Visceral hypersensitivity and impaired gastric accommodation may be even more important than delayed emptying in the symptomatology of gastroparesis [26] which is likely why the results of gastric emptying scintigraphy do not predict symptom severity or quality of life (Fig. 68.2)

Summary

In summary, gastroparesis is a chronic and often debilitating condition characterized by a delay in gastric emptying without mechanical obstruction. The disease often presents with nausea, vomiting, bloating, and/or abdominal pain. Many etiologies exist, the most common being diabetes, postsurgical, and idiopathic, although rarer neurologic, post-infectious, and autoimmune causes exist. After ruling out mechanical obstruction with cross-sectional imaging and endoscopy, the diagnosis of gastroparesis is made with gastric emptying scintigraphy. However, gastric emptying study results do not predict symptom severity, which can often be severely life-limiting and carry significant social and economic implications.

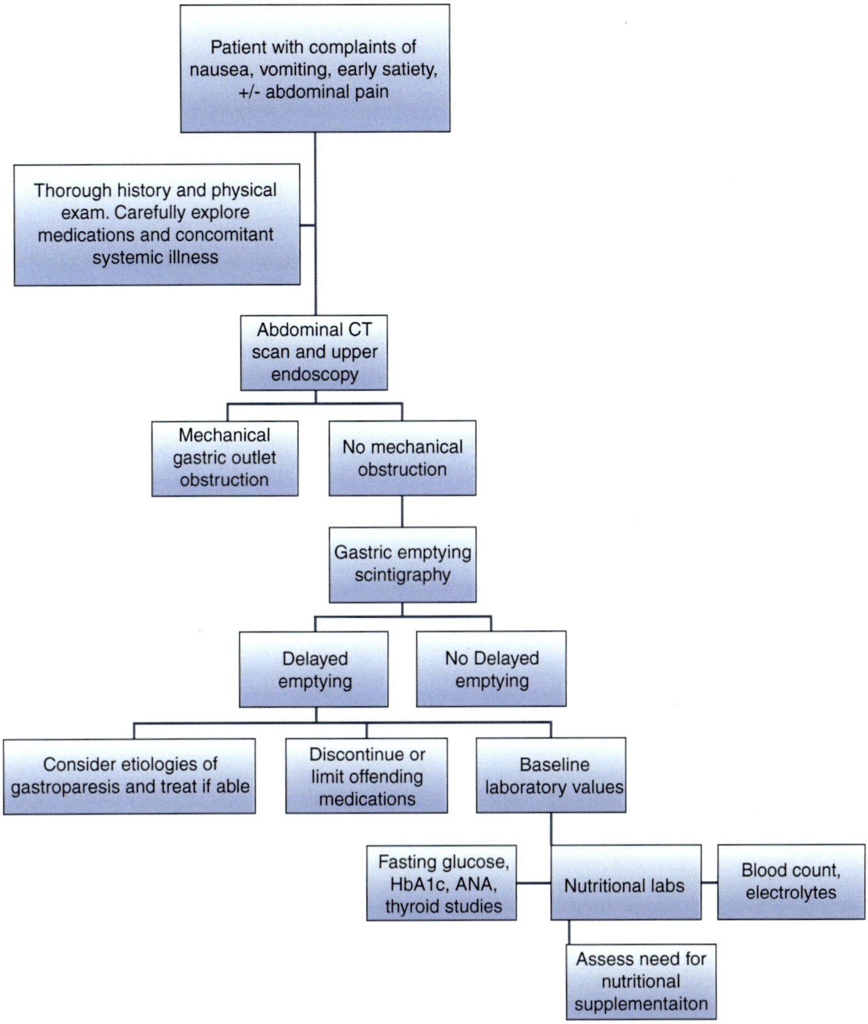

Fig. 68.2 Diagnosis and workup of a gastroparesis

References

1. Jung HK, Choung RS, Locke GR 3rd, et al. The incidence, prevalence, and outcomes of patients with gastroparesis in Olmsted County, Minnesota, from 1996 to 2006. Gastroenterology. 2009;136:1225.
2. Stein B, Everhart KK, Lacy BE. Gastroparesis: a review of current diagnosis and treatment options. J Clin Gastroenterol. 2015;49(7):550–8.
3. Lacy BE, Crowell MD, Mathis C, Bauer D, Heinberg LJ. Gastroparesis: quality of life and health care utilization. J Clin Gastroenterol. 2018;52:20–4. [Epub ahead of print].

4. Carbone F, Tack J. Gastroduodenal mechanisms underlying functional gastric disorders. Dig Dis. 2014;32(3):222–9.
5. Camilleri M, Malagelada JR, Brown ML, et al. Relation between antral motility and gastric emptying of solids and liquids in humans. Am J Phys. 1985;249(5 Pt 1):G580–5.
6. Mearin F, Camilleri M, Malagelada JR. Pyloric dysfunction in diabetics with recurrent nausea and vomiting. Gastroenterology. 1986;90(6):1919–25.
7. Fraser RJ, Horowitz M, Maddox AF, et al. Postprandial antropyloroduodenal motility and gastric emptying in gastroparesis–effects of cisapride. Gut. 1994;35(2):172–8.
8. Kumar A, Attaluri A, Hashmi S, et al. Visceral hypersensitivity and impaired accommodation in refractory diabetic gastroparesis. Neurogastroenterol Motil. 2008;20(6):635–42.
9. Camilleri M, Parkman HP, Shafi MA, et al. Clinical guideline: management of gastroparesis. Am J Gastroenterol. 2013;108:18–37.
10. Harberson J, Thomas R, Harbison S, et al. Gastric neuromuscluar pathology of gastroparesis: analysis of full-thickness antral biopsies. Dig Dis Sci. 2010;55:359–70.
11. Parkman HP, Yates K, Hasler WL, et al. Similarities and differences between diabetic and idiopathic gastroparesis. Clin Gastroenterol Hepatol. 2011;9(12):1056–64.
12. Soykan I, Sivri B, Sarosiek I, et al. Demography, clinical characteristics, psychological and abuse profiles, treatment, and long-term follow-up of patients with gastroparesis. Dig Dis Sci. 1998;43:2398.
13. Vittal H, Farrugia G, Gomez G, Pasricha PJ. Mechanisms of disease: the pathological basis of gastroparesis--a review of experimental and clinical studies. Nat Clin Pract Gastroenterol Hepatol. 2007;4:336.
14. Hasler WL, Wilson LA, Parkman HP, et al. Bloating in gastroparesis: severity, impact, and associated factors. Am J Gastroenterol. 2011;106:1492–502.
15. Sarosiek I, Davis B, Eichler E, McCallum RW. Surgical approaches to treatment of gastroparesis: gastric electrical stimulation, pyloroplasty, total gastrectomy and enteral feeding tubes. Gastroenterol Clin N Am. 2015;44(1):151–67. https://doi.org/10.1016/j.gtc.2014.11.012. Review.
16. Parkman HP, Yates K, Hasler WL, et al. Clinical features of idiopathic gastroparesis vary with sex, body mass, symptom onset, delay in gastric emptying, and gastroparesis severity. Gastroenterology. 2011;140:101–15.
17. Pasricha PJ, Parkman HP. Gastroparesis: definitions and diagnosis. Gastroenterol Clin N Am. 2015;44(1):1–7. https://doi.org/10.1016/j.gtc.2014.11.001. Review.
18. Nguyen LA, Snape WJ Jr. Clinical presentation and pathophysiology of gastroparesis. Gastroenterol Clin N Am. 2015;44(1):21–30. https://doi.org/10.1016/j.gtc.2014.11.003. Review.
19. Cherian D, Sachdeva P, Fisher RS, Parkman HP. Abdominal pain is a frequent symptom of gastroparesis. Clin Gastroenterol Hepatol. 2010;8:676.
20. Tougas G, Eaker EY, Abell TL, et al. Assessment of gastric emptying using a low fat meal: establishment of international control values. Am J Gastroenterol. 2000;95:1456.
21. Shin AS, Camilleri M. Diagnostic assessment of diabetic gastroparesis. Diabetes. 2013;62(8):2667–73. https://doi.org/10.2337/db12-1706. Review.
22. Parkman HP. Assessment of gastric emptying and small-bowel motility: scintigraphy, breath tests, manometry, and SmartPill. Gastrointest Endosc Clin N Am. 2009;19:49–55.
23. Cassilly D, Kantor S, Knight L, et al. Gastric emptying of a nondigestible solid: assessment with simultaneous SmartPill pH and pressure capsule, antroduodenal manometry, gastric emptying scintigraphy. Neurogastroenterol Motil. 2008;20(4):311–9.
24. Kuo B, McCallum RW, Koch K, et al. Comparison of gastric emptying of a nondigestible capsule to a radiolabeled meal in healthy and gastroparetic subjects. Aliment Pharmacol Ther. 2008;27(2):186–96.
25. Szarka LA, Camilleri M, Vella A, et al. A stable isotope breath test with a standard meal for abnormal gastric emptying of solids in the clinic and in research. Clin Gastroenterol Hepatol. 2008;6(6):635–43.
26. Hasler WL. Gastroparesis: pathogenesis, diagnosis, and management. Nat Rev Gastroenterol Hepatol. 2011;8:438–53.

Medical Management of Gastroparesis: Diet and Medications

69

Deepti Jacob and Michael Camilleri

Introduction

In this chapter, we review the role of diet and medications in the medical management of gastroparesis. The rationale for the recommendations requires a brief discussion of the definition, epidemiology, physiology of gastric emptying, as well as the etiology and pathogenesis of gastric emptying disorders, which may impact the choice of therapies.

Definition

Gastroparesis is defined as a syndrome characterized by delayed gastric emptying with associated symptoms in the absence of mechanical obstruction [1]. The cardinal symptoms are nausea, postprandial fullness, bloating, upper abdominal pain, early satiety and, with more severe disease, vomiting. Weight loss, malnutrition, dehydration, electrolyte imbalance, bezoar formation, and aspiration pneumonia may be apparent in severe cases [2, 3]. These symptoms may also be seen with other etiologies such as peptic ulcer disease, functional dyspepsia, and gastritis secondary to *Helicobacter pylori* [1]; hence, accurate documentation of delayed gastric emptying is essential before initiating treatment [1, 4, 5]. Symptoms generally do not predict the degree of delay in gastric emptying; therefore, the prevalence of gastroparesis cannot be estimated solely based on symptoms [6, 7]. For example, Maleki et al. documented symptoms such as nausea and vomiting occurred in ~15% of patients with type 1 or 2 diabetes in an epidemiological study in southeastern Minnesota [8]. In contrast, based on studies in the same community (Olmsted County, MN), the

D. Jacob · M. Camilleri (✉)
Division of Gastroenterology and Hepatology, Mayo Clinic, Rochester, MN, USA
e-mail: camilleri.michael@mayo.edu

J. Grams et al. (eds.), *The SAGES Manual of Foregut Surgery*,
https://doi.org/10.1007/978-3-319-96122-4_69

population-based incidence of definite gastroparesis ranged from 6.3 to 17.2 cases per 100,000 person-years when adjusted for age and sex [6], and the prevalence of gastroparesis was estimated to be 5% among patients with type 1 diabetes, 1% among patients with type 2 diabetes, and 0.2% in the nondiabetic controls [9].

Physiology of Normal Gastric Emptying

Normal gastric emptying is a complex process that is dependent on the coordinated interaction between the smooth muscles of the gastric fundus, antrum, pylorus, and duodenum, the enteric (intrinsic) and central (extrinsic) nervous systems, and specialized pacemaker cells called the interstitial cells of Cajal (ICC) [10, 11]. Gastric accommodation effectively increases the gastric volume without raising the intragastric pressure [10, 12], which in turn allows for the food to be transferred to the gastric antrum. In the antrum, food is broken down to 1–2 mm particles in order to pass through the pylorus [10, 13].

Gastric emptying of food (solids and liquids) is also dependent on the physical consistency [14, 15], the fat content, and the total caloric load of a meal [14] (Fig. 69.1). Liquids of low caloric density empty exponentially from the stomach under the pressure gradient between fundic tone and pylorus and with minimal motor action by the distal stomach [14]. Higher caloric liquids or homogenized solids empty in a linear fashion under the pressure gradient from the fundus and with the coordinated antropyloroduodenal motility [14]. For digestible food of more solid consistency, gastric emptying occurs in two periods: the lag period and the post-lag period [13, 14, 16]. During the lag period, food is initially retained in the proximal stomach and transferred to the antrum where trituration occurs, reducing solid food particle size to <2 mm. Following this trituration, solid food empties linearly from the stomach during the post-lag period, similar to a homogenized solid meal. Nondigestible solids require the interdigestive migrating motor complex [MMC] [14, 15] in order to be emptied from the stomach. However, since there is a

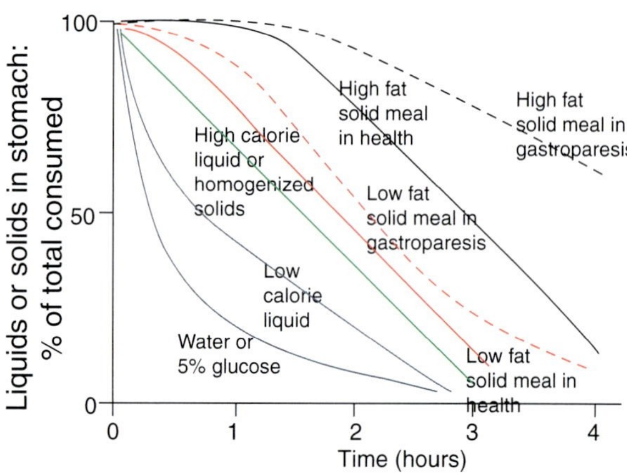

Fig. 69.1 Gastric emptying curves for different consistency and content of meals used in gastric emptying studies. (Reproduced from Camilleri [14])

wide range of the number of MMCs throughout the day and because about one third of the MMCs are not associated with an antral component even in healthy humans [14], it is possible for nondigested solids to remain in the healthy stomach for several hours [14]. Thus, residual nondigestible food at endoscopy after overnight fasting does not imply gastric motor dysfunction [14].

Etiology

There are many causes of gastroparesis; however, the most common forms are idiopathic (36%), diabetic (29%), and postsurgical (13%) [1] in a tertiary care center. Other etiologies include post-viral, iatrogenic (post-vagotomy or vagal injury), collagen vascular disorders, Parkinson's disease, and medications (GLP-1 agonists, amylin analogs, cyclosporine, opioids) [1, 17]. A particular form of gastroparesis manifests as feeding intolerance in patients admitted to the ICU who are critically ill and receiving enteral nutrition; this form of gastroparesis is usually multifactorial. Contributing factors include medications and the underlying diverse diseases that may result in inhibition of gastric emptying. Regardless of etiology, a female predominance of gastroparesis has been noted in multiple studies [6, 18, 9, 19].

Pathogenesis of Gastroparesis

Pathogenesis of gastroparesis includes extrinsic autonomic neuropathy affecting the vagus nerve, intrinsic or enteric neuropathy, pathology of the interstitial cells of Cajal, and myopathy.

Extrinsic

The central nervous system controls digestion through the autonomic nervous system; parasympathetic control is mediated through the vagus, and sympathetic control is mediated through the spinal cord at T5 to T10 via the celiac ganglia [10, 11, 20]. The myenteric ganglia innervating the pyloric sphincter are supplied by splanchnic efferents in the celiac ganglia [21, 22]. The vagus nerve affects gastric motility indirectly via the enteric nervous system, through vagal efferents that arise from the dorsal motor nucleus and terminate in the myenteric plexus [10]. Vagus nerve dysfunction decreases antral contractile frequency and pyloric relaxation and, thus, prevents the passage of food. These dysfunctions have been demonstrated post subdiaphragmatic vagotomy, as demonstrated in rats [23, 24] and in humans [25]. Additionally, in response to sham feeding (which stimulates brainstem vagal nuclei), gastric acid output is decreased by two thirds in long-standing, insulin-dependent diabetics, again suggestive of vagal neuropathy [26].

Variable degrees of myelin degeneration have been documented in the vagus nerves of patients with diabetes affected by gastroparesis [27–29].

Intrinsic Dysfunctions

The enteric nervous system (ENS) integrates the signals from the central nervous system to the effector systems: motor, vascular, and secretory. The ENS is organized in ganglia in the myenteric, deep mucosal and submucosal plexi. In patients with gastroparesis, there is a decrease in the number of enteric nerve fibers [30] and in the interstitial cells of Cajal (ICCs) [31]. Interstitial cells of Cajal serve as a non-neuronal pacemaker system that aids in gastric propulsion, in sensation, and in generating an electrical rhythm for the contractile activity [32, 33]. Reduced numbers of nerves and ICCs were observed particularly in diabetic gastroparesis; however, these losses did not correlate with symptom severity [30]. Neuronal deficiencies affect both the excitatory and inhibitory innervation.

Nitric oxide induces smooth muscle relaxation and consequently, with gastric accommodation, relaxation of the pylorus and gastric emptying [24, 34]. It is synthesized by neuronal nitric oxide synthase (nNOS) which is expressed in the enteric nerves [19, 24]. Loss of nNOS has been found to be associated with the pathogenesis of gastroparesis in multiple studies [28, 35, 36] and more often in patients with idiopathic gastroparesis than in diabetic gastroparesis [30]. Loss of nNOS is also related to a loss of ICCs in the stomach [24]; however sildenafil, which induces the same intracellular increase in cGMP as does NO, did not improve gastric emptying in humans [37].

Recent evidence suggests that there is a reduction in M2 macrophages and an increase in proinflammatory M1 macrophages, resulting in depletion of ICCs as a result of immune injury and oxidative stress [38, 39].

Management of Gastroparesis (Fig. 69.2)

General Measures

All medications that decrease GI motility should be discontinued, if possible. These include narcotics (including tramadol and tapentadol), tricyclic antidepressants, dopamine agonists, calcium channel blocking medications, α2-adrenergic agonists, lithium, progesterone-containing medications, and muscarinic cholinergic receptor antagonists. In patients with diabetes and gastroparesis, incretin-based medications (e.g., the amylin analog, pramlintide) and GLP-1 analogs (e.g., exenatide, liraglutide) may decrease gastric emptying [40–42], and the risk/benefit ratio should be discussed with the patient's diabetologist.

While diabetes is a common cause of gastroparesis, there is conflicting evidence whether long-term glycemic control improves gastric emptying rates and symptoms of gastroparesis [43, 44]. However, acute hyperglycemia can certainly slow gastric emptying in both patients with diabetes and healthy controls [45, 46].

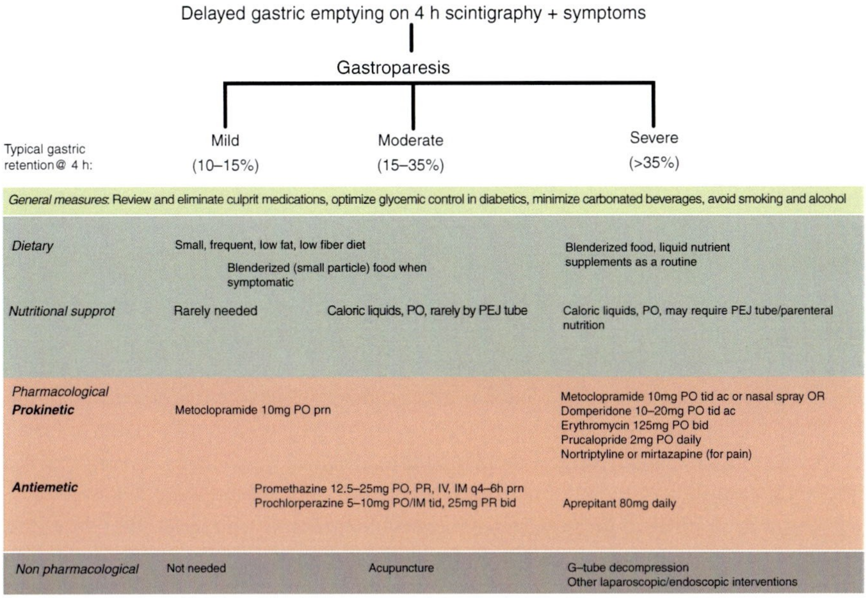

Fig. 69.2 Summary of strategies in the management of gastroparesis. (Adapted from Camilleri [113])

Dietary Interventions

Little research has been done in this area, to date. Gastroparesis is known to cause poor oral intake, resulting in deficiencies in calories, vitamins, and minerals [47, 48]. The general principles of dietary management are based on measures that optimize gastric emptying while meeting the patient's nutritional requirements. The approximate caloric requirement of a patient can be estimated by multiplying 25 kcal by their current body weight in kilograms [49], though more formal calculations based on Harris-Benedict equations may be required in patients with significant gastroparesis.

Oral Nutrition

Both fat and fiber delay gastric emptying, and the stomach only empties at a rate of 1–2 kcal/minute [1]. Hence, patients with gastroparesis should consume small, frequent meals that are low in fat and fiber [1, 48]. Blenderized solids or nutrient liquids (which aid in meeting the nutrient and caloric goals without aggravating symptoms) can be used, since gastric emptying of nutrient liquids is often preserved in gastroparesis [1]. In a recent study involving patients with diabetic gastroparesis, patients on a small-particle diet (compared to those on a standard diet) had decreased symptoms of nausea, vomiting, postprandial fullness, bloating [50], regurgitation, heartburn, and anxiety levels, but abdominal pain was not affected [50]. A liquid multivitamin should also be prescribed [51]. Poor tolerance of liquids is predictive of poor outcome with oral nutrition [48]. In those circumstances, enteral nutrition can be considered.

Patients should also be counseled to minimize carbonated beverages and to avoid smoking and alcohol, as the former can aggravate gastric distension and the latter can delay gastric emptying [52–55].

Enteral Nutrition

In patients with gastroparesis unable to tolerate oral intake, jejunal feeding can be considered, as long as the small bowel function is normal. This approach improves symptoms and reduces hospitalizations while maintaining nutrition [56, 57]. Regulated enteral nutrition may also improve glycemic control in diabetic patients [1]. Prior to the placement of a jejunal tube, successful nasojejunal feeding should be demonstrated, as occasionally patients with gastroparesis can also have small bowel dysfunction which renders them unable to tolerate jejunal feeds. Complications of enteral feeding include infection, tube migration, tube dislodgement, and pulmonary aspiration [58]. In general, enteral feeding should be delivered directly to the proximal jejunum through a feeding tube placed directly into the small bowel with the aid of endoscopy, radiology, or laparoscopy. Enteral feeding is preferred over parenteral nutrition due to decreased potential for complications, lesser cost, and more ease of delivery [1]. Patients may also require venting gastrostomy for relief of gastroparesis symptoms. Usually, such a vent is placed through a separate percutaneous endoscopic gastrostomy (PEG). Our experience is that PEG with jejunal tube extensions are associated with displacement of the latter into the stomach, and, therefore, we recommend separate gastrostomy and jejunostomy tubes, if both venting and feeding are required. In addition, it is unlikely that, in patients with gastroparesis, the delivery of nutrient liquid via gastrostomy will restore hydration and nutrition will be more successful compared to the ingestion of the same fluids orally, as long as there are no difficulties with swallowing.

Parenteral Nutrition

This should be coordinated by experts in home parenteral nutrition with attention given to hydration, electrolytes, mineral, and vitamin deficiencies, as well as calorie and nitrogen supplementation. Further discussion is beyond the scope of this chapter.

Medications

This section considers current medications, most of which are used off-label (apart from metoclopramide) and promising experimental medications.

Prokinetics

Prokinetic medications promote the antegrade movement of luminal GI contents through increased contractility of the GI tract [2]. In a recent systematic review and meta-analysis on the efficacy and safety of prokinetics in critically ill patients receiving enteral nutrition, moderate-quality evidence indicated that prokinetic agents were associated with decreased feeding intolerances, the risk of developing high gastric residual volumes, and increased the success of post-pyloric feeding tube placement [59]. In a prior systematic analysis that reviewed the role of prokinetics in patients with gastroparesis, erythromycin was the most efficacious in stimulating gastric emptying, while both erythromycin and domperidone were noted to improve overall symptoms of gastroparesis [60]. However, this analysis did not consider the tachyphylaxis associated with longer-term use of motilin agonists, such as the macrolide antibiotics including erythromycin, which result in failed therapy of dropouts beyond 4 weeks of treatment [61].

Prokinetic agents can be grouped into four broad classes: dopamine receptor antagonists, motilin receptor agonists, $5HT_4$ receptor agonists, and the (experimental) ghrelin receptor agonists.

Dopamine Receptor Antagonists

Dopamine which is present in significant amounts in the GI tract has several inhibitory effects on gastrointestinal motility. This is thought to be secondary to the suppression of neuronal acetylcholine release by D2 receptor agonists [62].

Metoclopramide is the only FDA-approved medication for the treatment of gastroparesis; it targets both D1 and D2 dopamine receptors [1, 62] with a peripheral gastrointestinal prokinetic effect (predominantly in the stomach) and central action in the chemoreceptor trigger zone on the floor of the fourth ventricle to antagonize dopamine receptors, inducing antiemetic effect [62]. It is recommended that metoclopramide be started at the lowest possible dose (5 mg, 15 min before meals and at bedtime) and then titrated to the lowest efficacious dose up to a maximum of 40 mg/day. When possible, dose reductions (such as 5 mg before two main meals of the day) or drug holidays should be considered, in order to minimize potential side effects [63, 64].

Metoclopramide is available as a tablet, orally disintegrating sublingual formulation, nasal spray, liquid, and injectable form [65, 66]. Wherever possible, liquid, sublingual, or nasal formulations of the medication should be used in patients with gastroparesis to enhance drug pharmacokinetics. Metoclopramide as a nasal spray decreased symptoms of gastroparesis in women (not in men) with diabetic gastroparesis [66]. The side effects of metoclopramide include akathisia, restlessness, insomnia, and agitation that usually occur 1–2 weeks into therapy [65]. Most of these acute side effects are treatable with diphenhydramine and resolve with cessation of the drug [65]. Major side effects include irreversible tardive dyskinesia (FDA black box warning) and corrected QT prolongation [14]. The risk of irreversible tardive dyskinesia from prolonged (>3 months) use of metoclopramide was estimated to be 1–10% from data acquired in a referral clinic for involuntary movements [63]. However, more relevant studies of population- and prescription-based data suggest a much lower risk of tardive dyskinesia, that is, <1% [59]. This risk appears to be increased in patients with advanced age, female gender, diabetes, cirrhosis, alcoholism, schizophrenia, known organic CNS pathology, and concomitant use of neuroleptics that affect the dopaminergic pathways.

Another less appreciated side effect of metoclopramide is depression that can either be induced or worsened [65]. Potential side effects should be discussed in detail with patients and clearly documented in the medical record before prescribing. There is a black box warning from the FDA to prescribers advising against prescription of metoclopramide for longer than 3 months. Therefore, unless patients have therapeutic benefits that outweigh the potential risks, it is recommended that this medication should not be used for more than 12 weeks [1].

Domperidone, another D2 receptor antagonist, is as efficacious as metoclopramide in the treatment of gastroparesis and has less central side effects [2]. The recommended dose is 10 mg tid before meals. It is not approved for general prescription in the United States, given its propensity to cause prolongation of corrected QT, cardiac arrhythmias, and sudden cardiac death [67, 68]. It can only be prescribed in the United States through the FDA's expanded access to investigational drugs [14]. A baseline electrocardiogram (ECG) should be obtained prior to treatment, and the drug should be withheld if the corrected QTc is greater than 470 ms in male and 450 ms in female patients [1]. Follow-up ECGs are also recommended to check for QTc prolongation once patients are started on domperidone.

In a recent systematic review, increased risk for cardiac events was noted in patients older than 60 years of age or in those receiving doses more than 30 mg/day [68]. The European Medicines Agency also recommends that this medication not be used for more than 1 week at a time. In a recent prospective study in patients with symptoms of refractory gastroparesis, there was symptomatic improvement of postprandial fullness, nausea, vomiting, and stomach fullness in 68% of patients, with at least moderate improvement of symptoms in 45% of patients [69]. Response tended to be better in those with normal or mildly decreased gastric emptying (<30% retention at 4 h); 12% of patients had to discontinue treatment due to side effects, and the most common side effects included headache, tachycardia, palpitations, and diarrhea. Other reported side effects were increased prolactin levels, potential for breast discharge, and altered menstrual cycles [69].

Drug interactions can occur when dopamine receptor antagonists are prescribed with certain antiemetics and antidepressants which may also be prescribed for the treatment of gastroparesis. These interactions are typically due to influence on the functions of CYP450-2D6 or CYP450-3A4, and, hence, caution must be exercised while prescribing these medications [1].

Motilin Receptor Agonists

Motilin is a gastrointestinal hormone synthesized and secreted by specific endocrine cells, mostly in the upper small intestine and smaller amounts in the gastric antrum [70, 71]. This is released in the fasting state during migrating motor complexes that begin in the upper gut [71]. This release of motilin, coinciding with phase III of the migrating motor complex, is thought to aid with clearing the stomach and intestine from undigested material, preventing bacterial overgrowth in the upper gut and possibly initiating the sensation of hunger [70].

Macrolide antibiotics (e.g., erythromycin, clarithromycin, azithromycin [14]) are motilin receptor agonists that are often used off-label in patients with gastroparesis. The efficacy of motilin receptor agonists to increase gastric emptying is dependent on their ability to stimulate cholinergic receptors on smooth muscle [70] in addition to stimulation of cholinergic mechanisms [72] . Erythromycin and azithromycin stimulate gastric emptying and antral pressure activity [73]. Erythromycin, however, has the potential to interact with other medications metabolized by cytochrome P450 CYP 3A4 [14], thereby increasing plasma erythromycin concentrations which, in turn, can result in cardiac (ventricular) arrhythmias and sudden death [73, 74]. Compared to erythromycin, azithromycin has less drug-to-drug interactions [75] and might be a more feasible option. Regardless, they are both associated with tachyphylaxis caused by downregulation of the motilin receptor that occurs approximately 2 weeks after initiation of therapy [76]. A lower dose of erythromycin at 125 mg twice daily might delay the onset of downregulation of the motilin receptors [65]. There is also a theoretical risk of antibiotic resistance and antibiotic-associated diarrhea with use of these antibiotics; however, in the context of gastroparesis, these antibiotics are typically prescribed at lower doses, usually below the levels associated with antimicrobial activity [65].

An experimental non-macrolide motilin agonist, *RQ-00201894*, selectively activates the motilin receptor and causes long-lasting cholinergic activity in the human stomach, which, in turn, is thought to aid in gastric emptying [71]. More studies are needed to evaluate this as a potential treatment for gastroparesis.

$5HT_4$ Receptor Agonists

$5HT_4$ receptor agonists facilitate the release of acetylcholine from the myenteric plexus by activating the $5HT_4$ receptors, thereby resulting in smooth muscle contractions and accelerated gastric emptying. In the past, cisapride was widely used to treat gastroparesis. However, due to its risk of cardiotoxicity associated with effects on the hERG channel rather than effects on cardiac $5HT_4$ receptors, it is no longer being used.

In a recent study by Florencia Carbone et al. [77], *prucalopride*, a highly selective, high-affinity $5HT_4$ receptor agonist with no effects on hERG channel, was found to significantly decrease gastric half-emptying time and improve symptoms and quality of life in patients with idiopathic gastroparesis. Prucalopride, though not available in the United States, is already approved for the treatment of chronic idiopathic constipation in most countries.

Two experimental $5HT_4$ receptor agonists are *velusetrag* and *YKP10811*. Velusetrag is undergoing clinical trials in patients with gastroparesis. It is relatively well tolerated [78] and has been shown to accelerate gastric emptying after 4–9 days of treatment in healthy controls [79].

YKP10811, a new selective $5HT_4$ receptor agonist and benzamide derivative, accelerated gastric emptying in patients with functional constipation at doses of 10 and 20 mg [80]. Further research is needed to document its efficacy in gastroparesis.

Ghrelin Receptor Agonist

Ghrelin, a 28-amino acid motilin-related peptide produced in the stomach, plays an important role in the control of food intake and energy balance [81]. Studies have shown that administration of synthetic ghrelin increased gastric emptying and improved meal-related symptoms in patients with idiopathic gastroparesis [81].

In recent studies, *relamorelin*, a pentapeptide ghrelin receptor agonist, has shown promise in patients with type 1 or type 2 diabetes. Relamorelin accelerated gastric half-emptying time of solids in type 1 and type 2 diabetic patients with prior documentation of delayed gastric emptying [14, 82, 83] and increased frequency of distal antral motor contractions without inhibiting gastric accommodation or inducing satiation [84]. In a large phase 2A randomized, controlled trial in patients with diabetic gastroparesis, relamorelin significantly accelerated gastric emptying, decreased vomiting (by~ 60%), and decreased other symptoms such as nausea, abdominal pain, bloating, and early satiety [85].

Antiemetics

Very often the treatment for gastroparesis is focused on symptom management. The most commonly prescribed agents include *phenothiazines* (e.g., prochlorperazine) or *antihistamine agents* (promethazine). However, co-administration of antiemetics and prokinetics can result in drug interactions, especially if the drugs are metabolized via the CYP450 pathway. This could result in high blood levels and drug toxicity and can potentially cause ventricular arrhythmias and sudden death [1, 14]. Other medications that have been used to help with symptoms of nausea and vomiting (but with limited research) include *5HT$_3$ receptor antagonists*, such as ondansetron or granisetron, transdermal scopolamine, and dronabinol (a synthetic cannabinoid) [1]. It is important to note that scopolamine and cannabinoid agents may inhibit gastrointestinal contractility.

Recent preliminary reports suggest efficacy of the *neurokinin 1 (NK1) receptor antagonist*, aprepitant. When released from enteric afferents or extrinsic primary afferent neurons, tachykinins have the potential to influence both nerve and muscles by interacting with different types of tachykinin receptors, including NK1 receptors. Tachykinins have an excitatory effect on gastrointestinal motor activity but can also inhibit motor activity by stimulating either inhibitory neuronal pathways or by interrupting excitatory relays. Aprepitant acts by counteracting the activity of substance P, the preferred ligand at NK1 receptors [86]. It has been widely used in the setting of chemotherapy-induced nausea and vomiting in combination with other agents [87]. In a recent randomized, controlled trial of 4-week duration involving 126 patients with gastroparesis and related disorders associated with symptoms of chronic nausea and vomiting, aprepitant resulted in overall symptom relief compared to placebo [88]. No significant adverse effects were reported. There have also been two case reports [89, 90] in the literature in which aprepitant was used successfully to treat symptoms of nausea and vomiting in patients with gastroparesis. More research is required to tease out the nuances, mechanism of action, and longer-term efficacy of this medication in patients with documented delayed gastric emptying.

Neurosensory Modulation and Pain Management

The management of pain is an important aspect of caring for patients with gastroparesis. In clinical practice, low-dose tricyclic antidepressants (TCAs) and selective serotonin reuptake inhibitors (SSRIs) have been used with anecdotal success. TCAs have shown some benefit in patients with functional nausea and vomiting [91] and also in diabetic patients with chronic nausea and vomiting [92]. Given that *nortriptyline* has less anticholinergic effects compared to amitriptyline, it was tested in a large randomized, controlled trial and resulted in no benefit over placebo on composite or individual scores in relief of symptoms [93].

There have been multiple case reports [94–98] showing that the antidepressant, *mirtazapine*, helps to ameliorate symptoms in both diabetic and nondiabetic gastroparesis. Mirtazapine acts by blocking both $5HT_2$ and $5HT_3$ receptors as well as by antagonizing the adrenergic alpha$_2$-autoreceptors and alpha$_2$-heteroreceptors [99]. In canine studies, mirtazapine has been shown to improve gastric emptying and colonic transit and to normalize delay in gastric emptying induced by rectal distension [100]. Further clinical studies are warranted to study the effect of mirtazapine on gastric emptying in humans.

Opioids should be avoided for treatment of pain in gastroparesis, given their potential to decrease gastric motility. *Tapentadol*, a μ-opioid receptor agonist and a norepinephrine reuptake inhibitor, was shown to retard gastric emptying [101].

Although *tramadol* was reported not to retard gastric emptying of solids or liquids in a crossover study of 12 healthy participants, the study showed 40% slower orocecal transit and significant delay in colonic transit [102] and tramadol-induced dose-related inhibition of gastrointestinal transit in mice [103].

The GABA-ergic agents, *gabapentin* and *pregabalin*, are possible alternatives for pain relief [1], but they need to be formally studied in gastroparesis.

Intra-Pyloric Injection of Botulinum Toxin

Botulinum toxin inhibits pyloric smooth muscle contractility by two mechanisms: inhibition of acetylcholine release and by direct smooth muscle inhibition at higher doses [104]. Multiple small observational studies have suggested that intra-pyloric botulinum toxin can improve gastric emptying and symptoms [105–108] in patients with diabetic and nondiabetic gastroparesis. In one retrospective analysis of almost 150 patients (female gender, age <50 years, increased botulinum toxin dose), those with idiopathic gastroparesis responded better; 73.4% of evaluable patients had a clinical response to a second injection [109]. However, two sham-controlled trials of Botox were negative [110, 111].

Complementary and Alternative Therapy

Many patients seek alternative therapy to help with their symptoms of gastroparesis. In a single-blinded, randomized study involving 19 patients with type 2 diabetes and symptoms of gastroparesis, 9 patients showed improvement in gastric half-emptying time following treatment with *electroacupuncture* [112]. Symptom scores also improved significantly at the end of treatment as well as at 2 weeks. More studies are needed before recommending these modalities of treatment; however, given the chronicity of this illness, it is important to keep an open mind when patients choose alternative and complementary therapies.

Conclusion

There is still considerable unmet need in the field of medical management of gastroparesis. Novel pharmacotherapy with prucalopride and relamorelin is promising, and endoscopic or laparoscopic interventions (considered elsewhere in this book) may change the landscape of therapeutic interventions for treatment of gastroparesis.

Acknowledgments We thank Mrs. Cindy Stanislav for excellent secretarial assistance.

References

1. Camilleri M, Parkman HP, Shafi MA, Abell TL, Gerson L. Clinical guideline: management of gastroparesis. Am J Gastroenterol. 2013;108(1):18–37. quiz 8
2. Abell TL, Bernstein RK, Cutts T, Farrugia G, Forster J, Hasler WL, et al. Treatment of gastroparesis: a multidisciplinary clinical review. Neurogastroenterol Motil. 2006;18(4):263–83.
3. Lacy BE, Weiser K. Gastric motility, gastroparesis, and gastric stimulation. Surg Clin North Am. 2005;85(5):967–87, vi-vii.
4. Bredenoord AJ, Chial HJ, Camilleri M, Mullan BP, Murray JA. Gastric accommodation and emptying in evaluation of patients with upper gastrointestinal symptoms. Clin Gastroenterol Hepatol. 2003;1(4):264–72.
5. Tack J, Bisschops R, Sarnelli G. Pathophysiology and treatment of functional dyspepsia. Gastroenterology. 2004;127(4):1239–55.
6. Jung HK, Choung RS, Locke GR, 3rd, Schleck CD, Zinsmeister AR, Szarka LA, et al. The incidence, prevalence, and outcomes of patients with gastroparesis in Olmsted County, Minnesota, from 1996 to 2006. Gastroenterology. 2009;136(4):1225–33.
7. Talley NJ, Locke GR 3rd, Lahr BD, Zinsmeister AR, Tougas G, Ligozio G, et al. Functional dyspepsia, delayed gastric emptying, and impaired quality of life. Gut. 2006;55(7):933–9.
8. Maleki D, Locke GR 3rd, Camilleri M, Zinsmeister AR, Yawn BP, Leibson C, et al. Gastrointestinal tract symptoms among persons with diabetes mellitus in the community. Arch Intern Med. 2000;160(18):2808–16.
9. Choung RS, Locke GR 3rd, Schleck CD, Zinsmeister AR, Melton LJ 3rd, Talley NJ. Risk of gastroparesis in subjects with type 1 and 2 diabetes in the general population. Am J Gastroenterol. 2012;107(1):82–8.
10. Nguyen LA, Snape WJ Jr. Clinical presentation and pathophysiology of gastroparesis. Gastroenterol Clin N Am. 2015;44(1):21–30.
11. Camilleri M, Bharucha AE, Farrugia G. Epidemiology, mechanisms, and management of diabetic gastroparesis. Clin Gastroenterol Hepatol. 2011;9(1):5–12. quiz e7.
12. Kindt S, Tack J. Impaired gastric accommodation and its role in dyspepsia. Gut. 2006;55(12):1685–91.
13. Camilleri M, Malagelada JR, Brown ML, Becker G, Zinsmeister AR. Relation between antral motility and gastric emptying of solids and liquids in humans. Am J Phys. 1985;249(5 Pt 1):G580–5.
14. Camilleri M. Novel diet, drugs, and gastric interventions for gastroparesis. Clin Gastroenterol Hepatol. 2016;14(8):1072–80.

15. Kelly KA. Gastric emptying of liquids and solids: roles of proximal and distal stomach. Am J Phys. 1980;239(2):G71–6.
16. Siegel JA, Urbain JL, Adler LP, Charkes ND, Maurer AH, Krevsky B, et al. Biphasic nature of gastric emptying. Gut. 1988;29(1):85–9.
17. Camilleri M, Grover M, Farrugia G. What are the important subsets of gastroparesis? Neurogastroenterol Motil. 2012;24(7):597–603.
18. Soykan I, Sivri B, Sarosiek I, Kiernan B, McCallum RW. Demography, clinical characteristics, psychological and abuse profiles, treatment, and long-term follow-up of patients with gastroparesis. Dig Dis Sci. 1998;43(11):2398–404.
19. Parkman HP, Yates K, Hasler WL, Nguyen L, Pasricha PJ, Snape WJ, et al. Similarities and differences between diabetic and idiopathic gastroparesis. Clin Gastroenterol Hepatol. 2011;9(12):1056–64. quiz e133-4.
20. Wood JD, Alpers DH, Andrews PL. Fundamentals of neurogastroenterology. Gut. 1999;45(Suppl 2):Ii6–ii16.
21. Gillespie JS, Maxwell JD. Adrenergic innervation of sphincteric and nonsphincteric smooth muscle in the rat intestine. J Histochem Cytochem. 1971;19(11):676–81.
22. Costa M, Gabella G. Adrenergic innervation of the alimentary canal. Zeitschrift fur Zellforschung und mikroskopische. Anatomie (Vienna, Austria : 1948). 1971;122(3):357–77.
23. Ishiguchi T, Nakajima M, Sone H, Tada H, Kumagai AK, Takahashi T. Gastric distension-induced pyloric relaxation: central nervous system regulation and effects of acute hyperglycaemia in the rat. J Physiol. 2001;533(Pt 3):801–13.
24. Oh JH, Pasricha PJ. Recent advances in the pathophysiology and treatment of gastroparesis. J Neurogastroenterol Motil. 2013;19(1):18–24.
25. Camilleri M, Brown ML, Malagelada JR. Relationship between impaired gastric emptying and abnormal gastrointestinal motility. Gastroenterology. 1986;91(1):94–9.
26. Feldman M, Corbett DB, Ramsey EJ, Walsh JH, Richardson CT. Abnormal gastric function in longstanding, insulin-dependent diabetic patients. Gastroenterology. 1979;77(1):12–7.
27. Forster J, Damjanov I, Lin Z, Sarosiek I, Wetzel P, McCallum RW. Absence of the interstitial cells of Cajal in patients with gastroparesis and correlation with clinical findings. J Gastrointest Surg. 2005;9(1):102–8.
28. Iwasaki H, Kajimura M, Osawa S, Kanaoka S, Furuta T, Ikuma M, et al. A deficiency of gastric interstitial cells of Cajal accompanied by decreased expression of neuronal nitric oxide synthase and substance P in patients with type 2 diabetes mellitus. J Gastroenterol. 2006;41(11):1076–87.
29. Feldman M, Richardson CT, Fordtran JS. Effect of sham feeding on gastric acid secretion in healthy subjects and duodenal ulcer patients: evidence for increased basal vagal tone in some ulcer patients. Gastroenterology. 1980;79(5 Pt 1):796–800.
30. Grover M, Farrugia G, Lurken MS, Bernard CE, Faussone-Pellegrini MS, Smyrk TC, et al. Cellular changes in diabetic and idiopathic gastroparesis. Gastroenterology. 2011;140(5):1575–85.e8.
31. Farrugia G. Interstitial cells of Cajal in health and disease. Neurogastroenterol Motil. 2008;20(Suppl 1):54–63.
32. Sanders KM, Koh SD, Ward SM. Interstitial cells of cajal as pacemakers in the gastrointestinal tract. Annu Rev Physiol. 2006;68:307–43.
33. Barajas-Lopez C, Berezin I, Daniel EE, Huizinga JD. Pacemaker activity recorded in interstitial cells of Cajal of the gastrointestinal tract. Am J Phys. 1989;257(4 Pt 1):C830–5.
34. Shah V, Lyford G, Gores G, Farrugia G. Nitric oxide in gastrointestinal health and disease. Gastroenterology. 2004;126(3):903–13.
35. He CL, Soffer EE, Ferris CD, Walsh RM, Szurszewski JH, Farrugia G. Loss of interstitial cells of cajal and inhibitory innervation in insulin-dependent diabetes. Gastroenterology. 2001;121(2):427–34.
36. Zarate N, Mearin F, Wang XY, Hewlett B, Huizinga JD, Malagelada JR. Severe idiopathic gastroparesis due to neuronal and interstitial cells of Cajal degeneration: pathological findings and management. Gut. 2003;52(7):966–70.

37. Dishy V, Cohen Pour M, Feldman L, Naftali T, Baumer M, Efrati S, et al. The effect of sildenafil on gastric emptying in patients with end-stage renal failure and symptoms of gastroparesis. Clin Pharmacol Ther. 2004;76(3):281–6.
38. Cipriani G, Gibbons SJ, Kashyap PC, Farrugia G. Intrinsic gastrointestinal macrophages: their phenotype and role in gastrointestinal motility. Cell Mol Gastroenterol Hepatol. 2016;2(2):120-30.e1.
39. Bernard CE, Gibbons SJ, Mann IS, Froschauer L, Parkman HP, Harbison S, et al. Association of low numbers of CD206-positive cells with loss of ICC in the gastric body of patients with diabetic gastroparesis. Neurogastroenterol Motil. 2014;26(9):1275–84.
40. Vella A, Lee JS, Camilleri M, Szarka LA, Burton DD, Zinsmeister AR, et al. Effects of pramlintide, an amylin analogue, on gastric emptying in type 1 and 2 diabetes mellitus. Neurogastroenterol Motil. 2002;14(2):123–31.
41. Drucker DJ, Nauck MA. The incretin system: glucagon-like peptide-1 receptor agonists and dipeptidyl peptidase-4 inhibitors in type 2 diabetes. Lancet. 2006;368(9548):1696–705.
42. Imeryuz N, Yegen BC, Bozkurt A, Coskun T, Villanueva-Penacarrillo ML, Ulusoy NB. Glucagon-like peptide-1 inhibits gastric emptying via vagal afferent-mediated central mechanisms. Am J Phys. 1997;273(4 Pt 1):G920–7.
43. Bharucha AE, Camilleri M, Forstrom LA, Zinsmeister AR. Relationship between clinical features and gastric emptying disturbances in diabetes mellitus. Clin Endocrinol. 2009;70(3):415–20.
44. Holzapfel A, Festa A, Stacher-Janotta G, Bergmann H, Shnawa N, Brannath W, et al. Gastric emptying in type II (non-insulin-dependent) diabetes mellitus before and after therapy readjustment: no influence of actual blood glucose concentration. Diabetologia. 1999;42(12):1410–2.
45. Fraser R, Horowitz M, Dent J. Hyperglycaemia stimulates pyloric motility in normal subjects. Gut. 1991;32(5):475–8.
46. Fraser RJ, Horowitz M, Maddox AF, Harding PE, Chatterton BE, Dent J. Hyperglycaemia slows gastric emptying in type 1 (insulin-dependent) diabetes mellitus. Diabetologia. 1990;33(11):675–80.
47. Ogorek CP, Davidson L, Fisher RS, Krevsky B. Idiopathic gastroparesis is associated with a multiplicity of severe dietary deficiencies. Am J Gastroenterol. 1991;86(4):423–8.
48. Parkman HP, Yates KP, Hasler WL, Nguyan L, Pasricha PJ, Snape WJ, et al. Dietary intake and nutritional deficiencies in patients with diabetic or idiopathic gastroparesis. Gastroenterology. 2011;141(2):486–98, 98.e1-7.
49. Bouras EP, Scolapio JS. Gastric motility disorders: management that optimizes nutritional status. J Clin Gastroenterol. 2004;38(7):549–57.
50. Olausson EA, Storsrud S, Grundin H, Isaksson M, Attvall S, Simren M. A small particle size diet reduces upper gastrointestinal symptoms in patients with diabetic gastroparesis: a randomized controlled trial. Am J Gastroenterol. 2014;109(3):375–85.
51. Abdalla SM, Kalra G, Moshiree B. Motility evaluation in the patient with inflammatory bowel disease. Gastrointest Endosc Clin N Am. 2016;26(4):719–38.
52. Camilleri M. Appraisal of medium- and long-term treatment of gastroparesis and chronic intestinal dysmotility. Am J Gastroenterol. 1994;89(10):1769–74.
53. Scott AM, Kellow JE, Eckersley GM, Nolan JM, Jones MP. Cigarette smoking and nicotine delay postprandial mouth-cecum transit time. Dig Dis Sci. 1992;37(10):1544–7.
54. Pfeiffer A, Hogl B, Kaess H. Effect of ethanol and commonly ingested alcoholic beverages on gastric emptying and gastrointestinal transit. Clin Investig. 1992;70(6):487–91.
55. Sanaka M, Anjiki H, Tsutsumi H, Abe K, Kawakami T, Saitoh M, et al. Effect of cigarette smoking on gastric emptying of solids in Japanese smokers: a crossover study using the 13C-octanoic acid breath test. J Gastroenterol. 2005;40(6):578–82.
56. Fontana RJ, Barnett JL. Jejunostomy tube placement in refractory diabetic gastroparesis: a retrospective review. Am J Gastroenterol. 1996;91(10):2174–8.
57. Parkman HP, Hasler WL, Fisher RS. American Gastroenterological Association technical review on the diagnosis and treatment of gastroparesis. Gastroenterology. 2004;127(5):1592–622.

58. Karamanolis G, Tack J. Nutrition and motility disorders. Best Pract Res Clin Gastroenterol. 2006;20(3):485–505.
59. Lewis K, Alqahtani Z, McIntyre L, Almenawer S, Alshamsi F, Rhodes A, et al. The efficacy and safety of prokinetic agents in critically ill patients receiving enteral nutrition: a systematic review and meta-analysis of randomized trials. Crit Care. 2016;20(1):259.
60. Sturm A, Holtmann G, Goebell H, Gerken G. Prokinetics in patients with gastroparesis: a systematic analysis. Digestion. 1999;60(5):422–7.
61. Richards RD, Davenport K, McCallum RW. The treatment of idiopathic and diabetic gastroparesis with acute intravenous and chronic oral erythromycin. Am J Gastroenterol. 1993;88(2):203–7.
62. Pasricha PJ, Pehlivanov N, Sugumar A, Jankovic J. Drug insight: from disturbed motility to disordered movement--a review of the clinical benefits and medicolegal risks of metoclopramide. Nat Clin Pract Gastroenterol Hepatol. 2006;3(3):138–48.
63. Rao AS, Camilleri M. Review article: metoclopramide and tardive dyskinesia. Aliment Pharmacol Ther. 2010;31(1):11–9.
64. Wijemanne S, Jankovic J, Evans RW. Movement disorders from the use of metoclopramide and other Antiemetics in the treatment of migraine. Headache. 2016;56(1):153–61.
65. Hejazi RA, McCallum RW, Sarosiek I. Prokinetics in diabetic gastroparesis. Curr Gastroenterol Rep. 2012;14(4):297–305.
66. Parkman HP, Carlson MR, Gonyer D. Metoclopramide nasal spray reduces symptoms of gastroparesis in women, but not men, with diabetes: results of a phase 2B randomized study. Clin Gastroenterol Hepatol. 2015;13(7):1256-63.e1.
67. van Noord C, Dieleman JP, van Herpen G, Verhamme K, Sturkenboom MC. Domperidone and ventricular arrhythmia or sudden cardiac death: a population-based case-control study in the Netherlands. Drug Saf. 2010;33(11):1003–14.
68. Marzi M, Weitz D, Avila A, Molina G, Caraballo L, Piskulic L. Cardiac adverse effects of domperidone in adult patients: a systematic review. Rev Med Chil. 2015;143(1):14–21.
69. Schey R, Saadi M, Midani D, Roberts AC, Parupalli R, Parkman HP. Domperidone to treat symptoms of gastroparesis: benefits and side effects from a large single-center cohort. Dig Dis Sci. 2016;61:3545.
70. Sanger GJ, Wang Y, Hobson A, Broad J. Motilin: towards a new understanding of the gastrointestinal neuropharmacology and therapeutic use of motilin receptor agonists. Br J Pharmacol. 2013;170(7):1323–32.
71. Broad J, Takahashi N, Tajimi M, Sudo M, Goralczyk A, Parampalli U, et al. RQ-00201894: a motilin receptor agonist causing long-lasting facilitation of human gastric cholinergically-mediated contractions. J Pharmacol Sci. 2016;130(2):60–5.
72. Coulie B, Tack J, Peeters T, Janssens J. Involvement of two different pathways in the motor effects of erythromycin on the gastric antrum in humans. Gut. 1998;43(3):395–400.
73. Larson JM, Tavakkoli A, Drane WE, Toskes PP, Moshiree B. Advantages of azithromycin over erythromycin in improving the gastric emptying half-time in adult patients with gastroparesis. J Neurogastroenterol Motil. 2010;16(4):407–13.
74. Ray WA, Murray KT, Meredith S, Narasimhulu SS, Hall K, Stein CM. Oral erythromycin and the risk of sudden death from cardiac causes. N Engl J Med. 2004;351(11):1089–96.
75. Moshiree B, McDonald R, Hou W, Toskes PP. Comparison of the effect of azithromycin versus erythromycin on antroduodenal pressure profiles of patients with chronic functional gastrointestinal pain and gastroparesis. Dig Dis Sci. 2010;55(3):675–83.
76. Thielemans L, Depoortere I, Perret J, Robberecht P, Liu Y, Thijs T, et al. Desensitization of the human motilin receptor by motilides. J Pharmacol Exp Ther. 2005;313(3):1397–405.
77. Florencia Carbone AR, Andrews CN, Holvoet L, Lukas VOTV, Bisschops R, Caenepeel P, Arts J, Athanasios P, Tack J. A controlled cross-over trial shows benefit of Prucalopride for symptom control and gastric emptying enhancement in idiopathic gastroparesis. Gastroenterology. 2016;150(4 Supplement 1):S-S1271.
78. Goldberg M, Li YP, Johanson JF, Mangel AW, Kitt M, Beattie DT, et al. Clinical trial: the efficacy and tolerability of velusetrag, a selective 5-HT4 agonist with high intrinsic activity,

in chronic idiopathic constipation - a 4-week, randomized, double-blind, placebo-controlled, dose-response study. Aliment Pharmacol Ther. 2010;32(9):1102–12.
79. Manini ML, Camilleri M, Goldberg M, Sweetser S, McKinzie S, Burton D, et al. Effects of Velusetrag (TD-5108) on gastrointestinal transit and bowel function in health and pharmacokinetics in health and constipation. Neurogastroenterol Motil. 2010;22(1):42–9, e7-8.
80. Shin A, Acosta A, Camilleri M, Boldingh A, Burton D, Ryks M, et al. A randomized trial of 5-hydroxytryptamine4-receptor agonist, YKP10811, on colonic transit and bowel function in functional constipation. Clin Gastroenterol Hepatol. 2015;13(4):701–8.e1.
81. Tack J, Depoortere I, Bisschops R, Verbeke K, Janssens J, Peeters T. Influence of ghrelin on gastric emptying and meal-related symptoms in idiopathic gastroparesis. Aliment Pharmacol Ther. 2005;22(9):847–53.
82. Shin A, Camilleri M, Busciglio I, Burton D, Stoner E, Noonan P, et al. Randomized controlled phase Ib study of ghrelin agonist, RM-131, in type 2 diabetic women with delayed gastric emptying: pharmacokinetics and pharmacodynamics. Diabetes Care. 2013;36(1):41–8.
83. Shin A, Camilleri M, Busciglio I, Burton D, Smith SA, Vella A, et al. The ghrelin agonist RM-131 accelerates gastric emptying of solids and reduces symptoms in patients with type 1 diabetes mellitus. Clin Gastroenterol Hepatol. 2013;11(11):1453–9.e4.
84. Nelson AD, Camilleri M, Acosta A, Busciglio I, Linker Nord S, Boldingh A, et al. Effects of ghrelin receptor agonist, relamorelin, on gastric motor functions and satiation in healthy volunteers. Neurogastroenterol Motil. 2016;28(11):1705–13.
85. Lembo A, Camilleri M, McCallum R, Sastre R, Breton C, Spence S, et al. Relamorelin reduces vomiting frequency and severity and accelerates gastric emptying in adults with diabetic gastroparesis. Gastroenterology. 2016;151(1):87–96.e6.
86. Rojas C, Slusher BS. Pharmacological mechanisms of 5-HT(3) and tachykinin NK(1) receptor antagonism to prevent chemotherapy-induced nausea and vomiting. Eur J Pharmacol. 2012;684(1-3):1–7.
87. Zhang Y, Yang Y, Zhang Z, Fang W, Kang S, Luo Y, et al. Neurokinin-1 receptor antagonist-based triple regimens in preventing chemotherapy-induced nausea and vomiting: a network meta-analysis. J Natl Cancer Inst. 2017;109(2):djw217.
88. Pasricha PJYK, Sarosiek I, et al. Aprepitant for symptoms of gastroparesis and related disorders: the APRON randomized clinical trial. Am J Gastroenterol. 2016;111:S480–1.
89. Chong K, Dhatariya K. A case of severe, refractory diabetic gastroparesis managed by prolonged use of aprepitant. Nat Rev Endocrinol. 2009;5(5):285–8.
90. Fahler J, Wall GC, Leman BI. Gastroparesis-associated refractory nausea treated with aprepitant. Ann Pharmacother. 2012;46(12):e38.
91. Prakash C, Clouse RE. Cyclic vomiting syndrome in adults: clinical features and response to tricyclic antidepressants. Am J Gastroenterol. 1999;94(10):2855–60.
92. Sawhney MS, Prakash C, Lustman PJ, Clouse RE. Tricyclic antidepressants for chronic vomiting in diabetic patients. Dig Dis Sci. 2007;52(2):418–24.
93. Parkman HP, Van Natta ML, Abell TL, McCallum RW, Sarosiek I, Nguyen L, et al. Effect of nortriptyline on symptoms of idiopathic gastroparesis: the NORIG randomized clinical trial. JAMA. 2013;310(24):2640–9.
94. Kim SW, Shin IS, Kim JM, Kang HC, Mun JU, Yang SJ, et al. Mirtazapine for severe gastroparesis unresponsive to conventional prokinetic treatment. Psychosomatics. 2006;47(5):440–2.
95. Johnstone M, Buddhdev P, Peter M, Diggory R. Mirtazapine: a solution for postoperative gastroparesis? BMJ Case Rep. 2009;2009.
96. Gooden JY, Takahashi PY. Mirtazapine treatment of diabetic gastroparesis as a novel method to reduce tube-feed residual: a case report. J Med Case Rep. 2013;7:38.
97. Song J, Lin N, Tian F, Li Y, Li Y. Successful treatment of gastroparesis with the antidepressant mirtazapine: a case report. J Nippon Medical School Nippon Ika Daigaku Zasshi. 2014;81(6):392–4.
98. Kundu S, Rogal S, Alam A, Levinthal DJ. Rapid improvement in post-infectious gastroparesis symptoms with mirtazapine. World J Gastroenterol. 2014;20(21):6671–4.

99. Anttila SA, Leinonen EV. A review of the pharmacological and clinical profile of mirtazapine. CNS Drug Rev. 2001;7(3):249–64.
100. Yin J, Song J, Lei Y, Xu X, Chen JD. Prokinetic effects of mirtazapine on gastrointestinal transit. Am J Physiol Gastrointest Liver Physiol. 2014;306(9):G796–801.
101. Jeong ID, Camilleri M, Shin A, Iturrino J, Boldingh A, Busciglio I, et al. A randomised, placebo-controlled trial comparing the effects of tapentadol and oxycodone on gastrointestinal and colonic transit in healthy humans. Aliment Pharmacol Ther. 2012;35(9):1088–96.
102. Maurer AH, Krevsky B, Knight LC, Brown K. Opioid and opioid-like drug effects on whole-gut transit measured by scintigraphy. J Nucl Med. 1996;37(5):818–22.
103. Dursteler C, Mases A, Fernandez V, Pol O, Puig MM. Interaction between tramadol and two anti-emetics on nociception and gastrointestinal transit in mice. Eur J Pain. 2006;10(7):629–38.
104. James AN, Ryan JP, Parkman HP. Inhibitory effects of botulinum toxin on pyloric and antral smooth muscle. Am J Physiol Gastrointest Liver Physiol. 2003;285(2):G291–7.
105. Miller LS, Szych GA, Kantor SB, Bromer MQ, Knight LC, Maurer AH, et al. Treatment of idiopathic gastroparesis with injection of botulinum toxin into the pyloric sphincter muscle. Am J Gastroenterol. 2002;97(7):1653–60.
106. Ezzeddine D, Jit R, Katz N, Gopalswamy N, Bhutani MS. Pyloric injection of botulinum toxin for treatment of diabetic gastroparesis. Gastrointest Endosc. 2002;55(7):920–3.
107. Lacy BE, Zayat EN, Crowell MD, Schuster MM. Botulinum toxin for the treatment of gastroparesis: a preliminary report. Am J Gastroenterol. 2002;97(6):1548–52.
108. Bromer MQ, Friedenberg F, Miller LS, Fisher RS, Swartz K, Parkman HP. Endoscopic pyloric injection of botulinum toxin a for the treatment of refractory gastroparesis. Gastrointest Endosc. 2005;61(7):833–9.
109. Coleski R, Anderson MA, Hasler WL. Factors associated with symptom response to pyloric injection of botulinum toxin in a large series of gastroparesis patients. Dig Dis Sci. 2009;54(12):2634–42.
110. Friedenberg FK, Palit A, Parkman HP, Hanlon A, Nelson DB. Botulinum toxin a for the treatment of delayed gastric emptying. Am J Gastroenterol. 2008;103(2):416–23.
111. Arts J, Holvoet L, Caenepeel P, Bisschops R, Sifrim D, Verbeke K, et al. Clinical trial: a randomized-controlled crossover study of intrapyloric injection of botulinum toxin in gastroparesis. Aliment Pharmacol Ther. 2007;26(9):1251–8.
112. Wang CP, Kao CH, Chen WK, Lo WY, Hsieh CL. A single-blinded, randomized pilot study evaluating effects of electroacupuncture in diabetic patients with symptoms suggestive of gastroparesis. J Altern Complement Med. 2008;14(7):833–9.
113. Camilleri M. Clinical practice. Diabetic gastroparesis. N Engl J Med. 2007;356:820–9.

Endoscopic Management: Interventions at the Pylorus

70

Andrew T. Strong and Matthew D. Kroh

Introduction

Gastroparesis is a functional disorder defined by delayed gastric emptying in the absence of mechanical obstruction and produces a myriad of symptoms for patients, including nausea, vomiting, early satiety, gastroesophageal reflux, abdominal bloating, and chronic abdominal pain [1]. Classically, gastroparesis is divided by etiology into medication-induced, postsurgical, diabetic, and idiopathic etiologies. Recent work has also associated gastroparesis with a number of additional neurological and connective tissue disease processes [2–4]. Gastroparesis is a spectrum of disease states unified by similar symptoms and objective finding of delayed gastric emptying. The development of new technologies to dynamically assess gastric neuromuscular function, innervation, and integration has enabled an understanding of the carefully choreographed array of myoelectric impulses, mechanical end effect, and neurohormonal regulation that together accommodate a food bolus and promote forward propulsive forces to empty the stomach. Delayed gastric emptying arises from perturbations of this choreography, impairing gastric accommodation, producing hypomotility of the gastric antrum, and generating intermittent pylorospasm [4].

Over the past decade, the convergence of three parallel developments has abetted the development of endoscopic treatments for gastroparesis at the pylorus. First, accumulated evidence about the beneficial role pyloric disruption has to correct gastric emptying in gastric conduits used for esophageal reconstruction and in mechanical gastric outlet obstruction. Second, the era of natural orifice transluminal

A. T. Strong
Department of General Surgery, Cleveland Clinic, Cleveland, OH, USA

M. D. Kroh (✉)
Digestive Disease Institute, Cleveland Clinic Lerner College of Medicine,
Department of General Surgery, Cleveland Clinic, Abu Dhabi, United Arab Emirates
e-mail: KrohM@ClevelandClinicAbuDhabi.ae; krohm@ccf.org

J. Grams et al. (eds.), *The SAGES Manual of Foregut Surgery*,
https://doi.org/10.1007/978-3-319-96122-4_70

endoscopic surgery (NOTES) ushered in a rapid development of new interventional endoscopic techniques and devices. And third is the renewed evidence that functional irregularities of the pylorus, including pylorospasm, contribute to delayed gastric emptying in patients with gastroparesis. This chapter will examine clinical outcomes and the technical conduct of endoscopic techniques aimed at the pylorus for treatment of gastroparesis.

Structure of the Pylorus

The pylorus is defined as the roughly 1.5–3 cm anatomic region between the distal antrum of the stomach and capacitive duodenal bulb, where longitudinal folds intermittently occlude the lumen. Structurally, it is bound by the proximal pyloric loop and distal pyloric loops. The proximal pyloric loop is a flattened, oblique muscular ring located near the duodenal bulb along the lesser curvature of the stomach, coursing several centimeters more proximal along the greater curvature. The distal pyloric loop is a more prominent muscle ring that restricts the lumen and defines the pyloric orifice. These two loops meet along the lesser curvature in the pyloric torus, a distinct ring comprised of a combination of fat, muscle, and a connective tissue. The collagenous component of this ring serves as the insertion of the longitudinal gastric muscle fibers, stabilizes the mucosa along the distal pyloric loop, and decouples myoelectric impulses from the stomach and duodenum [5].

Changes to the Neuromuscular Structure and Function of the Stomach Associated with Gastroparesis

Better understanding of gastroparesis and dyspepsia as disease processes has allowed for improved delineation that gastric neuromuscular function plays in both the normal and pathological state. For instance, the central role that interstitial cells of Cajal (ICC) play in both idiopathic and diabetic gastroparesis differentiates those disease states from postsurgical gastroparesis. As our understanding of these diseases has become more nuanced, disruption of particular sub-processes of gastric emptying has been associated with each etiology. As understanding increases, physicians may be better able to assess disease progression and match therapeutic interventions to the disease state.

Postsurgical Gastroparesis

A number of surgical procedures result in intentional or accidental vagal injury. Some examples include truncal, selective, and highly selective vagotomies, esophagectomy, and various fundoplications. Alterations in gastric emptying were often noted following vagotomy for peptic ulcer disease. In an attempt to allay problematic delays in gastric emptying, pyloroplasty was often performed prophylactically.

Gastroparesis that results from vagal injury is marked by antral hypomotility and poor antroduodenal coordination. Surprisingly, migrating motor complexes (MMC) are still noted in post-vagotomy patients, which are supported by the continued histological presence of ICCs. Perhaps for this reason, gastric function is sometimes recoverable after vagal nerve injuries. However, the lack of vagal cooperation with the MMCs and the duodenogastric reflex is more often irreversible. As a proportion of gastroparetic patients, a postsurgical etiology is explanatory in only a minority of patients, but poor motor function at the pylorus makes an attractive therapeutic target.

Idiopathic Gastroparesis

Idiopathic gastroparesis comprises those patients without a clear surgical or diabetic history as a primary etiology for their gastroparesis symptoms. There is a significant proportion of patients who recall a viral prodrome prior to the onset of gastroparesis symptoms. Histological evaluation of gastric tissue from idiopathic gastroparetic patients reveals a significant loss of ICCs [6, 7]. Some patients with a viral prodrome will experience reversal of their symptoms spontaneously over 6–24 months, despite similar histologic evidence of ICC dropout while symptomatic. Among patients with idiopathic gastroparesis, dysrhythmias are more common when compared to postsurgical gastroparesis [8]. It is worth noting that patients who were previously categorized as idiopathic have been found to have other causes for delayed gastric emptying, including several connective tissue and neurological disorders [9].

Diabetic Gastroparesis

In the United States, the incidence of diabetes is increasing rapidly. Chronic hyperglycemia that results from diabetes has systemic end-organ effects, including irreversible retinopathy, nephropathy, and neuropathy. Diabetic gastroparesis can be considered an enteric neuropathy that produces an array of perturbations in gross neuromuscular gastric function. While not all patients experience all manifestations, diabetic gastroparesis is marked by abnormal distribution of food particles within the stomach, impaired fundic relaxation, reduced incidence of antral conduction of MMCs, antral hypomotility and dilation, dysrhythmias, and smooth muscle cell (SMC) dysfunction [6, 10]. Increased resting pyloric tone and pylorospasm prematurely contract the pylorus, preventing peristaltic emptying [11]. Chronic hyperglycemia also reduces the prokinetic action of certain medications, making medical therapy challenging as well. Histological manifestations that underlie these changes include loss of ICCs, abnormal nerve termini, and abnormal connections to SMCs and other neurons [6, 10].

While hyperglycemia is likely responsible for these effects, differences exist between type 1 and type 2 diabetics [9]. In type 1 diabetes, gastroparesis generally occurs at a younger age and tends to produce more severe delays in gastric emptying. Type 2 diabetics, on the other hand, are more likely to be obese, tend to have a longer duration of hyperglycemia prior to onset of gastroparesis symptoms, experience more early satiety, have milder delays in gastric emptying, and more likely to have gastric dysrhythmias. Gastric emptying may actually be accelerated early in the diabetes disease course in type 2 diabetics. Dysregulation of gastric neuromuscular function can produce erratic values in blood glucose as delays in the delivery of nutrients to the duodenum do not match insulin delivery, resulting in hypoglycemia [12]. This is more common in patients that use exogenous insulin.

Indications for Pyloric Intervention

The mainstays of therapy for gastroparesis are initially antiemetic and prokinetic therapies, which are reviewed in Chap. 69. Unfortunately, due to either progressive disease or receptor downregulation or both, medications tend to loose efficacy over time. This is compounded by significant concerns regarding side effects for some medications used to treat gastroparesis [13]. With delayed gastric emptying, one or several of the sub-processes that together move mechanically digested food into the small intestine are altered. The principle of pyloric disruption is to maintain pyloric patency, removing pylorospasm as an obstructive pathology and rendering less significant the poor peristaltic food convection.

The treatment of gastroparesis occurs within a multidisciplinary clinic at the authors' institution. Patients with confirmed diagnoses of gastroparesis are generally trialed on medical therapies initially, as well as assessment and management of other associated comorbidities. If medical therapies produce undesirable side effects, lose efficacy, or are ineffective, collectively summarized as medically refractory, then referral is made to the surgical and surgical endoscopy providers for consideration of other therapeutic options. Patients with severe malnutrition are often referred earlier in order to establish enteral access to reach a minimum level of nutrition. The authors advocate that a diagnostic endoscopy precede any planned endoscopic intervention for gastroparesis to evaluate for other coincident pathologies, such as peptic ulcer disease or gastroesophageal reflux, and to rule out mechanical obstruction [14].

Pneumatic or Hydraulic Dilation

Pneumatic or hydraulic dilation of the pylorus has only recently been explored scientifically as a therapy for gastroparesis. Gourcerol and colleagues were the first to report on the effect of pyloric dilation in gastroparesis [15]. That study included 27 patients with gastroparesis, 21 healthy patients, and 5 patients who had undergone esophagectomy with gastric conduit reconstruction but who had not had a pyloroplasty. Baseline measurement of pyloric resting pressure and compliance was performed with an EndoFLIP® catheter (Crospon, Inc. Galway, Ireland), using impedance planimetry while fasting. For the ten gastroparetic patients with the lowest baseline compliance, pyloric dilation was performed using a hydraulic balloon dilated to 20 mm and 6.0 atmospheres of pressure. Impedance planimetry measurements were evaluated post procedure day 10 for these patients. All subjects completed the gastrointestinal quality of life index (GIQLI) prior to endoscopy and at follow-up. Their results confirm that gastroparesis is associated with decreased compliance (16.9 vs. 25.2 mm^2/mmHg, $p < 0.05$), but resting pressure was not different. Dilation was associated with an increase in compliance from 7.4 ± 0.4 mm^2/mmHg to 20.1 ± 4.9 mm^2/mmHg ($p < 0.01$). Dilation was also associated with significant decrease in $t_{1/2}$ for gastric emptying and GIQLI score compared to baseline [15].

In 2016, Wellington and colleagues published a retrospective case series of patients with gastroparesis accrued over 10 years with no prior pyloric interventions. Each of the patients included had normal gastric myoelectric activity (3.0 cycles per minute), as assessed by electrogastrogram. Patients either underwent injection with botulinum toxin A or balloon dilation to 20 mm at the pylorus. While 78% of patients in their series responded to pyloric intervention, this was not stratified to intervention [16].

These studies are insufficient to support any recommendation about pyloric dilation as a treatment modality. However, since both studies include measurements of physiologic parameters of gastric function as part of their criteria, this underscores the need for further studies to help discriminate these patients and route them to appropriate therapeutic interventions. Potentially, pneumatic/hydraulic dilation may be most useful as a screening tool to determine what patients are most likely to benefit from more permanent pyloric disruption.

Transpyloric Stenting

Self-expanding metal stents (SEMS) are composed of metal alloys, either with or without a polymeric covering for part or all of their length. Stents are constrained on a delivery catheter either delivered through or alongside the endoscope and then expand with deployment. Some stents can be delivered and deployed using only endoscopic guidance, while others require or benefit from fluoroscopic guidance. Some commercially available stents are approved for transpyloric application in the presence of malignant obstructions; however, transpyloric stenting for gastroparesis is off-label in most cases. A comprehensive review of stent technology is outside the scope of this chapter, but it has been reviewed elsewhere [17].

Clarke and colleagues made the first report of transpyloric stenting in gastroparetic patients [18]. In that series a through-the-scope double-layered, covered nitinol stent was placed across the pylorus under endoscopic guidance (Niti-S™, Taewoong Medical South Korea), with the proximal end within the gastric antrum. Each of the three patients experienced significant symptomatic relief and improvement of gastric emptying studies at greater than 90-day follow-up. One of the patients experienced stent migration requiring re-intervention and stent replacement.

Stent migration is the greatest challenge to transpyloric stenting, and retrieval may require deep endoscopic techniques and may not be possible endoscopically.

One case series reviewed 48 transpyloric stents placed in 30 patients, secured with endoscopic suturing (OverStitch®, Apollo Endosurgery, Austin, Texas), over the scope clip (OTSC®, Ovesco, Tubingen Germany), through the scope clip, or no fixation [19]. Endoscopic suturing was the best technique for securement in that series, with an average of two sutures placed per stent. However, nearly half (48%) of suture-secured stents still migrated [19]. Despite that, 75% of the patients experienced clinical improvement in symptoms, and 11 of 16 (68.8%) with post-procedural gastric emptying studies had an objective improvement in gastric emptying. This series is too small to ascertain what fixation technique is superior. Moreover, the OverStitch® device, currently the only endoscopic suturing device available in the United States, requires a double-lumen endoscope and represents an increased cost in consumable supplies for the case. Similarly, OTSC® clips are more costly single-use devices, and placement requires removal and reintroduction of the endoscope.

Endoscopic Injection of Botulinum Toxin at the Pylorus

Early studies of botulinum toxin were driven by three factors. First, botulinum toxin had shown efficacy in relaxing the lower esophageal sphincter in achalasia [20]. Second, apart from establishing enteral access, endoscopic therapy for gastroparesis was relatively unexplored. And third was evidence that pyloric disruption aids gastric emptying for gastric interposition grafts when used for esophageal reconstruction.

Botulinum toxin A is one of seven biochemically distinct neurotoxins produced by the anaerobic bacteria of the *Clostridium* genus. Despite differences in polypeptide molecular structure, each of the botulinum toxins has the same net effect, binding to cholinergic peripheral nerves, preventing exocytosis of acetylcholine and other neurotransmitters [21, 22]. This produces a chemodenervation, but not cell death. Nanogram quantities of botulinum toxin can be fatal. Both botulinum toxin A (Botox®, Allergan, Dublin, Ireland, and Dysport® Ipsen Biopharmacetuicals, Binding Ridge, New Jersey) and botulinum toxin B (NeuroBloc®, Elan Pharmaceuticals, Dublin, Ireland) are commercially available.

At the pylorus, acetylcholine is released by both ICCs and vagal efferent neurons that collectively control antroduodenal coordination. Botulinum toxin is highly specific for these peripheral cholinergic nerves and produces smooth muscle paralysis following injection, reducing pyloric tone and allowing greater gastric emptying. The first report of pyloric injection of botulinum toxin in the pylorus as a treatment for gastroparesis was on six patients with diabetic gastroparesis [23]. Using a 25G injection needle, a total of 100 units of botulinum toxin A were injected in 4 quadrants of the pylorus. Each of the patients showed at least mild improvement in symptom scores at 2 and 6 weeks following injection. A 2-h solid-phase scintigraphic gastric emptying study was completed at 48 h and 6 weeks after injection, which were all also objectively improved from baseline [23]. A similar report was made shortly thereafter, including 10 patients with medically refractory idiopathic gastroparesis, and using 100 units of botulinum toxin A injected in the pylorus [24].

Symptoms and gastric emptying both improved in that case series and were highly correlated [24]. A third publication that same year showed similar results of pyloric injection of botulinum toxin A, but authors used a higher dose of 200 units [25]. All three patients included in that series had symptom improvement; however, objective gastric emptying was improved in only two out of three patients included. Additional open-label studies followed that further confirmed these findings [26–28]. The use of 100 and 200 unit dosing reflects the size of the commercially available vials of Botox® (Allergan, Dublin, Ireland) used in each study.

Two randomized, double-blind, placebo-controlled trials followed these retrospective cases series. The first was performed in Belgium, and included 23 patients, with a crossover design [29]. All patients underwent endoscopic injection of 100 units of botulinum toxin A or saline and then a second endoscopy with the other medication 4 weeks later. Symptoms were evaluated at baseline, 4 and 8 weeks with the Gastroparesis Cardinal Symptom Index (GCSI) [30], and subjects underwent gastric emptying study with a breath test at the same time points. There was symptom improvement and objective improvement in gastric emptying with both treatments, but the effects were not different statistically. A second study randomized 32 patients to either saline or 200 units of botulinum toxin A injection at the pylorus [31]. GSCI and scintigraphic gastric emptying studies were performed at baseline and 4 weeks. An improvement in GCSI of ≥9 points was defined as a response. At 4 weeks follow up, symptoms improved in 37.5% of the botulinum toxin group and 56.3% of the saline placebo group ($p = 0.29$) [31]. Two-hour solid-phase scintigraphic gastric emptying time was statistically different from baseline in the botulinum toxin A (−16.3 ± 22.9%, $p = 0.02$), but not different in the placebo group (−10.8 ± 20.6%, $p = 0.08$); these changes were not statistically different from each other ($p = 0.052$) [31]. These two negative results and prior case series were enumerated in a systematic review, which concluded that based on current evidence, botulinum toxin is not recommended as a treatment for gastroparesis [32].

Despite this, botulinum toxin continues to be used to treat gastroparesis. It is now recognized that poor patient selection partially accounted for negative results in the randomized controlled trials. Neither randomized controlled trial assessed for alterations in pyloric tone or function prior to randomization and thus likely included patients without this pathology [32, 33]. They were also both underpowered to assess the conclusions they sought to investigate. A large retrospective case series was published in 2009 to attempt to ascertain what subgroups responded to botulinum toxin therapy [34]. They identified that a greater proportion of patients had symptom improvement with higher doses of botulinum toxin (54.2% at 100 units, 76.7% at 200 units; odds ratio of 2.79, 95%CI 1.20–6.51) [34]. Further, most who had symptom improvement with a first injection had similar results with a second injection (73.4%) [34]. In their analysis, female gender, age less than 50 years, and postsurgical gastroparesis etiology were favorably associated with symptom improvement [34]. This underscores that selectivity is warranted and greater study, likely in a prospective design, is needed [35]. Similar to hydraulic dilation of the pylorus and transpyloric stenting, injection of botulinum toxin may be best suited as a screening test for patients who would benefit from more permanent pyloric disruption.

Peroral Endoscopic Pyloromyotomy (POP)

An accumulating amount of evidence exists for surgical pyloric disruption to augment gastric emptying in gastroparetic patients [36–38]. Compared to the previously discussed therapies, the major advantage of pyloroplasty or pyloromyotomy is the durability of procedure. The endoscopic approach presents a less invasive approach compared to the open or even laparoscopic techniques.

The origins of peroral endoscopic pyloromyotomy (POP) can be traced to two other pyloric pathologies. Endoscopic pyloromyotomy has been reported as a therapy for recalcitrant peptic strictures and hypertrophic pyloric stenosis in infants and been effective in reducing pyloric obstruction in small case series and case reports [39, 40]. In both cases, a linear mucosotomy was made, and the muscle fibers divided. The mucosotomy was not closed. Since those reports, per oral endoscopic myotomy (POEM) was introduced and is now widely regarded as an effective therapy for esophageal achalasia, a disease marked by hypertonicity of the lower esophageal sphincter. The submucosal tunneling technique used in a POEM to approach the muscle fibers of the distal esophagus was first adapted to the pylorus by Kawai and colleagues in a pig model [41]. In these four pigs, the median resting pressure of the pylorus was immediately reduced by 63%, which was durable over 2 weeks duration. A nearly identical technique was outlined in a second study by Chaves et al. [42]. Necropsy confirmed complete division of the circular muscles of the pylorus was achieved but noted two small perforations [42].

The first human application of submucosal tunnel used to complete an endoscopic pyloromyotomy was published by Khashab and colleagues [43]. While the authors introduced the term gastric peroral endoscopic myotomy (G-POEM), this procedure has since become known more commonly as peroral pyloromyotomy (POP), our preferred nomenclature. This initial case report detailed a female patient with diabetic gastroparesis from long-standing type 1 diabetes. She had previously responded to transpyloric stenting, but repeated stent migration had proven problematic. She was either not a candidate for or declined other surgical options. Following endoscopic pyloromyotomy, symptom improvement persisted for the 12-week follow-up period despite little change in objective gastric emptying on repeat imaging [43]. This report was followed by a case report of successful performance of endoscopic pyloromyotomy by a second group in a patient with postsurgical gastroparesis [44].

A few prospective series of POP therapy have been published since those case reports. Shlomovits et al. performed seven POP procedures including two patients with postsurgical gastroparesis and five patients with idiopathic gastroparesis [45]. The first six cases completed were performed simultaneous with another laparoscopic foregut operation, allowing not only laparoscopic observation of the POP procedure but the ability to intervene, laparoscopically if necessary [45]. There were two complications, one bleeding 2 weeks post procedure and the other pneumonia. Six patients had improvement in symptoms (85.7%). The patient that did not have symptom improvement with POP subsequently underwent a laparoscopic pyloroplasty and again failed to improve. At 3 months follow-up, four patients had objective improvement or normalization of gastric emptying [45]. Other groups have published additional small case series [46–49]. The first multicenter trial was published in 2016 and included 30 patients across 5 centers [48]. These patients were split relatively evenly among the major gastroparesis etiologies (11 diabetic, 12 postsurgical, 7 idiopathic). Two adverse events occurred, capnoperitoneum and gastric ulceration, each in one patient. The latter was attributed to patient failure to comply with post-procedural proton pump inhibitor therapy. At a median follow-up of 5.5 months, 26 patients had improved symptoms (86.7%). Only 17 had gastric emptying studies available, but 8 had normalized gastric emptying, and 6 had improvement in gastric emptying time.

Despite these promising early results, some caveats are necessary. First, endoscopists that were already skilled in POEM procedures performed all of the POP procedures that have currently been reported. Fine control of the endoscope can be difficult in the distal stomach, which is why some authors position the mucosotomy along the greater curve, where the curvature of the stomach can help stabilize the endoscope. An overtube may be used for stabilization as well. A number of sizeable blood vessels also enter the distal antrum, mainly along the greater curve, and can be difficult to control, especially for the endoscopist not familiar with endoscopic control of hemorrhage within a submucosal tunnel. Finally, though the distal extent of the pylorus is often easily identified, the duodenum presents no clear demarcation, and is thin-walled, presenting the possibility of injury [37].

Technique: Peroral Endoscopic Pyloromyotomy (POP)

POP is performed in the operating room or in the endoscopy suite under general anesthesia. The patient is positioned supine on the table, general anesthesia is induced, and the patient is endotracheally intubated. Antibiotic prophylaxis is routinely administered, including coverage for enteric bacteria, anaerobes, and fungus. A standard length, high-definition, forward-viewing gastroscope is used, fitted with an oblique or tapered-tipped endoscopic dissection cap (Barrx™ RFA Cleaning Cap, Covidien, Mansfield, MA) secured with a tape. Carbon dioxide insufflation is used throughout the procedure. An electrosurgical generator (Vio® 300D, Erbe Elektromedizin GmbH, Tubingen, Germany) is used to apply energy for both cutting and coagulation (Endo Cut effect 2 and Spray coag effect 2). A full diagnostic upper endoscopy is performed, with careful attention to pathology in the antrum, pylorus, and duodenum, as well as lavage and evacuation of the stomach if needed. A location for the mucosotomy is located 3–4 cm proximal to the pylorus. We prefer to select a site along the lesser curvature, though other publications also describe the use of a greater curvature site. The lesser curve position allows for the mucosa to reside below the scope in the tunnel, similar to the typical orientation in a POEM procedure. A mucosal lift is performed using an aliquot of a solution of 5–15 mL of 1% methylene blue dye and 1 mL of 1:1000 epinephrine mixed in 500 mL of 0.9% sodium chloride (see Fig. 70.1a). A triangular tip knife (KD-640 L, Olympus, Tokyo, Japan) is used to make a transverse mucosotomy 1.5–2 cm in length using

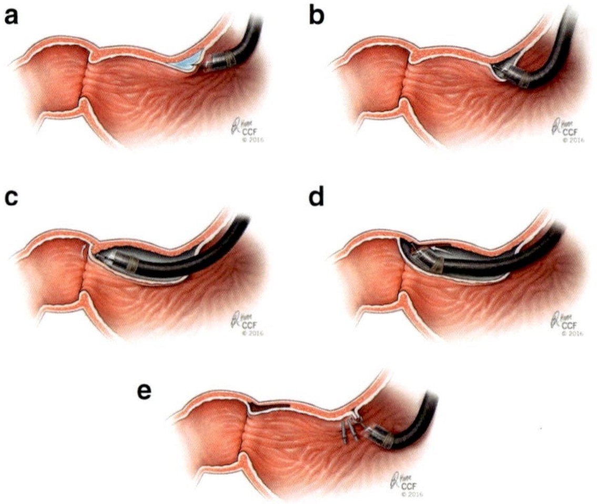

Fig. 70.1 Steps of a peroral pyloromyotomy (POP). (**a**) Submucosal fluid injection to produce mucosal lift, located 3–4 cm proximal to the pylorus along the lesser curve of the stomach; (**b**) Entrance into the submucosal plane and beginning of submucosal tunnel; (**c**) Completion of submucosal tunnel and visualization of the muscle of the pylorus; (**d**) Division of the pyloric muscle to complete pyloromyotomy; (**e**) Closure of the mucosotomy with hemostatic through the scope clips

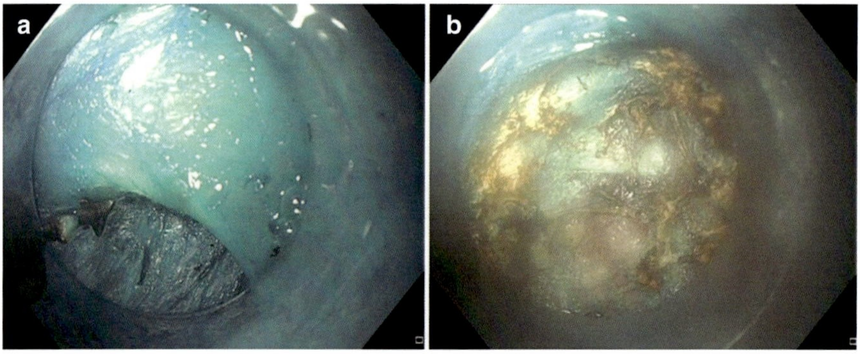

Fig. 70.2 Intraprocedural image from peroral pyloromyotomy (POP): (**a**) Complete visualization of the pyloric muscle prior to division; (**b**) Completed pyloromyotomy seen from within the submucosal tunnel. (Images Courtesy of Dr. Matthew Kroh, Cleveland Clinic Foundation)

cutting current. Use of a round-tip knife has also been described (DualKnife™, Olympus, Tokyo, Japan). The endoscope is advanced into the mucosotomy, and a submucosal tunnel is created with spray cautery to the point that the pylorus is visualized and mobilized up to the duodenal bulb (see Figs. 70.1b, c, and 70.2a). The pylorus is divided completely using cautery in a retrograde manner back toward the stomach for 2 cm (see Figs. 70.1d and 70.2b). Following division of the pyloric muscle fibers, visual inspection of the pylorus is completed, and typically there is already an increase in the pyloric diameter. The mucosotomy is then closed with through-the-scope clips (see Fig. 70.1e).

Post-procedure Management

Our protocol is to admit patients overnight, and they are kept *nil* per os after the procedure. On post-procedure day 1, a contrast-enhanced fluoroscopic upper gastrointestinal series is obtained to verify that there is no obstruction or leak. Following this, a clear liquid diet is introduced. The patient is advanced to a pureed diet prior to discharge and instructed to maintain this diet for 2 weeks. Proton pump inhibitors and sucralfate are maintained through the perioperative period and for 4 weeks postdischarge.

Gastroparesis is a challenging and increasingly prevalent disease with many options for treatment. The success of any technique is dependent on the etiology of the disease, and treatment failures are not uncommon. Endoscopic treatments for gastroparesis that target the pylorus are evolving techniques that hold promise in early studies. The success of these endoscopic treatments will depend on the conduct and reporting of larger series demonstrating efficacy and durability over the long term.

References

1. Hasler WL. Gastroparesis: symptoms, evaluation, and treatment. Gastroenterol Clin N Am. 2007;36:619–647, ix. https://doi.org/10.1016/j.gtc.2007.07.004.
2. Camilleri M, Bharucha AE, Farrugia G. Epidemiology, mechanisms, and management of diabetic gastroparesis. Clin Gastroenterol Hepatol. 2011;9:5–12.; quiz e7. https://doi.org/10.1016/j.cgh.2010.09.022.
3. Parkman HP, Hasler WL, Fisher RS, American Gastroenterological Association. American Gastroenterological Association medical position statement: diagnosis and treatment of gastroparesis. Gastroenterology. 2004;127:1589–91.
4. Nguyen LA, Snape WJ. Clinical presentation and pathophysiology of gastroparesis. Gastroenterol Clin N Am. 2015;44:21–30. https://doi.org/10.1016/j.gtc.2014.11.003.
5. Ramkumar D, Schulze KS. The pylorus. Neurogastroenterol Motil. 2005;17(Suppl 1):22–30. https://doi.org/10.1111/j.1365-2982.2005.00664.x.
6. Grover M, Farrugia G, Lurken MS, Bernard CE, Faussone-Pellegrini MS, Smyrk TC, Parkman HP, Abell TL, Snape WJ, Hasler WL, Ünalp-Arida A, Nguyen L, Koch KL, Calles J, Lee L, Tonascia J, Hamilton FA, Pasricha PJ, NIDDK Gastroparesis Clinical Research Consortium. Cellular changes in diabetic and idiopathic gastroparesis. Gastroenterology. 2011;140:1575–1585.e8. https://doi.org/10.1053/j.gastro.2011.01.046.
7. Grover M, Bernard CE, Pasricha PJ, Lurken MS, Faussone-Pellegrini MS, Smyrk TC, Parkman HP, Abell TL, Snape WJ, Hasler WL, McCallum RW, Nguyen L, Koch KL, Calles J, Lee L, Tonascia J, Ünalp-Arida A, Hamilton FA, Farrugia G, NIDDK Gastroparesis Clinical Research Consortium (GpCRC). Clinical-histological associations in gastroparesis: results from the gastroparesis clinical research consortium. Neurogastroenterol Motil. 2012;24:531–539, e249. https://doi.org/10.1111/j.1365-2982.2012.01894.x.

8. Chen JD, Lin Z, Pan J, McCallum RW. Abnormal gastric myoelectrical activity and delayed gastric emptying in patients with symptoms suggestive of gastroparesis. Dig Dis Sci. 1996;41:1538–45.
9. Koch KL. Chapter 49: gastric neuromuscular function and neuromuscular disorders. In: Sleisenger Fordtrans Gastrointest. Liver Dis. 10th ed: Philadelphia, PA: Saunders Elsevier; 2016. p. 811–38.
10. Faussone-Pellegrini MS, Grover M, Pasricha PJ, Bernard CE, Lurken MS, Smyrk TC, Parkman HP, Abell TL, Snape WJ, Hasler WL, Unalp-Arida A, Nguyen L, Koch KL, Calles J, Lee L, Tonascia J, Hamilton FA, Farrugia G, NIDDK Gastroparesis Clinical Research Consortium (GpCRC). Ultrastructural differences between diabetic and idiopathic gastroparesis. J Cell Mol Med. 2012;16:1573–81. https://doi.org/10.1111/j.1582-4934.2011.01451.x.
11. Mearin F, Camilleri M, Malagelada JR. Pyloric dysfunction in diabetics with recurrent nausea and vomiting. Gastroenterology. 1986;90:1919–25.
12. Koch KL. Diabetic gastropathy: gastric neuromuscular dysfunction in diabetes mellitus: a review of symptoms, pathophysiology, and treatment. Dig Dis Sci. 1999;44:1061–75.
13. Ehrenpreis ED, Deepak P, Sifuentes H, Devi R, Du H, Leikin JB. The metoclopramide black box warning for tardive dyskinesia: effect on clinical practice, adverse event reporting, and prescription drug lawsuits. Am J Gastroenterol. 2013;108:866–72. https://doi.org/10.1038/ajg.2012.300.
14. ASGE Standards of Practice Committee, Fukami N, Anderson MA, Khan K, Harrison ME, Appalaneni V, Ben-Menachem T, Decker GA, Fanelli RD, Fisher L, Ikenberry SO, Jain R, Jue TL, Krinsky ML, Maple JT, Sharaf RN, Dominitz JA. The role of endoscopy in gastroduodenal obstruction and gastroparesis. Gastrointest Endosc. 2011;74:13–21. https://doi.org/10.1016/j.gie.2010.12.003.
15. Gourcerol G, Tissier F, Melchior C, Touchais JY, Huet E, Prevost G, Leroi AM, Ducrotte P. Impaired fasting pyloric compliance in gastroparesis and the therapeutic response to pyloric dilatation. Aliment Pharmacol Ther. 2015;41:360–7. https://doi.org/10.1111/apt.13053.
16. Wellington J, Scott B, Kundu S, Stuart P, Koch KL. Effect of endoscopic pyloric therapies for patients with nausea and vomiting and functional obstructive gastroparesis. Auton Neurosci. 2016;202:56. https://doi.org/10.1016/j.autneu.2016.07.004.
17. ASGE Technology Committee, Varadarajulu S, Banerjee S, Barth B, Desilets D, Kaul V, Kethu S, Pedrosa M, Pfau P, Tokar J, Wang A, Song L-MWK, Rodriguez S. Enteral stents. Gastrointest Endosc. 2011;74:455–64. https://doi.org/10.1016/j.gie.2011.04.011.
18. Clarke JO, Sharaiha RZ, Kord Valeshabad A, Lee LA, Kalloo AN, Khashab MA. Through-the-scope transpyloric stent placement improves symptoms and gastric emptying in patients with gastroparesis. Endoscopy. 2013;45(Suppl 2 UCTN):E189–90. https://doi.org/10.1055/s-0032-1326400.
19. Khashab MA, Besharati S, Ngamruengphong S, Kumbhari V, El Zein M, Stein EM, Tieu A, Mullin GE, Dhalla S, Nandwani MC, Singh V, Canto MI, Kalloo AN, Clarke JO. Refractory gastroparesis can be successfully managed with endoscopic transpyloric stent placement and fixation (with video). Gastrointest Endosc. 2015;82:1106–9. https://doi.org/10.1016/j.gie.2015.06.051.
20. Leyden JE, Moss AC, MacMathuna P. Endoscopic pneumatic dilation versus botulinum toxin injection in the management of primary achalasia. Cochrane Database Syst Rev. 2014:CD005046. https://doi.org/10.1002/14651858.CD005046.pub3.
21. Montecucco C, Molgó J. Botulinal neurotoxins: revival of an old killer. Curr Opin Pharmacol. 2005;5:274–9. https://doi.org/10.1016/j.coph.2004.12.006.
22. Vittal H, Pasricha PF. Botulinum toxin for gastrointestinal disorders: therapy and mechanisms. Neurotox Res. 2006;9:149–59.
23. Ezzeddine D, Jit R, Katz N, Gopalswamy N, Bhutani MS. Pyloric injection of botulinum toxin for treatment of diabetic gastroparesis. Gastrointest Endosc. 2002;55:920–3.
24. Miller LS, Szych GA, Kantor SB, Bromer MQ, Knight LC, Maurer AH, Fisher RS, Parkman HP. Treatment of idiopathic gastroparesis with injection of botulinum toxin

into the pyloric sphincter muscle. Am J Gastroenterol. 2002;97:1653–60. https://doi.org/10.1111/j.1572-0241.2002.05823.x.
25. Lacy BE, Zayat EN, Crowell MD, Schuster MM. Botulinum toxin for the treatment of gastroparesis: a preliminary report. Am J Gastroenterol. 2002;97:1548–52. https://doi.org/10.1111/j.1572-0241.2002.05741.x.
26. Lacy BE, Crowell MD, Schettler-Duncan A, Mathis C, Pasricha PJ. The treatment of diabetic gastroparesis with botulinum toxin injection of the pylorus. Diabetes Care. 2004;27:2341–7.
27. Bromer MQ, Friedenberg F, Miller LS, Fisher RS, Swartz K, Parkman HP. Endoscopic pyloric injection of botulinum toxin a for the treatment of refractory gastroparesis. Gastrointest Endosc. 2005;61:833–9.
28. Arts J, van Gool S, Caenepeel P, Verbeke K, Janssens J, Tack J. Influence of intrapyloric botulinum toxin injection on gastric emptying and meal-related symptoms in gastroparesis patients. Aliment Pharmacol Ther. 2006;24:661–7. https://doi.org/10.1111/j.1365-2036.2006.03019.x.
29. Arts J, Holvoet L, Caenepeel P, Bisschops R, Sifrim D, Verbeke K, Janssens J, Tack J. Clinical trial: a randomized-controlled crossover study of intrapyloric injection of botulinum toxin in gastroparesis. Aliment Pharmacol Ther. 2007;26:1251–8. https://doi.org/10.1111/j.1365-2036.2007.03467.x.
30. Revicki DA, Rentz AM, Dubois D, Kahrilas P, Stanghellini V, Talley NJ, Tack J. Gastroparesis cardinal symptom index (GCSI): development and validation of a patient reported assessment of severity of gastroparesis symptoms. Qual Life Res. 2004;13:833–44.
31. Friedenberg FK, Palit A, Parkman HP, Hanlon A, Nelson DB. Botulinum toxin a for the treatment of delayed gastric emptying. Am J Gastroenterol. 2008;103:416–23. https://doi.org/10.1111/j.1572-0241.2007.01676.x.
32. Bai Y, Xu M-J, Yang X, Xu C, Gao J, Zou D-W, Li Z-S. A systematic review on intrapyloric botulinum toxin injection for gastroparesis. Digestion. 2010;81:27–34. https://doi.org/10.1159/000235917.
33. Clarke JO, Snape WJ. Pyloric sphincter therapy: botulinum toxin, stents, and pyloromyotomy. Gastroenterol Clin N Am. 2015;44:127–36. https://doi.org/10.1016/j.gtc.2014.11.010.
34. Coleski R, Anderson MA, Hasler WL. Factors associated with symptom response to pyloric injection of botulinum toxin in a large series of gastroparesis patients. Dig Dis Sci. 2009;54:2634–42. https://doi.org/10.1007/s10620-008-0660-9.
35. Ukleja A, Tandon K, Shah K, Alvarez A. Endoscopic botox injections in therapy of refractory gastroparesis. World J Gastrointest Endosc. 2015;7:790–8. https://doi.org/10.4253/wjge.v7.i8.790.
36. Toro JP, Lytle NW, Patel AD, Davis SS, Christie JA, Waring JP, Sweeney JF, Lin E. Efficacy of laparoscopic pyloroplasty for the treatment of gastroparesis. J Am Coll Surg. 2014;218:652–60. https://doi.org/10.1016/j.jamcollsurg.2013.12.024.
37. Lebaras C, Swanstrom LL. Per-oral Pyloromyotomy (POP): an emerging application of submucosal tunneling for the treatment of refractory gastroparesis. Gastrointest Endosc Clin N Am. 2016;26:257–70. https://doi.org/10.1016/j.giec.2015.12.012.
38. Hibbard ML, Dunst CM, Swanström LL. Laparoscopic and endoscopic pyloroplasty for gastroparesis results in sustained symptom improvement. J Gastrointest Surg. 2011;15:1513–9. https://doi.org/10.1007/s11605-011-1607-6.
39. Hagiwara A, Sonoyama Y, Togawa T, Yamasaki J, Sakakura C, Yamagishi H. Combined use of electrosurgical incisions and balloon dilatation for the treatment of refractory post-operative pyloric stenosis. Gastrointest Endosc. 2001;53:504–8. https://doi.org/10.1067/mge.2001.113281.
40. Ibarguen-Secchia E. Endoscopic pyloromyotomy for congenital pyloric stenosis. Gastrointest Endosc. 2005;61:598–600.
41. Kawai M, Peretta S, Burckhardt O, Dallemagne B, Marescaux J, Tanigawa N. Endoscopic pyloromyotomy: a new concept of minimally invasive surgery for pyloric stenosis. Endoscopy. 2012;44:169–73. https://doi.org/10.1055/s-0031-1291475.
42. Chaves DM, Gusmon CC, Mestieri LHM, de Moura EGH, Veras MM, Pessorrusso FCS, Sakai P. A new technique for performing endoscopic pyloromyotomy by gastric

submucosal tunnel dissection. Surg Laparosc Endosc Percutan Tech. 2014;24:e92–4. https://doi.org/10.1097/SLE.0b013e31829cec0e.

43. Khashab MA, Stein E, Clarke JO, Saxena P, Kumbhari V, Chander Roland B, Kalloo AN, Stavropoulos S, Pasricha P, Inoue H. Gastric peroral endoscopic myotomy for refractory gastroparesis: first human endoscopic pyloromyotomy (with video). Gastrointest Endosc. 2013;78:764–8. https://doi.org/10.1016/j.gie.2013.07.019.
44. Chaves DM, de Moura EGH, Mestieri LHM, Artifon EL, Sakai P. Endoscopic pyloromyotomy via a gastric submucosal tunnel dissection for the treatment of gastroparesis after surgical vagal lesion. Gastrointest Endosc. 2014;80:164. https://doi.org/10.1016/j.gie.2014.03.045.
45. Shlomovitz E, Pescarus R, Cassera MA, Sharata AM, Reavis KM, Dunst CM, Swanström LL. Early human experience with per-oral endoscopic pyloromyotomy (POP). Surg Endosc. 2015;29:543–51. https://doi.org/10.1007/s00464-014-3720-6.
46. Gonzalez J-M, Lestelle V, Benezech A, Cohen J, Vitton V, Grimaud J-C, Barthet M. Gastric per-oral endoscopic myotomy with antropyloromyotomy in the treatment of refractory gastroparesis: clinical experience with follow-up and scintigraphic evaluation (with video). Gastrointest Endosc. 2016;85:132. https://doi.org/10.1016/j.gie.2016.07.050.
47. Mekaroonkamol P, Li LY, Dacha S, Xu Y, Keilin SD, Willingham FF, Cai Q. Gastric per-oral endoscopic pyloromyotomy (G-POEM) as a salvage therapy for refractory gastroparesis: a case series of different subtypes. Neurogastroenterol Motil. 2016;28:1272–7. https://doi.org/10.1111/nmo.12854.
48. Khashab MA, Ngamruengphong S, Carr-Locke D, Bapaye A, Benias PC, Serouya S, Dorwat S, Chaves DM, Artifon E, de Moura EG, Kumbhari V, Chavez YH, Bukhari M, Hajiyeva G, Ismail A, Chen Y-I, Chung H. Gastric per-oral endoscopic myotomy for refractory gastroparesis: results from the first multicenter study on endoscopic pyloromyotomy (with video). Gastrointest Endosc. 2016;85:123. https://doi.org/10.1016/j.gie.2016.06.048.
49. Gonzalez J-M, Vanbiervliet G, Vitton V, Benezech A, Lestelle V, Grimaud J-C, Barthet M. First European human gastric peroral endoscopic myotomy, for treatment of refractory gastroparesis. Endoscopy. 2015;47(Suppl 1 UCTN):E135–6. https://doi.org/10.1055/s-0034-1391821.

Endoscopic Management: Decompression and Feeding

71

Jeffrey Marks, Luis A. Martin del Campo, Shreya Gupta, Terence Jackson, Jennifer A. Kalil, and Aric Wogsland

Introduction

Gastroparesis is a complex disorder and has a significant impact on quality of life, healthcare costs, and morbidity/mortality [1]. Diabetes is the most commonly recognized etiology of gastroparesis. Other etiologies include postsurgical, iatrogenic, connective tissue disorders and idiopathic gastroparesis. Symptoms of gastroparesis include nausea, vomiting, abdominal bloating, and pain. These symptoms can lead to poor oral intake and caloric and nutritional deficits. For patients with severe gastroparesis who are unable to maintain nutrition via oral intake, and those with normal small bowel function, a feeding tube not only helps maintain metabolic needs but also improves symptoms and reduces hospitalization rates [2]. Gastrostomy tubes can also be used for decompression for relief of symptoms and provide better quality of life [3]. This review describes endoscopic methods of providing enteral access for feeding and decompression in patients with gastroparesis.

Endoscopic Feeding

Gastroduodenal dysmotility disorders are associated with weight loss, recurrent episodes of dehydration, and electrolyte disturbances. Enteral nutrition must be considered in patients with such disorders prior to parenteral routes. Enteral nutrition helps maintain mucosal integrity of the gastrointestinal tract and prevents bacterial translocation. It is also cheaper and less morbid compared to parenteral nutrition. Refractory gastroparesis is a challenging disorder and is one of the most common indications for

J. Marks · L. A. Martin del Campo (✉) · S. Gupta · T. Jackson · J. A. Kalil · A. Wogsland
Department of Surgery, University Hospitals Cleveland Medical Center, Cleveland, OH, USA

J. Grams et al. (eds.), *The SAGES Manual of Foregut Surgery*,
https://doi.org/10.1007/978-3-319-96122-4_71

post-pyloric feeding. Other indications for enteral post-pyloric feeding include severe acute and chronic pancreatitis, recurrent aspiration, severe gastroesophageal reflux, severe hyperemesis, and persistent nutritional compromise [4, 5] (Table 71.1).

Absolute contraindications for endoscopic enteral access include anatomic inability to perform an endoscopy (pharyngeal or esophageal obstruction), inability to bring the gastric/jejunal wall in apposition with the abdominal wall, and limited life expectancy of less than 4 weeks. Relative contraindications include coagulopathy, severe cardiopulmonary illness, previous gastric surgery, and ascites [6].

Options for post-pyloric feeding (Fig. 71.1) include intraduodenal tube feeding, nasojejunal tube (NJ), percutaneous endoscopic gastrostomy tube with jejunal extension (PEG-J), direct percutaneous endoscopic jejunostomy (PEJ) tube, surgical jejunostomy tube, and radiologic assisted enteral access. Intraduodenal feeding is no longer routinely used secondary to significant reflux of feeds back into the stomach. It is also contraindicated in the settings of recurrent aspiration and pancreatitis [7]. In this chapter we will concentrate on endoscopic techniques for jejunal access.

Nasojejunal Tube

Nasojejunal feeding trial should be the first step when initiating enteral feeds on a patient with gastraparesis [1]. Concomitant small bowel dysfunction may occur with gastroparesis and can be easily detected with a nasojejunal feeding trial. Being smaller in size compared to nasogastric tubes, NJ tubes cause less discomfort but clog more often, may get dislodged back into the stomach, and are not useful for decompression purposes.

NJ tubes can be placed manually, fluoroscopically, and endoscopically [8]. Manual placement involves the use of a 8–9 French tube with a guidewire and weighted tip. The technique of insertion is similar to that of a nasogastric tube. Post-pyloric passage is facilitated by placing the patient in a right lateral decubitus position, air insufflation of the stomach, pH sensory feeding tube guidance, prokinetic agents, and electromagnetic sensor-guided systems [7, 8]. The most significant

Table 71.1 Indications and contraindications of endoscopic enteric/post-pyloric feeding

Indications	Absolute contraindications	Relative contraindications
Gastroparesis/outlet obstruction	Diffuse peritonitis	Coagulopathy
Oropharyngeal malignancy	Lack of gastric/jejunal apposition	Ascites
Neurologic disorders/dysphagia	Limited life expectancy	Severe cardiopulmonary illness
Recurrent aspiration/reflux	Oropharyngeal obstruction	Previous abdominal surgery
Pancreatitis		Small bowel motility disorder
Persistent nutritional deficiency		Obesity

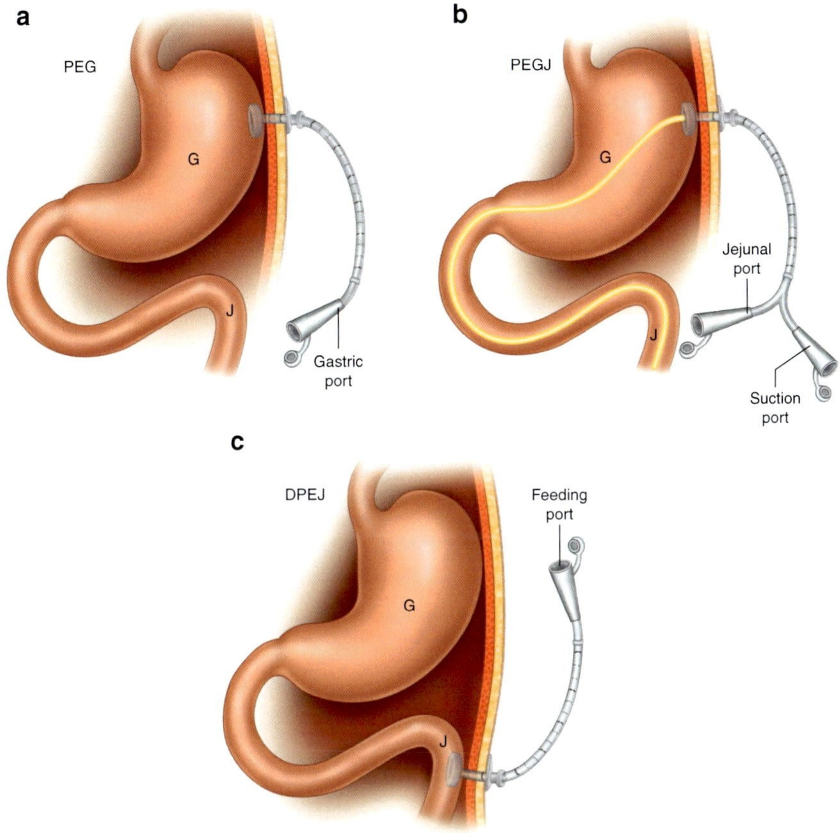

Fig. 71.1 Endoscopic-assisted percutaneous enteral access options: (**a**) Percutaneous endoscopic gastrostomy (PEG). (**b**) Percutaneous endoscopic gastrostomy with jejunal extension (PEG-J). (**c**) Direct percutaneous endoscopic jejunostomy tube (PEJ)

complication of bedside, blind or semi blind placement of an NJ tube, relates to misplacement and failure to recognize misplacement. These include vocal cord injury, bronchopleural fistula, aspiration pneumonia, tracheal perforation, hydrothorax, and mediastinitis [9]. Other complications of NJ tube placement are listed in Table 71.2. NJ tubes can also be placed with the help of endoscopy with a high success rate (80–90%) [10].

Techniques

1. Through the scope technique: After placing a standard gastroscope or a therapeutic upper endoscope in the duodenum, a flexible unweighted 7–10 French NJ tube with a guidewire is advanced through a working channel and pushed deep

Table 71.2 Complications of NJ tube placement [8, 10]

Nasopharyngeal complications	Epistaxis
	Nasal mucosal ulceration
	Pyriform sinus perforation
	Nasal trauma
Misplacement complications	Pulmonary intubation
	Tube feeding in pulmonary tree
	Pneumothorax
	Tracheobronchial trauma
	Pulmonary aspiration
	Tracheoesophageal fistula
Enteric complications	Gastric perforation
	Gastrointestinal bleeding
	Duodenal perforation
	Reflux esophagitis
Other complications	Clogging
	Dislodgement
	Knotted tube
	Arrhythmia
	Empyema
	Otitis media
	Myocardial infarction

into the jejunum, beyond the tip of the endoscope while simultaneously withdrawing the endoscope. After withdrawal of the endoscope, the feeding tube is passed from the mouth to the nose with the help of a plastic device. A success rate of 90% has been reported with an average procedure time of 19 min [11].

2. Push technique: A 12 French weighted flexible NJ tube is used with a 0.035 guidewire inserted from the back but not beyond the tip of the tube. A separate Savary guidewire can be inserted in a similar fashion beside the previous guidewire to provide increased stiffness. A standard upper endoscopy is then performed. With the endoscope in the stomach, the NJ tube is blind inserted via the patient's nasal cavity. Once advanced to the stomach, the tip of the endoscope or a biopsy forceps can be used to direct the NJ tube toward the pylorus. After getting past the pylorus, the NJ tube and the endoscope are advanced simultaneously; keep the tube 3–4 cm ahead of the endoscope, maintaining direct visualization of the tip of the tube. Once the tube is satisfactorily advanced, the endoscope is withdrawn taking care not to dislodge the NJ tube. The guidewires are then removed, and the NJ tube is secured externally. A success rate of 97% has been reported with a procedure time of 5–26 min [10].
3. Pull technique: In the presence of a gastroscope in the stomach, a feeding tube with a suture attached at its tip is inserted via the patient's nasal cavity. Once in the stomach, the suture is grasped with biopsy forceps to guide and "pull" the NJ tube to the correct location. A success rate of 80–93% has been reported for this method and about 15–50 min of procedure time. This procedure may often be

challenging secondary to difficulty grasping the suture as it adheres to the side of the NJ tube in the stomach's moist environment and difficulty releasing it after completion of the procedure [10, 12].

4. Via nasal endoscopy/through the scope technique: A 6 mm endoscope with a 3.2 mm instrument channel is inserted through the nose, advanced through the esophagus into the stomach. It is then advanced beyond the pylorus into the jejunum. Once in the jejunum, an 8 French feeding tube is advanced through the instrument channel into the jejunum. The endoscope is then withdrawn taking care that the feeding tube is not withdrawn from its desired location. This procedure may be complicated by the presence of high gastric residue making visualization through the small scope challenging. A success rate of 82% has been reported with a procedure time of 16–40 min [13].
5. Over the guidewire technique: After placing an upper endoscope into the jejunum, a guidewire is inserted into the biopsy channel and advanced into the small bowel. While maintaining visualization of the wire and taking care not to dislodge it, the endoscope is withdrawn. An oronasal transfer of the wire is then performed. Fluoroscopy is then required to ensure the appropriate positioning of the wire. A feeding tube is then advanced over the wire under fluoroscopy [12]. This procedure may also be performed with a nasal endoscopy and insertion of wire. Success rates of 82–93% have been reported [10].

Post procedure Care

Following placement of the tube and confirmation of appropriate positioning, dilute feed may be started at low infusion rates. After ensuring that the patient is able to tolerate diluted infusions, feeds are gradually advanced to iso-osmolar preparations and slowly increased to goal infusion rate.

Troubleshooting

Inadvertent removal of the NJ tube is the most frequently encountered complication, therefore evaluating for appropriate location of the tube must be a part of troubleshooting. A plain X-ray of the abdomen can be used to satisfactorily ensure proper location of the tube. The other most commonly encountered complication is a clogged tube. A clogged tube may be declogged using water flushes, enzyme instillation (Clog Zapper® CORPAK Medsystems), and mechanical declogging devices like the Bard Brush® or the Bionix DeClogger®. [14]

Jejunostomy Tube

For patients requiring long-term (>30d) [15] enteral access, who are found to have normal small bowel function after a successful trial of nasojejunal feeding, a jejunostomy feeding tube must be considered. It has been shown to improve symptoms and reduce hospitalizations in patients with gastroparesis [2]. Usually placed at 20–30 cm from the ligament of Treitz, a jejunostomy tube (J tube) may be inserted endoscopically, surgically (open or laparoscopic), and radiographically. In this chapter we will review the endoscopic methods of J tube placement. A J tube can be placed endoscopically either directly (percutaneous endoscopic jejunostomy, PEJ) or indirectly via a pre-existing or immediately placed gastrostomy tube (percutaneous endoscopic gastrostomy with jejunostomy extension, PEG-J).

Indications for placement of an endoscopically placed jejunostomy tube are similar to those of a NJ tube but also include patients with surgically altered gastric anatomy. Contraindications are absolute, e.g., diffuse peritonitis and esophageal or pharyngeal obstruction, and relative, e.g., coagulopathy, prior laparotomies, and ascites.

Percutaneous Endoscopic Gastrostomy

For placement of PEG-J, the patient must first have a prior gastrostomy. This gastrostomy may be a prior surgically (open or laparoscopic), radiographically, or endoscopically placed gastrostomy tube. If the patient does not have a prior gastrostomy tube, one will need to be placed for the purposes of placing a PEG-J. We will briefly review the different endoscopic techniques of percutaneous endoscopic gastrostomy (PEG) tube placement [6].

1. Pull PEG technique: First introduced by Gauderer and Ponsky in 1980 [16], this is a commonly used method for gastric access. With the patient in supine position, in the presence of continuous cardiopulmonary monitoring, sedation, analgesics, and antibiotic prophylaxis is administered. The procedure is performed by an endoscopist and a bedside assistant. A diagnostic upper endoscopy is first performed, and the stomach is fully insufflated with the light pointing toward the anterior abdominal wall. Room lights are turned down to look for transillumination. Manual palpation of the anterior abdominal wall is performed to look for finger indentation of the stomach endoscopically. By the use of transillumination and finger indentation, an appropriate location for the PEG tube is chosen about a finger breath below the costal margin. Recommended site is on the anterior aspect of the stomach, proximal to the incisura and midway between the greater and lesser curve. Short-acting local anesthetic is used to infiltrate the skin at that location using a half-filled syringe and a small-gauge needle (23G). Following infiltration, the needle is slowly advanced, while suctioning on the syringe, toward the peritoneal cavity. There should be synchrony between aspiration of air in the syringe and the appearance of the needle on the endoscopic camera with the bedside assistant and the endoscopist vocalizing "air" and "needle" synchronously. This method is known as the "safe tract" technique [17]. This allows confirmation of safe gastric access. The small-gauge needle is now taken out, and an incision approximately 1.5 times the diameter of the PEG tube is made. The endoscopist advances a polypectomy

snare and opens it at the anticipated entry site on the gastric wall. A large bore needle with a sheath around it is then inserted into the stomach. The snare is used to tightly encircle the sheath, and the needle is removed. A looped wire is inserted through the sheath. The sheath is then withdrawn, and the wire is tightly caught by the snare. The snare with the wire and the endoscope are now withdrawn together. Once brought out of the oral cavity, the looped wire is released from the snare, and the PEG tube is looped through it. Next, the assistant, while maintaining steady pressure around the skin puncture site, gently pulls looped wire out through the abdominal wall. The tapered end of the PEG tube emerges from the skin and then the tube. Reinsertion of the endoscope at this point is not mandatory but allows for confirmation of the location and tightness of the PEG tube. The polypectomy snare in the endoscope can be used to grasp the internal bumper as it is pulled by the assistant to facilitate reinsertion. This repeat endoscopy also allows to assess for hemostasis. The external bumper is then placed to secure the tube. Approximately 1 cm gap should be allowed between the internal bumper and the mucosa and the external bumper and skin.

2. Push PEG technique: This technique is similar to the "pull" method in terms of gaining access to the stomach using the "safe tract" technique. Following this, a stiff wire is introduced into the stomach and pulled out through the mouth. A gastrostomy tube is then advanced over this wire and "pushed" out through the stomach and abdominal wall. The endoscope is then reinserted to confirm adequate positioning of the gastrostomy tube.
3. Introducer PEG technique: First introduced in 1984, this tube uses the Seldinger technique to insert a balloon gastrostomy tube into the stomach [18]. The procedure starts with a diagnostic endoscopy and identification of the ideal location for placement of the PEG tube by transillumination, finger indentation, and "safe tract" technique. Next, the area of choice is infiltrated with local anesthetic, and an incision for the passage of the PEG tube is made. A needle is advanced through this incision into the stomach, and a stiff wire is advanced into the stomach. The needle is then withdrawn leaving in the wire. A dilator and then a sheath are then introduced over this wire under direct endoscopic vision. The sheath with the ballooned tube must be fully inserted into the stomach. The sheath is then peeled away from the tube and the balloon inflated. The tube is then secured in place. This technique has been shown to have a more complications including accidental dislodgement, surgical site infection, and gastrointestinal perforation [19] but can be performed with an endoscope without a biopsy channel or when an oropharyngeal obstruction prevents the "pull" or "push" of a PEG tube.
4. Laparoscopic-assisted PEG (LA-PEG): This technique offers a minimally invasive option for those patients in whom a PEG tube placement was not successful either because of lack of transillumination/good finger indentation or because of the inability to gain gastric access [20]. With the patient in a supine position, under general anesthesia, laparoscopy is begun with a 5 mm umbilical port. The abdomen is examined for reasons for unsuccessful PEG. An upper endoscopy is then performed, and the stomach is insufflated. The PEG is then inserted using the "pull" PEG technique under laparoscopic visualization [21, 22].

Postoperative Care

Following placement, the authors allow medication administration via the PEG immediately and for infusion of feeds 3 h after the procedure. Dry dressing is used on top of the external bumper to minimize soakage from any initial drainage, and tape is used as a mesentery to keep the tube perpendicular to the skin and relatively immobile. The tube is flushed before and after feeds to prevent clogging.

Complications

The overall complication rate from PEG tube placement is low with the most common complication being infection. It varies from 5% to 25% in different studies [15, 23]. Other common complications include tube dislodgement which occurs in up to 12.8% of patients [24] and leakage around the tube. Some rare but major complications include bleeding (1%), aspiration pneumonitis, visceral perforation, or injury [15, 23]. Among the involved organs, colon and small bowel [25, 26] are most likely injured, rarely spleen and liver. Other complications of PEG tube placement are listed in Table 71.3.

Management of these complications depends on its severity and acuity. A rapidly spreading necrotizing infection or peritonitis with evidence of hollow viscus perforation may need an urgent operative intervention, but most PEG complications can be treated nonoperatively. Early dislodgement of the tube (<1–2 weeks) without peritonitis is managed by placing a nasogastric tube to suction, starting antibiotics, and attempting a PEG rescue [27]. Bleeding around the PEG site can be controlled

Table 71.3 Complications of PEG tube placement [6, 15]

Intraprocedural	Bleeding
	Cardiopulmonary compromise
	Aspiration
Early	Bleeding
	Tube dislodgement
	Wound infection/necrotizing infection
	Visceral perforation/injury
	Aspiration pneumonitis
Late	Peristomal drainage
	Tube dislodgement
	Clogging
	Tube degradation
	Skin ulceration/granulation around PEG
	Persistent gastric fistula after removal of PEG
	Gastric outlet obstruction
	Buried bumper syndrome
	Gastrocolic fistula
	Metastatic seeding

by briefly tightening the external bumper to the skin or by placing a temporary U-shaped stitch to allow hemostasis. Buried bumper syndrome is defined as the extrusion of the head of the tube from the gastric lumen into the subcutaneous tissue. This can further lead to leakage and infection around the surgical site as well as in the peritoneal cavity. It is managed by removing the PEG tube and allowing the gastrostomy to heal. Other rarer complications include gastrocolic fistula [28] which are managed by allowing the fistulous tract to mature and then removing the tube to allow for the tract to heal.

Percutaneous Endoscopic Gastrostomy with Jejunal Extension (PEG-J)

A PEG-J tube can be placed as an extension to a previously placed PEG tube, or the existing PEG can be replaced completely with an "all-in-one" PEG-J kit with gastric and jejunal ports. This PEG-J tube can be placed using several techniques [6, 29]. Being smaller-caliber tubes, they are more prone to dislodgment and clogging when compared to larger bore PEJ tubes.

1. A guidewire is inserted into the pre-existing PEG and guided beyond the pylorus and into the jejunum by the endoscope. The jejunal extension tube is then advanced over the wire under endoscopic visualization. Fluoroscopy may be used to help assess for appropriate positioning as well.
2. Pull technique: Similar to a NJ pull technique, a jejunal tube with a string at its tip is advanced through a pre-existing PEG tube. The string is then grasped with biopsy forceps and advanced into the jejunum. Once it is positioned appropriately, the strings are released, and the endoscope is withdrawn taking care not to dislodge the PEG-J tube. Clips may be used to secure the string to jejunal mucosa to prevent early dislodgement.
3. Another technique uses a small-caliber endoscope through the pre-existing PEG. The endoscope is advanced into the jejunum. A wire is advanced into the jejunum through the working channel. The endoscope is then exchanged over the wire with the jejunal tube. Its final location is confirmed using fluoroscopy. This method was found to be a faster method and sometimes did not require conscious sedation [30].

Percutaneous Endoscopic Jejunostomy (PEJ) Tube

Described by Shike et al. [31], a PEJ tube can be a durable enteral access for long-term feeding. The advantages offered by direct PEJ placement include longer durability compared to the PEG-J tubes and less invasiveness compared to surgically placed jejunostomy tubes. In comparison to PEG-J tubes, PEJ tubes have been found to have a longer patency, less migration and less re-intervention. It also provides similar patient satisfaction [29, 32, 33]. As with other forms of jejunal feeding, PEJ tubes have also shown a trend toward decreased aspiration risks [32].

Indications for a PEJ tube are similar to other indications for jejunal feeding. Specific indications include patients with possible need for an esophagectomy where the integrity of the gastric conduit needs to be preserved and a h/o prior gastrectomy [34]. Contraindications for PEJ tube placement are also similar to those for a PEG placement.

Technique

PEJ tube placement can be performed under conscious sedation or with general anesthesia. Preprocedural prophylactic antibiotics are used. This procedure is commonly performed with a pediatric colonoscope but can be performed with a dedicated balloon or non-balloon enteroscope as well. PEJ placement uses the same principles of finger indentation, transillumination, and "safe-track" that are used for PEG placement. With an endoscope in the jejunum and an endoscopic snare ready, an appropriate site of puncture is selected using transillumination and finger indentation. The site is prepped and infiltrated with local anesthetic. A small-gauge needle is inserted at the selected spot. As soon as the needle is seen in the jejunum, it is snared tightly. A stab incision is made adjacent to the needle, and a larger bore needle with a sheath is inserted in the same track as the first needle. The snare is now transferred to the larger bore needle, and the first needle is removed. From this point on, the procedure follows a similar approach to the endoscopic pull PEG technique. Reinsertion of the endoscope to confirm location of the tube is not mandatory but may be performed at the operator's discretion. Variations of this procedure include using a longer needle [35] and using ultrasound to help delineate the target loop of jejunum in cases where transillumination cannot be easily achieved [36].

Complications of PEJ tubes have been reported in ~2–6% of cases and include jejunal volvulus, necrotizing infections, bowel perforations, and bleeding. Obesity, previous abdominal operations, and ascites may decrease success rates and increase complications. Use of T-fasteners may decrease the risk of jejunal volvulus by providing additional fixation points [37].

Endoscopic Gastrojejunostomy

The concept of creating a gastrojejunal bypass endoscopically to address the caveats of enteral stents for gastric outlet obstruction has been recently studied in humans [38]. Using endoscopic ultrasound and fluoroscopic assistance, the jejunum is located from the gastric lumen in order to advance a guidewire through a needle and create a tract for placement of a lumen-apposing metal stent.

Although a promising technique, this procedure is technically demanding and is still in its initial stages. It has only been studied in gastric obstruction (both malignant and benign) and is yet to be studied in the context of gastroparesis. Among the present concerns are safety and long-term patency.

Decompression

Indications for enteric decompression include chronic small bowel obstruction, peritoneal and intraperitoneal malignancy, gastric outlet obstruction, and gastroparesis.

Severe gastroparesis has debilitating symptoms of abdominal distension, nausea, and vomiting. Lack of relief of these symptoms has a profound effect on patient weight and lifestyle. Gastrostomy tubes have been shown to provide excellent (90%) symptomatic relief when placed for decompressive purposes [3, 39]. Venting gastrostomy or venting enterostomy also reduce hospitalization rates [40, 41]. Decompressive gastrostomy tubes can be placed endoscopically, surgically, or radiographically. Endoscopic and radiographic gastrostomy offers a minimally invasive approach compared to surgical gastrostomy. Percutaneous radiographic gastrostomy placement has been shown to have a higher complication rate compared to PEG tubes over a 30-day period [42]. A PEG-J tube with 28 French gastrostomy tube and a 8–10 French feeding jejunal extension can be used to simultaneously drain the stomach and feed the jejunum [43]. Techniques for placement of PEG and PEG-J tubes have already been discussed in this chapter.

In situations where an endoscopic or radiographic gastrostomy is technically difficult or not possible, percutaneous transesophageal access to the stomach or jejunum may be used for decompression. Percutaneous transesophageal gastrostomy (PTEG) tube was first described in 1998 [44] and is a promising option for decompression and feeding; however, this is not yet an FDA-approved method. Placement involves the use of ultrasound, fluoroscopy, and a balloon inflated in the cervical esophagus to help delineate anatomy. This is performed under intravenous sedation and local anesthetic, with the use of prophylactic antibiotics. Procedure begins with the passage of a wire through a nostril into the esophagus. A rupture free balloon is inserted into the esophagus via the nostril over the guidewire and then inflated with contrast. Fluoroscopy is used to position this inflated balloon above the clavicle. Under ultrasound guidance, an access site on the left side of the neck is selected. The left side of the neck is prepped and draped. A 22 gauge needle is used to access the balloon. A wire is then inserted through the needle into the balloon. The balloon and the wire are then advanced as a unit into the stomach. The wire is then retracted from the balloon and advanced into the stomach. The deflated balloon is then removed. The neck access to the esophagus is then dilated with a sheath and dilator over the wire, a catheter is then advanced through the sheath into the esophagus and subsequently into the stomach or jejunum. The catheter is then sutured to the skin. The procedure time varied from 6 to 60 min [45]. A complication rate of 16–20% has been noted, including an esophageal leak, a catheter dislodgement, and a tracheoesophageal fistula [45, 46]. PTEG can also be performed under endoscopic guidance [47].

Summary

Endoscopy is an invaluable tool in obtaining enteral access for nutrition and decompression. What was limited to guiding feeding tubes into the gastrointestinal tract in the 1970s, advanced to getting direct access to the stomach in the 1980s. Since then advancement in endoscopic and surgical techniques have allowed us direct access to the small bowel and allowed for innovative techniques like PTEG and endoscopic gastrojejunostomy (not FDA approved). This variety of endoscopic approaches to establish enteral access for nutrition and decompression establishes endoscopy as a vital adjunct to modern clinical practice.

References

1. Camiller M, Parkman HP, Shafi MA, Abell TL, Gerson L. Clinical guideline: management of gastroparesis. Am J Gastroenterol. 2013;108(1):18–38. https://doi.org/10.1038/ajg.2012.373. Clinical.
2. Fontana R, Barnett J. Jejunostomy tube placement in refractory diabetic gastroparesis: a retrospective review. Am J Gastroenterol. 1996;91(10):2174–8.
3. Kim CH, Nelson DK. Venting percutaneous gastrostomy in the treatment of refractory idiopathic gastroparesis. Gastrointest Endosc. 1998;47(1):67–70. https://doi.org/10.1016/S0016-5107(98)70301-3.
4. Jain R, Maple JT, Anderson MA, et al. The role of endoscopy in enteral feeding. Gastrointest Endosc. 2011;74(1):7–12. https://doi.org/10.1016/j.gie.2010.10.021.
5. Russell M, Stieber M, Brantley S, et al. American Society for Parenteral and Enteral Nutrition and American Dietetic Association: standards of practice and standards of professional performance for registered dieticians (generalist, specialty, and advanced) in nutrition support. J Am Diet Assoc. 2007;107(10):1815–22. https://doi.org/10.1016/j.jada.2007.08.024.
6. Ibrahim S, El-Hayek K, Chand B. Endoscopic techniques of enteral access. In: Principles of flexible endoscopy for surgeons. New York: Springer; 2013. p. 119–28.
7. Niv E, Fireman Z, Vaisman N. Post-pyloric feeding. World J Gastroenterol. 2009;15(11):1281–8. https://doi.org/10.3748/wjg.15.1281.
8. Kirby DF, DeLegge MH, Fleming CR. American Gastroenterological Association technical review on tube feeding for enteral nutrition. Gastroenterology. 1995;108(4):1282–301. https://doi.org/10.1016/0016-5085(95)90231-7.
9. Smithard D, Barrett NA, Hargroves D, Elliot S. Electromagnetic sensor-guided enteral access systems: a literature review. Dysphagia. 2015;30(3):275–85. https://doi.org/10.1007/s00455-015-9607-4.
10. Wiggins TF, DeLegge MH. Evaluation of a new technique for endoscopic nasojejunal feeding-tube placement. Gastrointest Endosc. 2006;63(4):590–5. https://doi.org/10.1016/j.gie.2005.10.043.
11. Bosco JJ, Gordon F, Zelig M. A reliable method for the endoscopic placement of a nasoenteric feeding tube. Gastrointest Endosc. 1994;40:740–3.
12. Stark S, Sharpe J, Larson G. Endoscopically placed nasoenteral feeding tubes. Indications and techniques. Am Surg. 1991;57(4):203–5.
13. Zick G, Frerichs A, Ahrens M, et al. A new technique for bedside placement of enteral feeding tubes: a prospective cohort study. Crit Care. 2011;15(1):R8. https://doi.org/10.1186/cc9407.
14. Fisher C, Blalock B. Clogged feeding tubes: a clinician's Thorn. Nutr Issues Gastroenterol. 2014;38:16–22.
15. Rahnemai-Azar AA, Rahnemaiazar AA, Naghshizadian R, Kurtz A, Farkas DT. Percutaneous endoscopic gastrostomy: indications, technique, complications and management. World J Gastroenterol. 2014;20(24):7739–51. https://doi.org/10.3748/wjg.v20.i24.7739.
16. Gauderer M, Ponsky J, Izant R. Gastrostomy without laparotomy: a percutaneous endoscopic technique. J Pediatr Surg. 1980;15(6):872–5.
17. Foutch P, Talbert G, Waring J, Sanowski R. Percutaneous endoscopic gastrostomy in patients with prior abdominal surgery: virtues of the safe tract. Am J Gastroenterol. 1988;83(2):147–50.

18. Russell TR, Brotman M, Norris F. Percutaneous gastrostomy. A new simplified and cost-effective technique. Am J Surg. 1984;148(1):132–7. https://doi.org/10.1016/0002-9610(84)90300-3.
19. Van Dyck E, Macken EJ, Roth B, Pelckmans PA, Moreels TG. Safety of pull-type and introducer percutaneous endoscopic gastrostomy tubes in oncology patients: a retrospective analysis. BMC Gastroenterol. 2011;1(1):23. https://doi.org/10.1186/1471-230X-11-23.
20. Gupta A, Manejwala A. Laparoscopic assisted percutaneous endoscopic gastrostomy (LAPEG): a simple and safe technique of gastrostomy tube placement in patients with failed PEG by surgeons with basic laparoscopy skills. Available at: http://www.sages.org/meetings/annual-meeting/abstracts-archive/laparoscopic-assisted-percutaneous-endoscopic-gastrostomy-lapeg-a-simple-and-safe-technique-of-gastrostomy-tube-placement-in-patients-with-failed-peg-by-surgeons-with-basic-laparoscopy-skills/.
21. Thaker AM, Sedarat A. Laparoscopic-assisted percutaneous endoscopic gastrostomy. Curr Gastroenterol Rep. 2016;18(9):1–7. https://doi.org/10.1007/s11894-016-0520-2.
22. Lopes G, Salcone M, Neff M. Laparoscopic-assisted percutaneous endoscopic gastrostomy tube placement. J Soc Laparoendosc Surg Soc Laparoendosc Surg (JSLS). 2010;14(1):66–9. https://doi.org/10.4293/108680810X12674612014662.
23. Richter-Schrag H-J, Richter S, Ruthmann O, Olschewski M, Hopt UT, Fischer A. Risk factors and complications following percutaneous endoscopic gastrostomy: a case series of 1041 patients. Can J Gastroenterol. 2011;25(4):201–6. Available at: http://www.embase.com/search/results?subaction=viewrecord&from=export&id=L362757264\n; http://www.pulsus.com/journals/pdf_frameset.jsp?jnlKy=2&atlKy=10055&isArt=t&jnlAdvert=Gastro&adverifHCTp=&sTitle=Riskfactorsandcomplicationsfollowingpercutaneousendoscopi.
24. Rosenberger LH, Newhook T, Schirmer B, Sawyer RG. Late accidental dislodgement of a percutaneous endoscopic gastrostomy tube: an underestimated burden on patients and the health care system. Surg Endosc. 2011;25(10):3307–11.
25. Guloglu R, Taviloglu K, Alimoglu O. Colon injury following percutaneous endoscopic gastrostomy tube insertion. J Laparoendosc Adv Surg Tech A. 2003;13(1):69–72. https://doi.org/10.1089/109264203321235520.
26. Karhadkar A, Schwartz H, Dutta S. Jejunocutaneous fistula manifesting as chronic diarrhea after PEG tube replacement. J Clin Gastroenterol. 2006;40(6):560–1.
27. Marks JM, Ponsky JL, Pearl JP, McGee MF. PEG "rescue": a practical NOTES technique. Surg Endosc Other Interv Tech. 2007;21(5):816–9. https://doi.org/10.1007/s00464-007-9361-2.
28. Fortunato JE, Troy AL, Cuffari C, et al. Outcome after percutaneous endoscopic gastrostomy in children and young adults. J Pediatr Gastroenterol Nutr. 2010;50(4):390–3. https://doi.org/10.1097/MPG.0b013e3181aed6f1.
29. Fan AC, Baron TH, Rumalla A, Harewood GC. Comparison of direct percutaneous endoscopic jejunostomy and PEG with jejunal extension. Gastrointest Endosc. 2002;56(6):890–4. https://doi.org/10.1016/S0016-5107(02)70366-0.
30. Adler D, Gostout C, Baron T. Percutaneous transgastric placement of jejunal feeding tubes with an ultrathin endoscope. Gastrointest Endosc. 2002;55(1):106–10.
31. Shike M, Schroy P, Ritchie M, Lightdate C, Morse R. Percutaneous endoscopic jejunostomy in cancer patients with previous gastric resection. Gastrointest Endosc. 1987;33:372–4.
32. Zopf Y, Rabe C, Bruckmoser T, Maiss J, Hahn E, Schwab D. Percutaneous endoscopic jejunostomy and jejunal extension tube through percutaneous endoscopic gastrostomy: a retrospective analysis of success, complications and outcome. Digestion. 2009;79(2):92–7.
33. DeLegge M, Buck G, Fang J, et al. Randomized prospective comparison of direct percutaneous endoscopic jejunostomy vs percutaneous endoscopic gastrostomy with jejunal extension feeding tube placement for enteral feeding [abstract]. Gastrointest Endosc. 2004;59(AB):158.
34. Maple JT, Petersen BT, Baron TH, Gostout CJ, Wong Kee Song LM, Buttar NS. Direct percutaneous endoscopic jejunostomy: outcomes in 307 consecutive attempts. Am J Gastroenterol. 2005;100(12):2681–8. https://doi.org/10.1111/j.1572-0241.2005.00334.x.
35. Fisher NC, Moran GW. Direct percutaneous endoscopic jejunostomy: high completion rates with selective use of a long drainage access needle. Diagn Ther Endosc. 2009;2009:1. https://doi.org/10.1155/2009/520879.

36. Sharma VK, Close T, Bynoe R, Vasudeva R. Ultrasound-assisted direct percutaneous endoscopic jejunostomy (DPEJ) tube placement. Surg Endosc. 2000;14(2):203–4. https://doi.org/10.1007/s004649900102.
37. Murphy C, Fang J, Adler D. Direct percutaneous endoscopic jejunostomy: who, when, how, and what to avoid. Pract Gastroenterol. 2014;38(Series 9):24–36.
38. Tyberg A, Perez-Miranda M, Sanchez-Ocaña R, et al. Endoscopic ultrasound-guided gastrojejunostomy with a lumen-apposing metal stent: a multicenter, international experience. Endosc Int Open. 2016;4:276–81. https://doi.org/10.1055/s-0042-101789.
39. Pothuri B, Montemarano M, Gerardi M, et al. Percutaneous endoscopic gastrostomy tube placement in patients with malignant bowel obstruction due to ovarian carcinoma. Gynecol Oncol. 2005;96(2):330–4. https://doi.org/10.1016/j.ygyno.2004.09.058.
40. Murr M, Sarr M, Camilleri M. The surgeon's role in the treatment of chronic intestinal pseudoobstruction. Am J Gastroenterol. 1995;90(12):2147–51.
41. Pitt HA, Mann LL, Berquist WE, Ament ME, Fonkalsrud EW, DenBesten L. Chronic intestinal pseudo-obstruction. Management with total parenteral nutrition and a venting enterostomy. Arch Surg. 1985;120(5):614–8. https://doi.org/10.1001/archsurg.1985.01390290090015.
42. Silas AM, Pearce LF, Lestina LS, et al. Percutaneous radiologic gastrostomy versus percutaneous endoscopic gastrostomy: a comparison of indications, complications and outcomes in 370 patients. Eur J Radiol. 2005;56(1):84–90. https://doi.org/10.1016/j.ejrad.2005.02.007.
43. Shike M, Wallach C, Bloch A, Brennan MF. Combined gastric drainage and jejunal feeding through a percutaneous endoscopic stoma. Gastrointest Endosc. 1990;36(3):290–2. https://doi.org/10.1016/S0016-5107(90)71026-7.
44. Oishi H, Murata J, Kameoka S. Percutaneous transesophageal gastric-tube drainage—development of the balloon catheter and future prospects [Japanese]. Nippon Geka Gakkai Zasshi. 1998;99:275.
45. Aramaki T, Arai Y, Inaba Y, et al. Phase II study of percutaneous transesophageal gastrotubing for patients with malignant gastrointestinal obstruction; JIVROSG-0205. J Vasc Interv Radiol. 2013;24(7):1011–7. https://doi.org/10.1016/j.jvir.2013.04.005.
46. Udomsawaengsup S, Brethauer S, Kroh M, Chand B. Percutaneous transesophageal gastrostomy (PTEG): a safe and effective technique for gastrointestinal decompression in malignant obstruction and massive ascites. Surg Endosc Other Interv Tech. 2008;22(10):2314–8. https://doi.org/10.1007/s00464-008-9984-y.
47. Murakami M, Nishino K, Takaoka Y, et al. Endoscopically assisted percutaneous transesophageal gastrotubing: a retrospective pilot study. Eur J Gastroenterol Hepatol. 2013;25(8):989–95.

Surgical Management: Gastric Neurostimulation

72

Brian Richard Davis

Introduction

Symptoms of gastroparesis (GP) are non-specific resulting in misdiagnosis and low access to specialist care. The GP Cardinal Symptom Index (GCSI) is composed of postprandial fullness, early satiety, nausea, vomiting, bloating, and upper abdominal pain. Patients often present in a progressive state of malnutrition and dehydration with debilitation from repeat hospital admissions, serial courses of total parenteral nutrition (TPN), and frequent narcotic dependence.

Selection criteria for surgical therapy include presence of symptoms over a year, demonstrated delayed gastric emptying on radiolabeled studies at 2- and 4-hour intervals, and weight loss of between 5% and 10% of normal body weight. Gastric emptying scintigraphy is performed with 99 m technetium sulfur colloid-labeled egg sandwich with standard imaging at 0, 1, 2, and 4 hours. Delayed emptying consistent with GP is defined as gastric retention of equal to or greater than 60% at 2 hours and equal to or greater than 10% at 4 hours. Candidates for surgery must be carefully evaluated to exclude rumination syndrome, cyclical vomiting syndrome, and bulimia. Medication-induced GP should also be excluded resulting from narcotic analgesics, anticholinergic agents, and some diabetes medications.

Classification of GP falls into three categories: diabetic, idiopathic, and postsurgical. Diabetics demonstrate a high prevalence of GP: reported in 40% of type 1 and 10–20% of type 2. The 10-year incidence is reported as 5.2% in diabetes type 1 and 1% in type 2. Pathology demonstrates depletion of the interstitial cells of Cajal that serve to regulate gastric slow waves in the stomach and pylorus. Idiopathic GP most commonly presents in young or middle-aged women with symptoms that overlap with functional dyspepsia. Symptoms can present following viral prodrome suggesting a post-viral GP. Complications of autonomic

B. R. Davis (✉)
Department of Surgery, Texas Tech Paul L. Foster School of Medicine, El Paso, TX, USA
e-mail: br.davis@ttuhsc.edu

J. Grams et al. (eds.), *The SAGES Manual of Foregut Surgery*,
https://doi.org/10.1007/978-3-319-96122-4_72

neuropathy can lead to GP from infection with cytomegalovirus, Epstein-Barr virus, and varicella zoster. Pathology demonstrates chronic inflammation and infiltration of the gastric muscularis propria with polymorphonuclear cells. Postsurgical GP occurs in 10% of Nissen fundoplication cases with inadvertent injury to the vagus nerve. GP results in 50% of operations with known transection of the vagus to include Billroth I and II and vagotomy with pyloroplasty. Postsurgical cases respond best to pyloroplasty and gastrectomy.

Surgical Management: Gastric Neurostimulation

Gastric neurostimulation (invented in 1963) currently has two manifestations resulting in differing results. High-energy stimulation has been utilized (up to four leads) to entrain slow waves of the stomach and improve gastric emptying. This pacemaker function has become impractical for routine implantation secondary to extreme energy requirements. Gastric electrical stimulation (GES) has been approved for the treatment of gastroparesis (GP) by the FDA since 2000 (Humanitarian Device Exemption). The Enterra Therapy System (Medtronic, Minneapolis, MN, USA) delivers high-frequency low-energy stimulation to the region of vagal afferent nerve fibers in the antrum of the stomach (Fig. 72.1). The stimulation pulse width is a few hundred microseconds, and frequency is three to four times higher than physiologic rates of gastric slow waves.

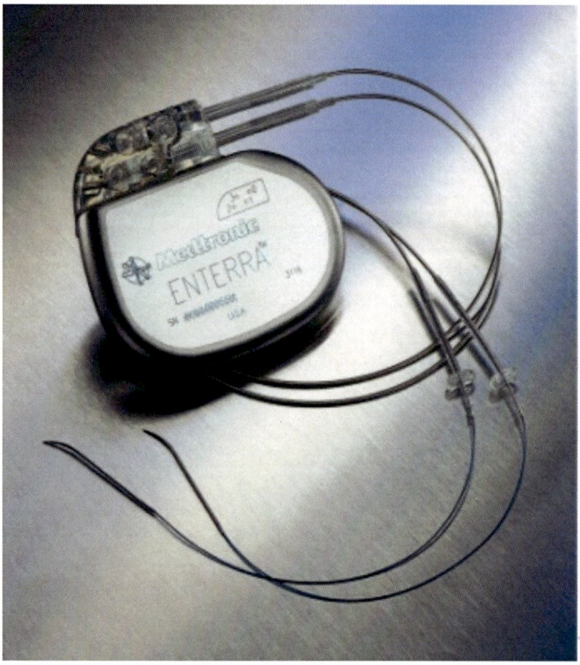

Fig. 72.1 Gastric electrical stimulator (GES) electrodes and pulse generator (Enterra, Medtronic, Minneapolis, MN, USA)

The Worldwide Anti-Vomiting Electrical Stimulation Study [1], a double-blind crossover study, demonstrates significant reductions in weekly vomiting and improvement in total symptom scores in greater than 50% of patients. McCallum et al. [2] demonstrate the largest series with a 10-year follow-up where Enterra produces significant and sustained improvement in total symptom scores of patients with gastroparesis: 60% in diabetic GP, 59% in postsurgical GP, and 49% in idiopathic GP. Investigators agree that diabetic GP represents the best indication for GES. Factors that impair response to GES include narcotic dependence, peripheral neuropathy, migraine headaches, menstrual cycle-driven vomiting, and endometriosis-induced abdominal pain. Proposed mechanisms include efferent vagal feedback to the thalamus that interrupts cyclical vomiting. Increased autonomic/vagal function may result in improved gastric accommodation, capacitance, and relaxation following meals.

GES electrodes are implanted deep to the serosa and into the muscularis propria during laparotomy, laparoscopic, or robot-assisted surgery. Laparoscopic and robot-assisted techniques utilize port placements that facilitate triangulation to accurately suture leads into the antrum (Fig. 72.2). Two electrodes are placed 10 cm proximal to the pylorus along the greater curvature of the stomach. Leads are sutured in place parallel to each other 1 cm apart (9.5 and 10.5 cm from the pylorus). The surgeon verifies lead placement with upper endoscopy to prevent full thickness mucosal perforation of the stomach. The leads (35 cm length) are connected to a subdermal pocket containing a pulse generator that is programmed to

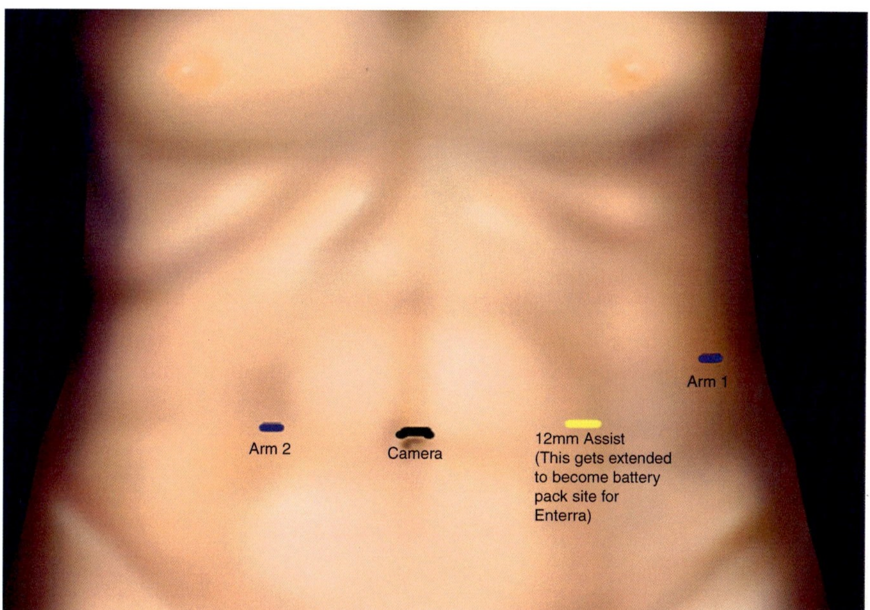

Fig. 72.2 Robot-assisted and laparoscopic port configuration for GES electrode insertion

standard parameters (5 milliamps, 14 Hertz, 330 microseconds, cycle on 0.1 second, cycle off 5 seconds) using a handheld programmer (Model 7432 or Model 8840, Medtronic, Minneapolis, MN, USA). Impedance (resistance between the two electrodes) at the time of electrode placement should be between 400 and 800 Ohms to ensure delivery of adequate current. Voltage is adjusted approximately 3 months after surgery to maintain a 5-milliamp current.

Complications of GES therapy include pulse generator subdermal pocket infection (6%), lead migration (1%), lead penetration into the stomach (3%), pulse generator migration (1%), and small bowel obstruction (1%). Other indications for repeat surgery for GP include total gastrectomy secondary to treatment failure (4%) and lack of symptomatic improvement (2%). Depleted pulse generator batteries are replaced every 10 years without changing electrodes.

GES demonstrates symptomatic relief of nausea and emesis without normalization of gastric emptying times on follow-up studies. Sarosiek et al. [3, 4] propose the addition of pyloroplasty (PP) to GES therapy with demonstration of an overall 64% improvement in gastric emptying times at 4 hours compared to 7% observed in GES alone. Davis et al. [5] demonstrate long-term results of simultaneous GES and PP with reduction in total symptom scores in 71% of GP patients and normalization of gastric emptying time in 60%. Combined simultaneous GES and PP leads to significant reductions hospital length of stay (LOS) and overall weight gain with no noted increased incidence of pulse generator infections. Robot-assisted approaches to simultaneous combined GES and PP are also described by Davis et al. [5] with demonstration of technical feasibility and significant contribution to decreased hospital LOS.

Summary

1. Postsurgical or idiopathic GP patients should be offered surgical or endoscopic PP as an initial option to improve gastric emptying.
2. Symptomatic individuals presenting with primary nausea and emesis should be offered gastric electrical neurostimulation (GES).
3. Individuals with gastric feeding intolerance manifested by cyclical nausea and emesis should have nutritional rehabilitation followed by combined GES therapy and PP that can safely be performed simultaneously.
4. GP patients who have failed therapy with GES and PP should be prepared for a subtotal or total gastrectomy after nutritional rehabilitation to reduce perioperative complications.

References

1. Abell T, McCallum R, Hocking M, Koch K, Abrahamsson H, LeBlanc I, Lindberg G, Konturek J, Nowak T, Quigley EMM, Tougas G, Starkebaum W. Gastric electrical stimulation for medically refractory gastroparesis. Gastroenterology 2003;125(2):421–28.
2. McCallum RW, Lin Z, Forster J, Roesser K, Hou Q, Sarosiek I. Gastric electrical stimulation improves outcomes for patents with gastroparesis for up to 10 years. Clin Gastroenterol Hepatol. 2011;9(4):314–9.

3. Sarosiek I, Davis B, Eichler E, McCallum RW. Surgical approaches to treatment of gastroparesis: gastric electrical stimulation, pyloroplasty, total gastrectomy and enteral feeding tubes. Gastroenterol Clin N Am. 2015;44:151–67.
4. Sarosiek I, Forster J, Lin Z, Cherry S, Sarosiek J, McCallum R. The addition of pyloroplasty as anew surgical approach to enhance effectiveness of gastric electrical stimulation therapy in patients with gastroparesis. Neurogastroenterol Motil. 2013;25(2):134–80.
5. Davis BR, Sarosiek I, Bashashati M, Alvarado B, McCallum RW. The long-term efficacy and safety of pyloroplasty combined with gastric electrical stimulation therapy in gastroparesis. J Gastrointest Surg. 2017;21(2):222–7.

Surgical Management: Pyloroplasty

73

Benjamin R. Veenstra and Minh B. Luu

Indications

(a) Pyloroplasty is an excellent treatment modality for patients with gastroparesis, whether diabetic, idiopathic, or postsurgical. While numerous treatment modalities exist, including gastric stimulator implantation and gastrectomy, pyloroplasty allows for effective treatment without precluding future treatment modalities.

Patient Position and Port Placement

(a) Patient setup and positioning is similar to that of laparoscopic anti-reflux surgery (LARS) (see previous chapter). Both a standard supine and split leg configuration can be used. In the standard configuration, the surgeon is positioned on the patient's left side, along with the camera operator, while the first assistant is situated on the patient's right. In the split leg configuration, the surgeon stands between the patient's legs, while the first assistant is on the patient's left, and the camera operator is on the patient's right. We prefer the split leg configuration as it allows for a more direct view of the pylorus by the surgeon and is ergonomically favorable for suturing.

B. R. Veenstra (✉)
Department of Surgery, Division of MIS and Bariatrics, Rush University Medical Center, Chicago, IL, USA
e-mail: Benjamin_Veenstra@Rush.Edu

M. B. Luu
Departments of General and Upper GI Surgery, Rush University Medical Center, Chicago, IL, USA

J. Grams et al. (eds.), *The SAGES Manual of Foregut Surgery*,
https://doi.org/10.1007/978-3-319-96122-4_73

(b) Monitors are placed at both sides of the head of the table, allowing for unobstructed and convenient viewing for all parties.
(c) Suction and irrigation connections come off the head of the table on the patient's right, while electrocautery and insufflation connections come off the head of the table on the patient's left. Special instruments include atraumatic Debakey (hunter) graspers, 5 mm needle drivers, park instrument, diamond-flex liver retractor, ultrasonic dissection device, and scissors.
(d) Ideal port placement is dependent on triangulation of the pylorus, allowing for easy visualization as well as comfortable suturing. We place our camera in between the right and left working hand ports. Our preference for entry into the abdomen is via Veress technique in the left upper quadrant at Palmer's point. Once insufflation is achieved, we OptiView in our designated camera port site.
(e) With improved optics, a 5 mm port for the camera is sufficient, allowing passage of a 5 mm 30 ° laparoscope. The camera port is placed just off the left of midline, ~15 cm inferior to the xiphoid, akin to LARS placement. Placement of the camera too high risks awkward downward visualization and difficult angles for suturing, while a lower camera placement is usually better tolerated. Four more ports are placed to allow for adequate retraction and assistance. A 5 mm port is placed in the far right lateral subcostal region for the liver retractor. Another 5 mm port is placed ~ 5 cm inferior and right of the subxiphoid for the left working hand. A 10 mm port is placed in the left subcostal region for the right-hand working port to allow for easy passage of an SH needle. Finally a 5 mm assistant port can be placed in the far left lateral subcostal region.

Operative Technique

Exposure and Identification of the Pylorus

(i) Once visual entrance into the abdomen is achieved, the body of the stomach is identified. Following the lesser curvature of the stomach caudally leads the operator to the region of the pylorus. To aid in visualization, we place a self-retaining liver retractor through the right most lateral port to fully expose the pylorus and duodenum. Confirmation of the pylorus can generally be achieved by the use of a blunt instrument over the suspected region with a gentle sweeping motion, appreciating the fullness of the associated muscle. Alternatively, since endoscopy is routinely used at the completion of the case for a leak test, the location of the pylorus can be confirmed in this manner as well.

Placement of Stay Sutures and Orientation

(i) With the pylorus identified, we place two stay sutures (2–0 Vicryl), one at the superior and another at the inferior boundary of the visualized pylorus (Fig. 73.1).

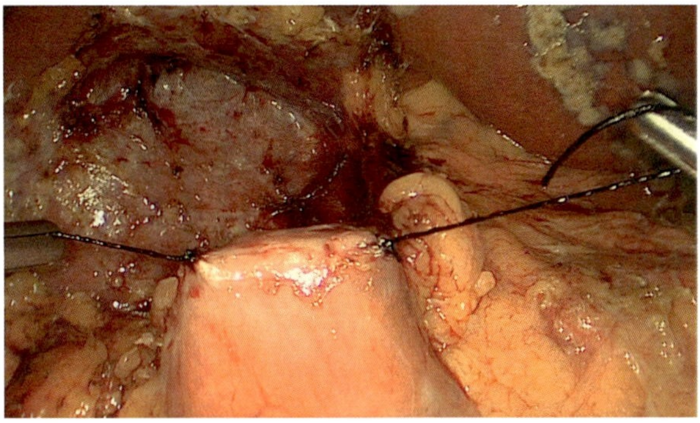

Fig. 73.1 Placement of stay sutures allows for easy retraction and orientation of the pylorus

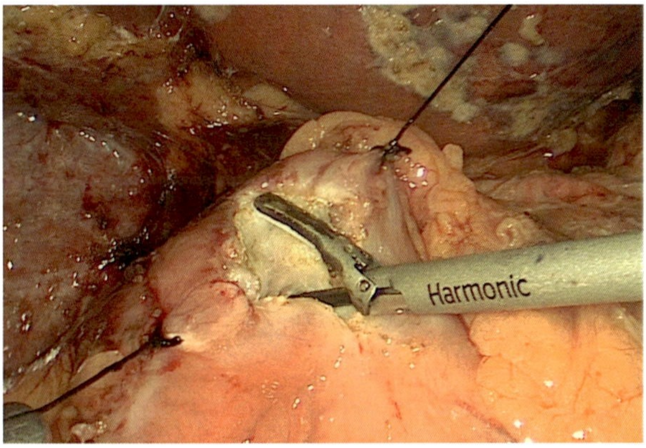

Fig. 73.2 Use of ultrasonic shears for transection of the pylorus. Note the thickness of the muscle, requiring division in "packets" of tissue

These aid in retraction during pyloroplasty, as well as keep the proper orientation during transection of the pylorus.

Transection of the Pylorus

(i) Although numerous energy devices can be used to transect the pylorus, our preference is an ultrasonic dissection device. This device has the advantage of an easy "pop in" with the active blade of the device, as well as excellent hemostasis. The key to an ideal transection is keeping proper orientation and dividing the pylorus at a completely perpendicular angle. To facilitate this, the assistant holds the superior stay suture and retracts this medially. The surgeon uses his/her left hand to grasp the inferior stay suture and retracts this laterally, while the right hand of the surgeon operates the ultrasonic device. While applying the "fast" setting of the device, the active blade is used to "pop" into the stomach, just on the gastric side of the pylorus. This is done in such a manner that the continued trajectory is directly in the middle of the exposed pyloric ring. Once the gastrotomy is made, subsequent bites of the pylorus are taken. Often, the pylorus needs to be taken in vertical "packets" due to its thickness (Fig. 73.2). The transection is carried out through the entire pylorus and onto the duodenum for approximately 1–2 cm.

HM Pyloroplasty

(i) With the pylorus transected (Fig. 73.3), a Heineke-Mikulicz pyloroplasty is performed using 2–0 Vicryl sutures on an SH needle. We begin by placing two to three sutures in an interrupted fashion at the superior portion of the transection, bringing the horizontally oriented transection of the pylorus together in the standard vertical manner. These first sutures are tied down after each placement with care to dunk the mucosa. Two to three interrupted sutures are then placed at the inferior portion of the transection, also tying after each

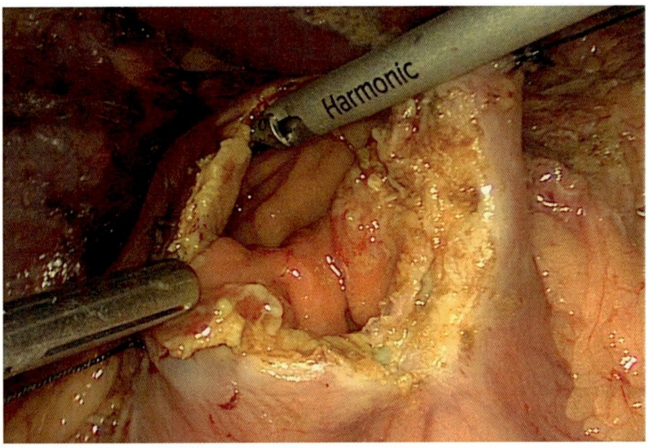

Fig. 73.3 Fully transected pylorus

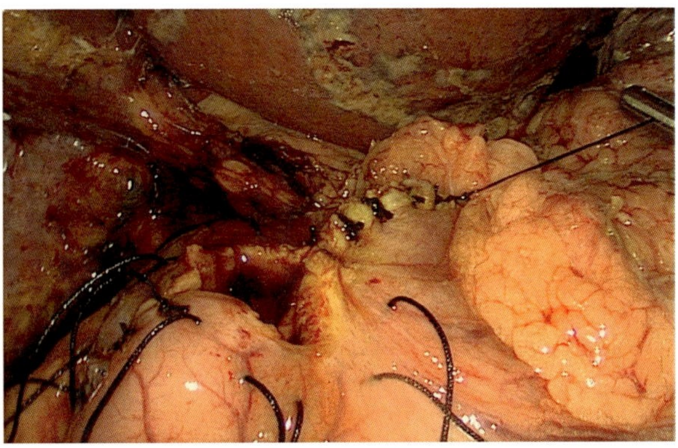

Fig. 73.4 Partially completed pyloroplasty with final sutures placed prior to tying

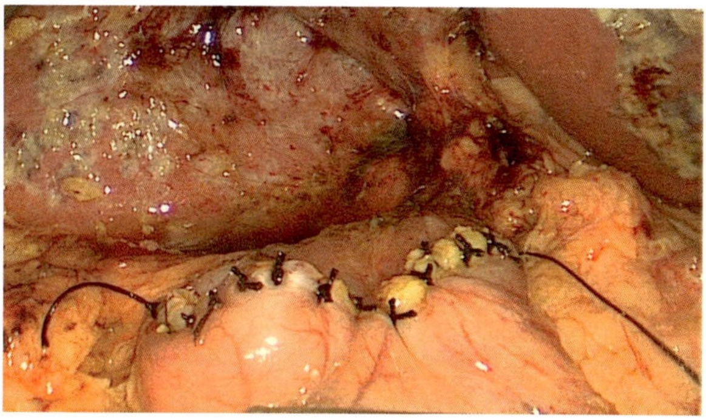

Fig. 73.5 Completed pyloroplasty

placement. Subsequent sutures are placed in an alternating manner between the superior and inferior portions of the transection. As the center is reached, the last five to six sutures are placed but not tied down immediately, allowing for accurate placement with secure bites of tissue (Fig. 73.4). Once all sutures are placed, the remaining sutures are tied down. Generally, spacing between sutures is 0.3 cm.

Leak Test with Endoscopy

(i) Once the pyloroplasty is completed (Fig. 73.5), we perform a leak test to ensure an airtight closure. The assistant performs endoscopy navigating the scope into the distal stomach. The surgeon uses the left-hand grasper to compress and occlude the duodenum distal to the pyloroplasty. The right-hand port is used to instill saline and to submerge the closure. Using insufflation on the scope, the integrity of the closure is tested. If any bubbles are noted, additional interrupted stitches are placed until an airtight closure is achieved.

Postoperative Management

(a) A nasogastric tube is not commonly left in place. IV antiemetics are used aggressively to minimize postoperative nausea and emesis.
(b) An upper GI or other imaging studies are not routinely obtained unless clinically warranted (unexplained tachycardia, change in exam).
(c) Patients are started on a clear liquid diet the first postoperative day and advanced to a full liquid or pureed diet as tolerated. Patients remain on this diet for 1 week and advance to a soft diet at home. Advancement to an unrestricted diet is typically achieved 1 month postop.
(d) Hospital stay is 2–3 days.

Postoperative Complications and Outcomes

(a) Suture line leak is the most worrisome complication of laparoscopic pyloroplasty. However, the incidence of this in the literature is low, ranging from 0 to 1.1% [1]. Depending on the timing of the leak, management may be operative or non-operative (percutaneous drain placement and NPO status). Overall morbidity of the procedure is ~8% with a 14% readmission rate [2]. In addition to subjective improvement in symptoms, objective improvement has also been demonstrated. A significant decrease in the T1/2 on postoperative gastric emptying scintigraphy has been found in multiple studies [3]. In conclusion, laparoscopic pyloroplasty provides a safe and effective treatment modality for gastroparesis.

References

1. Shada AL, Dunst CM, Pescarus R, Speer EA, Cassera M, Reavis KM, Swanstrom LL. Laparoscopic pyloroplasty is a safe and effective first-line surgical therapy for refractory gastroparesis. Surg Endosc. 2016 Apr;30(4):1326–32.
2. Toro JP, Lytle NW, Patel AD, Davis SS Jr, Christie JA, Waring JP, Sweeney JF, Lin E. Efficacy of laparoscopic pyloroplasty for the treatment of gastroparesis. J Am Coll Surg. 2014 Apr;218(4):652–60.
3. Hibbard ML, Dunst CM, Swanström LL. Laparoscopic and endoscopic pyloroplasty for gastroparesis results in sustained symptom improvement. J Gastrointest Surg. 2011 Sep;15(9):1513–9.

Gastrectomy for Gastroparesis

74

Mary Hawn and Matthew Cooper

Introduction

Gastroparesis is a chronic disorder characterized by delayed gastric emptying in the absence of mechanical obstruction. The first-line treatment is dietary and lifestyle modification followed by medical therapy consisting primarily of prokinetic agents and antiemetics for symptom management. Management of gastroparesis is often frustrating for both physician and patient and is associated with significant morbidity as well as large financial burden on the healthcare system.

Symptoms of gastroparesis are often difficult to distinguish from other abdominal complaints, and patients frequently have undergone multiple abdominal operations (fundoplication, cholecystectomy, etc.), which have failed due to not addressing the underlying issue of delayed gastric emptying.

The role of surgery in the management of gastroparesis is not very well defined with research studies ongoing. The majority of large society guidelines either fail to mention gastrectomy or include it as a passing afterthought [1, 2]. Surgical therapy is available for patients for whom medical management has been unsuccessful and includes venting gastrostomy, pyloroplasty, and gastric stimulators [3]. These less invasive surgical interventions that preserve normal anatomy should be considered prior to embarking on a larger surgical adventure such as gastrectomy. Patients with severe gastroparesis refractory to medical treatment can be thought of as having complete end-organ failure of the stomach. Often the best treatment for a nonfunctioning end organ is removal of said organ; such is the case in gastroparetic patients and gastrectomy.

M. Hawn (✉) · M. Cooper
Department of Surgery, Stanford Hospital and Clinics, Stanford, CA, USA
e-mail: mhawn@stanford.edu

J. Grams et al. (eds.), *The SAGES Manual of Foregut Surgery*,
https://doi.org/10.1007/978-3-319-96122-4_74

Preoperative Considerations

A complete workup for the diagnosis of gastroparesis including gastric emptying study is necessary to ensure correct diagnosis and management of these complex patients. EGD to assess for any mechanical sources of obstruction and to evaluate the stomach and esophagus are important. Preoperative imaging such as UGI and CT with oral contrast can be helpful to define anatomy, especially in the setting of prior abdominal surgery.

Many patients with gastroparesis referred for surgery may have severe nutritional deficiencies due to chronic nausea and vomiting. CBC, electrolytes, albumin, prealbumin, and LFTs are useful in identifying electrolyte abnormalities or the need for supplemental nutrition. Nutrition may be achieved by TPN or by enteral feeding via jejunostomy. As many patients with gastroparesis are diabetic, preoperative, intraoperative, and postoperative glycemic management is paramount. A significantly elevated preoperative glycosylated hemoglobin (greater than10) warrants referral to an endocrinologist prior to surgery and close follow-up in the perioperative period.

Gastroparesis has historically been a disease of normal to underweight patients due to the decreased oral intake from symptoms. However, as the number of obese patients worldwide continues to increase, the number of obese patients suffering from gastroparesis rises as well. Currently there are a growing number of obese patients presenting with diabetic and idiopathic gastroparesis. For this subset of patients, gastric bypass offers the relief from their gastroparesis symptoms as well as the added benefit of weight loss. Understanding pre-, intra-, and postoperative management of obese patients is paramount. Patients should undergo comprehensive preoperative multidisciplinary evaluation with attention to dietary and psychological issues that will impact the patient postoperatively. Obesity-related comorbidities such as HTN, diabetes, sleep apnea, COPD, etc. should be evaluated and treated prior to undergoing surgery. For obese patients with gastroparesis, we strongly recommend consultation with dietitian to assist with pre- and postoperative diet and nutrition concerns. Patients will need to be instructed on the requirement to take vitamin supplements as well as the importance of adequate protein intake and hydration for the duration of their life after surgery.

Obese patients often have fatty liver making exposure of the proximal stomach difficult during surgery. Because of this, it is advisable to place patients on a liver shrinking diet (high-protein liquid diet) for at least 2 weeks before surgery. As little as 5–10 pound weight loss can reduce the liver size thus facilitating a smooth and uncomplicated surgery. All patients undergoing surgery should receive pharmacological and mechanical DVT prophylaxis in the perioperative period.

Bhayani and colleagues found 100% of patients with retained gastric contents on intraoperative endoscopy despite 24–48 h of clear liquids and 12+ h of nil per os. This is not surprising given the nature of the disease. If a patient is able to tolerate an even longer period of liquid diet, this is advisable to decrease the chance of aspiration at the time of surgery. The presence of likely retained gastric contents should be clearly communicated to the anesthesia team so they can take proper precautions against aspiration during intubation. We recommend assuming that all patients will have some degree of retained gastric contents and to proceed accordingly. Before making any incisions, EGD with lavage can be utilized to remove any retained gastric contents. Taking this into consideration, antifungal prophylaxis in addition to antibacterial prophylaxis may be warranted depending on the situation. All obese patients are given prophylactic blood thinners prior to surgery.

Intraoperative Considerations

Patients can be positioned in either split leg position or supine depending on surgeon preference. We prefer split leg for better ergonomics when performing foregut procedures. Use of a beanbag, footboard, and secure strapping of the patient is essential to ensure the patient will not move when placed in steep reverse Trendelenburg position. As many of these patients have other obesity-related comorbidities such as hypertension, heart disease, etc., close communication with anesthesia is of utmost importance.

Entry to the abdominal cavity is achieved by the use of a Veress needle at Palmer's point. However, it is important to note that given the vague nature symptoms associated with gastroparesis, many patients have undergone previous surgery, so great caution must be exercised with entry to the abdominal cavity.

After completion of pneumoperitoneum, a 30° laparoscope is inserted using a 12 mm visual port 14 cm below the xiphoid just to the left of the midline. A complete survey of the peritoneal cavity is performed. Additional ports are placed as follows: two in the LUQ and two in the RUQ approximately 8 cm apart in a V-shaped line with the camera port at the apex.

A Nathanson or other type of liver retractor is then placed centered over the caudate lobe to facilitate exposure of the proximal stomach.

The lesser sac is entered by entering the gastrocolic ligament in an avascular plane using ultrasonic shears or electrocautery. Care is taken to stay close to the stomach to avoid bleeding. Frequently adhesions between the pancreas and posterior wall of the stomach can hamper the dissection. These can be taken down using shears or electrocautery to better free the stomach. When dissecting up the proximal one third of the greater curve, it is helpful to grasp the anterior wall of the stomach and roll it laterally while also grasping the posterior side of the stomach. This exposes the proximal short gastric vessels. Exercise caution when retracting the fundus as excess traction can cause the fragile splenic capsule to tear and bleed. The greater curvature is then dissected-free laterally using ultrasonic shears all the way to the angle of His. At the completion of dissection, the left crus and hiatus should be visible.

Attention is then turned to the distal stomach, and the greater curve is taken down toward the pylorus. Firm anterior retraction of the stomach aids in duodenal dissection. The antrum is retracted toward the abdominal wall, and the duodenum is dissected off the head of the pancreas using endoshears. The duodenum only needs to be mobilized just past the pylorus. Typically the gastroduodenal artery marks the extent of the dissection, and the right gastroepiploic artery is identified at its takeoff from the GDA. The right gastroepiploic artery is isolated and divided between clips or vascular stapler load. Next retract the duodenum caudally, and visualize the right gastric artery anteriorly at its takeoff from the common hepatic. Once dissected-free, the right gastric is divided.

We then turn our attention to creating the gastric pouch. Approximately 5–7 cm is measured distally from the GE junction along the lesser curve. The lesser sac is entered by using ultrasonic dissector to take down branches of the left gastric artery. A horizontal fire of an appropriately sized 45 mm stapler load starts the creation of the pouch.

We prefer a stapled anastomosis using a 25 mm EEA stapler. After the horizontal fire of the 45 mm stapler, a gastrotomy is made on the anterior wall of the stomach using ultrasonic shears. The anvil of the EEA is then brought through the lower left port site after being attached to an 5 mm esophageal retractor. The anvil and esophageal are then placed through the gastrotomy and proximal to the staple line. Using the esophageal retractor, an anterior gastrotomy on the pouch is made using electrocautery, and the anvil is brought out through the incision. The suture connecting the anvil and esophageal retractor is then cut and the retractor removed. It is important to only make a large enough enterotomy for just the tip of the anvil so as to not compromise the circular-stapled anastomosis. It is important at this time to remove all tubes from the mouth except for the ET tube. The gastric pouch is then completed using sequential fires of staple loads aiming at the angle of His. After the stomach pouch has been created, the remainder of the stomach should be detached and can be placed into an endocatch bag and moved to the side of the abdomen.

The table is taken out of reverse Trendelenburg position. The omentum is retracted cephalad thus exposing the transverse mesocolon. The transverse colon is retracted cephalad exposing the proximal jejunum, which is followed proximally to the ligament of Treitz.

Starting at the ligament of Treitz, 40 cm of jejunum is measured out. At this point the jejunum is stretched to the anterior abdominal wall to ensure the mesentery is long enough for the Roux limb to reach the stomach. If it is not long enough we proceed distally until a suitable section of jejunum is found. The jejunum is divided using an appropriately sized 60 mm staple load. The mesentery is divided until the small bowel can be brought up to the anterior abdominal wall. A stitch is placed on the distal jejunum to identify the Roux limb. In nonobese patients, a 75 cm Roux limb is measured out. In obese patient, a 150 cm Roux limb is created. Once the Roux limb has been measured, the biliopancreatic and Roux limbs are placed parallel to each other and stay sutures placed approximately 1 cm away from another. Enterotomies are made using electrocautery on the antimesenteric border of each limb between the stay sutures. A 60 mm stapler is then placed into the enterotomies and fired. The staple line is inspected for hemostasis, and then a single stitch is placed across the middle of the enterotomy. The stay sutures are then elevated, and the common enteromy is closed with a fire of the 60 mm stapler. The mesenteric defect is closed using interrupted nonabsorbable suture.

The omentum is divided vertically using the ultrasonic shears. The Roux limb is brought into the left upper quadrant. Another stay suture is placed approximately 2 cm proximal to the stay suture on the end of the cut bowel. An enterotomy is made using ultrasonic shears compromising approximately 50% of the bowel circumference. The EEA stapler is then brought through the left-sided port. This port site often needs to be dilated manually with a Pean clamp prior to inserting the stapler. The stapler is then placed into the small bowel and the spike advanced at the antimesenteric border. The spike is then placed into the anvil and the stapler closed and fired. The stapler is removed and excess jejunum resected with a 60 mm staple load. Staple lines are inspected for hemostasis. The Roux limb is then occluded with a bowel clamp and submerged with saline. An EGD is advanced into the stomach pouch into the Roux limb assessing for hemostasis, patency, and integrity. The scope is withdrawn into the pouch which is inflated with air, and the submerged areas are inspected for any bubbles which would indicate a leak. The scope is then removed after suctioning out the air. The stomach is then removed through the left lower quadrant incision. We recommend placing drains around the gastrojejunostomy.

The fascia of the left-sided incision is closed with a Carter-Thomason device. The remainder of the 10–12 mm ports do not need to be closed as the radially dilating trocars are used off the midline. Skin incisions are closed using subcuticular stitches of 4–0 absorbable monofilament suture and sterile dressings applied.

As with any gastric bypass or other foregut surgery, laparoscopic approach provides good visualization for dissection and performance of the surgery. Robotic-assisted surgery can also be considered depending on surgeon preference.

If the patient has had a previous fundoplication, then it should be left intact at the time of gastrectomy and the anastomosis performed just distal to the fundoplication.

Although we describe removal of the gastric remnant, it is also feasible to leave it in place. If it is very large, a decompressing gastrotomy tube can be placed at the time of surgery. Depending on the patient's nutrition status and ability to tolerate diet preoperatively, a feeding jejunostomy can be placed at the time of surgery as well to facilitate proper postoperative nutrition.

Postoperative Care

Early ambulation after surgery is crucial in preventing DVT particularly in obese patients. Immediately after surgery, patients are instructed to use an incentive spirometer. Heparin or lovenox is given for the duration of the hospital stay. If a Foley catheter was placed at the time of surgery it should be removed on POD 1. Patients are started on a non-carbonated, low caloric post-bariatric clear liquid diet on POD1. If they tolerate this diet, they are advanced to a full liquid diet upon discharge.

Long-term dietary goals include 50–80 g of protein/day as well as at least 64 oz. of water daily. Continued dietary counseling is helpful after surgery to help patients adjust to the new dietary restriction. Dietary supplementation with a multivitamin which includes iron (ferrous fumarate or ferrous sucrate preferred due to better absorption post-bypass) and B12 is critical in these patients. Bypass patients are seen in follow-up at 2 weeks, 3 months, 6 months, and yearly to assess degree of weight loss and check labs.

Complications

Early postoperative complications include intraluminal and extraluminal bleeds, anastomotic leak, intraabdominal abscess, bowel obstruction, PE, DVT, and wound infection. Late complications include bowel obstruction, internal hernia, marginal ulceration, GI bleed, cholelithiasis, gastro-gastro fistula (if remnant stomach left in place), and vitamin deficiencies.

Outcomes

One study found that despite careful patient selection, disease optimization, and preoperative preparation, 17% of patients undergoing gastrectomy for gastroparesis suffered major postoperative morbidity requiring surgical intervention [4]. Complications requiring reoperation were GJ/EJ leak, JJ leak, and duodenal stump leak. They also found a higher incidence of surgical site infection. 80% of patients with belching/bloating had improvement or resolution of their symptoms (Figs. 74.1 and 74.2), 60% had improvement or resolution of nausea, and 50% of patients demonstrated improvement or resolution of their chronic abdominal pain (Fig. 74.1).

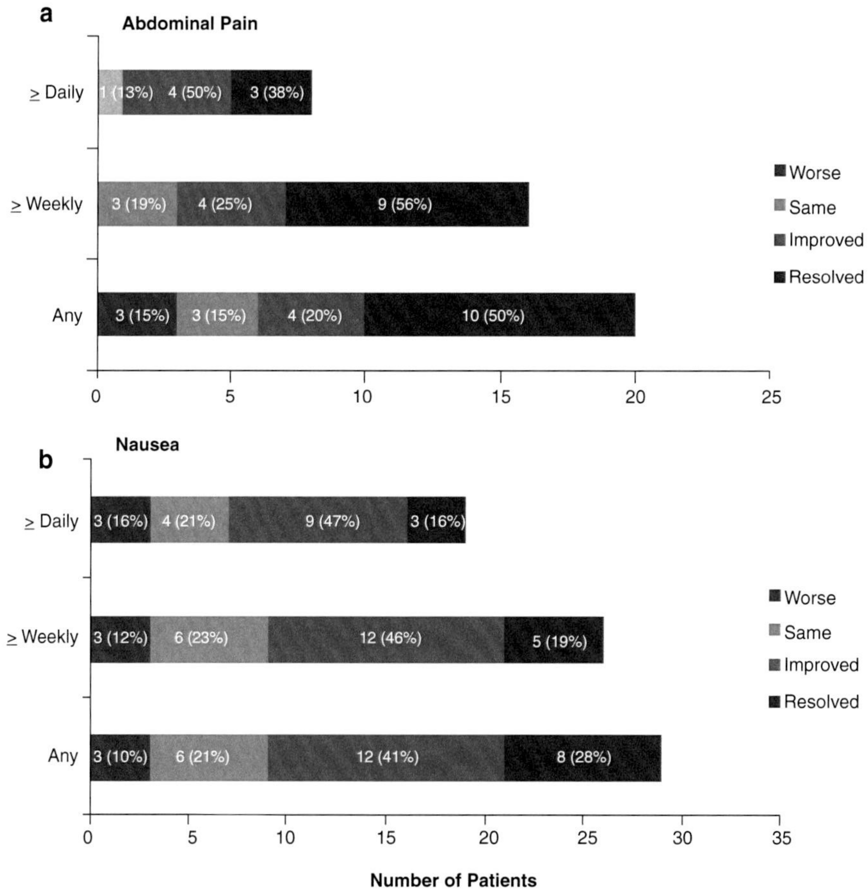

Fig. 74.1 Change in symptoms with preoperative abdominal pain (**a**) or nausea (**b**). (From: Bhayani et al. [4])

Fig. 74.2 Pre- and postoperative symptoms. (From: Bhayani et al. [4])

	Preoperative score (median)	Postoperative score (median)	*p* value
Abdominal pain	1	1	0.3[a]
Nausea	3	1	0.002[a]
Any symptoms, *n* (%)			
Belching	14 (40)	6 (17)	0.03[b]
Bloating	18 (51)	4 (11)	0.0005[b]

[a]Wilcoxon signed-rank *p* value

[b]McNemar's *p* value

Conclusion

Gastroparesis remains a chronic disease with debilitating symptoms and often ineffective treatments. When medical therapy and other less invasive surgical treatments fail, it is appropriate to consider gastrectomy if the patient continues to be symptomatic and is willing to accept the risks. Some studies have shown gastrectomy to be superior to gastric electronic stimulation in the treatment of gastroparesis [5]. Roux-en-Y gastric bypass with or without remnant gastrectomy offers a safe, effective treatment for many patients with gastroparesis refractory to medical treatment.

References

1. Jones M, Maganti K. A systematic review of surgical therapy for gastroparesis. Am J Gastroenterol. 2003;98:2122–9.
2. Smith DS, Williams CS, Ferris CD. Diagnosis and treatment of chronic gastroparesis and chronic intestinal pseudo-obstruction. Gastroenterol Clin N Am. 2003;32:619–58.
3. Sun Z, Rodriguez J, McMichael J, Chand B, Nash D, Brethauer S, Schauer P, El-Hayek K, Kroh M. Surgical treatment of medically refractory gastroparesis in the morbidly obese. Surg Endosc. 2015;29(9):2683–9.
4. Bhayani NH, Sharata AM, Dunst CM, Kurian AA, Reavis KM, Swanstrom LL. End of the road for a dysfunctional end organ: laparoscopic gastrectomy for refractory gastroparesis. J Gastrointest Surg. 2015;19(3):411–7.
5. Zehetner J, Ravari F, Ayazi S, Skibba A, Darehzereshki A, Pelipad D, Mason RJ, Katkhouda N, Lipham JC. Minimally invasive surgical approach for the treatment of gastroparesis. Surg Endosc. 2013;27:61–6.

Expert Commentary: Algorithm for the Treatment of Gastroparesis

75

Vic Velanovich

Gastroparesis is a vexing problem that is becoming increasingly common. Gastroparesis is more than just delayed gastric emptying. It is delayed gastric emptying associated with symptoms. Delayed gastric emptying by itself does not require treatment. It is the symptoms of gastroparesis that require treatment. These symptoms include nausea, vomiting, bloating, abdominal pain, acid reflux, regurgitation, weight loss/malnutrition, and abdominal heaviness. Some patients will progress to a food fear. Improvement of gastric emptying may or may not be necessary to improve symptoms. In fact, it is common that patient-perceived symptoms correlate very poorly with objective measurements of physiological function. The focus of the clinician is symptomatic improvement.

Although diabetes is one of the most common causes, there are a variety of other causes (Table 75.1). It is very important to determine the cause of the gastroparesis because this will determine therapy. One must never fall into the trap that just because you have a hammer, the whole world is a nail. It is frequent that gastroparesis is the presenting problem for an underlying systemic disease. Treating gastroparesis in isolation of the systemic disease is doing the patient a disservice. The clinician needs to be aware and question the patient carefully for the associated symptoms that will provide clues that a systemic disease exists. If such symptoms exist, then appropriate referral to another specialist may be in order. The clinician evaluating patients with gastroparesis needs to develop a disciplined, systematic approach to their evaluation before embarking on treatment (Fig. 75.1).

The first issue that needs to be addressed is whether or not the symptoms are related to a surgically correctable cause (Fig. 75.1). Of the causes of symptoms suggestive of gastroparesis, surgically correctable causes are mechanical obstruction, isolated gastroparesis, or postvagotomy or gastrectomy gastroparesis. Nonsurgically

V. Velanovich
Department of Surgery, University of South Florida, Tampa, FL, USA
e-mail: vvelanov@health.usf.edu

J. Grams et al. (eds.), *The SAGES Manual of Foregut Surgery*,
https://doi.org/10.1007/978-3-319-96122-4_75

Table 75.1 Causes of gastroparesis

Causes of gastroparesis
Diabetes mellitus
Idiopathic
Upper gastrointestinal surgery
Partial gastrectomy
Vagotomy/vagal nerve injury
Systemic sclerosis
Scleroderma
Amyloidosis
Systemic lupus erythematous
Ischemic-related
Celiac axis stenosis
Median arcuate ligament syndrome
Pan-gastrointestinal dysmotility
Small bowel pseudo-obstruction
Colonic inertia
Diffuse autonomic nervous system dysfunction
Other neurologic disorders (migraine, Parkinson's)
Cyclical vomiting syndrome
Eating disorders
Medication-related

correctable causes include gastroparesis associated with systemic diseases (e.g., neurological or infiltrative diseases), functional disorders (e.g., functional dyspepsia, nausea, irritable bowel syndrome, etc.), and psychogenic causes (e.g., eating disorders). Sadly, up to 30% of women with "idiopathic" gastroparesis have been sexually abused, and the emotional consequences of this abuse may need specialized care. One must not assume that the referring physician has done a thorough evaluation assessing for these causes. Once the nonsurgically correctable causes have been ruled out, the clinician then needs to evaluate the potential surgically correctable causes.

This first requires a careful evaluation for a mechanical cause of gastric outlet or downstream duodenal or jejunal obstruction. An esophagogastroduodenoscopy is not sufficient to rule out a mechanical cause as a mechanical obstruction, such as a tumor, may be present in the third or fourth portion of the duodenum or proximal jejunum. An upper gastrointestinal contrast series or computed tomographic scan is useful for this purpose. Once a mechanical cause is ruled out, the clinician can proceed with an evaluation of the presence of delayed gastric emptying with gastric emptying scintigraphy.

After documentation of delayed gastric emptying, the clinician needs to pinpoint the cause. First is to determine if the gastroparesis is related to prior gastric surgery. Postgastrectomy or postvagotomy gastroparesis generally can respond to medical and dietary management (Table 75.2). However, if it does not and the symptoms are severe, then completion of gastrectomy in the case of postgastrectomy gastroparesis or improved drainage in the case of postvagotomy gastroparesis may be considered.

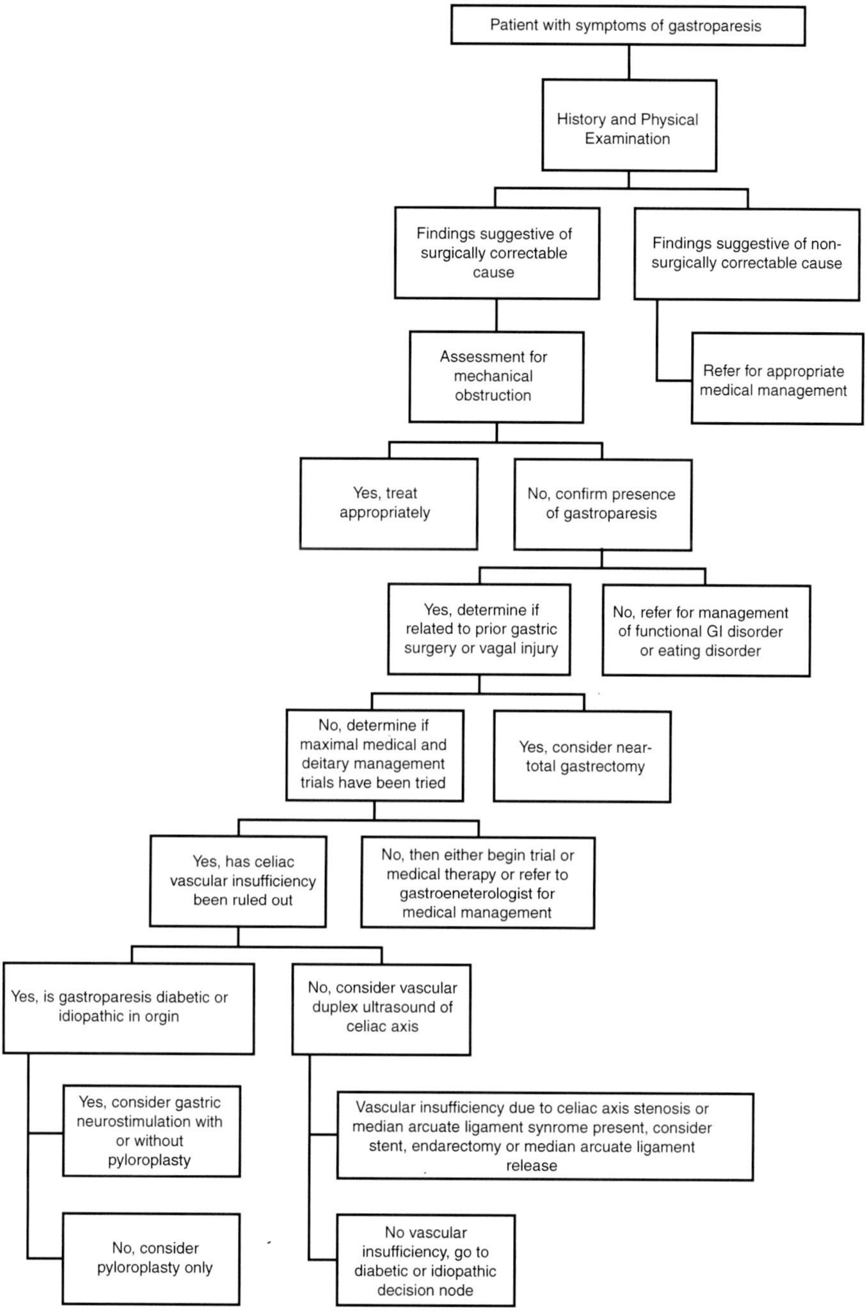

Fig. 75.1 Algorithm for assessment and management of gastroparesis

Table 75.2 Gastroparesis diet

Food groups	Foods recommended	Foods not recommended
Breads, cereal, and grains	White flour products White rice Grains <2 gm fiber	Whole grains, brown rice, popcorn, granola
Vegetables	Most well-cooked or canned vegetables, potatoes, lettuce	Raw vegetables, cruciferous vegetables, corn
Fruits	Most canned fruit, fruit juice without pulp, bananas, melon	Raw fruits, dried fruits, juice with pulp
Meat	Well-cooked meat, poultry, fish, eggs, or soy foods	Fried meats, lunch meats, dry beans, nuts, peanut butter
Milk and milk products	Skim milk, soy milk, reduced fat cheese, yogurt	Whole milk, cream, regular ice cream, sour cream
Fats and oils	Less than 3–5 servings/day of any oils	Most fats

Once isolated gastroparesis in the intact stomach has been determined, then the clinician needs to determine if maximal medical therapy has been achieved. In addition to dietary counseling (Table 75.2), the organization G-Pact.org provides a cookbook of meals which are appropriate for patients with gastroparesis. However, most will require some type of medication. Firstly, the patient needs to be weaned off of narcotics, if he or she is using this medication for pain. Secondly, prokinetic and antiemetic medications may be used to ease symptoms. It is not the purpose of this chapter to go into detail as to medication options, but the clinician needs to be aware of them. Although endoscopic treatments, such as pyloric balloon dilation or injection of the pylorus with botulinum toxin, have been used, these have generally been found to be ineffective. I would not recommend endoscopic therapy for gastroparesis as a general rule, save for peroral endoscopic pyloromyotomy in a controlled setting.

A cause of gastroparesis that is becoming increasingly recognized is vascular insufficiency. My suspicion for this is particularly high in patients who have a significant postprandial pain component to their gastroparesis. This can be evaluated with vascular duplex ultrasound to determine celiac axis stenosis or median arcuate ligament syndrome is present. I have increasingly used this test in my routine preoperative evaluation of gastroparesis. If vascular insufficiency is found, then it should be treated appropriately. Celiac axis stenosis needs to be referred to a vascular surgeon for either a stent or endarterectomy. If median arcuate ligament syndrome is present, then median arcuate ligament release should be considered before proceeding with treatment of the gastroparesis.

Once vascular insufficiency has been ruled out or treated, then the clinician needs to determine if the cause of the gastroparesis is from diabetes mellitus or idiopathic and not some other cause. This is a crucial distinction. The Food and Drug

Administration has approved the gastric neurostimulator for only diabetic or idiopathic gastroparesis under the Humanitarian Device Exemption. The neurostimulator should not be placed in any other circumstance. Also, there is data to suggest that continued use of narcotics for underlying pain will reduce the effectiveness of this device. It is my practice not to offer the gastric neurostimulator to patients who are taking narcotic pain medication. However, in patients who have gastroparesis from a cause other than diabetes or idiopathic, pyloroplasty can be considered. This is most commonly done as a laparoscopic pyloroplasty, but investigations into peroral pyloroplasty have shown promise. In patients with diabetic or idiopathic gastroparesis, gastric neurostimulation can be considered for patients whose primary symptoms are nausea and vomiting. However, it has been my experience that gastric neurostimulation is relatively ineffective in patients whose primary symptoms are pain and bloating. In those patients, I advised against a neurostimulator. In fact, I generally think of the neurostimulator as an antiemetic device rather than a prokinetic device. Patients can have improvement in symptoms of nausea and vomiting with relatively little change in gastric emptying as measured objectively by gastric emptying scintigraphy. Occasionally, patients may also benefit from a pyloroplasty as an adjunct to neurostimulation.

With respect to post-implant patient care, expectations management is critical for success. Only about 25% of patients will notice symptomatic improvement immediately. It is more common that patients will require multiple adjustments of what I refer to as the "electrical dosing." The managing physician can make adjustments on the device in the following areas: voltage, pulse width (measured in microseconds), rate (measured in Hertz), time on (measured in seconds), and time off (measured in seconds). The voltage is converted to ampere depending on the resistance between the electrodes in the gastric wall. Although there is no official measure of electrical dosing, when one combines the units of the adjustable variables, the "unit of measure" is V-pulse-s/day. In practicality, however, this unit is not easy to measure. Usually, adjustments are made incrementally beginning with voltage, rate, time on, and time off. Pulse width, in general, has the least effect on effectiveness. The patient needs to understand that it may take several weeks to months to find the right "electrical dosing" which maximizes symptom relief at the least electrical dosing possible. The importance of this has to be with battery life—the higher the electric dosing, the shorter the battery life. In addition, patients need to understand that they may still require antiemetic and prokinetic medications. Nevertheless, despite careful patient selection and diligent follow-up, about 20% of patients will not note any symptomatic improvement.

Patients need to be aware that gastroparesis is a fluctuating disease. Physiologic and emotional stress can lead to less symptomatic relief than desired. For example, any type of infection, either bacterial or viral, injury or surgery, hypothyroidism, hypoadrenalism, hyperglycemia, and even menses in female, can lessen the effects of the neurostimulator.

Conclusion

Patients with gastroparesis suffer tremendously. By the time they see the surgeon, they are usually at the end of their rope. However, it is incumbent on the clinician to provide a thorough evaluation. With this, the patients who can be helped with surgery can be sorted from the ones who cannot. The surgical approach is generally pyloroplasty or gastric neurostimulation. Despite careful selection, many patients will have persistent symptoms. However, most will have some measure of relief.

Index

J. Grams et al. (eds.), *The SAGES Manual of Foregut Surgery*,
https://doi.org/10.1007/978-3-319-96122-4

H